McDonald and Avery's

Dentistry
for the Child *and*
Adolescent

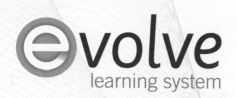

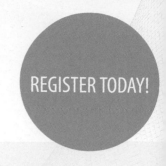
REGISTER TODAY!

To access your resources, visit:

http://evolve.elsevier.com/DeanMcDonaldAvery/

Evolve Learning Resources for *McDonald and Avery's Dentistry for the Child and Adolescent*, ninth edition, offers the following features:

- **Testbank questions and answers for each chapter**
- **Case studies**
- **Image Collection**
- **Suggested Readings**
- **Weblinks**

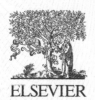
ELSEVIER

McDonald and Avery's
Dentistry
for the Child *and*
Adolescent

Jeffrey A. Dean, DDS, MSD

Ralph E. McDonald Professor of Pediatric Dentistry and
Professor of Orthodontics
Indiana University School of Dentistry
James Whitcomb Riley Hospital for Children
Indianapolis, Indiana

David R. Avery, DDS, MSD

Ralph E. McDonald Professor Emeritus of Pediatric Dentistry
Indiana University School of Dentistry
James Whitcomb Riley Hospital for Children
Indianapolis, Indiana

Ralph E. McDonald, DDS, MS, LLD

Dean Emeritus and Professor Emeritus of Pediatric Dentistry
Indiana University School of Dentistry
Indianapolis, Indiana

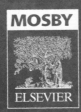

MOSBY

ELSEVIER

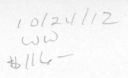

3251 Riverport Lane
Maryland Heights, Missouri 63043

Notice

Knowledge and best practice in this field are constantly changing. As new research and experience broaden our knowledge, changes in practice, treatment, and drug therapy may become necessary or appropriate. Readers are advised to check the most current information provided (i) on procedures featured or (ii) by the manufacturer of each product to be administered, to verify the recommended dose or formula, the method and duration of administration, and contraindications. It is the responsibility of the practitioner, relying on their own experience and knowledge of the patient, to make diagnoses, to determine dosages and the best treatment for each individual patient, and to take all appropriate safety precautions. To the fullest extent of the law, neither the Publisher nor the Authors assumes any liability for any injury and/or damage to persons or property arising out of or related to any use of the material contained in this book.

The Publisher

ISBN: 978-0-323-05724-0

Acquisitions Editor: John Dolan
Developmental Editor: Joslyn Dumas
Publishing Services Manager: Julie Eddy
Senior Project Manager: Andrea Campbell
Design Direction: Karen Pauls

Printed in China

Last digit is the print number: 9   8   7   6   5   4   3   2   1

Working together to grow libraries in developing countries

www.elsevier.com | www.bookaid.org | www.sabre.org

ELSEVIER   BOOK AID International   Sabre Foundation

Contributors

Christopher Edward Belcher, MD
Director
Pediatric Infectious Diseases
Infectious Diseases of Indiana
Indianapolis, Indiana

Ronald A. Bell, DDS, Med
Professor of Pediatric Dentistry and Orthodontics
College of Dental Medicine
Medical University of South Carolina
Charleston, South Carolina

Jeffrey D. Bennett, DMD
Professor and Chair
Department of Oral Surgery and Hospital Dentistry
Indiana University School of Dentistry
Indianapolis, Indiana
Diplomate, American Board of Oral and Maxillofacial
    Surgeons (ABOMS)
Diplomate, National Dental Board of Anesthesiology
Fellow, American Association of Oral and Maxillofacial
    Surgeons (AAOMS)
Fellow, American Dental Society of Anesthesiology
    (ADSA)

David T. Brown, DDS, MS
Chair and Professor
Department of Restorative Dentistry
Indiana University School of Dentistry
Indianapolis, Indiana

David A. Bussard, DDS, MS
Associate Clinical Professor
Department of Oral and Maxillofacial Surgery
Indiana University School of Dentistry
Indiana Oral and Maxillofacial Surgery Associates
Indianapolis, Indiana

Judith R. Chin, DDS, MS
Associate Professor
Department of Pediatric Dentistry
Indiana University School of Dentistry
Indianapolis, Indiana

Robert J. Cronin, Jr., DDS, MS
Professor and Director, Graduate Division
Department of Prosthodontics
The University of Texas Health Science Center at
San Antonio Dental School
San Antonio, Texas

Murray Dock, DDS, MSD, RPh
Associate Professor of Clinical Pediatrics
University of Cincinnati, School of Medicine
Division of Pediatric Dentistry
Cincinnati Children's Hospital Medical Center
Cincinnati, Ohio

Burton L. Edelstein, DDS, MPH
Professor of Dentistry and Health Policy Management
Department of Community Health
College of Dental Medicine
Columbia University Medical Center
New York, New York

Robert J. Feigal, DDS, PhD*
Professor and Chair, Department of Preventive
    Sciences
School of Dentistry, University of Minnesota
Minneapolis, Minnesota

Donald J. Ferguson, DMD, MSD
Dean and Professor of Orthodontics
Nicolas and Asp College of Postgraduate Dentistry
Dubai Healthcare City
Dubai, United Arab Emirates

Elie M. Ferneini, DMD, MD, MHS
Oral and Maxillofacial Surgeon
Clinical Instructor, University of Connecticut
Private Practice
Greater Waterbury OMS
Waterbury, Connecticut

Charles J. Goodacre, DDS, MSD
Professor and Dean
School of Dentistry
Loma Linda University
Loma Linda, California

Ann Page Griffin, BA
Clinical Associate Professor
Department of Family Medicine
East Carolina University School of Medicine
Co-Chairman, Board
Practicon, Inc.
Greenville, North Carolina

---

*Deceased

James K. Hartsfield, Jr., DMD, MS, MMSc, PhD, FACMG
Professor and E. Preston Hicks Endowed Chair in Orthodontics and Oral Research
University of Kentucky College of Dentistry
Lexington, Kentucky

Roberta A. Hibbard, MD
Professor of Pediatrics
Indiana of University School of Medicine
Indianapolis, Indiana

Randy A. Hock, MD, PhD, MMM
Presbyterian Blume Pediatric Hematology & Oncology Clinic
Presbyterian Novant Medical Group
Charlotte, North Carolina

Donald V. Huebener, DDS, MS, MAEd
Professor, Plastic and Reconstructive Surgery
Department of Surgery, School of Medicine
Washington University, St. Louis, Missouri
Professor, Pediatric Dentistry
School of Dental Medicine
Southern Illinois University
Alton, Illinois

Christopher V. Hughes, DMD, PhD
Associate Professor and Chair
Department of Pediatric Dentistry
Henry M. Goldman School of Dental Medicine
Boston University
Boston, Massachusetts

Charles E. Hutton, DDS
Emeritus Professor of Oral and Maxillofacial Surgery
Indiana University School of Dentistry
Indianapolis, Indiana

Vanchit John, DDS, MSD, MDS, BDS
Chairperson, Associate Professor and Director
Department of Predoctoral Periodontics
Indiana University School of Dentistry
Indianapolis, Indiana

James E. Jones, DMD, MSD, EdD, PhD
Professor and Chair
Department of Pediatric Dentistry
Indiana University School of Dentistry
James Whitcomb Riley Hospital for Children
Indianapolis, Indiana

Joan E. Kowolik, BDS, LDS, RCS
Associate Professor of Pediatric Dentistry
Department of Pediatric Dentistry
Indiana University School of Dentistry
Indianapolis, Indiana

John T. Krull, DDS
Assistant Professor
Department of Pediatric Dentistry
Indiana University School of Dentistry
Private Practice of Orthodontics
Indianapolis, Indiana

George E. Krull, DDS
Private Practice of Pediatric Dentistry
Clarkston, Michigan

Thomas H. Lapp, DDS, MS
Clinical Assistant Professor of Oral and Maxillofacial Surgery
Indiana University School of Dentistry
Oral and Maxillofacial Surgeon
Private Practice
Indianapolis, Indiana

Jasper L. Lewis, DDS, MS
Clinical Assistant Professor
Department of Pediatric Dentistry
University of Tennessee College of Dentistry
Memphis, Tennessee
Clinical Professor, Department of Surgery
Chief of the Division of Dentistry
Clinical Assistant Professor
Department of Family Medicine
School of Medicine, East Carolina University
Private Practice of Pediatric Dentistry
Greenville, North Carolina

James L. McDonald, Jr., PhD
Emeritus Professor of Oral Biology
Indiana University School of Dentistry
Indianapolis, Indiana

John S. McDonald, DDS, MS, FACD
Volunteer Professor
Departments of Surgery and Anesthesia
Volunteer Associate Professor
Department of Pediatrics
Division of Pediatric Dentistry
College of Medicine, University of Cincinnati
Cincinnati, Ohio
Private Practice of Oral and Maxillofacial Pathology/Head and Neck Pain
Cincinnati, Ohio

Dale A. Miles, BA, DDS, MS, FRCD(C), Dip. ABOM, Dip. ABOMR
Adjunct Professor
University of Texas Health Science Center at San Antonio
San Antonio, Texas
Adjunct Professor
Arizona School of Dentistry and Oral Health
Mesa, Arizona
CEO, Digital Radiographic Solutions
Fountain Hills, Arizona

B. Keith Moore, PhD
Professor Emeritus
Indiana University School of Dentistry
Division of Dental Materials
Department of Restorative Dentistry
Indianapolis, Indiana

Edwin T. Parks, DMD, MS
Professor of Diagnostic Sciences
Indiana University School of Dentistry
Indianapolis, Indiana

Laura Romito, DDS, MS
Associate Professor of Oral Biology
Indiana University School of Dentistry
Indianapolis, Indiana

Alan Michael Sadove, MD
Private Practice of Esthetic Surgery
Meridian Plastic Surgeons and Medical Skin
    Care
Indianapolis, Indiana

Brian J. Sanders, DDS, MS
Professor of Pediatric Dentistry
Director, Riley Dental Clinic
Director, Advanced Education Program in Pediatric
    Dentistry
Indianapolis, Indiana

Amy D. Shapiro, MD
Co-Medical Director and Pediatric Hematologist
Indiana Hemophilia and Thrombosis Center
Indianapolis, Indiana

Jenny I. Stigers, DMD
Associate Professor
University of Kentucky College of Dentistry
Lexington, Kentucky

George K. Stookey, MSD, PhD
Distinguished Professor Emeritus of Preventive
    and Community Dentistry
Indiana University School of Dentistry
Indianapolis, Indiana

James A. Weddell, DDS, MSD
Associate Professor of Pediatric Dentistry
Indiana University School of Dentistry
James Whitcomb Riley Hospital for Children
Indianapolis, Indiana

**Gerald Z. Wright, DDS, MSD, FRCD(C),
    Dip. Amer. Brd**
Professor Emeritus
University of Western Ontario
London, Ontario, Canada
Secretary General
International Association of Paediatric Dentistry

Karen M. Yoder, MSD, PhD
Professor and Director
Division of Community Dentistry
Department of Preventative and Community Dentistry
Indiana University School of Dentistry
Indianapolis, Indiana

Preface

The ninth edition of *Dentistry for the Child and Adolescent* presents current diagnostic and treatment recommendations based on research, clinical experience, and current literature. The newest edition follows the same basic structure and format of the previous eight editions. The contributors who joined us in the preparation of this latest revision express a coordinated philosophy and the approach to the most modern concepts of dentistry for the child and adolescent. The information contained herein is relevant to the contemporary science and practice of pediatric dentistry. This textbook is designed to help undergraduate dental students and postdoctoral pediatric dental students provide efficient and superior comprehensive oral health care to infants, children, teenagers, and medically compromised patients. It also provides experienced dentists with reference information regarding new developments and techniques.

This ninth edition represents a significant revision, with three main areas of enhancement. Perhaps most notable is the addition of color illustrations throughout the textbook, which significantly enhance the esthetic quality of the material. In addition, the book is connected with Elsevier's Evolve website, which will provide advantages for both students and faculty of pediatric dentistry in utilizing the information from the text, as well as providing additional features. Finally, multiple significant areas of improvement in individual chapters were accomplished during this revision. Specific notable chapter improvements include:

- Chapter 3 underwent a significant rewrite with the addition of a new author and provides our contemporary knowledge of nonpharmacologic behavioral guidance.
- Chapter 5 has been enhanced in the digital radiography section with material regarding three-dimensional cone-beam computed tomography, an exciting new area in dental diagnostics.
- Chapter 6, in addition to discussing the increasing link between dental disease and genetics, includes an interesting discussion regarding the link between tooth agenesis and the diagnosis of cancer.
- Chapter 8 contains substantial new information regarding childhood oral pathologies.
- Two new authors have contributed to the rewriting of Chapter 10, this most important chapter regarding dental caries, and Chapter 12, on nutritional considerations for the pediatric dental patient.
- Chapters 13, 20, and 21 have new authors added to the list of contributors, which has provided enhanced insight to these chapter topics.
- Chapter 20 in particular has several new cases regarding trauma to the dentition.
- Chapter 27, about the management of the developing occlusion, has undergone a significant rewrite, with many new cases added to illustrate the basic principles involved.
- Chapters 29 and 30, both about practice management and community oral health, were significantly revised. In addition, a new author was added to chapter 30, providing significant revisions and enhancements regarding access to dental care for children.
- Finally, Chapter 31 is a revision of a pediatric oral surgery chapter from several editions ago that has returned at the request of our readers.

Again, thanks to our author contributors for all of their dedication and work on this ninth edition!

Ralph E. McDonald
David R. Avery
Jeffrey A. Dean

Acknowledgments

A textbook can be planned and written only with the supportive interest, encouragement, and tangible contributions of many people. Therefore, it is a privilege to acknowledge the assistance of others in the preparation of this text. First of all, we would like to thank the many authors and co-authors who have made this ninth edition possible. Donna Bumgardner provided manuscript preparation and valuable editorial assistance. Mark Dirlam, Kyla Jones, Terry Wilson, and Tim Centers provided assistance with new illustrations. Our excellent library staff was eager to help in any way possible, and the assistance of Janice Cox, Barbara Gushrowski, Keli Schmidt, Mike Delporte, and Sue Hutchinson is much appreciated. We also gratefully acknowledge the professional staff at Elsevier who has provided valuable assistance and superb guidance in the publication of this ninth edition; special thanks to John Dolan, Executive Editor; Joslyn Dumas, Associate Developmental Editor; and Andrea Campbell, Senior Project Manager.

The faculties of pediatric dentistry and other disciplines at Indiana University have contributed substantially to this work in many ways. We truly appreciate their willingness to share information relevant to scientific accuracy of the manuscripts. In particular, we gratefully acknowledge Drs. Michael Baumgartner, John Emhardt, Margherita Fontana, Gopal Krishna, Dongmei Liu, Charles Palenik, Phillip Pate, Jeffrey Platt, Paul Walker, and Susan Zunt. Many pediatric dentistry postdoctoral students and auxiliary staff have also assisted in numerous ways. The encouragement and support of all members of our families sustained our resolve to complete this task when it seemed that it would not get done. We extend our heartfelt thanks to all who played a role in helping us bring this project to a successful conclusion.

Contents

*Deceased

CHAPTER 1

Examination of the Mouth and Other Relevant Structures

▲ Ralph E. McDonald, David R. Avery, and Jeffrey A. Dean

CHAPTER OUTLINE

A dentist is traditionally taught to perform a complete oral examination of the patient and to develop a treatment plan from the examination findings. The dentist then makes a case presentation to the patient or parents, outlining the recommended course of treatment. This process should include the development and presentation of a prevention plan that outlines an ongoing comprehensive oral health care program for the patient and establishment of the "dental home."

The plan should include recommendations designed to correct existing oral problems (or halt their progression) and to prevent anticipated future problems. It is essential to obtain all relevant patient and family information, to secure parental consent, and to perform a complete examination before embarking on this comprehensive oral health care program for the pediatric patient. *Anticipatory guidance* is the term often used to describe the discussion and implementation of such a plan with the patient and/or parents. The American Academy of Pediatric Dentistry has published guidelines concerning the periodicity of examination, preventive dental services, and oral treatment for children as summarized in Table 1-1.

Each pediatric patient should be given an opportunity to receive complete dental care. The dentist should not attempt to decide what the child, parents, or third-party agent will accept or can afford. If parents reject a portion or all of the recommendations, the dentist has at least fulfilled the obligation of educating the child and the parents about the importance of the recommended procedures. Parents of even moderate income usually find the means to have oral health care completed if the dentist explains that the child's future oral health and even general health are related to the correction of oral defects.

INITIAL PARENTAL CONTACT WITH THE DENTAL OFFICE

The parent usually makes the first contact with the dental office by telephone. This initial conversation between the parent and the office receptionist is very important. It provides the first opportunity to attend to the parent's concerns by pleasantly and concisely responding to questions and by offering an office appointment. The receptionist must have a warm, friendly voice and the ability to communicate clearly. The receptionist's responses should assure the parent that the well-being of the child is the chief concern.

The information recorded by the receptionist during this conversation constitutes the initial dental record for the patient. Filling out a patient information form is a convenient method of collecting the necessary initial information (see Fig. 29-3). Additional discussion of the initial communication with parents is presented in Chapter 29.

THE DIAGNOSTIC METHOD

Before making a diagnosis and developing a treatment plan, the dentist must collect and evaluate the facts associated with the patient's or parents' chief concern and any other identified problems that may be unknown to the patient or parents. Some pathognomonic signs may lead to an almost immediate diagnosis. For example, obvious gingival swelling and drainage may

Table 1-1

Recommendations for Preventive Pediatric Oral Health Care

Because each child is unique, these recommendations are designed for the care of children who have no contributing medical conditions and are developing normally. These recommendations will need to be modified for children with special health care needs or if disease or trauma manifests variations from normal. The American Academy of Pediatric Dentistry (AAPD) emphasizes the importance of very early professional intervention and the continuity of care based on the individualized needs of the child. Refer to the text of this guideline for supporting information and references.

	AGE				
	6–12 mo	12–24 mo	2–6 yr	6–12 yr	12+ yr
Clinical oral examination[1,2]	•	•	•	•	•
Assess oral growth and development[3]	•	•	•	•	•
Caries-risk assessment[4]	•	•	•	•	•
Radiographic assessment[5]	•	•	•	•	•
Prophylaxis and topical fluoride[4,5]	•	•	•	•	•
Fluoride supplementation[6,7]	•	•	•	•	•
Anticipatory guidance counseling[8]	•	•	•	•	•
Oral hygiene counseling[9]	Parent	Parent	Patient/parent	Patient/parent	Patient
Dietary counseling[10]	•	•	•	•	•
Injury prevention counseling[11]	•	•	•	•	•
Counseling for nonnutritive habits[12]	•	•	•	•	•
Counseling for speech/language development	•	•	•	•	•
Substance abuse counseling				•	•
Counseling for intraoral/perioral piercing				•	•
Assessment and treatment of developing malocclusion			•	•	•
Assessment for pit and fissure sealants[13]			•	•	•
Assessment and/or removal of third molars					•
Transition to adult dental care					•

[1]First examination at the eruption of the first tooth and no later than 12 months. Repeat every 6 months or as indicated by child's risk status/susceptibility to disease.
[2]Includes assessment of pathology and injuries.
[3]By clinical examination.
[4]Must be repeated regularly and frequently to maximize effectiveness.
[5]Timing, selection, and frequency determined by child's history, clinical findings, and susceptibility to oral disease.
[6]Consider when systemic fluoride exposure is suboptimal.
[7]Up to at least 16 years.
[8]Appropriate discussion and counseling should be an integral part of each visit for care.
[9]Initially, responsibility of parent; as child develops, jointly with parent; then, when indicated, only child.
[10]At every appointment; initially discuss appropriate feeding practices, then the role of refined carbohydrates and frequency of snacking in caries development and childhood obesity.
[11]Initially play objects, pacifiers, cars seats; then when learning to walk, sports and routine playing, including the importance of mouthguards.
[12]At first, discuss the need for additional sucking; digits vs. pacifiers; then the need to wean from the habit before malocclusion or skeletal dysplasia occurs. For school-aged children and adolescent patients, counsel regarding any existing habits such as fingernail biting, clenching, or bruxism.
[13]For caries-susceptible primary molars, permanent molars, premolars, and anterior teeth with deep pits and fissures; placed as soon as possible after eruption.

be associated with a single, badly carious primary molar. Although the collection and evaluation of these associated facts are performed rapidly, they provide a diagnosis only for a single problem area. On the other hand, a comprehensive diagnosis of all of the patient's problems or potential problems may sometimes need to be postponed until more urgent conditions are resolved. For example, a patient with necrotizing ulcerative gingivitis or a newly fractured crown needs immediate treatment, but the treatment will likely be only palliative, and further diagnostic and treatment procedures will be required later.

The importance of thoroughly collecting and evaluating the facts concerning a patient's condition cannot be overemphasized. A thorough examination of the pediatric dental patient includes assessment of:

- General growth and health
- Chief complaint, such as pain
- Extraoral soft tissue and temporomandibular joint evaluation
- Intraoral soft tissue
- Oral hygiene and periodontal health
- Intraoral hard tissue
- Developing occlusion
- Caries risk
- Behavior

Additional diagnostic aids are often also required, such as radiographs, study models, photographs, pulp tests, and, infrequently, laboratory tests.[1]

In certain unusual cases, all of these diagnostic aids may be necessary to arrive at a comprehensive diagnosis. Certainly no oral diagnosis can be complete unless the diagnostician has evaluated the facts obtained by medical and dental history taking, inspection, palpation, exploration (if teeth are present), and often imaging (e.g., radiographs). For a more thorough review of evaluation of the dental patient, refer to the chapter by Glick, Greenberg, and Ship in *Burket's Oral Medicine*.[2]

PRELIMINARY MEDICAL AND DENTAL HISTORY

It is important for the dentist to be familiar with the medical and dental history of the pediatric patient. Familial history may also be relevant to the patient's oral condition and may provide important diagnostic information in some hereditary disorders. Before the dentist examines the child, the dental assistant can obtain sufficient information to provide the dentist with knowledge of the child's general health and can alert the dentist to the need for obtaining additional information from the parent or the child's physician. The form illustrated in Fig. 1-1 can be completed by the parent. However, it is more effective for the dental assistant to ask the questions informally and then to present the findings to the dentist and offer personal observations and a summary of the case. The questions included on the form will also provide information about any previous dental treatment.

Information regarding the child's social and psychological development is important. Accurate information reflecting a child's learning, behavioral, or communication problems is sometimes difficult to obtain initially, especially when the parents are aware of their child's developmental disorder but are reluctant to discuss it. Behavior problems in the dental office are often related to the child's inability to communicate with the dentist and to follow instructions. This inability may be attributable to a learning disorder. An indication of learning disorders can usually be obtained by the dental assistant when asking questions about the child's learning process; for example, asking a young school-aged child how he or she is doing in school is a good lead question. The questions should be age-appropriate for the child.

A notation should be made if a young child was hospitalized previously for general anesthetic and surgical procedures. Shaw reported that hospitalization and a general anesthetic procedure can be a traumatic psychological experience for a preschool child and may sensitize the youngster to procedures that will be encountered later in a dental office.[3] If the dentist is aware that a child was previously hospitalized or the child fears strangers in clinic attire, the necessary time and procedures can be planned to help the child overcome the fear and accept dental treatment.

Occasionally, when the parents report significant disorders, it is best for the dentist to conduct the medical and dental history interview. When the parents meet with the dentist privately, they are more likely to discuss the child's problems openly and there is less chance for misunderstandings regarding the nature of the disorders. In addition, the dentist's personal involvement at this early time strengthens the confidence of the parents. When there is indication of an acute or chronic systemic disease or anomaly, the dentist should consult the child's physician to learn the status of the condition, the long-range prognosis, and the current drug therapy.

Current illnesses or histories of significant disorders signal the need for special attention during the medical and dental history interview. In addition to consulting the child's physician, the dentist may decide to record additional data concerning the child's current physical condition, such as blood pressure, body temperature, heart sounds, height and weight, pulse, and respiration. Before treatment is initiated, certain laboratory tests may be indicated and special precautions may be necessary. A decision to provide treatment in a hospital and possibly under general anesthesia may be appropriate.

The dentist and the staff must also be alert to identify potentially communicable infectious conditions that threaten the health of the patient and others. Knowledge of the current recommended childhood immunization schedule is helpful. It is advisable to postpone nonemergency dental care for a patient exhibiting signs or symptoms of acute infectious disease until the patient recovers. Further discussions of management of dental patients with special medical, physical, or behavioral problems are presented in Chapters 2, 3, 14, 15, 23, 24, and 28.

The pertinent facts of the medical history can be transferred to the oral examination record (Fig. 1-2) for easy reference by the dentist. A brief summary of important medical information serves as a convenient reminder to the dentist and the staff, because they refer to this chart at each treatment visit.

The patient's dental history should also be summarized on the examination chart. This should include a record of previous care in the dentist's office and the facts related by the patient and the parent regarding previous care in another office. Information concerning the patient's current oral hygiene habits and previous and current fluoride exposure helps the dentist develop an effective dental disease prevention program. For example, if the family drinks well water, a sample may be sent to a water analysis laboratory to determine the fluoride concentration.

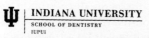

UNIVERSITY PEDIATRIC DENTISTRY ASSOCIATES
Riley Hospital for Children • Outpatient Center • Dental MSA
702 Barnhill Drive, Room #4205
Indianapolis, IN 46202-5200
(317) 274-3865 • (317) 274-9653 Fax

Place Patient Label Here

OFFICE USE ONLY

Patient Name: _____
                         Last   First   MI

DOB_____   Record #: _____

MEDICAL – DENTAL HISTORY

Child's name: _____ Sex: _____ Race: _____ Height: _____ Weight: _____ Birth Date: _____

Date of last medical examination: _____ Child's physician/ pediatrician: _____ Place of birth: _____ Telephone: _____

Physicians address: _____

GROWTH AND DEVELOPMENT:

Any learning, behavioral, excessive nervousness, or communication problems? YES☐ NO☐
Has child had psychological counseling or is counseling being considered for the near future? YES☐ NO☐
Were there any complications during pregnancy or was child premature at birth? YES☐ NO☐

CENTRAL NERVOUS SYSTEM:

Any history of cerebral palsy, seizures, convulsions, fainting, or loss of consciousness? YES☐ NO☐
Any history of injury to the head? YES☐ NO☐
Any sensory disorders? (Seeing, Hearing) YES☐ NO☐

CARDIOVASCULAR SYSTEM:

Any history of congenital heart disease, heart murmur, or heart damage from rheumatic fever? YES☐ NO☐
Has any heart surgery been done or recommended? YES☐ NO☐
Any history of chest pains or high blood pressure? YES☐ NO☐

HEMATOPOIETIC AND LYMPHATIC SYSTEMS:

Has your child ever had a blood transfusion or blood products transfusion? YES☐ NO☐
Any history of anemia or sickle cell disease? YES☐ NO☐
Does your child bruise easily, have frequent nosebleeds, or bleed excessively from small cuts? YES☐ NO☐
Is your child more susceptible to infections than other children ? YES☐ NO☐
Is there any history of tender or swollen lymph nodes or glands? YES☐ NO☐

RESPIRATORY SYSTEM:

Any history of pneumonia, cystic fibrosis, asthma, shortness of breath, or difficulty in breathing? YES☐ NO☐

GASTROINTESTINAL SYSTEM:

Any history of stomach, intestinal or liver problems? YES☐ NO☐
Any history of hepatitis or jaundice? YES☐ NO☐
Any history of eating disorders, such as anorexia nervosa (binge) or bulimia (binge/purge)? YES☐ NO☐
Any history of unintentional weight loss? YES☐ NO☐

GENITOURINARY SYSTEM:

Any history of urinary tract infections, bladder or kidney problems? YES☐ NO☐
Is the patient pregnant or possibly pregnant? YES☐ NO☐

ENDOCRINE SYSTEM:

Any history of diabetes? YES☐ NO☐
Any history of thyroid disorders or other glandular disorders? YES☐ NO☐

SKIN:

Any history of skin problems? YES☐ NO☐
Any history of cold sores (herpes) or canker sores (aphthae)? YES☐ NO☐

EXTREMITIES:

Any limitations of use of arms or legs? YES☐ NO☐
Any arthritis, joint bleeding, joint replacements, or other joint problems? YES☐ NO☐
Any problems with muscle weakness or muscular dystrophy? YES☐ NO☐

ALLERGIES:

Is your child allergic to any medications? YES☐ NO☐
Any hay fever, hives, or skin rashes caused by allergies? YES☐ NO☐
Any other allergies? YES☐ NO☐

MEDICATIONS AND TREATMENTS:

Is your child currently taking any medication (prescription or non-prescription medicine)? YES☐ NO☐
If yes, Medication(s)   Dosage (mg.)   Times Per Day

_____   _____   _____
_____   _____   _____
_____   _____   _____

Has your child ever received therapy (x-ray treatments) or is it planned? YES☐ NO☐
Has your child ever received chemotherapy or is it planned? YES☐ NO☐

HOSPITALIZATIONS:

Has your child been hospitalized? YES☐ NO☐
Hospital   (1) _____ (2) _____ (3) _____
Date   _____   _____   _____
Reason   _____   _____   _____

Figure 1-1 Form used in completing the preliminary medical and dental history. (Printed with permission from Indiana University–University Pediatric Dentistry Associates.)

University Pediatric Dentistry Associates   702 Barnhill Drive, RM #4205 • Indianapolis, IN 46202-5200 • (317) 274-3865 • (317) 274-9653 Fax

MEDICAL – DENTAL HISTORY   Date of Birth: _____   ACT#:_____

IMMUNIZATIONS: Is your child presently protected by Immunization against:

DTaP/DTP/DT/Td: diphtheria, whooping cough (pertussis), tetanus?   YES☐ NO☐
IPV: inactive poliovirus or poliomyelitis?   YES☐ NO☐
MMR: measles (rubeola), mumps, and German measles (rubella)?   YES☐ NO☐
Hib: (Haemophilus b vaccine)?   YES☐ NO☐
PCV: Pneumococcal vaccine?   YES☐ NO☐
HepB: Hepatitis B vaccine ?   YES☐ NO☐
Varicella: Varicella vaccine or history of Chicken Pox?   YES☐ NO☐

PLEASE CHECK ANY OF THE ILLNESSES THAT YOUR CHILD HAS NOW, HAS RECENTLY BEEN EXPOSED TO, OR HAS HAD IN THE PAST:

Chicken Pox (Varicella)   NOW☐ EXPOSED☐ PAST☐
Eye infection (conjunctivitis)   NOW☐ EXPOSED☐ PAST☐
German measles or 3-day measles (rubella)   NOW☐ EXPOSED☐ PAST☐
Glandular fever or mono (infectious mononucleosis)   NOW☐ EXPOSED☐ PAST☐
HIV/AIDS   NOW☐ EXPOSED☐ PAST☐
Lead poisoning   NOW☐ EXPOSED☐ PAST☐
Measles (rubella)   NOW☐ EXPOSED☐ PAST☐
Mumps (parotitis)   NOW☐ EXPOSED☐ PAST☐
Scarlet fever (scarlatina)   NOW☐ EXPOSED☐ PAST☐
Sore throat (tonsillitis or pharyngitis)   NOW☐ EXPOSED☐ PAST☐
Substance abuse, alcoholism, drug addiction   NOW☐ EXPOSED☐ PAST☐
Tuberculosis   NOW☐ EXPOSED☐ PAST☐
Upper respiratory infection (URI), or common cold (pharyngitis, rhinitis, sinusitis, or tonsillitis)   NOW☐ EXPOSED☐ PAST☐
Venereal disease (genital herpes, gonorrhea, syphilis or other)   NOW☐ EXPOSED☐ PAST☐

DENTAL HISTORY:

Does your child have a **toothache** or other **immediate dental problem**?   YES☐ NO☐
Has your child ever had a **toothache**?   YES☐ NO☐
Has your child had any injury to the mouth, teeth or jaws (fall, blow, etc.)? When: _____   YES☐ NO☐
Is this your child's first dental visit?   YES☐ NO☐
    *If no, please tell us: First visit date: _____ Dentist: _____ Reason: _____
                            Last visit date: _____ Dentist: _____ Reason: _____
Has your child ever had an unfavorable dental experience?   YES☐ NO☐
Is (was) your child nourished by nursing beyond one year of age?   YES☐ NO☐
    Please tell us, how was your child nursed? ☐ Breast ☐ Nursing Bottle ☐ Both To what age? _____
Does your child fail to eat a well-balanced diet?   YES☐ NO☐
    Please describe your child's diet on a typical day: _____
Does (or has) your child have (or had) sucking habit beyond one year of age?   YES☐ NO☐
    *If yes, please check all that apply: ☐ Thumb   ☐ Finger   ☐ Pacifier   ☐ Other: _____
Does (or has) your child have (or had) any other oral habits beyond one year of age?   YES☐ NO☐
    *If yes, please check all that apply: ☐Lip Biting ☐Mouth Breather ☐Nail Biting ☐Teeth Grinding ☐Other: _____
Does (or has) your child have (or had) difficulty opening their mouth, or does their jaw sometimes lock or stick in a certain position?   YES☐ NO☐
Does (or has) your child have (or had) popping or clicking noises or pain during chewing or yawning?   YES☐ NO☐
Does (or has) your child have (or had) frequent headaches or pain in or about the ears, eyes, or cheeks?   YES☐ NO☐

DENTAL DISEASE PREVENTION:

How often does your child brush? _____   Times per:_____ / _____
Does someone assist your child with brushing and cleaning the teeth?   Who helps: _____   YES☐ NO☐
Does someone inspect for thoroughness after the procedure?   Who inspects: _____   YES☐ NO☐
Does your child use a fluoride toothpaste?   What brand: _____   YES☐ NO☐
Does your child use dental floss? _____   How often: _____   YES☐ NO☐
Has your child ever had a fluoride treatment?   When: _____   YES☐ NO☐
Has your child ever taken fluoride supplement or vitamins with fluorides?   When: _____   YES☐ NO☐

Drinking water source:

CITY WATER   ☐   Name of city _____
PRIVATE WELL   ☐   Has a fluoride analysis been done?   Date of analysis: _____   Fluoride content: _____
OTHER   ☐   Please Describe: _____

▶ SIGNATURE (Parent or Legal Guardian only)   ▶ SIGNATURE PEDIATRIC DENTISTRY RESIDENT   ▶ DATE

RESIDENT   Medical Consultations Recommended? Yes / No   Purpose for Consultation: _____
COMMENTS: Date Requested? _____

SEMI-ANNUAL REVIEW of Medical-Dental History: If history remains essentially unchanged, sign below.
DATE: _____   PARENT/GUARDIAN: _____   RESIDENT: _____
DATE: _____   PARENT/GUARDIAN: _____   RESIDENT: _____
DATE: _____   PARENT/GUARDIAN: _____   RESIDENT: _____

A new history form must be completed every 2 years for Essentially Negative or every 1 year for Positive History

Figure 1-1 Cont'd

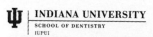

INDIANA UNIVERSITY
SCHOOL OF DENTISTRY
IUPUI

UNIVERSITY PEDIATRIC DENTISTRY ASSOCIATES
Riley Hospital for Children • Outpatient Center • Dental MSA
702 Barnhill Drive, Room #4205
Indianapolis, IN 46202-5200
(317) 274-3865 • (317) 274-9653 Fax

Place Patient Label Here

OFFICE USE ONLY

Patient Name:
_____
Last   First   MI

DOB_____   Record #: _____

ORAL EXAMINATION RECORD

Address: Same ☐ New ☐ _____   Telephone: Same☐ New☐ _____
**** New address and/or phone number must be noted here and updated in practice software.

MEDICAL HISTORY SUMMARY

Last History Completed: _____   Update Due: _____   Weight: _____

Current Medication Status & Medication Usage:

DENTAL HISTORY SUMMARY

Date of Last Exam: _____   Last Radiographs: B.W.: _____ A.O.:_____ P.A.:_____ F.M.:_____

Appliances: _____   Last Cemented: _____   Last Replaced: _____

Description of Present Problem:

Summary of Prior Treatment:

EXTRA ORAL FINDINGS

Head: Neck:

Face: Lips: Hands:

INTRA ORAL FINDINGS

Palate and Oropharynx: Airway: I   II   III   IV

Tongue and Floor of Mouth: Buccal Mucosa:

Frena: Gingivae and Periodontium:

OCCLUSION REVIEW

Facial Profile: _____

Molar Relationship:

PRIMARY (Terminal Plane):	R	L		PERMANENT:	R	L
Straight	☐	☐		Molar		
Mes. Step	☐	☐		End to End	☐	☐
Dist. Step	☐	☐		Class	___	___
Primate Space	☐	☐		Canine		
Canine Relationship	___	___		Relationship	___	___

Incisor Relationship:
Overjet   _____mm
Overbite   _____%
Openbite   _____mm

Arch Length: (General Impression)

Maxilla		Mandible	
Adequate	☐	Adequate	☐
Inadequate	☐	Inadequate	☐

Midline: Normal ☐   Deviated ☐
Maxilla   _____mm   R☐ L☐
Mandible   _____mm   R☐ L☐
Mandibular:
Shift R☐ L☐ Ant. ☐_____mm

Eruption Sequence & Timimg:
Normal ☐   Describe ☐
_____
_____

TMJ and Function:

Opening Path:	Normal	☐	Deviated	☐
Closing Path:	Normal	☐	Deviated	☐
Opening: ___mm	Normal	☐	Limited	☐

Joint Sounds:	None	Left	Right
Opening	☐	☐	☐
Closing	☐	☐	☐
Crepitus	☐	☐	☐

Muscle Tenderness:

Tongue Function: Supernumerary Teeth/ Congenitally Missing Teeth:

Crossbite: Ectopic Eruption:

Oral Habits: Other Anomalies:

Analysis Recommended: YES☐   NO☐

Figure 1-2 Chart used to record the oral findings and the treatment proposed for the pediatric patient. See legend on opposite page. (Printed with permission from Indiana University–University Pediatric Dentistry Associates.)

University Pediatric Dentistry Associates 702 Barnhill Drive RM #4205 • Indianapolis IN 46202-5200 • (317) 274-3865 • (317) 274-9653 Fax

ORAL EXAM RECORD

Patient Name: _____

Date of Birth: _____ ACT#: _____

HARD TISSUE EXAMINATION

		Clinical	Radiographic			Clinical	Radiographic
A	1			J	16		
B	2			I	15		
C	3			H	14		
D	4			G	13		
E	5			F	12		
	6				11		
	7				10		
	8				9		
P	25			O	24		
Q	26			N	23		
R	27			M	22		
S	28			L	21		
T	29			K	20		
	30				19		
	31				18		
	32				17		

Plaque Score: A B C D F
Prior Score:

Fluoride Status:

Brushing / Flossing:

Habits:

Periodontal:

Periodontal Screening _____|_____|_____
& Recording: _____|_____|_____

DIAGNOSTIC SUMMARY

Behavior:

Eruption sequence:

Occlusion:

Caries:

Caries Risk Assessment: ☐Low ☐Moderate ☐High

Upper Right   **TREATMENT PROPOSED**   **Upper Left**

Lower Right   **Lower Left**

Treatment sequence, additional notations:

1.
2.
3.
4.
5.

Instructions given:

_____ _____ _____
Assistant   Resident   Faculty Instructor

Figure 1-2 Cont'd

CLINICAL EXAMINATION

Most facts needed for a comprehensive oral diagnosis in the young patient are obtained by a thorough clinical and radiographic examination. In addition to examining the structures in the oral cavity, the dentist may in some cases wish to note the patient's size, stature, gait, or involuntary movements. The first clue to malnutrition may come from observing a patient's abnormal size or stature. Similarly, the severity of a child's illness, even if oral in origin, may be recognized by observing a weak, unsteady gait of lethargy and malaise as the patient walks into the office. All relevant information should be noted on the oral examination record (see Fig. 1-2), which becomes a permanent part of the patient's chart.

The clinical examination, whether the first examination or a regular recall examination, should be all inclusive. The dentist can gather useful information while getting acquainted with a new patient. Attention to the patient's hair, head, face, neck, and hands should be among the first observations made by the dentist after the patient is seated in the chair.

The patient's hands may reveal information pertinent to the comprehensive diagnosis. The dentist may first detect an elevated temperature by holding the patient's hand. Cold, clammy hands or bitten fingernails may be the first indication of abnormal anxiety in the child. A callused or unusually clean digit suggests a persistent sucking habit. Clubbing of the fingers or a bluish color in the nail beds suggests congenital heart disease that may require special precautions during dental treatment.

Inspection and palpation of the patient's head and neck are also indicated. Unusual characteristics of the hair or skin should be noted. The dentist may observe signs of head lice (Fig. 1-3), ringworm (Fig. 1-4), or impetigo (Fig. 1-5) during the examination. Proper referral is indicated immediately, because these conditions are contagious. After the child's physician has supervised the treatment to control the condition, the child's dental appointment may be rescheduled. If a contagious condition is identified but the child also has a dental emergency,

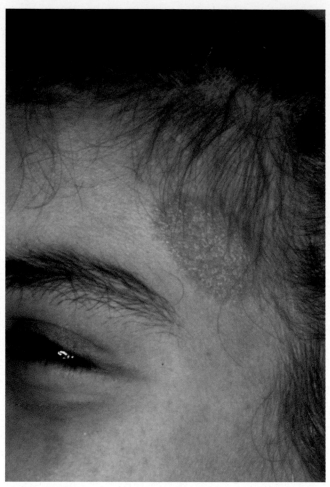

Figure 1-4 Lesion on forehead above left eyebrow is caused by ringworm infection. Several fungal species may cause the lesions on various areas of the body. The dentist may identify lesions on the head, face, or neck of a patient during a routine clinical examination. (Courtesy Dr. Hala Henderson.)

the dentist and the staff must take appropriate precautions to prevent spread of the disease to others while the emergency is alleviated. Further treatment should be postponed until the contagious condition is controlled.

Variations in size, shape, symmetry, or function of the head and neck structures should be recorded. Abnormalities of these structures may indicate various syndromes or conditions associated with oral abnormalities.

TEMPOROMANDIBULAR EVALUATION

Okeson[4] published a special report on temporomandibular disorders in children. Okeson indicated that, although several studies include children 5 to 7 years of age, most observations have been made in young adolescent. Studies have placed the findings into the categories of symptoms or signs—those reported by the child or parents and those identified by the dentist during the examination.

One should evaluate TMJ function by palpating the head of each mandibular condyle and observing the patient while the mouth is closed (teeth clenched), at rest, and in various open positions (Fig. 1-6A, B). Movements

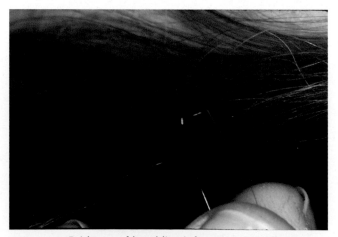

Figure 1-3 Evidence of head lice infestation. Usually the insects are not seen, but their eggs, or nits, cling to hair filaments until they hatch. (Courtesy Dr. Hala Henderson.)

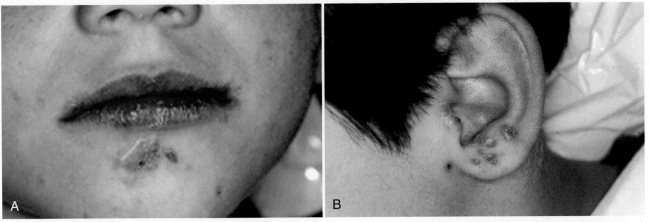

Figure 1-5 Characteristic lesions of impetigo on the lower face **(A)** and on the right ear **(B).** These lesions occur on various skin surfaces, but the dentist is most likely to encounter them on upper body areas. The infections are of bacterial (usually streptococcal) origin and generally require antibiotic therapy for control. The child often spreads the infection by scratching the lesions. (Courtesy Dr. Hala Henderson.)

of the condyles or jaw that are not smoothly flowing or deviate from the expected norm should be noted. Similarly, any crepitus that may be heard or identified by palpation, or any other abnormal sounds, should be noted. Sore masticatory muscles may also signal TMJ dysfunction. Such deviations from normal TMJ function may require further evaluation and treatment. There is a consensus that temporomandibular disorders in children can be managed effectively by the following conservative and reversible therapies: patient education, mild physical therapy, behavioral therapy, medications, and occlusal splints.[5]

Discussion of the diagnosis and treatment of complex TMJ disorders is available from many sources; we suggest Okeson's *Management of Temporomandibular Disorders and Occlusion* (2008).[6]

The extraoral examination continues with palpation of the patient's neck and submandibular area (see Fig. 1-6C, D). Again, deviations from normal, such as unusual tenderness or enlargement, should be noted and follow-up tests performed or referrals made as indicated.

If the child is old enough to talk, speech should be evaluated. The positions of the tongue, lips, and perioral musculature during speech, while swallowing, and while at rest may provide useful diagnostic information.

The intraoral examination of a pediatric patient should be comprehensive. There is a temptation to look first for obvious carious lesions. Certainly controlling carious lesions is important, but the dentist should first evaluate the condition of the oral soft tissues and the status of the developing occlusion. If the soft tissues and the occlusion are not observed early in the examination, the dentist may become so engrossed in charting carious lesions and in planning for their restoration that other important anomalies in the mouth are overlooked. Any unusual breath odors and abnormal quantity or consistency of saliva should also be noted.

The buccal tissues, lips, floor of the mouth, palate, and gingivae should be carefully inspected and palpated (Fig. 1-7). The use of the periodontal screening and

recording program (PSR) is often a helpful adjunct in children. PSR is designed to facilitate early detection of periodontal diseases with a simplified probing technique and minimal documentation. Clerehugh and Tugnait[7] recommend initiation of periodontal screening in children following eruption of the permanent incisors and the first molars. They suggest routine screening in these children at the child's first appointment and at regular recare appointments so that periodontal problems are detected early and treated appropriately. Immunodeficient children are especially vulnerable to early loss of bone support.

A more detailed periodontal evaluation is occasionally indicated even in young children. Periodontal disorders of children are discussed further in Chapter 20.

The tongue and oropharynx should be closely inspected. Enlarged tonsils accompanied by purulent exudate may be the initial sign of a streptococcal infection, which can lead to rheumatic fever. When streptococcal throat infection is suspected, immediate referral to the child's physician is indicated. In some cases it may be helpful to the physician and convenient for the dentist to obtain a throat culture specimen while the child is still in the dental office, which contributes to an earlier definitive diagnosis of the infection. The diagnosis and treatment of soft tissue problems are discussed throughout this book; see Chapters 7, 8, and 20.

After thoroughly examining the oral soft tissues, the dentist should inspect the occlusion and note any dental or skeletal irregularities. The dentition and resulting occlusion may undergo considerable change during childhood and early adolescence. This dynamic developmental process occurs in all three planes of space, and with periodic evaluation the dentist can intercept and favorably influence undesirable changes. Monitoring of the patient's facial profile and symmetry; molar, canine, and anterior segment relationships; dental midlines; and relation of arch length to tooth mass should be routinely included in the clinical examination. More detailed evaluation and analysis are indicated when significant discrepancies are found during

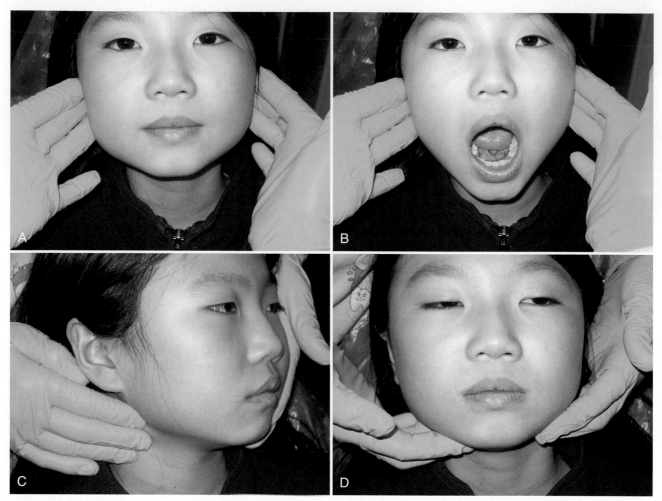

Figure 1-6 A and **B,** Observation and palpation of temporomandibular joint function. **C** and **D,** Palpation of the neck and submandibular areas.

critical stages of growth and development. Diagnostic cast and cephalometric analyses may be indicated relatively early in the mixed dentition stage and sometimes in the primary dentition. Detailed discussions of analyses of developing occlusions and interceptive treatment recommendations are presented in Chapters 25 through 27.

Finally, the teeth should be inspected carefully for evidence of carious lesions and hereditary or acquired anomalies. The teeth should also be counted and identified individually to ensure recognition of supernumerary or missing teeth. Identification of carious lesions is important in patients of all ages but is especially critical in young patients because the lesions may progress rapidly in early childhood caries if not controlled. Eliminating the etiology of the carious activity, preventive management of the caries process, and restoration of cavitated lesions as needed will prevent pain and the spread of infection and will contribute to the stability of the developing occlusion.

If the dentist prefers to perform the clinical examination of a new pediatric patient before the radiographic and prophylaxis procedures, it may be necessary to correlate radiographic findings or other initially questionable findings with the findings of a second brief oral

examination. This is especially true when the new patient has poor oral hygiene. Detailed inspection and exploration of the teeth and soft tissues cannot be performed adequately until the mouth is free of extraneous debris.

During the clinical examination for carious lesions, each tooth should be dried individually and inspected under a good light. A definite routine for the examination should be established. For example, a dentist may always start in the upper right quadrant, work around the maxillary arch, move down to the lower left quadrant, and end the examination in the lower right quadrant. Morphologic defects and incomplete coalescence of enamel at the base of pits and fissures in molar teeth can often be detected readily by visual and explorer examination after the teeth have been cleaned and dried. The decision whether to place a sealant or to restore a defect depends on the patient's history of dental caries, the parents' or patient's acceptance of a comprehensive preventive dentistry program (including dietary and oral hygiene control), and the patient's dependability in returning for recare appointments.

In patients with severe dental caries, caries activity tests and diet analysis may contribute to the diagnostic process

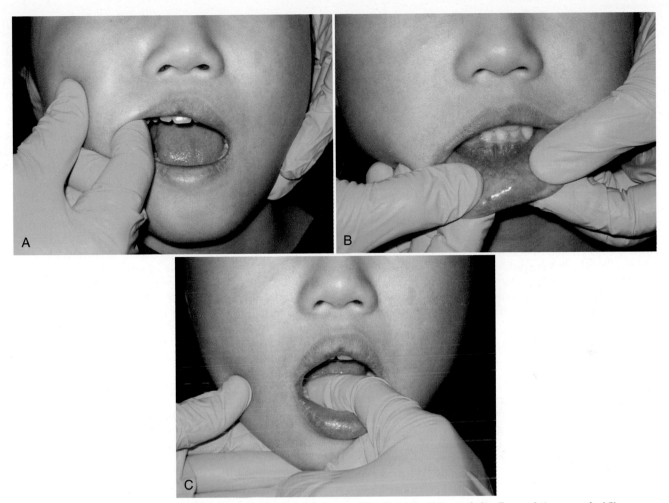

Figure 1-7 Inspection and palpation of the buccal tissues **(A)**, the lips **(B)**, and the floor of the mouth **(C)**.

by helping define specific etiologic factors. These procedures probably have an even greater value in helping the patient or parents understand the carious disease process and in motivating them to make the behavioral changes needed to control the disease. The information provided to the patient or parents should include instruction in plaque control and the appropriate recommendations for fluoride exposure. Dental caries susceptibility, the caries disease process, caries activity tests, diet analysis, and caries control are discussed in Chapter 10. Plaque control procedures and instructions are presented in detail in Chapter 11.

The dentist's comprehensive diagnosis depends on the completion of a number of procedures but requires a thorough, systematic, and critical clinical examination. Any deviation from the expected or desired size, shape, color, and consistency of soft or hard tissues should be described in detail. The severity of associated problems and their causes must be clearly identified to the parents or the patient before success of a comprehensive oral health care program can be expected.

During the initial examination and at subsequent appointments, the dentist and auxiliary staff members should be alert to signs and symptoms of child abuse and neglect. These problems are increasing in prevalence, and the

dentist can play an important role in detecting their signs and symptoms; Chapter 2 is devoted to this subject.

UNIFORM DENTAL RECORDING

Many different tooth charting systems are currently in use, including the universal system illustrated in the hard tissue examination section of Fig. 1-2. This system of marking permanent teeth uses the numbers 1 to 32, beginning with the upper right third molar (No. 1) and progressing around the arch to the upper left third molar (No. 16), down to the lower left third molar (No. 17), and around the arch to the lower right third molar (No. 32). The primary teeth are identified in the universal system by the first 20 letters of the alphabet, A through T.

The Fédération Dentaire International Special Committee on Uniform Dental Recording has specified the following basic requirements for a tooth charting system:
1. Simple to understand and teach
2. Easy to pronounce in conversation and dictation
3. Readily communicable in print and by wire
4. Easy to translate into computer input
5. Easily adaptable to standard charts used in general practice

The committee found that only one system, the two-digit system, seems to comply with these requirements. According to this system, the first digit indicates the quadrant and the second digit the type of tooth within the quadrant. Quadrants are allotted the digits 1 to 4 for the permanent teeth and 5 to 8 for the primary teeth in a clockwise sequence, starting at the upper right side; teeth within the same quadrant are allotted the digits 1 to 8 (primary teeth, 1 to 5) from the midline backward. The digits should be pronounced separately; thus the permanent canines are teeth one-three, two-three, three-three, and four-three.

In the "Treatment Proposed" section of the oral examination record (see Fig. 1-2), the individual teeth that require restorative procedures, endodontic therapy, or extraction are listed. Gingival areas requiring follow-up therapy are also noted. A check mark can be placed beside each listed tooth and procedure as the treatment is completed. Additional notations concerning treatment procedures completed and the date are recorded on supplemental treatment record pages.

RADIOGRAPHIC EXAMINATION

When indicated, radiographic examination for children must be completed before the comprehensive oral health care plan can be developed, and subsequent radiographs are required periodically to allow detection of incipient carious lesions or other developing anomalies.

A child should be exposed to dental ionizing radiation only after the dentist has determined the radiographic requirement, if any, to make an adequate diagnosis for the individual child at the time of the appointment.

Obtaining isolated occlusal, periapical, or bite-wing films is sometimes indicated in very young children (even infants) because of trauma, toothache, suspected developmental disturbances, or proximal caries. Carious lesions appear smaller on radiographs than they actually are.

As early as 1967, Blayney and Hill[8] recognized the importance of diagnosing incipient proximal carious lesions with the appropriate use of radiographs. If the pediatric patient can be motivated to adopt a routine of good oral hygiene supported by competent supervision, many of these initial lesions would be arrested.

Radiographic techniques for the pediatric patient are described in detail in Chapter 5.

EARLY EXAMINATION

Historically, dental care for children has been designed primarily to prevent oral pain and infection, the occurrence and progress of dental caries, the premature loss of primary teeth, the loss of arch length, and the development of an association between fear and dental care. The dentist is responsible for guiding the child and parent, resolving oral disorders before they can affect health and dental alignment, and preventing oral disease. The goals of pediatric dental care therefore are primarily preventive. The dentist's opportunity to conduct an initial oral examination and parental consultation during the patient's infancy is a key element in achieving and maintaining these goals.

Some dentists, especially pediatric dentists, like to counsel expectant parents before their child is born. They consider it appropriate to discuss with expectant mothers the importance of good nutrition during pregnancy and practices that can influence the expected child's general and dental health.

It is also appropriate to inquire about medication that the expectant mother is taking. It is known that the prolonged ingestion of tetracyclines may result in discolored, pigmented, and even hypoplastic primary teeth.

The expectant mother should be encouraged to visit her dentist and to have all carious lesions restored. The presence of active dental caries and accompanying high levels of *Streptococcus mutans* can lead to transmission by the mother to the infant and may be responsible for the development of carious lesions at a very early age.

It is not intended that the pediatric dentist should usurp the responsibility of the expectant mother's physician in recommending dietary practices; rather, the dentist should reinforce good nutritional recommendations provided by medical colleagues.

INFANT DENTAL CARE

The infant oral health care visit should be seen as the foundation on which a lifetime of preventive education and dental care can be built to help assure optimal oral health into childhood. Oral examination, anticipatory guidance including preventive education, and appropriate therapeutic intervention for the infant can enhance the opportunity for a lifetime of freedom from preventable oral disease. The 2008 American Academy of Pediatric Dentistry guidelines on infant oral health care include the following recommendations:

1. All primary health care professionals who serve mothers and infants should provide parent/caregiver education on the etiology and prevention of early childhood caries (ECC).
2. The infectious and transmissible nature of bacteria that cause ECC and methods of oral health risk assessment (e.g., Caries Assessment Tool [CAT]), anticipatory guidance, and early intervention should be included in the curriculum of all medical, nursing, and allied health professional programs.
3. Every infant should receive an oral health risk assessment from his or her primary health care provider or qualified health care professional by 6 months of age.
4. Parents or caregivers should establish a dental home for infants by 12 months of age.
5. Health care professionals and all stakeholders in children's health should support the identification of a dental home for all infants at 12 months of age.

Thus it is appropriate for a dentist to perform an oral examination for an infant of any age, even a newborn, and an examination is recommended anytime the parent or physician calls with questions concerning the appearance of an infant's oral tissues. Even when there are no known problems, the child's first dental visit and oral examination should take place by at least 1 year of age. This early dental visit enables the dentist and parents to discuss ways to nurture excellent oral health before any serious problems have had an opportunity to develop. An adequate oral examination for an infant is generally simple and brief, but it may be the important first step toward a lifetime of excellent oral health.

Some dentists may prefer to "preside" during the entire first session with the infant and parents. Others may wish to delegate some of the educational aspects of the session to auxiliary members of the office staff and then conduct the examination and answer any unresolved questions. In either case, it is sometimes necessary to have an assistant available to help hold the child's attention so that the parents can concentrate on the important information being provided.

It is not always necessary to conduct the infant oral examination in the dental operatory, but it should take place where there is adequate light for a visual examination. The dentist may find it convenient to conduct the examination in the private consultation room during the initial meeting with the child and the parents. The examination procedures may include only direct observation and digital palpation. However, if primary molars have erupted or if hand instruments may be needed, the examination should be performed in an area where instrument transfers between the dental assistant and the dentist may proceed smoothly.

The parents should be informed before the examination that it will be necessary to gently restrain the child and that it is normal for the child to cry during the procedure. The infant is held on the lap of a parent, usually the mother. This direct involvement of the parent provides emotional support to the child and allows the parent to help restrain the child. Both parents may participate or at least be present during the examination.

The dentist should make a brief attempt to get acquainted with the infant and to project warmth and caring. However, many infants and toddlers are not particularly interested in developing new friendships with strangers, and the dentist should not be discouraged if the infant shuns the friendly approach. Even if the child chooses to resist (which is common and normal), only negligible extra effort is necessary to perform the examination procedure. The dentist should not be flustered by the crying and resistant behavior and should proceed unhurriedly but efficiently with the examination. The dentist's voice should remain unstrained and pleasant during the examination. The dentist's behavior should reassure the child and alleviate the parents' anxiety concerning this first dental procedure.

One method of performing the examination in a private consultation area is illustrated in Fig. 1-8A. The dentist and the parent are seated face to face with their knees touching. Their upper legs form the "examination table" for the child. The child's legs straddle the parent's body, which allows the parent to restrain the child's legs and hands. An assistant is present to record the dentist's examination findings as they are dictated and to help restrain the child if needed. If adequate space is available in the consultation area, the approach illustrated in Fig. 1-8B may be useful. The dental assistant is seated at a desk or writing stand near the child's feet. The dental assistant and the parent are facing the same direction side by side and at a right angle to the direction that the dentist is facing. The dental assistant is in a good position to hear and record the dentist's findings as they are dictated, even if the child is crying loudly. These positions (see Fig. 1-8) are also convenient for demonstrating oral hygiene procedures to the parents.

The positions of the dentist, parent, child, and dental assistant during the examination at the dental chair are illustrated in Fig. 1-9. The dental assistant is seated higher to permit good visibility and to better anticipate the dentist's needs. The assistant is also in a good position to hear and record the dentist's findings. The parent and the dental assistant restrain the child's arms and legs. The child's head is positioned in the bend of the parent's arm. The dentist establishes a chairside position so that not only the

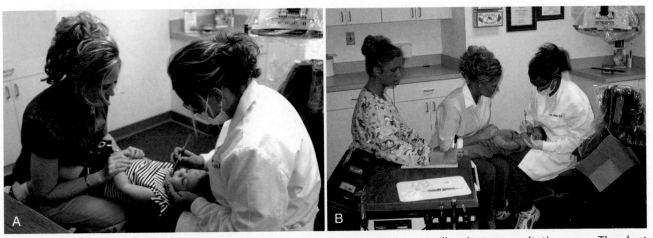

Figure 1-8 A, One method of positioning a child for an oral examination in a small, private consultation area. The dental assistant is nearby to record findings. **B,** If space allows three people to sit in a row, this method may be used to make it easier for the dental assistant to hear the findings dictated by the dentist. The dental assistant also helps restrain the child's legs.

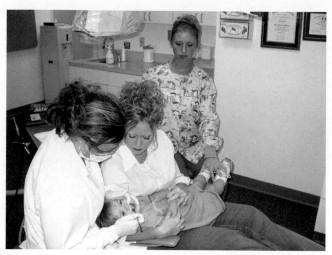

Figure 1-9 Oral examination of a very young child in the dental operatory.

dentist's hands but also the lower arms and abdomen may be available for support of the child's head if necessary.

The infant oral examination may often be performed by careful direct observation and digital palpation. The dentist may need only good lighting for visibility and gauze for drying or debriding tissues. Sometimes a tongue depressor and a soft-bristled toothbrush are also useful. At other times, as previously mentioned, the dentist will want the complete operatory available. The examination should begin with a systematic and gentle digital exploration of the soft tissues without any instruments. The child may find this gentle palpation soothing, especially when alveolar ridges in teething areas are massaged. The digital examination may help relax the child and encourage less resistance. If hand instruments are needed, the dentist must be sure to have a stable finger rest before inserting an instrument into the child's mouth.

Although there is little or no effective communication between the dentist and patient, the child realizes at the conclusion of the examination that nothing "bad" happened. The child also realizes that the procedure was permitted by the parents, who remained and actually helped with the examination. The child will not hold a lasting grudge against anyone, and the experience will not have a detrimental effect on future behavior as a dental patient. On the contrary, our experiences suggest that such early examinations followed by regular recall examinations often contribute to the youngsters' becoming excellent dental patients without fear at very young ages. These children's chances for enjoying excellent oral health throughout life are also enhanced.

DETECTION OF SUBSTANCE ABUSE

It is within the scope of pediatric dentistry to be concerned with life-threatening habits and illnesses such as alcoholism and drug addiction that may occur in the older child.

Rosenbaum[9,10] has reported that abusers in the teen years and younger are as common as adult addicts. Drug abuse problems interact directly with the dental care of a

patient. Obtaining and maintaining a satisfactory history is important. The office health questionnaire, as presented in this chapter, must be worded to allow the patient or parent to give some indication of a drug problem. It is often difficult to detect addiction from casual observation. Therefore input from the patient giving an indication of addiction is needed. At subsequent visits, the dentist must also consider changes in the general health history as well as answers to specific questions.

It is also important to know if the patient is taking drugs at the time of the dental visit because there could be an interaction with drugs, such as nitrous oxide, that may be given in the dental office. If the patient is under the influence of an abused substance, dental treatment should be postponed until a time when the patient is not "high."

Symptoms of substance abuse may include depression, feelings of inadequacy, frustration, helplessness, immaturity, self-alienation, poor object relations, and major deficiencies in ego structure and functioning. Heavy drug users tend to have poor impulse control. Hygiene in general and oral hygiene specifically are frequently neglected by those with a drug problem. In addition, because a patient is taking drugs that affect normal thought processes, the pain from untreated dental conditions may be masked. This combination of factors results in a patient with very little dental interest who is practicing unsatisfactory prevention. The result is increased oral disease.

Identification of substance abusers is difficult, even for an experienced observer. There are specific clues, however, that can be sought when one is attempting to draw general conclusions. Abrupt changes in behavior are common, as are signs of depression and moodiness. Interest in the opposite sex often decreases. Without any apparent consumption of alcohol, a drug-addicted person can appear intoxicated. There may be a desperate need for money, as well as a loss of appetite and loss of weight. The presence of scars along veins could be indicative of drug injection. Addicts frequently wear long-sleeved shirts, regardless of the weather, in an effort to cover identifying scars.

Fletcher and colleagues[11] state that use of illegal drugs and volatile substances is common among young people in developed countries, such as the United States and the United Kingdom. As well as presenting direct health risks, drug use is associated with accidental injury, self-harm, suicide, and other "problem" behaviors, such as alcohol misuse, unprotected sex, and antisocial behavior. Drug use at an early age is also associated with future use of particularly harmful drugs, such as heroin or cocaine. In turn, dependence on these drugs is associated with high rates of morbidity and mortality, social disadvantage, and crime. It is because of these health and social problems that reducing teenage drug use is a priority.

Their review of the literature however, suggests that positive ethos and overall levels of strong school relationships and engagement are associated with lower rates of drug use, and that, at the individual level, negative behaviors and attitudes relating to school are also associated with drug use.

MacDonald[12] reports that experimentation is a normal adolescent learning tool, but when combined with normal adolescent curiosity and fearlessness, it may be dangerous. Tobacco smoking is an example of a common teenage experiment. In a study by the National Survey on Drug Use and Health, 12% of adolescents age 12 to 17 years had smoked one or more cigarettes in the past month and of those who had never smoked, more than 22 % were considered susceptible to start smoking.[13]

ETIOLOGIC FACTORS IN SUBSTANCE ABUSE

Drug abuse in young people can be traced to many causes, the most important of which is considered to be rebellion against parents and society. Other factors may include a need to forget the pressures of daily living, a desire for pleasure, and a need to conform to the group with which young people want to be associated. Through drugs young people obtain a momentary feeling of independence and power because they have disobeyed the rules of their parents and society. The satisfaction gained through rebelling against parents can give adolescents a reinforcing motive for persisting in drug abuse.

Children of wealthy parents are increasingly recognized as a high-risk group for the development of such traits as narcissism, poor impulse control, poor tolerance of frustration, depression, and poor coping ability. Therefore it is not surprising that a large number of children within this group use drugs to cope with frustrations, boredom, anxiety, and depression.

In general, drug users have been found to be less interested in formal education, less involved in organized activities such as athletics, and less likely to have well-defined goals than youngsters who do not use drugs. Adolescents who use drugs heavily have been described as manifesting more psychological problems than nonusers do. Significantly higher percentages of nonusers of drugs reported close relationships with their parents. Children involved in abusing drugs are more often found to have experienced the loss of a parent or have parents that are divorced.

SPECIFIC SUBSTANCES AND FREQUENCY OF USE

For more than 33 years, the University of Michigan's Institute for Social Research, funded by the National Institute of Drug Abuse, has collected data on past month, past year, and lifetime drug use among 12th graders. It was expanded in 1991 to include eighth and 10th graders. The most recent report(http://www.drugabuse.gov/Infofacts/HSYouthtrends.html) breaks the information down into positive and negative trends in abuse. Positive trends since 2001 include a decrease in past year prevalence of reported lifetime use of any illicit drug by 32%, 25%, and 13% amongst eighth, 10th, and 12th graders, respectively. Peak years for all three grades occurred in the mid-1990s, but have fallen since then. Although the trends are not consistent among all three grades, some positive trends were seen in abuse of the following drugs: marijuana, methamphetamine, sedatives/barbiturates, inhalants, cigarettes/nicotine, crack/cocaine, anabolic steroids, and alcohol. Some of the positive trends were only mild changes in reported use, and there was no significant increase over the past year. For example, after some increases in years past, there were no significant

increases in positive trends for inhalants in the most recent year reported.

Negative trends included an "unacceptably high" use of prescription drugs, with 15% of high school seniors reporting nonmedical use of at least one prescription medication within the past year. For 3 years in a row, eighth graders' perception of the harmfulness in taking MDMMA (Ecstasy) decreased. In addition, the use of Ecstasy increased among 10th and 12th graders for the last 3 and 2 years, respectively. Similar negative trends were also seen for hallucinogens. Finally, the use of heroin/opiates continued. Even though the prevalence of heroin use among high school students is lower than most of the other drugs discussed here (between 0.2% and 1% depending on the student's type of abuse and their grade in school), its use was increased in the past year. Also in the past year, the use of OxyContin increased from 1.8% for eighth graders to 5.2% for 12th graders, and the use of Vicodin increased from 2.7% for eighth graders to 9.6% for 12th graders.

Suppose the dentist identifies a person who needs help. What can be done? Unless the dentist is exceptionally well qualified to handle problems of addiction, the answer is direct or indirect referral to a treatment center. If the person expresses a need, the dentist may directly inform that person or the parents about agencies in the area that provide assistance. However, addicts may react defensively, even with hostility, if a direct approach is used. As with any problem related to general or dental health, preventive efforts must begin with the young. Children at a very young age need to be helped to develop a positive self-image, a sense of self-worth, and a separate identity.

SUICIDAL TENDENCIES IN CHILDREN AND ADOLESCENTS

During the examination of the child, the pediatric dentist should be alert to signs and symptoms of suicidal tendencies. How prevalent is suicide in the young child and adolescent? According to the American Academy of Child and Adolescent Psychiatry (http://www.aacap.org), thousands of teenagers commit suicide each year. It is the sixth leading cause of death in 5- to 14-year-olds and the third leading cause of death in 15- to 24-year-olds. Suicidal tendencies follow a pattern and background that can be observed by the astute professional or parent. The following excerpt is from the *American Academy of Child and Adolescent Psychiatry*, May 2008[14]:

> Teenagers experience strong feelings of stress, confusion, self-doubt, pressure to succeed, financial uncertainty, and other fears while growing up. For some teenagers, divorce, the formation of a new family with step-parents and step-siblings, or moving to a new community can be unsettling and can intensify self-doubts. For some teens, suicide may appear to be a solution to their problems and stress.

Depression and suicidal feelings are treatable mental disorders. The child or adolescent needs to have his or her illness recognized and diagnosed, and appropriate treatment plans developed. When parents are in doubt whether their child has a serious problem, a psychiatric examination can be helpful. Many of the signs and symptoms of suicidal feelings are similar to those of depression.

- Parents should be aware of the following signs of adolescents who may try to kill themselves:
  - Change in eating and sleeping habits
  - Withdrawal from friends, family, and regular activities
  - Violent actions, rebellious behavior, or running away
  - Drug and alcohol use
  - Unusual neglect of personal appearance
  - Marked personality change
  - Persistent boredom, difficulty concentrating, or a decline in the quality of schoolwork
  - Frequent complaints about physical symptoms, often related to emotions, such as stomachaches, headaches, or fatigue
  - Loss of interest in pleasurable activities
  - Not tolerating praise or rewards
- A teenager who is planning to commit suicide may also:
  - Complain of being a bad person or feeling rotten inside
  - Give verbal hints with statements such as, "I won't be a problem for you much longer," "Nothing matters," "It's no use," and "I won't see you again."
  - Put his or her affairs in order, for example, give away favorite possessions, clean his or her room, or throw away important belongings
  - Become suddenly cheerful after a period of depression
  - Have signs of psychosis (hallucinations or bizarre thoughts)

Children who say they want to kill themselves or that they are going to commit suicide should not be ignored, and further expressions of concern and discussion with the child is important. In addition, assistance from a mental health professional should be actively sought. With appropriate counseling and family support, intervention can be successful.

It should be recognized that the pediatric dentist and the orthodontist are in a unique position to recognize early warning signs of adolescent suicide. Loochtan and Cole[15] surveyed 1000 practicing orthodontists and 54 department chairs of postdoctoral programs. Of those surveyed, 50% had at least one patient who had attempted suicide, and 25% had at least one young patient who actually did commit suicide.

INFECTION CONTROL IN THE DENTAL OFFICE

The dental team is exposed to a wide variety of microorganisms in the saliva and blood of their patients. These may include hepatitis B and C, herpesviruses, cytomegalovirus, measles virus, mumps virus, chickenpox virus, human immunodeficiency virus, *Mycobacterium* tuberculosis, streptococci, staphylococci, and other non–vaccine-preventable infections. Because it is impossible to identify all of those

patients who may harbor dangerous microorganisms, it is necessary to use standard precautions and practice infection control procedures routinely to avoid spread of disease. The following infection control procedures as described by Miller and Palenik[16] are based on those recommended for dentistry by the Centers for Disease Control and Prevention (CDC) in the Public Health Service of the U.S. Department of Health and Human Services[17]:

Always obtain (and update) a thorough medical history, as discussed previously in this chapter, and include questions about medications, current illnesses, hepatitis, unintentional weight loss, lymphadenopathy, oral soft tissue lesions, or other infections.

Clean all reusable instruments in an ultrasonic cleaner or washer/disinfector, and minimize the amount of hand scrubbing performed. Wear heavy rubber gloves, mask, and protective clothing and eyewear to protect against puncture injuries and splashing.

Sterilize all reusable instruments that penetrate or come into contact with oral tissues or that become contaminated with saliva or blood. Metal or heat-stable instruments should be sterilized in a steam autoclave, a dry heat oven, or an unsaturated chemical vapor sterilizer. Heat-sensitive items may require up to 10 hours' exposure time for sterilization in a liquid chemical agent approved by the U.S. Food and Drug Administration as a disinfectant/sterilant, followed by rinsing with sterile water. High-level disinfection may be accomplished by submersion in the disinfectant/sterilant chemical for the exposure time recommended on the product label, followed by rinsing with water.

Monitoring of sterilization procedures should include a combination of process parameters, including mechanical, chemical, and biological. These parameters evaluate both the sterilizing conditions and the procedure's effectiveness. Biological monitoring must occur weekly.

Dental instruments must be wrapped before sterilization. Unwrapped instruments have no shelf life and must be used immediately after processing.

Wearing of personal protective equipment (gloves, masks, protective eyewear, and clinical attire) is required when treating patients.

Contamination of clinical contact surfaces with patient materials can occur by direct spray or spatter generated either during dental procedures or by contact with gloved hands. Barrier protection of surfaces and equipment can prevent contamination of clinical contact surfaces, but is particularly effective for those that are difficult to clean. Barriers include clear plastic wrap, bags, sheets, tubing, and plastic-backed paper or other materials impervious to moisture. If barriers are not used, cleaning and disinfection of surfaces between patients should employ an EPA-registered hospital disinfectant with a tuberculocidal claim (i.e., intermediate-level disinfectant).

Hand hygiene (e.g., handwashing, hand antisepsis, or surgical hand antisepsis) substantially reduces potential pathogens on the hands. Evidence indicates that proper hand hygiene is the single most critical measure for reducing the risk of transmitting organisms. For routine dental examinations and nonsurgical procedures, handwashing and hand antisepsis is achieved by using either a plain or antimicrobial soap and water. If the hands are not visibly soiled, an alcohol-based hand rub is adequate.

Regulated medical waste is only a limited subset of waste: 9% to 15% of total waste in hospitals and 1% to 2% of total waste in dental offices. Regulated medical waste requires special storage, handling, neutralization, and disposal and is covered by federal, state, and local rules and regulations. Examples of regulated waste found in dental practice settings are solid waste soaked or saturated with blood or saliva (e.g., gauze saturated with blood after surgery), extracted teeth, surgically removed hard and soft tissues, and contaminated sharp items (e.g., needles, scalpel blades, and wires.)

Dental prostheses, appliances, and items used in their fabrication (e.g., impressions, occlusal rims, and bite registrations) are potential sources for cross-contamination and require handling in a manner that prevents exposure of practitioner and patients.

BIOFILM

The goal of infection control in dentistry is to reduce or eliminate exposure of patients and dental team members to microorganisms. Potential pathogens usually can come from patients and practitioners. Another source, however, could be from the environment, such as air or water.

Dental unit water lines contain relatively small amounts of water, much of which is in continuous contact with the inner surfaces of the tubing. The water is not in constant motion with extended dormant periods. Movement of water varies with greatest flow being in the middle of the tubing. Dental unit water lines readily become colonized by a variety of microorganisms, including bacteria, viruses, and protozoa. Water entering dental units usually contains few microorganisms. However, water coming out of the unit is often highly contaminated. Proliferation of microorganisms occurs within biofilms that adhere to internal surfaces of dental unit water lines.

Most waterborne organisms are of low pathogenicity or are opportunistic pathogens causing harmful infections only under special conditions or among immunocompromised individuals. Microorganisms of greatest concern are the species of *Pseudomonas*, *Legionella*, and *Mycobacterium*.

Biofilms form quickly and serve as continuous sources of contamination for dental unit water lines water. Flushing of lines temporarily reduces microbial emissions, but does not remove biofilm. Use of sterile water does not reduce the level of microorganisms released. The only remedy is to remove effectively the biofilms through the application of certain chemicals. Routine use of additional chemicals helps retard biofilm development. There is no evidence of widespread public health problems from exposure to dental unit water lines emissions. However, sources of microbes causing low levels of infectious diseases are difficult to identify. The presence of microorganisms in dental unit water lines water is of concern and is contrary to the goals of infection control. Because exposure to microorganisms can cause infections, it is the responsibility of dental health care practi-

tioners to use water that has the lowest level of microbial contamination.

EMERGENCY DENTAL TREATMENT

All too often a patient's initial dental appointment is prompted by an emergency situation. The diagnostic procedures necessary for an emergency dental appointment are outlined in this chapter previously, but the emergency appointment tends to focus on and resolve a single problem or a single set of related problems rather than provide a comprehensive oral diagnosis and management plan for the patient. Once the emergency problem is under control, the dentist should offer comprehensive services to the patient or parents.

The remainder of this book presents information for dentists and dental students to augment their diagnostic and management skills in providing oral health care services to children and adolescents during both emergency and preplanned dental visits.

REFERENCES

1. American Academy of Pediatric Dentistry. Guideline on periodicity of examination, preventive dental services, anticipatory guidance/counseling, and oral treatment for infants, children and adolescents, *Pediatr Dent* 29:102-108, 2008. [Suppl: Reference manual 2008-2009].
2. Glick M, Greenberg MS, Ship JA. Introduction to oral medicine and oral diagnosis: Evaluation of the dental patient. In Greenberg MS, Glick, M Ship JA, eds: *Burket's oral medicine*, ed 11, Hamilton, Ontario, 2009, BC Decker.
3. Shaw O. Dental anxiety in children, *Br Dent J* 139:134-139, 1975.
4. Okeson JP. Temporomandibular disorders in children, *Pediatr Dent* 11(12):325-333, 1989
5. American Academy of Pediatric Dentistry. Guideline on acquired temporomandibular disorders in infants, children and adolescents, *Pediatr Dent* 24:189-191, 2008. [Suppl: Reference manual 2008-2009]
6. Okeson JP. *Management of temporomandibular disorders and occlusion*, ed 6, St. Louis, 2008, Mosby.
7. Clerehugh V, Tugnait A. Diagnosis and management of periodontal diseases in children and adolescents, *Periodontology* 26:146-168, 2000-2001.
8. Blayney JR, Hill IN. Fluorine and dental caries, *J Am Dent Assoc* 74:233-302, 1967.
9. Rosenbaum CH. Dental precautions in treating drug addicts: A hidden problem among teens and preteens, *Pediatr Dent* 2:94-96, 1980.
10. Rosenbaum CH. Did you treat a drug addict today? *Int Dent J* 31:307-312, 1981.
11. Fletcher A, Bonell C, Hargreaves J. School effects on young people's drug use: A systematic review of interventional and observational studies, *J Adolesc Health* 42:3 (209-220), 2008.
12. MacDonald DI. Drugs, drinking and adolescence, *Am J Dis Child* 138:117-125, 1984.
13. Centers for Disease Control and Prevention. Racial/ethnic differences among youths in cigarette smoking and susceptibility to start smoking–United States, 2002-2004, *MMWR Morb Mortal Wkly Rep* 55:1275-1277, 2006.
14. American Academy of Child and Adolescent Psychiatry. Teen suicide, *Facts for Families*, issue 10, 2008.

15. Loochtan RM, Cole RM. Adolescent suicide in orthodontics: Results of a survey, *Am J Orthod Dentofacial Orthop* 1010:180-187, 1991.

16. Miller CH, Palenik CJ. *Infection control and hazardous materials management for the dental team*, ed 4, St. Louis, 2009, Mosby.

17. Centers for Disease Control and Prevention: guidelines for infection control in dental health care settings-2003, *MMWR Morb Mortal Wkly Rep* 52(RR17):1-78, 2003.

SUGGESTED READINGS

American Academy of Pediatric Dentistry. Infant oral health care, *Pediatr Dent* (supplemental issue: reference manual 2002-2003) 24:47, 2002.

American Academy of Pediatric Dentistry. Periodicity of examination, preventive dental services, anticipatory guidance and oral treatment for children, *Pediatr Dent* (supplemental issue: reference manual (2002-2003) 24:52-53, 2002.

Depaola LG, et al. A review of the science regarding dental unit waterlines, *J Am Dent Assoc* 133(9):1199-1206, 2002.

Glick M, Greenberg MS, Ship JA. Introduction to oral medicine and oral diagnosis: evaluation of the dental patient. In Greenberg MS, Glick M, and Ship JA, eds. *Burket's oral medicine,* ed 11, Hamilton, Ontario, 2008, BC Decker.

Okeson JP. Management of temporomandibular disorders and occlusion, ed 6, St Louis, 2008, Mosby.

Palenik CJ. Strategic planning for infection control, *J Contemp Dent Pract* 1(4):103, 2000.

CHAPTER 2

Child Abuse and Neglect

▲ Roberta A. Hibbard and Brian J. Sanders

CHAPTER OUTLINE

Child abuse and neglect affect millions of children in the United States each year. The health harms from child maltreatment are long reaching and clearly correlate with morbidity in adulthood. Health care and dental professionals are in unique positions to identify the possibly abused child and must be knowledgeable in the recognition, documentation, treatment, and reporting of suspected child abuse cases. To appropriately intervene, professionals must be willing to consider abuse or neglect as a possibility—if it is not considered, it cannot be diagnosed.[1] This chapter includes a discussion of the types of child maltreatment frequently encountered, the clinical presentation and management of such issues, and the documentation and reporting of suspected child abuse.

IS IT CHILD ABUSE?

Child abuse and neglect encompass a variety of experiences that are threatening or harmful to the child and are the result of acts of commission or omission on the part of a responsible caretaker. Child maltreatment is usually divided into categories of physical abuse, sexual abuse, emotional or psychological abuse, and neglect in its many forms. Children living in violent homes are increasingly recognized as victims of maltreatment. Many gray areas exist in the determination of threat or harm, and disagreements about the "abusive" nature of some experiences are common. No one individual is responsible for deciding what is abuse or neglect. Identification, treatment, and intervention are the tasks of professionals from multidisciplinary backgrounds working together to provide care and evaluation in the best interests of the child.

Maltreatment is not always willful; that is, the harm or injury inflicted is not always the intent of the act. Emotion expressed actively or passively against the child is often unplanned, but nonetheless can result in significant harm or death. Education and prevention efforts may teach parents to redirect their actions and explore more appropriate discipline techniques and ways to manage anger or frustration.

PHYSICAL ABUSE

Physical abuse is often the most easily recognized form of child maltreatment. The battered child syndrome was initially described by Kempe and colleagues in 1962 and elaborated further by Kempe and Helfer in 1972 as the clinical picture of physical trauma in which the explanation of injury was not consistent with the severity and type of injury observed.[2,3] These injuries are inflicted and not accidental; some result from punishment that is inappropriate for the child's age, condition, or level of development. Some result from a parent's frustration and lack of control in acting out anger. Physical abuse is usually recognized by the pattern of injury and/or its inconsistency with the history related. Bruises, welts, fractures, burns, and lacerations are commonly inflicted physical injuries. Approximately 50% of physical abuse results in facial and head injuries that could be recognized by the dentist; 25% of physical abuse injuries occur in or around the mouth.

SEXUAL ABUSE

Sexual abuse and sexual misuse are frequently interchanged terms that denote any sexually stimulating activity that is inappropriate for the child's age, level of cognitive development, or role within the family. Many definitions incorporate the desire for sexual gratification on the part of one of the participants. In the spectrum of child sex play, sexual experimentation, and parent-child physical-sexual contact, it may be difficult to distinguish normal behavior from lustful intrusion. Sexually abusive acts may range from exhibitionism or kissing to fondling, intercourse, pornography, or rape. Trauma to the mouth may result from sexual contact. In some states, statutes may include age criteria or an age differential in the legal definition of some forms of sexual abuse. Practitioners should be aware that there are differences in state definitions.

NEGLECT

Inattention to the basic needs of a child, such as food, clothing, shelter, medical care, education, and supervision, may constitute neglect. Whereas physical abuse tends to be episodic, neglect tends to be chronic. Determination of neglect also depends on the child's age and level of development as it relates to periods of time without supervision, the parents' whereabouts, parental intention, and responsibilities of the child when the child is not supervised or not attending school. The American Academy of Pediatric Dentistry defines dental neglect as "willful failure of parent or guardian to seek and follow through with treatment necessary to ensure a level of oral health essential for adequate function and freedom from pain and infection."[4] Level of medical and dental care, adequate nutrition, and adequate food and clothing must be considered in light of cultural and religious differences, poverty, community requirements and standards, and the impact of such neglect on the physical well-being of the child.

EMOTIONAL OR PSYCHOLOGICAL ABUSE

Emotional abuse has been a concern for many years, but definitions and standards for identifying such abuse have been extremely difficult to establish. It is often difficult to demonstrate the direct or causal link between the emotional and verbal abuse and the harm to the child. Such harm is usually seen as abnormal behaviors or mental health problems that are multifactorial in origin. Emotional and verbal abuse involve interactions or lack of interactions on the part of the caretaker that inflict damage on the child's personality, emotional well-being, or development. Harm to the child generally occurs in various ways over a prolonged period. Continuous isolation, rejection, degradation, terrorization, corruption, exploitation, or denial of affection are examples of behaviors that frequently have damaging effects on the child.

CHILD ABUSE IN THE MEDICAL SETTING

Perhaps the most difficult form of child maltreatment to identify and treat is a factitious disorder. Initially called *Munchausen syndrome by proxy*, then *pediatric condition falsification*, the problem is one of child abuse in the medical setting. These are conditions in which the perpetrator (usually the mother) relates a fictitious history, produces false signs or symptoms, and fabricates illnesses in the child that result in extensive medical evaluations, testing, and often prolonged hospitalizations. The fabrication may be deliberate to gain medical attention, the result of parental psychosis, or simply fraudulent to obtain money or services. Because health care providers are often dependent on the parental history of the child's illness, it takes some time for the practitioner to realize the inconsistencies and possibly fabricated or exaggerated nature of the complaints. These children may present with persistent and recurrent illnesses that cannot be explained, with signs and symptoms that do not make sense clinically. The bizarre nature of many of these cases makes them almost unbelievable to professionals involved, and an unbelieving social and legal system has considerable difficulty protecting a child.

LEGAL REQUIREMENTS

Every state has legal statutes requiring that suspected child abuse or neglect be reported to authorities. Statutes vary somewhat from state to state regarding detailed definitions of child abuse and neglect, but all states mandate that health care providers (including dentists) report child abuse or neglect when it is suspected. It is important to emphasize that one is required to report suspicions of child maltreatment and one need not have proof. Once reported it is the responsibility of social and legal authorities to determine the needs of the child and family, whether maltreatment has occurred, and what intervention or service is legally allowable or necessary.

WHO IS ABUSED

Children from all walks of life may be victims of child abuse or neglect—no age, race, gender, or socioeconomic level is spared. Statistics on child abuse reflect only those cases known or suspected, and all studies struggle with the component of the unknown. In 2006, the U.S. Department of Health and Human Services reported almost 65% of child maltreatment encompasses neglect, 16% involves physical abuse; 9% involves sexual abuse, and 7% involves emotional abuse. A little more than 2% of victims experienced medical neglect. Children who are victims of one form of maltreatment often are maltreated in other ways as well.

Sociodemographic characteristics of maltreated children vary somewhat by type of abuse or neglect. The average age of identification of maltreatment victims is 7.4 years; 48% are male; 49% are white, 23% are black, and 18% are Hispanic. Females are slightly overrepresented as abuse victims because sexual abuse is more prevalent among females. The youngest children (infants to 2 years) tend to be neglected most often and sexually or emotionally abused least often. Older children (12 to 17 years) are the least neglected, but the most sexually and emotionally abused. Family characteristics overrepresented among families of maltreated children and therefore considered risk factors include the presence of more children in the home, lower socioeconomic status, spousal abuse, drug or alcohol abuse, and significant health or economic stresses. Risk factors play a role, but ultimately every child is a potential victim.

IDENTIFICATION OF POSSIBLE CHILD ABUSE

As stated earlier, child abuse and neglect are not identified if they are not considered as a diagnostic possibility. One must be willing to consider the diagnosis of abuse to make the diagnosis. A number of characteristics of the child, parent, or story given to explain the child's condition may lead a professional to suspect child maltreatment.

Indicators of child abuse and neglect are those signs or symptoms that should raise one's suspicions of the possibility of child maltreatment. The presence of such indicators does not "prove" maltreatment, but should lead one to be more thorough in thinking through a medical versus abusive or neglectful etiology. Many of the signs and symptoms are nonspecific and may be present for a variety of reasons—child abuse is only one of those reasons. Indicators of abuse and neglect often depend on the child's age and developmental level, and vary with the child's experiences and resiliency.

PHYSICAL INDICATORS

Situations raising the strongest suspicions and the most easily recognized maltreatment cases are those in which the pattern of injury is not consistent with the account history offered to explain it. The history should be consistent with the injury as it relates to mechanism of the injury, the timing of the injury, and the developmental level of the child. For example, a 3-month-old (nonambulatory) child is not going to sustain a spiral femur fracture from crawling. A bruise in the shape of a hand print on the cheek does not result from a fall down the stairs (Fig. 2-1). Accounts from two or more individuals

(e.g., parents or a parent and child) that conflict with each other or that change over time are also very suspicious. Any significant injury that is reportedly "unwitnessed" should raise concerns of possible abuse.

Physical indicators of child maltreatment tend to be somewhat more objective but must also be considered with the history. Unexplained bruises or welts in places not routinely subject to the child's rough-and-tumble lifestyle are those that become suspicious. Shin bruises and forehead bumps are expected in toddlers; bruises in the small of the back or torso are not. Unexplained injuries on the face, mouth, or lips; bruises clustering to form regular patterns or reflecting the shape of an article used to inflict the injury; and scattered significant bruises on different surface areas at various stages of healing are all suspicious. Similarly, unexplained fractures of the skull, multiple fractures in varying stages of healing, injuries to growth centers in the bone, and fractures in children younger than 2 years of age should raise concerns. Such injuries can be unintentional, but a clear explanation must be sought. Skull fractures may result from a short fall, but accompanying severe multilayer retinal hemorrhages or subdural hematoma with brain injury would make that explanation untenable. Burns are another form of recognizable child abuse; intentional cigarette (Fig. 2-2) and immersion burns are readily distinguishable from accidental splash burns, and immersion burns require a careful history and scene investigation to determine the etiology.

BEHAVIORAL INDICATORS

Significant behavioral changes often linked to child maltreatment include withdrawal, depression, poor school performance, regression in developmentally appropriate

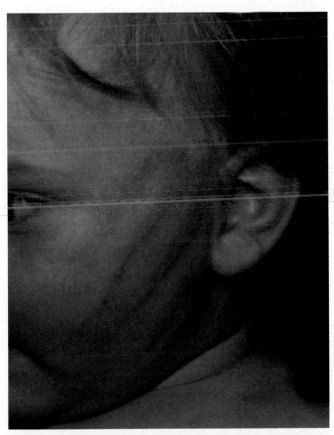

Figure 2-1 Bruise in the shape of a hand print on the cheek. (From Hobbs CJ, Wynne JM: *Physical signs of child abuse: A colour atlas*, ed 2, London, 2001, WB Saunders/Harcourt Publishers.)

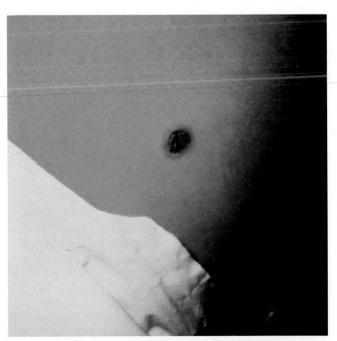

Figure 2-2 Intentional cigarette burn. (From Zitelli BJ, Davis HW: *Atlas of pediatric physical diagnosis*, ed 5, Philadelphia, 2008, Mosby.)

behavior, acting out, clinginess, and somatic complaints. Young maltreated children may show inappropriate affection toward others or may be extremely wary and distant in social interactions. Many children demonstrate affection toward an abusive parent; this should not be construed as evidence against maltreatment. Children, who are afraid to go home, are frightened by their parents, or report injury by caretakers should be taken seriously. Extensive lists can be found describing behavioral indicators of possible maltreatment. These should be considered in light of the child's entire clinical history and presentation and not in isolation. When other explanations for such behaviors are not found, maltreatment is an appropriate consideration.

Behavioral indicators also may be present in caretakers. Lack of concern or inappropriately high levels of concern in relation to the severity of the child's injury are not unusual observations. Parents may be defensive and hostile when questioned, or may refuse hospitalization and testing for the child. The explanation for the injury may be inconsistent with the pattern of the injury or the child's abilities, or the explanation may change when the perpetrator realizes that the first story is not believed. Poor judgment, jealousy or extreme protectiveness, child abandonment, violent behavior, or erratic behavior (which suggests drug or alcohol use, or psychiatric illness) are other clues to possible maltreatment by caretakers.

Indications of possible neglect include a delay in seeking medical care for a child's obvious injury, doctor or emergency department "shopping," or excessive use of medical care for an apparently well child. The child may be seen for repeated ingestions of harmful substances or have repeated hospitalizations. Children whose basic needs for medical and dental care, food, clothing, shelter, or education are not being met may be victims of neglect.

EVALUATION

Trauma to the orofacial structures is a frequent manifestation of child abuse. Studies have indicated that the incidence is as high as 50% in child physical abuse. Because abusive parents do not always show the same caution when visiting the dentist as when visiting the physician, the dental practitioner may be the first person to identify the abused child. Therefore the dentist must learn to recognize an abused child and make the appropriate referral.[5]

THE HISTORY

The dentist who suspects child abuse or neglect needs to complete a thorough dental and general physical examination. The combination of information is what influences or creates the suspicion of possible child maltreatment. The history should be a complete dental and medical history. Details regarding any trauma should be complete and obtained separately from more than one source (e.g., parent and child) if possible. Open-ended questions should be used; "yes" or "no" questions should be avoided. Often, the best question is, "What happened?" The dentist need only ask for a level of detail that would indicate suspicions of abuse or neglect that would

be reported. Details might include who witnessed the injury and who was with the child when the injury occurred, where the child and supervising adults were, and what happened. Questions should include how and when the incident occurred. A description of present and past injuries, as well as the child's developmental abilities, may be helpful. If information is obtained that makes the dentist suspicious of child maltreatment, detailed questioning about the incident should be suspended.

COMMUNICATION WITH THE PATIENT

Professionals who are identifying and reporting suspected child maltreatment will have to talk to children in most circumstances to clarify a possible suspicion. They should not, however, be conducting investigative interviews of children to learn all the details or sort out the truthfulness of comments. A suggested guideline is the following: if based on your knowledge and experience you have reason to believe the child may have been abused or neglected, report it. Further detailed interviewing about maltreatment by a noninvestigating professional is neither necessary nor appropriate; that is the job of child protective service agencies. If, however, the child is talking and wants to disclose more, it is appropriate to listen and provide support. Avoiding "investigative" questions does not preclude taking a complete dental and medical history.

PHYSICAL EXAMINATION

The examination of the patient by a dentist should include the entire body that is exposed without undressing the child. The examination begins before the patient is in the operatory. Observations should be assessed in the context of the age, developmental level, and known history of the child. Observe the patient's posture, gait, and clothing. The dental staff should be trained in recognizing abuse and neglect so that they may alert the dentist if they become concerned. Inappropriate dress may be an indication of neglect and/or abuse. For example, a child who appears with a long-sleeved shirt in the middle of the hot summer may be dressed in this manner to cover old injuries. The child or parent's behavior may be inappropriate. A lack of spontaneous smiling and avoidance of eye contact by the child may be an indicator, as could be the parents' behavior of being overly watchful and vigilant.

The dentist should start the examination at the top, beginning with the hair and scalp, and systematically work down. Alopecia without an underlying medical cause may be an indicator of malnutrition or hair pulling. Continue the examination by looking at the nose and nasal septum. A deviated septum or clotted blood may be an indicator of previous trauma. Look for periorbital ecchymosis, ptosis, and deviated or unequal pupils, which indicate significant facial trauma. Bruises inside and behind the ears are worrisome. In cases of suspected head trauma, a neurologic assessment (history and physical) by the dentist can ensure that the child receives immediate necessary attention. If there is any question of abnormality, the child should be referred to a pediatrician or neurosurgeon familiar with child abuse as soon as possible.

Any bruise in the shape of an object, such as a belt, looped cord, hand print, or hanger, should alert the practitioner to inflicted trauma. The varying color of bruises should be particularly noted to identify the several stages of resolution that would indicate ongoing trauma. The neck should be examined for evidence of rope burns or bruises (Fig. 2-3) that may indicate attempted strangulation. Severe shaking can result in large bruises on the back of the neck that may also indicate brain damage. Physical trauma to the child's chest or ribs may elicit a painful response from the child if a lifting motion is used to slide the child up to the top of the dental chair during the examination. The presence of adult bite marks (Fig. 2-4) may be a sign of physical abuse, sexual abuse, or neglect. They may also be helpful in identifying the abuser. Bite marks should be clearly documented and photographed, if possible, when they are first observed, because they tend to fade rapidly. A forensic dentist or bite mark expert should be consulted as soon as possible when adult bite marks are suspected. Any visible patterns of injury should be photographed if possible; most law enforcement agencies will dispatch a photographer if requested in child abuse cases.

On completion of the general physical examination, the dentist should examine the teeth and supporting structures. Note any missing teeth or previously traumatized teeth (avulsions, luxations, intrusions, or fractures) and pay especially close attention to any soft tissue injuries. The mandible should be examined for any deviation on opening, range of motion, trismus, and occlusion at rest. The maxilla should also be examined for any mobility indicating a facial fracture. Bleeding under the tongue may indicate a fracture of the body of the mandible.

Note the condition of the maxillary labial frenum and the lower lingual frenum. A torn maxillary frenum on a child who is immobile may indicate possible trauma to the mouth from a slap, fist blow, or forced feeding. A torn lingual frenum could be indicative of sexual abuse or forced feeding (Figs. 2-5 and 2-6).

Bruising or petechia of the soft and hard palate may indicate sexual abuse in the form of oral penetration (Fig. 2-7). If evidence of infection or ulceration is noted, specimens should be cultured for evidence of a sexually transmitted disease, such as gonorrhea, syphilis, or venereal warts. The child who presents with extensive, untreated dental caries, untreated infection, or dental pain may be considered a victim of physical neglect if the parents are not attending to the child's basic medical and dental needs. Before filing a report, the dentist should determine whether the failure to provide dental care is willful or due to a lack of awareness or finances. Taking a good medical and dental history and making repeated

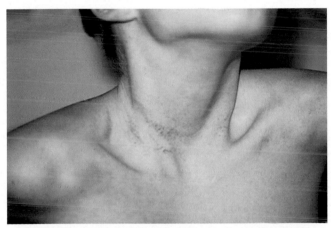

Figure 2-3 Attempted strangulation marks on the neck of an adolescent. (From Hobbs CJ, Wynne JM: *Physical signs of child abuse: A colour atlas,* ed 2, London, 2001, WB Saunders/Harcourt Publishers.)

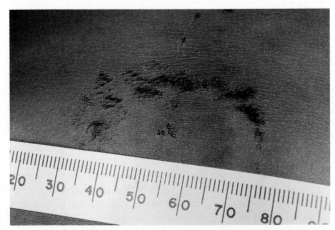

Figure 2-4 The presence of an adult bite mark may be a sign of physical or sexual abuse or neglect. (From Swartz MH: *Textbook of physical diagnosis: History and examination,* ed 5, Philadelphia, 2006, Saunders.)

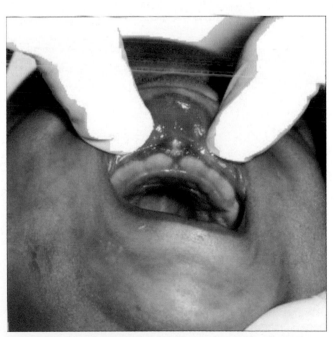

Figure 2-5 Torn frenulum from blunt force trauma to the mouth. Upon further investigation, this child was found to have 17 fractures.

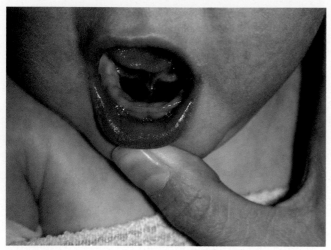

Figure 2-6 Sublingual hemorrhage in an infant with signs of genital and abdominal trauma.

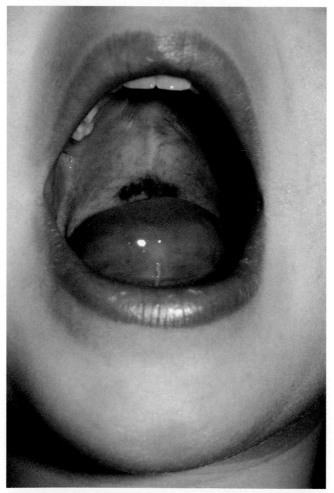

Figure 2-7 Palatal hemorrhage from oral-genital contact.

attempts to obtain appropriate treatment for the child help sort out these issues. A call to a child protective service agency is indicated if repeated attempts to address the cause of the dental neglect are not met with success, because dental neglect can cause significant pain, discomfort, and possible disability.

It is the combination of a complete history and physical examination that combine to form the basis for suspicion of child maltreatment while considering the differential diagnosis.

MANAGEMENT: DOCUMENTATION AND REPORTING

Clinical and medicolegal management of suspected child abuse and neglect involve several basic steps: medical and dental management, documentation (including photographs), and reporting. As health care professionals, dentists should be especially sensitive to the need for protecting children from abuse or neglect. They must, of course, treat dental conditions and injuries.

TREATMENT

Any medical or dental treatment that is indicated by the child's condition should be provided. A referral for a complete pediatric history-taking and physical examination will assist in identifying and treating other possibly associated conditions (e.g., failure to thrive, anemia). Medical evaluation should include assessment for medical conditions that can mimic or be confused with child abuse. The child's primary care physician or a child abuse pediatrician may assist in considering the complete differential diagnosis and any additional medical evaluation necessary.[6] Referral to a physician does not eliminate the dentist's obligation to make a report to authorities if maltreatment is suspected.

DOCUMENTATION

All data collected in the medical history and physical examination must be documented in a complete and objective manner. Pertinent positive and negative findings should be included. Actual comments and behaviors should be recorded; opinions about those behaviors should be avoided. For visible injuries, photographs should be taken if possible. The child's name and the date of the photograph should be included in the picture. Most law enforcement officials will take photographs if requested to do so when suspected child abuse is reported. When suspected maltreatment is reported to authorities, the time, date, and method of reporting (telephone or written report) should be documented in the medical and dental record.

REPORTING

The dentist is obligated by law to report suspected findings of child abuse to the appropriate authorities, that is, child protective service agencies and/or law enforcement officials. Failure to do so may result in the filing of civil or criminal charges against the dentist. Reports of suspected child maltreatment to local authorities mandated to investigate allegations are allowable without parental consent under Health Insurance Portability and Accountability Act regulations. With increased public awareness and inclusion of courses on child abuse in the dental curriculum, ignorance of the laws of child abuse is not an acceptable excuse.

Reporting is initiated simply with a telephone call to the appropriate child protective service or law enforcement agency, depending on local statutes. The telephone call initiates a response by appropriately trained professionals. The reasons for the suspicion with supporting documentation should be communicated verbally and in writing. Dentists are mandated to report based on "reasonable suspicion," and they are not responsible for any further investigation. If the concern is dental neglect, the dentist must work with the authorities to educate them on the diagnosis and need for care, then establish and follow through on a plan of treatment. It is possible to report suspected child abuse anonymously, but it is preferred that you give your name so that the agency can contact you if there are any further questions. There should be no reluctance on the part of the dentist to report suspected child abuse because of concern that it will require a great deal of time. In most cases after the initial report has been filed, no further involvement is necessary on the part of the dentist, and few cases require a court appearance. Detailed documentation in the dental record may lessen the likelihood of need for a personal appearance.

PARENTAL CONCERNS

In most situations, parents should be told of the concerns about possible child abuse or neglect and the legal requirement to report it to local authorities. This can help maintain the relationship with the patient and family. It also can be helpful to ask the parent if there has ever been a concern that someone might have hurt the child. Health care professionals should not make any accusations about who may have caused the harm. Simple statements such as the following should be used: "Because of an injury like this in a child of this age, we have to think about all of the possible causes. The nature of the child's condition means I am required by law to make a report to Child Protective Services."

In those situations in which a child is suspected to have been significantly harmed in the home, in which the parent is expected to be violent, or in which possible retribution against the child for having told is a concern, it may be more prudent to contact authorities and have them present to protect the child before parents are told. Discuss the severity of the situation with the authorities and make a plan with them to determine whether you should release the child from the office or await their arrival. The dental professional has no legal obligation to inform parents that abuse or neglect is suspected or will be reported; some situations may best be handled by not telling the parents at the time a report is filed.

The major concern must be for the welfare of the patient, and any concerns about losing a patient from a practice should be secondary. Individuals are protected from civil and criminal liability if the report is made in good faith. When the dentist's action is presented to parents as motivated by concern for the child and by an attitude of "let's figure out what is going on," many parents are eventually appreciative and will continue to seek support and care from the reporting professional.

OBLIGATION OF THE DENTIST

The privileged quality of communication between the caretakers or the patient and the practitioner is not grounds for excluding evidence in a judicial proceeding resulting from a report or for failing to make a report as required by law.

Strict confidentiality of records is maintained. Reports and any other information obtained in reference to a report are confidential and available only to persons authorized to examine them by the juvenile code. Some state statutes stipulate that a mandated reporter who fails to make a report when abuse or neglect is suspected may be liable for proximate damages caused by the failure to report. Criminal liability is another possibility for failing to report.

The health care professional must remember that it is suspicions of child abuse or neglect that must be reported; proof is not required. It is the responsibility of child protective service agencies and law enforcement officials to investigate suspicions and determine whether intervention is necessary. The health care professional can assist by providing as much information as possible through communication and coordination. Investigating professionals cannot do their jobs if the health care professional does not share detailed information regarding why the suspicions exist. Health care professionals who are unhappy with the outcome of system intervention (e.g., nothing was done) are usually those who would not or did not provide the information available that would assist authorities in making the best-informed decisions. If the health care professional believes that a bad decision is being made, a follow-up telephone call to the assigned case worker or case worker's supervisor to clarify concerns and interventions is appropriate. Many misperceptions exist about what interventions are possible legally. Communication and coordination can improve everyone's knowledge and understanding about a child's needs and what can be done to meet them.

Child abuse and neglect are identifiable in the dental office. Knowledgeable practitioners must be able and willing to identify, document, and report suspicions of child maltreatment. Awareness of local child protective community resources and professionals can facilitate interaction with the legal system and improve the ability to appropriately protect abused or neglected children.

REFERENCES

1. Jones R et al. Clinicians' description of factors influencing their reporting of suspected child abuse: Report of the child abuse reporting experience study research group, *Pediatrics* 112(2):259-266, 2008.
2. Kempe CH et al. The battered child syndrome, *JAMA* 181:17-24, 1962.
3. Kempe C, Helfer R. *Helping the battered child and his family*, Philadelphia, 1972, JB Lippincott.
4. American Academy of Pediatric Dentistry. Definition of dental neglect, *Pediatr Dent* 29(7):11, 2007-2008.
5. Harris JC, Sidebotham PD, Welbury RR. Safeguarding children in dental practice, *Primary Care Dentistry* 34:508-517, 2007.
6. Kellogg N, AAP Committee on Child Abuse and Neglect. Oral and dental aspects of child abuse and neglect, *Pediatrics* 116(6):1565-1568, 2005.

SUGGESTED READINGS

American Academy of Pediatric Dentistry. Guidelines on oral and dental aspects of child abuse and neglect, *Pediatr Dent* 29(7):77-79, 2007-2008.
American Dental Association Council on Dental Practice. *The dentist's responsibility in identifying and reporting child abuse*, Chicago, 1987, The Association.

Becker DB, Needleman HL, Kotelchuck M. Child abuse and dentistry: orofacial trauma and its recognition by dentists, *J Am Dent Assoc* 97:24-28, 1978.

Blain SM. Abuse and neglect as a component of pediatric treatment planning, *J Calif Dent Assoc* 19(9):16-24, 1991.

Brassard MR, Germain R, Stuart N. *Psychological maltreatment of children and youth,* New York, 1987, Pergamon Press.

Bross D et al, editors. *The new child protection team handbook,* New York, 1988, Garland Publishing.

Bross DC. Managing pediatric dental patients: issues raised by the law and changing views of proper child care, *J Pediatr Dent* 26(2):125-130, 2004.

Burgess AW et al. *Sexual assault of children and adolescents,* Lexington, Mass, 1978, DC Heath.

Carrotte PV. An unusual case of child abuse, *Br Dent J* 168: 444-445, 1990.

Croll TP, Menna VJ, Evans CA. Primary identification of an abused child in a dental office: a case report, *Pediatr Dent* 3: 339-342, 1981.

Croll TP et al. Rapid neurologic assessment and initial management for the patient with traumatic dental injuries, *J Am Dent Assoc* 100:530-534, 1980.

Daro D. *Confronting child abuse: theory, policy and practice,* New York, 1987, Free Press.

Davis GR, Domoto PK, Levy RL. The dentist's role in child abuse and neglect, *J Dent Child* 46:185-192, 1979.

Davis MJ, Vogel L. Neurological assessment of the child with head trauma, *J Dent Child* 62:93-96, 1995.

Faller K, editor. *Social work with abused and neglected children: a manual of interdisciplinary practice,* New York, 1981, Free Press.

Giangrego E. Child abuse: recognition and reporting, *Spec Care Dent* 6:62-67, 1986.

Golden MH, Samuels MP, Southall DP. How to distinguish between neglect and deprivational abuse, *Arch Dis Child* 88:105-107, 2003.

Indiana State Department of Health, Division of Maternal and Child Health. Child abuse and neglect identifying and reporting for the health care provider, 1991.

Kempe C, Helfer R. *Helping the battered child and his family,* Philadelphia, 1972, JB Lippincott.

Kittle PE, Richardson DS, Parker JW. Two child abuse/child neglect examinations for the dentist, *J Dent Child* 48:175-180, 1981.

Malecz RE. Child abuse, its relationship to pedodontics: a survey, *J Dent Child* 46:193-194, 1979.

Myers JE, Wendell PD. Child abuse reporting legislation in the 1980s, Denver, 1987, The American Humane Association.

Needleman HL. Orofacial trauma in child abuse: types, prevalence, management and the dental profession's involvement, *Pediatr Dent* 8:71-80, 1986.

Perspectives on child maltreatment in the 80's, DHHS Pub No (OHDS) 84-30338, Washington, DC, US Department of Health and Human Services, National Center on Child Abuse and Neglect.

Sanger RG, Bross DC. *Clinical management of child abuse and neglect,* Chicago, 1984, Quintessence Publishing.

Saxe MD, McCourt JW. Child abuse: a survey of ASDC members and diagnostic data assessment for dentists, *J Dent Child* 58:361-366, 1991.

Sheridan MS. The deceit continues: an updated literature review of Munchausen syndrome by proxy, *Child Abuse Negl* 27:431-451, 2003.

Sidebotham P, Golding J, ALSPAC Study Team. Child mal treatment in the "children of the nineties." A longitudinal study of parental risk factors, *Child Abuse Negl* 25:1177-1200, 2001.

Stanley RT. Child abuse—what's a dentist to do, *Ohio Dent J* 55(9):16-27, 1981.

Wissow LS. Child abuse and neglect, *N Engl J Med* 332(21): 1425-1431, 1995.

CHAPTER 3

Nonpharmacologic Management of Children's Behaviors

▲ Gerald Z. Wright and Jenny I. Stigers

CHAPTER OUTLINE

The foundation of practicing dentistry for children is the ability to guide them through their dental experiences. In the short term, this ability is a prerequisite to providing for their immediate dental needs. More long-lasting beneficial effects also can result when the seeds for future dental health are planted early in life. The process of leading a child through a dental appointment had for many years been termed "behavior management." In 2003, the American Academy of Pediatric Dentistry (AAPD) sponsored a national symposium on behavior management that focused on clinical techniques as well as the changing environment and trends of contemporary pediatric dental practices. Following this conference, the AAPD introduced the term "behavior guidance" in its clinical guidelines to emphasize that the goals are not to "deal with" a child's behavior but rather to enhance communication and partner with the child and parent to promote a positive attitude and good oral health.

A professional goal is to promote positive dental attitudes and improve the dental health of society. Logically, children are keys to the future.

A major difference between the treatment of children and the treatment of adults is the relationship. Treating adults generally involves a one-to-one relationship, that is, a dentist-patient relationship. Treating a child, however, usually relies on a one-to-two relationship among dentist, pediatric patient, and parents or guardians. Fig. 3-1, which illustrates this relationship, is known as the *pediatric dentistry treatment triangle*. Recently, society has been centered in the triangle. Management methods acceptable to society and the litigiousness of society have been factors influencing treatment modalities. Note that the child is at the apex of the triangle and is the focus of attention of both the family and the dental team. Although mothers' attitudes have been shown to significantly affect their children's

behaviors in the dental office, the roles of families have been changing, and the entire family environment must be considered. Because changes are constantly occurring within each personality, one must remember that there is an ever-changing, dynamic relationship among the corners of the triangle—the child, the family, and the dental team. The arrows placed on the lines of communication also remind us that communication is reciprocal.

The importance of this unifying concept will become evident as behavior guidance techniques are described. However, this concept also serves as the basis of organization for this chapter, whose goal is to discuss the nonpharmacologic approaches to managing children's behavior in dentistry.

PEDIATRIC DENTAL PATIENTS

Child development involves the study of all areas of human development from conception through young adulthood. It involves more than physical growth, which often implies only an increase in size. *Development* implies a sequential unfolding that may involve changes in size, shape, function, structure, or skill.

Over the years, numerous child development theories have evolved. Summarizing them, Alpern stated that the most important general principle concerning development is that human development is not unitary.[1] He contended that there were several relatively important aspects of child development and that no single aspect could be used to assess development. He cautioned about relating to children through a single developmental label and suggested that a basic appreciation of child development knowledge could be helpful to the dentist.

Early child development study linked changes to specific chronologic ages. The initial work gathered age

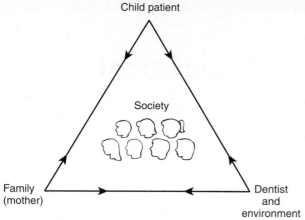

Child patient

Society

Family
(mother)

Dentist
and
environment

Figure 3-1 The pediatric treatment triangle illustrates basic relationships in pediatric dentistry.

norms for physiologic developmental tasks. Eventually personality description principles also evolved. One of the pioneering and most notable groups, headed by Arnold Gesell, was at Yale University. Typical personality characteristics related to specific chronologic ages that have relevance to dentistry are listed in Box 3-1. These can help when developing behavioral guidance strategies. For example, if the dentist knows the limitation of a 2-year-old's vocabulary, it becomes apparent that communication must occur through the sense of touch and

voice modulation rather than through the spoken word. Recognizing also the close symbiotic relationship with parents, dentists generally try to keep the parent-child pair intact.

Relating personality characteristics to chronologic ages has led to some interesting labeling. For example, a non-compliant 2-year-old often is referred to as in the stage of the "terrible twos." Dentists sometimes refer to such children as being in the *precooperative stage.* Unfortunately, this has led in some instances to using the age of the child, rather than the child's ability, as a reason for non-compliance.

The broad area of physical development involves changes that occur in children's size, strength, motor coordination, functioning of body systems, and so forth. Thus the child's total physical growth and efficiency from the moment of conception until adulthood is termed *physical development.* Because a child's physical development is relatively independent of other major areas of development, subareas of physical development have to be relatively independent. A child's coordination cannot be judged by physical size, nor is physical strength related to dental development.

Relating physical changes to specific chronologic ages led to the establishment of developmental milestones that became a means of assessing individual children. Classic developmental milestones are listed in Table 3-1. From these milestones, ranging from infancy through early childhood, two pieces of information are derived: (1) the average age at which a child acquires particular skills and (2) the normal range of ages at which a skill is acquired. A general principle is that, the earlier a skill emerges, the narrower is the range. On the other hand, developmental tasks tend to occur with wider ranges of normality as age increases. For the dentist, this holds practical importance. For example, consider the task of teaching children how to floss their teeth. Because the ability to floss occurs later in life (9 to 12 years of age),

Box 3-1

Age-Related Psychosocial Traits and Skills for 2- to 5-Year-Old Children

TWO YEARS
Geared to gross motor skills, such as running and jumping
Likes to see and touch
Very attached to parent
Plays alone; rarely shares
Has limited vocabulary; shows early sentence formation
Becoming interested in self-help skills

THREE YEARS
Less egocentric; likes to please
Has very active imagination; likes stories
Remains closely attached to parent

FOUR YEARS
Tries to impose powers
Participates in small social groups
Reaches out—expansive period
Shows many independent self-help skills
Knows "thank you" and "please"

FIVE YEARS
Undergoes a period of consolidation; deliberate
Takes pride in possessions
Relinquishes comfort objects, such as a blanket or thumb
Plays cooperatively with peers

Based on the work of Dr. A. Gesell.[5]

Table 3-1

Average Age and Age Range of Selected Physical Developmental Milestones

Developmental Task	Average Age	Normal Age Range
Focuses on light	2 wk	1 to 4 wk
Lies on stomach, lifts chin	3 wk	1 to 10 wk
Birth weight doubles	6 mo	5 to 7 mo
Rolls from back to stomach	7 mo	5½ to 11 mo
Sits alone	7 mo	6 to 11 mo
Stands with support	10 mo	7½ to 14 mo
Stands alone	13½ mo	9 to 18 mo
Walks alone	14 mo	10 to 20 mo
Bowel control attained	18 mo	1 to 2½ yr
First menstruates	12 yr, 9 mo	10 to 17 yr

there is a wide performance range. Knowing the general developmental principle reminds the clinician to consider the ability or readiness of the individual to perform a given task.

Another area that has received great attention from psychologists is the socialization of children. As with physical development, age-specific skills have been derived for social development; these take into account both interpersonal relationships and independent functioning skills. Some of the key personality characteristics are identified in Box 3-1.

An important process for dentists is the child's growth toward independent functioning. For their survival, infants are dependent on others to clothe, feed, and nurture them. As children grow and their ability to care for themselves improves, they gain social independence. Recognizing that the change from functional dependency to functional autonomy is a normal process in social development can assist the dentist. Many young children want to brush their own teeth, but lack digital dexterity. Parents, on the other hand, understand the lack of digital skills and often insist on attending to their children's oral health care. Appreciating that this tug-of-war is a normal part of social maturation allows the dentist to intercede and make appropriate conciliatory recommendations.

Intellectual development is probably the area most comprehensively studied, beginning in the early 1900s with the work of Alfred Binet.[2] The method that he employed quantified mental abilities in relation to chronologic age. It led to the concept of the IQ (intelligence quotient), which was measured by tasks examining memory, spatial relationships, reasoning, and a variety of other primary mental skills. By determining the average age required to pass each task, he derived age norms. This enabled an examiner to determine a child's mental age based on performance. For health care providers, viewing children in terms of their mental ages can be a helpful approach.

The IQ formula used by Binet follows:

$$IQ = \frac{Mental\ age}{Chronologic\ age} \times 100$$

Thus a child who performs tasks accomplished by a 10-year-old and who has the chronologic age of 8 years has an IQ of 125 (10/8 × 100 = 125). Quantification of intelligence has led to various classification guides. Since the time of Binet, more than 300 tests have been devised to measure intellectual development. The best known and best standardized of these tests are the Wechsler intelligence scales. These are individualized as opposed to group tests, and separate forms of the test are available for preschoolers (Wechsler Preschool and Primary Scale of Intelligence, or WPPSI), children (Wechsler Intelligence Scale for Children-Revised, or WISC-R), and adults (Wechsler Adult Intelligence Scale, or WAIS).

Currently, IQ is obtained by assessment with one or more standardized, individually administered intelligence tests such as the Wechsler Intelligence Scales for Children or the Revised, Stanford–Binet. Those judged to be of normal intelligence may span categories ranging from very superior or genius to dull or borderline deficiency. Significantly subaverage intellectual functioning is defined as an IQ of about 70 or less (approximately two standard deviations below the mean). However, retardation or *intellectual disability* (a term now recommended by the American Association on Intellectual and Developmental Disabilities) would not be diagnosed in an individual with an IQ of less than 70 without significant limitations in adaptive function in at least two domains. These might include communication, self-care, social/interpersonal skills, and adaptation to home living, use of community resources, functional academic skills, and as an adult, work/leisure skills and safety. A measure of adaptive functioning is obtained from a developmental and medical history and one or more reliable collateral sources (e.g., caregiver, educator). Scales have been designed to quantify adaptive functioning, such as the Vineland Adaptive Behaviour Scales, whose measures provide a composite score reflective of subscores in several adaptive skill domains.

It is those individuals with intelligence deficiency that concern the dentist because they may require special behavior guidance. Four degrees of severity of mental retardation are specified according to the level of intellectual impairment (and with the proviso of a deficit in adaptive functioning).[3] They are listed in Table 3-2.

Table **3-2**	
Degrees of Severity of Mental Retardation	
Mild mental retardation	IQ level 50-55 to approximately 70
Moderate retardation	IQ level 35-40 to 50-55
Severe mental retardation	IQ level 20-25 to 35-40
Profound mental retardation	IQ level 20 or 25

From American Psychiatric Association, DSM-IV.[3]

Mild Mental Retardation: This category is roughly equivalent to what used to be referred to as *educable*. It is the largest group and comprises 85% of people with mental retardation. As a group, individuals with mild mental retardation develop social and communication skills in the preschool years, and with appropriate support can usually live successfully in the community as adults.

Moderate Mental Retardation: This group is roughly equivalent to the outmoded term *trainable* and constitutes about 10% of people with mental retardation. Individuals in this group profit from vocational training and can attend to their personal care with moderate supervision. With support and supervision, they generally adapt well to life in the community.

Severe Mental Retardation: About 3% to 4% of people with mental retardation may be severely retarded. As adults, they may be able to perform simple tasks in supported settings and can adapt well to life in the community, such as a group home or family environment unless they have a complicating associated handicap requiring special care.

Profound Mental Retardation: This group comprises approximately 1% to 2% of people with mental retardation. This group generally has an identifiable neurologic disorder accounting for the condition. A highly structured setting with individualized care giving and supervision is generally required.

Scores from tests, even the highly standardized ones, are only estimates and may not be a fair appraisal for a given child on a given day. The younger the child, the less reliable the test scores. The more delayed the child, the less reliable the test scores. The more an individual's cultural and educational opportunities differ from the norm, the less reliable and valid that test is for that individual. However, the information from psychometric assessments can alert a dentist to the possibility that a child may need an individualized approach in the dental office, as well as elsewhere.

The environment is such a crucial factor in the development of a human being that it can be discussed as an independent factor only on the theoretic level. The fact that each child appears to have a characteristic temperament from his or her earliest age has been suggested by Sigmund Freud and by Gesell and Ilg.[4,5] In recent years, however, some psychiatrists and psychologists have emphasized the influence of the child's early environment when discussing the origin of human personality. Whether personality is developed by "nature" (genetic influence) or "nurture" (environmental influence) is an age-old, unresolved question. However, if these two influences are in harmony, healthy development of the child can be expected; if they are dissonant, behavioral problems are almost sure to ensue.

VARIABLES INFLUENCING CHILDREN'S DENTAL BEHAVIORS

The responses of children to the dental environment are diverse and complex. Children present for treatment with differences in age, maturity, temperament, experience, family background, culture, and oral health status. Klingberg and Broberg,[6] in a review of literature from 1982 to 2006, reported dental fear/anxiety and dental behavior management problems were relatively common for pediatric dental patients, each affecting 9% of children and adolescents. Girls exhibited more dental anxiety and dental behavior management problems than did boys. Dental fear/anxiety was more closely associated with temperamental traits such as shyness, inhibition, and negative emotionality, whereas behavioral problems were connected with activity and impulsivity.

Most dentists readily recognize children with dental behavior management problems, whereas dental fear and anxiety may be more subtle. Fear is best understood in context of personal, environmental, and situational influences. It can be a normal reaction for young children, especially in unfamiliar situations where they lack control or perceive the potential for pain. As children age, with increasing ability to anticipate, understand, and control impulses, fears may be expected to decline. But if fear or anxiety is disproportionate to the situation, an unpleasant experience is likely and the child may become uncooperative, displaying disruptive behavior.

Dental fear/anxiety is not synonymous with dental behavior management problems. In a study of more than 3200 Swedish children, Klingberg and Berggren[7] found that 27% of patients with dental behavior management problems showed dental fear and anxiety, whereas 61% of those with fear/anxiety reacted with behavioral problems. The key to successful outcomes (ie, compliance, relief of anxiety, completion of quality care, development of trusting relationship) is appropriately assessing the child and family to prepare them to actively participate in a positive manner in the child's oral health care. Dentistry has had some difficulty identifying the stimuli that lead to misbehavior in the dental office, although several variables in children's backgrounds have been related to it.

Parental Anxiety

With few exceptions, investigations indicate a significant correlation between maternal anxiety and a child's cooperative behavior at the first dental visit. High anxiety on the part of parents tends to affect their children's behavior negatively. Although the scientific data reveal that children of all ages can be affected by their mothers' anxieties, the effect is greatest with those younger than 4 years of age. This might be anticipated because of the child-parent symbiosis that begins in infancy and gradually diminishes.

Medical Experiences

The importance of medical experiences, a highly complex variable, has been debated over the years. There is general agreement, however, that children who view medical experiences positively are more likely to be cooperative with the dentist. The emotional quality of past visits rather than the number of visits is significant.

Pain during previous medical visits is another consideration in a child's medical experiences. The pain may have been moderate or intense, real or imaginary. Nonetheless, parental beliefs about past medical pain also are significantly correlated with their children's cooperative behavior in the dental environment. Study also has shown that previous surgical experiences adversely influence behavior at the first dental visit, but this was not the case in subsequent visits.

Awareness of Dental Problem

Some children may approach their dentist knowing that they have a dental problem. The problem may be as serious as a chronic dental abscess or as simple as extrinsic staining of the dentition. However, there is a tendency toward negative behavior at the first dental visit when the child believes that a dental problem exists. Their concern about having caries also may lead to missed appointments. Such considerations provide the dentist greater motivation for educating the parents about the value of establishing a dental home early, before any dental problems develop.

General Behavior Problems

Klingberg and Broberg[6] found some support for a relationship between general behavioral problems and dental behavior management problems. Children who have difficulty focusing attention and or adjusting activities to their general environment have increased problems complying with behavioral expectations in the dental environment. General fears can be important etiologic factors in development of dental fears. Some children, however, have behavioral problems only in the dental environment; this may be due to previous negative experiences with dental care.

CLASSIFYING CHILDREN'S COOPERATIVE BEHAVIOR

Numerous systems have been developed for classifying the behavior of children in the dental environment. An understanding of them holds more than academic interest. The knowledge of these systems can be an asset to the dentist in several ways: it can assist in directing the behavior guidance approach, it can provide a means for systematically recording behaviors, and it can assist in evaluating the validity of current research.

Wright's clinical classification places children in three categories[8]:
- Cooperative
- Lacking in cooperative ability
- Potentially cooperative

During examination of a child, the cooperative behavior of the patient is taken into account because it is a key to rendering treatment. Most children seen in the dental office cooperate. Cooperative children are reasonably relaxed. They have minimal apprehension. They may be enthusiastic. They can be treated by a straightforward, behavior-shaping approach. When guidelines for behavior are established, they perform within the framework provided.

In contrast is the child lacking in cooperative ability. This category includes very young children with whom communication cannot be established and of whom comprehension cannot be expected. Because of their age, they lack cooperative abilities. Another group of children who lack cooperative ability is those with specific debilitating or disabling conditions. The severity of the child's condition prohibits cooperation in the usual manner. At times, special behavior guidance techniques are used for these children. Although their treatment is accomplished, immediate major positive behavioral changes cannot be expected. Characteristically, the nomenclature applied to a potentially cooperative child is behavior problem. This type of behavior differs from that of children lacking cooperative ability because these children have the capability to perform cooperatively. This is an important distinction. When a child is characterized as potentially cooperative, clinical judgment is that the child's behavior can be modified; that is, the child can become cooperative.

The dental literature is filled with descriptions of potentially cooperative patients. Moreover, the adverse reactions have been given specific labels, such as uncontrolled, defiant, timid, tense-cooperative, and whining. Dentists often use these labels because they convey, in as few words as possible, the essence of the clinical problem.

Another system, which has been used in behavioral science research, is referred to as the Frankl Behavioral Rating Scale.[9] The scale divides observed behavior into four categories, ranging from definitely positive to definitely negative. Following is a description of the scale:
- *Rating 1: Definitely negative.* Refusal of treatment, forceful crying, fearfulness, or any other overt evidence of extreme negativism
- *Rating 2: Negative.* Reluctance to accept treatment, uncooperativeness, some evidence of negative attitude but not pronounced (sullen, withdrawn)
- *Rating 3: Positive.* Acceptance of treatment; cautious behavior at times; willingness to comply with the dentist, at times with reservation, but patient follows the dentist's directions cooperatively
- *Rating 4: Definitely positive.* Good rapport with the dentist, interest in the dental procedures, laughter and enjoyment.

Although the Frankl method of classification has been a popular research tool, it also lends itself to a shorthand form that can be used for recording children's behavior in the dental office. One can identify those children displaying a positive cooperative behavior by jotting down "+" or "++." Conversely, uncooperative behavior can be noted by "−" or "−−." A shortcoming of this method is that the scale does not communicate sufficient clinical information regarding uncooperative children. If a child is judged as "−," the user of this classification system must qualify as well as categorize the reaction. By recording "−, tearful," a better description of the clinical problem is made.

THE FUNCTIONAL INQUIRY

Before the dentist treats a child, medical and dental histories are essential. However, a functional inquiry, from a behavioral viewpoint, also should be conducted. During the inquiry, there are two primary goals: (1) to learn about patient and parental concerns and (2) to gather information enabling a reliable estimate of the cooperative ability of the child. Coupling the findings from the functional inquiry with the clinical experience, the dentist is in a much better position to meet the patient's needs and to apply appropriate behavior guidance strategies to treat individual pediatric patients than by simply proceeding inadequately informed.

Usually, functional inquiries are conducted in two ways: (1) by a paper and pencil questionnaire completed by the parent and (2) by direct interview of child and parent. In some offices one method may predominate, whereas in others both techniques are used. Each method has specific merits.

Written questionnaires can be important tools for gaining information, because probing questions can uncover critical facts about child-rearing practices in the home, a child's school experiences, or the patient's developmental status. Four questions with clinical relevance that can be added to history forms are listed in Box 3-2.

The responses to these questions, originally from behavioral science research, can alert the clinician to a potential behavioral problem. If a parent responds

Box 3-2

Clinically Relevant Questions That Can Be Added to History Forms

(CIRCLE ONE)	
How do you think your child has reacted to past medical procedures?	Very well Moderately well Moderately poorly Very poorly
How would you rate your own anxiety (fear, nervousness) at this moment?	High Moderately high Moderately low Low
Does your child think there is anything wrong with his or her teeth, such as a chipped tooth, decayed tooth, gum boil?	Yes No
How do you expect your child to react in the dental chair?	Very well Moderately well Moderately poorly Very poorly

negatively to more than one question, the chance of encountering a behavior problem rises considerably. An unlimited list of questions could be prepared for paper and pencil questionnaires, but from the dentist's viewpoint, a lengthy list is impractical.

Most practicing dentists recognize the merits of personal contact with parents. For the personal interview to serve as an efficient functional inquiry tool, a structured framework is necessary. The paper and pencil questionnaire is a starting point. It provides general information or clues that help guide the personal interview. Consider the following question:

Do you consider your child to be (check one):
___ advanced in learning?
___ progressing normally?
___ a slow learner?

If the parent has indicated that the child is a slow learner, more factual information is necessary. A leading question in the personal interview might be, "What school does your child attend?" A child may attend a special education class or a special school. Knowledge of the child's class or special school can offer a clue about the functional level of the patient. There is no limit to the depth of the personal interview, but if it is to be efficient, questioning must be thoughtful. Other avenues that can be explored include rewards and consequences used in the home environment. These provide insight into the type of behavior guidance techniques that would be acceptable to a parent.

PARENTS OF PEDIATRIC PATIENTS

From the moment of their children's birth, parents shape children's behaviors by selective encouragement and discouragement of particular behaviors, by their disciplinary

techniques, and by the amount of freedom they allow. In early years, at least, it is mainly from parents that children learn what they are supposed to do and what behavior is forbidden. Unfortunately, societal changes in the latter part of the twentieth century have created dynamics that can indirectly affect the behavior of children in dental offices. For example, a center of social policy reported that one in 10 children lives in a household not headed by a parent. Often these children are brought to dental offices by caretakers or child care workers who are unfamiliar with the children's histories. Reconstituted or blended families, same-sex families, and single-parent families all have their special sets of circumstances. Considering 218 children of teenaged mothers from birth to 5 years, Stier and colleagues[10] found them at greater risk for maltreatment than children of older mothers. When providing dental care for children, it is important that dentists understand parents' expectancies. In dentist-parent relationships, a difficult question is, "What does a parent or caregiver consider an acceptable behavioral guidance technique?" Considering the previously mentioned societal changes and that North America is a cultural mosaic with many parents having dental attitudes deeply rooted in their heritage, it is not an easy question to answer.

Despite the acknowledged importance of the parental role in the pediatric treatment triangle and the necessity of gaining parental cooperation, it is only recently that the dental literature has provided dentists with advice for dealing with parents. Three notable works on parental acceptance are by Murphy and colleagues,[11] Lawrence and associates,[12] and Eaton and coworkers.[13] The three studies are similar in design: Parents are shown videotapes of different behavioral guidance methods and instructed to indicate their acceptability of them on a rating scale. The studies span 2 decades and provide interesting information as well as showing how parental attitudes change. In the earlier study,[11] 10 techniques were videotaped. Four of the techniques found to be acceptable were tell-show-do, positive reinforcement, voice control, and use of a mouth prop. Six techniques found to be unacceptable involved restraint methods, sedation, and general anesthesia.

The latter two studies[12,13] used the same videotape and demonstrated eight behavior guidance methods. All studies showed tell-show-do as the most acceptable technique. Nitrous oxide sedation was found to be the next most acceptable technique in the latter two studies. All studies were able to establish a hierarchy of parental acceptance based upon the mean ratings of parent responses allowing the observation of two interesting changes. Hand-over-mouth became the least accepted technique, whereas general anesthesia became the third most accepted method for behavior guidance.

Caution has to be exercised when applying the results of these investigations to clinical practice. Eaton noted considerable variability in parental attitudes to all techniques. The studies also require replication using the same videotapes in different locales. Do New England parents, Spanish speaking parents in Florida or New Mexico, Native American parents, and West Coast parents all hold the same views as Midwestern Americans where these studies were performed?

There is not complete agreement as to what formulates parental attitudes. Eaton and colleagues[13] found that parental gender, age, and social status were unrelated to attitudes. However, an earlier study by Fields, Machen and Murphy[14] showed that social status correlated negatively with general anesthesia. Those parents in the higher socioeconomic group frowned on general anesthesia. This points out again how things have changed over 2 decades in that the Eaton study showed much greater acceptance of general anesthesia.

Parents of pediatric patients often require understanding and have to be led through their children's dental experiences. We live in a litigious society, and it is critical to develop rapport with parents.

Casamassimo and Wilson reported on a survey of diplomates of the American Board of Pediatric Dentistry.[15] Most diplomates indicated that there has been a change in parental demographics. There are more single parents, increased mobility, and more dual-income families. The findings from this report found that children's behaviors in dental offices were strongly related to parenting styles, preferences, and demands. Failure of parents to set limits on their children's behaviors was the main parental child-rearing problem. They also found that parental expectations often were unattainable.

Dentists in practice have to anticipate these types of problems and learn to contend with them. The diplomates suggested several methods of coping with parent's and children's behaviors; however, one recommendation, the improvement of communication, dwarfed all others in frequency. Communication can mean many things, but in this instance it refers to the dentist's getting his or her message across to the parents and having them work with the dentist.

STRATEGIES OF THE DENTAL TEAM

A primary objective during dental procedures is to lead children step by step so that they develop a positive attitude toward dentistry. Fortunately, most children progress easily and pleasantly through their dental visits without undue pressure on themselves or the dental team. These successes can be attributed to a number of factors, such as a child's confident personality, a parent's proper preparation of the child for the appointment, or a dental team's excellent communicative skills. On the other hand, some children's dental office experiences cause anxiety and the beginning of a negative dental attitude. Sometimes these controllable but apprehensive children are managed without medication, as long as appropriate nonpharmacologic psychologic techniques are used.

Because behavior guidance techniques are used daily and come naturally to many persons, their importance is sometimes overlooked or they are taken for granted. This increases the potential for avoidable behavior problems. However, fully understanding and consciously implementing strategies can lead to recognizable improvements in child management skills. Although this section heightens awareness of various techniques commonly used in dental offices today, it should be regarded as only a start to the study of behavior guidance strategies.

PREAPPOINTMENT BEHAVIOR MODIFICATION

Psychologists have developed many techniques for modifying patients' behaviors by using the principles of learning theory. These techniques are called *behavior modification*. Usually they are thought about in conjunction with dentist-patient intraoperatory relationships. However, preappointment behavior modification, as it is used here, refers to anything that is said or done to positively influence the child's behavior before the child enters a dental operatory. The merit of this strategy is that it prepares the pediatric patient and eases the introduction to dentistry. It has received a great deal of attention because the first dental visit is crucial in the formation of the child's attitude toward dentistry. If the first visit is pleasant, it paves the road for future successes.

Several methods of preappointment behavior modification are recognized. Films or videotapes have been developed to provide a model for the young patient. The goal is to have the patient reproduce behavior exhibited by the model. On the day of the appointment, or perhaps at a previous visit, the new pediatric patient views the presentation.

Most modeling studies indicate that there is merit in introducing children to dentistry in this way, but not all studies show statistically improved cooperative behavior on the part of the children. The lack of replication may be the result of differences in experimental design, dental teams, or videotapes or films. It suggests a necessity for careful videotape or film selection for office use.

Preappointment behavior modification can also be performed with live patient models such as siblings, other children, or parents. Many dentists allow young children into the operatory with parents to preview the dental experience. Because the observing child likely will be initiated into dental care with a dental examination, a parent's recall visit offers an excellent modeling opportunity. On these occasions, many young children climb into the dental chair after their parents' appointments. These previews should be selected carefully. Young children are sometimes frightened by loud noises, as from a high-speed handpiece.

The merits of modeling procedures, commonly using audiovisual or live models, are recognized by psychologists. Rimm and Masters[16] summarized them as follows: (1) stimulation of new behaviors, (2) facilitation of behavior in a more appropriate manner, (3) disinhibition of inappropriate behavior due to fear, and (4) extinction of fears. These procedures offer the practicing dentist some interesting ways to modify children's behavior before their dental visit.

Another behavior modification method involves preappointment parental education via mailings, prerecorded messages, or customized Web pages. Precontact with the parent can provide directions for preparing the child for an initial dental visit and therefore can increase the likelihood of a successful first appointment. Beneficial effects of preappointment mailings were demonstrated in a controlled

---

Dear Parent:

Children who have pleasant dental appointments when they are very young are likely to have a favorable outlook toward dental care throughout life. The first appointment is very important in this attitude formation. That is the reason I am writing to you.

At our first appointment we will examine your child's teeth and gums and take any necessary x-ray films. For most children this will be an interesting and even happy occasion. All the people on our staff enjoy children and know how to work with them, but you, parents, play an important role in getting children started with a good attitude toward dental care. One of the useful things that you can do is to be completely natural and easygoing when you tell your child about the appointment with the dentist. This approach enables children to view their dental visit as an opportunity to meet some new people who want to help them stay healthy.

Your cooperation is appreciated. Remember, good general health depends partly on the development of good habits, such as sensible eating, sleeping routines, and exercise. Dental health also depends on good habits, such as proper toothbrushing, regular dental visits, and a good diet. We will have a chance to further discuss these points during your child's appointment.

Sincerely,

Figure 3-2 Letter to assist parents in preparing children for first dental visit. (Adapted from Wright GZ, Alpern GD, Leake JL. The modifiability of maternal anxiety as it relates to children's cooperative dental behavior, *J Dent Child* 40:265-271, 1973.)

study by Wright, Alpern, and Leake.[17] Children seemed better prepared by their mothers, and the dentist saw more cooperative pediatric patients. Almost all parents understood the letter's contents, acknowledged the dentist's thoughtfulness, and welcomed the concern for the proper presentation to their children. A similar letter is shown in Fig. 3-2. Dentists using preappointment educational materials should be selective. Over-preparation could confuse a parent or provoke anxiety.

FUNDAMENTALS OF BEHAVIOR GUIDANCE

Behavior guidance involves the total dental health team. Indeed, many dental auxiliaries are invaluable when it comes to providing care for children. All of the personnel have a stake in guiding a child through the dental experience.

Over the years, behavior guidance has meant different things to different people. In 1895, McElroy wrote, "Although the operative dentistry may be perfect, the appointment is a failure if the child departs in tears."[18] This was the first mention in dental literature of measuring the success or failure of a child's appointment by anything other than technical proficiency. Pediatric dentistry has progressed since that time, and one definition is the following:

Behavior guidance is the means by which the dental health team effectively and efficiently performs treatment for a child and, at the same time, instills a positive dental attitude.

Effectively in this definition refers to providing high-quality dental care. Efficient treatment is a necessity in private practice today. Quadrant dentistry, or perhaps half-mouth dentistry, using auxiliary personnel is vital in delivering efficient service to children. Finally, the development of a pediatric patient's positive attitude is an integral part

of this definition. In the past many practitioners have considered "getting the job done" to be behavior management. The current definition suggests a great deal more.

What has been omitted from the definition of behavior guidance also is interesting. There is no mention of any specific techniques or modalities of treatment. The definition allows the exercise of individuality. The challenge to the dentist is to satisfy the elements of the definition as frequently as possible and as safely as possible for each child in a dental practice.

Although various methods in managing pediatric dental patients have evolved over the years, certain practices and concepts remain fundamental to successful behavior guidance. These are basic to establishing good dental team–pediatric patient relationships. These practices increase the chances for success when providing care for children. They should be considered inviolate. The following fundamentals of behavior guidance center on the attitude and integrity of the entire dental team.

Positive Approach

There is general agreement that the attitude or expectations of the dentist can affect the outcome of a dental appointment. The child will respond with the type of behavior expected. In essence, the child fulfills the dentist's prophecy. Thus positive statements increase the chances of success with children. They are more effective than thoughtless questions or remarks. To obtain success with children, it is important to anticipate success.

Team Attitude

Personality factors such as warmth and interest that can be conveyed without a spoken word are critical when treating children. A pleasant smile tells a child that an adult cares. Children respond best to a natural and friendly attitude. Often this can be conveyed immediately to the pediatric patient through a casual greeting. Children also can be made to feel comfortable in the dental office by the use of nicknames, which can be placed on a patient's record. Noting school accomplishments or extracurricular activities such as Cub Scouts, baseball, hockey, or other hobbies helps in initiating future conversations and demonstrates a friendly, caring attitude to a pediatric patient.

Organization

Plans in the dental office have many dimensions, beginning, for example, with the reception area. Who summons the new patient? The dentist, the dental assistant, the dental hygienist, or the receptionist? If a child creates a disturbance in the reception area, who will address the problem? Each dental office must devise its own contingency plans, and the entire office staff must know in advance what is expected of them and what is to be done. Such plans are key features of many pediatric dental offices because they increase efficiency and contribute to successful dental staff–pediatric patient relationships. Also, a well-organized, written treatment plan must be available for the dental office team. Delays and indecisiveness can build apprehension in young patients.

Truthfulness

Unlike adults, most children see things as either "black" or "white." The shades between are difficult for them to discern. To youngsters the dental health team is either truthful or not. Because truthfulness is extremely important in building trust, it is a fundamental principle in caring for children.

Tolerance

A seldom-discussed concept, tolerance level varies from person to person. It refers to the dentist's ability to rationally cope with misbehaviors while maintaining composure. Recognizing individual tolerance levels is especially important when treating children. As well as varying from person to person, tolerance levels fluctuate for a given individual. For example, an upsetting experience at home can affect the clinician's mood in the dental office. Some people are in a better frame of mind early in the morning, whereas the coping abilities of others improve as the day progresses. Thus afternoon people should instruct receptionists not to book children with behavior problems the first thing in the morning. Learning to recognize factors that overtax tolerance levels is another fundamental, because it prevents loss of self-control.

Flexibility

Because children are children, lacking in maturity, the dental team must be prepared to change its plans at times. A child may begin fretting or squirming in the dental chair after half an hour, and the proposed treatment may have to be shortened. On the other hand, a dentist may plan an indirect temporary pulp treatment, but because the child is difficult, the plan may have to be altered to complete treatment at a single session. Many

dentists, following accepted four-handed dentistry practices, work at the 11-o'clock or 12-o'clock position. Treatment of small children may demand a change in operating position. Thus the dental team must be flexible as the situation demands.

COMMUNICATING WITH CHILDREN

Several effective communication techniques can be suggested. These key points are guidelines, not inflexible rules, because in the unpredictable world of pediatric health care, one must always be prepared to improvise.

Establishment of Communication

Previous editions of this textbook have stated that the first objective in the successful management of the young child is to establish communication. It is generally agreed that involving a child in a conversation not only enables the dentist to learn about the patient but also may relax the child. There are many ways of initiating verbal communication, and the effectiveness of these approaches differs with the age of the child. Generally, verbal communication with younger children is best initiated with complimentary comments, followed by questions that elicit an answer other than "yes" or "no."

Establishment of the Communicator

Members of the dental team must be aware of their roles when communicating with a pediatric patient. Generally the dental assistant talks with the child during the transfer from reception room to operatory and during preparation of the child in the dental chair. When the dentist arrives, the dental assistant usually takes a more passive role, because the child can listen to only one person at a time. It is important that communication occur from a single source. When both dentist and dental assistant provide directions, the result may be a response that is undesirable simply because the child becomes confused.

Message Clarity

Communication is a complex, multisensory process. It includes a transmitter, a medium, and a receiver. The dentist or dental health team is the transmitter, the spoken word frequently is the medium, and the pediatric patient is the receiver. The message must be understood in the same way by both the sender and the receiver. As Chambers indicates, there has to be a "fit" between the intended message and the understood one.[19]

Very often, to improve the clarity of messages to young patients, dentists use euphemisms to explain procedures. For pediatric dentists, euphemisms or word substitutes are like a second language. Examples of word substitutes that can be used to explain procedures to children are given in Box 3-3.

It is important to be careful in selecting words and phrases used to indoctrinate the new pediatric dental patient, because for the young child, language labels are the basis for many generalizations. The classic example is the language label for "doctor," which confuses many youngsters. This is known as *mediated generalization*. Eventually, as a result of experiences, the child learns that the "dentist doctor" is different from the "physician doctor" and that

Box 3-3

Word Substitutes for Explaining Procedures to Children

DENTAL TERMINOLOGY	WORD SUBSTITUTES
Rubber dam	Rubber raincoat
Rubber dam clamp	Tooth button
Rubber dam frame	Coat rack
Sealant	Tooth paint
Fluoride varnish	Tooth vitamins
Air syringe	Wind gun
Water syringe	Water gun
Suction	Vacuum cleaner
Alginate	Pudding
Study models	Statues
High speed	Whistle
Low speed	Motorcycle

the physician's office and the dentist's office are different environments. The process of sorting out such differences is referred to as *discrimination*.

Voice Control

Throughout the dental literature, reference is made to voice control. It is difficult to describe this effective communicative technique using the written word. Sudden and firm commands are used to get the child's attention or to stop the child from whatever is being done. Another form of voice control is a slow and deliberate cadence that can function like music set to a mood. In both cases, what is heard is more important because the dentist is attempting to influence behavior directly, not through understanding.

Although dentists have always recognized the merit of properly employing voice control when children's behaviors have been disruptive, Greenbaum and colleagues have given it scientific credence.[20] Considering the use of loud commands as a punishment technique, they compared the effects of loud and normal voice commands given to 40 children with potential behavior problems. Their findings demonstrated that loud commands reduced disruptive behaviors.

Chambers' theory is that voice control is most effective when used in conjunction with other communications.[19] A sudden command of "Stop crying and pay attention!" may be a necessary preliminary measure for future communication. The same message spoken in a foreign language probably would be equally effective in stopping disruptive patient behavior that was preventing communication. Used properly in correct situations, voice control is an effective behavior guidance tool.

Multisensory Communication

In verbal communications, the focus is on what to say or how it is said. However, nonverbal messages also can be sent to patients or received from them. Body contact can be a form of nonverbal communication. The dentist's simple act of placing a hand on a child's shoulder while sitting on a chairside stool conveys a feeling of warmth

and friendship. Greenbaum and colleagues found that this type of physical contact helped children to relax, especially those 7 to 10 years of age.[20]

Eye contact is also important. The child who avoids it often is not fully prepared to cooperate. Apprehension can be conveyed without a spoken word. Detecting a rapid heartbeat or noticing beads of perspiration on the face are observations that alert the dentist to a child's nervousness. When the dentist talks to children, every effort should be made not to tower above them. Sitting and speaking at eye level allows for friendlier and less authoritative communications.

Problem Ownership

In difficult situations, dentists sometimes forget that they are guiding the behavior of children. They begin by sending "you" messages. For example, "You must sit still!" These are negative messages and only undermine the rapport between a pediatric patient and dentist. "You" messages carry the implication that the child is wrong. An alternative is to send "I" messages. These messages establish the focus of the problem, such as "I can't fix your teeth if you don't open your mouth wide." This is one of the techniques discussed by Wepman and Sonnenberg that is particularly well suited to increase the flow of information between the dentist and the pediatric patient.[21] These techniques are incorporated into the Parent Effectiveness Training Program, which was popularized in the early 1970s.

Active Listening

Listening also is important in the treatment of children. However, listening to the spoken words may be more important in establishing rapport with the older child than guiding the behavior of a younger child, for whom attention to nonverbal behavior often is more crucial. Active listening is the second step in encouraging the kind of genuine communication cited by Wepman and Sonnenberg.[21] The patient is stimulated to express feelings, and the dentist does the same, as necessary processes in communication.

Appropriate Responses

Another principle in communicating with children is that "the response should be appropriate to the situation." The appropriateness of the response depends primarily on the extent and nature of the relationship with the child, the age of the child, and evaluation of the motivation of the child's behavior. An inappropriate response would be a dentist's displaying extreme displeasure with an anxious young child on the first visit when there has been insufficient time to establish a good rapport. On the other hand, if a dentist has made inroads with a child, who then displays unacceptable behavior, a dentist may well express disapproval without losing personal control. The response is then appropriate.

BEHAVIOR SHAPING

Behavior shaping is a common nonpharmacologic technique. It is a form of behavior modification; hence, it is based on the established principles of social learning. By definition, it is that procedure which very slowly develops behavior by reinforcing successive approximations of the desired behavior until the desired behavior comes to be. Proponents of the theory hold that most behavior is learned and that learning is the establishment of a connection between a stimulus and a response. For this reason, it is sometimes called stimulus-response (S-R) theory.

When shaping behavior, the dental assistant or dentist is teaching a child how to behave. Young children are led through these procedures step by step. They have to be communicative and cooperative to absorb information that may be complex for them. The following is an outline for a behavior-shaping model:

1. State the general goal or task to the child at the outset.
2. Explain the necessity for the procedure. A child who understands the reason is more likely to cooperate.
3. Divide the explanation for the procedure. Children cannot always grasp the overall procedure with a single explanation; consequently, they have to be led through the procedure slowly.
4. Give all explanations at a child's level of understanding. Use euphemisms appropriately.
5. Use successive approximations. Since its introduction in 1959, tell-show-do has remained a cornerstone of behavior guidance. Tell-show-do is a series of successive approximations. It is a component of behavior shaping that should be routinely used by all members of the dental team who work with children. Dental assistants, dental hygienists, and dentists should demonstrate various instruments step by step before their application by telling, showing, and doing. When the dentist works intraorally, a pediatric patient should be shown as much of the procedure as possible. Only when the child has a view of the procedures being undertaken are successive approximations being performed properly (Fig. 3-3).
6. Reinforce appropriate behavior. Be as specific as possible, because specific reinforcement is more effective than a generalized approach. This advice is supported by the clinical research of Weinstein and colleagues, who studied dentists' responses to children's behavior and found that immediate and specific reinforcements were most consistently followed by reductions in children's fear-related behaviors.[22]
7. Disregard minor inappropriate behavior. Ignored minor misbehavior tends to extinguish itself when it is not reinforced.

Behavior shaping is regarded as a learning model. A general rule about learning models is that the most efficient learning models are those that follow the learning theory model most closely. Deviations from the model create less efficiency in terms of learning. One way to improve consistency in this area is to record various clinical sessions with pediatric patients, using a tape recorder or videotape system, and then to review the tapes, keeping in mind the basics of the behavior-shaping learning model.

Although tell-show-do is similar to behavior shaping, the two differ. As well as demanding the reinforcement of

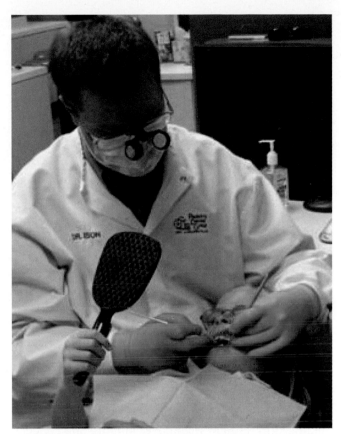

Figure 3-3 Child views intraoral procedure with hand mirror. If mirror blocks light to oral cavity, smaller mirror is used. With fiberoptic handpieces, blockage of light is not a problem.

cooperative behavior, behavior shaping also includes the need to retrace steps if misbehavior occurs. For example, if a child is shown an instrument and looks away, the dentist must revert to the explanatory portion of the procedure. Behavior shaping requires that the "desired behavior" be observed along the way. If the dentist proceeds along the sequential steps and begins performing treatment when the desired behavior is not present, there is deviation from the learning model and a greater likelihood of increased misbehavior.

RETRAINING

Children who require retraining approach the dental office displaying considerable apprehension or negative behavior. The demonstrated behavior may be the result of a previous dental visit or the effect of improper parental or peer orientation. Determining the source of the problem is helpful, because then the problem can be avoided through another technique or deemphasized, or a distraction can be used. These ploys begin the retraining program, which eventually leads to behavior shaping.

When encountering negative behavior, the dentist should always have in mind that an objective is to build a new series of associations in the child's mind. If a child's expectation of being hurt is not reinforced, a new set of expectations is learned. The dentist can be trusted! The child develops a new perception of the dental office and a new relationship to dentistry. Unacceptable behavior learned previously becomes extinguished. It is critical to remember that the stimulus must be altered to elicit a change in the response.

Individuals respond to stimuli to which they have been preconditioned. If the original stimulus and the new one are very similar, then the response will be similar. This is known as *stimulus generalization*. If a child has had an unpleasant experience in the dental office and then is taken to a different office where there is a different dentist and an entirely different staff and surroundings, the child still tends to generalize that an unpleasant event will occur in this new dental office. There are enough similar stimuli to produce this response. To offset the generalization, the dental team must demonstrate a "difference." This is one of the reasons why the use of nitrous oxide–oxygen sedation often works when retraining children. It offers a difference.

AVERSIVE CONDITIONING

The behavior modification method of aversive conditioning is also known as hand-over-mouth exercise, or by the acronym HOME.[23] Its purpose is to gain the attention of a highly oppositional child so that communication can be established and cooperation obtained for a safe course of treatment. The technique fits the rules of learning theory: maladaptive acts (screaming, kicking) are linked to restraint (hand over mouth), and cooperative behavior is related to removal of the restriction and the use of positive reinforcement (praise). It is important to stress that aversive conditioning is not used routinely but as a method of last resort, usually with children 3 to 6 years of age who have appropriate communicative abilities. In recent years, attitudes toward HOME have changed. Surveys of pediatric dentistry diplomates in 1972 and 1981 demonstrated acceptance by a substantial portion of the profession. In both instances, more than 80% of the pediatric dentists indicated that they used aversive therapy at times. However, Adair[24] reported HOME was used by a distinct minority of pediatric dentists. The greatest frequency of use was by older men, likely reflecting attitudes and training during their residency programs.

Inquiring into acceptance of the technique by dental educators, Davis and Rombom found 83% of respondents to their survey taught aversive conditioning in advanced training programs.[25] Adair found that 54% thought the technique was unacceptable, and 18% did not teach it at all. Some parents, too, have disapproved of the technique (Eaton[13] found it the only technique rated unacceptable by parents), and another concern has been a legal one. Bowers points out that acceptance of aversive conditioning by the dental professional is not an absolute assurance of the legality of the technique and that until a court rules on its legitimacy there remains some degree of uncertainty.[26] He also contends that the dentist who uses aversive conditioning in accordance with the standards of the prudent dentist in the locale and who obtains the requisite consent to treatment should not fear liability for battery or malpractice.

Aversive conditioning can be a safe and effective method of managing a child with an extremely difficult behavior problem. However, any departure from the accepted application of aversive conditioning may expose the dentist to liability. Those dentists or dental students who contemplate using it should consult detailed writings beforehand. Dentists should be aware of the acceptability of the technique in their practice location. Once a technique is found to be legally unacceptable in one instance, a legal risk to the dentist arises from failing to gain full consent or from using the procedure.[27]

PRACTICAL CONSIDERATIONS

Some procedural aspects of dental practice help guide children through their dental experiences successfully. Like many of the techniques described previously, they have evolved over the years without experimental testing. Nevertheless, these practical considerations form an integral part of present-day dental practice. They also would be fruitful areas for future research.

Scheduling

Children are bundles of energy. Lacking the patience of adults, many children become restless and tired when faced with long delays in a reception area. This should be taken into account when designing an office schedule. A good general rule is that a child should not be kept waiting in the reception area and that every effort should be made to be on time.

Morning appointment times have been suggested for children. It is a practice that has guided scheduling in many dental offices, because children are more alert and the dental team is fresher in the morning. Many dentists also believe that when age groups are kept together (preschoolers in the morning and older children in the afternoon), the peer group has a positive influence, with children serving as models for each other. Another advantage is that the dental office may run more smoothly with less psychological change of pace.

Sometimes expediency rather than a realistic evaluation of a child's behavior may predispose the dentist toward morning appointments for preschool children. Frequently it is easier to persuade parents to take younger children out of nursery school or kindergarten than to arrange morning appointments for elementary or junior high school children. From a behavioral standpoint, other factors seem important when deciding the appointment time. Patient-related concerns include patient age, presence of a handicapping condition, and need for any sedation. The dentist's attitude also is important. Some dentists avoid seeing children with behavior problems first thing in the morning. A policy regarding scheduling should be formulated by the dentist, and scheduling should not be left to chance.

Another scheduling concern has been appointment length. Historically, writers have agreed that the nature of childhood precludes giving the sustained attention that may be required for long dental visits. Generally, a long visit is defined as any period in excess of half an hour. Most of these views were expressed more than 30 years ago, and appointments have increased in duration. Improved technology, the application of time and motion studies by efficiency experts, and the current trend toward quadrant or half-mouth dentistry have altered contemporary practices. Whether this affects children adversely remains a question for researchers. In Lenchner's study, the behavior of 43 children between 3 and 5½ years of age who were undergoing operative dentistry was examined in both short and long appointments.[28] Short appointments ranged from 16 to 30 minutes, whereas longer appointments were 48 to 125 minutes. The investigator found no significant difference in children's behavior during long dental appointments compared with shorter ones. On the other hand, Getz and Weinstein, studying videotapes of 36 children between 3 and 5 years of age who were undergoing restorative treatment, found the opposite.[29] The longer the restorative phase, the greater the likelihood of a stress-fear reaction. Thus current evidence on appointment duration is divided.

Parent-Child Separation

Today's parents actively participate in health care services through the process of informed consent, and increasingly many accompany their children during their health care experiences. Until recently, parental presence in the dental operatory was minimal. Some practitioners find that excluding the parent from the operatory can contribute toward development of positive behavior on the part of the child. Starkey suggested that the policy of requiring the parent to remain in the reception room could be justified for many reasons, which include parental interference and limitations on dentist-child interactions.[30]

Another reason for advocating a separation policy is that the dentist may be more relaxed and comfortable when the parent remains in the reception area, so as not to be "performing." As a consequence of this more relaxed manner, the dentist's actions are likely to have a more positive effect on the child's behavior.

Adair and colleagues[31] found that a clear majority of pediatric dentists in all age/gender groups allowed parents to be present in the operatory for a variety of procedures. Feigal[32] suggested that the parental presence could be used to the dentist's advantage. Informed consent and communication can be streamlined into the normal office flow. Parental presence can reassure both the parent and the child. Parents can witness the dentist's compassionate approach and hear the educational instructions provided to the children. At the same time, the dentist obtains rapid feedback on parental attitudes and beliefs. When an office policy is formed, many dentists who exclude parents from the operatory make exceptions. A parent can be a major asset in supporting and communicating with a disabled child, often providing important information and interpretation. Another important exception relates to age. Very young children (those who have not reached the age of understanding and full verbal communication) have a close symbiotic relationship with parents; consequently, they usually are accompanied by them. The age factor was studied by Frankl and associates, who investigated the effect of a parent's presence in the operatory.[9] In their study, the intact group (parent present with child) reacted more favorably than the separated group. It should be noted that children 3½ to 4 years of age appeared to benefit most from the parent's presence. Those older than 4 years demonstrated similar levels of response to dental care regardless of parental presence. Thus dentists who contemplate admitting only parents of infants and toddlers to the operatory might consider extending the age level somewhat.

The separation procedure warrants serious consideration. The dentist must develop an office policy, notify the office staff of it, and assume responsibility to train office personnel in reception room strategies. In this age of accountability, the dentist may also have to explain the policy to a parent. Establishment of the policy therefore should be based on a rationale that takes into account the benefits and drawbacks resulting from separation, the benefits to the individual child, as well as the dental team's personal comfort level. Because some dentists become tense when parents are present and others enjoy having parents in the operatory, to some extent an office policy becomes an individual decision.

Tangible Reinforcements

Giving gifts to children has become a fact of commercial life in North America. There is general agreement on the merit of this practice in the dental office; gift giving can serve as a reward. If the gift has a dental significance (e.g., a toothbrush kit), so much the better. In these situations the gift is also used as a reinforcement for dental health.

Various trinkets in a toy chest should be used as tokens of affection for children, not as bribes. Finn made the following distinction between rewards and bribes: "A bribe is promised to induce the behavior. A reward is recognition of good behavior after completion of the operation, without previously implied promise."[33] The gift giving practice can have spectacular results. Many children who seem tense during operative procedures suddenly perk up on completion and scurry for a gift. These gifts provide a pleasant reminder of the appointment.

LIMITATIONS

Children today differ from those of 20 or 30 years ago. The child begins school earlier. Through the media, the child is more aware than children were years ago. We hear more of children facing poverty, experiencing learning disorders, and developing poor coping skills, and are more aware of children with eating disorders and drug use. Children also have legal and social advocates who have influenced management techniques. Limitations on the dentist exist today that were unheard of previously.

Parenting also has changed. Much of the behavioral science research was done with traditional families in the 1960s and 1970s. Single-parent homes were less common, and terms such as *reconstituted families* and *partner relationships* were unknown. What about the child-rearing practices in these families? Two decades ago, when "father" came to the office, it usually meant that the child had a behavior problem and "father" was the enforcer. With both parents working in many homes, it is not unusual for a father to accompany a child to the dental office.

Have parental expectations changed in the dental office? Yes. This chapter discusses the reasons why parents might be excluded from the operatory, but it also urges reviewing the policy periodically. Years ago parents did not expect to enter the operatory. Currently, many parents insist on their right to accompany their child. Societal changes influence our management methods, and there is a need to review past research carefully and assess its applicability to the present.

The dentist has societal limitations, too, and they are changing approaches to management. Years ago, the HOME technique might have been used to subdue a 3-year-old so that the dentist could perform an examination. This chapter does not describe the technique in detail because today it is not used by most dentists. Indeed, Carr and colleagues report decreased or discontinued use of controversial techniques like HOME because of parental influences and legal and ethical concerns.[34] Dental students rarely have the opportunity to use the technique.

The corners of the pediatric treatment triangle have been changing rapidly, which influences the practice of dentistry for children. Recognizing these changing times, the Council on Clinical Affairs of the American Academy of Pediatric Dentistry has produced guidelines for behavior guidance.[35] The techniques recommended in this chapter conform to these guidelines. However, there are limitations to written standards; these standards change. Dental students and dentists must remember to keep abreast of the times in this highly dynamic area.

REFERENCES

1. Alpern GD. Child development: Basic concepts and considerations. In Wright GZ: *Behavior management in dentistry for children*, Philadelphia, 1975, WB Saunders.
2. Binet A. New methods for the diagnosis of the intellectual level of subnormals, *L'Année Psycholgique* 12:191-244, 1905.
3. *Diagnostic and statistical manual of mental disorders*, ed 4, Washington, DC, 1994, American Psychiatric Association.
4. Freud S. *The problem of anxiety*, New York, 1936, WW Norton and Co.[Originally published in 1923 in German.]
5. Gesell A, Ilg FL. *Child development: an introduction to the study of human growth*, New York, 1949, Harper & Row.
6. Klingberg G, Broberg AG. Dental fear/anxiety and dental behaviour management problems in children and adolescents: a review of prevalence and concomitant psychological factors, *Int J Paediatr Dent* 17(6):391-406, 2007.
7. Klingberg G, Berggren U, Carlsson SG, Noren JG. Child dental fear: cause-related factors and clinical effects, *Eur J Oral Sci* 103(6):405-412, 1995.
8. Wright GZ. *Behavior management in dentistry for children*, Philadelphia, 1975, WB Saunders.
9. Frankl SN, Shiere FR, Fogels HR. Should the parent remain in the operatory? *J Dent Child* 29:150-163, 1962.
10. Stier DM et al. Are children born to young mothers at increased risk of maltreatment? *Pediatrics* 91:642-648, 1993.
11. Murphy ML, Fields HW Jr, Machen JB. Parental acceptance of pediatric dentistry behavior techniques, *Pediatr Dent* 6:193-198, 1984.
12. Lawrence SM et al. Parental attitudes toward behavior management techniques in pediatric dentistry, *Pediatr Dent* 13:151-155, 1991.
13. Eaton JJ et al. Attitudes of contemporary parents toward behavior management techniques used in pediatric dentistry, *Pediatr Dent* 27:107-113, 2005.
14. Fields HW Jr et al. The acceptability of various behavior management techniques relative to types of treatment, *Pediatr Dent* 6:199-203, 1984.
15. Casamassimo P, Wilson S. Effects of changing US parenting styles on dental practice: perceptions of diplomates of the American Board of Pediatric Dentistry, *Pediatric Dent* 24:18-22, 2002.
16. Rimm DC, Masters JC. *Behavior therapy: techniques and empirical findings*, New York, 1974, Academic Press.
17. Wright GZ, Alpern GD, Leake JL. The modifiability of maternal anxiety as it relates to children's cooperative dental behavior, *J Dent Child* 40:265-271, 1973.
18. McElroy CM. Dentistry for children, *Calif Dent Assoc Trans* 85, 1895.
19. Chambers DW. Behavior management techniques for pediatric dentists: an embarrassment of riches, *J Dent Child* 44:30-34, 1977.
20. Greenbaum PE, et al. Dentist's reassuring touch: effects on children's behavior, *Pediatr Dent* 15:20-24, 1993.
21. Wepman BJ, Sonnenberg EM. Effective communication with the pedodontic patient, *J Pedod* 2:316-321, 1979.
22. Weinstein P et al. The effect of dentists' behaviors on fear-related behaviors in children, *J Am Dent Assoc* 104:32-38, 1982.
23. Levitas TC. HOME—Hand over mouth exercise, *J Dent Child* 41:178-182, 1974.
24. Adair SM, et al. A survey of members of the American Academy of Pediatric Dentistry on their use of behavior management techniques, *Pediatr Dent* 26:159-166, 2004.
25. Davis MJ, Rombom HM. Survey of the utilization and rationale for hand-over-mouth (HOM) and restraint in post-doctoral pedodontic education, *Pediatr Dent* 1:87-90, 1979.
26. Bowers LT. The legality of using hand-over-mouth exercise for management of child behavior, *J Dent Child* 49: 257-265, 1982.
27. Bross DC. Managing pediatric dental patients: issues raised by the law and changing views of proper child care, *Pediatr Dent* 26(2):125-130, 2004.
28. Lenchner V. The effect of appointment length on behavior of the pedodontic patient and his attitude toward dentistry, *J Dent Child* 33:61-74, 1966.
29. Getz T, Weinstein P. The effect of structural variables on child behavior in the operatory, *Pediatr Dent* 3:262-266, 1981.
30. Starkey PE. Training office personnel to manage children. In Wright GZ: *Behavior management in dentistry for children*, Philadelphia, 1975, WB Saunders.
31. Adair SM, Schafer TE, Waller JL, Rockman RA. Age and gender differences in the use of behavior management techniques by pediatric dentists, *Pediatr Dent* 29:403-408, 2007.
32. Feigal RJ. Guiding and managing the child dental patient: a fresh look at old pedagogy, *J Dent Education* 65:1369-1377, 2001.
33. Finn SB. *Clinical pedodontics*, ed 4, Philadelphia, 1973, WB Saunders.
34. Carr KR et al. Behavior management techniques among pediatric dentists practicing in the southeastern United States, *Pediatr Dent* 21:347-353, 1999.
35. American Academy of Pediatric Dentistry. Guideline on Behavior Guidance for the Pediatric Dental Patient, *Pediatr Dent* (supplemental issue: reference manual 2008-2009) 30:125-133, 2008.

CHAPTER 4

Development and Morphology of the Primary Teeth

▲ Ralph E. McDonald and David R. Avery

CHAPTER OUTLINE

This chapter presents a brief review of the development of the teeth. An accurate chronology of primary tooth calcification is of clinical significance to the dentist. It is often necessary to explain to parents the time sequence of calcification in utero and during infancy. The common observation of tetracycline pigmentation, developmental enamel defects, and generalized hereditary anomalies can be explained if the calcification schedule is known. A brief discussion of the morphology of the primary teeth is also appropriate before considering restorative procedures for children.

A complete review is available in the reference texts on oral histology, dental anatomy, and developmental anatomy listed at the end of the chapter. Furthermore, contemporary scientists are rapidly gaining knowledge of tooth development at the molecular level. We suggest that readers with a special interest in the molecular events of tooth development study the listed references by Smith[1] and by Miletich and Sharpe.[2]

LIFE CYCLE OF THE TOOTH

INITIATION (BUD STAGE)

Evidence of development of the human tooth can be observed as early as the sixth week of embryonic life. Cells in the basal layer of the oral epithelium proliferate at a more rapid rate than do the adjacent cells. The result is an epithelial thickening in the region of the future dental arch that extends along the entire free margin of the jaws. This thickening is called the *primordium* of the ectodermal portion of the teeth and what results is called the *dental lamina*. At the same time, 10 round or ovoid swellings occur in each jaw in the position to be occupied by the primary teeth.

Certain cells of the basal layer begin to proliferate at a more rapid rate than do the adjacent cells (Fig. 4-1A). These proliferating cells contain the entire growth potential of the teeth. The permanent molars, like the primary teeth, arise from the dental lamina. The permanent incisors, canines, and premolars develop from the buds of their primary predecessors. The congenital absence of a tooth is the result of a lack of initiation or an arrest in the proliferation of cells. The presence of supernumerary teeth is the result of a continued budding of the enamel organ.

PROLIFERATION (CAP STAGE)

Proliferation of the cells continues during the cap stage. As a result of unequal growth in the different parts of the bud, a cap is formed (see Fig. 4-1B). A shallow invagination appears on the deep surface of the bud. The peripheral cells of the cap later form the outer and inner enamel epithelium.

As with a deficiency in initiation, a deficiency in proliferation results in failure of the tooth germ to develop and in less than the normal number of teeth. Excessive proliferation of cells may result in epithelial rests. These

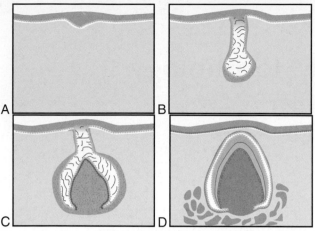

Figure 4-1 Life cycle of the tooth. **A**, Initiation (bud stage). **B**, Proliferation (cap stage). **C**, Histodifferentiation and morphologic differentiation (bell stage). **D**, Apposition and calcification. (Adapted from Bath-Balogh M, Fehrenbach MJ: *Illustrated dental embryology, histology, and anatomy*, ed 2, Philadelphia, 2006, Saunders.)

rests may remain inactive or become activated as a result of an irritation or stimulus. If the cells become partially differentiated or detached from the enamel organ in their partially differentiated state, they assume the secretory functions common to all epithelial cells, and a cyst develops. If the cells become more fully differentiated or detached from the enamel organ, they produce enamel and dentin, which results in an odontoma (see Fig. 7-5) or a supernumerary tooth. The degree of differentiation of the cells determines whether a cyst, an odontoma, or a supernumerary tooth develops (see Fig. 27-56).

HISTODIFFERENTIATION AND MORPHODIFFERENTIATION (BELL STAGE)

The epithelium continues to invaginate and deepen until the enamel organ takes on the shape of a bell (see Fig. 4-1C). It is during this stage that there is a differentiation of the cells of the dental papilla into odontoblasts and of the cells of the inner enamel epithelium into ameloblasts.

Histodifferentiation marks the end of the proliferative stage as the cells lose their capacity to multiply. This stage is the forerunner of appositional activity. Disturbances in the differentiation of the formative cells of the tooth germ result in abnormal structure of the dentin or enamel. One clinical example of the failure of ameloblasts to differentiate properly is amelogenesis imperfecta (see Figs. 7-32 and 7-33). The failure of the odontoblasts to differentiate properly, with the resultant abnormal dentin structure, results in the clinical entity dentinogenesis imperfecta (see Fig. 7-31).

In the morphodifferentiation stage, the formative cells are arranged to outline the form and size of the tooth. This process occurs before matrix deposition. The morphologic pattern of the tooth becomes established when the inner enamel epithelium is arranged so that the boundary between it and the odontoblasts outlines the future

dentinoenamel junction. Disturbances and aberrations in morphodifferentiation lead to abnormal forms and sizes of teeth. Resulting conditions include peg teeth, other types of microdontia, and macrodontia.

APPOSITION

Appositional growth is the result of a layer-like deposition of a nonvital extracellular secretion in the form of a tissue matrix. This matrix is deposited by the formative cells, ameloblasts, and odontoblasts, which line up along the future dentinoenamel and dentinocemental junction at the stage of morphodifferentiation. These cells deposit the enamel and dentin matrix according to a definite pattern and at a definite rate. The formative cells begin their work at specific sites that are referred to as *growth centers* as soon as the blueprint, the dentinoenamel junction, is completed (see Fig. 4-1D).

Any systemic disturbance or local trauma that injures the ameloblasts during enamel formation can cause an interruption or an arrest in matrix apposition, which results in enamel hypoplasia (see Fig. 7-16). Hypoplasia of the dentin is less common than enamel hypoplasia and occurs only after severe systemic disturbances (see Fig. 7-15).

CALCIFICATION

Calcification (mineralization) takes place following matrix deposition and involves the precipitation of inorganic calcium salts within the deposited matrix. The process begins with the precipitation of a small nidus about which further precipitation occurs. The original nidus increases in size by the addition of concentric laminations. There is an eventual approximation and fusion of these individual calcospherites into a homogeneously mineralized layer of tissue matrix. If the calcification process is disturbed, there is a lack of fusion of the calcospherites. These deficiencies are not readily identified in the enamel, but in the dentin they are evident microscopically and are referred to as interglobular dentin.

EARLY DEVELOPMENT AND CALCIFICATION OF THE ANTERIOR PRIMARY TEETH

Kraus and Jordan found that the first macroscopic indication of morphologic development occurs at approximately 11 weeks in utero.[3] The maxillary and mandibular central incisor crowns appear identical at this early stage as tiny, hemispheric, moundlike structures.

The lateral incisors begin to develop morphologic characteristics between 13 and 14 weeks. There is evidence of the developing canines between 14 and 16 weeks. Calcification of the central incisor begins at approximately 14 weeks in utero, with the maxillary central incisor slightly preceding the lower central. The initial calcification of the lateral incisor occurs at 16 weeks and of the canine at 17 weeks.

The developmental dates listed precede by 3 to 4 weeks the dates that appear in the chronology of the human dentition, as developed by Logan and Kronfeld.[4] This observation has been confirmed by Lunt and Law.[5]

EARLY DEVELOPMENT AND CALCIFICATION OF THE POSTERIOR PRIMARY TEETH AND THE FIRST PERMANENT MOLAR

The maxillary first primary molar appears macroscopically at 12½ weeks in utero. Kraus and Jordan[3] observed that as early as 15½ weeks the apex of the mesiobuccal cusp may undergo calcification. At approximately 34 weeks the entire occlusal surface is covered by calcified tissue. At birth, calcification includes roughly three fourths of the occlusal gingival height of the crown.

The maxillary second primary molar also appears macroscopically at about 12½ weeks in utero. There is evidence of calcification of the mesiobuccal cusp as early as 19 weeks. At birth, calcification extends occlusogingivally to include approximately one fourth of the height of the crown.

The mandibular first primary molar initially becomes evident macroscopically at about 12 weeks in utero. Calcification may be observed as early as 15½ weeks at the apex of the mesiobuccal cusp. At birth, a completely calcified cap covers the occlusal surface.

The mandibular second primary molar also becomes evident macroscopically at 12½ weeks in utero. According to Kraus and Jordan, calcification may begin at 18 weeks.[3] At the time of birth, the five centers have coalesced and only a small area of uncalcified tissue remains in the middle of the occlusal surface. There are sharp conical cusps, angular ridges, and a smooth occlusal surface, all of which indicate that calcification of these areas is incomplete at birth. Thus there is a calcification sequence of central incisor, first molar, lateral incisor, canine, and second molar.

The work of Kraus and Jordan indicates that the adjacent second primary and the first permanent molars undergo identical patterns of morphodifferentiation but at different times and the initial development of the first permanent molar occurs slightly later. Their research has also shown that the first permanent molars are uncalcified before 28 weeks of age; at any time thereafter calcification may begin. Some degree of calcification is always present at birth.

MORPHOLOGY OF INDIVIDUAL PRIMARY TEETH

MAXILLARY CENTRAL INCISOR

The mesiodistal width of the crown of the maxillary central incisor is greater than the cervicoincisal length. Developmental lines are usually not evident in the crown; thus the labial surface is smooth. The incisal edge is nearly straight even before abrasion becomes evident. There are well-developed marginal ridges on the lingual surface and a distinctly developed cingulum (Figs. 4-2 and 4-3). The root of the incisor is cone shaped with tapered sides.

MAXILLARY LATERAL INCISOR

The outline of the maxillary lateral incisor is similar to that of the central incisor, but the crown is smaller in all dimensions. The length of the crown from the cervical to the incisal edge is greater than the mesiodistal width. The root outline is similar to that of the central incisor but is longer in proportion to the crown.

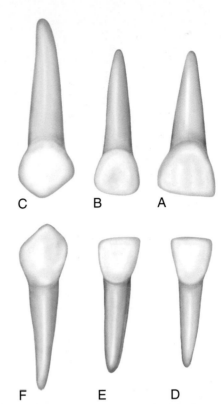

Figure 4-2 Primary right anterior teeth, labial aspect. **A,** Maxillary central incisor. **B,** Maxillary lateral incisor. **C,** Maxillary canine. **D,** Mandibular central incisor. **E,** Mandibular lateral incisor. **F,** Mandibular canine. (From Nelson SJ: *Wheeler's dental anatomy, physiology, and occlusion,* ed 9, Philadelphia, 2010, WB Saunders.)

MAXILLARY CANINE

The crown of the maxillary canine is more constricted at the cervical region than are the incisors, and the incisal and distal surfaces are more convex. There is a well-developed sharp cusp rather than a relatively straight incisal edge. The canine has a long, slender, tapering root that is more than twice the length of the crown. The root is usually inclined distally, apical to the middle third.

MANDIBULAR CENTRAL INCISOR

The mandibular central incisor is smaller than the maxillary central, but its labiolingual measurement is usually only 1 mm less. The labial aspect presents a flat surface without developmental grooves. The lingual surface presents marginal ridges and a cingulum. The middle third and the incisal third on the lingual surface may have a flattened surface level with the marginal ridges, or there may be a slight concavity. The incisal edge is straight and bisects the crown labiolingually. The root is approximately twice the length of the crown.

MANDIBULAR LATERAL INCISOR

The outline of the mandibular lateral incisor is similar to that of the central incisor but is somewhat larger in all dimensions except labiolingually. The lingual surface may have greater concavity between the marginal ridges. The incisal edge slopes toward the distal aspect of the tooth.

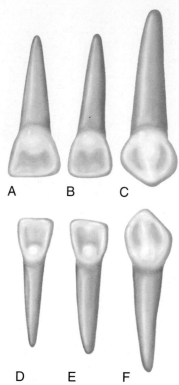

Figure 4-3 Primary right anterior teeth, lingual aspect.
A, Maxillary central incisor. **B**, Maxillary lateral incisor.
C, Maxillary canine. **D**, Mandibular central incisor.
E, Mandibular lateral incisor. **F**, Mandibular canine.
(From Nelson SJ: *Wheeler's dental anatomy, physiology,
and occlusion*, ed 9, Philadelphia, 2010, WB Saunders.)

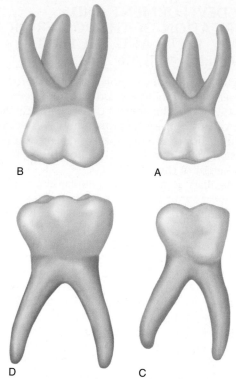

Figure 4-4 Primary right molars, buccal aspect. **A**, Maxillary
first molar. **B**, Maxillary second molar. **C**, Mandibular first
molar. **D**, Mandibular second molar. (From Nelson SJ: *Wheeler's
dental anatomy, physiology, and occlusion*, ed 9, Philadelphia,
2010, WB Saunders.)

MANDIBULAR CANINE

The form of the mandibular canine is similar to that of
the maxillary canine, with a few exceptions. The crown
is slightly shorter, and the root may be as much as 2 mm
shorter than that of the maxillary canine. The mandibular canine is not as large labiolingually as its maxillary
opponent.

MAXILLARY FIRST MOLAR

The greatest dimension of the crown of the maxillary first
molar is at the mesiodistal contact areas, and from these
areas the crown converges toward the cervical region
(Figs. 4-4 through 4-6).

The mesiolingual cusp is the largest and sharpest. The
distolingual cusp is poorly defined, small, and rounded.
The buccal surface is smooth, with little evidence of developmental grooves. The three roots are long, slender,
and widely spread.

MAXILLARY SECOND MOLAR

There is considerable resemblance between the maxillary
primary second molar and the maxillary first permanent
molar. There are two well-defined buccal cusps, with a
developmental groove between them. The crown of the
second molar is considerably larger than that of the first
molar.

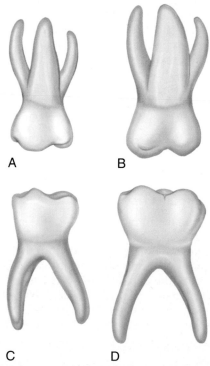

Figure 4-5 Primary right molars, lingual aspect. **A**, Maxillary
first molar. **B**, Maxillary second molar. **C**, Mandibular first
molar. **D**, Mandibular second molar. (From Nelson SJ: *Wheeler's
dental anatomy, physiology, and occlusion*, ed 9, Philadelphia,
2010, WB Saunders.)

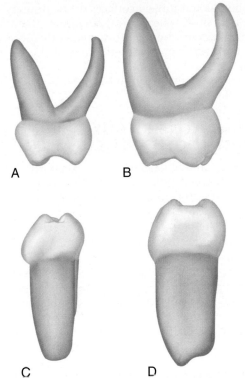

The bifurcation between the buccal roots is close to the cervical region. The roots are longer and heavier than those of the first primary molar, and the lingual root is large and thick compared with the other roots (see Figs. 4-4 and 4-5).

The lingual surface has three cusps: a mesiolingual cusp that is large and well developed, a distolingual cusp, and a third and smaller supplemental cusp (cusp of Carabelli). A well-defined groove separates the mesiolingual cusp from the distolingual cusp. On the occlusal surface a prominent oblique ridge connects the mesiolingual cusp with the distobuccal cusp (Fig. 4-7).

MANDIBULAR FIRST MOLAR

Unlike the other primary teeth, the first primary molar does not resemble any of the permanent teeth. The mesial outline of the tooth, when viewed from the buccal aspect, is almost straight from the contact area to the cervical region. The distal area of the tooth is shorter than the mesial area.

The two distinct buccal cusps have no evidence of a distinct developmental groove between them; the mesial cusp is the larger of the two.

There is a pronounced lingual convergence of the crown on the mesial aspect, with a rhomboid outline present on the distal aspect. The mesiolingual cusp is long and sharp at the tip; a developmental groove separates this cusp from the distolingual cusp, which is rounded and well developed. The mesial marginal ridge is well developed, to the extent that it appears as another

Figure 4-6 Primary right molars, mesial aspect. **A**, Maxillary first molar. **B**, Maxillary second molar. **C**, Mandibular first molar. **D**, Mandibular second molar. (From Nelson SJ: *Wheeler's dental anatomy, physiology, and occlusion*, ed 9, Philadelphia, 2010, WB Saunders.)

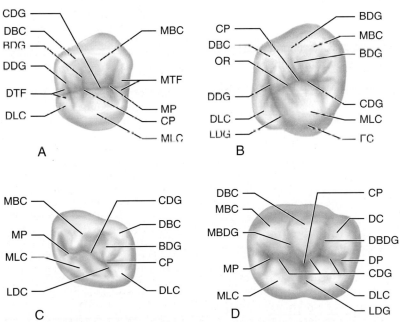

Figure 4-7 Primary right molars, occlusal aspect. **A**, Maxillary first molar. **B**, Maxillary second molar. **C**, Mandibular first molar. **D**, Mandibular second molar. *BDG,* Buccal developmental groove; *CDG,* central developmental groove; *CP,* central pit; *DBC,* distobuccal cusp; *DBDG,* distobuccal developmental groove; *DC,* distal cusp; *DDG,* distal developmental groove; *DLC,* distolingual cusp; *DP,* distal pit; *DTF,* distal triangular fossa; *FC,* fifth cusp; *LDG,* lingual developmental groove; *MBC,* mesiobuccal cusp; *MBDG,* mesiobuccal developmental groove; *MLC,* mesiolingual cusp; *MP,* mesial pit; *MTF,* mesial triangular fossa; *OR,* oblique ridge. (From Nelson SJ: *Wheeler's dental anatomy, physiology, and occlusion*, ed 9, Philadelphia, 2010, WB Saunders.)

small cusp lingually. When the tooth is viewed from the mesial aspect, there is an extreme curvature buccally at the cervical third. The crown length is greater in the mesiobuccal area than in the mesiolingual area; thus the cervical line slants upward from the buccal to the lingual surface.

The longer slender roots spread considerably at the apical third, extending beyond the outline of the crown. The mesial root, when viewed from the mesial aspect, does not resemble any other primary root. The buccal and lingual outlines of the root drop straight down from the crown, being essentially parallel for more than half their length. The end of the root is flat and almost square.

MANDIBULAR SECOND MOLAR

The mandibular second molar resembles the mandibular first permanent molar, except that the primary tooth is smaller in all its dimensions. The buccal surface is divided into three cusps that are separated by a mesiobuccal and distobuccal developmental groove. The cusps are almost equal in size. Two cusps of almost equal size are evident on the lingual surface and are divided by a short lingual groove.

The primary second molar, when viewed from the occlusal surface, appears rectangular with a slight distal convergence of the crown. The mesial marginal ridge is developed to a greater extent than the distal marginal ridge.

One difference between the crown of the primary molar and that of the first permanent molar is in the distobuccal cusp; the distal cusp of the permanent molar is smaller than the other two buccal cusps.

The roots of the primary second molar are long and slender, with a characteristic flare mesiodistally in the middle and apical thirds.

MORPHOLOGIC DIFFERENCES BETWEEN PRIMARY AND PERMANENT TEETH

Nelson has listed the following differences in form between the primary and permanent teeth[6]:
1. The crowns of the primary teeth are wider mesiodistally in comparison with crown length than are those of the permanent teeth.
2. The roots of primary anterior teeth are narrow and long compared with crown width and length.
3. The roots of the primary molars are relatively longer and more slender than the roots of the permanent teeth. There is also a greater extension of the primary roots mesiodistally. This "flaring" allows more room between the roots for the development of the premolar tooth crowns.
4. The cervical ridge of enamel at the cervical third of the anterior crowns is much more prominent labially and lingually in the primary than in the permanent teeth.
5. The crowns and roots of primary molars are more slender mesiodistally at the cervical third than are those of the permanent molars.
6. The cervical ridge on the buccal aspect of the primary molars is much more definite, particularly on the maxillary and mandibular first molars, than that on the permanent molars.
7. The buccal and lingual surfaces of the primary molars are flatter above the cervical curvatures than those of the permanent molars, which makes the occlusal surface narrower compared with that of the permanent teeth.
8. The primary teeth are usually lighter in color than the permanent teeth.

SIZE AND MORPHOLOGY OF THE PRIMARY TOOTH PULP CHAMBER

Considerable individual variation exists in the size of the pulp chamber and pulp canal of the primary teeth. Immediately after the eruption of the teeth, the pulp chambers are large, and in general they follow the outline of the crown. The pulp chamber decreases in size as age increases and under the influence of function and of abrasion of the occlusal and incisal surfaces of the teeth.

No attempt is made here to describe in detail each pulp chamber outline; rather, it is suggested that the dentist examine critically the bite-wing radiographs of the child before undertaking operative procedures. Just as there are individual differences in the calcification time of teeth and in eruption time, so are there individual differences in the morphology of the crowns and the size of the pulp chamber. However, radiographs do not demonstrate completely the extent of pulp horn into the cuspal area.

Finally, the cementoenamel junction of primary teeth presents three interesting morphologic relationships in which the cementum is over enamel, the cementum and enamel are edge to edge, or there is a gap between the cementum and enamel with dentin exposure. This irregularity in the cementoenamel junction may indicate the need to take care during restorative and other procedures to avoid damage.[7]

REFERENCES

1. Smith CE. Cellular and chemical events during enamel maturation, *Crit Rev Oral Biol Med* 9:128-161, 1998.
2. Miletich I, Sharpe PT. Normal and abnormal dental development, *Hum Mol Genet* 12:R69-R73, 2003.
3. Kraus BS, Jordan RE. *The human dentition before birth*, Philadelphia, 1965, Lea & Febiger.
4. Logan WHG, Kronfeld R. Development of the human jaws and surrounding structures from birth to the age of fifteen years, *J Am Dent Assoc* 20:379-427, 1933.
5. Lunt RC, Law DB. A review of the chronology of calcification of deciduous teeth, *J Am Dent Assoc* 89:599-606, 1974.
6. Nelson SJ. *Wheeler's dental anatomy, physiology, and occlusion*, ed 9, Philadelphia, 2010, WB Saunders.
7. Francischone LA, Consolaro A. Morphology of the cementoenamel junction of primary teeth, *J Dent Child* 75:252-259, 2008.

SUGGESTED READINGS

Avery J, Chiego D. *Essentials of oral histology and embryology*, ed 3, St Louis, 2006, Mosby.
Nanci A. *Ten Cate's oral histology*, ed 7, St Louis, 2008, Mosby.
Schour I, Massler M. Studies in tooth development: the growth pattern of human teeth, *J Am Dent Assoc* 27:1778-1793, 1940.

CHAPTER 5

Radiographic Techniques

▲ Dale A. Miles and Edwin T. Parks

Roentgen's discovery of the x-ray in 1895 provided one of the most important diagnostic aids in dentistry. Radiographs are essential if we are to treat children successfully. Evidence indicates that, unless carious lesions are discovered early, the primary teeth will not be retained until normal exfoliation.

Early diagnosis of caries prevents the pediatric patient from experiencing dental pain, extraction, and emotional stress. In addition, eruptive or developmental problems can be discovered with the use of radiographic images, and early treatment of these problems may reduce the need for prolonged orthodontic procedures. Some restorative procedures require an accurate registration of the pulpal outline that only a radiograph can reveal.

The selection of appropriate radiographs for the pediatric patient depends on the age of the child, the size of the oral cavity, and the level of patient cooperation. These are determined by a careful clinical examination of the patient before ordering the radiographic survey. The examination determines the need for radiographs and the type to be taken. Ideal technique should expose the patient to a minimum amount of radiation, require as few radiographs as possible, take as little time as possible, and provide a diagnostically accurate examination of the dentition and supporting structures. The child's cooperation is as essential to radiographic examination as is the selection of correct radiographic technique. Both increase the probability of success and reduce additional radiographic exposure.

Dental radiographic equipment can be threatening or can generate curiosity, depending on the child. It is wise to allow the patient to run a hand over the x-ray machine head and become acquainted with the "camera." The patient might hold one of the films and be shown where it will be placed. If it is a film that requires biting pressure, the patient should be shown how to bite on the film.

Show-and-tell goes a long way in gaining cooperation. Careful wording of the description of the procedure is essential to gain patient cooperation. The potential cooperation of a patient may be lost when the patient hears the phrase "shooting a couple of films." Imaging the easiest region first may ensure success in other areas. This is particularly important if the child has an exaggerated gag reflex or objects to the placement of the film. The use of topical anesthetic agents may be beneficial in both situations.

The dentist should be patient with the child in obtaining radiographs. Repeated attempts at film placement may be necessary before the actual radiation exposure is made. If the child is uncooperative, firmness, voice control, and tender loving care are often effective. Emotionally, mentally, and physically disabled children require special handling.

RADIATION SAFETY AND PROTECTION

One characteristic of x-radiation is its ability to impart some of its energy to the matter it traverses. If that matter is living tissue, then some biologic injury may occur. Much information about high levels of radiation and subsequent damage is available. The effects of low levels of x-radiation (as used in diagnostic radiology) on biologic systems are virtually unknown. Our assumptions of damage are based on extrapolation of data from high levels to lower levels of radiation.

Still, dental health professionals must be concerned about any risk that the patient may encounter during therapy. Concern is focused on three primary biologic effects of low-level radiation: (1) carcinogenesis, (2) teratogenesis (malformations), and (3) mutagenesis. Carcinogenesis and malformations are a response of somatic tissues and in most instances are believed to have a threshold response; that is, a certain amount of radiation is necessary before the response is seen. Mutation may occur as a response of genetic tissue (gonads) to x-radiation and is believed to have no threshold. In general, younger tissues and organs are more sensitive to radiation, with the sensitivity decreasing from the period before birth until maturity. It must also be recognized that far higher doses of radiation can be withstood by localized areas than by the whole body. We know that we live in a world that exposes us to natural background radiation averaging 360 mrem per year (3.60 millisievert) in the United States. Medical and dental radiographic examinations add to that exposure and so must be ordered judiciously.

With regard to patient protection, evidence has shown that there are critical organs vulnerable to possible development of late effects. These organs should be shielded when possible. These critical organs and the associated adverse biologic effects are the following: (1) the skin (cancer), (2) red bone marrow (leukemia), (3) the gonads (mutation, infertility, and fetal malformations), (4) the eyes (cataracts), (5) the thyroid (cancer), (6) the breasts (cancer), and (7) possibly the salivary glands (cancer).

The practitioner and staff can physically protect the patient and indirectly protect themselves from unnecessary exposure to radiation by using correct technique. The most obvious method of protecting the patient is to shield those areas not being evaluated. This is easily accomplished using a lead apron and thyroid collar (Fig. 5-1).

The apron and collar may be incorporated as a single unit or used separately. The apron protects the gonads and chest from the primary beam and scatter radiation whereas the collar shields the thyroid. This method does not provide complete protection, particularly of the thyroid, but it does provide a great reduction in exposure. Aprons used in panoramic radiography have a front and back because the source of radiation is from the side and the rear of the patient.

Faster film speeds have contributed most significantly to the reduction in radiation to the patient. Film speeds of the D and F groups are available for intraoral radiography. Faster film also reduces error from patient movement, a consideration with the pediatric patient. Extraoral

(panoramic) radiography uses film-screen combinations that also have reduced exposure times. Recently, there has been an increased use of beam-positioning devices (Fig. 5-2), which virtually eliminate some of the technical errors, particularly film cone cuts. Using different lengths and shapes of the cone (Fig. 5-3) has also aided in the reduction of patient radiation exposure. Use of a long rectangular collimator reduces the area unnecessarily exposed to radiation by almost 4 square inches compared with a round collimator. The use of higher kilovolt peak techniques reduces patient exposure to radiation and lowers contrast, thus increasing the number of shades of gray on the film. An additional benefit of using high kilovolt peak technique is that the exposure time is shortened, which potentially reduces retakes caused by patient movement.

Finally, quality control (and thus patient protection) begins with proper processing. With the shift toward using digital radiography, this concern becomes reduced. However, the majority of dental practices still use traditional film and wet tank chemical processing. If the processing does not function at an optimal level, retakes will be required, necessitating additional patient exposure. The dentist must insist on time-temperature developing and the use of proper-strength chemicals if wet tanks are used. The processing area should be clean and free of white light (light leaks). If automatic processing is used, chemical parameters must be continuously monitored and the unit must be cleaned weekly.

SELECTION CRITERIA AND RADIOGRAPHIC EXAMINATIONS

The decision to make radiographs is based on a thorough evaluation and examination of the patient. Radiographs should be made only when there is an expectation that

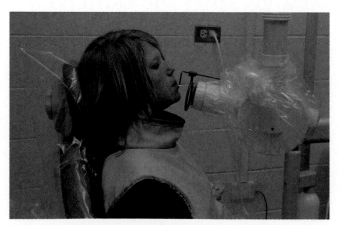

Figure 5-1 Lead apron and thyroid collar in place.

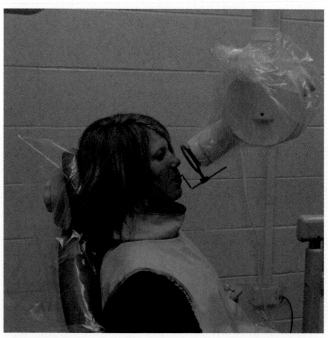

Figure 5-2 Use of the Rinn XCP positioning device.

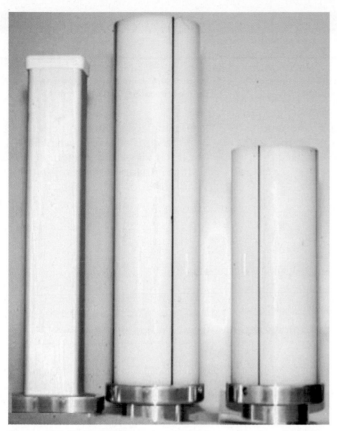

Figure 5-3 Rectangular and round cones of various lengths.

disease is present or when an undetected condition left untreated could adversely affect the patient's dental health. Therefore the decision to use ionizing radiation is based on professional judgment (Table 5-1).

Selection criteria are clinical signs or symptoms that allow the practitioner to identify patients who will benefit from a radiographic examination. Two important considerations when deciding whether to perform a radiographic examination for children are (1) the stage of dentition development and (2) the risk of dental caries.

The criteria for making radiographs, developed in part by the Conference on Radiation Exposure in Pediatric Dentistry, were summarized by Nowak and colleagues[1] as follows.

CRITERIA FOR EXPOSING OF RADIOGRAPHS IN ASYMPTOMATIC CHILDREN

The criteria for exposing radiographs assume that the child is asymptomatic and that the dentist finds no specific clinical indications for radiographic examination. Exceptions to this rule include those conditions in which there is clinical evidence of injury, disease such as caries, pulpal pathosis, delayed or accelerated eruption or exfoliation of teeth, swelling, hemorrhage, pain, or ulceration, or those conditions in which there is a need to evaluate treatment. In such cases, taking appropriate radiographs is indicated to confirm the diagnosis and facilitate and evaluate treatment.

DEVELOPMENT OF THE DENTITION AS CRITERION

Dental radiographs are indicated in the following situations.

Primary Dentition
If the proximal surfaces of the primary teeth cannot be visually and tactilely inspected, and the child can be expected to cooperate, then dental radiographs should be made to determine the presence of interproximal caries. If all surfaces of all primary teeth can be examined clinically because of open contact, then radiographs are not indicated.

If the child's behavior is such that obtaining films of adequate diagnostic quality is doubtful, then radiographs should be deferred until behavior improves.

Early Transitional Dentition (After Appearance of Permanent First Molars or Permanent Mandibular Incisors, or Both)
Radiographs are obtained to evaluate the presence of interproximal caries, developmental anomalies of teeth, and pathologic conditions of the hard and soft tissues of the mouth, jaws, and associated structures.

Early Permanent Dentition (After Puberty; After Patients Have Achieved Most of Their Adult Stature; Late Adolescence)
Radiographs are obtained to evaluate the same tissues as in the early mixed dentition and to check the position and developmental status of the third molars.

No other dental radiographs are routinely needed in children. Other radiographs would be prescribed for diagnostic purposes. For example, diagnostic bite-wing radiographs are obtained to detect the presence of interproximal caries if the risk of caries activity is high for that individual. Occlusal caries, detected clinically, and discolored marginal ridges are indications of high risk of caries activity. Periapical films of the canine areas could be obtained if these teeth were not clinically palpable by 9 years of age. The dentist must use clinical judgment and evaluate such factors as oral hygiene practices, diet, attitude and compliance, fluoride history, alignment of teeth, and morphology of teeth to determine the necessity for, the extent of, and the type and frequency of diagnostic radiographs.

RISK OF THE PATIENT FOR DENTAL CARIES AS CRITERION

A high risk of dental caries may be associated with poor oral hygiene, fluoride deficiency, prolonged nursing (bottle or breast), high-carbohydrate diet, poor family dental health, developmental enamel defects, developmental disability, acute or chronic medical history, and genetic abnormality.

The child with a high risk of dental caries should have bite-wing radiographs made as soon as posterior primary teeth are in proximal contact. The age of the patient is not an important variable. If interproximal caries is detected, then follow-up radiographs are indicated semiannually until the child is caries-free and therefore is classified as having a low risk for dental caries.

Table 5-1

Guideline for Prescribing Dental Radiographs

Patient Category	Child	
	Primary Dentition (before eruption of first permanent tooth)	**Transitional Dentition (after eruption of first permanent tooth)**
***New Patient** All new patients to assess dental diseases and growth and development	Posterior bite-wing examination if proximal surfaces of primary teeth cannot be visualized or probed	Individualized radiographic examination consisting of periapical/occlusal views and posterior bite-wings *or* panoramic examination and posterior bite-wings
***Recall Patient** Clinical caries or high-risk factors for caries†	Posterior bite-wing examination 6-month intervals *or* until no carious lesions are evident	
No clinical caries and no high-risk factors for caries†	Posterior bite-wing examination at 12- to 14-month intervals if proximal surfaces of primary teeth cannot be visualized or probed	Posterior bite-wing examination at 12- to 24-month intervals
Periodontal disease or a history of periodontal treatment	Individualized radiographic examination consisting of selected periapical and/or bite-wing radiographs for areas where periodontal disease (other than nonspecific gingivitis) can be demonstrated clinically	
Growth and development assessment	Usually not indicated	Individualized radiographic examination consisting of a periapical/occlusal *or* panoramic examination

The recommendations contained in this table were developed by an expert dental panel comprised of representatives from the Academy of General Dentistry, American Academy of Dental Radiology, American Academy of Oral Medicine, American Academy of Pediatric Dentistry, American Academy of Periodontology, and American Dental Association under the sponsorship of the Food and Drug Administration (FDA). Courtesy Carestream Health, Inc.

Adolescent Permanent Dentition (before eruption of third molars)	Adult Dentulous	Edentulous
Individualized radiographic examination consisting of posterior bite-wings and selected periapicals. A full mouth intraoral radiographic examination is appropriate when the patient presents with clinical evidence of generalized dental disease or a history of extensive dental treatment.		Full mouth intraoral radiographic examination *or* panoramic examination
Posterior bite-wing examination at 6- to 12-month intervals *or* until no carious lesions are evident	Posterior bite-wing examination at 12- to 18-month intervals	Not applicable
Posterior bite-wing examination at 18- to 36-month intervals	Posterior bite-wing examination at 24- to 36-month intervals	Not applicable
Individualized radiographic examination consisting of selected periapical and/or bite-wing radiographs for areas where periodontal disease (other than nonspecific gingivitis) can be demonstrated clinically		Not applicable
Periapical *or* panoramic examination to assess developing third molars	Usually not indicated	Usually not indicated

*Clinical situations for which radiographs may be indicated include the following:

A. Positive Historical Findings
1. Previous periodontal or endodontic therapy
2. History of pain or trauma
3. Familial history of dental anomalies
4. Postoperative evaluation of healing
5. Presence of implants

B. Positive Clinical Signs/Symptoms
1. Clinical evidence of periodontal disease
2. Large or deep restorations
3. Deep carious lesions
4. Malposed or clinically impacted teeth
5. Swelling
6. Evidence of facial trauma
7. Mobility of teeth
8. Fistula or sinus tract infection
9. Clinically suspected sinus pathology
10. Growth abnormalities
11. Oral involvement in known or suspected systemic disease
12. Positive neurologic findings in the head and neck
13. Evidence of foreign objects
14. Pain and/or dysfunction of the temporomandibular joint
15. Facial asymmetry
16. Abutment teeth for fixed or removable partial prosthesis
17. Unexplained bleeding
18. Unexplained sensitivity of teeth
19. Unusual eruption, spacing, or migration of teeth
20. Unusual tooth morphology, calcification, or color
21. Missing teeth with unknown reason

†Patients at high risk for caries may demonstrate any of the following:
1. High level of caries experience
2. History of recurrent caries
3. Existing restoration of poor quality
4. Poor oral hygiene
5. Inadequate fluoride exposure
6. Prolonged nursing (bottle or breast)
7. Diet with high sucrose frequency
8. Poor family dental health
9. Developmental enamel defects
10. Developmental disability
11. Xerostomia
12. Genetic abnormality of teeth
13. Many multisurface restorations
14. Chemo/radiation therapy

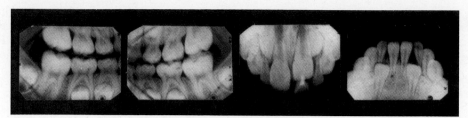

Figure 5-4 Four-film series.

A child who has a low risk for dental caries may be defined as a normal, healthy, asymptomatic patient exposed to optimal levels of fluoride (preferably since birth), who performs daily preventive techniques and consumes a diet with few exposures to retentive carbohydrates between meals. Posterior bite-wing radiographs should be made for the low-risk patient with closed proximal contacts. If no evidence of caries is found, then radiographs may be retaken every 12 to 18 months if primary teeth are in contact or after up to 24 months if permanent teeth are in contact. Bite-wing radiographs may be obtained more frequently if the child enters the high-risk category.

The more rapid progression of caries in primary teeth should be considered in determining the time interval between bite-wing radiographs.

TYPES OF FINDINGS ANTICIPATED AS CRITERIA

Bite-wing radiographs are indicated when a clinical examination discloses posterior tooth contact. Bite-wing examinations are recommended at the first clinical evidence of caries. Bite-wing radiographs are usually taken every 12 to 18 months in the absence of dental caries with primary tooth contact or every 24 months with permanent tooth contact.

By the time the first permanent tooth has erupted (posterior or anterior), an anterior occlusal radiograph should be made. This allows detection of conditions such as supernumerary teeth, missing teeth, and dens in dente. A radiographic examination that includes the tooth-bearing areas of the mandible and maxilla is recommended at approximately the time of the early mixed dentition to assess the dental age of the patient and to aid in the early diagnosis of congenital and developmental anomalies.

The radiographic examination may consist of one of the following: posterior periapical radiographs, panoramic radiograph, or lateral jaw 45-degree projections. Another similar radiographic examination may be made within 2 years after the eruption of the permanent second molars.

To check on growth and development, a cephalometric radiograph may be prescribed by the practitioner who is providing the orthodontic diagnosis or treatment.

RADIOGRAPHIC EXAMINATIONS

When a new patient is seen at the dental office and no previous radiographs are available, it may be necessary to obtain a baseline series of radiographs. Again, we emphasize that the decision to make a radiographic examination is based on the criteria previously outlined. These examinations include the following.

Four-Film Series

This series consists of a maxillary and mandibular anterior occlusal and two posterior bite-wings (Fig. 5-4).

Eight-Film Survey

This survey includes a maxillary and mandibular anterior occlusal (or periapicals), a right and left maxillary posterior occlusal (or periapicals), right and left primary mandibular molar periapicals, and two posterior bite-wings (Fig. 5-5).

Twelve-Film Survey

This examination includes four primary molar-premolar periapical radiographs, four canine periapical radiographs, two incisor periapical radiographs, and two posterior bite-wing radiographs (Fig. 5-6).

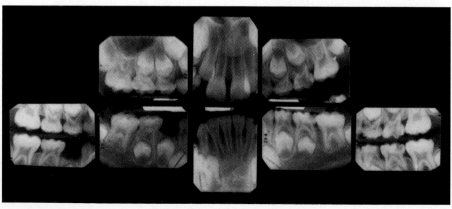

Figure 5-5 Eight-film survey.

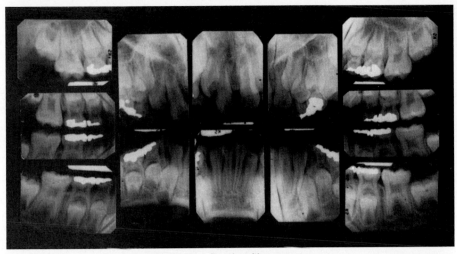

Figure 5-6 Twelve-film survey.

Sixteen-Film Survey

This examination consists of the 12-film survey and the addition of four permanent molar radiographs (Fig. 5-7).

COMMONLY USED RADIOGRAPHIC TECHNIQUES

Several techniques are commonly used to radiograph a child's dentition. The technique used depends primarily on the size of the oral cavity, the number of teeth present, and patient cooperation. The procedures commonly used by the private practitioner include the following:

1. Bite-wing
2. Periapical
3. Occlusal
4. Panoramic

BITE-WING TECHNIQUE

A No. 0 bite-wing film is usually the most suitable size for the smaller patient. However, some children's mouths are large enough to receive a No. 2 bite-wing film. The head is positioned so that the midsagittal plane is perpendicular and the ala-tragus line is parallel to the floor. The inferior edge of the bite-wing film packet is placed in the floor of the mouth between the tongue and the lingual aspect of the mandible and the bite-tab or positioning device is placed on the occlusal surfaces of the mandibular teeth (Fig. 5-8). The anterior edge of the film packet is located as far anteriorly as possible in the region of the canine so that the distal aspect of the canine will be recorded. The lower anterior corner of the film packet is bent slightly toward the lingual to facilitate film placement and to decrease possible patient discomfort. The anteroinferior corner of the film packet usually lies near or at the attachment of the lingual frenum in the midline. In addition, the posterosuperior corner may be bent to prevent the gag reflex.

The dentist holds the bite-tab against the occlusal surfaces of the patient's mandibular teeth with an index finger, and the patient is instructed to "close slowly." The finger is rolled out of the way onto the buccal surfaces of the teeth as the patient closes in centric occlusion. The central ray enters through the occlusal plane at a point below the pupil of the eye. The vertical angle is +8 to +10 degrees. The horizontal diameter of the open-end cone is parallel to the end of the bite-tab or to the mean tangent of the buccal surfaces of the posterior teeth being radiographed.

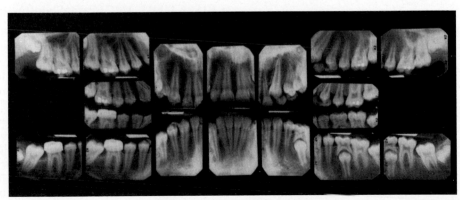

Figure 5-7 Sixteen-film survey.

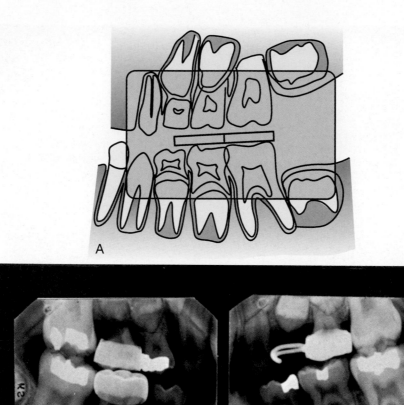

Figure 5-8 Posterior bite wing. **A,** Film placement. **B,** Radiograph.

PARALLELING TECHNIQUE

In principle, the paralleling technique requires the object (long axis of the tooth) and the film to be parallel in all dimensions. To achieve this, the film packet is placed farther away from the object, particularly the maxilla. This tends to magnify the image. This undesirable effect is offset when a longer cone is used, which thus reduces magnification. Use of a longer cone also increases image sharpness by decreasing the penumbra. Striving for true parallelism will enhance image accuracy.

Because the film is placed farther away from the object, a film holder is necessary (Fig. 5-9). Some of those

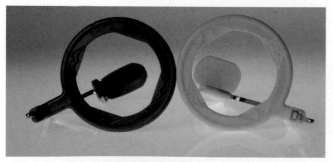

Figure 5-9 Rinn XCP positioning devices and film holders cut down to accommodate child patient's mouth.

holders also have beam-aligning devices to help ensure parallelism and reduce partial exposure of the film; thus unwanted cone cuts are eliminated. For the smaller child, the film holder may need to be reduced in size to accommodate the film and the child's mouth. Film-holding devices with cone alignment guides reduce operator error and thus reduce exposure of the patient to radiation. Because of the shallowness of the child's palate and floor of the mouth, film placement is somewhat compromised. Even so, the resulting films are satisfactory.

BISECTING ANGLE TECHNIQUE

The bisecting angle technique is based on a principle called the *rule of isometry*, which basically states that two triangles are equal if they have two equal angles and a common side. The clinical application of this rule has the central ray directed perpendicularly to a plane that bisects the angle created by the long axis of the tooth and the film (Fig. 5-10). This technique is not as accurate as the paralleling technique and should be used as an accessory technique when paralleling technique is uncomfortable.

Positioning devices and film holders are also available for this technique. If the beam-aligning devices are not used, prescribed head positions are necessary, which may

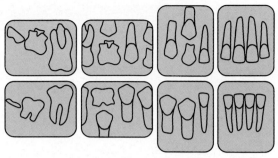

Figure 5-11 Positioning landmarks for film placement. (Courtesy Mark Dirlam.)

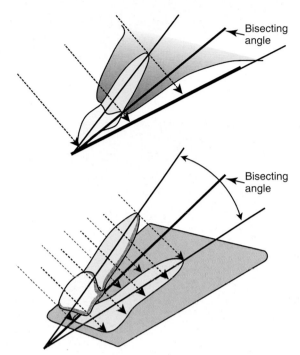

Figure 5-10 The bisecting angle. (Courtesy Mark Dirlam.)

increase operator error. Even though there are limitations to this technique, in some situations it may be the only usable one.

SPECIFIC DENTAL PROJECTIONS

Periapical Technique

There are essentially two methods of taking periapical radiographs: paralleling and bisecting angle techniques. Each has benefits and limitations when used with the pediatric patient. It is not within the scope of this chapter to describe these techniques in detail. Thorough understanding will allow the practitioner to use them to the best advantage in any given situation.

Regardless of which technique is used, film positioning for the two techniques is identical. In general, films are positioned so that all areas of concern can be visualized, and there are usually multiple views of a particular area. This is beneficial when minor technical errors exclude an area of importance on one film, because it can be visualized on another.

Regional film positions for the maxilla and mandible are identical; that is, film position for the maxillary molar projection is identical to that for the mandibular molar. Therefore only the regional positions are explained (Fig. 5-11). In all cases the identification dot is placed toward the occlusal surface.

Molar Projection

The unfolded film packet is positioned so that all of the third molar, the second molar, and all or part of the first molar are recorded. Thus the anterior edge of the film packet is usually located at the mesial contact of the first molar. The plane of the packet should be parallel to the buccal surfaces of the molars.

Premolar or Primary Molar Projection

The packet may be folded anteriorly for relief in the palate or floor of the mouth and positioned so that the first molar, the first and second premolars or first and second primary molars, and the distal surface of the canine are recorded. The film packet is placed parallel to the buccal surfaces of the premolars or primary molars.

Permanent or Primary Canine Projection

The film packet is usually bent, particularly for a younger child, by a long narrow bend of the part of the packet that will be toward the midline. The canine and lateral incisors are recorded in their entirety. The film should be positioned so that the central beam of x-rays is parallel to the proximal surfaces of the canine and lateral incisor and therefore perpendicular to the film.

Permanent or Primary Incisor Projection

If the film packet must be folded because of the narrowness of the arch, a ⅛-inch bend should be made on each edge throughout the entire length of the film that parallels the long axis of the teeth. The film packet is positioned so that the central incisors are centered mesiodistally on the film. The central ray is parallel to the contacts of the proximal surfaces and perpendicular to the film.

Anterior Maxillary Occlusal Technique

In the anterior maxillary occlusal technique, the patient's occlusal plane should be parallel to the floor, and the sagittal plane should be perpendicular to the floor (Fig. 5-12). A No. 2 periapical film is placed in the patient's mouth so that the long axis of the film runs from left to right rather than anteroposteriorly and the midsagittal plane bisects the film. The patient is instructed to bite lightly to hold the film. The anterior edge of the film should extend approximately 2 mm in front of the incisal edge of the central incisors. The central ray is directed to the apices of the central incisors and a centimeter (half-inch) above the tip of the nose and through the midline. The vertical angle is +60 degrees. This film is exposed at the usual setting for maxillary incisor periapical films.

Posterior Maxillary Occlusal Technique

In the posterior maxillary occlusal technique, the patient's occlusal plane should be parallel to the floor, and the sagittal plane should be perpendicular to the floor (Fig. 5-13). A No. 2 periapical film is placed in the patient's mouth so

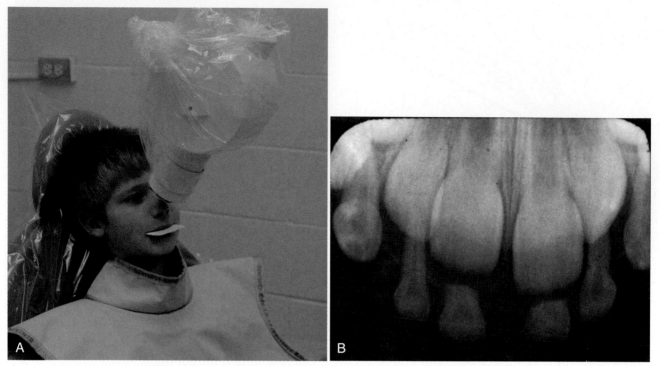

Figure 5-12 Anterior maxillary occlusal. **A,** Technique. **B,** Radiograph.

that the long axis of the film is parallel to the floor. The anterior edge of the film should extend just mesial to the canine. The outer buccal edge of the film should extend approximately 2 mm beyond the primary molar crowns. The patient is instructed to bite lightly to hold the film. The central ray is directed toward the apices of the primary molars as well as interproximally. The vertical angle is +50 degrees. The film is exposed at the usual setting for maxillary premolar periapical films.

Anterior Mandibular Occlusal Technique

The film placement for the anterior mandibular occlusal technique is identical to that for the anterior maxillary occlusal technique, except that the film must be placed so that the tube side faces the x-ray source

(Fig. 5-14). In addition, when the patient occludes on the film, the anterior edge of the film is 2 mm beyond the incisal edge of the lower incisors. The patient's head is positioned so that the occlusal plane is at a −45-degree angle. The cone is then aligned at a −15-degree vertical angle, and the central ray is directed through the symphysis.

PANORAMIC RADIOGRAPHY

Numerous panoramic x-ray units are available to the dental profession (Fig. 5-15). Body-section radiography uses a mechanism by which the x-ray film and the source of the x-rays move simultaneously in opposite directions at the same speed. Refer to textbooks by Langland et al (1989) and Miles et al (1999) for a more definitive discussion of

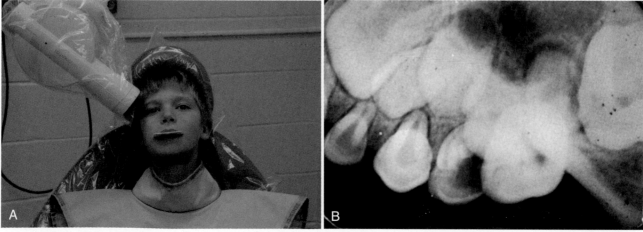

Figure 5-13 Posterior maxillary occlusal. **A,** Technique. **B,** Radiograph.

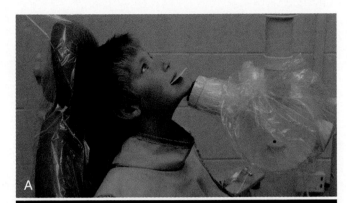

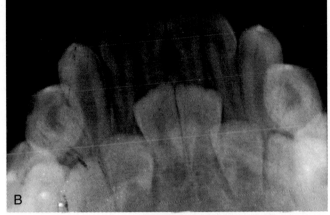

Figure 5-14 Anterior mandibular occlusal. **A,** Technique. **B,** Radiograph.

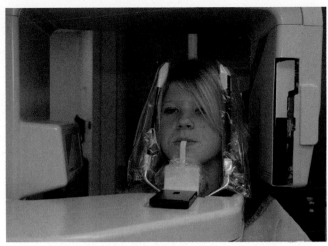

Figure 5-15 Patient positioned in a panoramic unit.

the principles of panoramic imaging. The most contemporary panoramic machines can now "open" the interproximal contacts because of the use of a C-arm on the top of the machine. This allows the robotic path of the machine to direct the central beam at right angles through the bicuspid region contacts (Fig. 5-16). The use of such a machine with a digital receptor allows a very low dose and means that the operator, in many cases, may not even need to place an image receptor in the mouth. This would

be a very big advantage in some cases in which the child is not tolerant of an intraoral image acquisition. Note that these oversized "bite-wing" images have a spatial resolution of 6 to 7 line pairs/mm. This is exceptionally high for panoramic machines. While this technique may not eliminate intraoral bite-wing images completely, it could be used in an initial patient examination and follow-up imaging if there is a low caries risk and give more information for clinical decisions with very low patient dose.

A panoramic radiographic unit can be used for examination of children. Because the examination is obtained without placement of the film in the mouth, it does not alarm the anxious child who may refuse an intraoral film. Moreover, the young patient may find the movement entertaining or fun. The diversion of being momentarily entertained usually invites cooperation. However, staying completely immobile for 15 seconds may not be possible for some very young children.

Although panoramic radiography is considered a supplement to, rather than a substitute for, the intraoral

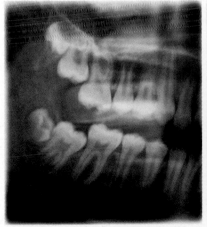

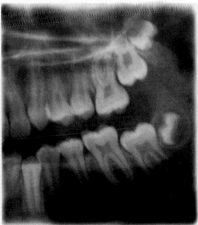

Figure 5-16 Digital panoramic radiograph of a 10-year-old boy. This image was acquired directly from the panoramic machine using a special program that collimates the image at a reduced exposure and "opens" the contacts by using a different "start" position to eliminate most of the overlapping of contacts in the premolar region seen with other panoramic machines. (Image courtesy Planmeca, Inc., Roselle, IL.)

periapical radiographic series, it does provide excellent coverage of the structures that are viewed during pediatric dental diagnosis. A typical diagnostic film or digital panoramic image includes the teeth, the supporting structures, the maxillary region extending to the superior third of the orbit, and the entire mandible including the temporomandibular joint region. Pediatric dentists who have used panoramic radiographic technique have discovered condylar fractures, traumatic cysts, and anomalies that might have gone undetected with the routine periapical series of radiographs (Fig. 5-17).

Panoramic radiology can be valuable when disabled patients are examined if the patient can sit in a chair and hold his or her head in position. It may be necessary to administer relaxants or sedatives to palsied or spastic patients, who are more difficult to control when they are emotionally charged by the dental visit.

The only inherent drawback to panoramic radiography is lack of image detail for diagnosing early carious lesions. Adjunct bite-wing radiographs and selected periapical radiographs are required for that task.

Lateral Jaw Technique

A 5- × 7-inch x-ray film is used for the lateral jaw technique (Fig. 5-18). The film is marked with a right or left lead identification letter placed on the film packet slightly anterior and superior to the central portion of the film. When the film is finally positioned, this letter should be located in the area of the orbit.

The patient's head is positioned so that the occlusal plane is parallel and the sagittal plane is perpendicular to the floor. The long axis of the film, also perpendicular to the floor, rests on the patient's shoulder and against the face. The patient is instructed to rotate the head toward the film until the nose rests against it. Then the chin is raised and the head tilted approximately 15 degrees toward the film. The patient secures the film with the palm of the hand and with fingers extended. The cone is

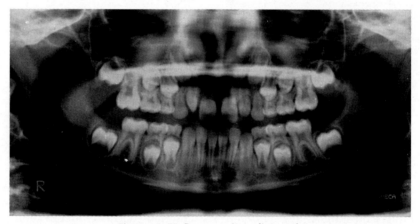

Figure 5-17 Panoramic radiograph

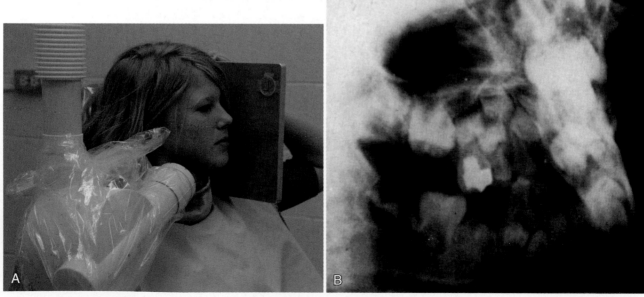

Figure 5-18 Lateral view of jaw. **A,** Technique. **B,** Radiograph.

positioned so that the central x-ray beam enters at a point a half-inch behind and below the angle of the mandible on the side opposite the film. The vertical angle is 17 degrees. The central x-ray beam is perpendicular to the horizontal plane of the film. With specialized panoramic views this technique is slowly becoming obsolete, however for some significantly medically compromised patients, it still remains a helpful tool.

LOCALIZATION TECHNIQUES

One method of localizing embedded or unerupted teeth uses the buccal object rule, which states that the image of any buccally oriented object appears to move in the opposite direction from a moving x-ray source. On the other hand, the image of any lingually oriented object appears to move in the same direction as a moving x-ray source (Fig. 5-19).

Using this principle for localization, the practitioner makes two radiographs of the unerupted tooth. The technique consists of positioning the patient's head so that the sagittal plane is perpendicular to the floor and the ala-tragus line is parallel to the floor. An intraoral periapical film is placed in the mouth and then exposed. A second film is placed in the mouth in the same position as the first film, with the patient's head position remaining the same. The second film is then exposed. The vertical angulation should be the same for each exposure. However, the horizontal angle is shifted either anteriorly or posteriorly, depending on the area being examined, for the second view.

Fig. 5-20A illustrates an unerupted maxillary permanent canine. The shadow of this tooth is superimposed over the central incisor root. When the horizontal angle of the x-ray tube is shifted posteriorly (see Fig. 5-20B), the crown of the unerupted canine also seems to move posteriorly, and the image of the canine crown is no longer superimposed over the central incisor root. If the buccal object rule is applied, it can be seen that the embedded canine is oriented lingually to the erupted teeth.

Fig. 5-21A illustrates an embedded maxillary permanent canine. The shadow of the crown of this tooth covers a small portion of the lateral incisor root on its distal

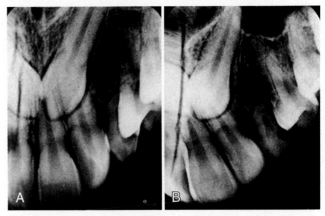

Figure 5-20 A, Shadow of the maxillary permanent canine is superimposed over the central incisor root. **B,** When the horizontal angle of the x-ray tube is shifted posteriorly, the crown of the unerupted canine appears to move posteriorly. The canine is lingually placed.

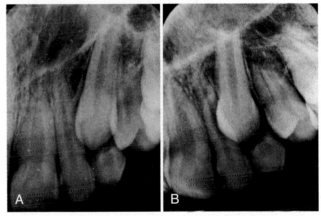

Figure 5-21 A, Shadow of the maxillary permanent canine covers a small portion of the lateral incisor root on its distal aspect. **B,** When the horizontal angle of the x-ray tube is shifted posteriorly, the canine appears to move anteriorly. The canine lies buccal to the erupted teeth.

aspect. When the horizontal angle is shifted posteriorly (see Fig. 5-21B), the unerupted crown appears to move anteriorly or in a direction opposite to the shift of the x-ray source. Thus the unerupted canine is oriented buccally to the erupted teeth.

Another localization technique is the cross-section occlusal radiograph. Depending on the size of the child's mouth, either the adult occlusal or a No. 2 periapical film may be used. To obtain a cross-section occlusal radiograph of the maxilla, the patient's sagittal plane is perpendicular to the floor, and the ala-tragus line is parallel to the floor. The patient is asked to occlude lightly on the film. The central ray is projected through the midsagittal plane and enters the skull 1 cm posterior to bregma. (Bregma is the point at which the sagittal suture meets the coronal suture.) The proper vertical angulation is determined when the central ray is directed through the long axis of the maxillary central incisor roots (Fig. 5-22).

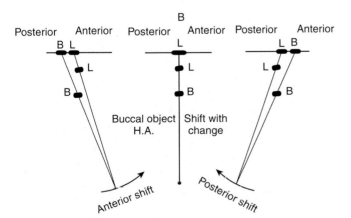

Figure 5-19 The buccal object rule. *B,* Buccal; *L,* lingual; *H.A.,* horizontal angle.

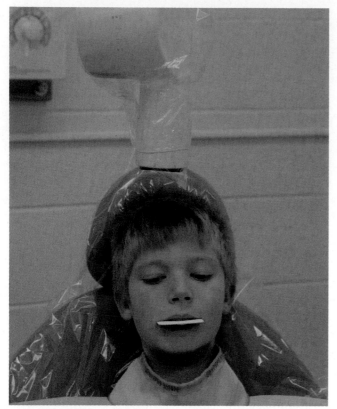

Figure 5-22 Cross-sectional maxillary occlusal technique demonstrating the proper head position and central-ray entry point. The central ray is directed coincidentally with the long axis of the central incisor roots.

A maxillary central incisor periodical radiograph demonstrating a grossly dilacerated central incisor may be seen in Fig. 5-23A. It is important to determine, before a surgical procedure, if the crown of such a tooth is in a labial or a lingual position. In this instance, the crown is positioned labially (see Fig. 5-23B).

The cross-section occlusal film can be employed for localization of anomalies in the mandible. Either the adult occlusal or a No. 2 periapical film can be used.

The patient's head is tilted backward sufficiently to direct the central ray through the long axis of the erupted teeth (Fig. 5-24). The patient's head must be tilted on its long axis to accommodate positioning of the x-ray tube. If determination of the buccal or lingual position of an impacted mandibular third molar is desired, the central ray should be projected through the long axis of the mandibular second molar. If it is necessary to localize an unerupted second premolar, the central ray should be directed through the long axis of the first premolar. Fig. 5-25A, reveals an unerupted mandibular premolar that has been displaced by an ossifying fibroma. In Fig. 5-25B, a cross-section occlusal radiograph demonstrates that the crown of the premolar is lingually placed.

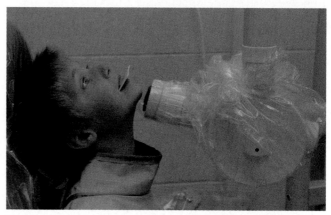

Figure 5-24 Cross-section mandibular occlusal technique demonstrating the proper head position and vertical angulation of the x-ray head.

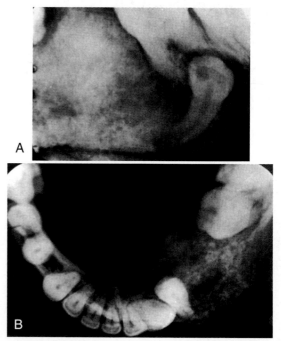

Figure 5-25 A, Unerupted mandibular premolar displaced by an ossifying fibroma. **B,** The crown of the unerupted premolar is lingually oriented.

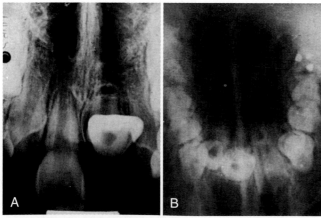

Figure 5-23 A, Dilacerated maxillary central incisor. **B,** The crown of the dilacerated central incisor lies labially.

DIGITAL RECEPTORS FOR PEDIATRIC PATIENTS

Digital x-ray systems use solid-state detector technology such as CCD (charge-coupled devices) or CMOS (complementary metal oxide semiconductors) for image acquisition. Most of these systems have electronic wires attached to the sensor. Children younger than 4 or 5 years of age may not tolerate these wired sensors, may damage the cables because they do not understand the procedure and may "chew" on the cable, or may be more fearful just of the appearance of a wired system. For these reasons a phosphor-based digital x-ray system may be ideal for the pediatric patient. There is one "wireless" solid-state image detector from Schick Technologies, the Schick CDR Wireless sensor (Fig. 5-26).

Photostimulable phosphors (PSPs) or storage phosphors are used for digital imaging for image acquisition. Unlike panoramic or cephalometric screen materials, PSPs do not fluoresce instantly to produce light photons. Instead, these materials store the incoming x-ray photon information like a latent image in conventional film-based radiography until the plates are scanned by a laser beam in a drum scanner. The laser scanning excites the phosphor to give up the stored energy as an electronic signal, which is then digitized, with various gray levels assigned to points on the curve to create the image information. The currently available phosphor imaging systems (Table 5-2) are from Soredex (OpTime), AirTechniques (ScanX), and Gendex (DenOptix).

These phosphor plates have no wire to the computer and resemble intraoral film in every way, including size, thickness, rigidity, and receptor placement. They are soft and flexible much like film, and as with conventional x-ray film techniques, infection control procedures must be employed. The plates must be wrapped, exposed, and unwrapped and then carefully shaken out of the barrier envelope onto a clean surface, wiped with a disinfectant, and fed into the laser scanner. After use, the plates must be exposed to light to eliminate any latent image before they are placed into new barrier envelopes for the next patient. Thus the total time to process each image can take several minutes. Unlike film, however, the plates should not be curved or bent,

Table 5-2

Photostimulable Phosphor Systems

Company	System	Phosphor Type	Resolution (line pairs/mm)
Soredex	OpTime	Agfa	>6
AirTechniques	ScanX	Fuji	6 to 8
Gendex	DenOptix	Fuji	~9

because a permanent defect or artifact will be created in the phosphor coating. The plate would then need to be replaced.

In some machines like the DenOptix system, the plates are put into a template holder that is then placed into the drum scanner (Fig. 5-27). After the scanning process is completed, the resultant digital image can then be viewed on a monitor in about 30 seconds to 2.5 minutes depending on the system. This is called *analog-to-digital conversion* and it is how the phosphor imaging system becomes "digital." The technology is not new. This type of signal readout by laser scanning has been used in the laboratory industry for reading biologic fluid samples for decades. This "digital" imaging technique requires two steps to retrieve the final image, just like film. The technique also requires the same two-stage infection control procedures

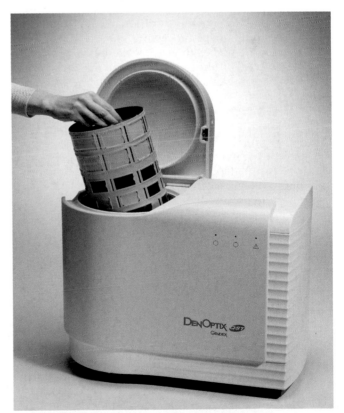

Figure 5-27 The Dentsply-Gendex DenOptix phosphor plate scanner.

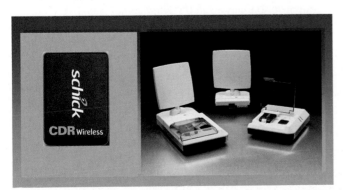

Figure 5-26 The Schick Technologies CDR Wireless system showing the sensor *(left)* and the charging unit and wireless RF antennas *(right)*.

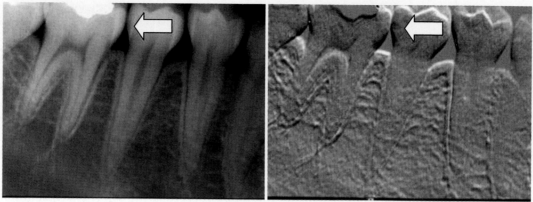

Figure 5-28 An interproximal carious lesion on the distal surface of tooth No. 29 *(left)* made more apparent by electronic image processing *(right)*.

as for film. But the final image is digital and can be subjected to electronic image processing to extract disease features more readily for treatment decision making. An excellent explanation of the PSP process appears in the April 2000 issue of *Dental Clinics of North America*.

The advantage of these digital-like phosphors is really in the image processing that can be applied after the image is acquired. Although electronic image processing can be performed on conventional x-ray film, the film must first be converted to digital information by scanning the image. Storage phosphors (PSPs) and true digital images from solid-state detectors like CCD and CMOS receptors provide a virtually instantaneous digital image and require no additional data conversion before electronic image processing.

If the dentist wishes to employ these digital systems, either solid-state or phosphor, he or she must use a good paralleling instrument system and paralleling technique to be successful.

CONE BEAM VOLUMETRIC IMAGING

The newest technique available to dentists is a type of computed tomography (CT) technique called cone beam volumetric imaging (CBVI). Using exposure factors not dissimilar to conventional x-ray generators (low kV and low mA), these devices allow two- and three-dimensional gray scale and color reconstruction of the maxilla and mandible. Some machines, such as the Planmeca ProMax CBVT and the Carestream (formerly Kodak) 9000D, can do both panoramic and CBVT images using the same basic radiographic platform. This is a significant advance for dentistry and for evaluation of the pediatric patient.

For example, if a pediatric dentist has a machine that takes a digital panoramic for evaluation of the "mixed dentition," then the x-ray absorbed dose is minimal. If there is an anomaly like an impacted permanent cuspid or mesiodens, these dual-purpose machines can use the "cone beam" detector to more fully characterize and visualize the clinical problem. Fig. 5-28 graphically illustrates this concept.

INTERPRETATION

When interpreting radiographs, the dentist must develop a systematic approach so that no areas of the radiographs are missed. No one way is necessarily better than another, as long as the approach is consistently followed. Viewing conditions should be adjusted so that the maximum information can be obtained from the radiographs. The radiographs should be placed in a mount that does not allow light to be transmitted through the periphery, only through the film itself. Other extraneous light from around the mount should also be masked out. It is preferable for the room in which the radiographs are reviewed to have subdued lighting. Finally, it is recommended that a magnifying glass be used. If these viewing conditions are followed, more information will be obtained, and thus better care will be provided for the patient.

REFERENCE

1. Nowak AJ et al. Summary of the Conference on Radiation Exposure in Pediatric Dentistry, *J Am Dent Assoc* 103: 426-428, 1981.

SUGGESTED READINGS

Alcox RW, Jameson WR. Patient exposures from intraoral radiographic examinations, *J Am Dent Assoc* 88:568-579, 1974.
Block AJ, Goepp RA, Mason EW. Thyroid radiation dose during panoramic and cephalometric dental x-ray examinations, *Angle Orthod* 47:17-24, 1977.
Brooks SL, Joseph LP. US Department of Health and Human Services. Basic concepts in the selection of patients for dental x-ray examinations, Food and Drug Administration Pub No 85-8249, Washington, DC, 1985, US Government Printing Office.
Council on Dental Materials, Instruments and Equipment, American Dental Association. Recommendations in radiographic practices, *J Am Dent Assoc* 109:764-765, 1984.
Gibbs SJ et al. Patient risk from intraoral dental radiography, *Dentomaxillofac Radiol* 17:15-23, 1988.
Gibbs SJ et al. Patient risk from rotational panoramic radiograph, *Dentomaxillofac Radiol* 17:25-32, 1988.

Hildebolt CF et al. Dental photostimulable phosphor radio
graphy, *Dent Clin North Am* 44(2):273-299, 2000.

Joseph LP. US Department of Health and Human Services.
The selection of patients for x-ray examinations: dental
radiographic examinations, Food and Drug Administration
Pub No 88-8273, Washington, DC, 1987, US Government
Printing Office.

Kasle MJ. Radiograph: cross-fire localization technic, *Dent Surv*
45:29-31, 1969.

Kasle MJ. Radiographic technique for difficult maxillary third
molar views, *J Am Dent Assoc* 83:1104-1105, 1971.

Kasle MJ, Langlais RP. *Basic principles of oral radiology, vol 4, Exercises in dental radiology,* Philadelphia, 1981, WB Saunders.

Langland OE et al. *Panoramic radiology,* ed 2, Philadelphia, 1989,
Lea & Febiger.

Miles DA et al. *Radiographic imaging for dental auxiliaries,*
ed 3, Philadelphia, 1999, WB Saunders.

Myers DR et al. Radiation exposure during panoramic radio
graphy in children, *Oral Surg* 46:588-593, 1978.

National Council on Radiation Protection and Measurements.
Dental x-ray protection, Report No 35, Washington, DC,
1970, The Council.

National Council on Radiation Protection and Measurements.
Radiation protection in pediatric radiology, Report No 68,
Washington, DC, 1981, The Council.

Smith QW et al. Radiation exposure in the dental setting: an
update, *Radiol Technol* 55:546, 1983.

Valachovic RW, Lurie AG. Risk-benefit considerations in pedodontic radiology, *Pediatr Dent* 2:128-146, 1980.

White SC, Rose TC. Absorbed bone marrow dose in certain
dental radiographic techniques, *J Am Dent Assoc* 98:553-558,
1979.

CHAPTER 6

Clinical Genetics for the Dental Practitioner

▲ **James K. Hartsfield, Jr.** and **David Bixler**

CHAPTER OUTLINE

*T*he purpose of this chapter is twofold: to review genetic principles and to mention a few examples of the influence of genetic factors on major craniofacial, oral, and dental conditions. As the basis for relatively rare developmental dysplasias, diseases, and syndromes that show a genetic cause or marked genetic influence becomes known, increasing attention is being paid to those genetic factors that influence (or are associated with) more common conditions. An increased appreciation of how genetic factors interact with environmental (nongenetic) factors to influence growth and pathology will lead to an increased understanding of pathogenesis and the recognition that some groups or individuals may be more susceptible, or that they may respond differently to treatment.[1] Further information may be found online in the Genetics Home Reference Your Guide to Understanding Genetic Conditions at http://ghr.nlm.nih.gov.

REVIEW OF GENETIC PRINCIPLES

The *genome* contains the entire genetic content of a set of chromosomes present within a cell or an organism. Within the genome are genes that represent the smallest physical and functional units of inheritance that reside in specific sites (called loci, or locus for a single location). A *gene* can be defined as the entire DNA sequence necessary for the synthesis of a functional polypeptide molecule (production of a protein via a messenger RNA intermediate) or RNA molecule (transfer RNA and ribosomal RNA). *Genotype* generally refers to the set of genes that an individual

carries and, in particular, usually refers to the specific pair of alleles (alternative forms of a particular gene) that a person has at a given location (locus) of their total collection of DNA, called their *genome*. In contrast, *phenotype* is the observable properties and physical characteristics of an individual, as determined by the individual's genotype and the environment in which the individual develops over a period of time.

Remarkable advances in the biochemical techniques that are used to study cell molecular biology and DNA have taken researchers to the threshold of understanding the regulation of cell functions. To illustrate, not so long ago DNA analyses were performed on minute amounts (picograms) of DNA. This limitation was necessary because there was so little DNA available for study in samples. When the DNA polymerase enzyme was discovered that could replicate DNA through the polymerase chain reaction and make it by the gram, this sample problem disappeared. This advance facilitated completion of the human genome project, which resulted not only in definition of a single human genome sequence composed of overlapping parts from many humans, but also in an expanding catalogue of more than 1 million sites of variation in the human genome sequence. These variations (or polymorphisms) may be used as markers to perform genetic analysis (including analysis of genetic-environmental interaction) in human beings.[2] The genome varies from one individual to the next, most often in terms of single base changes of the DNA, called *single nucleotide polymorphisms* (SNPs, pronounced "snips"). The main use of this human SNP map will be to determine the contributions of genes to diseases (or non-disease phenotypes) that have complex, multifactorial bases.[3]

CELL DIFFERENTIATION AND DEVELOPMENTAL BIOLOGY

It is fascinating that a single fertilized ovum contains within itself the potential for development of the incredibly complicated human organism. Cellular differentiation is a critical component of this developmental process, and aside from the development of antibody diversity, typically occurs in the absence of genetic alteration or mutation. Different types of cells gain their specific identities by using a particular subset of the approximately 30,000 or more genes present within the genome. The types of polypeptides that a cell can synthesize include enzymes, which catalyze various activities of cellular metabolism and homeostasis; structural proteins, which form the intracellular and extracellular scaffolding or cellular matrix; and regulatory proteins, which convey signals from the outside of the cell to the nucleus and modulate or control specific gene expression. In a developing embryo, cells reside in a three-dimensional environment and are responsive to signals from themselves (autocrine), from nearby sources (paracrine), and from anatomically distant sources (endocrine). Many of these signals are mediated by soluble molecules (either peptide or nonpeptide in origin) that bind to specific receptors (proteins) that are present on the surface or on the inside of cells. In addition to signals from soluble factors, cells can respond to cell-to-cell or cell-to-extracellular matrix signals.[4]

The action of "turning on" or "turning off" specific genes, referred to as *regulation of gene expression*, is carefully orchestrated and remains a critical element in determining cell specificity and tissue morphogenesis. Transcription factors bind to DNA and either facilitate or suppress initiation of gene transcription, the most common control point of gene expression. In the development of the craniofacial complex there is increasing evidence for the role of homeobox-containing gene families that encode transcription factors. These then are critical for the control of complex interactions between genes that are subsequently expressed during development.[5]

In summary:
1. The genetic message lies in the DNA itself, which is coded and transmitted from cell generation to cell generation when these DNA molecules are replicated (or duplicated).
2. A given cell type and function is defined by what specific RNA molecules are made from the DNA master. These RNA molecular copies direct protein synthesis in the cell.
3. Transcription factors determine which genes are expressed through the production of the RNA and subsequent protein.
4. Development occurs through the action of specific transcription factors and other regulators of protein production on specific genes that need to be expressed next in time.

CHROMOSOMES

DNA is grouped into units called *chromosomes*. Humans have 46 chromosomes that contain an estimated 30,000 genes, including numerous duplicates. Of the 46 chromosomes, the sex chromosomes are the X and Y, with the remaining 44 chromosomes referred to as *autosomes*. Each autosome has a paired mate that is referred to as its *homologue*. Therefore, with the exception of some of the genes on the X and Y chromosomes in males, there are at least two copies of each gene unless a piece of DNA is deleted. Thus the human chromosome complement consists of 23 pairs of chromosomes (one pair of sex chromosomes and 22 pairs of autosomes).

One area of special interest to the clinician is cytogenetics, the study of chromosomes. This interest has been stimulated by the development of techniques in which cells are grown in culture and the chromosomes are examined under a microscope for changes in size, shape, and fine structure. This is called *karyotyping*. Fig. 6-1 shows the karyotypes of a normal human male and female. By applying this technique, Lejeune and colleagues demonstrated that the fundamental cause in Down syndrome is the presence of an extra specific chromosome (number 21) in the affected individual's karyotype.[6] When an entire extra chromosome is present, the condition is called a *trisomy* of the chromosome in question, for example, trisomy 21 for Down syndrome. Fig. 6-2 shows the karyotype of a male who has Down syndrome. The extra chromosome in the group of number 21 and number 22 chromosomes is readily apparent.

Since this report in 1959, many disease states have been shown to be associated with an incorrect chromosome complement. By using this approach with considerable refinement, it was shown that alterations in the fine structure of chromosomes, as well as in their number, could be present. Monosomy of an autosome, or a missing autosomal chromosome, had not been believed to be compatible with life, but several monosomies in live-born children have now been reported. Monosomy of the sex chromosomes can be compatible with life and typically affects development of both internal and external sex organs of the individuals. The best known example of this is Turner syndrome, which occurs in approximately 1 in every 5000 live female births. These persons are phenotypic females who are usually missing one of the X chromosomes and are chromosomally designated as 45, X. Other aberrations of the X chromosome may also cause Turner syndrome. Affected individuals are typically short of stature, lack secondary sex characteristics, and are sterile. The Turner syndrome karyotype is shown in Fig. 6-3. Table 6-1 lists common chromosomal aberrations that produce clinical disease, including examples of translocations (the attachment of a broken piece from one chromosome to another, but not homologous, chromosome) and deletions (the absence of a piece of chromosome).

Chromosome abnormalities are an important cause of spontaneous abortion. About 15% of all recognized pregnancies end in spontaneous abortion, and the incidence of chromosome abnormalities in such abortions is greater

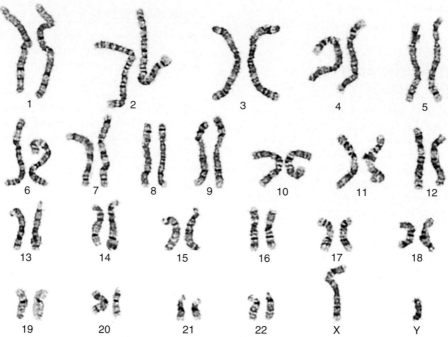

Figure 6-1 Banded karyotypes of a normal human male *(left)* and female *(right)*. Group designations according to Denver nomenclature are also indicated. (Courtesy Cytogenetic Laboratories, Indiana University School of Medicine.)

than 50%. Only 0.3% to 0.5% of all live-born infants have a chromosome abnormality that is detectable with standard microscopic karyotyping. Microdeletions and microduplications of DNA, not visible by routine chromosome karyotype analysis, are a major cause of human malformation and mental retardation. A complementary analysis called *comparative genomic hybridization* (CGH) or *array comparative genomic hybridization* (arrayCGH or aCGH) can improve the diagnostic detection rate of these small chromosomal abnormalities. This technique attains such a high-resolution screening by hybridizing differentially labeled test and reference ("normal") DNAs to arrays consisting of thousands of genomic clones. In this way, relatively small differences between the test and reference DNA sequences may be discovered and investigated further if indicated.[7,8]

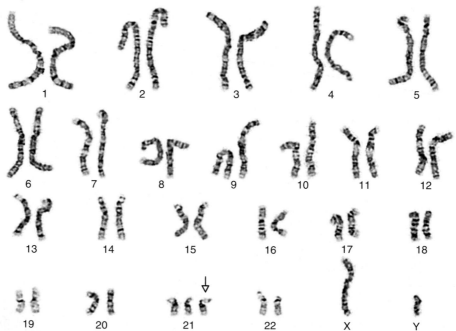

Figure 6-2 Banded karyotype of a male with trisomy of chromosome 21 (Down syndrome). (Courtesy Cytogenetic Laboratories, Indiana University School of Medicine.)

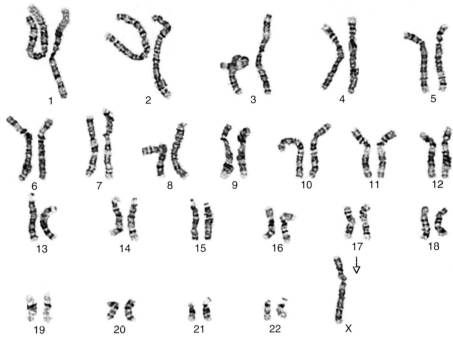

Figure 6-3 Banded karyotype of a female with missing X chromosome (Turner syndrome). (Courtesy Cytogenetic Laboratories, Indiana University School of Medicine.)

Table **6-1**

Common Chromosomal Aberrations

Type	Specific Alteration	Clinical Result
Aneuploidy	Trisomy 21	Down syndrome
	Trisomy 18	Edwards syndrome
	Trisomy 13	Patau syndrome
	Extra X chromosomes	In females: XXX, XXXX, XXXXX syndromes
		In males: Klinefelter syndrome—XXY, XXXY, and XXXXY
	Monosomy, autosomal	Usually nonviable
	Monosomy, X chromosome	In females: Turner syndrome, 45,X
		In males: nonviable, 45,Y
Translocation	14/21, 21/21 or 21/22	Translocation carrier (normal phenotype) or Down syndrome
Deletion	Ring chromosome	Variable
	Short arm chromosome No. 5	Cri du chat syndrome
	Philadelphia chromosome (No. 22)	Chronic myeloid leukemia

HEREDITARY TRAITS IN FAMILIES

Heritability is the proportion of the total phenotypic variance in a sample that is contributed by genetic variance.[9] On an individual basis for a binary trait (i.e., a disease or trait that an individual either has or does not have), heritability is not the proportion of disease or the trait attributable to, or caused by, genetic factors. For a quantitative trait, heritability is not a measure of the proportion of an individual's score attributable to genetic factors.[10] A trait with a heritability of 1 is said to be expressed without any environmental influence, whereas a trait with a heritability of 0.5 has half its variability (from individual to individual) influenced by environmental factors and half by genotypic factors. Values greater than 1 may occur because the methodology provides an estimate of heritability under several simplifying assumptions that may be incorrect.

There is the common perception that knowing a trait's heritability will somehow affect how a patient should be treated (e.g., for malocclusion) or that it will define the limits of tooth movement or the manipulation of jaw growth. This is not true. The ability of the patient to respond to changes in the environment (including treatment), which has nothing to do with heritability, defines these limits. Heritability estimates imply nothing about trait size or treatment limits based upon a presumed genetic "predetermination."[11] Even so, the estimation of heritability can provide an indication of the relative importance of genetic factors on a trait in a group at that time. Confirming that there is a certain degree of genetic influence on a trait is a preliminary step to performing further specific genetic linkage studies (using DNA markers) to determine areas of the genome that appear to be associated with the characteristics of a given trait.[12]

When hereditary traits in families are to be studied, it is convenient to think of three classes of genetically influenced traits:.(1) monogenic, (2) polygenic, and (3) multifactorial. Recently the polygenic and multifactorial classes have often been combined into what are referred to as *complex traits* rather than Mendelian traits.[13] Monogenic traits are produced and regulated by a single gene locus. Usually they are relatively rare in the general population (occurrence in fewer than 1 per 1000 individuals). However, if the appearance of an affected person is striking, there may be instant recognition of the disease, as with patients having albinism, achondroplasia, or neurofibromatosis. Monogenetic conditions often occur in families and show transmission characteristics of the Mendelian (dominant or recessive) traits.

Polygenic traits, too, are hereditary and typically exert influence over common characteristics such as height, skin, and intelligence. This influence takes place through many gene loci collectively asserting their regulation of the trait. Although each gene involved has a minimal effect by itself, the effect of all the genes involved is additive. The associated phenotype is rarely discrete and is most commonly continuous or quantitative. Because these traits show a quantitative distribution of their phenotypes in a population, they do not show Mendelian inheritance patterns. It is important to note that the very nature of their influence (multiple genes each with a small additive effect) dictates that their environment may readily influence them. Monogenic traits are not readily amenable on a large scale to environmental modification, although there can be variation, presumably secondary to other genetic and environmental factors. By contrast, one can easily think of a dozen environmental factors known to influence height and intelligence quotient.

Finally, multifactorial traits or conditions are influenced by multiple genes but differ significantly from polygenic traits in that the influence is achieved through an interaction of multiple genes and environmental factors, and occurs when a liability threshold is exceeded. Although typically the number of genes involved is many, occasionally a few genes, sometimes only two or three, influence the trait. The effect of these genes on the phenotype is therefore a net effect, not necessarily a simple additive one. Furthermore, phenotypic expression approaches that of a discrete Mendelian trait and therefore cannot be readily classed as a quantitative trait. Likewise, the effect of a gene influencing the phenotype may not be as great as that of a gene associated with a monogenic trait, but the gene may be referred to as having a major effect. Among the well-known hereditary types of conditions designated as multifactorial are many of the severe nonsyndromic congenital malformations such as cleft lip and palate (CLP), neural tube defects such as spina bifida-anencephaly, and hip dislocation. Multifactorial complex inheritance is discussed later.

The investigation of human heritable traits usually involves the observation of specific features in a family and the study of that family's pedigree. The affected individual in a family who first brings that family to the attention of the geneticist is called the *proband* or *propositus*. This individual is the index case. Brothers and sisters of the proband are *siblings* or sibs. Thus a sibship consists of all the brothers and sisters in a nuclear family unit (parents and their offspring). The clinical appearance in an individual of a given trait, such as eye color or height, is that individual's phenotype, whereas the specific genetic makeup that influences or is associated with the phenotype is the genotype.

In an earlier section, the point is made that the human chromosome complement has 22 homologous pairs of autosomes and one pair of sex chromosomes. Because of homologue pairing (excluding the X and Y chromosomes in the male), there are at least two copies of each gene, one located at the same position (locus) on each member of the homologous pair. Genes at the same locus on a pair of homologous chromosomes are *alleles*. When both members of a pair of alleles are identical, the individual is *homozygous* for that locus. When the two alleles at a specific locus are different, the individual is *heterozygous* for that locus.

A gene that results in the expression of a particular phenotype in single dose (i.e., heterozygous) is a dominant gene. If the gene must be present in double dose (homozygous) to express the phenotype, it is a recessive gene. It is actually the phenotype that is dominant or recessive and not the gene itself. The terms *dominant gene* and *recessive gene*, though, are commonly used to describe these types of inherited traits in families.

Construction of a pedigree, which is a shorthand method of classifying the family data, conveniently summarizes the family data for the study of inherited traits. The symbols used in constructing a pedigree are shown in Fig. 6-4. The observable inheritance patterns followed by such monogenic traits within families are determined by (1) whether the trait is dominant or recessive, (2) whether the gene is autosomal (on one of the autosomes) or X linked (on the X chromosome), and (3) the chance distribution in the offspring of those genes passed from parents in their gametes (sperm and ova). Pedigree construction is a valuable tool for the clinician who is concerned with the diagnosis of and counseling regarding hereditary traits. Every dentist should be able to construct and interpret a pedigree, because it is a certainty that patients will come to the dentist's office with heritable oral diseases that need diagnosing before treatment is begun.

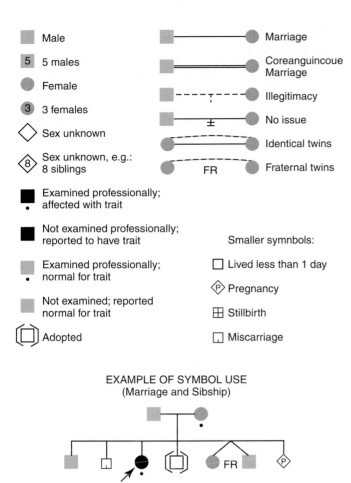

Figure 6-4 Pedigree symbols used in family studies.

The simple patterns of monogenic inheritance seen in families are described in the following discussion. Because all the Mendelian modes of inheritance are found in the amelogenesis imperfecta (AI) disorders, these are used to illustrate basic genetic principles.

DEVELOPMENTAL BIOLOGY OF ENAMEL

For a review of how molecular biologists are studying the genetic factors involved in dental development, there is a paper by Tucker and Sharpe.[14] The two developmentally different cell layers involved in dentinogenesis, inner enamel epithelium (enamel) and neural crest (dentin), are separated by an extracellular matrix.[15] Specific tooth development is then mutually dependent on reciprocal cell-to-cell signaling between these two developmentally different cell layers.[16] The genes involved in the development of these tissues are candidates for DNA mutation analysis, especially if they are in a chromosome location that has been associated with or linked to an inherited defect of enamel or dentin. The most intriguing dental research today is (1) the attempt to localize the genes for these proteins to specific loci and (2) the biochemical identification of a specific defect in the protein that prevents it from functioning normally. The following is a discussion of genetic principles best exemplified by the

heritable disorders of enamel. Further discussion of the molecular basis of the heritable disorders of dentin and enamel appears in Chapter 7.

Based on the clinical appearance, radiographic characteristics, and microscopic features, oral pathologists have recognized three major types of inherited enamel defects: hypoplasia, hypocalcification, and hypomaturation.[17] These terms also provide the general description of the disease phenotypes. For example, in type 1, enamel hypoplasia, the enamel is hard and well calcified but defective in amount, so the teeth appear small. Two types of deficient enamel phenotypes are seen: generalized (all the enamel) and localized (pits and grooves in specific areas). Type 2, hypocalcification disorders, are those in which the enamel matrix is so drastically altered that normal calcification cannot occur, with the result that the clinical phenotype is a soft, mushy enamel that easily wears away. Type 3 defect, hypomaturation, involves the process of maturation of the enamel crystal. This occurs after an essentially normal enamel matrix has been established. The enamel is of normal thickness (not hypoplastic) and relatively normal hardness (slightly hypocalcified) with reduced radiographic density and discoloration.

From this collection of enamel diseases we can now draw out four examples of AI that illustrate the four major Mendelian modes of inheritance: autosomal dominant (AD), autosomal recessive (AR), X-linked dominant (XLD), and X-linked recessive (XLR).

One characteristic of inherited dental defects is that both dentitions (primary and permanent) are affected. Occasionally, the defect is expressed differently in the two dentitions, as in the case of dentin dysplasia type II.[18] However, it is much more common to see the same clinical and radiographic picture in both dentitions. Both dentitions are affected in the AI disorders.

AUTOSOMAL DOMINANT INHERITANCE

From pedigrees such as that shown in Fig. 6-5, the following criteria for AD inheritance may be deduced:
1. The phenotype occurs in successive generations, that is, it shows vertical inheritance.
2. On the average, 50% of the offspring of an affected parent will also be affected.

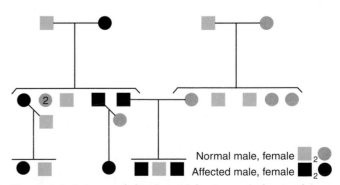

Figure 6-5 Autosomal dominant inheritance in hypocalcified amelogenesis imperfecta.

3. Normal parents have normal offspring. The following causes of exceptions to this rule are worth noting:
   • Nonpenetrance of the trait (defined later).
   • A mutation in either the sperm or egg.
   • Germinal mosaicism. This is an increasingly invoked explanation for this situation. In this case, one of the parents is mosaic in the germ cell line and the sperm or eggs are of two types—one cell line with and one cell line without the mutation. Chance determines which sperm cell line will be selected. However, as the molecular basis of genetic traits becomes evident, mutation analysis may show that a parent believed to not be affected may actually also have the somatic mutation found in affected children.
   • Nonpaternity. Although this is not strictly a genetic problem, the illegitimacy rate in the U.S. population is high enough to make this a likely explanation when a normal couple has a child affected with a completely penetrant dominant trait.
4. Males and females are equally likely to be affected.

The hypocalcification type of AI provides an excellent example of AD inheritance. For diagnosing this trait, several criteria are employed. First, enamel matrix is susceptible to abrasion. The clinical picture is typical—gross accumulation of plaque on teeth that are hypersensitive because of the exposed dentin. Second, radiographs show enamel of varying thickness interproximally but with a Swiss cheese appearance because of loss of mineral. Thus severe abrasion of this soft enamel is common.

AUTOSOMAL RECESSIVE INHERITANCE

Recessively inherited traits require that both genes of a given pair at a single locus code for defective proteins. Thus, of the two alleles at this genetic locus for AI, both must be mutants to show the trait. The following three gene pairs are recognized: AA—normal; Aa—heterozygote, showing an unaffected phenotype; aa—homozygous-affected. The most common genetic situation producing an affected child is that in which both parents are heterozygous at this genetic locus (Fig. 6-6).

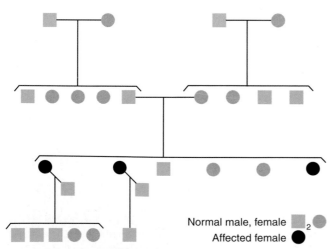

Figure 6-6 Autosomal recessive inheritance in pigmented amelogenesis imperfecta.

Normal male, female
Affected female

The following significant points about recessive inheritance must be noted:
1. The concept of a gene carrier is used here. The carrier is heterozygous for a recessive gene, and this single gene has only subtle, if any, expression. Parents of an affected child are typically heterozygous (carriers) and are then interpreted as being normal. Sometimes the carrier state can be detected, as in the case of phenylketonuria or Tay-Sachs disease. In these conditions a test is available for carrier identification to detect the presence of the single mutant gene. This greatly improves the precision of genetic counseling.
2. The rarer the recessive gene, the more likely that normal parents who have an affected child will be blood relatives. This is a consanguineous mating. Given that both parents who produce an AR-affected child are heterozygotes, it is easy to see that only one out of the four possible combinations of parents' genes results in the homozygous-affected genotype. Hence, the recurrence risk for an affected child in this case is 25%. Note that transmission of the phenotype in a pedigree is horizontal (typically present only in sibs) and not vertical as with a dominant trait.

Of several AR types of AI, the one chosen for discussion here is the pigmented hypomaturation form. In this instance, the genetic defect probably lies in the protein needed in late tooth development to produce mature, hard, and dense enamel. The defective enamel present is softer than normal but not nearly as soft and easily abraded as in the hypocalcification defect. Remarkably, a brown pigment is found in these outer layers of enamel that are formed last, imparting a dark brown, unsightly appearance that necessitates restorative treatment. A pedigree illustrating AR inheritance of this hypomaturation defect is shown in Fig. 6-6.

X-LINKED OR SEX-LINKED INHERITANCE

Genes on the sex chromosomes are unequally distributed to males and females. This inequality is the result of the following facts: (1) males have one X and one Y chromosome, whereas females have two X chromosomes and (2) the genes active on the Y chromosome are essentially concerned with the development of the male reproductive system. For these reasons, then, males are hemizygous for X-linked genes, meaning that they have only half (or one each) of the X-linked genes. Because females have two X chromosomes, they may be either homozygous or heterozygous for X-linked genes, just as with autosomal genes.

Interesting genetic combinations are made possible by the male hemizygous condition. Because only one gene locus of each kind in the X chromosome is represented in the male, all recessive genes in single dose express themselves phenotypically and thereby behave as though they were dominant genes. On the other hand, X-linked recessive (XLR) genes must be present in double dose (homozygous) in females to fully express themselves. Consequently, full expression of rare XLR diseases in practice is restricted to males and is seen infrequently in females.

To this point we have considered heritable defects in two of the three major types of enamel disorders. The third type—AI, hypoplastic type—shows both autosomal and X-linked modes of inheritance, but only one X-linked type is described here.

X-LINKED DOMINANT

Fig. 6-7 is the pedigree of a family with an X-linked dominant (XLD) form of AI, hypoplastic type.[19] The clinical features are diagnostic and in some females can be quite striking.

Once again, both dentitions are affected similarly. The surface defect has been described as being granular, lobular, or even pitted. Conceivably, all these different forms of expression are the result of the action of a single gene (or at least its alleles). The enamel is hard but because of its thinness is more susceptible to fracture and abnormal wear. Under the appropriate conditions, this trait resembles a hypocalcification defect. However, radiographs quickly resolve this diagnostic problem and show enamel of normal density but with greatly reduced thickness.

X-LINKED RECESSIVE

A pedigree of a family with the X-linked recessive form of enamel hypomaturation is shown in Fig. 6-8. The genetic criteria for diagnosing an XLR trait are summarized as follows:

1. Because the gene cannot be passed from father to son, affected fathers almost never have affected sons. A son could be affected if the mother is a carrier of the XLR trait.
2. All daughters of an affected male receive his X-linked genes. Therefore affected males transmit the trait to their grandsons if they are affected through their daughters.
3. The incidence of the trait is much higher in males than in females. This is typified by the disease hemophilia, which is also caused by an XLR gene.

The clinical features of XLR hypomaturation type AI are most striking. The enamel has a somewhat reduced hardness but is not soft. However, the crowns of the teeth look like mountains with snow on them. Hence the name given has been "snow-capped teeth." Radiologically the

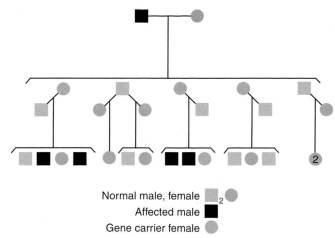

Normal male, female
Affected male
Gene carrier female

Figure 6-8 X-linked recessive inheritance in hypomaturation amelogenesis imperfecta.

enamel is hypomature; it shows a lack of contrast between enamel and dentin even though the enamel is of normal thickness.

It should be noted that heterozygous females occasionally show significant clinical expression of a single XLR gene. The reason for this apparent contradiction is the process of X-inactivation, termed *lyonization* after geneticist Mary Lyon. This occurs only in females. All normal female cells have two X chromosomes, but most of the genes on one of the two X chromosomes are inactivated approximately at the blastula stage of development. This has the effect of making the total number of active, X-linked genes about the same in both males and females. If the female is heterozygous for an X-linked trait, two populations of cells result. One cell population has genes on one X chromosome that are active, while the other cell population has genes on the other X chromosome that are active. When by chance the X chromosome with the deleterious gene is active in a significant proportion of the cells, its expression may be observed in that female. Chance dictates that this imbalance does not occur frequently, but because all females are, by

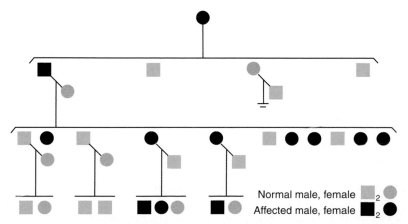

Normal male, female
Affected male, female

Figure 6-7 X-linked dominant inheritance in hypoplastic amelogenesis imperfecta.

definition of lyonization, mosaic with regard to X-linked traits, phenotypic expression of heterozygous genes may occur in them.

The previous statements concerning the distribution of XLR genes in males and females apply equally as well to XLD genes. The principal difference lies in the fact that when the gene is dominant more females than males will show the trait (see pedigree in Fig. 6-8). Because all XLR genes behave as dominant genes in males, no new criteria are made for their inheritance in males. The following criteria distinguish an XLD trait in families:

1. Affected males must transmit the trait to all of their daughters (as with XLR traits), but all of them are affected, because fathers give their X chromosome to their daughters and their Y chromosome to their sons.
2. Affected males cannot transmit the trait to their sons (just as with XLR traits).
3. Heterozygous females transmit the trait on the average to 50% of their children of both sexes, whereas homozygous-affected females will have only affected children. The latter situation is exceptionally rare for a dominant trait and is practically never observed. Thus all females affected with a dominantly inherited X-linked trait are considered to be heterozygotes until proven otherwise.

Two points are emphasized here. First, transmission of XLD genes by females follows a pattern indistinguishable from that of autosomal transmission. Thus these two types of dominant inheritance can be differentiated only by observation of the offspring of affected males. Second, it was noted that XLR disorders are much less common in females than in males. The reverse is true for XLD traits. An XLD trait should appear about twice as often in females as in males, because females have twice as many X chromosomes as males.

VARIATION IN GENE EXPRESSION

The patterns of inheritance shown in traits determined by genes at a single locus are usually easy to recognize. However, many factors may modify the expression of a gene in a family in such a way that a typical monogenic pattern of inheritance is not discernible. Two concepts related to modification of gene action are discussed here: penetrance and expressivity.

PENETRANCE

When a person with a given genotype fails to demonstrate the phenotype characteristic for the genotype, the gene is said to show reduced penetrance. This is a situation most commonly seen with dominant traits. Dentinogenesis imperfecta, an AD trait, is practically 100% penetrant, because all individuals who carry that gene show its phenotype. On the other hand, osteogenesis imperfecta shows incomplete penetrance, because pedigree studies demonstrate individuals who must carry the gene but who do not appear to be affected. Another relevant example is found in the CLP trait. Consider the following family history: a grandfather and his grandson both have CLP but the boy's mother (also the grandfather's daughter) does

not. The probability is very high that her son's cleft liability came from his grandfather and therefore was passed through the mother without being expressed as an overt cleft. Possibly the subtle action or predisposition of a clefting gene or genes may be found using measurements of facial structures, or variation in other structures such as the orbicularis oris muscle may be identified. This could increase the power of linkage analysis of the predisposing genotype. With the spectacular advances in the understanding of the human genome, we may be able to locate a gene that regulates clefting before its action at the molecular level is known or how it shows this action as a clinical trait.

EXPRESSIVITY

If a single gene trait can show different phenotypes in the affected members of kindred, it shows variable expressivity. Osteogenesis imperfecta also provides an illustration of variable gene expression. The cardinal signs of this disease are (1) multiple fractures, (2) blue sclera, (3) dentinogenesis imperfecta, and (4) otosclerosis, which results in a hearing deficit. Affected persons in a single family may show any one or a combination of these signs, which illustrates the considerable variation in gene expression. The minimum expression of the gene observed in a family might then be only a blue color to the sclera, which could be unnoticed by the clinician. In this case, highly variable gene expression may fade into nonpenetrance.

The craniosynostosis syndromes are AD traits associated with single gene mutations. They also provide good examples of how, even with the strong influence of a single gene, the phenotype can vary markedly. Although it was once thought that a particular mutation in a given gene would always result in a specific syndrome, several identical mutations in the fibroblast growth factor receptor 2 (FGFR2) gene have been found in patients diagnosed with the three different clinical craniosynostosis syndrome entities of Crouzon, Pfeiffer, and Jackson-Weiss syndrome.[20,21]

Another example of the individual variability of these single gene mutation autosomal dominant phenotypes occurred when two individuals in the same family had the classic phenotypes of Pfeiffer and Apert syndromes. In addition, seven other family members had unusually shaped heads and facial appearance reminiscent of Crouzon syndrome.[22] The phenotype may be so variable that this individual may appear to be clinically normal, yet have the same gene mutation associated with Crouzon syndrome in three of his children and two of his grandchildren. Only through the analysis of radiographic measurements was a minimal expression of features suggestive of Crouzon syndrome evident.[23]

EPIGENETICS

The influence of one or more modifying genes through their protein products in reducing or enhancing the effect of another gene has been referred to as *epigenetics*, but is now commonly referred to as *epistasis*. Now *epigenetics* refers to changes in gene expression that are inherited but not caused by alteration in the sequence of the gene. Examples of epigenetics include gene expression that is altered by methylation or acetylation, and by inhibition of messenger RNA expression by interfering RNA or microRNA binding.[24] Although monozygotic (identical) twins are epigenetically indistinguishable during the early years of life, older monozygous twins exhibit remarkable differences in their overall content and genomic distribution of 5-methylcytosine DNA and histone acetylation, which can create differences in gene expression between the twin pairs.[25] These epigenetic factors can help explain the relationship between an individual's genetic background, the environment, aging, and disease. It can do so because the epigenetic state varies among tissues and during a lifetime, whereas the DNA sequence remains essentially the same. As cells adapt to a changing internal and external environment, epigenetic mechanisms can "remember" these changes in the normal programming and reprogramming of gene activity.[26] This is leading to a new way of thinking on how the genome and environment interact, with a tremendous impact on the study of developmental biology, cancer, and other diseases.

MULTIFACTORIAL INHERITANCE

The following features typify multifactorial inheritance, in contrast to monogenic inheritance: (1) multiple genes (polygenes) at different loci are involved in expressing the phenotype, and (2) the phenotype produced is a summation of the effects of polygenes interacting with their environment. The phenotypic result is often a continuously varying spectrum of that trait (e.g., height) rather than presentation as a discrete (trait present or absent) phenotype.

Many common diseases, such as dental caries, have continuous variation with no sharp distinction between normal (average) and abnormal (extremes). However, there may be a specific measurement point beyond which that disease is arbitrarily regarded by the clinician as abnormal.

Multifactorial inheritance is troublesome to analyze genetically; in fact, geneticists often arrive at a diagnosis of multifactorial inheritance for a given trait only after the monogenic forms of inheritance have been considered and found to be unlikely. Certain techniques for studying it have been developed. The simplest is the method of resemblance between relatives, which states that the more closely related two individuals are, the more closely they resemble each other concerning the specific trait in question. It is important to stress, though, the continuous phenotypic variation that is characteristic of inheritance patterns resulting from polygenes.

This issue of continuous variation is emphasized because the most common diseases with which the dentist must deal (i.e., periodontal disease, dental caries, and malocclusion) are multifactorial traits. Only the extremes of variation are readily apparent to the dentist, such as in the child with rampant caries or the adult who is caries free. In this latter instance, if one did not understand the concept of multifactorial inheritance, one might conclude that such individuals represent a discrete phenotype influenced by a single gene in a Mendelian manner. This is frequently not the case.

A most important feature of traits produced by polygenes is that they are susceptible to environmental modification. A phenotype resulting from the concerted action of 100 genes is much more likely to be altered and modified by the existing environment than a trait controlled by only one or even several genes. Even so, this does not mean that a trait resulting from only one or even several genes cannot be influenced by environmental factors. The change in phenotype depends on the individual's ability to respond to the environmental factor, which may be heavily influenced by the same gene(s) originally influencing the phenotype or by other genes.

An example of a polygenic trait that is markedly influenced by environmental factors is dental caries, which is the interaction product of three essential factors: a cariogenic diet, a caries-producing bacterial flora, and a susceptible tooth. These three factors encompass a variety of biologically complicated entities, such as saliva, plaque, tooth matrix formation, and crystallization. It should be easy to see that the development of these complex elements must involve a great number of genes. Environmental modification, such as properly timed systemic fluoride supplementation, produces a considerable alteration in the phenotype without changing the genetic constitution of the individual. The reader can probably think of additional environmental modifications that can produce a greatly altered dental caries experience without changing an individual's genes. Some conditions that are attributed to a multifactorial inheritance because they tend to occur in particular families may be greatly influenced by a gene or genes that predispose to the condition, depending on what other genetic or environmental factors are involved.

MULTIFACTORIAL (COMPLEX) INHERITANCE IN HUMAN DISEASES

For many common disorders, such as diabetes and hypertension, and even for the major common congenital malformations (i.e., spina bifida, hydrocephalus, and CLP), there is a definite familial tendency. This is shown by the fact that the proportion of affected near relatives is greater than the incidence in the general population. However, this proportion is much lower than what is expected for a monogenic trait, and the explanation most commonly offered for major congenital malformations is that they are multifactorial traits. As previously stated, one definition of a complex trait is that it represents the summation of the effects of many genes (polygenes) interacting with the environment, which is why it has also been termed multifactorial. Environment is defined as those nongenetic circumstances that render an individual more or less susceptible to a disease state. In contrast to so-called simple monogenic traits, whose characteristics have been summarized in preceding paragraphs, multifactorial complex diseases show the following characteristics:

1. Each person has a liability for a given disease, and that liability represents a sum of the genetic and environmental liabilities.
2. The multifactorial-threshold model is a mathematical way of expressing these liabilities. For polygenic

traits, the model is simply a gaussian curve. As already noted, for multifactorial traits, a threshold must be added to allow the continuous polygenic model to be used in describing noncontinuous or discrete traits. For many human congenital malformations, a multifactorial model with threshold is appropriate for describing discrete traits such as CLP. Such a threshold means that all persons with sufficient gene dosage and environmental interaction will be above the threshold of expression and show the cleft lip. Those with less will not show a cleft lip. A graphic representation of this idea is shown in Fig. 6-9.

3. Because of the differing dosage of polygenes in groups that show a specific phenotype (e.g., CLP), the overall incidence of this trait will vary in near relatives of those affected. For example, a dominantly inherited trait has a gene dosage of 1 in 2 (50%). Assuming that several polygenes may be involved in CLP, this figure decreases at least 10-fold to about 1% to 5%. The incidence in a random population is even lower, or about 1 per 1000. Therefore increasing gene dosage for a multifactorial complex trait in a family is associated with an increased incidence of that trait in near relatives of the affected individuals. The nature of this system with a threshold permits large numbers of persons at risk for showing that phenotype (CLP) to carry the liability for clefting without expressing it clinically. Based on current research findings regarding traits that are multifactorial with a threshold, it appears that it will be difficult to relate these mathematical observations to cellular biologic function.

Toward the end of the nineteenth century, Galton recognized that twins could be useful for evaluating the nature-nurture argument that was raging at that time. Interest in the twin method for study of the relative importance of heredity and environment in humans has been increasing. One explanation for this interest is that many human traits are complex, are susceptible to environmental modification, and therefore are difficult to study by conventional methods. The twin method allows an approach to the study of such traits and is based on

the principle that human twins are of two basic types: monozygotic (or identical) twins, resulting from a single ovum fertilized by a single sperm, and dizygotic (or fraternal) twins, resulting from fertilization of two ova by two sperm. It is axiomatic that monozygotic twins have identical genotypes, whereas dizygotic twins are no more closely related to each other than are any two siblings.[27] It also follows that differences between monozygotic twins result from environmental differences (although as previously mentioned, epigenetics could be a factor), whereas those between dizygotic twins result from differences in both heredity and environment.

To use the twin method, one must distinguish between the two types of zygosity. If both twins are identical for the trait in question (regardless of their zygosity), they are described as *concordant*. If they are unlike for the trait, they are *discordant*. Such intrapair differences are usually expressed in percentage figures for a group of twins being evaluated. For example, monozygous twins show a 33% concordance for CLP, whereas dizygous twins show only a 5% concordance.

Another method to estimate the heritability of a trait and to evaluate evidence of linkage of a phenotype with DNA polymorphisms is by sib-pair analysis. Heritability estimates can be generated from within- and between-sibship variance quantified by generalized linear models, with confounding factors controlled for where indicated. Polymorphic DNA markers may be tested for genetic linkage (proximity) to a gene influencing a particular phenotype by testing whether the magnitude of the phenotypic difference between two siblings is correlated with the alleles they share that are identical by descent (IBD). An allele is considered to be IBD if both members of a sibling pair inherited the same marker allele from the same parent. If a marker is linked to a gene contributing to the phenotype in question, then siblings with a similar (if quantitative) or the same (if discrete) phenotype would be expected to share more alleles IBD, whereas siblings with widely differing phenotypes would be expected to share few if any alleles IBD near any gene(s) influencing the phenotype.[28] In addition, another method of looking for DNA markers is the linkage disequilibrium or association analysis. In its simplest terms, this refers to a nonrandom association of alleles at two or more loci. It was found that some sections of DNA do not tend to change through generations, in what are called *haplotype blocks*. Because of this, testing one SNP within each block for significant association with a disease or trait is possible when an influencing locus for that disease or trait is located in or at least close to that haplotype block.[29] Partly because these haplotype blocks occur in populations, these analyses can be performed on unrelated individuals (affected and controls), as opposed to linkage analyses.

However, if the control individuals are from a different genetic background than the affected individuals, then there may be a bias. One way to deal with that problem is to use the quantitative transmission disequilibrium test. This analysis calculates the difference between the value of the quantitative trait in the offspring and the average value of the quantitative trait in all offspring in all families studied, while simultaneously

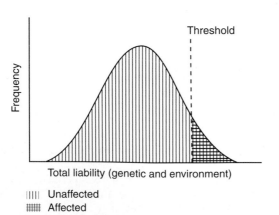

Figure 6-9 Multifactorial model for inheritance of cleft lip and palate.

considering the allele transmission from parent to offspring.[30] Thus, whereas the sib-pair linkage analysis involves two or more siblings, the quantitative transmission disequilibrium test involves trios of parents and one or more siblings.

INFLUENCE OF GENETIC FACTORS ON MAJOR CRANIOFACIAL, ORAL, AND DENTAL CONDITIONS

GENETICS AND DENTAL CARIES

It is clear from many dietary studies that variation in susceptibility to dental caries exists even under identical, controlled conditions.[31] This implies that, because of genetic differences, certain environmental factors are potentially more cariogenic for some people than for others. This is not to say that dental caries is an inherited disease; rather, genetic influences may modify the overt expression of this disease in the individual.

Fifty years ago, dental caries was presented to dental students as a disease that was so common that more than 99% of the general population was afflicted by it. Although it is still recognized as a common disease, the use of systemic and topical fluorides and persistence by organized dentistry to bring about changes in dietary habits and oral hygiene practices have contributed significantly to a remarkable decrease in the prevalence of this disorder, especially noted in children. Currently, it is not unusual for a prepubertal-age child to be caries free. However, there is individual variation in caries that is not fully explained by hygiene or fluoride exposure.

Three essential interacting elements comprise the model system for dental caries that is most commonly used to discuss its etiology. These factors are microorganisms, substrate (fermentable carbohydrates), and host factors, such as tooth anatomy. It is in the last area of the host factors that genetics exerts a major influence on dental caries initiation.

Several investigators have studied the genetic aspects of dental caries in humans, using both the twin and the family pedigree approaches. Because dental caries is an age-dependent process, much of the reported data cannot be compared because of age differences in the various population groups studied. Nevertheless, the family observations by Klein and Palmer[32] and Klein[33] are worth noting. Their findings indicated that children have a caries experience remarkably similar to that of their parents when the susceptibility of both parents is the same (either high or low). When caries susceptibility of the two parents is dissimilar, however, the children's susceptibility tends to be more like that of the mother than that of the father. This finding was particularly evident in daughters.

Because dental caries is an infectious communicable disease, however, familial clustering may to some degree reflect familial environmental contact, with transmission of cariogenic bacteria to children at certain ages. Li and Caufield found that mothers are the principal source of mutans streptococci to their infants, with a greater rate of transmission to female than male infants.[34]

The more common a genetic trait is, the more difficult it is to demonstrate its genetic character. Several authors have attempted to do this for dental caries by the study of twins. Book and Grahnen attempted to maximize differences in caries experience within families by selecting caries-free 20-year-old men and comparing caries experience within their families.[35] Results showed that parents and siblings of caries-free propositi had significantly lower rates of decayed, missing, and filled teeth than the control families. The authors concluded that the observed differences are hereditary and probably polygenic in nature.

Studies of twins by Dahlberg and Dahlberg,[36] Mansbridge,[37] Horowitz and colleagues,[38] Caldwell and Finn,[39] and Bretz and colleagues[40] indicated that genetic factors make a significant contribution to individual differences in caries susceptibility. However, most authors agree that this genetic component of dental caries is overshadowed by the overall effect of environmental factors in most subjects. Although it appears that genetic factors significantly contribute to the colonization of specific oral bacteria,[41] or the levels of *Streptococcus mutans* specifically,[42] the conclusion from clinical twin and familial correlation studies and estimation of heritability studies regarding the degree of genetic influence on caries may be confounded by familial factors such as oral hygiene habits, diet, and the already mentioned transmission of cariogenic bacteria within the family.

A review of inherited risks for susceptibility to caries found evidence of an association between altered dental enamel development in defined populations and an increased risk of caries, as well as a relationship between host immune complex genes and different levels of cariogenic bacteria and enamel defects.[43] This is further supported by the finding of a significant interaction between tuftelin SNP genotypes and *S. mutans* levels,[44] and variation in the amelogenin gene and caries susceptibility.[45] Thus the individual's genotype may influence the likelihood of intraoral colonization of cariogenic bacteria, which further exemplifies the complexity of caries development. Genetic studies on well-characterized populations with clearly defined caries experience will help define those host factors that have the greatest influence on the incidence of caries.[35]

For example, the first genome wide association (GWAS) study on human caries suggested that loci for low caries susceptibility were located on chromosomes 5q13.3, 14q11.2, and Xq27.1, whereas loci for high caries susceptibility were located on chromosomes 13q31.1 and 14q24.3.[46] Further work to define the genes involved, which may for example be related to saliva flow, plaque formation, and diet preferences, are underway. Bretz and colleagues found that genetic factors contributed independently to both dental caries and sucrose sweetness preference,[47] although it is likely that an increased preference for sweets would affect the caries rate.

The foundation for looking for different individual susceptibilities to caries is based upon animal studies. Hunt and colleagues succeeded in establishing caries-resistant and caries-susceptible strains of rats using inbreeding techniques.[48] Although the resistant strain was challenged by oral inoculation of cariogenic bacteria, the resistant phenotype was maintained. These were the first studies to confirm the presence of important genetic elements influencing dental caries susceptibility.

From this information, it is clear that heredity plays an important but complex role in the cause of dental caries. Studies done largely since the 1970s have examined the influence of saliva proteins on dental plaque formation. A group of saliva proteins designated as the proline-rich proteins (PRPs) because of their high content of the amino acid proline have been linked to early plaque and pellicle formation.[49,50] PRPs closely resemble enamel matrix proteins in both composition and structure, which accounts for why they bond so tightly to hydroxylapatite crystals. Furthermore, the ability to produce these several types of PRPs is inherited as a group of autosomal codominant traits. At least eight different polymorphic PRPs are known, and all these proteins are coded for by a block of genes called the salivary protein complex, located on the short arm of human chromosome 12.[50,51] These polymorphic acidic PRPs in saliva are encoded at two loci, PRH1 and PRH2. Pa, Db, and PIF are alleles at the PRH1 locus,[52] and PRH2 codes for Pr.[53] Only a few studies have attempted to associate these salivary protein phenotypes with oral disease states. Yu and colleagues reported significant association between Pa+ and Pr22 and an increase in dental caries scores in the permanent teeth of children 5 to 15 years of age.[54] This result suggested that persons with either or both of these two genotypes (Pa+ and/or Pr22) may be at significant risk for increased susceptibility to dental caries, whereas the allelic genes, Pa- and Pr11 or Pr12, appear to confer caries resistance. The mechanism of action could be related to the formation of a caries-susceptible plaque. Zakhary and colleagues found that presence or absence of the Db allele of PRH1 may affect caries; in their study, all caucasians had significantly greater *S. mutans* colonization than did African-Americans, but only Db-negative caucasians had significantly more caries.[55]

In summary, susceptibility to human dental caries is influenced to a significant but variable degree by genetic factors in most individuals.[56] This genetic influence control is undoubtedly complex in nature and strongly implies considerable environmental influence. However, there are likely individuals in whom the genetic susceptibility is markedly greater than that of most of the population. Specific types of dental caries susceptibility representing the extremes of variation of this trait may ultimately prove to be monogenic or major gene traits, but at present the evidence is insufficient for a clear statement of such inheritance.

GENETICS AND PERIODONTAL DISEASE

The periodontal disease state is often described as a local inflammatory disease with possible underlying systemic factors. This disease is so widespread in human populations and has such widely varying clinicohistopathologic features that it seems certain that multiple diseases with multiple causes are being lumped together as a single entity. Periodontists suggest that there is evidence for the

existence of several variant types of periodontal disease generally subclassified by the age of onset, severity of bone loss, oral hygiene status, and presence or absence of local factors. One might visualize a continuum of disease expression ranging from a localized gingivitis to a generalized periodontitis with severe bone and tooth loss. Such a complex disease shows both inflammatory and degenerative pathologic features.

It is easy to understand why genetic studies of this common problem have been neglected. As is true for dental caries, periodontal disease is common, occurs with a continuum of expressivity, and is greatly influenced by environmental conditions, such as diet, occlusion, and oral hygiene habits. All of these features fit the description of a complex type of disease or at least of disease susceptibility.

Most genetic studies of a trait make use of families with multiple affected individuals or twins. A carefully designed study of twins with periodontal disease by Ciancio and colleagues was reported in 1969.[57] Using the Ramfjord index, which evaluates gingival inflammation, calculus formation, tooth mobility, and tooth loss in all four quadrants of the mouth, the authors examined seven monozygotic and 12 dizygotic pairs of teenaged twins. They concluded that there was no evidence in these twins for significant heritability of any of these dental parameters.

Alternatively, Michalowicz and colleagues published a large study of adult twins (mean age, 40 years) of which there were 63 monozygotic and 33 dizygotic pairs.[58] Using elements of the Ramfjord index as criteria for diagnosis, heritability estimates were calculated. The authors state that from 38% to 82% of the periodontal disease identified in these twins was attributable to genetic factors.

Investigation by Kornman and colleagues into the association of different polymorphisms of inflammation-mediating genes and periodontal disease in adult nonsmokers indicated interleukin 1α and 1β (IL-1α and IL-1β) genotype may be a risk factor.[59] The IL-1β polymorphism was IL-1β +3953 and the IL-1α polymorphism was IL-1α -889. Nonsmokers aged 40 to 60 carrying the "2" allele (in either homozygous or heterozygous state) at both loci were observed to have nearly 19 times the risk of developing severe periodontitis as did subjects homozygous for the "1" allele at either or both of these loci. However, this association has been seen in other,[60] but not all populations.[60-63] Greenstein and Hart noted that the relationship of specific IL-1 genotypes and the level of crevicular fluid IL-1β is not clear, and that the ability of the genetic susceptibility test for severe chronic periodontitis based on the finding of Kornman and colleagues to forecast which patients will develop increased bleeding on probing, periodontitis, or loss of teeth or need for dental implants is ambiguous.[64] This illustrates the complexity of genetic association studies, and genetic counseling is based upon a marker that accounts for only a portion of phenotypic variation.[65,66]

Early-onset periodontitis has been the subject of most family studies. Because several forms of early-onset periodontitis (e.g., localized prepubertal periodontitis, localized juvenile periodontitis [JP], and generalized JP) can be found in the same family, the expression of the underlying genetic etiology appears to have the potential to be influenced by other genetic factors.[67]

Progress has been made in the study of rare genetic conditions or syndromes that can predispose to periodontal disease or have periodontal disease as a relatively consistent component of their pleiotropic effect. For example, leukocyte adhesion deficiency (LAD), type I and type II, are autosomal recessive (AR) disorders of the leukocyte adhesion cascade.[68] LAD type I has abnormalities in the integrin receptors of leukocytes resulting from mutations in the β2 integrin chain (ITGβ2) gene leading to impaired adhesion and chemotaxis, which results in an increased susceptibility for severe infections and early-onset (prepubertal) periodontitis.[69,70] LAD type II is also an AR disorder secondary to mutation in the SLC35C1 gene encoding a GDP-fucose transmembrane transporter (FucT1) located in the Golgi apparatus. The infectious episodes and the severity are much milder than those observed in LAD type I, and the only persistent clinical symptom is chronic severe periodontitis. The exact defect in the system is absence of the stalyl Lewis x (SleX) structure antigens, which are important ligands for the selectin on the leukocyte, which leads to a profound defect in leukocyte rolling, the first step in the adhesion cascade. This causes a marked decrease in chemotaxis accompanied by pronounced neutrophilia. Apart from the leukocyte defect, these patients suffer from severe growth and mental retardation and exhibit the rare Bombay blood group type.[68]

Ehlers-Danlos syndrome (EDS) is a collection of 10 types distinguished on the basis of clinical symptoms and inheritance pattern. In addition to consistent early-onset periodontal disease, patients with EDS type VIII have variable hyperextensibility of the skin, ecchymotic pretibial lesions, minimal bruising, minimal to moderate joint hypermobility of the digits, and cigarette paper scars. Inheritance is AD. Early-onset periodontal disease may also be found in patients with EDS type IV. These individuals are usually characterized by type III collagen abnormalities with hyperextensibility of the skin, ecchymotic pretibial lesions, easy bruisability, cigarette paper scars, joint hypermobility of digits, pes planus, and, of greatest concern, arterial and intestinal ruptures. Like type VIII, type IV also has AD inheritance.[71] The presence or absence of type III collagen abnormalities has been taken to be a differentiating factor between the two types, with EDS type IV showing abnormal type III collagen. The considerable overlap in phenotype of these two types warrants careful family and clinical evaluation, and biochemical studies of collagen when a patient with features of EDS and periodontal disease is evaluated.[72]

Chédiak-Higashi syndrome has frequently been linked with severe periodontitis.[70] This rare AR disorder is characterized by oculocutaneous hypopigmentation, severe immunologic deficiency with neutropenia and lack of natural killer cells, a bleeding tendency, and neurologic abnormalities. It is caused by mutations in the CHS1/LYST gene.[73]

Papillon-Lefèvre syndrome and Haim-Munk syndrome are two of the many different types of palmoplantar keratoderma, differing from the others by the occurrence of severe early-onset periodontitis with premature loss of the primary and permanent dentition. Haim-Munk syndrome is characterized in addition by arachnodactyly, acroosteolysis, and onychogryphosis.[74] Hart and colleagues[75] have shown that both of these AR syndromes are due to different mutations in the cathepsin C (CTSC) gene. A possible role for a mutation in this gene has also been reported in patients with generalized nonsyndromic aggressive periodontitis.[76]

EARLY-ONSET PERIODONTITIS

Early onset of periodontitis may occur in the primary dentition (prepubertal periodontitis), may develop during puberty (JP), or may be characterized by exceedingly rapid loss of alveolar bone (rapidly progressive periodontitis). Along with hypophosphatasia, prepubertal periodontitis appears to be the most commonly encountered cause of premature exfoliation of the primary teeth, especially in girls.[71]

JP has the following features:
1. An early onset of the breakdown of periodontal bone. This bone loss is of two types: chronic periodontitis in a generalized form affecting any dental area, and a localized form in which the molar or incisor regions of bone are the most severely affected.
2. Bone destruction that is rapid and vertical, with specific microorganisms associated with the periodontal lesion.
3. Familial aggregation, especially in the molar and incisor types. It seems probable that the generalized and localized types represent two different aspects of the same disorder; this discussion considers them as a complex entity called *familial JP*.

At least three different modes of inheritance have been proposed for JP. The early reports of Benjamin and Baer, and later that of Melnick and colleagues, offered support for an XLD trait.[77] This conclusion was based on the observation that twice as many females were observed to be affected as males (see preceding criteria for XLD inheritance). However, Hart and colleagues have shown that females are twice as likely as males to seek treatment.[78] When this biased ascertainment is considered, the male-to-female ratio is essentially unity. Saxen demonstrated that a clinical phenotype found in Finland closely resembling JP (if not actually JP) showed an AR mode of inheritance.[79] This disorder may be peculiar to Finland. Boughman and colleagues reported linkage of a gene in a single large family for an AD form of JP on chromosome 4 to another dental trait (dentinogenesis imperfecta, Shields type III).[80] Hart and colleagues, in a study of 19 unrelated families, strongly excluded linkage between an early-onset periodontitis susceptibility gene and chromosome region 4q12-q13 assuming locus homogeneity.[81] They concluded that the previous report of linkage was a false-positive, or that there are two or more unlinked forms of JP, with the form located in 4q12-q13 being less common. Dominant inheritance is probable for the type most prevalent in this country (Fig. 6-10).

Evaluation of the same IL-1α and IL-1β polymorphisms found by Kornman and colleagues[59] to be associated with

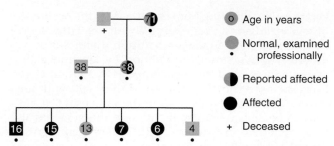

Figure 6-10 Pedigree of family with juvenile periodontitis, a dominant trait.

periodontitis in adult nonsmokers was performed in black and white families with two or more members affected with early-onset periodontitis by Diehl and colleagues.[82] Interestingly, they found the IL-1 alleles associated with high risk of early-onset periodontitis to be the ones suggested previously to be correlated with low risk for severe adult periodontitis. They concluded that early-onset periodontitis is a complex, oligogenic disorder (i.e., involving a small number of genes), with IL-1 genetic variation having an important but not exclusive influence on disease risk.

GENETICS OF MALOCCLUSION

The study of occlusion pertains to relationships between teeth in the same dental arch, as well as between the two dental arches when the teeth come together. Many factors are involved in the definition of normal occlusion. Some of the most important orofacial parameters of occlusion are airway function, soft tissue anatomy and function, size of the maxilla, size of the mandible (both rami and body), arch form, anatomy of teeth (including malformation), congenitally missing teeth, and rotation of teeth. All of these important elements must be included in the concept of occlusion.

Malocclusion is perhaps somewhat easier to define. One may simply say that malocclusion is a significant deviation from normal occlusion. However, this description is useful only if one considers the multiple aspects implicit in such a definition. Normal occlusion and malocclusion are dynamic concepts that involve the interrelationships of many factors, not a few of which have been shown to be influenced by genetic factors. For example, in a study of the association of the Pro561Thr (P56IT) variant in the growth hormone receptor (GHR) gene with craniofacial measurements on lateral cephalometrics radiographs by Yamaguchi and colleagues, those who did not have the GHR P56IT allele had a significantly greater mandibular ramus length (condylion-gonion) than did those with the GHR P56IT allele in a normal Japanese sample of 50 men and 50 women.[83] The average mandibular ramus height in those with the GHR P56IT allele was 4.65 mm shorter than the average for those without the GHR P56IT allele. This significant correlation between the GHR P56IT allele and shorter mandibular ramus height was confirmed in an additional 80 women.

Theoretically, there are two general ways in which predisposing or causative factors for malocclusion could be due to heritable characteristics.[84] One would be inheritance of a disproportion between the size of the teeth and the jaws, resulting in crowding or spacing, whereas the other would be inheritance of a disproportion in the position, size, or shape of the mandible and maxilla. Genetic influences on each of these traits are rarely due to a single gene, which would be necessary for malocclusion to be due to the simple inheritance of discrete skeletal and dental characteristics. Instead they are often polygenic with the potential for environmental influence. Part of the practice of orthodontics is to use environmental (i.e., nongenetic) influences for the correction of malocclusion. Dental anthropologists would say that malocclusion is uncommon in pure racial populations. However, it has been debated whether this is due to the lack of procreation with other populations or the less refined diet often eaten by these typically isolated groups.

The experiments of Stockard and colleagues in dogs have been cited as evidence that crossbreeding among inbred strains increases the incidence of malocclusion.[85] However, the anomalies they produced may have been due in part to the influence of a major gene or genes that have been bred to be part of specific breeds. It seems improbable that racial crossbreeding in humans could resemble the condition of these experiments and thereby result in a synergistic increase of orofacial malrelations. An exception may occur on an individual basis in the child of an individual a dominant trait or syndrome that results in a malocclusion child. Depending on whether it is autosomal or X-linked, the dominant gene, if transmitted to an offspring, may also affect the offspring's occlusal development in a similar fashion as in the affected parent.

Studies of occlusion in twins have also been made. Lundstrom performed an intensive analysis of specific dentofacial attributes in twins and concluded that heredity played a significant role in determining the following characteristics: tooth size, width and length of the dental arch, height of the palate, crowding and spacing of teeth, and degree of overbite.[86] Kraus and colleagues made a cephalometric study of triplets in an attempt to assign an inherited basis to specific craniofacial morphologic features.[87] The authors looked at the lateral profile of the head and cranial vault, the outline of the calvaria, the cranial base, and the facial complex, which included both the upper and lower face and the maxillomandibular relationship. In addition, they selected 17 individual measurements of single portions of a given bone (e.g., posterior border of ramus). They concluded that morphology of an individual bone is under strong genetic control but that the environment plays a major role in determining how various bony elements are combined to achieve a harmonious or disharmonious craniofacial skeleton. This observation at least partly explains the remarkable differences sometimes seen in the facial patterns of identical twins and emphasizes the important role of environment in their development.

Class III malocclusion morphology is heterogeneous, with varying incidence among different ethnic groups, and various facial patterns may as a composite result in the condition.[88,89] There is a strong heritable component in class III malocclusion in general, with modes of inheritance being reported to be polygenic,[90] autosomal dominant in a Libyan sample,[91] and autosomal dominant with incomplete penetrance with a multifactorial component in a Brazilian sample.[92] The variation in ethnic incidence may also reflect variation in genes involved in these groups as suggested by the finding of linkage to chromosomes 1p36, 6q25, and 19p13.2 in Korean and Japanese patients primarily with mandibular prognathism,[93] and to 1p22.1, 3q26.2, 11q22, 12q13.13, and 12q23 in Colombian patients primarily with maxillary hypoplasia.[94]

Harris has shown that the craniofacial skeletal patterns of children with class II malocclusions are heritable and that there is a high resemblance to the skeletal patterns in their siblings with normal occlusion. From this he concluded that the genetic basis for this resemblance is probably polygenic. Interestingly, Harris used the family skeletal patterns as predictors for treatment prognosis of the child with a class II malocclusion.[95]

King and colleagues noted that many studies that which estimate heritability of craniofacial structures may have a bias because they have generally involved subjects who had not undergone orthodontic treatment, and that often subjects judged to have an extreme malocclusion were excluded. They found that, in contrast to the relatively high heritability of cephalometric variables and low heritability of occlusal variables in subjects with naturally occurring good occlusion, the heritability estimates for craniofacial skeletal variables in subjects with overt malocclusions were significantly lower and the heritability estimates for occlusal variations were significantly higher. This observation supports the idea that everyone does not react to specific environmental factors in the same manner, although those who are related are more likely to react in a similar fashion. To quote King and colleagues[96]:

> We propose that the substantive measures of intersib similarity for occlusal traits reflect similar responses to environmental factors common to both siblings. That is, given genetically influenced facial types and growth patterns, siblings are likely to respond to environmental factors (e.g., reduced masticatory stress, chronic mouth breathing) in similar fashions. Malocclusions appear to be acquired, but the fundamental genetic control of craniofacial form often diverts siblings into comparable physiologic responses leading to development of similar malocclusions.

Although we have some information about genetic influence on specific traits (e.g., missing teeth, occlusal patterns, tooth morphology, and even mandibular prognathism), these cases are exceptions, and we do not have sufficient information to make accurate predictions about the development of occlusion simply by studying the frequency of its occurrence in parents or even siblings. Admittedly, family patterns of resemblance are frequently obvious, but predictions must be made cautiously because of the genetic and environmental variables and their interaction, which are unknown and difficult to evaluate.

Currently, the results of studies on the genetic and environmental factors that influence the development of malocclusion are representative of the samples studied, not necessarily of any particular individual. In addition, the extent that a particular trait is influenced by genetic factors may have little if any effect on the success of environmental (treatment) intervention. Even so, it may be that genetic factors that influenced a trait will also influence the response to intervention to alter that trait, or other genetic factors may be involved in the response. Therefore the possibility of altering the environment to gain a more favorable occlusion theoretically exists even in individuals in whom the malocclusion does have a relatively high genetic influence. However, the question of how environmental and genetic factors interact is most relevant to clinical practice, because it may explain why a particular alteration of the environment (treatment) may be successful in one compliant patient and not in another.[97]

Multiple factors and processes contribute to the individual response to treatment. Some patients exhibit unusual untreated growth patterns, treatment outcomes, or reactions to medications linked to polymorphic genes. Analysis of overall treatment response requires a systems analysis using informatics for integration of all relevant information. The influence of genetic factors on treatment outcome must be studied and understood in quantitative terms for it to be applied effectively for each patient. Conclusions from retrospective studies must be evaluated by prospective testing to truly evaluate their value in practice. Genetic studies are necessary to further the evidence base for practice. Only then will we begin to truly understand how nature (genetic factors) and nurture (environment factors, including treatment) together affect treatment of our patients.[1]

EXTERNAL APICAL ROOT RESORPTION

Basic descriptors of root resorption are based on the anatomic region of occurrence; that is, designations are *internal root resorption* and *external root resorption* (cervical root resorption and external apical root resorption [EARR]). EARR is a frequent iatrogenic outcome associated with orthodontic treatment and may also occur in the absence of orthodontic treatment.[98,99] Although orthodontic treatment is associated with some maxillary central incisor EARR in most patients, and more than one third of those treated experience greater than 3 mm of loss, severe EARR (>5 mm) occurs in 2% to 5%.[100,101]

Currently, there are no reliable markers to predict which patients will develop EARR nor how severe EARR will be following orthodontic tooth movement,[102] although the shape of the root does appear to be associated with the likelihood of EARR and is best examined on periapical rather than panoramic radiographs.[103] Even when duration of treatment is a factor, it along with several significant dentofacial structural measurements (e.g., overjet) do not account for enough of the observed variability to be useful as predictors of EARR by themselves.[101]

Although orthodontic tooth movement, or *biomechanics*, has been found to account for approximately one tenth to one third of the total variation in EARR,[104-106]

Owman-Moll and colleagues showed that individual variation overshadowed the force magnitude and the force type in defining the susceptibility to histologic root resorption associated with orthodontic force.[107] Individual variations were considerable regarding both extension and depth of histologic root resorption within individuals, and these were not correlated to the magnitude of tooth movement achieved.[108]

The degree and severity of EARR associated with orthodontic treatment is multifactorial, involving host and environmental factors,[109] with genetic factors accounting for at least 50% of the variation overall and approximately two thirds of the variation seen in maxillary central incisor EARR.[110,111] In addition, studies in a panel of different inbred mice also supported a genetic component involving multiple genes in histologic root resorption.[112,113]

A polymorphism in the IL-1β gene in orthodontically treated individuals account for 15% of the variation in maxillary central incisor EARR. Individuals homozygous for the IL-1β allele 1 have a 5.6-fold (95% confidence interval, 1.9 to 21.2) increased risk of EARR greater than 2 mm compared with individuals who are not homozygous for the IL-1β allele 1.[114] The potential for IL-1β to have an effect on root resorption was supported by the increase in orthodontically induced histologic root resorption in the absence of IL-1β cytokine in a knockout mouse model,[115,116] and a P2rx7 knockout mouse model,[117,118] because a lack of the P2rx7 receptor results in a lack of interleukin-1β. In both of these mouse knockout models, there was no difference at baseline between the wild-type ("normal") and knockout mice histologic root resorption, whereas the application of force resulted in a significant increase in histologic root resorption in the wild-type mice. There was in addition a significant ($P < .02$) increase in histologic root resorption in both types of knockout mice with force applied over the force applied wild-type mice. Thus there was a significant interaction between the genotype and environment (orthodontic force) on histologic root resorption.

Although IL-1β is the first genetic marker suggested to be associated with EARR, it accounts for too small an amount of the total variation to be predictive. Additional genetic studies such as the one that found genetic linkage for EARR with a marker on chromosome 18 near the RANK gene are needed to determine what other genes influence EARR.[119] Other candidate genes include P2RX7, the genes for other proteins involved in the maturation and release of IL-1β, and those involved in the RANK/RANKL/OPG pathway of osteoclastogenesis.[116] Future estimation of susceptibility to EARR will likely require the analysis of a number of genes, root morphology, dental and facial measurement values, and the amount of tooth movement planned for treatment.

GENETICS OF CLEFT LIP AND PALATE

Studies of the CLP phenotype in twins indicate that monozygous twins have a 35% concordance rate, whereas dizygous twins show less than 5% concordance.[120] Information from two sources (families and twins) then establishes a genetic basis for CLP, but despite many extensive investigations, no simple pattern of inheritance has been demonstrated. This has led to proposal of a variety of genetic modes of inheritance for CLP, including dominance, recessiveness, and sex linkage, and has led ultimately to the documentation of modifying conditions that may be present, such as incomplete penetrance and variable gene expressivity.[121] There are three important reasons for the failure to resolve the question of a hereditary basis for clefts: (1) some clefts are of a nongenetic origin and should not be included in a genetic analysis; such cases are seldom recognized and are difficult to prove; (2) individuals who have increased genetic liability for having a child with CLP often fail to be recognized, but because they do not have CLP themselves they cannot be identified with certainty; this latter situation defines the problem of nonpenetrance for genes that control CLP[122]; and (3) CLP, although sometimes appearing to be relatively simple in origin, is undoubtedly a complex of diseases with different etiologies lumped together because of clinical disease resemblance (they all show clefting).

There are two clearly recognized groups of etiologically different clefts—cleft lip either with or without cleft palate (CL(P)) and isolated cleft palate (cleft palate only, or CPO). These two entities, CL(P) and CPO, occur as single cases in a family and as multiple cases in a family. In the former they are called *sporadic*, and in the latter they are called *familial* or *multiplex*. Some researchers refer to multiplex cases as those individuals with findings in addition to an oral cleft, even if a specific syndrome is not recognized. It should also be noted that the CPO that occurs without a cleft of the lip is different from the palatal cleft that occurs as a part of CL(P). The embryology and developmental timing are both different, and CPO is more commonly part of a syndrome than is CL(P). CPO is less common, with a prevalence of approximately 1 per 1500 to 2000 births in caucasians, whereas CL(P) is more common, 1 to 2 per 1000 births. The prevalence of CPO does not vary in different racial backgrounds, but the prevalence of CL(P) varies considerably, with Asian and American Indians having the highest rate and Africans the lowest. There are also gender ratio differences, with more males having CL(P) and more females having CPO. Except in a small number of syndromes such as Van der Woude syndrome, families with one type of clefting segregating in the family do not have the other cleft type occur at a rate higher than the population prevalence.

When all potential study groups for CL(P) and CPO are considered, the minimum number is six: three subgroups for CL(P) and three for CPO. These three for each type of cleft are the sporadic and the familial groups, and a group of syndromes that feature CL(P) and/or CPO. Approximately 30% of CL(P) and 50% of CPO patients have one of more than 400 described syndromes.[123]

As noted earlier, it is probable that minor and subtle facial changes are more likely to produce the best-correlated phenotype needed to pinpoint the cleft genotype. Part of the reason for this view is the suspicion that certain facial shapes are more predisposed to developing CL(P) than others[124,125] and that subepithelial defects of the upper lip musculature are part of the phenotypic spectrum of oral clefts and may represent an occult, subclinical manifestation of the anomaly.[126] Although this approach seems best for producing an accurately generated clefting phenotype, further study is needed of the developmental anatomy of the head and face.

Recurrence risks for CL(P) and CPO have been reported in which penetrance was not considered. These data are frequently cited by genetic counselors as illustrating the lesser risk associated with a multifactorial than with a monogenic trait. These data consider CL(P) and CPO without regard to the three groups discussed previously. These data, therefore, are average risk figures (Table 6-2).

The published data on nonsyndromic cleft populations comes from around the world (Japan, China, Hawaii, Denmark, Sweden, Great Britain, and North America). These studies make it clear that both CL(P) and CPO are heterogeneous diseases. That is, there are multiple causes for the single phenotypes, CL(P), and CPO. To summarize the generally accepted hereditary basis for CL(P) and CPO: Single, nonsyndromic cases of CL(P) and CP, or sporadic clefts, are believed to be the result of a complex interaction between multiple genetic and environmental factors. Hence, their etiology is multifactorial in the true sense of the word, and the chance that these multiple factors would interact to produce a cleft phenotype in relatives is small, probably less than 1%.

The ?other nonsyndromic group consists of multiple cases of clefts that occur in a single family. These are called familial (or multiplex) and have been viewed by researchers as the "true" genetic cases. Familial occurrences of CL(P) and CPO seem most likely to be accounted for by the action of a single major gene, but the influence of multifactorial (complex) trait factors is difficult to rule out. Thus we are left with the idea that both multifactorial and single major gene elements may have a role in producing sporadic and familial cases of CL(P) and CPO. For an overview of genetic factors in orofacial clefting, the reader is referred to the papers by Lidral and colleagues and Vieira and colleagues.[123,127]

An example of an environmental (dietary) factor that is associated with a decrease in neural tube defects such as spina bifida, as well as orofacial clefting, is the maternal intake of folate (folic acid), now a common component in prenatal vitamins. To be effective, such vitamins or other dietary supplements must be used at least around the time of conception because of the embryologic timing of neural tube closure, and lip and palate formation. Because of the public health importance and critical need before a woman may realize that she is pregnant, folic acid fortification of grains in the United States became mandatory January 1, 1998, specifically to reduce the occurrence of neural tube defects, which has happened. This has also to a lesser degree reduced the occurrence of orofacial clefting. Interestingly, however it did not decrease the occurrence of orofacial clefting in the children whose mothers smoke cigarettes, a risk factor associated with an increase in the occurrence of orofacial clefting.[128]

Although some genetic and environmental risk factors for CL(P) have been identified, many nonsyndromic clefts are not linked to any of these factors. Furthermore, there is a paucity of information available on the long-term consequences for children born with CL(P) or CPO. To address these concerns the National Center on Birth Defects and Developmental Disabilities at the Centers for Disease Control and Prevention conducted a workshop entitled "Prioritizing a Research Agenda for Orofacial Clefts." Experts in the fields of epidemiology, public health, genetics, psychology, speech pathology, dentistry, health economics, and others participated in this workshop to review the state of knowledge on orofacial clefts, identify knowledge gaps that need additional public health research, and create a prioritized public health research agenda based on these gaps. Their report is recommended to the reader as an excellent summary of the current knowledge and future research priorities for orofacial clefting.[129]

Table 6-2

Recurrence Risks for Cleft Lip with or without Cleft Palate (CL[P]) and Isolated Cleft Palate (CP)

	MATING TYPE		
Fogh-Andersen[76,121]	4%	2%	14%
CL(P)	12%	7%	17%
CP*			
Curtis and Walker[130]	4%	4%	19%
CL(P)	2%	6%	14%
CP*			
Curtis, Fraser, and Warburton[131]	4%	—	17%
CL(P)	7%	—	15%
CP*			

*Isolated cleft palate data were obtained from families with cleft individuals, in addition to the immediate family unit.

REFERENCES

1. Hartsfield JK Jr. Personalized orthodontics, the future of genetics in practice, *Semin Orthod* 14:166-171, 2008.
2. Pemberton TJ, Gee J, Patel PI. Gene discovery for dental anomalies: a primer for the dental professional, *J Am Dent Assoc* 137(6):743-752, 2006.
3. Chakravarti A. To a future of genetic medicine, *Nature* 409(6822):822-823, 2001.
4. Everett ET, Hartsfied JK Jr. Mouse models for craniofacial anomalies. In *Biological mechanisms of tooth movement and craniofacial adaptation*. Boston, 2000, Harvard Society for the Advancement of Orthodontics.
5. Cobourne MT. Construction for the modern head: current concepts in craniofacial development, *J Orthod* 27(4):307-314, 2000.
6. Lejeune J, Turpin R, Gautier J. Le mongolisme; premier exemple d'aberration et autosomique humaine, *Ann Genet* 1959;1:41-49, 1959.
7. Vissers LE et al. Array-based comparative genomic hybridization for the genomewide detection of submicroscopic chromosomal abnormalities, *Am J Hum Genet* 73(6):1261-1270, 2003.
8. Slavotinek AM. Novel microdeletion syndromes detected by chromosome microarrays, *Hum Genet* 124(1):1-17, 2008.
9. Goodenough U. *Genetics*, 3rd ed. Philadelphia, 1984, WB Saunders.
10. Hopper JL. *Heritability in biostatistical genetics and genetic epidemiology.* New York, 2002, Wiley.
11. Harris EF. Interpreting heritability estimates in the orthodontic literature, *Semin Orthod* 14:125-134, 2008.
12. LaBuda MC, Gottesman II, Pauls DL. Usefulness of twin studies for exploring the etiology of childhood and adolescent psychiatric disorders, *Am J Med Genet* 1993;48(1):47-59.
13. Abass S, Hartsfield JK Jr. Investigation of genetic factors affecting complex traits using external apical root resorption as a model, *Semin Orthod* 14:115-124, 2008.
14. Tucker A, Sharpe P. The cutting-edge of mammalian development; how the embryo makes teeth, *Nat Rev Genet* 5(7):499-508, 2004.
15. Croissant R, Guenther H, Slavkin H. How are embryonic pre-ameloblasts instructed by odontoblasts to synthesize enamel. In Slavkin HC, Greulich RC, eds. *Extracellular matrix influences on gene expression*. New York, 1975, Academic Press.
16. Sharpe PT. Neural crest and tooth morphogenesis, *Adv Dent Res* 15:4-7, 2001.
17. Witkop CJ, Sauk JJ. Defects of enamel. In Stewart R, Prescott G, eds. *Oral facial genetics*. St. Louis, 1976, Mosby.
18. Dean JA et al. Dentin dysplasia, type II linkage to chromosome 4q, *J Craniofac Genet Dev Biol* 17(4):172-177, 1997.
19. Schulze C, Lenz F. Uber Zahnschmelzhypoplasie von unvollstandig dominatem geschlechtgebundenen Erbang, *Z Mensch Vererb Konstitutionsl* 31:14-114, 1952.
20. Mulvihill JJ. Craniofacial syndromes: no such thing as a single gene disease, *Nat Genet* 9(2):101-103, 1995.
21. Park WJ, Bellus GA, Jabs EW. Mutations in fibroblast growth factor receptors: phenotypic consequences during eukaryotic development, *Am J Hum Genet* 57(4):748-754 1995.
22. Escobar V, Bixler D. On the classification of the acrocephalosyndactyly syndromes, *Clin Genet* 12(3):169-178, 1977.
23. Everett ET et al. A novel FGFR2 gene mutation in Crouzon syndrome associated with apparent nonpenetrance, *Cleft Palate Craniofac J* 36(6):533-541, 1999.
24. Rosenberg RN, Stuve O, Eagar T. 200 years after Darwin, *JAMA* 301(6):660-662, 2009.
25. Fraga MF et al. Epigenetic differences arise during the lifetime of monozygotic twins, *Proc Natl Acad Sci U S A* 102(30):10604-10609, 2005.
26. Feinberg AP. Epigenetics at the epicenter of modern medicine, *JAMA* 299(11):1345-1350, 2008.
27. Smith SM, Penrose LS. Monozygotic and dizygotic twin diagnosis, *Ann Hum Genet* 19(4):273-289, 1955.
28. Kruglyak L, Lander ES. Complete multipoint sib-pair analysis of qualitative and quantitative traits, *Am J Hum Genet* 57(2):439-454, 1995.
29. Slatkin M. Linkage disequilibrium—understanding the evolutionary past and mapping the medical future, *Nat Rev Genet* 9(6):477-485, 2008.
30. Abecasis GR, Cardon LR, Cookson WO. A general test of association for quantitative traits in nuclear families, *Am J Hum Genet* 66(1):279-292, 2000.
31. Gustafsson BE, et al. The Vipeholm dental caries study; the effect of different levels of carbohydrate intake on caries activity in 436 individuals observed for five years, *Acta Odontol Scand* 11(3-4):232-264, 1954.
32. Klein H, Palmer CE. Studies of dental caries. V. Familial resemblance in caries experience in siblings, *Public Health Rep* 53:1353-1364, 1938.
33. Klein H. The family and dental disease. IV. Dental disease (DMF) experience in parents and offspring, *J Am Dent Assoc* 33:735-743, 1946.
34. Li Y, Caufield PW. The fidelity of initial acquisition of mutans streptococci by infants from their mothers, *J Dent Res* 74(2):681-685, 1995.
35. Book JA, Grahnen H. Clinical and genetical studies of dental caries. II. Parents and sibs of adult highly resistant (caries-free) proposition, *Odontol Rev* 4:1-53, 1953.
36. Dahlberg G, Dahlberg B. Uber Karies und andere Zahnveranderungen bei Zwillingen, *Uppsala Lakerf Forh* 47:395-416, 1942.
37. Mansbridge JN. Heredity and dental caries, *J Dent Res* 38(2):337-347, 1959.
38. Horowitz SL, Osborne RH, Degeorge FV. Caries experience in twins, *Science* 128(3319):300-301, 1958.
39. Caldwell RC, Finn SB. Comparisons of the caries experience between identical and fraternal twins and unrelated children, *J Dent Res* 39:693-694, 1960.
40. Bretz WA et al. Dental caries and microbial acid production in twins, *Caries Res* 39(3):168-172, 2005.
41. Corby PM et al. Heritability of oral microbial species in caries-active and caries-free twins, *Twin Res Hum Genet* 10(6):821-828, 2007.
42. Corby PM, Bretz WA, Hart TC et al. *Mutans* streptococci in preschool twins, *Arch Oral Biol* 50(3):347-351, 2005.
43. Shuler CF. Inherited risks for susceptibility to dental caries, *J Dent Educ* 65(10):1038-1045, 2001.
44. Slayton RL, Cooper ME, Marazita ML. Tuftelin, mutans streptococci, and dental caries susceptibility, *J Dent Res* 84(8):711-714, 2005.
45. Deeley K, Letra A, Rose EK et al. Possible association of amelogenin to high caries experience in a Guatemalan-Mayan population, *Caries Res* 42(1):8-13, 2008.
46. Vieira AR, Marazita ML, Goldstein-McHenry T. Genome-wide scan finds suggestive caries loci, *J Dent Res* 87(5):435-439, 2008.
47. Bretz WA, Corby PM, Melo MR et al. Heritability estimates for dental caries and sucrose sweetness preference, *Arch Oral Biol* 51(12):1156-1160, 2006.
48. Hunt HR, Hoppert CA, Rosen S. Genetic factors in experimental rat caries. In Sognnaes RF, ed. *Advances in experimental caries research*. Washington, DC, 1995, American Associates for the Advancement of Science.

49. Mayhall CW. Concerning the composition and source of the acquired enamel pellicle of human teeth, *Arch Oral Biol* 15(12):1327-1341, 1970.
50. Bennick A, Chau G, Goodlin R et al. The role of human salivary acidic proline-rich proteins in the formation of acquired dental pellicle in vivo and their fate after adsorption to the human enamel surface, *Arch Oral Biol* 28(1): 19-27, 1983.
51. Mamula PW et al. Localization of the human salivary protein complex (SPC) to chromosome band 12p13.2, *Cytogenet Cell Genet* 39(4):279-284, 1985.
52. Azen EA et al. Alleles at the PRH1 locus coding for the human salivary-acidic proline-rich proteins Pa, Db, and PIF, *Am J Hum Genet* 41(6):1035-1047, 1987.
53. Maeda N. Inheritance of the human salivary proline-rich proteins: a reinterpretation in terms of six loci forming two subfamilies, *Biochem Genet* 23(5-6):455-464, 1985.
54. Yu PL, et al. Human parotid proline-rich proteins: correlation of genetic polymorphisms to dental caries, *Genet Epidemiol* 3(3):147-152, 1986.
55. Zakhary GM, Clark RM, Bidichandani SI et al. Acidic proline-rich protein Db and caries in young children, *J Dent Res* 86(12):1176-1180, 2007.
56. Dawson DV. Genetic factors appear to contribute substantially to dental caries susceptibility, and may also independently mediate sucrose sweetness preference, *J Evid Based Dent Pract* 8(1):37-39, 2008.
57. Ciancio SG, Hazen SP, Cunat JJ. Periodontal observations in twins, *J Periodontal Res* 4(1):42-45, 1969.
58. Michalowicz BS, Aeppli D, Virag G et al. Periodontal findings in adult twins, *J Periodontol* 62(5):293-299, 1991.
59. Kornman KS, Crane A, Wang HY et al. The interleukin-1 genotype as a severity factor in adult periodontal disease. *J Clin Periodontol* 24(1):72-77, 1997.
60. Wagner J, Kaminski WE, Aslanidis C et al. Prevalence of OPG and IL-1 gene polymorphisms in chronic periodontitis, *J Clin Periodontol* 34(10):823-827, 2007.
61. Sakellari D, Katsares V, Gerogiadou M et al. No correlation of five gene polymorphisms with periodontal conditions in a Greek population, *J Clin Periodontol* 33(11):765-770, 2006.
62. Fiebig A, et al: Polymorphisms in the interleukin-1 (IL1) gene cluster are not associated with aggressive periodontitis in a large Caucasian population, *Genomics* 92(5):309-315, 2008.
63. Nikolopoulos GK, Dimou NL, Hamodrakas SJ et al. Cytokine gene polymorphisms in periodontal disease: a meta-analysis of 53 studies including 4178 cases and 4590 controls, *J Clin Periodontol* 35(9):754-767, 2008.
64. Greenstein G, Hart TC. Clinical utility of a genetic susceptibility test for severe chronic periodontitis: a critical evaluation, *J Am Dent Assoc* 133(4):452-459, 492-453, 2002.
65. Kinane DF, Hart TC. Genes and gene polymorphisms associated with periodontal disease, *Crit Rev Oral Biol Med* 14(6):430-449, 2003.
66. Kinane DF, Shiba H, Hart TC. The genetic basis of periodontitis, *Periodontol 2000* 39:91-117, 2005.
67. Schenkein HA. Inheritance as a determinant of susceptibility for periodontitis, *J Dent Educ* 62(10):840-851, 1998.
68. Etzioni A, Tonetti M. Leukocyte adhesion deficiency II-from A to almost Z, *Immunol Rev* 178:138-147, 2000.
69. Arnaout MA et al. Point mutations impairing cell surface expression of the common beta subunit (CD18) in a patient with leukocyte adhesion molecule (Leu-CAM) deficiency, *J Clin Invest* 85(3):977-981, 1990.
70. Meyle J, Gonzales JR. Influences of systemic diseases on periodontitis in children and adolescents, *Periodontology 2000* 26:92-112, 2001.
71. Hartsfield JK Jr. Premature exfoliation of teeth in childhood and adolescence, *Adv Pediatr* 41:453-470, 1994.
72. Hartsfield JK Jr, Kousseff BG. Phenotypic overlap of Ehlers-Danlos syndrome types IV and VIII, *Am J Med Genet* 37(4):465-470, 1990.
73. Nagle DL et al. Identification and mutation analysis of the complete gene for Chediak-Higashi syndrome, *Nat Genet* 14(3):307-311, 1996.
74. Hart TC et al. Genetic studies of syndromes with severe periodontitis and palmoplantar hyperkeratosis, *J Periodontal Res* 32(1 Pt 2):81-89, 1997.
75. Hart TC et al. Haim-Munk syndrome and Papillon-Lefevre syndrome are allelic mutations in cathepsin C, *J Med Genet* 37(2):88-94, 2000.
76. Noack B et al. Cathepsin C gene variants in aggressive periodontitis, *J Dent Res* 87(10):958-963, 2008.
77. Melnick M, Shields ED, Bixler D. Periodontosis: a phenotypic and genetic analysis, *Oral Surg Oral Med Oral Pathol* 42(1):32-41, 1976.
78. Hart TC et al. Re-interpretation of the evidence for X-linked dominant inheritance of juvenile periodontitis, *J Periodontol* 63(3):169-173, 1992.
79. Saxen L. Heredity of juvenile periodontitis, *J Clin Periodontol* 7:279-288, 1989.
80. Boughman JA et al. An autosomal-dominant form of juvenile periodontitis: its localization to chromosome 4 and linkage to dentinogenesis imperfecta and Gc, *J Craniofac Genet Dev Biol* 6(4):341-350, 1986.
81. Hart TC et al. Reevaluation of the chromosome 4q candidate region for early onset periodontitis, *Hum Genet* 91(5):416-422, 1993.
82. Diehl SR et al. Linkage disequilibrium of interleukin-1 genetic polymorphisms with early-onset periodontitis, *J Periodontol* 70(4):418-430, 1999.
83. Yamaguchi T, Maki K, Shibasaki Y. Growth hormone receptor gene variant and mandibular height in the normal Japanese population, *Am J Orthod Dentofacial Orthop* 119(6):650-653, 2001.
84. Proffit WR. *Contemporary orthodontics*, ed 3, St. Louis, 1999, Mosby.
85. Stockard CR. The genetic and endocrine basis for differences in form and behavior, *Am Anat Memoirs* 19, 1941.
86. Lundstrom A. *Tooth size and occlusion in twins*, Stockholm, 1948, AB Fahlcrantz Boktryckeri.
87. Kraus BS, Wise WJ, Frei RA. Heredity and the craniofacial complex, *Am J Orthod* 45:172-217, 1959.
88. Singh GD. Morphologic determinants in the etiology of class III malocclusions: a review, *Clin Anat* 12(5):382-405, 1999.
89. Bui C, King T, Proffit W et al. Phenotypic characterization of class III patients, *Angle Orthod* 76(4):564-569, 2006.
90. Litton SF, Acermann LV, Isaacson RJ et al. A genetic study of Class 3 malocclusion, *Am J Orthod* 58(6):565-577, 1970.
91. El-Gheriani AA, Maher BS, El-Gheriani AS et al. Segregation analysis of mandibular prognathism in Libya, *J Dent Res* 82(7):523-527, 2003.
92. Cruz RM, Krieger H, Ferreira R et al. Major gene and multifactorial inheritance of mandibular prognathism, *Am J Med Genet A* 146A(1):71-77, 2008.
93. Yamaguchi T, Park SB, Narita A et al. Genome-wide linkage analysis of mandibular prognathism in Korean and Japanese patients, *J Dent Res* 84(3):255-259, 2005.
94. Frazier-Bowers S, Rincon-Rodriguez R, Zhou J et al. Evidence of linkage in a Hispanic cohort with a class III dentofacial phenotype, *J Dent Res* 88(1):56-60, 2009.

95. Harris JE. Genetic factors in the growth of the head. Inheritance of the craniofacial complex and malocclusion, *Dent Clin North Am* 19(1):151-160, 1975.

96. King L, Harris EF, Tolley EA. Heritability of cephalometric and occlusal variables as assessed from siblings with overt malocclusions, *Am J Orthod Dentofacial Orthop* 104(2):121-131, 1993.

97. Hartsfield JKJ. Development of the vertical dimension: Nature and nurture, *Semin Orthod* 8:113-119, 2002.

98. Harris EF, Butler ML. Patterns of incisor root resorption before and after orthodontic correction in cases with anterior open bites, *Am J Orthod Dentofacial Orthop* 101(2): 112-119, 1992.

99. Harris EF, Robinson QC, Woods MA. An analysis of causes of apical root resorption in patients not treated orthodontically, *Quintessence Int* 24(6):417-428, 1993.

100. Killiany DM. Root resorption caused by orthodontic treatment: an evidence-based review of literature, *Semin Orthod* 5(2):128-133, 1999.

101. Taithongchai R, Sookkorn K, Killiany DM. Facial and dentoalveolar structure and the prediction of apical root shortening, *Am J Orthod Dentofacial Orthop* 110(3):296-302, 1996.

102. Vlaskalic V, Boyd RL, Baumrind S. Etiology and sequelae of root resorption, *Semin Orthod* 4(2):124-131, 1998.

103. Sameshima GT, Asgarifar KO. Assessment of root resorption and root shape: periapical vs panoramic films, *Angle Orthod* 71(3):185-189, 2001.

104. Linge L, Linge BO. Patient characteristics and treatment variables associated with apical root resorption during orthodontic treatment, *Am J Orthod Dentofacial Orthop* 99(1):35-43, 1991.

105. Baumrind S, Korn EL, Boyd RL. Apical root resorption in orthodontically treated adults, *Am J Orthod Dentofacial Orthop* 110(3):311-320, 1996.

106. Horiuchi A, Hotokezaka H, Kobayashi K. Correlation between cortical plate proximity and apical root resorption, *Am J Orthod Dentofacial Orthop* 114(3):311-318, 1988.

107. Owman-Moll P, Kurol J, Lundgren D. Continuous versus interrupted continuous orthodontic force related to early tooth movement and root resorption. *Angle Orthod* 65(6):395-401, 1995.

108. Kurol J, Owman-Moll P, Lundgren D. Time-related root resorption after application of a controlled continuous orthodontic force, *Am J Orthod Dentofacial Orthop* 110(3):303-310, 1996.

109. Ngan DC, Kharbanda OP, Byloff FK et al. The genetic contribution to orthodontic root resorption: a retrospective twin study, *Aust Orthod J* 20(1):1-9, 2004.

110. Harris EF, Kineret SE, Tolley EA. A heritable component for external apical root resorption in patients treated orthodontically, *Am J Orthod Dentofacial Orthop* 111(3):301-309, 1997.

111. Hartsfield JK Jr, Everett ET, Al-Qawasmi RA. Genetic factors in external apical root resorption and orthodontic treatment, *Crit Rev Oral Biol Med* 15(2):115-122, 2004.

112. Al-Qawasmi RA, Harsfield JK Jr, Everett ET et al. Root resorption associated with orthodontic force in inbred mice: Genetic contributions, *Eur J Orthod* 28(1):13-19, 2006.

113. Abass SK, Hartsfield JK Jr, Al-Qawasmi RA et al. Inheritance of susceptibility to root resorption associated with orthodontic force in mice, *Am J Orthod Dentofacial Orthop* 134:742-750, 2008.

114. Al-Qawasmi RA Hartsfield JK Jr, Everett ET, et al. Genetic predisposition to external apical root resorption, *Am J Orthod Dentofacial Orthop* 123(3):242-252, 2003.

115. Al-Qawasmi RA et al. Root resorption associated with orthodontic force in IL-1Beta knockout mouse, *J Musculoskelet Neuronal Interact* 4(4):383-385, 2004.

116. Hartsfield JK Jr. Pathways in external apical root resorption associated with orthodontia, *Orthod Craniofac Res* 12: 236-242, 2009.

117. Viecilli RF, Katona TR, chen J et al. Three-dimensional mechanical environment of orthodontic tooth movement and root resorption, *Am J Orthod Dentofacial Orthop* 133(6):791 e711-726, 2008.

118. Viecilli RF et al. Orthodontic mechanotransduction and the role of the P2X7 receptor, *Am J Orthod Dentofacial Orthop* 135:694.e1-694.e16, 2009.

119. Al-Qawasmi RA, Hartsfield JK JR, Everett ET et al. Genetic predisposition to external apical root resorption in orthodontic patients: linkage of chromosome-18 marker, *J Dent Res* 82(5):356-360, 2003.

120. Shields ED, Bixler D, Fogh-Andersen P. Facial clefts in Danish twins, *Cleft Palate J* 16(1):1-6, 1979.

121. Fogh-Andersen P. *Incidence of harelip and cleft palate*, Copenhagen, 1942, *Nyt Nordisk Forlag*.

122. Metrakos JD, Metrakos K, Baxter H. Clefts of the lip and palate in twins; including a discordant pair whose monozygosity was confirmed by skin transplants, *Plast Reconstr Surg Transplant Bull* 22(2):109-122, 1958.

123. Lidral AC, Moreno LM, Bullard SA. Genetic factors and orofacial clefting, *Semin Orthod* 14:103-114, 2008.

124. Ward RE, Moore ES, Hartsfield JKJ. Morphometric characteristics of subjects with oral facial clefts and their relatives. In Wyszynski DF, ed. *Cleft lip and palate from origin to treatment.* New York, 2002, *Oxford University Press*.

125. Weinberg SM, Neiswanger K, Richtsmeier JT et al. Three-dimensional morphometric analysis of craniofacial shape in the unaffected relatives of individuals with nonsyndromic orofacial clefts: a possible marker for genetic susceptibility, *Am J Med Genet A* 146A(4):409-420, 2008.

126. Weinberg SM, Brandon CA, McHenry TH et al. Rethinking isolated cleft palate: evidence of occult lip defects in a subset of cases, *Am J Med Genet A* 146A(13):1670-1675, 2008.

127. Vieira AR, McHenry TG, Daack-Hirsch S et al. Candidate gene/loci studies in cleft lip/palate and dental anomalies finds novel susceptibility genes for clefts, *Genet Med* 10(9):668-674, 2008.

128. Yazdy MM, Honein MA, Xing J. Reduction in orofacial clefts following folic acid fortification of the U.S. grain supply, *Birth Defects Res A Clin Mol Teratol* 79(1):16-23, 2007.

129. Yazdy MM, Honein MA, Rasmussen SA et al. Priorities for future public health research in orofacial clefts, *Cleft Palate Craniofac J* 44(4):351-357, 2007.

130. Curtis EJ, Walker NF. Etiological study of cleft lip and cleft palate, Toronto, 1961, The Research Institute of the Hospital for Sick Children, University of Toronto.

131. Curtis EJ, Fraser FC, Warburton D. Congenital cleft lip and palate, *Am J Dis Child* 102:853-857, 1961.

CHAPTER 7

Acquired and Developmental Disturbances of the Teeth and Associated Oral Structures

▲ Ralph E. McDonald, David R. Avery, and James K. Hartsfield, Jr.

CHAPTER OUTLINE

COMMON DISTURBANCES IN CHILDREN

Dental care services have become more readily available to children, and caries prevention programs have become more effective. There has been a steady decline in the incidence and prevalence of dental caries in permanent teeth among U.S. children (see Chapter 10). However, according to the first Surgeon General's report on oral health in America published in May 2000, dental caries is the single most common chronic childhood disease.[1]

Periodontal disturbances are also common. Although severe forms of periodontal disease are rare in children, all experience at least mild gingivitis on occasion. Both caries and periodontal disease are, for the most part, acquired and preventable disturbances of the teeth and jaws. Other chapters of this book are devoted to a more in-depth discussion of the cause, prevention, and management of dental caries (see Chapters 10, 17, 18, and 19) and periodontal disturbances (see Chapters 11 and 20).

Injuries to the teeth and supporting tissues represent another large category of acquired disturbances (see Chapter 21).

Many children have orthodontic conditions that justify corrective treatment, and for some of them the condition is serious enough to be categorized as deforming or crippling. Approximately 1 in 1000 children in the United States is born with a cleft lip or palate. These conditions are primarily developmental disturbances and are discussed in greater detail in Chapters 6 and 25 to 28.

ALVEOLAR ABSCESS

During the examination procedure, the dentist may observe evidence of an acute or chronic alveolar abscess. An alveolar abscess associated with the pulpless permanent tooth is usually a specific lesion localized by a fibrous capsule produced by fibroblasts that differentiate from the periodontal membrane. The primary tooth abscess is usually evident as a more diffuse infection, and the surrounding tissue is less able to wall off the process. The virulence of the microorganisms and the ability of the tissues to react to the infection probably determine whether the infection will be acute or chronic.

In the early stages, the acute alveolar abscess can be diagnosed based on radiographic evidence of a thickened periodontal membrane. The tooth is sensitive to percussion and movement, and the patient may have a slight fever. The acute symptoms of an alveolar abscess can be relieved by using antibiotic therapy. Relief of the symptoms is more efficient if drainage is also established (Fig. 7-1). Drainage may be established through the pulp chamber of the tooth and/or the associated gingiva or by extraction of the tooth. If extraction is selected as the best choice of treatment at the emergency appointment and the patient has an unremarkable medical history, concomitant antibiotic therapy is not always necessary. During this acute infection phase, however, it may be impossible to establish effective pain control for the extraction procedure with conventional outpatient techniques.

If establishing drainage through the pulp chamber is selected as part of the emergency treatment, a large opening should be made into the pulp chamber to permit drainage of the exudate. After initial débridement and rinsing, the opening to the chamber may be closed unless drainage persists to ooze indefinitely. If pain occurs during the excavation of tooth structure to establish drainage, the discomfort can be lessened if the tooth is stabilized by the dentist's fingers.

Warm saline mouth rinses often aid in localizing the infection and maintaining adequate drainage before endodontic treatment or extraction.

Chronic alveolar abscess, characterized by less soreness, is often a better-defined radiographic lesion. The patient will likely have some lymphadenopathy as well. Draining fistulas are also frequently associated with chronic alveolar abscesses. Usually, antibiotic therapy is unnecessary except in patients with an overriding systemic problem (e.g., patients susceptible to subacute bacterial endocarditis, patients with organ transplants, or those who are immunodeficient). Again, drainage and sterilization of the

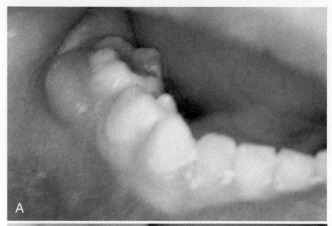
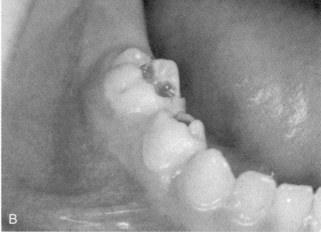

Figure 7-1 A, Acute alveolar abscess associated with a pulpless second primary molar. **B**, Removal of the roof of the pulp chamber to allow drainage resulted in immediate relief of pain. After the swelling is reduced, one can decide whether the tooth is to be treated or extracted.

infected local area are necessary through root canal therapy for the involved tooth or through extraction. If the lesion has only recently passed the acute stage, there may be a pointing soft tissue abscess. In this situation, incising and draining the soft tissue may be indicated in addition to opening the tooth, especially if the tooth is to be treated endodontically (Fig. 7-2). If the lesion is in an advanced chronic stage, drainage may already be established as a natural reaction (Fig. 7-3).

CELLULITIS

Cellulitis is a diffuse type of infection of the soft tissues that may be caused by a pulpless primary or permanent tooth. It often causes considerable swelling of the face or neck, and the tissue appears discolored.

Cellulitis is a very serious infection. It can be life threatening and is a potential complication of all acute dental infections. It is usually a result of severe untreated caries in patients who do not receive regular dental care or who may have had dental care only for treatment of dental emergencies. It is not unusual for the parents to take the child with dental cellulitis to the

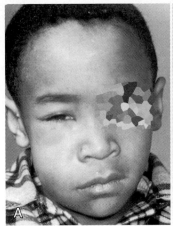
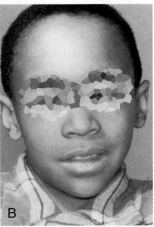

Figure 7-4 **A**, Patient appears to be acutely ill because of an infected permanent molar and resultant cellulitis. **B**, Use of broad-spectrum antibiotics reduced the acute symptoms of the disease and prevented extraoral drainage.

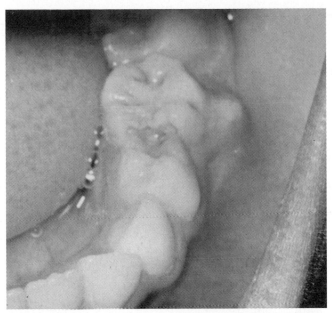

Figure 7-2 Chronic alveolar abscess associated with a pulpless second primary molar that is also a candidate for incision and drainage, in addition to removal of the roof of the pulp chamber to initiate root canal therapy if the tooth is to be saved.

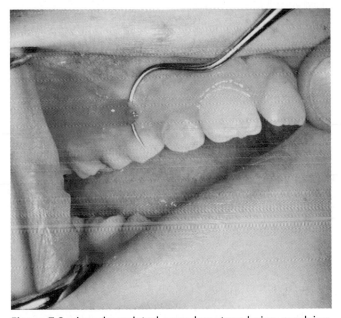

Figure 7-3 A pedunculated granulomatous lesion overlying the canine but associated with a chronic draining alveolar abscess of the maxillary right first primary molar.

hospital emergency department. The child appears acutely ill and may have an alarmingly high temperature with malaise and lethargy.

If a maxillary tooth is the problem, the swelling and redness may involve the eye (Fig. 7-4A). If cellulitis is treated too late, serious complications, such as involvement of the central nervous system or a cavernous sinus thrombosis, could occur. If cellulitis results from an infected mandibular tooth, the diffuse swelling and infection will spread to the floor of the mouth along fascial planes, nerves, and vessels. If the infection involves the submandibular, sublingual, and submental spaces, it is called *Ludwig angina*. In this condition the tongue and floor of the mouth become elevated to the extent that the patient's airway is obstructed and swallowing is impossible.

The establishment of drainage, if possible, by opening the pulp chamber of the affected tooth is helpful in reducing the acute symptoms of cellulitis. However, the child may have difficulty opening the mouth to permit the procedure. Incision of soft tissue to establish drainage is not indicated in the early stages of cellulitis because of the diffuse, nonlocalized nature of the infection.

The offending organisms in cellulitis from dental infections are usually capable of producing hyaluronidase and fibrinolysins. These agents break down the intercellular cementing substance (hyaluronic acid) and fibrin, which permits the rapid spread of the infection. One of the broad-spectrum antibiotics should be prescribed early to reduce the possibility of the infection localizing and draining on the outer surface of the face (see Fig. 7-4B). It should be emphasized to the parents or patient that antibiotics will not heal the condition completely and that follow-up treatment of the tooth is essential.

If the infection is already severe when the parent or patient seeks treatment, a blood culture or a culture of exudate may be performed to identify the infecting organisms. Then, if the infection does not respond to the initial antibiotic therapy, a second, more appropriate antibiotic may be selected after the causative organisms have been identified. Molinari has emphasized the continuing emergence of antibiotic-resistant bacterial strains that render many common antimicrobial agents ineffective.[2]

The child with cellulitis should be hospitalized if the clinical signs or symptoms warrant very close monitoring or if there is any question as to whether the parents or patient will follow through with the prescribed treatment. Hospitalization is recommended especially in the case of Ludwig angina, because maintenance of a patent airway may require the assistance of medical personnel. In these severe cases, parenteral administration of antibiotics is also recommended, at least initially.

DEVELOPMENTAL ANOMALIES OF THE TEETH

ODONTOMA

The abnormal proliferation of cells of the enamel organ may result in an odontogenic tumor, commonly referred to as an *odontoma*. An odontoma may form as a result of continued budding of the primary or permanent tooth germ or as a result of an abnormal proliferation of the cells of the tooth germ, in which case an odontoma replaces the normal tooth (Figs. 7-5 and 7-6). The anomaly is discussed in detail in Chapter 8. An odontoma should be surgically removed before it can interfere with eruption of teeth in the area. The presence of an odontoma should alert the practitioner to inquire about the concurrent presence of dysphagia or a family history of dysphagia that is perhaps due to hypertrophy of the smooth muscles of the esophagus as a part of the rare autosomal dominant odontoma-dysphagia syndrome.[3]

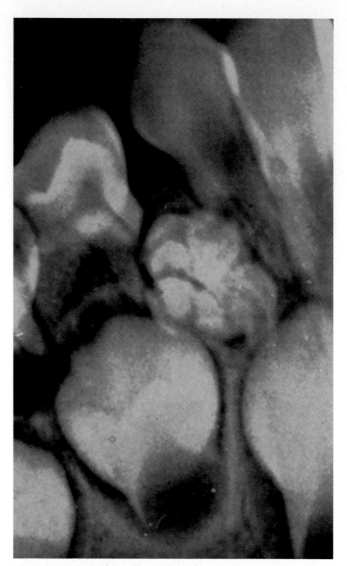

Figure 7-6 Complex composite odontoma.

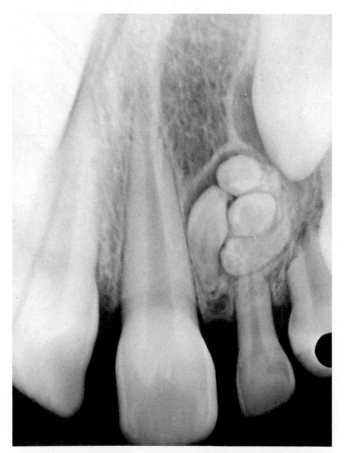

Figure 7-5 Compound composite odontoma. The anomalous structure consists of small structures resembling teeth.

FUSION OF THE TEETH

Fusion represents the union of two independently developing primary or permanent teeth. The condition is almost always limited to the anterior teeth and, like gemination (see the following discussion), may show a familial tendency.

The radiograph may show that the fusion is limited to the crowns and roots. Fused teeth will have separate pulp chambers and separate pulp canals (Fig. 7-7). Dental caries may develop in the line of fusion of the crowns, necessitating the placement of a restoration. A frequent finding in fusion of primary teeth is the congenital absence of one of the corresponding permanent teeth.

Delany and Goldblatt reported an interesting case that illustrates the multidisciplinary approach that may be indicated in the clinical management of certain problems associated with fused teeth.[4] The disciplines of pediatric dentistry, endodontics, surgery, restorative dentistry, and orthodontics were represented in the initial management of the case, and a post and core and a crown restoration

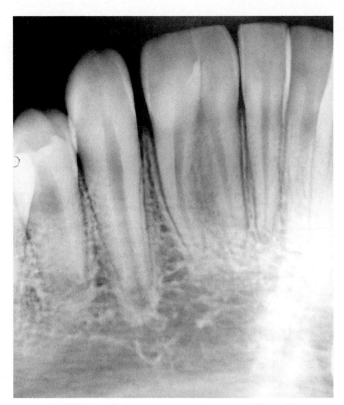

Figure 7-7 Fusion of a permanent central and lateral incisor.

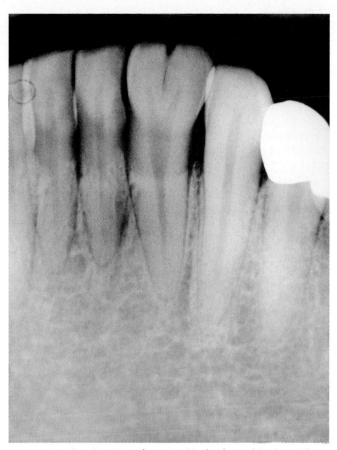

Figure 7-8 Gemination of a mandibular lateral incisor. The crown has a groove on the labial surface and is wider than normal.

were anticipated for the future. Yet excellent results were obtained in only 6 months with an organized approach to a complex problem that involved the fusion of a supernumerary tooth to a maxillary central incisor, severe crowding, and a palatally displaced lateral incisor. One root of the fused teeth was treated endodontically. The fused teeth were then hemisectioned, and the endodontically treated tooth was restored while the separated tooth was sacrificed. Orthodontic repositioning of the palatally displaced lateral incisor and alignment of the anterior segment concluded the management of the problem. A case of bilateral fusion of primary incisors has also been reported by Eidelman.[5]

The presence of a single primary and permanent maxillary central incisor may at first appear to be a product of fusion. However, if the single tooth is in the midline, and symmetric with normal crown and root shape and size, then it may be an isolated finding or may be part of the solitary median maxillary central incisor syndrome. This is a heterogeneous condition that may include other midline developmental abnormalities of the brain and other structures that can be due to mutation in the sonic hedgehog (SHH) gene, SIX3 gene, or other genetic abnormality.[6] The development of only one maxillary central incisor is an indication for further evaluation for other anomalies.

GEMINATION

A geminated tooth represents an attempted division of a single tooth germ by invagination occurring during the proliferation stage of the growth cycle of the tooth. The geminated tooth appears clinically as a bifid crown on a single root (Fig. 7-8). The crown is usually wider than normal, with a shallow groove extending from the incisal edge to the cervical region. The anomaly, which may follow a hereditary pattern of occurrence, is seen in both primary and permanent teeth, although it probably appears more frequently in primary teeth.

The treatment of a permanent anterior geminated tooth may involve reduction of the mesiodistal width of the tooth to allow normal development of the occlusion. Periodic disking of the tooth is recommended when the crown is not excessively large, as is eventual preparation of the tooth for restoration if dentin is exposed. Secondary dentin formation and pulpal recession will follow judicial periodic reduction of crown size. Devitalization of the tooth and root canal therapy followed by the construction of a postcrown may be needed when the geminated tooth is large and malformed.

DENS IN DENTE (DENS INVAGINATUS)

The diagnosis of dens in dente (tooth within a tooth) can be verified by a radiograph. The developmental anomaly has been described as a lingual invagination of the enamel. This condition can occur in primary and permanent teeth. Unusual cases of dens invaginatus have been reported in a mandibular primary canine,[7] a maxillary primary central incisor,[8] and a mandibular second primary molar.[9] Dens in dente is most often seen in the permanent maxillary lateral incisors. The condition should be suspected whenever deep lingual pits are observed in maxillary permanent lateral incisors. Grahnen and colleagues found in a study of 58 families that a similar anomaly was present in more than one third of the parents of children with dens in dente.[10] Within the same family, some had dens in dente and others had deep lingual pits, indicating that the condition may be inherited as an autosomal dominant trait with variable expressivity and possibly incomplete penetrance (see Chapter 6 for definitions).

Anterior teeth with dens in dente are usually of normal shape and size. In other areas of the mouth, however, the tooth can have an anomalous appearance. A dens in dente is characterized by an invagination lined with enamel and the presence of a foramen cecum with the probability of a communication between the cavity of the invagination and the pulp chamber (Fig. 7-9).

Application of sealant or a restoration in the opening of the invagination is the recommended treatment to prevent pulpal involvement. If the condition is detected before complete eruption of the tooth, the removal of gingival tissue to facilitate cavity preparation and restoration may be indicated.

The advisability of performing endodontic procedures on such a tooth with pulpal degeneration depends on its pulp morphology and the restorability of the crown (Fig. 7-10).

EARLY EXFOLIATION OF TEETH

Variations in the time of eruption of the primary teeth and in the time of exfoliation are frequently observed in pediatric patients. A variation of as much as 18 months in the exfoliation time of primary teeth may be considered normal. However, this pattern must be consistent with other aspects of the dental development. Exfoliation of teeth in the absence of trauma in children younger than 5 years of age merits special attention because it can be related to pathologic conditions of local and systemic origin.

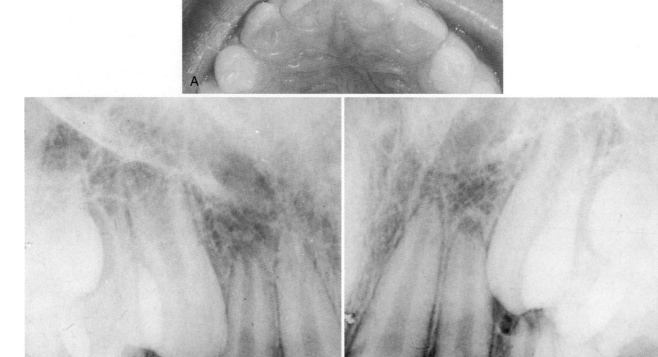

Figure 7-9 A, Small, "nonsticky" pits on the lingual surfaces of the maxillary lateral incisors are the only clues to the dens in dente condition of the teeth revealed radiographically in **B** and **C.**

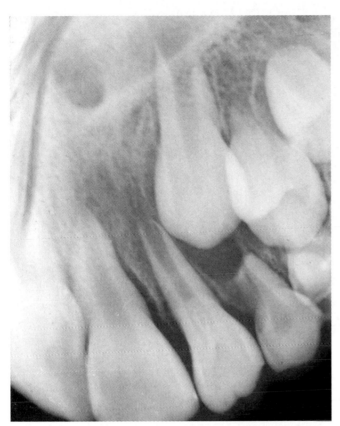

Figure 7-10 Dens in dente in a maxillary lateral incisor. A communication between the invagination and the pulp chamber apparently caused necrosis of the pulp.

The early exfoliation of primary teeth resulting from periodontitis has been observed occasionally in young children (see Chapters 6 and 20). Along with hypophosphatasia, prepubertal periodontitis appears to be the most common cause of premature exfoliation of the primary teeth, especially in girls.

HYPOPHOSPHATASIA

The clinical dental finding diagnostic of hypophosphatasia in children is premature exfoliation of the anterior primary teeth associated with deficient cementum. The loss of teeth in the young child may be spontaneous or may result from a slight trauma. Severe gingival inflammation will be absent. The loss of alveolar bone may be limited to the anterior region. The disease is characterized by improper mineralization of bone caused by deficient alkaline phosphatase activity in serum, liver, bone, and kidney (tissue nonspecific). Increased levels of urinary phosphoethanolamine are also seen.

Ongoing study into the etiology of hypophosphatasia indicates that the usually lethal autosomal recessive infantile type (I), as well as the usually autosomal recessive milder juvenile type (II) and the autosomal dominant adult type (III), are due to different mutations and heterozygosity versus homozygosity in the tissue-nonspecific alkaline phosphatase (TNSALP or ALPL) gene. Hu and colleagues state that, as a general rule, the earlier the appearance of the disease, the greater the severity.[11] Early exfoliation of the primary teeth is usually associated with the juvenile type (II), although such a history may also be present in the adult type (III).[11] Diagnostic tests should include the determination of serum alkaline phosphatase levels for parents and siblings.

Pseudohypophosphatasia, first described by Scriver and Cameron, is a rare disorder in which the child has the phenotype of juvenile hypophosphatasia and elevated levels of urinary phosphoethanolamine but plasma alkaline phosphatase activity is normal.[12] However, the clinical findings are similar to those of juvenile hypophosphatasia.

CHERUBISM (FAMILIAL FIBROUS DYSPLASIA)

Cherubism is a rare childhood disease affecting jaw development. Cherubism is usually inherited as an autosomal dominant trait with somewhat reduced penetrance in females. The expression may be so variable that a clinically normal-appearing parent may have a history of prominent facial swellings or radiographic evidence of abnormal bone pattern in the mandible. Although disease progression is expected to stabilize or even regress after puberty, a few very aggressive cases, sometimes producing morbid results, have been reported.[13-16] At least four cases of nonfamilial cherubism have been reported, which suggests occasional sporadic occurrences from spontaneous mutations.[17-19]

Two independent groups of investigators[20,21] have demonstrated that the gene for cherubism maps to chromosome 4p16. Follow-up work by Ueki and colleagues found that mutations in the gene encoding c-Abl binding protein SH3BP2 on chromosome 4p16.3 causes cherubism.[22] They found several different SH3BP2 gene mutations in patients with cherubism, which probably resulted in a gain of function or dominant-negative effect, although some other gene(s) may also cause cherubism in other patients. They postulated that the onset of cherubism and its anatomically circumscribed characteristics may be related to dental developmental processes in children, when signals unique to the mandible and maxilla are transmitted through the extracellular matrix, triggered by the eruption of secondary teeth.

A symmetric or asymmetric enlargement of the jaws may be noted at an early age. Numerous sharp, well-defined multilocular areas of bone destruction and thinning of the cortical plate are evident in the radiograph (Fig. 7-11). Teeth in the involved area are frequently exfoliated prematurely as a result of the loss of support or root resorption or, in permanent teeth, as a result of an interference in the development of roots. Spontaneous loss of the teeth may occur, or the child may pick the teeth out of the soft tissue.

McDonald and Shafer reported a case in which the mandible and maxilla of a 5-year-old girl were symmetrically enlarged.[23] Radiographs showed multilocular cystic involvement of both mandible and maxilla. A complete skeletal survey failed to reveal similar lesions in other bones. Microscopic examination of a segment of

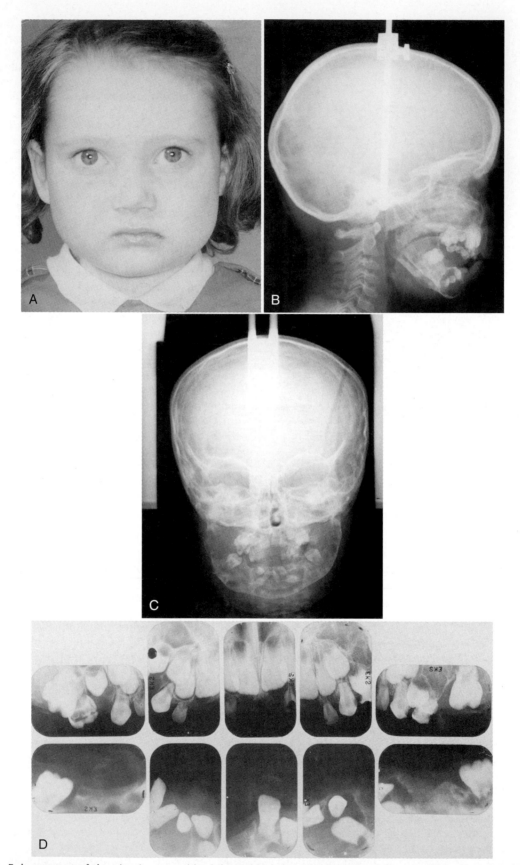

Figure 7-11 A, Enlargement of the cheeks caused by bilateral bulging of the bone of the mandible. **B** and **C**, lateral and anteroposterior cephalometric radiographs. Notice the displacement of the mandibular anterior teeth in a large area of bone destruction, the locular cystic involvement of the mandible and maxillae, and the number of missing teeth. **D**, Full-mouth radiographs demonstrating large areas of bone destruction and several missing teeth.

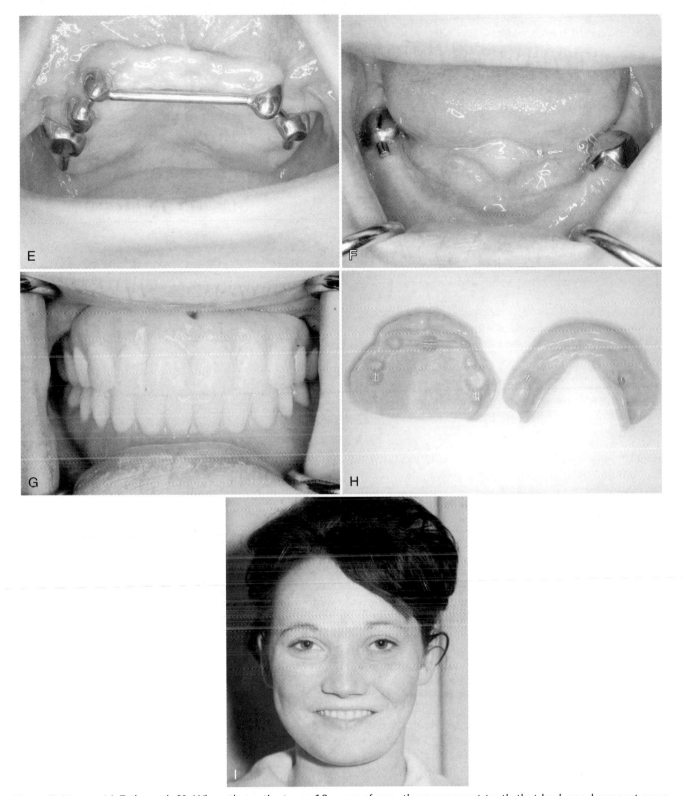

Figure 7-11. cont'd E through **H**, When the patient was 18 years of age, the permanent teeth that had good support were prepared for Baker attachments, and complete dentures were constructed. **I**, The restored mouth and improved appearance of the adult.

bone showed a large number of multinucleated giant cells scattered diffusely throughout a cellular stroma. The giant cells were large and irregular in shape and contained 30 to 40 nuclei. During a 10-year observation period, the bony lesions had not progressed appreciably.

The patient illustrated in Fig. 7-11 was followed into adulthood, and her mouth was restored in a very satisfactory manner. A comparison of the full-face photographs in Fig. 7-11 (A and I) illustrates that, as the face increases in height, the "cherubic" appearance caused by the bilateral bulging of the bone of the mandible is less apparent. Seven permanent teeth in the upper and lower arches were retained and prepared for Baker attachments. Complete dentures were constructed to restore function and improve appearance.

Pierce and colleagues have reported their dental management of a mother and two daughters with inherited craniofacial fibrous dysplasia over a 15-year period.[24] The daughters exhibited clinical and radiographic appearances similar to that of the patient just described, but the authors consider fibrous dysplasia and cherubism to be separate entities. Their treatment of the daughters, though more aggressive, resulted in nearly complete dentitions. Treatment included surgical autotransplantation of several teeth and bony recontouring. Orthodontic therapy was also provided for one child. Orthodontics was recommended for the other child but was declined; her dental alignment was acceptable 3 years after surgery.

Peters has reported a study of 20 cases of cherubism in one family that confirmed an autosomal dominant pattern of inheritance.[25] The author preferred a conservative approach in managing the giant cell lesions, because they tend to resolve with maturity. Von Wowern published an extensive review of the literature and a 36-year follow-up of families with cherubism.[26]

ACRODYNIA

The exposure of young children to minute amounts of mercury is responsible for a condition referred to as acrodynia or pink disease. Ointments and medications are the usual sources of the mercury. Weinstein and Bernstein recently reported on 20-month-old twin girls who presented to a hospital with the classic signs and symptoms of acrodynia.[27] Further investigation revealed that the girls had been receiving once- or twice-weekly doses of a mercury-containing teething powder during the preceding 4 months. Apparently such preparations are still available in some countries. Horowitz and colleagues reported on two young brothers who received a diagnosis of acrodynia after playing repeatedly with a broken sphygmomanometer.[28] Dental amalgam restorations do not cause acrodynia.

The clinical features of the disease include fever, anorexia, desquamation of the soles and palms (causing them to be pink), sweating, tachycardia, gastrointestinal disturbance, and hypotonia. The oral findings include inflammation and ulceration of the mucous membrane, excessive salivation, loss of alveolar bone, and premature exfoliation of teeth.

HYPOPHOSPHATEMIA (FAMILIAL OR X-LINKED HYPOPHOSPHATEMIC RICKETS OR VITAMIN D–RESISTANT RICKETS)

As reported by Hartsfield, hypophosphatemia is the most common inherited abnormality of renal tubular transport.[29] Clinical features become evident in the second year of life. They include short stature and bowing of the lower extremities in affected boys. Premature tooth exfoliation is sometimes also a feature. The inheritance pattern of the disease is usually X-linked dominant, and the disorder is twice as common in females as in males. The HYP Consortium of investigators found mutations in the PHEX (also called PEX) gene on the X chromosome in patients with this condition.[30]

Other dental manifestations often include apical radiolucencies, abscesses, and fistulas associated with pulp exposures in the primary and permanent teeth. The pulp exposures relate to the pulp horns extending to the dentinoenamel junction or even to the external surface of the tooth. The thin, hypomineralized enamel is abraded easily, which exposes the pulp. Dental radiographs show rickety bone trabeculations and absent or abnormal lamina dura.

McWhorter and Seale found that 25% of their patients with vitamin D–resistant rickets (VDRR) were affected with abscesses in primary teeth.[31] The results of their study indicated that the presence of one abscess is a predictor of future abscesses in the same patient. The authors suggested that early prophylactic treatment of all posterior primary teeth with pulpotomies and crown placement may be the most conservative therapy for a patient with VDRR who develops a spontaneous abscess. However, a follow-up retrospective study by Shroff and colleagues found the success rate for prophylactic pulpotomies in these patients to be only 44%.[32] They concluded that prophylactic pulpotomy therapy cannot be recommended for patients with VDRR based on the currently available data. They also suggested that a more aggressive approach using prophylactic pulpectomy as previously advocated by Rakocz and colleagues may be indicated in these patients and encouraged further investigation in this area.[33]

CYCLIC NEUTROPENIA (CYCLIC HEMATOPOIESIS)

Cyclic neutropenia is an autosomal dominant condition in which affected individuals are at risk for opportunistic infection during intervals of neutropenia that occur in a 21-day cycle concomitant with oscillation in bone marrow blood cell production. Levels of monocytes, platelets, lymphocytes, and reticulocytes also cycle with the same frequency. Horwitz and colleagues found several different single-base substitutions in the ELA2 gene encoding neutrophil elastase (also known as leukocyte elastase, elastase 2, and medullasin) in affected individuals, and hypothesized that a perturbed interaction between neutrophil elastase and serpins or other substrates may regulate mechanisms governing the clocklike timing of hematopoiesis.[34]

The condition occurs at any age. Numerous cases in children have been reported. The patients manifest a fever, malaise, sore throat, stomatitis, and regional lymphadenopathy, as well as headache, cutaneous infection, and conjunctivitis. Children exhibit a severe gingivitis with ulceration. With a return of the neutrophil count to normal, the gingiva may return to a nearly normal clinical appearance. Children experiencing repeated insults from the condition have a considerable loss of supporting bone around the teeth. A case report by da Fonseca and Fontes describes a young woman who had suffered from poor oral health throughout her lifetime, and as she approached 21 years of age, all her remaining permanent teeth were finally removed.[35] Soon after the extractions, the patient's blood counts improved to a level not previously seen by her hematologist.

OTHER DISORDERS

Premature exfoliation or marked mobility of teeth in childhood or adolescence has been associated in some cases with other systemic disorders, including acatalasia, Chédiak-Higashi syndrome, Coffin-Lowry syndrome, Down syndrome, Ehlers-Danlos syndrome types IV and VIII, Hajdu-Cheney syndrome, hyperpituitarism, hyperthyroidism, juvenile diabetes, Papillon-Lefèvre syndrome, progeria, Singleton-Merten syndrome, and some malignant diseases such as the histiocytosis X groups (see Chapter 8) and the leukemias (see Chapter 24).

ENAMEL HYPOPLASIA

Amelogenesis occurs in two stages. In the first stage, the enamel matrix forms, and in the second stage, the matrix undergoes calcification. Local or systemic factors that interfere with normal matrix formation cause enamel surface defects and irregularities called *enamel hypoplasia.* Factors that interfere with calcification and maturation of the enamel produce a condition termed enamel *hypocalcification.*

Enamel hypoplasia may be mild and may result in a pitting of the enamel surface or in the development of a horizontal line across the enamel of the crown. If ameloblastic activity has been disrupted for a long period, gross areas of irregular or imperfect enamel formation occur. Enamel hypoplasia is often seen as one component of many different syndromes.

Postnatal hypoplasia of the primary teeth is probably as common as hypoplasia of the permanent teeth, although the former usually does not occur in as severe a form. Hypoplasia of the primary enamel that forms before birth is rare, however (Fig. 7-12). In its mildest form, a prenatal disturbance is reflected as an accentuated neonatal ring in the primary tooth. In the severe type of neonatal disturbance, enamel formation is sometimes arrested at birth or during the neonatal period (Fig. 7-13). Postnatal amelogenesis is confined to the portion of the crown located cervically from the enamel area present at birth (Fig. 7-14).

Seow and colleagues have observed that enamel hypoplasia of the primary teeth is common in prematurely

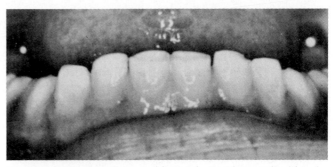

Figure 7-12 Prenatal enamel hypoplasia. The medical history revealed that the patient suffered from cerebral palsy as a result of premature birth (gestation, 6 months; birth weight, 2 lb, 5 oz). (Courtesy Dr. Stanley C. Herman.)

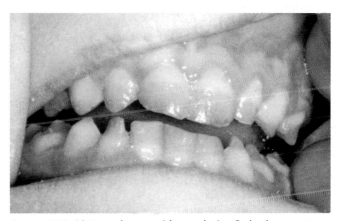

Figure 7-13 Neonatal enamel hypoplasia. Only the most cervical parts of the intrinsically stained areas are hypoplastic. The child experienced severe nutritional deficiency during the first month of extrauterine life. (Courtesy Dr. Stanley C. Herman.)

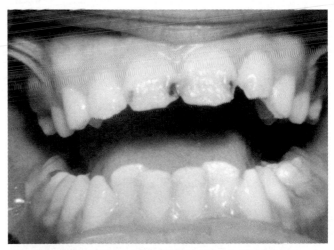

Figure 7-14 Enamel hypoplasia that occurred during infancy. A wide band of pitted enamel is evident on the maxillary and mandibular permanent incisors and first permanent molars. The child was severely affected with pneumonia at 6 months of age. (Courtesy Dr. Stanley C. Herman.)

born, very-low-birth-weight children; its pathogenesis is not understood clearly.[36] One likely mechanism is related to mineral deficiency, which may be diagnosed radiologically as demineralization of long bones. These authors believe that both local and systemic factors are involved. An important local factor is trauma from laryngoscopy and endotracheal intubation, which usually results in localized enamel hypoplasia involving only the left maxillary anterior teeth. Slayton and colleagues examined 698 well-nourished and healthy children 4 to 5 years of age and found that 6% had at least one primary tooth with enamel hypoplasia.[37]

HYPOPLASIA RESULTING FROM NUTRITIONAL DEFICIENCIES

Many clinical investigations have been undertaken to determine the relationship between hypoplastic defects of enamel and systemic disabilities. Relatively little importance has been placed on exanthematous fevers, but deficiency states, particularly those related to deficiencies in vitamins A, C, and D, calcium, and phosphorus, can often be related to the occurrence of enamel hypoplasia.

Sarnat and Schour observed that, in a group of 60 children who had adequate medical histories, two thirds of the hypoplastic disturbances occurred during infancy (birth to the end of the first year)[38] (Fig. 7-15). Approximately one third of enamel hypoplasia was found in the portion of teeth formed during early childhood (13 to 34 months) (Fig. 7-16). Less than 2% of enamel defects found originated in late childhood (35 to 80 months).

Sheldon and colleagues sought to determine whether defects in enamel were related to the occurrence of systemic ailments.[39] They examined ground sections of 95 teeth from 34 patients for whom detailed medical histories were available. In more than 70% of the individuals, a positive correlation was established between the time of formation of a band of defective enamel and the

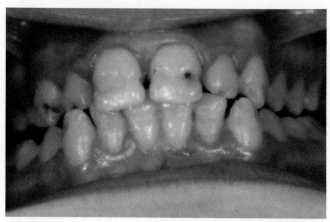

Figure 7-16 Enamel hypoplasia occurred during early childhood. Enamel formation on the incisal third of the lower incisors and the maxillary central incisors is normal.

existence of some systemic disability. However, defects in enamel occurred in 23% of patients who had no history of systemic conditions that might have produced enamel defects. No enamel changes occurred in 6% of patients who had histories of disabilities that had produced enamel changes in other patients. Deficiencies of vitamins A, C, and D, calcium, and phosphorus were the most common causes of defective enamel formation.

Purvis and colleagues, in a study of 112 infants with neonatal tetany in Edinburgh, observed that 63 (56%) later showed severe enamel hypoplasia of the primary teeth.[40] Histologic examinations revealed a prolonged disturbance of enamel formation in the 3 months before birth. An inverse relationship was demonstrated between the mean daily hours of bright sunshine in each calendar month and the incidence of neonatal tetany 3 months later. This observation suggested that enamel hypoplasia and neonatal tetany can be manifestations of vitamin D deficiency during pregnancy and are most likely the result of secondary hyperparathyroidism in the mother. A significantly higher mean maternal age and a preponderance of lower social class was also seen in the mothers of those in the tetany group. Another study in Edinburgh indicated that only 1% of pregnant mothers took vitamin D supplements.

Apparently in some children a mild deficiency state or systemic condition without clinical symptoms can interfere with ameloblastic activity and can produce a permanent defect in the developing enamel.

HYPOPLASIA RELATED TO BRAIN INJURY AND NEUROLOGIC DEFECTS

Herman and McDonald studied 120 children with cerebral palsy between 2½ and 10½ years of age (for whom complete medical records were available) to determine the prevalence of dental hypoplasia.[41] The researchers compared them with 117 healthy children in the same age group and observed enamel hypoplasia in 36% of the group with cerebral palsy and in 6% of the group without the disorder. A definite relationship between the time of occurrence of the possible factors that could have caused

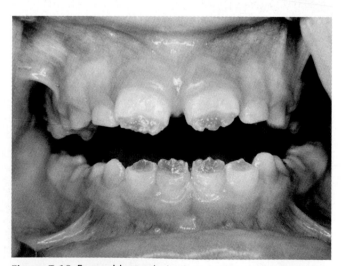

Figure 7-15 Enamel hypoplasia that developed as the result of a nutritional deficiency during infancy. The first permanent molars, maxillary central incisors, and mandibular incisors show hypoplastic enamel and dentin.

brain damage and the apparent time of origination of the enamel defect (based on its location in the enamel on the crown of the tooth) was established for 70% of the affected teeth of children with cerebral palsy (see Fig. 7-12). Evidence of enamel hypoplasia is an aid to the clinician and the research worker in determining when brain injury occurred in patients in whom the cause is not clearly defined.

Cohen and Diner observed that enamel defects occurred with greatest frequency in children with low intelligence quotients and a high incidence of neurologic defects.[42] They found that chronologically distributed enamel defects were a valuable aid in neurologic diagnosis, because they occur commonly in brain- damaged children. In addition, the defects indicate the time of insult to the developing fetus or infant even when the history is reportedly negative. Martinez and colleagues examined 170 children between 4 and 17 years of age (mean age, 12.03 years) with mental retardation and no history of dental trauma.[43] They found that 37% of these children had dental enamel defects.

HYPOPLASIA ASSOCIATED WITH NEPHROTIC SYNDROME

Oliver and Owings observed enamel hypoplasia in permanent teeth in a high percentage of children with nephrotic syndrome and found a correlation between the time of severe renal disease and the estimated time at which the defective enamel formation occurred.[44] Similarly, Koch and colleagues found a high incidence of enamel defects in the primary teeth of children were diagnosed with chronic renal failure early in infancy.[45]

HYPOPLASIA ASSOCIATED WITH ALLERGIES

Rattner and Myers discovered a correlation between enamel defects of the primary dentition and the presence of severe allergic reactions.[46] Enamel defects were present in 26 of 45 children with congenital allergies. The enamel lesions were localized in the occlusal third of the primary canines and first molars.

HYPOPLASIA ASSOCIATED WITH LEAD POISONING (PLUMBISM)

Lawson and Stout observed that in areas of Charleston, South Carolina, where there were very old frame buildings, the incidence of pitting hypoplasia was approximately 100% greater than published standards or the incidence in their control group of children.[47] They suggested that dentists treating children with unexplained pitting hypoplasia should consider previous exposure to lead as a part of their health evaluation, particularly if the child is from a family in a low economic stratum.

Pearl and Roland have pointed out that the fetus of a lead-poisoned mother can be affected because lead readily crosses the placenta during pregnancy.[48] They observed significant delays in development and eruption of the primary teeth in the child of a lead-poisoned mother. They also listed pica (ingestion of unusual objects to satisfy an abnormal craving) as a common sign of plumbism in children 1 to 6 years old, as well as in their mothers.

One mother admitted eating plaster from her apartment walls during several months of pregnancy.

HYPOPLASIA CAUSED BY LOCAL INFECTION AND TRAUMA

Enamel hypoplasia resulting from a deficiency state or a systemic condition will be evident on all the teeth that were undergoing matrix formation and calcification at the time of the insult. The hypoplasia will follow a definite pattern. Individual permanent teeth often have hypoplastic or hypocalcified areas on the crown that result from infection or trauma (Figs. 7-17 and 7-18).

Turner first described this localized type of hypoplasia.[49] He noted defects in the enamel of two premolars and traced the defects to apical infection of the nearest primary molar. Enamel hypoplasia resulting from local infection is called *Turner tooth*.

Bauer concluded from a study of autopsy material that the periapical inflammatory processes of primary teeth extend toward the buds of the pertinent permanent teeth and affect them during their prefunctional stage of

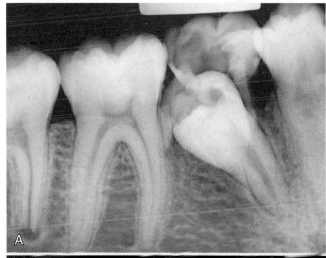

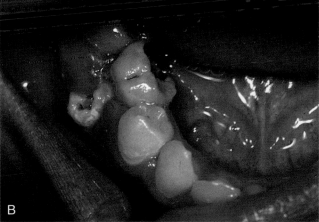

Figure 7-17 A, Infected mandibular second primary molar has caused hypoplasia of the second premolar and delayed eruption of the tooth. **B,** Hypoplasia is evident in the occlusal third of the second premolar.

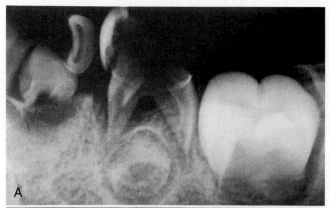

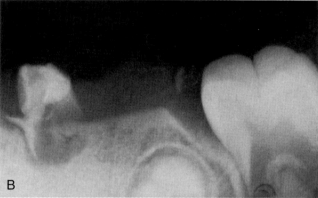

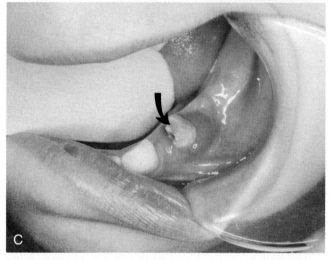

Figure 7-18 A, Only a root fragment remains as evidence of a pulpless first primary molar. The infection has affected the development of the first premolar. **B,** The second primary molar has been exfoliated prematurely. The first premolar is malformed as a result of the infection in the area. **C,** The malformed calcified mass *(arrow)* is surrounded by inflamed tissue.

eruption.[50] The infection fails to stimulate the development of a fibrous wall that would localize the lesion. Instead, the infection spreads diffusely through the bone around the buds of the successors and thereby affects the important protective layer of the young enamel, the united enamel epithelium.

Bauer found that in some cases the united enamel epithelium was destroyed and the enamel was exposed to inflammatory edema and to granulation tissue.[50] The granulation tissue later eroded the enamel and deposited a well-calcified, metaplastic, cementum-like substance on the surface of the deep excavation.

A traumatic blow to an anterior primary tooth that causes its displacement apically can interfere with matrix formation or calcification of the underlying permanent tooth. The trauma or subsequent periapical infection frequently produces defects on the labial surface of the permanent incisor (Fig. 7-19). The retention of infected primary teeth, even if they are asymptomatic, is unjustifiable. The development of hypoplastic defects on the permanent tooth, its deflection from the normal path of eruption, and even death of the developing tooth may result.

HYPOPLASIA ASSOCIATED WITH CLEFT LIP AND PALATE

Mink studied the incidence of enamel hypoplasia of the maxillary anterior teeth in 98 patients with repaired bilateral and unilateral complete cleft lip and palate; the individuals ranged in age from 1½ 18 years.[51] Among patients in the repaired unilateral and bilateral complete cleft lip and palate group, 66% of those with maxillary anterior primary teeth had one or more primary teeth affected with enamel hypoplasia; 92% of those with erupted maxillary anterior permanent teeth had one or more permanent teeth affected with enamel hypoplasia. Mink concluded that the permanent teeth are in earlier stages of development at the time of the surgical procedure and are more subject to damage.[51] Dixon also attributed many of the defects of tooth structure and formation observed in patients with cleft palate to the reparative surgery.[52] Vichi and Franchi, however, suggested that dental anomalies, including hypoplasia, probably result from multiple causes.[53] They emphasized the difficulty in understanding the role played by genetic factors, postnatal environment, nutrition, and surgical influences in the development of the dental anomalies.

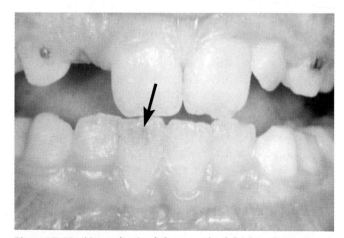

Figure 7-19 Hypoplastic defect on the labial surface of a mandibular permanent central incisor (arrow). There was a history of trauma to the primary tooth.

HYPOPLASIA CAUSED BY X-RADIATION AND CHEMOTHERAPY

Numerous dental abnormalities may result in surviving children who receive high-dose radiotherapy and chemotherapy during the time their teeth are forming. Kaste and colleagues reviewed clinical and radiographic records of 423 survivors of acute lymphoblastic leukemia.[54] Among these patients, they observed root stunting in 24.4%, microdontia in 18.9%, hypodontia in 8.5%, taurodontia in 5.9%, and overretention of primary teeth in 4%. The patients who were younger than 8 years old at diagnosis or who received cranial irradiation (in addition to chemotherapy) developed more dental abnormalities than those older than 8 years at diagnosis and those who did not receive cranial irradiation. They also noted that the resulting dental defects may affect the survivors' quality of life.

Maguire and Welbury point out that, as survival rates for children with cancer improve, the emphasis in therapy has moved from saving children at all costs to saving children at the least cost to the child, and therapy protocols are continually reviewed with this goal in mind.[55]

Children who receive high-dose x-radiation in the treatment of a malignancy are at risk for developing rampant caries in the irradiated area. The cause is generally believed to be associated with changes in salivary gland function and is discussed in Chapter 10.

Ameloblasts are somewhat resistant to x-radiation. However, a line of hypoplastic enamel that corresponds to the stage of development at the time of therapy may be seen (Fig. 7-20). Radiotherapy will have a more severe effect on the development of the dentin, and root formation will be stunted. Occasionally, development of the permanent teeth will be arrested (Fig. 7-21).

HYPOPLASIA RESULTING FROM RUBELLA EMBRYOPATHY

Musselman examined 50 children (average age, 2½ years) with congenital anomalies attributed to in utero infection with rubella.[56] Enamel hypoplasia was found in

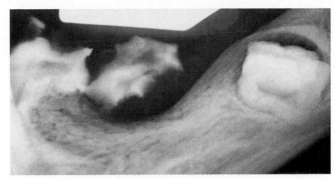

Figure 7-21 Absence of developing premolars and the malformed second permanent molar were caused by excessive x-radiation.

90% of the affected children, compared with only 13% of unaffected children in a control group. Tapered teeth also occurred in 78% of the children with a history of rubella (Fig. 7-22). Nine of the children in the study group had notched teeth, but this defect was not present in any of the children in the control group.

TREATMENT OF HYPOPLASTIC TEETH

The contention that hypoplastic teeth are more susceptible to dental caries than normal teeth has little supporting evidence. Carious lesions do develop, however, in the enamel defects and in areas of the clinical crown where dentin is exposed. Small carious and pre-carious areas can be restored with resin or glass ionomer. The restoration is usually confined to the area of involvement. The occlusal third of the first permanent molar often shows gross evidence of hypoplasia, and treatment is necessary before the tooth fully erupts.

Hypoplastic primary and permanent teeth with large areas of defective enamel and exposed dentin may be

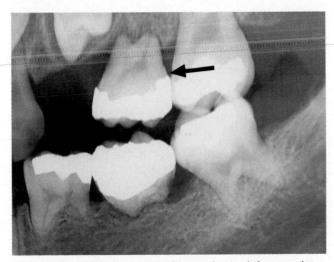

Figure 7-20 X-radiation caused hypoplastic defect on the crown of the first permanent molar *(arrow)* and stunting of root development.

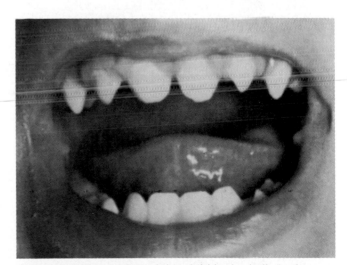

Figure 7-22 The mother of this child had rubella in the eighth week of pregnancy. The primary teeth were tapered and presented a rough hypoplastic surface. The child had a patent ductus arteriosus, pulmonary stenosis, and a cognitive disability. There was also a history of difficult feeding and dehydration at 2 months of age. (Courtesy Dr. Robert Musselman.)

sensitive as soon as they erupt. Satisfactory restoration may not be practical at this time. The topical application of fluoride has been found to decrease the sensitivity of the tooth. The application should be repeated as often as necessary to reduce sensitivity to thermal change and acid foods.

HYPOPLASIA CAUSED BY FLUORIDE (DENTAL FLUOROSIS)

Excess ingestion of fluoride can affect the ameloblasts during the tooth formation stage and can cause the clinical entity called dental fluorosis or mottled enamel. The appearance of enamel that is affected in its formation by excessive fluoride varies considerably. Although the more severe cases of dental fluorosis are associated with a high level of fluoride consumption, there is apparently a great deal of individual variation. The affected enamel is often limited superficially to the most outer surface and presents a white or brown opaque and/or pitted appearance.

Dental fluorosis is most often seen in permanent teeth, but it has also been observed in primary teeth. Levy and colleagues observed fluorosis of primary teeth in 12.1% of 504 children.[57] It was observed most often on second primary molars. The middle of the first year of life seemed to be the most important time with regard to the development of fluorosis in the primary dentition based on their estimates of fluoride ingestion prenatally and during the first year of life in these children.

The existence of a genetic influence on the development of fluorosis is supported by the finding that some inbred strains of mice are much more susceptible to fluorosis than other strains that receive the same fluoride dosage under identical conditions. Studies of these differing mouse strains should identify candidate genes for study in human cases of dental and skeletal fluorosis.[58]

ENAMEL MICROABRASION TO REMOVE SUPERFICIAL ENAMEL DISCOLORATIONS

For many years some dentists have advocated the application of hydrochloric acid as an effective method for destaining mottled enamel. McCloskey described a technique, originally advocated by Kane, that used 18% hydrochloric acid on the affected enamel surfaces.[59] Croll and Cavanaugh advocated a modified procedure that they called *enamel color modification* by controlled hydrochloric acid–pumice abrasion.[60,61] In their method, after the tooth or teeth are carefully isolated with a rubber dam and proper preparations have been made for safe use of the caustic agent, a slurry of fine pumice and 18% hydrochloric acid is applied under pressure and abrasion with a wooden stick. The slurry is rinsed away after each 5-second application until the desired color change has occurred. After a final rinsing with water, 1.1% neutral sodium fluoride gel is applied for 3 minutes. Next a fine fluoridated prophylactic paste is applied with a rotating rubber cup. Finally the enamel is polished with an aluminum oxide disk.

Dalzell and colleagues investigated the effects of the three variables of time, number of applications, and pressure on enamel loss when applying a slurry of 18% hydrochloric acid and pumice.[62] They found that enamel loss increased as the level of each variable increased and that a greater amount of enamel loss occurred when levels of two or three variables increased simultaneously. The combination of ten 10-second applications or fifteen 5-second applications with 20 g of pressure resulted in enamel loss of slightly less than 250 micrometers.

Croll proposed a modified procedure called *enamel microabrasion* in which a specially prepared abrasive compound (Prema, Premier Dental Products, King of Prussia, Pa) is applied to the discolored enamel areas, similarly to prophylaxis paste, using a synthetic rubber applicator in a 10:1 gear-reduction handpiece.[63] Frequent rinsing with water and reevaluation of the tooth for color correction are required. The instrumentation is continued until the undesirable coloration is removed or until a noticeable amount of enamel is being removed when the tooth is viewed from the incisal. Finally the abraded teeth are polished with a fine fluoridated prophylactic paste and given a 4-minute fluoride treatment (Fig. 7-23).

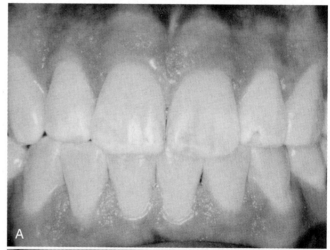

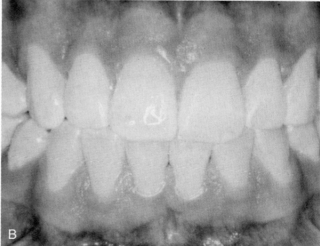

Figure 7-23 A, Mottled enamel. Because the brown pigmentation and white splotchy areas were objectionable, the teeth were treated by enamel microabrasion. **B**, Much of the pigment has been removed by enamel microabrasion.

Croll and Helpin have introduced a new delivery system for the microabrasion procedure.[64] A viscous, water-soluble abrasion slurry containing hydrochloric acid and silicon carbide microparticles (Opalustre, Ultradent Products, South Jordan, Utah) is conveniently applied to the tooth surface by a syringe. Vital tooth bleaching may be used in combination with enamel microabrasion to help remove deeper intrinsic discolorations. Bleaching is discussed later in this chapter.

PRE-ERUPTIVE "CARIES" (PRE-ERUPTIVE CORONAL RESORPTION OR PRE-ERUPTIVE INTRACORONAL RADIOLUCENCY)

Occasionally, defects on the crowns of developing permanent teeth are evident radiographically, even though no infection of the primary tooth or surrounding area is apparent (Fig. 7-24). Muhler referred to this condition as pre-eruptive "caries."[65] Such a lesion often does resemble caries when it is observed clinically, and the destructive lesion progresses if it is not restored. As soon as the lesion is reasonably accessible, the tooth should be uncovered by removal of the overlying primary tooth or by surgical exposure. The caries-like dentin is then excavated, and the tooth is restored with a durable temporary or permanent restorative material. In some cases, the lesion may be so extensive that indirect pulp therapy is justified (Fig. 7-25).

Mueller and colleagues reported caries-like resorption bilaterally in mandibular permanent second molars of a 12-year-old patient.[66] Both lesions were successfully treated in a fashion similar to the treatment illustrated in Fig. 7-25. Holan and colleagues reported three cases in which similar successful management of pre-eruptive tooth defects was performed.[67] Their experience and a review of other reported cases suggest that impacted teeth or teeth delayed in eruption may be at higher risk for developing the lesions. Savage and colleagues also published an informative literature review and case report relevant to this topic.[68]

Seow and associates[69,70] have published retrospective studies to determine the prevalence of pre-eruptive dentin

radiolucencies in permanent teeth using bite-wing and panoramic radiographs, respectively. In the study using bite-wing radiographs, the authors examined a set of films from 1959 subjects and observed 9919 unerupted permanent teeth. They found 126 subjects (6%) with 163 teeth (2%) exhibiting pre-eruptive dentin radiolucencies. In the study using panoramic radiographs, the investigators examined 1281 films of individual patients with 11,767 unerupted permanent teeth (incisors excluded). This study identified 42 subjects (3%) with 57 teeth (0.5%) exhibiting pre-eruptive dentin defects. The authors emphasize the importance of carefully studying radiographic images of unerupted teeth so that early detection and treatment are possible.

TAURODONTISM

Lysell credits Keith with giving the name to the phenomenon known as *taurodontism*.[71] This anomaly is characterized by a tendency for the body of the tooth to enlarge at the expense of the roots. The pulp chamber is elongated and extends deeply into the region of the roots (Fig. 7-26). A similar condition is seen in the teeth of cud-chewing animals such as the bull (Latin, *taurus*).

Jaspers and Witkop noted that taurodontism is found in about 2.5% of adult whites as an isolated trait, as well as in individuals with syndromes such as trichodento-osseous syndrome, otodental dysplasia, and X-chromosome aneuploidies.[72] Mena observed a mother and seven children, four of whom showed evidence of taurodontism in the permanent or primary teeth, or both.[73] This was probably the first report of taurodontism of the primary dentition as a definite family trait in black children. Gedik and Cimen reported taurodontism of six primary molars of a 7-year-old boy who had no syndromes or systemic disease.[74] Other pedigrees have been consistent with autosomal dominant or autosomal recessive inheritance. The inheritance may also be polygenic.

The clinical significance of the condition becomes apparent if vital pulp therapy or root canal therapy is necessary.

INHERITED DENTIN DEFECTS

Two broad categories of heritable dentin defects, dentinogenesis imperfecta and dentin dysplasia, are identifiable, each with distinct subtypes.

DENTINOGENESIS IMPERFECTA (HEREDITARY OPALESCENT DENTIN)

Dentinogenesis imperfecta is inherited as an isolated autosomal dominant trait ("isolated" in this use means that it occurs without other anomalies). Bixler and colleagues observed this pattern in a six-generation family in which 34 members were studied.[75] There was 100% penetrance and consistent gene expression within a sibship. In a survey of 96,000 Michigan children, Witkop reported a prevalence of 1 in 8000 with the trait.[76] The anomaly may be seen with osteogenesis imperfecta (Fig. 7-27). A decade later, Witkop suggested that there are two distinct diseases.[77] He recommended that the term *hereditary*

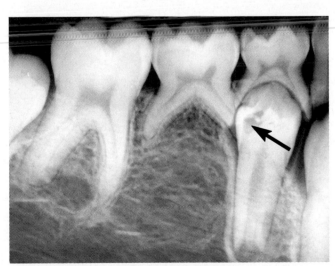

Figure 7-24 Pre-eruptive "caries" on the crown of an unerupted first premolar *(arrow)*.

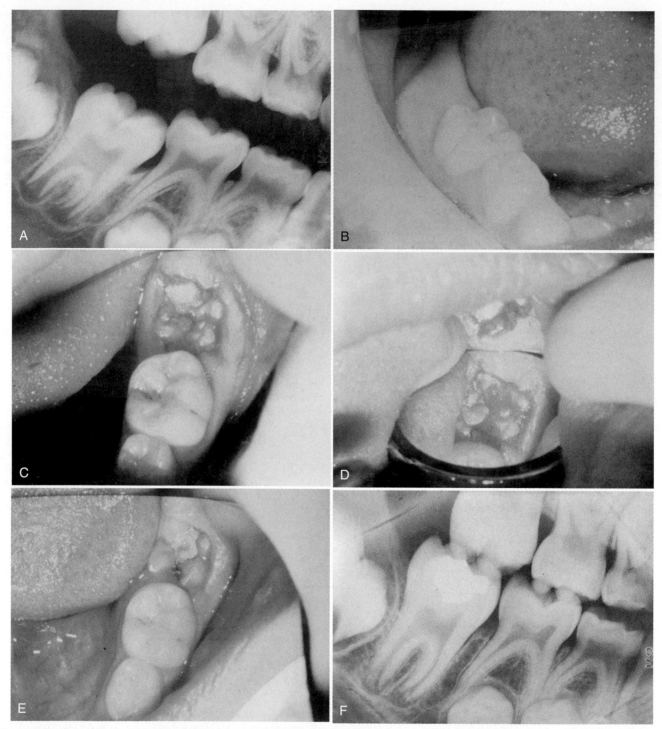

Figure 7-25 A and **B,** Pre-eruptive "caries" in a mandibular right first permanent molar that is still unerupted. **C,** Mirror view of the lesion on the occlusal surface of the unerupted tooth. **D,** Mirror view of excavated cavity after gross caries removal. **E,** Mirror view of temporary restoration 1 week postoperatively (dark spot on mesial marginal ridge area is an artifact). **F,** Nine months postoperatively, patient had continued normal root development and eruption of the tooth. The temporary restoration remained 3 months before the tooth was reentered and restored with amalgam. (Courtesy Drs. George E. Krull and James R. Roche.)

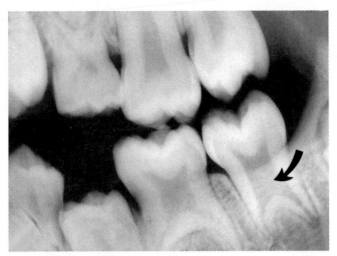

Figure 7-26 Taurodontism. Notice the elongated pulp chamber and short root canals (arrow).

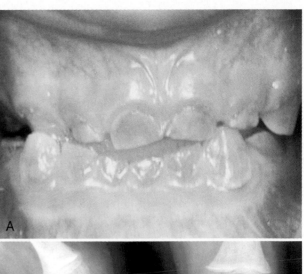

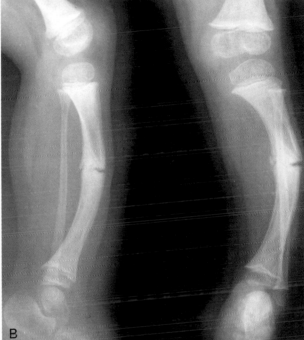

opalescent dentin be used for the disease that occurs as an isolated trait and the term *dentinogenesis imperfecta* be used for that which occurs in conjunction with osteogenesis imperfecta. Shields and colleagues recognized the difference and proposed a new classification: the dentin defect that occurs in association with osteogenesis imperfecta is termed (Shields) *type I dentinogenesis imperfecta* and that which occurs as an isolated trait is termed (Shields) *type II dentinogenesis imperfecta*.[78] In addition, the dentin defects seen in the isolated Brandywine triracial population in southern Maryland was termed (Shields) *type III dentinogenesis imperfecta*. These latter defects consisted of variable expression of the features of (Shields) type I (without osteogenesis imperfecta) and type II, shell-like teeth, and multiple pulp exposures (Fig. 7-28). In this condition, normal dentin formation is confined to a thin layer next to the enamel and cementum, followed by a layer of disorderly dentin containing a few tubules. The roots of shell teeth are short, and the primary teeth may be exfoliated prematurely.

Figure 7-27 A, Five-year-old girl with dentinogenesis imperfecta and osteogenesis imperfecta. The child had sustained numerous fractures of the long bones. **B,** A fracture of the tibia is evident in the radiograph.

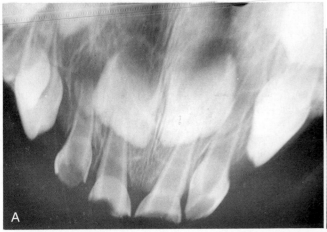

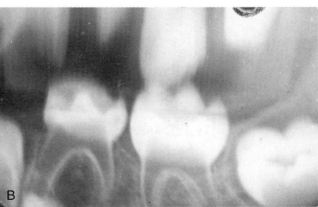

Figure 7-28 Shell teeth. The large size of the pulp cavities indicates the nonexistence of secondary dentin.

Mutations in the DSPP gene, which codes for the two major noncollagenous dentin matrix proteins, dentin sialoprotein (DSP) and dentin phosphoprotein (also known as phosphophorin), have been found in patients with (Shields) type II dentinogenesis imperfecta by Zhang and colleagues[79] and by Xiao and colleagues.[80] Sreenath and colleagues noted in the Dspp knockout mouse that the teeth have a widened predentin zone and develop defective dentin mineralization similar in phenotype to that in human (Shields) type III dentinogenesis imperfecta; these findings imply that this gene may also be involved in the latter condition.[81]

The clinical picture of dentinogenesis imperfecta is one in which the primary and permanent teeth are a characteristic reddish brown to gray opalescent color. Soon after the primary dentition is complete, enamel often breaks away from the incisal edge of the anterior teeth and the occlusal surface of the posterior teeth. The exposed soft dentin abrades rapidly, occasionally to the extent that the smooth, polished dentin surface is continuous with the gingival tissue (Fig. 7-29). Radiographs show slender roots and bulbous crowns. The pulp chamber is small or entirely absent, and the pulp canals are small and ribbon-like (Fig. 7-30). Periapical rarefaction in the primary dentition is occasionally observed. However, no satisfactory explanation has been offered, because

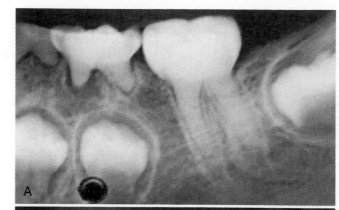

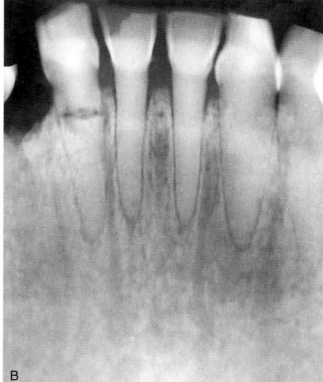

Figure 7-30 **A,** Slender roots with ribbon-like pulp canals and bulbous crowns are characteristic of dentinogenesis imperfecta. The primary molars show periapical rarefaction. **B,** Root fractures are common in older patients.

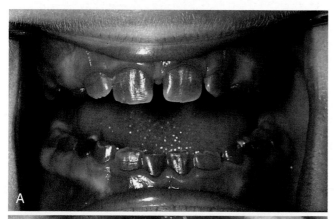

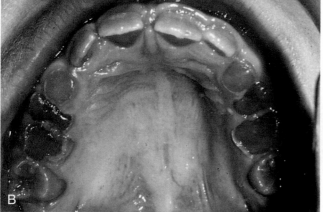

Figure 7-29 Dentinogenesis imperfecta. The primary teeth are severely abraded. Enamel is breaking away from the incisal edge of the lower permanent central incisors.

the condition apparently is not related to pulp exposures and pulpal necrosis. Multiple root fractures are often seen, particularly in older patients. Crowns of the permanent teeth often seem to be of better quality and have less destruction. Occasionally they appear essentially normal clinically (Fig. 7-31). There is some evidence of a genotype-phenotype correlation with Malmgren and colleagues showing one DSPP missense mutation being associated with a more severe phenotype in one family than what was seen in another affected family with a different DSPP missense mutation.[82]

The treatment of dentinogenesis imperfecta is difficult in both the primary and permanent dentitions. The

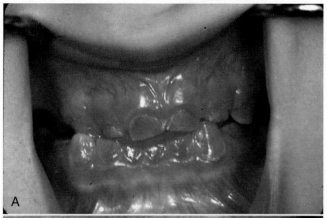

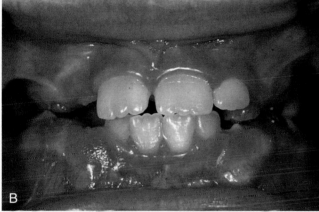

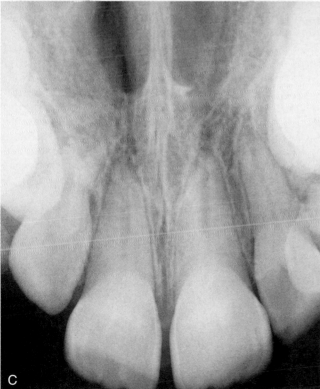

Figure 7-31 A, Four-year-old child with dentinogenesis imperfecta. **B,** The permanent teeth, in contrast to the primary teeth, are normal in color. **C,** The radiograph shows the typical picture of dentinogenesis imperfecta.

placement of stainless steel crowns on the primary posterior teeth may be considered as a means of preventing gross abrasion of the tooth structure. Full-coverage restorations may be placed on the permanent teeth if the crowns need protection in late adolescence or young adulthood. Bonded veneer restorations on anterior teeth have also been used successfully for esthetic improvement in patients with dentinogenesis imperfecta when full-coverage restorations are unnecessary.

Teeth that have periapical rarefaction and root fracture should be removed. Extraction of the affected teeth is difficult because of the brittleness of the dentin.

DENTIN DYSPLASIA

Dentin dysplasia is a rare disturbance of dentin formation that Shields and colleagues categorized into two types: radicular dentin dysplasia (type I) and coronal dentin dysplasia (type II).[78] Both primary and secondary dentitions are affected in dentin dysplasia type I, which is inherited as an autosomal dominant trait. Radiographically the roots are short and may be more pointed than normal. Usually the root canals and pulp chambers are absent except for a chevron-shaped remnant in the crown. The color and general morphology of the crowns of the teeth are usually normal, although they may be slightly opalescent and blue or brown. Periapical radiolucencies may be present at the apices of affected teeth.

Dentin dysplasia type II is inherited as an autosomal dominant trait in which the primary dentition appears opalescent and on radiographs has obliterated pulp chambers, similar to the appearance in dentinogenesis imperfecta. Unlike in dentinogenesis imperfecta, however, in dentin dysplasia type II the permanent dentition has normal color and radiographically exhibits a thistle tube pulp configuration with pulp stones.

Dean and colleagues, noting the phenotypic similarity of dentinogenesis imperfecta, Shields type II, to that in the primary dentition in dentin dysplasia type II, hypothesized that these conditions may be due to different alleles of the same gene.[83] Investigation of a family with 10 of 24 members affected in three generations showed that the candidate region for the dentin dysplasia type II gene overlaps the likely location of the gene for Shields type II dentinogenesis imperfecta. They suggested that a candidate gene for dentinogenesis imperfecta Shields type II and/or III should also be a candidate gene for dentin dysplasia type II. Subsequently Rajpar and colleagues showed that a DSPP missense mutation was present in a family with dentin dysplasia type II, thereby confirming the hypothesis of Dean and colleagues.[83,84] Further analysis of the DSPP gene in patients with Shields type II dentinogenesis imperfecta or dentin dysplasia type II suggests that these dominant phenotypes result from the disruption of signal peptide-processing and/or related biochemical events that interferes with protein processing.[85] This is consistent with the assertion that dentin dysplasia type II and Shields type II dentinogenesis imperfecta are milder and more severe forms, respectively, of the same developmental disease.[86]

AMELOGENESIS IMPERFECTA

As noted in Chapter 6, amelogenesis imperfecta is a developmental defect of the enamel with a heterogeneous etiology that affects the enamel of both the primary and permanent dentition. The anomaly occurs in the general population with an incidence of 1 in 14,000 to 1 in 16,000. Amelogenesis imperfecta has a wide range of clinical appearances with three broad categories observed: the hypocalcified type, the hypomaturation type, and the hypoplastic type. Although amelogenesis imperfecta can occur as a part of several syndromes, Cartwright and colleagues confirmed that the trait itself could also be associated with a skeletal anterior open bite,[87] although the pathophysiologic relationship between amelogenesis imperfecta and open bite remains unclear.[88]

Progress has been made in unraveling the molecular basis of the myriad clinical forms of amelogenesis imperfecta. Aldred and Crawford discussed the limitations of the existing classification systems and proposed an alternative classification based on the molecular defect, biochemical result, mode of inheritance, and phenotype.[89] Hart and colleagues recommended a standardized nomenclature for describing amelogenesis imperfecta that causes alterations at the genomic, complementary DNA, and protein levels.[90,91] Two clinically distinct forms of autosomal dominant amelogenesis imperfecta—smooth hypoplastic amelogenesis imperfecta and local hypoplastic amelogenesis imperfecta—are associated with mutations in the enamelin (ENAM) gene located at 4q21. In addition, autosomal dominant amelogenesis imperfecta can be associated with mutation in the Kallikrein-4 (KLK4) gene, and autosomal recessive pigmented hypomaturation amelogenesis imperfecta with an enamelysin (MMP-20) gene mutation, illustrating the heterogeneity of the condition. An X-linked form (AIH1) has been found to be associated with as many as 14 mutations in the amelogenin (AMELX) gene, located at Xp21.[92] However, at least one family has had the trait linked to another location on the chromosome Xq22-q28.[93]

The defective tooth structure is limited to the enamel. On radiographic examination the pulpal outline appears to be normal, and the root morphology is not unlike that of normal teeth. The difference in the appearance and quality of the enamel is thought to be attributable to the state of enamel development at the time the defect occurs. In the hypoplastic type, the enamel matrix appears to be imperfectly formed; although calcification subsequently occurs in the matrix and the enamel is hard, it is defective in amount and has a roughened, pitted surface (Fig. 7-32). In the hypocalcified type, matrix formation appears to be of normal thickness, but calcification is deficient and the enamel is soft (Fig. 7-33). In both of these more common types of the defect, the enamel becomes stained because of the roughness of the surface and the increased permeability.

In still another variant of amelogenesis imperfecta a thin, smooth covering of brownish yellow enamel is present. In this type the enamel does not seem excessively susceptible to abrasion or caries (Figs. 7-34 and 7-35).

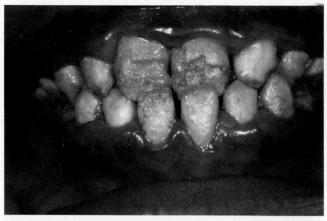

Figure 7-32 Both the primary and permanent teeth are affected by the hereditary anomaly amelogenesis imperfecta. The enamel is pitted but hard.

Congleton and Burkes reported three cases of amelogenesis imperfecta in which the patients also demonstrated taurodontism.[94] Others have identified cases with the clinical appearance of amelogenesis imperfecta and taurodontism along with strikingly curly hair and increased bone density (especially of the skull), which has been identified as trichodento-osseous syndrome (TDO). Seow has suggested that some cases reported as amelogenesis imperfecta with taurodontism were actually cases of trichodento-osseous syndrome.[95] Price and colleagues found that this autosomal dominant condition is caused by a mutation in the distal-less homeobox gene DLX3.[96] Even though the taurodontism and amelogenesis imperfecta traits in this condition are fully penetrant in affected individuals, the osseous and hair features are variably expressed even when the same deletion is present in a family—findings that indicate that the variable expression is influenced by other genes and/or environmental factors, although further studies by Price and colleagues indicated that trichodento-osseous syndrome and amelogenesis imperfecta of the hypomaturation-hypoplastic

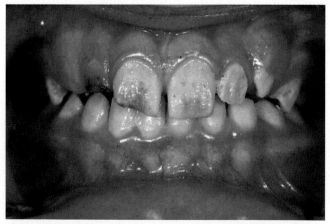

Figure 7-33 Hypocalcification type of amelogenesis imperfecta. The primary teeth were similarly affected. The enamel surface is soft.

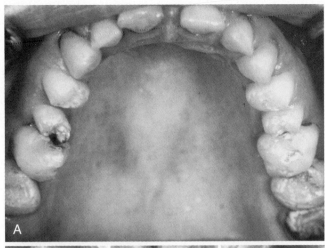

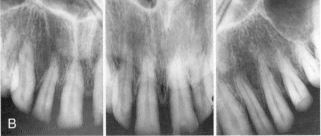

Figure 7-34 A, Case diagnosed as amelogenesis imperfecta. The permanent teeth have a thin covering of pigmented enamel. **B,** The radiographs show essentially normal root morphology. The crowns have a thin covering of enamel.

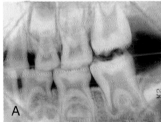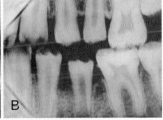

Figure 7-35 A and **B,** Left bite-wing radiographs of a patient with amelogenesis imperfecta. Radiograph in **B** was made 6 years after radiograph in **A** and demonstrates the maintenance of a caries free dentition despite the thin enamel.

type with taurodontism are two genetically distinct conditions.[97] Dong and colleagues found a mutation within the DLX3 gene homeodomain is associated with amelogenesis imperfecta (hypoplastic-hypomaturation type) with taurodontism (AIHHT). Because a DLX3 mutation outside the homeodomain is associated with trichodento-osseous syndrome (TDO), they suggested that TDO and some forms of AIHHT are allelic.[98]

The treatment of teeth with amelogenesis imperfecta– like defects depends on its severity and the demands of aesthetic improvement. When indicated, the teeth can be prepared for full-coverage restorations. For some cases of the hypomaturation and hypoplastic types, bonded veneer restorations may offer a more conservative alternative for management of the aesthetic problem of the anterior teeth. Patel and colleagues have reported successful treatment with porcelain laminate veneer restorations.[99]

ENAMEL AND DENTIN APLASIA

Teeth that have some characteristics of both dentinogenesis imperfecta and amelogenesis imperfecta have been described in the literature. Chaudhry and colleagues reported such a case and called the condition *odontogenesis imperfecta.*[100]

Schimmelpfennig and McDonald observed a similar dentition and termed it *enamel and dentin aplasia.*[101] The primary teeth were essentially devoid of enamel, and the smooth, severely abraded dentin was reddish brown. Radiographs showed normal alveolar bone around the roots of the teeth. Two teeth had pulp exposure and pulpal degeneration (Fig. 7-36). Radiolucent areas were present at the apices of the two primary teeth, with exposed and degenerated pulps. The pulp chambers and canals in all the primary teeth were extremely large, with no evidence that they were becoming obliterated. In ground sections of the primary teeth the dentinal tubules showed little evidence of a normal growth pattern. They were few and irregular, with a tendency toward branching. The cementum appeared normal and was acellular. No evidence of secondary dentin formation was found. A few fragments of enamel adhering to the dentin appeared thinner than normal, and few normal morphologic characteristics were present. The dentinoenamel junction was atypical in that it lacked the characteristic scalloping.

The permanent teeth, when they erupted, were partially covered with a thin, gray, poorly coalesced coating of enamel. Brown dentin could be seen on the labial aspect of the central incisors and at the base of the fissures of the first permanent molars. Stainless steel crown restorations were placed even before complete eruption to protect the teeth from continued abrasion.

AGENESIS OF TEETH

ANODONTIA

Anodontia, which implies complete failure of the teeth to develop, is a rare condition. Although agenesis of permanent teeth is often referred to as *congenital absence,* they would not, of course, be expected in the oral cavity at birth anyway. Gorlin and colleagues noted that, when agenesis occurs as an isolated trait, the primary dentition is not affected, and the inheritance is autosomal recessive.[102] Swallow reported on an 11-year-old boy who had a complete primary dentition but no permanent dentition.[103] Schneider also observed a 7-year-old white female with primary teeth but missing permanent teeth.[104] As is usually the case with presumed autosomal recessive inheritance, the hereditary background included no known consanguinity in the family or history of anodontia or ectodermal dysplasia in either the maternal or paternal

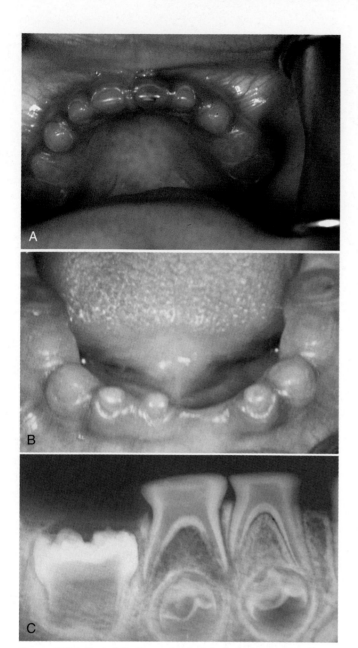

Figure 7-36 A and **B**, Severely abraded teeth are almost entirely devoid of enamel. The outline of a large pulp chamber can be seen through a thin covering of dentin. The mandibular second primary molars have pulp exposure. **C**, Radiograph shows large pulp canals and large pulp chambers. Apical rarefaction is associated with pulp exposure of the second primary molar.

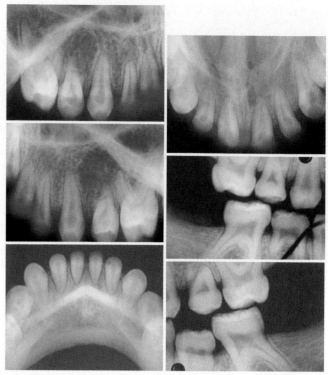

Figure 7-37 A complete primary dentition without evidence of permanent teeth in a 14-year-old girl.

lineages. Although consanguinity increases the likelihood that recessive traits or conditions will be expressed, most affected individuals do not have a family history of inbreeding. An overlay denture was constructed for the patient, which is often the treatment of choice. A comparable situation is shown in Fig. 7-37. Laird reported a similar patient in whom a complete primary dentition was present, but the only permanent teeth were maxillary first permanent molars.[105] Witkop studied two families in which both parents had peg or missing maxillary lateral incisors, which is an autosomal dominant trait with incomplete penetrance and variable expressivity, and concluded that agenesis of the permanent teeth can be an expression of the homozygous state of that gene.[106] This hypothesis is also supported by the findings in the family reported by Hoo.[107]

HYPODONTIA (OLIGODONTIA)

Agenesis of some teeth is referred to as *hypodontia*, which is preferable to the term *partial anodontia*. *Oligodontia* is sometimes used when only a few teeth develop. Hypodontia may occur without a family history of hypodontia, although it is often familial. It may also be found as a part of a syndrome, especially in an ectodermal dysplasia, although it usually occurs alone (isolated). Note that *isolated* in this usage means not occurring as part of a syndrome. It may still be familial.

Any one of the 32 permanent teeth may be missing. However, those most frequently missing in children are the mandibular second premolars, maxillary lateral incisors, and maxillary second premolars. This order of frequency has been confirmed in studies by Glenn[108] and by Grahnen.[109] The absence of teeth may be unilateral or bilateral. Glenn observed during an examination of 1702 children that 5% had a missing permanent tooth other than a third molar.[108] In 97% of the children, the formation of the second premolar could be detected radiographically at 5.5 years of age and that of the lateral incisor at 3.5 years of age.

In addition to the already mentioned autosomal dominant hypoplasia or agenesis of the maxillary lateral incisors, Vastardis and colleagues found absence of second premolars in one family showing an autosomal dominant pattern of inheritance to be caused by a mutation in the MSX1 gene located at 4p16.1.[110] In contrast, evidence for the genetic heterogeneity of hypodontia is provided by the finding of a frameshift mutation (resulting in premature termination of translation and a shortened protein) in the human PAX9 gene in a large family with autosomal dominant oligodontia.[111] X-linked inheritance of oligodontia or hypodontia through four generations of a family was described by Erpenstein and Pfeiffer.[112] Not only was there no male-to-male transmission, but males had oligodontia while females had hypodontia. Ahmad and colleagues demonstrated that hypodontia inherited in an autosomal recessive mode and associated with malformation of teeth, enamel hypoplasia, and failure of eruption could be linked to 16q12.1.[113]

Bennett and Ronk reported an unusual case of a 4-year-old boy with three missing primary teeth.[114] The mother related that the two missing mandibular central incisors erupted a few days after birth (neonatal teeth) and were removed because of a lack of root formation. The maxillary left first primary molar was congenitally missing as well. A panoramic radiograph of the patient also revealed the absence of multiple permanent tooth buds. The child did not exhibit any other signs or symptoms; he appeared normal in every other way, and there was no known familial history of missing teeth. A rare finding of nine congenitally missing primary teeth in a 3-year-old boy has been reported by Shashikiran and colleagues.[115] The boy's mother gave a history of consanguineous marriage. There was no known family history of missing teeth even among the patient's siblings. The primary teeth that were present appeared normal clinically and radiographically. The boy also exhibited ankyloglossia, and the frenum attachments were high in both arches. He did not show any evidence of other ectodermal disorders and otherwise appeared to be a normal young child.

Fleming and associates have reported that a missing maxillary central incisor may occur as an isolated dental finding.[116] This anomaly has also been reported to occur in association with growth retardation with or without growth hormone deficiency, in association with autosomal dominant holoprosencephaly, and occasionally in association with other midline developmental defects. As already stated in the discussion of fusion of teeth, children with this dental anomaly should be referred for medical follow-up unless a comprehensive evaluation for a diagnosis has already been performed. Growth hormone therapy or some other form of treatment may be indicated.

In addition to a number of syndromes including the ectodermal dysplasias in which tooth agenesis may be a feature, hypodontia may be associated with other dental anomalies such as small and short crowns and roots of the teeth that are present, conical crown shape, enamel hypoplasia, taurodontism, delayed eruption, prolonged retention of primary teeth, infraocclusion of primary teeth, ectopic eruption, transposition, lack of alveolar bone, reduced vertical dimensions, increased overbite, and tooth impaction (particularly palatally displaced canines).[117]

HYPODONTIA AND PALATALLY DISPLACED CANINES

The canine impacted or displaced palatally occurs in 85% of the cases and is not typically associated with dental crowding.[118] Palatally displaced canines are frequently, but not always, found in dentitions with various anomalies. These include small, peg-shaped or missing maxillary lateral incisors, hypodontia involving other teeth, dentition spacing, and dentitions with delayed development.[119] There is a greater likelihood of a palatally displaced canine on the same side of a missing or small maxillary lateral incisor, emphasizing a local environmental effect.[120] There are also cases in which a canine is palatally displaced without an apparent anomaly of the maxillary lateral incisors, and cases in which there are missing lateral incisors without palatal displacement of a canine. Adding to the complexity is the heterogeneity found in studies of cases of both bucally displaced canines,[121] and palatally displaced canines.[119] While the canine eruption theory of guidance by the lateral incisor root cannot explain all instances of palatally displaced canines, it does seem to play some role in some cases.[122]

Maxillary canine impaction or displacement is labial/buccal to the arch in 15% of the cases of maxillary canine impaction, and in contrast to palatal displacement being associated with small maxillary teeth,[123] is often associated with dental crowding.[118] Because there are varying degrees of genetic influence on these anomalies, there has been some discussion about palatally displaced canines themselves also being influenced by genetic factors to some degree. With apparent genetic and environmental factors playing some variable role in these cases, the etiology appears to be multifactorial.[124] This is supported by the occurrence of palatally displaced canines occurring in a higher percentage within families than in the general population.[125] Generally the phenotype is the result of some genetic influences (either or both directly or indirectly, e.g., though a primary effect on development of some or all of the rest of the dentition) interacting with environmental factors. Some of these cases may be examples of how primary genetic influences (which still interact with other genes and environmental factors) affect a phenotypic expression that is a variation in a local environment, such as the physical structure of the lateral incisor in relation to the developing canine.[126]

HYPODONTIA (OLIGODONTIA) AND CANCER

Recently it has been realized that hypodontia may be an indicator of susceptibility for developing cancer. A striking example of this was reported in a Finnish family in which oligodontia and colorectal cancer were associated with each other with autosomal dominant inheritance. The oligodontia and cancer predisposition were caused by a nonsense mutation in the AXIN2 gene, a Wnt-signaling regulator. Colorectal cancer or precancerous lesions in the family were found only in association with oligodontia and the AXIN2 mutation, and affected all those of the oldest generation who had the mutation. A different type of de novo mutation (frameshift) in the same gene was found in an unrelated young patient with oligodontia. Both mutations are expected to inactivate the AXIN2 protein function, leading to an increase in Wnt signaling, which may lead to cancer development. This change in AXIN2 protein function also clearly changes the network signaling involved in dental development.[127]

Further support for the proposition that hypodontia can be developmentally associated with cancer comes from the University of Kentucky report that women with epithelial ovarian cancer (EOC) are 8.1 times more likely to have hypodontia than are women without EOC. In contrast to the oligodontia reported with the specific mutations in the AXIN2 gene, the severity of hypodontia was similar between the two groups (affected and nonaffected) in the Kentucky study, with one or two teeth being agenic. Maxillary lateral incisors followed by second premolars were the most frequently affected teeth.[128] These findings are an example of how changes in the protein products of genes can have pleiotropic effects on different parts of the body at different times. Future studies into the family history and genotypes of individuals with hypodontia will help illustrate what the relative risk may be of individuals or family members developing cancer associated with hypodontia in the general population.

ECTODERMAL DYSPLASIAS

The congenital absence of primary teeth is relatively rare. When a number of the primary teeth fail to develop, other ectodermal deficiencies are usually evident. There are more than 100 types of ectodermal dysplasia with varying anomalies of ectodermal derivatives, including both the primary and permanent teeth, hair, nails, and skin. Children with a number of missing primary and permanent teeth may have some or all of the signs of a type of ectodermal dysplasia and should undergo further evaluation.

One of the more common types of ectodermal dysplasia is X-linked recessive hypohidrotic ectodermal dysplasia (XLHED), also called anhidrotic ectodermal dysplasia and Christ-Siemens-Touraine syndrome. A rare autosomal recessive form also occurs that is clinically indistinguishable from XLHED. Hypodontia and dental hypoplasia, as well as hypotrichosis, hypohydrosis/anhidrosis, and asteatosis are characteristic of XLHED. Secondary characteristics include a deficiency in salivary flow, protuberant lips, and a saddle-nose appearance. The skin is often dry and scaly, and there is fissuring at the corners of the mouth. Mutations in the EDA1 gene have been found in most patients with XLHED.[129]

Because the absence of teeth predisposes the child to a lack of alveolar process growth, the construction of dentures is complicated. However, as might be expected in at least most types of ectodermal dysplasia, skeletal structures are normal. Serial lateral cephalograms obtained during childhood and adolescence have shown that the sagittal development of the jaw occurs in an essentially normal manner. A deficiency in sweat glands causes a predisposition to increased body temperature,

and children with hypohidrosis/anhidrosis are extremely uncomfortable during hot weather. Many of them must reside in cool climates. Children with an ectodermal dysplasia usually have normal mentality and a normal life expectancy. Consanguinity increases the likelihood of expression of a trait or condition that is inherited in a recessive manner (Fig. 7-38) and may be one way a female with a normal karyotype can be affected.

The primary teeth that are present may be normal or reduced in size. The anterior teeth are often conical, which is characteristic of oligodontia associated with many types of ectodermal dysplasia. The primary molars without permanent successors have a tendency to become ankylosed.

The many types of ectodermal dysplasia with different modes of inheritance can be emphasized by describing a "tooth and nail" type of autosomal dominant ectodermal dysplasia, also called *Witkop syndrome*, reported by Giansanti and associates.[130] This ectodermal dysplasia is characterized by hypoplastic nails and hypodontia. A different mutation in the MSX1 gene than that found when only hypodontia is present has been reported in a family with tooth and nail syndrome by Jumlongras and colleagues.[131] In contrast to most nonsyndromic hypodontias, in which (excluding third molars) premolars and maxillary lateral incisors are most often missing, the mandibular incisors, second molars, and maxillary canines are most frequently absent. Overall, the teeth are generally not affected to the extent seen in XLHED, and there can be little involvement of the hair and sweat glands.[132]

For children with a large number of missing primary teeth, partial dentures can be constructed at an early age. Two-year-old and 3-year-old children have worn partial dentures successfully. Their ability to masticate food increases, and their nutritional status may improve. A partial denture can be adjusted or remade at intervals to allow for the eruption of permanent teeth. Denture construction at an early age may also reduce the psychologic problem of the child's feeling "different" (Fig. 7-39).

If the permanent teeth erupt in good position and in favorable relationship to each other, partial dentures may serve until the child is old enough for implants or a fixed partial denture as described in Chapter 22. Orthodontic and surgical procedures may be necessary before the prosthodontic treatment.

Bonding techniques have improved the ability to provide aesthetic interim restorations and greater function for patients with conical teeth with or without oligodontia or hypodontia. Nunn and colleagues published a series of five papers (monthly, beginning in the March 2003 *British Dental Journal*) that outline the management of patients with hypodontia by a coordinated interdisciplinary team of dentists and demonstrate the advantages of this approach.[133] Several dental specialties are represented on the team. Ideally, the initial responsibility for oversight and coordination of the patient's care begins in infancy with the services of a pediatric dentist. As the patient grows and develops through puberty, a general

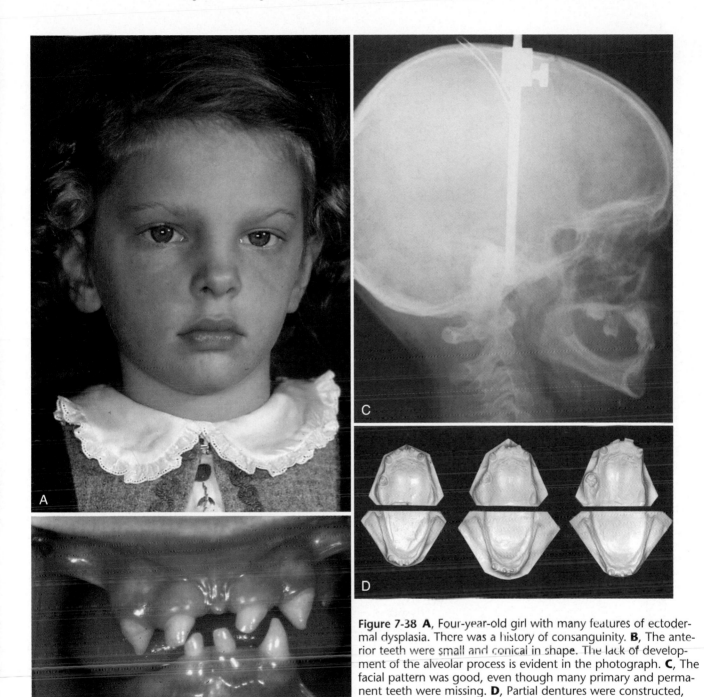

Figure 7-38 A, Four-year-old girl with many features of ectodermal dysplasia. There was a history of consanguinity. **B**, The anterior teeth were small and conical in shape. The lack of development of the alveolar process is evident in the photograph. **C**, The facial pattern was good, even though many primary and permanent teeth were missing. **D**, Partial dentures were constructed, modified, and remade as additional teeth erupted. The models show how growth has occurred in the mandible and maxilla.

family practitioner may assume the oversight and coordination responsibilities.

When maxillary lateral incisors are missing, the occlusion and arches must be analyzed carefully to determine whether there is sufficient room within the arch to maintain space and to provide fixed bridgework. If space for a normal-sized lateral incisor replacement is insufficient, the clinician may sometimes choose to move the canine forward into the lateral position and reshape it to make it appear more like a permanent lateral incisor.

INTRINSIC DISCOLORATION OF TEETH (PIGMENTATION OF TEETH)

The primary teeth occasionally have unusual pigmentation. Certain conditions arising from the pulp can cause the whole tooth to appear discolored. Factors causing these conditions include bloodborne pigment, blood decomposition within the pulp, and drugs used in procedures such as root canal therapy. Color changes in relation to trauma are discussed in Chapter 21.

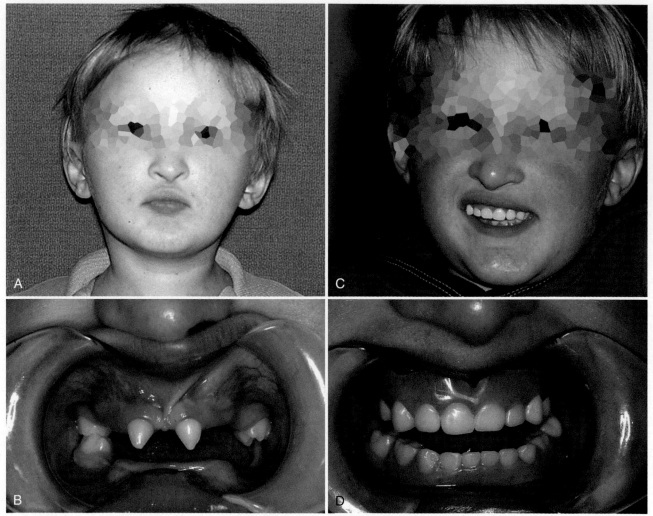

Figure 7-39 A, Four-year-old boy with characteristics of ectodermal dysplasia. Many primary and permanent teeth are congenitally missing. The skin is dry, and the hair is sparse. **B,** The anterior primary teeth are typically conical. **C** and **D,** A full maxillary overdenture and partial mandibular denture were constructed.

DISCOLORATION IN HYPERBILIRUBINEMIA

Excess levels of bilirubin are released into the circulating blood in a number of conditions.[134] If teeth are developing during periods of hyperbilirubinemia they may become intrinsically stained. The two most common disorders that cause this intrinsic staining are erythroblastosis fetalis and biliary atresia. Other less common causes are premature birth, ABO blood type incompatibility, neonatal respiratory distress, significant internal hemorrhage, congenital hypothyroidism, biliary hypoplasia, tyrosinemia, α1-antitrypsin deficiency, and neonatal hepatitis.

Erythroblastosis fetalis results from the transplacental passage of maternal antibody active against red blood cell antigens of the infant, which leads to an increased rate of red blood cell destruction.[135] It is a significant cause of anemia and jaundice in newborn infants despite the development of a method of prevention of maternal isoimmunization by Rh antigens; however, an infant from an Rh-negative mother's first pregnancy rarely contracts this hemolytic disease.

If an infant has had severe, persistent jaundice during the neonatal period, the primary teeth may have a characteristic blue-green color, although in a few instances brown teeth have been observed (Fig. 7-40). The color of the pigmented tooth is gradually reduced. The fading in color is particularly noticeable in the anterior teeth.

Cullen reported on the occurrence of erythroblastosis fetalis produced by Kell immunization.[136] In utero, the maternal antibodies coat the fetal red blood cells and cause hemolysis. The fetus develops anemia with a resultant increase in the bilirubin content of the amniotic fluid. The newborn appears pale and anemic. Shortly after birth, jaundice occurs as a result of the high bilirubin levels.

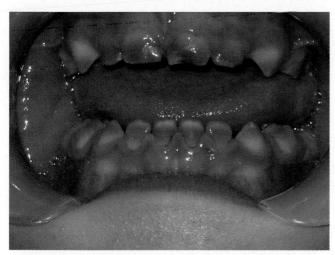

Figure 7-40 Characteristic blue-green discoloration of the primary teeth in an infant that suffered from persistent jaundice in the neonatal period.

DISCOLORATION IN PORPHYRIA

The porphyrias are inherited and acquired disorders in which the activities of the enzymes of the heme biosynthetic pathway are partially or almost completely deficient.[137] As a result, abnormally elevated levels of porphyrins and/or their precursors are produced, accumulate in tissues, and are excreted. Congenital erythropoietic porphyria (Günther disease) is a rare autosomal recessive form of the disease.

Children with congenital erythropoietic porphyria have red-colored urine, are hypersensitive to light, and develop subepidermal bullous lesions when their skin is exposed to sunlight. Their primary teeth are purplish brown as a result of the deposition of porphyrin in the developing structures. The permanent teeth also show evidence of intrinsic staining but to a lesser degree.

DISCOLORATION IN CYSTIC FIBROSIS

Cystic fibrosis is an inherited, chronic, multisystem, life-shortening disorder characterized primarily by obstruction and infection of the airways and poor digestion. It is autosomal recessive and is caused by mutations in both copies of the cystic fibrosis transmembrane regulator gene (CFTR). Zegarelli and colleagues have suggested that tooth discoloration in persons with cystic fibrosis is a result of the disease alone; of therapeutic agents, especially tetracyclines; or of a combination of the two factors.[138] The possibility that there is at least in part an intrinsic developmental enamel abnormality secondary to the disease is supported by the investigations of Wright and associates, who found abnormal enamel in the incisors of homozygous CFTR knockout mice.[139] Further studies by Arquitt and colleagues also strongly suggest that CFTR plays an important role in enamel formation.[140]

Although many patients with cystic fibrosis who lived during the latter half of the twentieth century endured unsightly discolorations of their teeth because they received tetracycline therapy during a period when their tooth crowns were forming, modern physicians rarely, if ever, prescribe tetracyclines for any patients during their tooth-forming years. During the era when tetracycline therapy for children was common, Primosch reported on tetracycline tooth discolorations, enamel defects, and dental caries in 86 young patients with cystic fibrosis.[141] The incidence of dental caries in these patients was compared to that in control subjects matched for sex, race, exposure to optimally fluoridated water, chronologic age, and dental age. The findings indicated a high prevalence of tooth discolorations and enamel defects but a significantly reduced caries experience in the patients with cystic fibrosis who had received the tetracycline drugs.

DISCOLORATION IN TETRACYCLINE THERAPY

Dentists and physicians have observed that children who have received tetracycline therapy during the period of calcification of the primary or permanent teeth show a degree of pigmentation of the clinical crowns of the teeth. As van der Bijl and Pitigoi-Aron pointed out, because the tetracyclines chelate calcium salts, the drugs are incorporated into bones and teeth during calcification.[142] The crowns of affected teeth are discolored, ranging from yellow to brown and from gray to black (Fig. 7-41). Currently most, if not all, infections in children can be treated effectively with antibiotics that do not cause tooth discoloration. Consequently this previously common problem is now rarely encountered.

Tetracycline is deposited in the dentin and to a lesser extent in the enamel of teeth that are calcifying during the time the drug is administered. The location of the pigment in the tooth can be correlated with the stage of development of the tooth and the time and duration of drug administration. The tetracyclines, which are yellow, fluoresce under ultraviolet light. When tetracyclines in the dental structures darken from yellow to brown, the fluorescence diminishes because of the destruction of the fluorophores.

The exposure of the teeth to light results in slow oxidation, with a change in color of the pigment from yellow

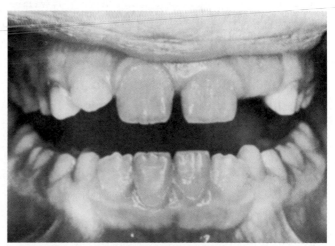

Figure 7-41 Pigmentation in tetracycline therapy. The permanent incisors that have erupted show a yellowish brown color.

to brown. The larger the dose of drug relative to body weight, the deeper the pigmentation. The duration of exposure to the drug may be less important than the total dose relative to body weight.

Because tetracyclines can be transferred through the placenta, the crowns of the primary teeth may also show noticeable discoloration if tetracyclines are administered during pregnancy. Moffitt and colleagues have observed that the critical period for tetracycline-related discoloration in the primary dentition is 4 months in utero to 3 months postpartum for maxillary and mandibular incisors and 5 months in utero to 9 months postpartum for maxillary and mandibular canines.[143]

The sensitive period for tetracycline-induced discoloration in the permanent maxillary and mandibular incisors and canines is 3 to 5 months postpartum to about the 7th year of the child's life. The maxillary lateral incisors are an exception because they begin to calcify at 10 to 12 months postpartum.

In addition to fluoride and the tetracyclines (including minocycline), ciprofloxacin has been associated with intrinsic staining. Medications that have been reported to cause extrinsic staining include chlorhexidine, oral iron salts, co-amoxiclav, and essential oils.[144]

BLEACHING OF INTRINSIC TOOTH DISCOLORATION

Vital bleaching of intrinsically discolored teeth became a popular dental cosmetic procedure during the late twentieth century (Fig. 7-42). Several safe techniques are available to achieve tooth bleaching. The accepted procedures incorporate the use of a peroxide compound placed on the tooth surface that bleaches the intrinsic tooth pigments to a lighter hue. Adding energy to the peroxide compound, as in the form of heat, light, or laser radiation, may accelerate this process.

Although many dilute tooth-bleaching products are available over the counter, the most efficient and effective systems are provided or prescribed by a dentist. To be safe, bleaching procedures must be carefully performed and monitored. Although these procedures are usually performed on permanent teeth, Brantley and associates reported successfully bleaching discolored primary teeth in a 4-year-old girl.[145]

Refer to current textbooks on endodontics or cosmetic dentistry for more information on bleaching techniques. Another valuable resource with considerable detailed information is the Special Supplement of the *Journal of the American Dental Association*, volume 128, April 1997. This supplement provides reports by numerous recognized bleaching experts presented during an international symposium on the subject of nonrestorative treatment of discolored teeth.

If the tooth discoloration is severe and bleaching does not adequately improve the condition, the dentist may consider masking the visible surfaces with bonded veneer restorations similar to those discussed in Chapter 18. Bleaching and enamel microabrasion may be used in combination for certain types of discoloration, and these procedures may also be used as adjunctive steps before placement of veneer restorations.

MICROGNATHIA

Micrognathia is usually considered a congenital anomaly; however, the condition may be acquired in later life. The mandible is most often affected (Fig. 7-43). The etiology of congenital micrognathia appears to be heterogeneous. Deficient nutrition of the mother and intrauterine injury resulting from pressure or trauma have been suggested as possible causes. In addition, micrognathia may be part of the Robin sequence, which also includes cleft palate (especially in the posterior with a rounded distal edge) and glossoptosis. Although this developmental sequence may be sporadic, it is often the pleiotropic expression of a gene for a condition such as Stickler syndrome or velocardiofacial syndrome and warrants a clinical genetic evaluation.[146]

Infants with mandibular micrognathia have difficulty breathing and experience episodes of cyanosis; they must be kept in a ventral position as much as possible. The anterior portion of the mandible is positioned so that the tongue has little if any support and can fall backward, causing an obstruction.

Based on longitudinal growth studies, Pruzansky and Richmond reported that, in most instances of congenital micrognathia, the increment in mandibular growth as related to total facial growth during infancy and early childhood is sufficient to overcome the extreme recessiveness of the chin at birth.[147] This is often referred to as "catch-up growth." Daskalogiannakis and colleagues performed 29 cephalometric measurements, taken at three different ages, on 96 patients with Robin sequence and compared them with similar measurements in 50 patients with isolated clefting of the palate (control group).[148] They found that patients with Robin sequence had significantly smaller mandibles than the control group from approximately 5.5 years of age to 17 years of age. This finding suggests that the mandibles of patients with Robin sequence do not really grow proportionately more than those in others not affected by the disorder.

The nursing bottle may be used in the treatment of congenital micrognathia to help promote adequate function of the mandible. Because the infant should be made to reach for the nipple of the nursing bottle, the bottle should never be allowed to rest against the mandible. The parent is instructed to sit the infant on his or her lap in an upright position and place gentle forward pressure on

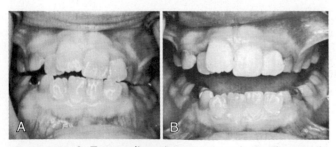

Figure 7-42 A, Tetracycline-pigmented teeth. **B,** The maxillary incisors have been bleached; the lower mandibular incisors are untreated.

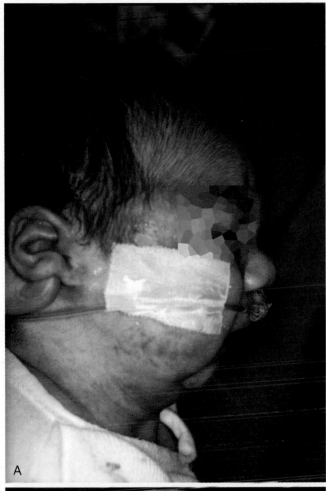

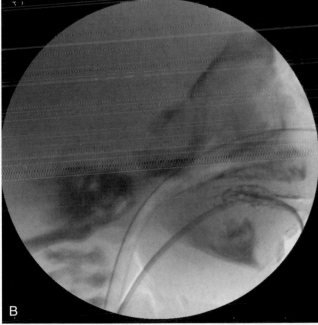

Figure 7-43 A, Micrognathia in a girl 1 month of age. The chin was noticeably recessive. **B**, The radiograph shows the extent of the development of the dentition at birth. When the patient was 1 year of age, the micrognathia was less noticeable.

the child's ramus with the thumb and fingers while offering the bottle. Thus the infant must extend the mandible to feed. Mandibular advancement by orthopedic force is sometimes recommended by Strohecker and Lahey.[149] Surgical mandibular reconstruction in some cases is another option proposed by James and Ma.[150]

Hotz and Gnoinski have described the use of a special palatal obturator appliance to help infants born with Robin sequence.[151] In addition to providing coverage to seal the cleft palate, the appliance includes a posterior extension to simulate the missing soft palate structures including the uvula. The appliance seems to stimulate the infant to maintain a more normal tongue position. The improved tongue position significantly reduces the tendency for the infant to experience life-threatening apneic episodes. Dean and colleagues also reported successful use of similar appliances in infants with Robin sequence.[152] Their study included 22 infants with severe airway obstruction. Their results supported the use of the obturator, but they also concluded that further study of treatment with these appliances was needed.

Acquired micrognathia may develop gradually and may not be evident until 4 to 6 years of age. This anomaly in growth is usually related to heredity. Ankylosis of the jaw caused by a birth injury or trauma in later life may result in an acquired type of micrognathia. Infection in the temporomandibular joint area can also cause arrested growth at the head of the condyle and lead to development of the acquired pattern of micrognathia. In cases of true ankylosis of the mandible, arthroplasty should be recommended.

ANOMALIES OF THE TONGUE

Pediatric patients with unremarkable medical histories rarely complain of symptomatic tongue lesions. However, the tongue should be inspected carefully during the examination. Several benign conditions may be evident that should be brought to the attention of the parents.

Burket described four main types of papillae of the tongue.[153] Large circumvallate papillae, 10 to 15 in number, may be found on the posterior border of the dorsum. These papillae have a blood supply and are the site of numerous taste buds. Fungiform (mushroom-shaped) papillae may be distributed over the entire dorsum of the tongue; however, they are present in greater numbers at the tip and toward the lateral margins of the tongue. Inflammatory and atrophic changes occurring on the dorsum of the tongue may involve the vascularized fungiform papillae. The most numerous papillae of the tongue are the filiform papillae, which are thin and hairlike, and evenly distributed over the dorsal surface. The filiform papillae are without a vascular core, and their continuous growth is slight. The foliate papillae represent a fourth type and are arranged in folds along the lateral margins of the tongue; the taste sensation is associated with these papillae.

MACROGLOSSIA

Macroglossia refers to a larger than normal size of the tongue. This condition may be either congenital or acquired. Congenital macroglossia, which is caused by an overdevelopment of the lingual musculature or vascular tissues, becomes increasingly apparent as the child develops.

An abnormally large tongue is characteristic of hypothyroidism, in which case the tongue is fissured and may extend from the mouth. Macroglossia is also commonly observed with type 2 glycogen-storage disease, neurofibromatosis type 1, and Beckwith-Wiedemann syndrome. It can be an isolated and sporadic (nonfamilial) trait or a familial (autosomal dominant) trait as studied by Reynoso and colleagues.[154] Macroglossia has also been cited as a characteristic of Down syndrome. Occasionally an allergic reaction causes a transitory enlargement of the tongue (angioneurotic edema). Both allergic reaction and injury can cause such severe enlargement of the tongue that a tracheotomy is necessary to maintain a patent airway.

A disproportionately large tongue may cause both an abnormal growth pattern of the jaw and malocclusion. Flaring of the lower anterior teeth and an Angle class III malocclusion are occasionally the result of macroglossia.

The treatment of macroglossia depends on its cause and severity. Surgical reduction of a portion of the tongue is occasionally necessary.

ANKYLOGLOSSIA (TONGUE-TIE)

In ankyloglossia a short lingual frenum extending from the tip of the tongue to the floor of the mouth and onto the lingual gingival tissue limits movements of the tongue and causes speech difficulties (Fig. 7-44). Stripping of the lingual tissues may occur if the tongue-tie is not corrected. Surgical reduction of the abnormal lingual frenum is indicated if it interferes with the infant's nursing (lingual frenectomy, frenotomy, or frenuloplasty). In the older child a reduction of the frenum should be recommended only if local conditions or speech problems warrant the treatment.

Ayers and Hilton reported a case of ankyloglossia in a 7-year-old boy who had been evaluated at his school for a speech problem.[155] The patient previously had routine dental examinations, but no treatment had been suggested by the dentist. Tongue mobility and speech patterns improved greatly after the frenum attachment was released surgically. The patient and parents reported very little postoperative discomfort.

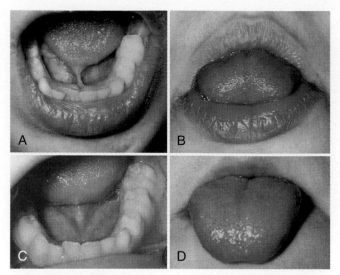

Figure 7-45 A, Ankyloglossia in a 6-year-old girl. **B**, Patient had limited tongue mobility and speech problems. **C**, Two weeks after surgical release. **D**, Tongue mobility and speech improved spontaneously.

This history and the results are similar to those of the 6-year-old girl with ankyloglossia illustrated in Fig. 7-45. Messner and Lalakea, after studying 30 children aged 1 to 12 years with ankyloglossia, concluded that tongue mobility and speech improve significantly after frenuloplasty.[156]

FISSURED TONGUE AND GEOGRAPHIC TONGUE (BENIGN MIGRATORY GLOSSITIS)

A fissured tongue is seen in a small number of children and may be of no clinical significance, although it is sometimes associated with hypothyroidism and Down syndrome. The fissures on the dorsum of the tongue usually have a symmetric pattern and may be longitudinal or at right angles to the margin of the tongue. Vitamin B–complex deficiency may be associated with the fissuring. Treatment of the fissured tongue is generally unnecessary unless a mild inflammation develops at the base of the fissures from an accumulation of food debris. Brushing of the tongue and improved oral hygiene aid in reducing the inflammation and soreness.

A wandering type of lesion and probably the most common tongue anomaly is known as *geographic tongue*. Rahamimoff and Muhsam observed a 14% prevalence of migratory glossitis in 5000 children 2 years old and younger.[157] Kleinman and colleagues reported a prevalence of geographic tongue of 0.6% in 39,206 children aged 5 to 17 years.[158] Meskin and colleagues observed the incidence of geographic tongue among college students to be 1.1%.[159]

Kullaa-Mikkonen studied the inheritance of fissured tongue in 31 families and concluded that fissured tongue with smooth-surfaced papillae is transmitted as an autosomal dominant trait with incomplete penetrance and is preceded by geographic tongue.[160] The severity of fissured tongue increased with age. Tongue fissuring with

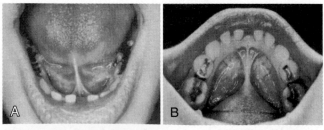

Figure 7-44 A, Ankyloglossia (tongue-tie). A short, heavy lingual frenum extends from the top of the tongue to the floor of the mouth and onto the lingual tissue. **B**, A mirror view of the abnormal frenum.

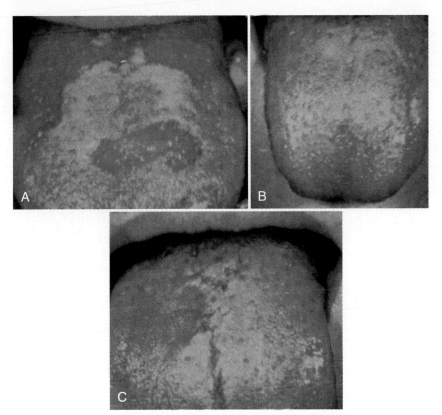

Figure 7-46 A, Geographic tongue. The smooth areas are devoid of filiform papillae. **B**, The pattern observed at the initial visit is indistinguishable 4 weeks later. **C**, In 1 year a new pattern is developing on the dorsum of the tongue.

normal-appearing filiform papillae was found not to be familial and was not associated with geographic tongue.

Geographic tongue is often detected during routine dental examination of pediatric patients who are unaware of the condition. Red, smooth areas devoid of filiform papillae appear on the dorsum of the tongue. The margins of the lesions are well developed and slightly raised. The involved areas enlarge and migrate by extension of the desquamation of the papillae at one margin of the lesion and regeneration at the other (Fig. 7-46). Every few days a change can be noted in the pattern of the lesions. The condition is self-limited, however, and no treatment is necessary.

Bánóczy and colleagues have indicated that gastrointestinal disturbances associated with anemia may be related to migratory glossitis.[161] In addition, a psychosomatic disorder should be considered as a possible etiologic factor. Histologically the process appears to be superficial, with desquamation of the keratin layers of papillae and inflammation of the corium.

COATED TONGUE

A white coating of the tongue is usually associated with local factors. The amount of coating on the tongue varies with the time of day and is related to oral hygiene and the character of the diet. The coating consists of food debris, microorganisms, and keratinized epithelium found on and around the filiform papillae (Fig. 7-47).

Children who have a congenital or acquired deficiency in salivary flow may have a coated tongue, occasionally to the extent that a dry crust appears on the dorsum of the tongue. Frequent rinsing with artificial saliva palliates the condition. Systemic disease with associated fever and dehydration may also cause a coating, which is usually

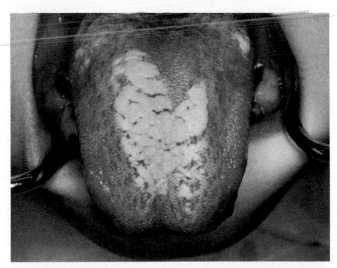

Figure 7-47 White coating of the tongue is usually associated with local factors.

white but may become stained with foods or drugs. In-creased ingestion of liquid is appropriate to alleviate this situation. Brushing the tongue with a toothbrush and dentifrice reduces the coating.

WHITE STRAWBERRY TONGUE

An enlargement of the fungiform papillae extending above the level of the white desquamating filiform pa-pillae gives the appearance of an unripe strawberry. The condition has been observed in cases of scarlet fever and Kawasaki disease in young children. During the course of scarlet fever and other acute febrile conditions the coating disappears, and the enlarged red papillae extend above a smooth denuded surface, which gives the appearance of a red strawberry or raspberry. The tongue returns to normal after recovery from the systemic condition.

BLACK HAIRY TONGUE

Black hairy tongue is rarely seen in children but occurs in young adults and has been related to the oral and sys-temic intake of antibiotics, smoking, and excessive inges-tion of dark drinks such as coffee and tea (Fig. 7-48). Ac-cumulations of keratin on the filiform papillae in the middle third of the tongue become elongated into hair-like processes, sometimes as long as 2.5 cm (1 inch). Neville and colleagues note that the cause is uncertain but that an apparent increase in keratin production or a decrease in normal keratin desquamation results.[134] It is a benign condition with no serious sequelae. Rigorous hy-gienic procedures such as brushing and scraping the tongue may help control it. When the condition appears during antibiotic therapy, it usually disappears again without specific treatment after the antibiotics are dis-continued.

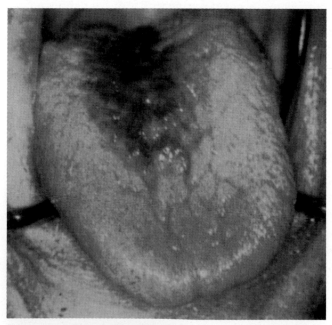

Figure 7-48 Black hairy tongue. This condition usually has no clinical significance.

INDENTATION OF THE TONGUE MARGIN (CRENATION)

During the examination of the pediatric patient, the den-tist may notice a scalloping or crenation along the lingual periphery. Careful examination will reveal the markings to be caused by the tongue's lying against the lingual surfaces of the mandibular teeth. Although usually no significance can be attached to these crenations, they have been related to pressure habits, macroglossia, vita-min B–complex deficiency, and systemic disease that causes a reduction of muscle tone.

MEDIAN RHOMBOID GLOSSITIS (CENTRAL PAPILLARY ATROPHY OF THE TONGUE)

Median rhomboid glossitis is an oval, rhomboid, or diamond-shaped reddish patch on the dorsal surface of the tongue immediately anterior to the circumvallate papillae. Flat, slightly raised, or nodular, it stands out distinctly from the rest of the tongue because it has no filiform papillae. This atrophic area is usually asymp-tomatic. Long believed to be a developmental anomaly, the condition is now recognized almost exclusively to represent a chronic, localized, and mild candidal infec-tion, as proposed by Cooke.[162]

Although median rhomboid glossitis occurs more of-ten in adults, it is sometimes seen in teenagers and even occurs infrequently in younger children. It has been observed with high prevalence in HIV-positive children by Barasch and colleagues.[163] Treatment with topical antifungal agents is appropriate.

TRAUMA TO THE TONGUE WITH EMPHASIS ON TONGUE PIERCING

A child may bite his or her tongue as a result of a traumatic blow or fall. The dentist may inadvertently traumatize the tongue with a cutting instrument during operative procedures. Deep laceration of the tongue re-quires suturing to minimize the scarring and to aid in hemorrhage control. In cases of severe injury, the tongue should be examined carefully to detect any enlargement that might interfere with the maintenance of an open airway.

Tongue piercing, a deliberate trauma, is one of the popular types of body piercing occurring in all parts of the world today, especially among teenagers and young adults (Fig. 7-49). Tongue piercing is of particular interest in dentistry because it carries a high risk of ad-verse intraoral sequelae and can have significant sys-temic effects as well. The scientific literature has ex-ploded with documented cases of complications following piercing procedures. Fractured teeth, dental abrasion, and gingival recession are reported to be com-mon sequelae.[164-166] Other observed complications with life-threatening potential include brain abscess,[167] ce-phalic tetanus,[168] endocarditis,[169] Ludwig angina,[170] and upper airway compromise.[171] Whenever appropriate, dentists should counsel their patients and other mem-bers of the community about the serious risks associated with this form of body art. If patients insist on wearing

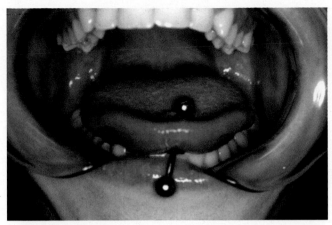

Figure 7-49 Tongue ornaments are popular among teenagers and young adults.

tongue ornaments and other such body jewelry, they should be advised at least to remove them during athletic activities in which the risk of injury is very high.[172]

ABNORMAL LABIAL FRENUM

A maxillary midline diastema is frequently seen in preschool children and in those in the mixed dentition stage. It is important to determine whether the diastema is normal for that particular time of development or is related to an abnormal maxillary labial frenum.

A midline diastema may be considered normal for many children during the time of eruption of the permanent maxillary central incisors. When the incisors first erupt, they may be separated by bone, and the crowns incline distally because of the crowding of the roots. With the eruption of the lateral incisors and the permanent canines, the midline diastema is reduced, and in most cases normal contact between the central incisors develops (see Fig. 27-55).

Insufficient tooth mass in the maxillary anterior region, the presence of peg lateral incisors, or the congenital absence of lateral incisors may cause a diastema. Other factors and anomalies, including a midline supernumerary tooth, an oral habit, macroglossia, and abnormally large mandibular anterior teeth, should be considered as possible causes (in addition to an abnormal labial frenum) of the midline diastema.

The labial frenum is composed of two layers of epithelium enclosing a loose vascular connective tissue. Muscle fibers, if present, are derived from the orbicularis oris muscle.

The origin of the maxillary frenum is at the midline on the inner surface of the lip. The origin is often wide, but the tissue of the frenum itself narrows in width and is inserted in the midline into the outer layer of periosteum and into the connective tissue of the internal maxillary suture and the alveolar process. The exact attachment site is variable. It can be several millimeters

above the crest of the ridge or on the ridge, or the fibers may pass between the central incisors and attach to the palatine papilla.

Many dentists delay considering an abnormal labial frenum as the cause of a diastema until all the maxillary permanent anterior teeth, including the canines, have erupted. This approach may be considered generally correct. However, other diagnostic points should be kept in mind.

One can carry out a simple diagnostic test for an abnormal frenum during mid to late mixed dentition by observing the location of the alveolar attachment when intermittent pressure is exerted on the frenum. If a heavy band of tissue with a broad, fanlike base is attached to the palatine papilla and produces blanching of the papilla, it is safe to predict that the frenum will unfavorably influence the development of the anterior occlusion (Fig. 7-50).

The abnormal labial frenum, in addition to causing a midline diastema, can produce other undesirable clinical conditions. The heavy band of tissue and low attachment can interfere with toothbrushing by making it difficult to place the brush at the proper level in the vestibule to brush in the conventional manner. If fibers of the frenum attach into the free marginal tissue, stretching of the lip during mastication and speech may cause stripping of the tissue from the neck of the tooth. Such attachment may also cause the accumulation of food particles and eventual pocket formation. The abnormal frenum may restrict movements of the lip, may interfere with speech, and may produce an undesirable cosmetic result (Fig. 7-51).

FRENECTOMY

The decision regarding treatment of the labial frenum should be made only after a careful evaluation to determine whether the result will be undesirable if the condition is allowed to remain.

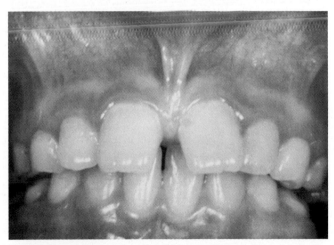

Figure 7-50 Abnormal labial frenum. There is blanching of the free marginal tissue between the central incisors and of the palatine papilla. A frenectomy is indicated.

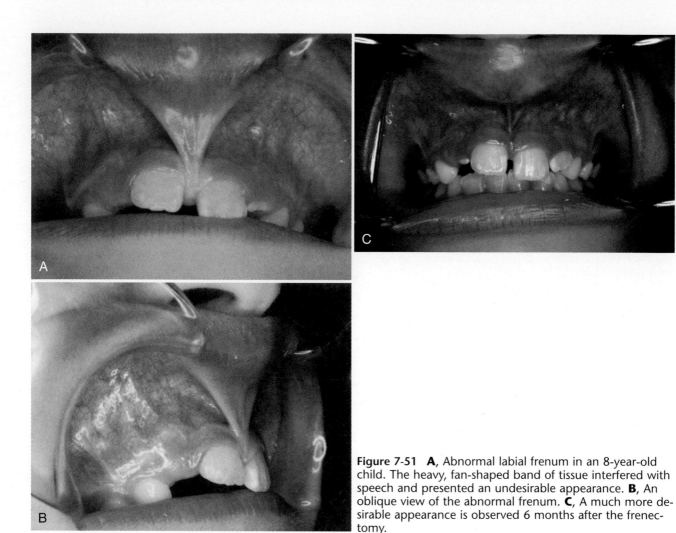

Figure 7-51 A, Abnormal labial frenum in an 8-year-old child. The heavy, fan-shaped band of tissue interfered with speech and presented an undesirable appearance. **B**, An oblique view of the abnormal frenum. **C**, A much more desirable appearance is observed 6 months after the frenectomy.

In the surgical technique, a wedge-shaped section of tissue is removed, including the tissue between the central incisors and the tissue extending palatally to the nasal palatine papilla (Figs. 7-51 and 7-52). Lateral incisions are made on either side of the frenum to the depth of the underlying bone. The free marginal tissue on the mesial side of the central incisors should not be disturbed. The wedge of tissue can be picked up with tissue forceps and excised with tissue shears at an area close enough to the origin of the frenum to provide a desirable cosmetic effect. Sutures are placed inside the lip to approximate the free tissue margins. It is generally unnecessary to suture or pack the tissue between the incisors.

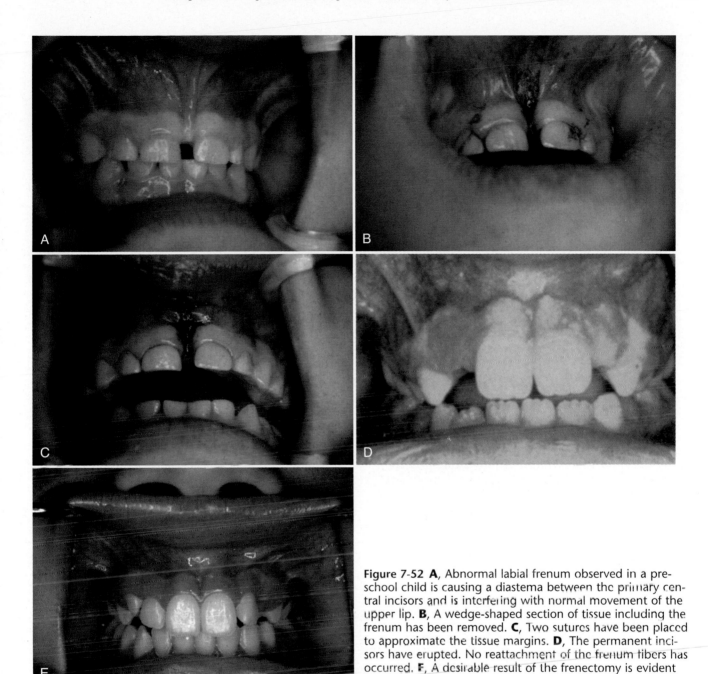

Figure 7-52 A, Abnormal labial frenum observed in a preschool child is causing a diastema between the primary central incisors and is interfering with normal movement of the upper lip. **B**, A wedge-shaped section of tissue including the frenum has been removed. **C**, Two sutures have been placed to approximate the tissue margins. **D**, The permanent incisors have erupted. No reattachment of the frenum fibers has occurred. **F**, A desirable result of the frenectomy is evident 5 years after the surgical procedure.

REFERENCES

1. US Department of Health and Human Services. Oral health in America: A report of the Surgeon General. Rockville, Md, US Department of Health and Human Services, National Institute of Dental and Craniofacial Research, National Institutes of Health, 2000.
2. Molinari JA. Microbial disease trends and acquired antibiotic resistance: Part 1, *Compend Contin Educ Dent* 18(2): 106-108, 1997.
3. Bader G. Odontomatosis (multiple odontomas), *Oral Surg Oral Med Oral Pathol* 23(6):770-773, 1967.
4. Delany GM, Goldblatt LI. Fused teeth: a multidisciplinary approach to treatment, *J Am Dent Assoc* 103(5): 732-734, 1981.
5. Eidelman E. Fusion of maxillary primary central and lateral incisors bilaterally, *Pediatr Dent* 3(4):346-347, 1981.
6. Nanni L et al. SHH mutation is associated with solitary median maxillary central incisor: a study of 13 patients and review of the literature, *Am J Med Genet* 102(1):1-10, 2001.
7. Holan G. Dens invaginatus in a primary canine: a case report, *Int J Paediatr Dent* 8(1):61-64, 1998.
8. Kupietzky A. Detection of dens invaginatus in a one-year old infant, *Pediatr Dent* 22(2):148-150, 2000.
9. Eden EK, Koca H, Sen BH. Dens invaginatus in a primary molar: report of case, *ASDC J Dent Child* 69(1): 49-53, 2002.
10. Grahnen H, Lindahl B, Omnell KA. Dens invaginatus. I. A clinical, roentgenological and genetical study of permanent upper lateral incisors, *Odont Rev* 10:115-137, 1959.

11. Hu CC et al. A clinical and research protocol for characterizing patients with hypophosphatasia, *Pediatr Dent* 18(1):17-23, 1996.
12. Scriver CR, Cameron D. Pseudohypophosphatasia, *N Engl J Med* 281(11):604-606, 1969.
13. Ayoub AF, el-Mofty SS. Cherubism: report of an aggressive case and review of the literature, *J Oral Maxillofac Surg* 51(6):702-705, 1993.
14. Silva EC et al. An extreme case of cherubism, *Br J Oral Maxillofac Surg* 40(1):45-48, 2002.
15. Timosca GC et al. Aggressive form of cherubism: report of a case, *J Oral Maxillofac Surg* 58(3):336-344, 2002.
16. Kalantar Motamedi MH. Treatment of cherubism with locally aggressive behavior presenting in adulthood: report of four cases and a proposed new grading system, *J Oral Maxillofac Surg* 56(11):1336-1342, 1998.
17. Grunebaum M, Tiqva P. Non familial cherubism: report of two cases, *J Oral Surg* 31(8):632-635, 1973.
18. DeTomasi DC, Hann JR, Stewart HM Jr. Cherubism: report of a nonfamilial case, *J Am Dent Assoc* 111(3):455-457, 1985.
19. Rattan V et al. Non-familial cherubism—a case report, *J Indian Soc Pedod Prev Dent* 15(4):118-120, 1997.
20. Mangion J et al. The gene for cherubism maps to chromosome 4p16.3, *Am J Hum Genet* 65(1):151-157, 1999.
21. Tiziani V et al. The gene for cherubism maps to chromosome 4p16, *Am J Hum Genet* 65(1):158-166, 1999.
22. Ueki Y et al. Mutations in the gene encoding c-Abl-binding protein SH3BP2 cause cherubism, *Nat Genet* 28(2):125-126, 2001.
23. McDonald RE, Shafer WG. Disseminated juvenile fibrous dysplasia of the jaws, *Am J Dis Child* 89(3):354-358, 1955.
24. Pierce AM et al. Fifteen-year follow-up of a family with inherited craniofacial fibrous dysplasia, *J Oral Maxillofac Surg* 54(6):780-788, 1996.
25. Peters WJ. Cherubism: a study of twenty cases from one family, *Oral Surg Oral Med Oral Pathol* 47(4):307-311, 1979.
26. Von Wowern N. Cherubism: a 36-year long-term follow-up of 2 generations in different families and review of the literature, *Oral Surg Oral Med Oral Pathol Oral Radiol Endod* 90(6):765-772, 2002.
27. Weinstein M, Bernstein S. Pink ladies: mercury poisoning in twin girls, *CMAJ* 168(2):201, 2003.
28. Horowitz Y et al. Acrodynia: a case report of two siblings, *Arch Dis Child* 86(6):453, 2002.
29. Hartsfield JK Jr. Premature exfoliation of teeth in childhood and adolescence, *Adv Pediatr* 41:453-470, 1994.
30. A gene (PEX) with homologies to endopeptidases is mutated in patients with X-linked hypophosphatemic rickets. The HYP Consortium, *Nat Genet* 11(2):130-136, 1995.
31. McWhorter AG, Seale NS. Prevalence of dental abscess in a population of children with vitamin D-resistant rickets, *Pediatr Dent* 13(2):91-96, 1991.
32. Shroff DV, McWhorter AG, Seale NS. Evaluation of aggressive pulp therapy in a population of vitamin D-resistant rickets patients: a follow-up of 4 cases, *Pediatr Dent* 24(4):347-349, 2002.
33. Rakocz M, Keating J 3rd, Johnson R. Management of the primary dentition in vitamin D-resistant rickets, *Oral Surg Oral Med Oral Pathol* 54(2):166-171, 1982.
34. Horwitz M et al. Mutations in ELA2, encoding neutrophil elastase, define a 21-day biological clock in cyclic haematopoiesis, *Nat Genet* 23(4):433-436, 1999.
35. da Fonseca MA, Fontes F. Early tooth loss due to cyclic neutropenia: long-term follow-up of one patient, *Spec Care Dentist* 20(5):187-190, 2000.
36. Seow WK et al. Mineral deficiency in the pathogenesis of enamel hypoplasia in prematurely born, very low birthweight children, *Pediatr Dent* 11(4):297-302, 1989.
37. Slayton RL et al. Prevalence of enamel hypoplasia and isolated opacities in the primary dentition, *Pediatr Dent* 23(1):32-36, 2001.
38. Sarnat BG, Schour I. Enamel hypoplasia (chronological enamel aplasia) in relation to systemic disease: a chronologic, morphologic and etiologic classification, *J Am Dent Assoc* 29:67-75, 1942.
39. Sheldon M, Bibby BG, Bales MS. Relationship between microscopic enamel defects and infantile disabilities, *J Dent Res* 24:109-116, 1945.
40. Purvis RJ et al. Enamel hypoplasia of the teeth associated with neonatal tetany: a manifestation of maternal vitamin-D deficiency, *Lancet* 2(7833):811-814, 1973.
41. Herman SC, McDonald RE. Enamel hypoplasia in cerebral palsied children, *J Dent Child* 30:46-49, 1963.
42. Cohen HJ, Diner H. The significance of developmental dental enamel defects in neurological diagnosis, *Pediatrics* 46(5):737-747, 1970.
43. Martínez A et al. Prevalence of developmental enamel defects in mentally retarded children, *ASDC J Dent Child* 69(2):151-155, 124, 2002.
44. Oliver WJ et al. Hypoplastic enamel associated with the nephrotic syndrome, *Pediatrics* 32:399-406, 1963.
45. Koch MJ et al. Enamel hypoplasia of primary teeth in chronic renal failure, *Pediatr Nephrol* 13(1):68-72, 1999.
46. Rattner LJ, Myers HM. Occurrence of enamel hypoplasia in children with congenital allergies, *J Dent Res* 41:646-649, 1962.
47. Lawson BF et al. The incidence of enamel hypoplasia associated with chronic pediatric lead poisoning, *S C Dent J* 29(11):5-10, 1971.
48. Pearl M, Roland NM. Delayed primary dentition in a case of congenital lead poisoning, *ASDC J Dent Child* 47(4):269-271, 1980.
49. Turner JG. Two cases of hypoplasia of enamel, *Br J Dent Sci* 55:227-228, 1912.
50. Bauer WH. Effect of periapical processes of deciduous teeth on the buds of permanent teeth, *Am J Orthod* 32:232-241, 1946.
51. Mink JR. Relationship of enamel hypoplasia and trauma in repaired cleft lip and palate. *In School of Dentistry.* Indianapolis, 1961 Indiana University.
52. Dixon DA. Defects of structure and formation of the teeth in persons with cleft palate and the effect of reparative surgery on the dental tissues, *Oral Surg Oral Med Oral Pathol* 25(3):435-446, 1968.
53. Vichi M, Franchi L. Abnormalities of the maxillary incisors in children with cleft lip and palate, *ASDC J Dent Child* 62(6):412-417, 1995.
54. Kaste SC et al. Dental abnormalities in children treated for acute lymphoblastic leukemia, *Leukemia* 11(6):792-796, 1997.
55. Maguire A, Welbury RR. Long-term effects of antineoplastic chemotherapy and radiotherapy on dental development, *Dent Update* 23(5):188-194, 1996.
56. Musselman RJ. *Dental defects and rubella embryopathy: a clinical study of fifty children.* Indianapolis: Indiana University, 1968 School of Dentistry.
57. Levy SM et al. Primary tooth fluorosis and fluoride intake during the first year of life, *Commun Dent Oral Epidemiol* 30(4):286-295, 2002.
58. Everett ET et al. Dental fluorosis: variability among different inbred mouse strains, *J Dent Res* 81(11):794-798, 2002.

59. McCloskey RJ. A technique for removal of fluorosis stains, *J Am Dent Assoc* 109(1):63-64, 1984.
60. Croll TP, Cavanaugh RR. Enamel color modification by controlled hydrochloric acid-pumice abrasion. I. Technique and examples, *Quintessence Int* 17(2):81-87, 1986.
61. Croll TP, Cavanaugh RR. Enamel color modification by controlled hydrochloric acid-pumice abrasion. II. Further examples, *Quintessence Int* 17(3):157-164, 1986.
62. Dalzell DP, Howes RI, Hubler PM. Microabrasion: effect of time, number of applications, and pressure on enamel loss, *Pediatr Dent* 17(3):207-211, 1995.
63. Croll TP. Enamel microabrasion: observations after 10 years, *J Am Dent Assoc* 128(Suppl):45-50, 1997.
64. Croll TP, Helpin ML. Enamel microabrasion: a new approach, *J Esthet Dent* 12(2):64-71, 2000.
65. Muhler JC. Effect of apical inflammation of the primary teeth on dental caries in the permanent teeth, *J Dent Child* 24:209-210, 1957.
66. Mueller BH et al. "Caries-like" resorption of unerupted permanent teeth, *J Pedod* 4(2):166-172, 1980.
67. Holan G, Eidelman E, Mass E. Pre-eruptive coronal resorption of permanent teeth: report of three cases and their treatments, *Pediatr Dent* 16(5):373-377, 1994.
68. Savage NW, Gentner M, Symons AL. Preeruptive intracoronal radiolucencies: review and report of case, *ASDC J Dent Child* 65(1):36-40, 1998.
69. Seow WK, Wan A, McAllan LH. The prevalence of pre-eruptive dentin radiolucencies in the permanent dentition, *Pediatr Dent* 21(1):26-33, 1999.
70. Seow WK, Lu PC, McAllan LH. Prevalence of pre-eruptive intracoronal dentin defects from panoramic radiographs, *Pediatr Dent* 21(6):332-339, 1999.
71. Lysell L. Taurodontism: a case report and a survey of the literature, *Odontol Rev* 13(2):158-174, 1962.
72. Jaspers MT, Witkop CJ Jr. Taurodontism, an isolated trait associated with syndromes and X-chromosomal aneuploidy, *Am J Hum Genet* 32(3):396-413, 1980.
73. Mena CA. Taurodontism, *Oral Surg Oral Med Oral Pathol* 32(5):812-823, 1971.
74. Gedik R, Cimen M. Multiple taurodontism: report of case, *ASDC J Dent Child* 67(3):216-217, 2000.
75. Bixler D, Conneally PM, Christen AG. Dentinogenesis imperfecta: genetic variations in a six-generation family, *J Dent Res* 48(6):1196-1199, 1969.
76. Witkop CJ Jr. *Genetics and dental health.* New York, 1961, McGraw-Hill.
77. Witkop CJ Jr. Manifestations of genetic diseases in the human pulp, *Oral Surg Oral Med Oral Pathol* 32(2):278-316, 1971.
78. Shields ED, Bixler D, el-Kafrawy AM. A proposed classification for heritable human dentine defects with a description of a new entity, *Arch Oral Biol* 18(4):543-553, 1973.
79. Zhang X et al. DSPP mutation in dentinogenesis imperfecta Shields type II, *Nat Genet* 27(2):151-152, 2001.
80. Xiao S et al. Dentinogenesis imperfecta 1 with or without progressive hearing loss is associated with distinct mutations in DSPP, *Nat Genet* 27(2):201-204, 2001.
81. Sreenath T et al. Dentin sialophosphoprotein knockout mouse teeth display widened predentin zone and develop defective dentin mineralization similar to human dentinogenesis imperfecta type III, *J Biol Chem* 278(27):24874-24880, 2003.
82. Malmgren B et al. Clinical, histopathologic, and genetic investigation in two large families with dentinogenesis imperfecta type II, *Hum Genet* 114(5):491-498, 2004.
83. Dean JA et al. Dentin dysplasia, type II linkage to chromosome 4q, *J Craniofac Genet Dev Biol* 17(4):172-177, 1997.
84. Rajpar MH et al. Mutation of the signal peptide region of the bicistronic gene DSPP affects translocation to the endoplasmic reticulum and results in defective dentine biomineralization, *Hum Mol Genet* 11(21):2559-2565, 2002.
85. McKnight DA et al. A comprehensive analysis of normal variation and disease-causing mutations in the human DSPP gene, *Hum Mutat* 29(12):1392-1404, 2008.
86. Beattie ML et al. Phenotypic variation in dentinogenesis imperfecta/dentin dysplasia linked to 4q21, *J Dent Res* 85(4):329-333, 2006.
87. Cartwright AR, Kula K, Wright TJ. Craniofacial features associated with amelogenesis imperfecta, *J Craniofac Genet Dev Biol* 19(3):148-156, 1999.
88. Ravassipour DB et al. Variation in dental and skeletal open bite malocclusion in humans with amelogenesis imperfecta, *Arch Oral Biol* 50(7):611-623, 2005.
89. Aldred MJ, Crawford PJ. Amelogenesis imperfecta— towards a new classification, *Oral Dis* 1(1):2-5, 1995.
90. Hart PS et al. A nomenclature for X-linked amelogenesis imperfecta, *Arch Oral Biol* 47(4):255-260, 2002.
91. Hart PS et al. Identification of the enamelin (g.8344delG) mutation in a new kindred and presentation of a standardized ENAM nomenclature, *Arch Oral Biol* 48(8):589-596, 2003.
92. Stephanopoulos G, Garefalaki ME, Lyroudia K. Genes and related proteins involved in amelogenesis imperfecta, *J Dent Res* 84(12):1117-1126, 2005.
93. Aldred MJ et al. Genetic heterogeneity in X-linked amelogenesis imperfecta, *Genomics* 14(3):567-573, 1992.
94. Congleton J, Burkes EJ Jr. Amelogenesis imperfecta with taurodontism, *Oral Surg Oral Med Oral Pathol* 48(6):540-544, 1979.
95. Seow WK. Taurodontism of the mandibular first permanent molar distinguishes between the tricho-dento-osseous (TDO) syndrome and amelogenesis imperfecta, *Clin Genet* 43(5):240-246, 1993.
96. Price JA et al. A common DLX3 gene mutation is responsible for tricho-dento-osseous syndrome in Virginia and North Carolina families, *J Med Genet* 35(10):825-828, 1998.
97. Price JA et al. Tricho-dento-osseous syndrome and amelogenesis imperfecta with taurodontism are genetically distinct conditions, *Clin Genet* 56(1):35-40, 1999.
98. Dong J et al. DLX3 mutation associated with autosomal dominant amelogenesis imperfecta with taurodontism, *Am J Med Genet A* 133A(2):138-141, 2005.
99. Patel RR et al. X-linked (recessive) hypomaturation amelogenesis imperfecta: a prosthodontic, genetic, and histopathologic report, *J Prosthet Dent* 66(3):398-402, 1991.
100. Chaudhry AP et al. Odontogenesis imperfecta. Report of a case, *Oral Surg Oral Med Oral Pathol* 14:1099-1103, 1961.
101. Schimmelpfennig CB, McDonald RE. Enamel and dentine aplasia; report of a case, *Oral Surg Oral Med Oral Pathol* 6(12):1444-1449, 1953.
102. Gorlin RJ, Herman NG, Moss SJ. Complete absence of the permanent dentition: an autosomal recessive disorder, *Am J Med Genet* 5(2):207-209, 1980.
103. Swallow JN. Complete anodontia of the permanent dentition, *Br Dent J* 107:143-145, 1959.
104. Schneider PE. Complete anodontia of the permanent dentition: case report, *Pediatr Dent* 12(2):112-114, 1990.
105. Laird GS. Congential anodontia, *J Am Dent Assoc* 51:722, 1955.

106. Witkop CJ Jr. Agenesis of succedaneous teeth: an expression of the homozygous state of the gene for the pegged or missing maxillary lateral incisor trait, *Am J Med Genet* 26(2):431-436, 1987.

107. Hoo JJ. Anodontia of permanent teeth (OMIM # 206780) and pegged/missing maxillary lateral incisors (OMIM # 150400) in the same family, *Am J Med Genet* 90(4): 326-327, 2000.

108. Glenn FB. A consecutive six-year study of the prevalence of congenitally missing teeth in private practice of two geographically separated areas, *J Dent Child* 31:269-270, 1964.

109. Grahnen H. Hypodontia in the permanent dentition, *Dent Abstr* 3:308-309, 1957.

110. Vastardis H et al. A human MSX1 homeodomain missense mutation causes selective tooth agenesis, *Nat Genet* 13(4):417-421, 1996.

111. Stockton DW et al. Mutation of PAX9 is associated with oligodontia, *Nat Genet* 24(1):18-19, 2000.

112. Erpenstein H, Pfeiffer RA. [Sex-linked-dominant hereditary reduction in number of teeth], *Humangenetik* 4(3):280-293, 1967.

113. Ahmad W et al. A locus for autosomal recessive hypodontia with associated dental anomalies maps to chromosome 16q12.1, *Am J Hum Genet* 62(4):987-991, 1998.

114. Bennett CG, Ronk SL. Congenitally missing primary teeth: report of case, *ASDC J Dent Child* 47(5):346-348, 1980.

115. Shashikiran ND, Karthik V, Subbareddy VV. Multiple congenitally missing primary teeth: report of a case, *Pediatr Dent* 24(2):149-152, 2002.

116. Fleming P, Nelson J, Gorlin RJ. Single maxillary central incisor in association with mid-line anomalies, *Br Dent J* 168(12):476-479, 1990.

117. Cobourne MT. Familial human hypodontia—is it all in the genes? *Br Dent J* 203(4):203-208, 2007.

118. McSherry PF. The ectopic maxillary canine: a review, *Br J Orthod* 25(3):209-216, 1998.

119. Becker A, Sharabi S, Chaushu S. Maxillary tooth size variation in dentitions with palatal canine displacement, *Eur J Orthod* 24(3):313-318, 2002.

120. Becker A, Gillis I, Shpack N. The etiology of palatal displacement of maxillary canines, *Clin Orthod Res* 2(2):62-66, 1999.

121. Chaushu S, Sharabi S, Becker A. Tooth size in dentitions with buccal canine ectopia, *Eur J Orthod* 25(5):485-491, 2003.

122. Becker A. In defense of the guidance theory of palatal canine displacement, *Angle Orthod* 65(2):95-98, 1995.

123. Paschos E et al. Investigation of maxillary tooth sizes in patients with palatal canine displacement, *J Orofac Orthop* 66(4):288-298, 2005.

124. Peck S, Peck L, Kataja M. The palatally displaced canine as a dental anomaly of genetic origin, *Angle Orthod* 64(4):249-256, 1994.

125. Pirinen S, Arte S, Apajalahti S. Palatal displacement of canine is genetic and related to congenital absence of teeth, *J Dent Res* 75(10):1742-1746, 1996.

126. Hartsfield JK Jr. Genetics and orthodontics. In Graber TM, Vanarsdall RL, Vig, KWL, eds. *Orthodontics: current principles and techniques.* St. Louis, 2005, Mosby.

127. Lammi L et al. Mutations in AXIN2 cause familial tooth agenesis and predispose to colorectal cancer, *Am J Hum Genet* 74(5):1043-1050, 2004.

128. Chalothorn LA et al. Hypodontia as a risk marker for epithelial ovarian cancer: a case-controlled study, *J Am Dent Assoc* 139(2):163-169, 2008.

129. Monreal AW, Zonana J, Ferguson B. Identification of a new splice form of the EDA1 gene permits detection of nearly all X-linked hypohidrotic ectodermal dysplasia mutations, *Am J Hum Genet* 63(2):380-389, 1998.

130. Giansanti JS, Long SM, Rankin JL. The "tooth and nail" type of autosomal dominant ectodermal dysplasia, *Oral Surg Oral Med Oral Pathol* 37(4):576-582, 1974.

131. Jumlongras D et al. A nonsense mutation in MSX1 causes Witkop syndrome, *Am J Hum Genet* 69(1):67-74, 2001.

132. Hudson CD, Witkop CJ. Autosomal dominant hypodontia with nail dysgenesis. Report of twenty-nine cases in six families, *Oral Surg Oral Med Oral Pathol* 39(3): 409-423, 1975.

133. Nunn JH et al. The interdisciplinary management of hypodontia: background and role of paediatric dentistry, *Br Dent J* 194(5):245-251, 2003.

134. Neville BW et al. *Oral and maxillofacial pathology,* 2nd ed. Philadelphia, 2002, WB Saunders.

135. Stoll BJ, Kliegman RM. Hemolytic disease of the newborn (erythroblastosis fetalis). In Behrman RE, Kliegman RM, Jenson HB, eds. *Nelson textbook of pediatrics.* Philadelphia, 2004, WB Saunders.

136. Cullen CL. Erythroblastosis fetalis produced by Kell immunization: dental findings, *Pediatr Dent* 12(6): 393-396, 1990.

137. Sassa S. The porphyrias. In In Behrman RE, Kliegman RM, Jenson HB, eds. *Nelson textbook of pediatrics.* Philadelphia, 2004, WB Saunders.

138. Zegarelli EV, et al. Discoloration of the teeth in a 24-year-old patient with cystic fibrosis of the pancreas not primarily associated with tetracycline therapy. Report of a case, *Oral Surg Oral Med Oral Pathol* 24(1):62-64, 1967.

139. Wright JT, Hall KI, Grubb BR. Enamel mineral composition of normal and cystic fibrosis transgenic mice, *Adv Dent Res* 10(2):270-274, 1996.

140. Arquitt CK, Boyd C, Wright JT. Cystic fibrosis transmembrane regulator gene (CFTR) is associated with abnormal enamel formation, *J Dent Res* 81(7):492-496, 2002.

141. Primosch RE. Tetracycline discoloration, enamel defects, and dental caries in patients with cystic fibrosis, *Oral Surg Oral Med Oral Pathol* 50(4):301-308, 1980.

142. van der Bijl P, Pitigoi-Aron G. Tetracyclines and calcified tissues, *Ann Dent* 54(1-2):69-72, 1995.

143. Moffitt JM et al. Prediction of tetracycline-induced tooth discoloration, *J Am Dent Assoc* 88(3):547-552, 1974.

144. Tredwin CJ, Scully C, Bagan-Sebastian JV. Drug-induced disorders of teeth, *J Dent Res* 84(7):596-602, 2005.

145. Brantley DH, Barnes KP, Haywood VB. Bleaching primary teeth with 10% carbamide peroxide, *Pediatr Dent* 23(6): 514-516, 2001.

146. Gorlin RJ, Cohen MM Jr, Hennekam RCM. *Syndromes of the head and neck,* 4th ed. New York, 2001, Oxford University Press.

147. Pruzansky S, Richmond JB. Growth of mandible in infants with micrognathia; clinical implications, *Am J Dis Child* 88(1):29-42, 1954.

148. Daskalogiannakis J, Ross RB, Tompson BD. The mandibular catch-up growth controversy in Pierre Robin sequence, *Am J Orthod Dentofacial Orthop* 120(3):280-285, 2001.

149. Strohecker B, Lahey D. Mandibular elongation by bone distraction: treatment for mandibular hypoplasia with Robin sequence, *Plast Surg Nurs* 17(1):8-10, 15, 1997.

150. James D, Ma L. Mandibular reconstruction in children with obstructive sleep apnea due to micrognathia, *Plast Reconstr Surg* 100(5):1131-1137, 1997.

151. Hotz M, Gnoinski W. Clefts of the secondary palate associated with the "Pierre Robin syndrome." Management by early maxillary orthopaedics, *Swed Dent J Suppl* 15:89-98, 1982.

152. Dean JA, et al. Prevention of airway obstruction in Pierre Robin sequence via obturator use, *Pediatr Dent* 24:173-174 (abstract), 2002.

153. Burket LW. *Oral medicine: diagnosis and treatment,* 7th ed. Philadelphia, 1977, JB Lippincott.

154. Reynoso MC et al. Autosomal dominant congenital macroglossia: further delineation of the syndrome, *Genet Couns* 5(2):151-154, 1994.

155. Ayers FJ, Hilton LM. Treatment of ankyloglossia: report of case, *ASDC J Dent Child* 44(3):237-239, 1977.

156. Messner AH, Lalakea ML. The effect of ankyloglossia on speech in children, *Otolaryngol Head Neck Surg* 127(6): 539-545, 2002.

157. Rahamimoff P, Muhsam HV. Some observations on 1246 cases of geographic tongue: the association between geographic tongue, seborrheic dermatitis, and spasmodic bronchitis; transition of geographic tongue to fissured tongue, *Am J Dis Child* 93(5): 519-525, 1957.

158. Kleinman DV, Swango PA, Pindborg JJ. Epidemiology of oral mucosal lesions in United States schoolchildren: 1986-87, *Commun Dent Oral Epidemiol* 22(4):243-253, 1994.

159. Meskin LH, Redman RS, Gorlin RJ. Incidence of geographic tongue among 3,668 students at the University of Minnesota, *J Dent Res* 42:895, 1963.

160. Kullaa-Mikkonen A. Familial study of fissured tongue, *Scand J Dent Res* 96(4):366-375, 1988.

161. Bánóczy J, Szabo L, Csiba A. Migratory glossitis. A clinical-histologic review of seventy cases, *Oral Surg Oral Med Oral Pathol* 39(1):113-121, 1975.

162. Cooke BE. Median rhomboid glossitis. Candidiasis and not a developmental anomaly, *Br J Dermatol* 93(4): 399-405, 1975.

163. Barasch A et al. Oral soft tissue manifestations in HIV-positive vs. HIV-negative children from an inner city population: A two-year observational study, *Pediatr Dent* 22(3):215-220, 2000.

164. Campbell A et al. Tongue piercing: impact of time and barbell stem length on lingual gingival recession and tooth chipping, *J Periodontol* 73(3):289-297, 2002.

165. De Moor RJ, De Witte AM, De Bruyne MA. Tongue piercing and associated oral and dental complications, *Endod Dent Traumatol* 16(5):232-237, 2000.

166. Ram D, Peretz B. Tongue piercing and insertion of metal studs: three cases of dental and oral consequences, *ASDC J Dent Child* 67(5):326-329, 2000.

167. Martinello RA, Cooney EL. Cerebellar brain abscess associated with tongue piercing, *Clin Infect Dis* 36(2): e32-34, 2003.

168. Dyce O et al. Tongue piercing. The new "rusty nail?" *Head Neck* 22(7):728-732, 2000.

169. Akhondi H, Rahimi AR. *Haemophilus aphrophilus* endocarditis after tongue piercing, *Emerg Infect Dis* 8(8): 850-851, 2002.

170. Perkins CS, Meisner J, Harrison JM. A complication of tongue piercing, *Br Dent J* 182(4):147-148, 1997.

171. Keogh IJ, O'Leary G. Serious complication of tongue piercing, *J Laryngol Otol* 115(3):233-234, 2001.

172. McGeary SP, Studen-Pavlovich D, Ranalli DN. Oral piercing in athletes: implications for general dentists, *Gen Dent* 50(2):168-172, 2002.

CHAPTER 8

Tumors of the Oral Soft Tissues and Cysts and Tumors of the Bone

▲ John S. McDonald

CHAPTER OUTLINE

*T*oo often, dental practitioners see their responsibility to the patient begin and end with the care and maintenance of the teeth and periodontium. Physicians do not give oral health the attention it deserves because they, for the most part, do not receive education and training from this perspective. This leaves the responsibility to the dental practitioner to monitor and help maintain the overall health and well-being of the patient as evidenced in the orofacial and head and neck structures that are so obviously within their purview. Even so, it remains easy to focus strictly on the dental needs of the patient and remain oblivious to, among other things, subtle or even not so subtle lumps, bumps, swellings, or changes in texture or color that may signify the presence of a reactive or a hamartomatous overgrowth of tissue, or a benign or malignant disease. These disorders occur within the oral and maxillofacial region too often for the dentist to take the attitude that they happen only in someone else's patients.

This chapter provides an overview of some of the more frequently encountered cysts and tumors in the oral and maxillofacial region soft tissues and bone in the pediatric age group.

BENIGN TUMORS OF THE ORAL SOFT TISSUE

SQUAMOUS PAPILLOMA AND VERRUCA VULGARIS

The squamous papilloma is a relatively common, benign neoplasm that arises from the surface epithelium. It is typically an exophytic lesion whose surface may vary from cauliflower-like to finger-like in appearance, and although it is generally a pedunculated lesion, it may arise from a sessile base. Although the average age of occurrence is in the fourth decade of life, nearly 20% of cases have been noted to occur before 20 years of age.[1,2] The most common sites of occurrence appear to be the tongue and palatal complex, followed by the buccal mucosa, gingiva, and lips. This lesion is also seen with some frequency on the mandibular alveolar ridge, floor of the mouth, and retromolar pad regions.[2]

Oral verruca vulgaris, or oral warts, are exophytic papillomatous lesions indistinguishable clinically from oral squamous cell papillomas. Like their skin counterpart, the common wart (verruca vulgaris), they are a viral

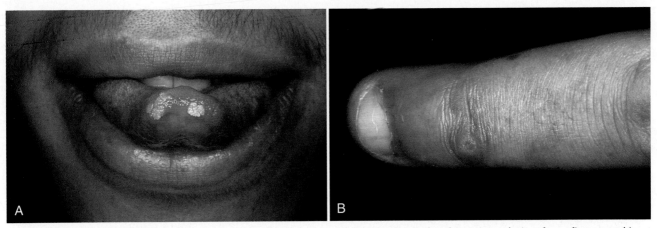

Figure 8-1 A, Verruca vulgaris on the anterior tip of the tongue. This is an example of autoinoculation from finger sucking. **B,** Notice the wart on this patient's finger from which he inoculated his tongue. (Courtesy Dr. Mark L. Bernstein.)

disorder associated with the human papillomavirus (HPV) and may be spread to the oral cavity in children through autoinoculation by finger or thumb sucking (Fig. 8-1). According to two reviews of HPV-associated diseases of oral mucosa, types 2 and 57 were most commonly found.[3,4] DNA types 6, 11, and 16 have also been demonstrated in oral verrucae.[5,6]

Although the histopathologic differences between squamous papilloma and verruca vulgaris are subtle, these lesions are distinguishable from one another. Histologically, the papilloma is seen as a proliferation of the spinous cell layer in a papillary pattern, often with hyperkeratosis, acanthosis, and basilar hyperplasia. Mitotic figures may be prominent. The supporting fibrous connective tissue stroma often contains prominent numbers of small blood vessels as well as an inflammatory cell infiltrate. HPV may, however, be seen in squamous cell papillomas. In 1982 the presence of HPV genus-specific antigens was demonstrated in two of five multiple papillomas.[7] In a subsequent review of the world literature analyzing 223 papillomas, the overall detection rate for HPV DNA was 49.8% with the most prevalent HPV types being HPV 6 and 11.4 HPV types 16 and 18 have also been detected in some squamous cell papillomas.[8]

The presence of papillomatosis often with convergence of rete ridges centrally, hyperkeratosis (either hyperparakeratosis or hyperorthokeratosis, or both) a coarse keratohyalin granular cell layer and vacuolated cells with pyknotic nuclei (koilocytes) may be used to differentiate verruca vulgaris from a squamous papilloma. Hence, from the above discussion both squamous papilloma and verrucous vulgaris should probably be considered benign, virus-induced epithelial hyperplasias and the identification of HPV does not appear to offer any diagnostic advantage because the histopathologic features alone allow for differentiation of one from the other.[9]

Treatment of either the oral squamous papilloma or verruca vulgaris is best accomplished by complete surgical excision of the lesion, including the base.

FIBROMA

The fibroma is the most common benign soft tissue tumor found in the oral cavity. It is characteristically a dome-shaped lesion with a sessile base and a smooth surface that is usually the color of the surrounding mucosa. It may vary from firm to flaccid in texture and most commonly occurs in sites predisposed to irritation or trauma, such as the buccal mucosa, lip, tongue, gingiva, and hard palate. It may occur at any age. Sometimes termed *focal fibrous hyperplasia*, a fibroma occurring in the oral cavity is reactive in nature, being basically either a reactive type of fibrous hyperplasia or in some cases a healed pyogenic granuloma that has undergone sclerosis.

Histologically the fibroma is a dome-shaped lesion composed of a fibrous connective tissue stroma that may vary from loose and delicate to quite dense in its appearance, with an overlying layer of stratified squamous epithelium. Treatment consists of simple surgical excision. There is little propensity for recurrence.

PYOGENIC GRANULOMA, PERIPHERAL OSSIFYING FIBROMA, PERIPHERAL ODONTOGENIC FIBROMA (WHO TYPE), AND PERIPHERAL GIANT CELL GRANULOMA

Pyogenic Granuloma

The pyogenic granuloma is a relatively common soft-tissue tumor that arises from the fibrous connective tissue of the skin or mucous membranes. Originally believed to be a botryomycotic infection, it is now known to be a reactive inflammatory process in which an exuberant fibrovascular proliferation of the connective tissue occurs secondary to some low-grade, chronic irritation.

Clinically the pyogenic granuloma is a raised lesion on either a sessile or a pedunculated base. Its surface may have a smooth, lobulated, or, occasionally, warty appearance that is erythematous and often ulcerated (Fig. 8-2). Depending on the age of the lesion, the texture varies from soft to firm and is suggestive of an ulcerated

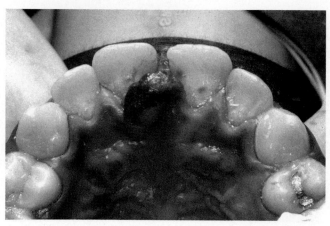

Figure 8-2 Pyogenic granuloma arising from the interdental papilla between the maxillary central incisors. The surface is lobulated with erythema and ulceration. There was poor oral hygiene with heavy accumulation of plaque on the lingual surfaces of the teeth.

fibroma. Because of the pronounced vascularity of these lesions, they often bleed easily when probed. A review of pyogenic granulomas of the oral cavity revealed a 65% to 70% incidence of occurrence on the gingiva, most commonly the maxillary anterior labial gingiva, followed by the lips, tongue, buccal mucosa, palate, mucolabial or mucobuccal fold, and alveolar mucosa of edentulous areas.[10] Twenty-seven percent of cases in this series of 46 patients were in individuals younger than 20 years of age. Another review of 38 cases reported an age range of 5 to 75 years (mean age, 33 years) with the most frequent site of occurrence also being on the gingiva (74%).[10,11]

Histologically the pyogenic granuloma presents as a remarkable proliferation of plump fibroblasts and endothelial cells with the formation of prominent numbers of thin-walled, endothelium-lined vascular channels. A polymorphous inflammatory cell infiltrate is present, and the overlying surface epithelium is often ulcerated. Treatment consists of surgical excision, with care being taken to completely remove any local irritant that may still be present that would predispose to recurrence of the lesion.

In addition to an ulcerated fibroma, which in fact may itself be a nearly healed or sclerosed pyogenic granuloma, both the peripheral ossifying fibroma and peripheral giant cell granuloma must be considered in the differential diagnosis of pyogenic granuloma because these lesions are clinically indistinguishable.

PERIPHERAL OSSIFYING FIBROMA AND PERIPHERAL ODONTOGENIC FIBROMA (WHO TYPE)

Peripheral Ossifying Fibroma

The peripheral ossifying fibroma is a reactive lesion believed to be of periodontal ligament origin that occurs exclusively on the gingiva. In the largest series of cases, 50% of the lesions were noted to occur in individuals between 5 and 25 years of age, with the peak incidence at 13 years.[12] The lesions were approximately equally divided between the maxilla and the mandible, with

more than 80% of the lesions in both jaws occurring anterior to the molar area.

Histologically the peripheral ossifying fibroma demonstrates a proliferation of plump fibroblasts in a characteristic stroma of delicate, interlacing collagen fibrils. Osteoid and calcified material varying from dystrophic calcification to spicules of lamellar bone may be found in the lesion. The surface epithelium is often ulcerated. Although simple surgical excision is the treatment of choice, recurrences are not uncommon and were reported by Cundiff and by Eversole and Rovin in 16% and 20% of cases, respectively.[12,13] In a more recent study of 134 cases of peripheral ossifying fibroma in patients aged 1 to 19 years, the overall recurrence rate was 8%. However, this was thought to represent the minimum rate of recurrence in that no attempt was made to determine how many patients with or without recurrent lesions were followed clinically, and if so, for how long.[14]

Peripheral Odontogenic Fibroma (WHO type)

Previously, the terms *peripheral ossifying fibroma* and *peripheral odontogenic fibroma* were used synonymously, which introduced considerable confusion into the literature. To clarify the confusion, the term *peripheral odontogenic fibroma* (World Health Organization [WHO] type) was proposed to denote the rare peripheral counterpart of the central odontogenic fibroma (WHO type), and the term *peripheral ossifying fibroma* was proposed to be retained and used to denote the relatively common reactive gingival lesion.[15] Clinically the peripheral odontogenic fibroma (WHO type) must be considered in the differential diagnosis of dome-shaped or nodular, usually nonulcerated, growths on the gingiva.

It is a rare odontogenic tumor characterized by a fibrous or fibromyxomatous stroma containing varying numbers of islands and strands of odontogenic epithelium. Cementum-like, bone-like, or dentinoid material may be present. Its age at presentation is strikingly similar to the peripheral ossifying fibroma. Even though treatment consists of local surgical excision, in one study recurrence was noted in 7 of 18 cases for which follow-up information was obtained.[16]

Peripheral Giant Cell Granuloma

The peripheral giant cell granuloma, like the peripheral ossifying fibroma, is a lesion unique to the oral cavity, occurring only on the gingiva. Unlike the peripheral ossifying fibroma, however, it may occur on the alveolar mucosa of edentulous areas. Like the pyogenic granuloma and peripheral ossifying fibroma, the peripheral giant cell granuloma may represent an unusual response to tissue injury. It is distinguishable from the pyogenic granuloma and peripheral ossifying fibroma only on the basis of its unique histomorphology, which is essentially identical to that of the central giant cell granuloma that is discussed later in this chapter. In a review of 720 cases, 33% were seen in patients younger than 20 years of age, which concurs with the findings of another study in which 33 of 97 cases (34%) occurred in individuals between 5 and 15 years of age.[17,18] There is a nearly 2:1 predilection of females to males, with the mandible being involved more often than the maxilla. Although it is rare, cervical root resorption may be seen in association with a peripheral giant cell granuloma.[19]

The peripheral giant cell granuloma is best treated by complete surgical excision, with care taken to excise it at its base. Little tendency for recurrence has been noted.

NEUROFIBROMA AND NEUROFIBROMATOSIS (VON RECKLINGHAUSEN'S DISEASE)

Neurofibroma is a benign neural neoplasm of Schwann cell origin of which several clinical forms are recognized. The solitary neurofibroma may present in the skin or oral mucous membranes as a soft tumor with a sessile or pedunculated base. Some neurofibromas are diffuse, presenting as a soft, nonspecific tissue mass or swelling. Although patients with neurofibromatosis may have either solitary or diffuse neurofibromas, the presence of either lesion does not in itself herald the diagnosis of this syndrome. The presence of a third form, the plexiform neurofibroma, is, however, considered to be diagnostic of neurofibromatosis. The plexiform neurofibroma differs from either the solitary or diffuse form in that it remains confined to the perineurium, presenting as a tortuous, fusiform enlargement of a nerve.

Neurofibromatosis type 1 (NF1), known as von Recklinghausen disease, is a relatively common disorder showing autosomal dominant inheritance with complete penetrance, variable clinical expressivity and pleiotropy, and age-dependent expression of clinical manifestations. It occurs in approximately 1 in 3000 live births with an equal sex predilection. The NF1 gene is carried on chromosome 17 and has tumor suppressor function, with the tumor-suppressing properties of neurofibromin (the NF1 gene product) then being impaired or lost. It is said to be the most common single-gene disorder to affect the human nervous system. The criterion for diagnosis is the presence of two or more of the following features: six or more café-au-lait spots (1.5 cm or larger in postpubertal individuals, 0.5 cm or larger in prepubertal individuals), two or more neurofibromas of any type or one or more plexiform neurofibromas, freckling in the axillary or inguinal region, optic glioma, two or more pigmented iris hamartomas or Lisch nodules, dysplasia of the sphenoid bone or dysplasia or thinning of long bone cortex with or without pseudoarthrosis, and a first-degree relative with NF1.

As previously noted, the NF1 gene is a tumor-suppressor gene, and thus patients with neurofibromatosis are at increased risk of developing benign and malignant tumors. Neurofibromatosis is a progressive condition with different presentations occurring at specific times with some complications worsening over time. While cutaneous or dermal neurofibromas are considered one of the characteristic features of this disorder and may appear in childhood, they more commonly develop in teenagers or adults. Although malignant peripheral nerve sheath tumors may be noted in pediatric patients with NF1, they usually develop in adulthood and are heralded by the presence of pain or rapid growth arising in a plexiform or deep nodular neurofibroma.[20]

Intraorally, neurofibromas may present as nodular lesions on either a sessile or pedunculated base, often

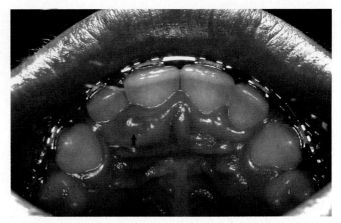

Figure 8-3 A 14-year-old boy undergoing orthodontic therapy was referred for evaluation of gingival hyperplasia on the lingual surfaces of the maxillary incisors and a firm swelling on the palatal side of tooth number 9 that was found after biopsy to be a neurofibroma *(arrow)*.

with a normal, pink mucosal color (Fig. 8-3); as a diffuse, ill-defined swelling with a firm to doughy consistency; or as a diffuse, noncompressible mass. They are most frequently found on the tongue and buccal mucosa but occasionally present as intraosseous lesions, which occur most commonly in the posterior mandible (Fig. 8-4).

The most common radiographic findings include an increase in bone density, enlarged mandibular foramen, lateral bowing of the mandibular ramus, increase in dimensions of the coronoid notch, and decrease in the mandibular angle.[21] Computed tomographic scans may reveal findings such as enlargement of the mandibular foramen and concavity of the medial surface of the ramus.

A great deal of histomorphologic variability may be noted, from relatively circumscribed but nonencapsulated solitary neurofibromas to diffuse and plexiform neurofibromas. The diffuse neurofibroma is characterized by its infiltrative growth pattern along connective planes and its Wagner and Meissner tactile corpuscles. Plexiform neurofibromas are characterized by fascicles of neoplastic Schwann cells and collagen within a myxoid matrix that is confined to the perineurium. Mast cells are common findings within neurofibromas.

Solitary lesions are best treated by simple surgical excision and show little propensity for recurrence. Surgical excision of diffuse neurofibromas is difficult because of their diffuse, infiltrating nature. Plexiform neurofibromas are also difficult to treat in that they have a tendency to grow along the course of a nerve, which results in frequent recurrences. It has been noted that (1) children younger than 10 years of age, (2) children with plexiform neurofibromas in the head, face, and neck, and (3) those with tumors that cannot be almost completely removed are at particular risk for progression of their lesions.[22]

HEMANGIOMA

Vascular anomalies are commonly encountered lesions of childhood and may be divided into hemangiomas and vascular malformations.[23] Hemangiomas are differentiated from vascular malformations as they demonstrate

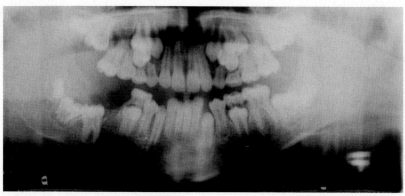

Figure 8-4 Neurofibroma involving the molar region and ramus of the right mandible in a child with neurofibromatosis. (Courtesy Dr. Robin Cotton.)

proliferative activity while vascular malformations grow commensurately with the child.[24] The hemangioma is a common, benign, vasoformative tumor that frequently occurs in the head and neck in children. It is generally believed to be hamartomatous rather than neoplastic in nature. Most hemangiomas are either present at birth or develop within the first year of life. It is believed that even those lesions that do not appear until adult life may have been present but not clinically evident until they began to enlarge.

Hemangiomas arising in the oral soft tissues most commonly affect the tongue, lips, and buccal mucosa. Clinically, they may be flat or raised and may vary from deep red to blue in color. Their histologic classification is based on the size of the vascular spaces. A capillary hemangioma is the most common type and is composed of many tiny capillaries with a pronounced endothelial cell proliferation. The cellular or juvenile hemangioma consists principally of a proliferation of endothelial cells with only small numbers of discernible capillaries. A cavernous hemangioma is characterized by large, blood-filled sinusoidal spaces lined by endothelial cells and supported by a fibrous stroma. Hemangiomas may also occur centrally within either the mandible or maxilla.

Vascular malformations most frequently involve the skin but also may affect visceral organs or bone. They may be categorized as fast-flow lesions and slow-flow lesions.[25] Fast flow lesions include arterial malformations, arteriovenous malformations, and arteriovenous fistulas. Slow-flow lesions include capillary malformations, lymphatic malformations, and venous malformations. Vascular malformations of the mandible (i.e., arteriovenous malformations or central hemangioma of the mandible as they were sometimes called) are potentially dangerous in that a biopsy or simple event such as a tooth extraction may lead to a catastrophic hemorrhage possibly leading to death.[26] These lesions may be asymptomatic, picked up only as incidental radiographic findings, or they may cause pain and swelling. They are typically well-circumscribed radiolucent lesions with no characteristic radiographic pattern to denote their underlying nature. Occasionally, loose or displaced teeth may be seen. Arteriovenous malformations bear a radiographic

similarity to any number of other relatively well-circumscribed unilocular or multilocular radiolucent lesions in the jaws. Therefore it is advisable to aspirate such lesions with a needle before surgery or dental extraction to avoid the possibility of severe blood loss or exsanguination caused by the inability to control the resultant profuse bleeding.

The treatment for hemangiomas varies with the type, location, and size of the lesion involved. Many lesions spontaneously involute with age, especially those that are noted early and cease growing during the first year of life. Others require no treatment because of their small size and innocuous nature.

LYMPHANGIOMA

Lymphangiomas are relatively rare benign congenital tumors of the lymphatic system. Even though the embryologic events leading to their development remain unclear, they are thought to arise as a benign hamartomatous proliferation of sequestered lymphatic rests. Forming along tissue planes or penetrating adjacent tissue, they become canalized and, in the congenital absence of venous drainage, accumulate fluid. The head and neck region is most commonly involved with up to two thirds of cases being present at birth and as many as 90% being present by the second year of life; a small number may not be manifest for a number of years.[27]

Lymphangiomas are classified on a histologic basis into three types: capillary lymphangiomas, cavernous lymphangiomas, and cystic hygroma. The capillary lymphangioma is typically composed of a proliferation of thin-walled, endothelium-lined channels primarily devoid of erythrocytes. The cavernous lymphangioma is characterized by the presence of dilated sinusoidal endothelium-lined vascular channels devoid of erythrocytes. The cystic hygroma is a macroscopic form of the cavernous lymphangioma, with large sinusoidal spaces lined with a single layer of endothelial cells that form multilocular cystic masses of varying sizes. Lymphangiomas of the oral soft tissues occur most commonly on the tongue, lips, and buccal mucosa. They are often elevated and nodular in appearance and may have the same color as the surrounding mucosa. Treatment is generally not indicated for small oral mucosal lymphangiomas; partial or complete spontaneous involution is occasionally noted.

Although cystic hygromas may be found in sites in the oral cavity, such as the tongue, they most frequently appear as a mass in the neck, occasionally extending into the mediastinum. Most commonly presenting as an asymptomatic soft tissue mass, they are usually slow growing; however, they may undergo sudden enlargement in the presence of trauma, inflammation, internal hemorrhage, or respiratory tract infection. Large cystic hygromas may encroach on the airway and esophagus, leading to difficulty in swallowing and even causing airway obstruction.

CONGENITAL EPULIS (GINGIVAL GRANULAR CELL LESION) OF THE NEWBORN

The congenital epulis of the newborn is a rare lesion of uncertain histogenesis that occurs exclusively in newborn infants, chiefly on the maxillary anterior alveolar ridge and less commonly on the mandibular anterior alveolar ridge. Although usually solitary lesions, they may be multiple, most often affecting both the maxilla and mandible although rare simultaneous occurrence of lesions on the maxillary anterior alveolar ridge and tongue have been reported. Clinically the lesion presents at birth as a pink, smooth to lobulated, pedunculated mass that may vary in size from a few millimeters to more than 7 cm in diameter. More than 90% of cases occur in girls (Fig. 8-5).

While typically considered a lesion of uncertain histogenesis, immunohistochemical studies have revealed strong and diffuse cytoplasmic staining for neuron-specific enolase and vimentin, which suggests that the congenital epulis may be derived from uncommitted nerve-related mesenchymal cells.[28]

Although histologic similarities to the granular cell tumor have long been noted, the epithelium over the congenital epulis is generally thin without rete ridge formation, whereas the granular cell tumor is characterized by pseudoepitheliomatous hyperplasia of the overlying epithelium; distinct differences are obvious on both ultrastructural and immunohistochemical evaluation. One differentiating factor between the congenital epulis and granular cell tumor tumors is the absence of S100 in the former and its presence in the latter lesion.[29]

Although the clinical presence of the congenital epulis may frighten parents, it ceases to grow following birth and is entirely benign, with some cases undergoing spontaneous involution. The usual treatment is simple surgical excision, with care taken not to interfere with the developing dentition. There is no propensity for recurrence, even in those cases in which the lesion is incompletely removed.

MUCOCELE

The mucocele, or *mucus retention phenomenon,* as it is often called, is a salivary gland lesion of traumatic origin that forms when the main duct of a minor salivary gland is torn with subsequent extravasation of mucus into the fibrous connective tissue so that a cystlike cavity is produced. The wall of this cavity is formed by compressed bundles of collagen fibrils, and its lumen contains inspissated mucin.

Mucoceles are noted to occur most commonly on the lower lip, with the floor of the mouth and buccal mucosa being the next most frequent sites of involvement. Mucoceles are only rarely seen on the upper lip, retromolar pad, or palate. Although they may occur at any age and have been reported to be present at birth, they tend to be noted most frequently in the second and third decades of life. No obvious sex predilection is noted.

A mucocele may be located either in the superficial mucosa, where it is typically seen as a fluid-filled vesicle or blister (Fig. 8-6), or deep within the connective tissue as a fluctuant nodule with the overlying mucosa normal

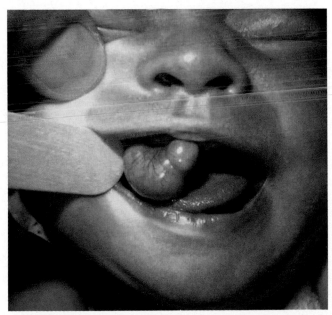

Figure 8-5 Congenital epulis of the newborn. (Courtesy Dr. Robin Cotton.)

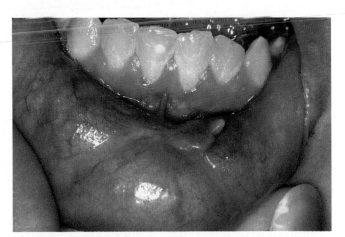

Figure 8-6 Mucocele on the lower lip. Notice the small white area of fibrosis where the mucocele has spontaneously drained with healing on the roof of the lesion, only to have the mucocele recur.

in color. There may be spontaneous drainage of the inspissated mucin with temporary resolution, especially in superficial lesions, and subsequent recurrence as the mucous saliva continues to drain into the connective tissue at the site of the torn duct. Fibrosis may be observed over the surface of long-standing lesions where chronic periodic drainage has taken place.

Treatment is by surgical excision, with removal of the involved accessory salivary gland. Marsupialization will only result in recurrence.

RANULA

Ranula is the clinical term for a mucocele occurring on the floor of the mouth after trauma to components of the sublingual glands. Two varieties of ranula exist: cystic (mucus retention cyst) and pseudocystic (mucus retention phenomenon or mucocele). In the cystic type, there is partial obstruction of the distal end of a sublingual gland duct that results in a small epithelial lined cyst usually less than 1 cm in diameter. However, the most common variety of ranula (which is pseudocystic) forms as a result of extravasation of mucus into the fibrous connective tissue after a tear in a sublingual gland duct and, as in the case of a mucocele, arises as a result of the escape of mucus into the adjacent connective tissue. The clinical term *plunging ranula* is used when extravasated mucus dissects through the mylohyoid muscle and along the fascial planes of the neck, producing a swelling evident in the floor of the mouth.

Ranulas are typically slowly enlarging, fluctuant masses occurring to one side of the midline of the floor of the mouth and are so named because of their resemblance to the bloated underside of a frog's belly (Fig. 8-7). Lesions are usually treated by marsupialization, with occasional recurrence being noted. Chronic recurrence may require excision of the entire involved gland.

BENIGN TUMORS OF BONE

FIBRO-OSSEOUS LESIONS OF THE JAWS

The fibro-osseous lesions of the jaws include a diverse group of lesions sharing as a common denominator the replacement of normal bone architecture by a benign fibrous stroma containing varying amounts of mineralized material, including woven bone, lamellar bone, and curvilinear trabeculae or spherical calcifications. The mineralized material may histologically resemble bone and/or cementum. Because of the similar histomorphology of these lesions, diagnosis is best made on the basis of distinguishing clinical and radiographic as well as histologic features. This group of lesions includes fibrous dysplasia (considered a developmental process), reactive or dysplastic processes grouped under the collective term *cemento-osseous dysplasia*, and ossifying fibroma, which is a benign neoplasm. Because of the frequency of occurrence of fibrous dysplasia and ossifying fibroma of bone in the jaws of children, and the relative lack of occurrence of the cemento-osseous dysplasia group of lesions in this age group, only the former two are discussed here.

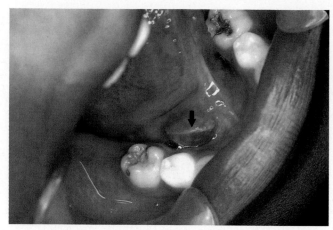

Figure 8-7 Ranula on the floor of the mouth *(arrow)*.

FIBROUS DYSPLASIA

Fibrous dysplasia of the jaws is a distinct clinicopathologic entity that is generally considered to be a nonneoplastic developmental lesion of bone. One of a variety of disease entities included in the spectrum of benign fibroosseous lesions of the jaws, it is distinguished from the others by its clinical and radiographic features. In the child and adolescent, it has most often been confused with the ossifying and cementifying fibroma, which is a benign neoplasm believed to be of periodontal ligament origin. Fibrous dysplasia is caused by a somatic activating mutation of the alpha subunit of the G protein (Gs-alpha) that ultimately results in abnormalities of osteoblast differentiation and therefore abnormal bone.

The two forms of fibrous dysplasia are (1) the relatively rare polyostotic form of the disease and (2) the considerably more common monostotic fibrous dysplasia. A severe form of polyostotic fibrous dysplasia called *McCune-Albright syndrome* is associated with café-au-lait macules on the skin and a variety of endocrine disorders, most commonly precocious puberty, but also including Cushing's syndrome, hyperthyroidism, hyperparathyroidism, and diabetes mellitus.

Monostotic fibrous dysplasia tends to develop early in life with lesions being detected late in the first and early second decades.[30] It is seen with approximately equal frequency in males and females, with the maxilla being involved more frequently than the mandible. Maxillary involvement can be an especially serious form of the disease, frequently involving contiguous bones across suture lines, including the maxillary sinus, floor of the orbit, sphenoid bone, base of the skull, and occiput. This form of the disease has been called *craniofacial fibrous dysplasia* and is not truly monostotic in its nature.

The most common clinical manifestation is a painless swelling of the jaws characterized by a smooth, uniform, fusiform expansion of the involved alveolar ridge. Obliteration of the mucobuccal or mucolabial fold is a common feature, with the overlying mucosa being normal in appearance. When the maxilla is involved, elevation of the eye may be noted.

Radiographically, maxillary lesions most often show a ground-glass appearance of the bone, whereas mandibular lesions usually show either a ground-glass or a mixed radiolucent-radiopaque appearance (Fig. 8-8). Their borders are typically poorly defined, except for the anterior portion of some maxillary lesions, which may appear to be well circumscribed. Divergence of roots may be noted, and in children in whom developing permanent teeth are present there may be displacement of teeth with noneruption (see Fig. 8-8). Other potential distinguishing radiographic findings include superior displacement of the mandibular canal and a fingerprint bone pattern as well as displacement of the maxillary sinus cortex, alteration of the lamina dura because of the abnormal bone pattern, and narrowing of the periodontal ligament space.[31]

Histologically there is a benign fibrous stroma with bony trabeculae varying from woven to lamellar in appearance, proportionate to the relative maturity of the lesion.

Monostotic fibrous dysplasia of the jaws is typically a slow-growing, painless, progressive enlargement of bone whose growth pattern often stabilizes with time as maturation in skeletal growth is reached. Conservative therapy is indicated because of the benign nature of this lesion and because surgically the margins are ill defined and blend into the surrounding normal bone. Surgery, chiefly in the form of osseous recontouring, should be considered only when there is functional or significant cosmetic deformity and then usually only after stabilization of the disease process. Because this is a benign lesion of bone, radiation therapy is contraindicated because of the possibility of development of a postradiation sarcoma in the area. In symptomatic cases in which pain control and disease stabilization are needed, bisphosphonates have been used, resulting in pain relief and, in a number of patients, disease stabilization as well.[32] Little, however, is known about the long-term skeletal effects of childhood bisphosphonate use and it has been recommended that its use be limited to experienced pediatric units.[32]

OSSIFYING AND CEMENTIFYING FIBROMA

The ossifying fibroma is a benign neoplasm of bone grouped with fibrous dysplasia and other benign nonodontogenic tumors under the broad category of benign fibro-osseous lesions of the jaws. As with other benign fibro-osseous lesions, it is characterized histologically by a benign fibrous stroma, with formation of variable amounts of woven-appearing bone, lamellar bone, and spherical to annular to amorphous cementum-like calcifications. Although it was traditionally considered to be an odontogenic neoplasm of periodontal ligament origin affecting the tooth-bearing areas of the jaws, the occurrence of histologically identical neoplasms in the temporal, frontal, ethmoid, and sphenoid bones leaves this concept in doubt. When the cementum or cementum-like calcifications predominate, the term is *cementifying fibroma*. When both bone and cementum-like tissues are present, the lesions are termed *cemento-ossifying fibromas*. Although there is a predilection for occurrence in the third and fourth decades of life, the ossifying fibroma is found with some frequency in patients younger than 20 years of age. The mandible is involved more often than the maxilla, with the molar and premolar region of the mandible being the most common site of occurrence.

The ossifying fibroma may be entirely asymptomatic, being discovered on routine radiographic examination, or may present as a painless expansion of bone. Radiographically the ossifying fibroma is a well-circumscribed lesion, often with a well-demarcated sclerotic border (Fig. 8-9). Beyond this, the radiographic features are quite variable.[33] It most frequently presents as a unilocular radiolucency with or without radiopaque foci, which may be superimposed over teeth, may be interposed between contiguous teeth, or may reside in edentulous regions. Aggressively expansile lesions with or without radiopaque foci as well as multilocular expansile lesions may also be noted. Tooth displacement or divergence of roots of teeth and/or root resorption may be seen with varying degrees of frequency with tooth displacement or root divergence

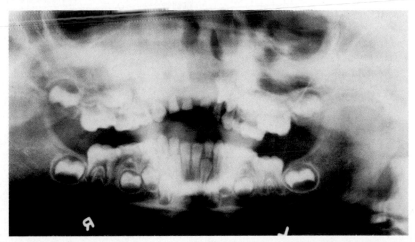

Figure 8-8 Panelipse radiograph for a child with fibrous dysplasia presenting as a uniformly radiodense lesion crossing the midline with poorly defined borders blending into the surrounding bone. Notice the displacement of the developing teeth.

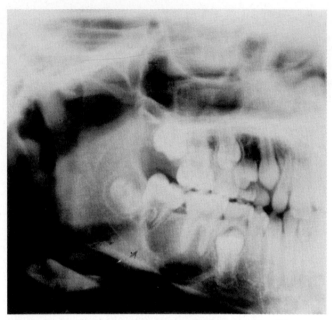

Figure 8-9 Ossifying fibroma in a 10-year-old boy. The radiograph shows a well-circumscribed, expansile, radiolucent lesion with thinning of the inferior cortical plate of bone. (Courtesy Dr. Mark L. Bernstein.)

being reported in from 17% to 33% of cases and root resorption being seen between 11% and 44% of the time.[33,34] Cortical thinning and bony expansion with clinical deformity have been reported in as many as 91% of cases.

Initial treatment is by enucleation or curettage where possible, with the frequency of recurrence varying from 0% to 28%.[33,35]

JUVENILE OSSIFYING FIBROMA

The term *juvenile ossifying fibroma* (JOF), also known as juvenile active ossifying fibroma and juvenile aggressive ossifying fibroma, encompasses two distinct clinicopathologic variants of ossifying fibroma involving the craniofacial bones: the trabecular juvenile ossifying fibroma (TrJOF) and the psammomatoid juvenile ossifying fibroma (PsJOF). The TrJOF affects both the maxilla and the mandible with the maxilla being involved slightly more frequently.[36] Occurrence in extragnathic locations is extremely rare.[30] The reported mean age ranges from 8{½} to 12 years (range, 2 to 12 years). The PsJOF was noted to occur predominantly in the sinonasal and orbital bones in patients with a mean age range of 16 to 33 years (range, 3 months to 72 years). Aggressive growth was noted to occur in some cases of both types with a high recurrence rate after excision (30% to 56% of cases). It has been proposed that despite some similarities in biologic behavior, differences in histologic, demographic, and clinical presentation between PsJOF and TrJOF warrants their separation into two distinct clinicopathologic entities.[36]

CENTRAL GIANT CELL GRANULOMA

First described in 1953 as *giant-cell reparative granuloma,* the central giant cell granuloma (CGCG) of the jaws is a relatively uncommon benign lesion of bone.[37] The

CGCG of the jaws occurs most commonly during the first 30 years of life, with more than 60% of lesions noted before 20 years of age and nearly 50% occurring in patients younger than 16 years of age. The CGCG occurs more often in females than in males. It may be found in either jaw, but the mandible is involved twice as often as the maxilla. Although it was traditionally accepted that the majority of lesions occur anterior to the first permanent molar, a study of 80 cases of CGCG, found that nearly 50% of cases occurred in the molar, ramus, and tuberosity regions.[38] Usually asymptomatic, CGCG may present with aggressive growth, pain, and swelling. Radiographically the CGCG may vary from a unilocular radiolucency to a multilocular expansile bone-destructive lesion with displacement and noneruption of teeth, root resorption, and cortical perforation (Fig. 8-10). Histologically the CGCG is composed of a few too many monocyte-derived multinucleated giant cells in a fibrous connective tissue stroma of ovoid to spindle shaped, probably fibroblast-related, mesenchymal cells and round monocyte-macrophages. Prominent numbers of extravasated red blood cells with associated hemosiderin pigment are often scattered throughout the fibrous connective tissue. Varying amounts of osteoid and trabeculae of bone are also noted.

The pathogenesis of CGCG of the jaws remains unknown with lesions, as a group, exhibiting features of both reactive and neoplastic disease. There is also considerable discussion in the literature as to its relationship to giant cell tumor of bone. It has been suggested by a number of authors that the CGCG and giant cell tumor of other bones represent a spectrum of a single disease process, with the differences in clinical behavior partially accounted for by differences in age

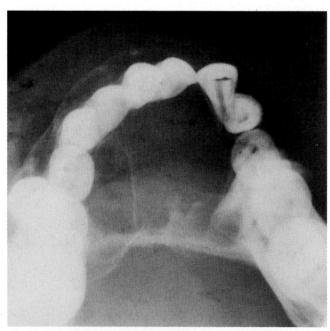

Figure 8-10 Central giant cell granuloma involving the anterior mandible presenting radiographically as a multilocular, radiolucent lesion with expansion and thinning of the cortical plates. Notice also the faint trabeculation within the lesion.

distribution and by the site of occurrence among other factors.[39-41]

As originally described, the CGCG was a rather indolent process that yielded readily to therapy with the therapeutic procedure of choice being surgical curettage.[37] It was subsequently reported that there is a range of biologic behavior of CGCGs from quiescent to aggressive, expansile bone-destructive lesions.[42] Lesions in CGCG have since been classified as *nonaggressive* and *aggressive*, based on their clinical presentation. Nonagressive lesions are characterized by a slow, asymptomatic growth without perforation of the cortical plate of bone or root resorption. Features of aggressive lesions may include rapid growth, expansion and or perforation of the cortical plate of bone with soft tissue extension, pain, and root resorption.[38,40-42] It has also been suggested that younger age at presentation may be associated with more aggressive behavior. In one series, for example,[40] recurrence developed in five of the 25 patients for whom follow-up information was available, with the average age of these five patients being 11 years compared with an average age of 29 years for patients without recurrence. In a study of 31 cases of CGCG of the jaws in 29 patients, seven lesions demonstrated cortical perforation and soft tissue extension.[41] Lesions recurred in five cases, all of which showed microscopically confirmed cortical perforation at the time of first occurrence.

Surgical curettage is the most commonly used therapy for CGCG, although in aggressive cases resection may be indicated. Alternative treatments to surgical curettage have been suggested, including injections of corticosteroid, calcitonin, and interferon (INF-α) as well as some others.[43] Radiation therapy is contraindicated.

ODONTOGENIC CYSTS

Odontogenic cysts are so named because it is believed that they are derived from epithelium that arose from the dental lamina during odontogenesis. They may be developmental or inflammatory in origin. Even though the pathogenesis of the developmental types of odontogenic cysts is not clearly understood, it is known that inflammatory cysts such as the periapical cyst (apical periodontal cyst, radicular cyst) result from proliferation of epithelial rests of Malassez secondary to inflammation from pulpal necrosis of an associated tooth.[44]

Because of their relative potential for occurrence in the pediatric dental population, four types of developmental odontogenic cysts — the primordial cyst, dentigerous cyst, eruption cyst, and odontogenic keratocyst — are discussed in this chapter. The odontogenic keratocyst is also discussed in relation to the nevoid basal cell carcinoma syndrome (Gorlin syndrome).

PRIMORDIAL CYST

Traditionally the primordial cyst was considered to be an uncommon type of odontogenic cyst formed by cystic degeneration of the enamel organ (primordium) before the formation of enamel or dentin. Primordial cysts are usually asymptomatic and are most likely to be found on routine radiographic examination. Although they begin

to evolve when the enamel organ is developing before the formation of the enamel or dentin, they may not be noticed or become clinically evident for many years.

Radiographically, the primordial cyst may be a well-circumscribed, unilocular- or multilocular-appearing radiolucent lesion in a location where a permanent tooth failed to develop and where none has been extracted. Such cysts are more commonly found in the third molar region but may occur in any location where a permanent tooth would have formed.

Although more typically lined by nonkeratinizing, stratified squamous odontogenic cyst-lining epithelium with a fibrous connective tissue wall, the primordial cyst may present as a histologically distinct type of odontogenic cyst, the odontogenic keratocyst. In one large series of cases, 60 of 135 (44.4%) primordial cysts were histologically odontogenic keratocysts.[45] Some authors have concluded that all primordial cysts are odontogenic keratocysts and use the two terms synonymously. However, taking into the consideration that, in the study cited here, in which greater than 55% of cysts that clinically and radiographically fit the traditional criteria for a primordial cyst were not histologically odontogenic keratocysts, the concept that the two terms are synonymous ignores the histologic evidence to the contrary.

Appropriate treatment for the primordial cyst is surgical removal unless an extremely large bone-destructive lesion is present, in which case cystotomy with placement of a polyethylene drain followed by cystectomy when the cyst has reached a manageable size is the treatment of choice. If the lesion is found histologically to be an odontogenic keratocyst, the chance for recurrence is high.

DENTIGEROUS CYST

The dentigerous cyst, the most common type of odontogenic cyst, is found in association with the crown of an impacted, embedded, or otherwise unerupted tooth. The incidence of dentigerous cysts has been shown as 1.44 per every 100 unerupted teeth.[46] Even though the dentigerous cyst is considered to be a developmental type of odontogenic cyst, it has been speculated that some may have an inflammatory origin from a source such as periapical inflammation from a nonvital deciduous tooth.[47] Although dentigerous cysts are typically asymptomatic and are usually found on routine radiographic examination, they may be large, destructive, expansile lesions of bone. The radiographic appearance is that of a well-defined radiolucent lesion that may be unilocular or multilocular in its appearance. The lesion may vary in size from one in which the differentiation from an enlarged dental follicle is somewhat arbitrary (a pericoronal radiolucency of 2.5 mm or greater from the crown of the tooth has been generally accepted as differentiating a dentigerous cyst from a dental follicle)[48] to a large, bone-destructive lesion that may resorb the roots of primary teeth, cause the divergence of or completely displace permanent teeth, and produce large areas of bone destruction in either the mandible or the maxilla (Fig. 8-11).

In addition to its potential for bone destruction and because of the multipotential nature of this epithelium

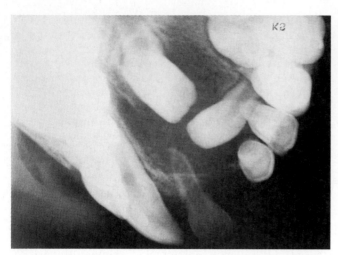

Figure 8-11 A dentigerous cyst in an 8-year-old girl associated with the developing maxillary central incisor with bone destruction and expansion, as well as displacement of the lateral incisor.

derived from the dental lamina, several entities may arise in or be associated with the wall of a dentigerous cyst. For example, 8.5% of cysts that clinically appear as dentigerous cysts have been found histologically to be odontogenic keratocysts.[45] Although these cysts are relatively uncommon in children and adolescents, it is believed that the majority of ameloblastomas in this age group are associated with dentigerous cysts with 50% to 80% of cases of cystic ameloblastoma appearing radiographically as dentigerous cysts.[49-51] It has been concluded, based on histopathologic features, that these ameloblastomatous changes occurred in a preexisting cyst rather than representing cystic degeneration of a solid tumor.[50] Mucus-secreting cells, and more significantly mucoepidermoid carcinoma, may also arise in the wall of a dentigerous cyst.

The treatment of choice for dentigerous cysts is surgical removal. Large bone-destructive lesions are, however, best treated initially by cystotomy and the placement of a polyethylene drain in the lesion, which facilitates shrinkage with healing around the periphery to the point where the lesion becomes amenable to more simple surgical removal. Because of the potential for occurrence of an odontogenic keratocyst or the development of an ameloblastoma or more rarely mucoepidermoid carcinoma, all such lesions, when removed, should be submitted for histopathologic evaluation.

ERUPTION CYST OR ERUPTION HEMATOMA

The eruption cyst or eruption hematoma is a type of dentigerous cyst associated with an erupting primary or permanent tooth in its soft tissue phase after erupting through bone. The lesion is usually a translucent, smooth, painless swelling over the erupting tooth. If bleeding occurs into the cystic space, it may appear blue to blueblack and is then called an *eruption hematoma*. In most cases, no treatment is indicated because the tooth usually erupts into the oral cavity undelayed and in a normal fashion.

ODONTOGENIC KERATOCYST

The odontogenic keratocyst is a distinct clinicopathologic entity with a clearly identifiable histologic appearance. Clinically it is characterized by a high rate of recurrence after treatment and the potential to become an aggressive, bone-destructive lesion. In a review of 312 cases, the peak incidence was found to be in the second and third decades of life, with 17% occurring before 20 years of age (only two cases were noted in children younger than 10 years of age).[45] The mandible is involved twice as frequently as the maxilla, with the most common site of origin being the mandibular third molar region and ramus of the mandible, followed by the maxillary third molar region, mandibular first and second molar area, maxillary canine area, and mandibular premolar region. Half of the patients were symptomatic, with swelling and drainage being the most common clinical findings.

Radiographically, the odontogenic keratocyst may be a unilocular or multilocular lesion, almost always with a well-defined sclerotic border (Fig. 8-12). Tooth displacement, particularly of unerupted teeth, root resorption, root divergence, and extrusion of erupted teeth may be seen. Although radiographic evaluation typically includes a panoramic radiograph, in the case of large lesions, especially those in the maxilla, computed tomography studies should be performed preoperatively to accurately define margins and soft tissue extension that may be present.

The histologic appearance is pathognomonic. The lesion has a thin, generally uniform lining epithelium, usually 6 to 10 cells in thickness, with palisading and hyperchromasia of the basal layer of cells and a corrugated parakeratin layer. Often parakeratotic squames are shed into the lumen of the cyst cavity. Occasionally a cyst is lined by orthokeratin with a subjacent granular cell layer. These cysts have been termed *orthokeratinized odontogenic cysts* and should be differentiated clinically from the odontogenic keratocyst because the orthokeratinized odontogenic cyst shows little clinical aggressiveness and rarely recurs.[52]

There is no uniform agreement as to the most appropriate method of treatment of odontogenic keratocysts. Recommendations vary from enucleation, with or without adjunctive therapy such as application of Carnoy solution, to marsupialization or decompression, to marginal or segmental resection. This is partly because of their variable clinical presentation, which includes differences in size and the multilocular nature of many odontogenic keratocysts, as well as their benign nature coupled with the high frequency of recurrence that has been recorded for these lesions. A review of 22 reports citing 1592 cases of odontogenic keratocysts revealed a recurrence rate varying from 3% to 62% and an average rate of recurrence of 30.8%.[53] Seventy percent of recurrences have been shown to take place within 5 years of treatment.[54] Although these lesions should be surgically excised, enucleation is difficult because the cyst lining is

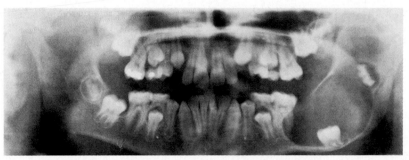

Figure 8-12 An odontogenic keratocyst in a 9-year-old girl involving the angle and ramus of the left mandible with displacement of the developing second and third molar teeth. (Courtesy Dr. Steven Reubel.)

often extremely thin and friable, and it has been suggested that disruption of the epithelial lining in the resected specimen may be a primary determinant of recurrence.[55] It has also been shown that odontogenic keratocysts that are completely enucleated recur significantly less often than those removed piecemeal.[56] Patients with documented or suspected nevoid basal cell carcinoma syndrome have a higher rate of recurrence than patients without the syndrome.[56,57] Enucleation followed by application of Carnoy solution, and decompression followed by enucleation have been associated with low recurrence rates and resulted in significantly less morbidity than resection.[58] The radiograph in Fig. 8-13 shows a large odontogenic keratocyst in which decompression was performed with placement of a polyethylene drain, followed by cystectomy as the lesion became more surgically manageable.

NEVOID BASAL CARCINOMA (GORLIN) SYNDROME

The nevoid basal carcinoma syndrome is a trait with autosomal dominant inheritance with complete penetrance and remarkably variable expressivity.[59] It is caused by a mutation of the Patched (PTCH) gene, which is thought to be crucial for proper embryonic development and for tumor suppression. Traditionally characterized by a symptom complex of multiple basal cell carcinomas of the skin, odontogenic keratocysts and rib abnormalities (bifid, fused, or splayed ribs), a variety of other abnormalities may accompany this disorder. Patients may have characteristic facies with cranial enlargement, frontal and parietal bossing with overdevelopment of the supraorbital ridges, hypertelorism, and a broad nasal root and mild mandibular prognathism. Calcification of the falx cerebri is evident radiographically in the majority of adult patients. In addition to the basal cell carcinomas, palmar and plantar pits and epidermal cysts of the skin are commonly seen. Congenital malformations such as cleft lip and cleft palate and polydactyly or syndactyly may be present. Spina bifida occulta of the cervical or thoracic vertebrae may occur and marfanoid habitus may be seen. A variety of benign and malignant neoplasms have been reported to occur, including medulloblastoma, meningioma, ovarian fibroma, and fetal rhabdomyoma along with quite a number of miscellaneous other tumors.[59] Neurologic abnormalities, including cognitive disabilities, may be noted, and some patients may be hyporesponsive to parathyroid hormone. Because of the association of the odontogenic keratocyst with the basal cell nevus syndrome, all patients with single or multiple odontogenic keratocysts should be evaluated medically with this condition in mind. This is especially true when an odontogenic keratocyst is found in a young patient because the median age of appearance is younger in syndromic than nonsyndromic patients.[59]

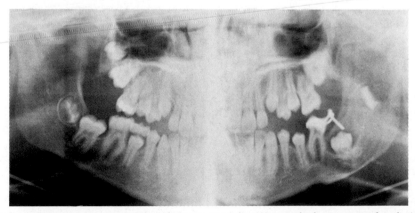

Figure 8-13 Same patient as in Fig. 8-12, 9 months after marsupialization and placement of a drain. Notice shrinkage of the cyst with bone fill in the area. Notice also inferior displacement of the inferior alveolar nerve. (Courtesy Dr. Steven Reubel.)

Also, as previously stated, there is an apparent increase in the rate of recurrence of odontogenic keratocysts in patients with the syndrome.

ODONTOGENIC TUMORS

The odontogenic tumors are so named because of their presumed origin from the tissues derived from the developing odontogenic elements, that is, epithelium ultimately derived developmentally from the dental lamina and/or ectomesenchymally derived mesenchymal cells. The word *tumor* is used in its broadest sense, which here includes neoplastic and hamartomatous processes.

AMELOBLASTOMA

Ameloblastoma, the most common odontogenic neoplasm, is an aggressive, benign odontogenic neoplasm of ectodermal origin. Usually an asymptomatic lesion, its initial presentation may be facial swelling. It may present with symptoms of pain and occasionally with lip/facial numbness. Ameloblastoma may be discovered on routine radiographic evaluation or may show features such as bony expansion, mobility, or divergence of teeth. The average age of patients with ameloblastoma is approximately 36 years, with more than 80% of the lesions occurring in the mandible and more than 70% occurring in the molar-ramus area.

At first glance, with the average age of occurrence of ameloblastomas in the fourth decade of life, the discussion of this entity in a pediatric context would not appear to be particularly relevant to this chapter. In 1977, however, the unicystic ameloblastoma was described, which was thought to be a prognostically distinct entity.[60] In the 20 patients studied, the average age was 21 years with half of patients being younger than 20 years. Clinically and radiographically the lesions were described as having the features of a nonneoplastic cyst, with the majority mimicking dentigerous cysts. A critical review of 193 cases of unicystic ameloblastoma in the literature found that the mean age at the time of diagnosis of unicystic ameloblastoma was most closely related to one clinical feature: the presence of an impacted tooth. Cases associated with an impacted tooth have been termed the *dentigerous* type and those not associated with an impacted tooth the *nondentigerous* type. The mean age at diagnosis of the dentigerous variant was 16.5 years, whereas that of the nondentigerous type was 35.2 years.[61] There is a strong predilection for mandibular involvement, particularly the molar-ramus region.[62,63]

Not all cases of ameloblastoma in children and adolescents are of the unicystic variety. In a clinicopathologic analysis of 37 cases of ameloblastoma in individuals 19 years old and younger, the average age at diagnosis was 10.4 years with no obvious sex predilection. Whereas 31 of these cases were unicystic (radiographically unilocular or multilocular), five were conventional ameloblastomas, all of which were multilocular radiographically. All of the cases reported in this study occurred in the mandible, with 80% occurring in the molar-ramus area.

Radiographically, ameloblastomas may present as either unilocular or multilocular radiolucent lesions, with or without bony expansion. Cystic-appearing spaces may be compartmentalized by separate, distinct septa of bone. Unicystic ameloblastoma, which is considered a distinct prognostic entity, occurs almost exclusively in the mandible, predominantly in the posterior part. Although most commonly found in association with the crowns of impacted teeth, unicystic ameloblastomas may be seen in interradicular, periapical, or edentulous regions.

Histologically, they are distinguished by their histologic resemblance to the enamel organ. Regardless of age or location, ameloblastomas demonstrate singly or in combination a variety of distinct histologic patterns. They are frequently characterized by discrete islands of neoplastic odontogenic epithelium with a peripheral layer of columnar to cuboidal epithelial cells that are palisaded in their appearance with polarization of the nuclei away from the basement membrane. The central portions of these islands of neoplastic odontogenic epithelium are composed of cells that resemble the stellate reticulum. In some lesions, these central areas may take on an acanthomatous or granular appearance. The plexiform pattern is the one most frequently encountered in the pediatric age group, with arrangement of tumor cells as a network of interconnecting strands of cells. An important histologic finding in the unicystic form, other than the observation of ameloblastic change in the cyst lining itself, is the presence of a significant luminal and/or mural component characterized by a proliferation of ameloblastic odontogenic epithelium into the lumen of the cyst, the fibrous cyst wall, or both. Mural invasion of the cyst wall portends a higher risk of recurrence for this lesion.

Therapy is by surgical removal, the method of which varies according to the location and clinical and radiographic extent of the lesion. Although a recurrence rate of 55% to 90% has been found for ameloblastomas of all types that have been treated by curettage, it has been believed that the cystic form, which is the type found most commonly in children, potentially carried a lower potential for recurrence.[51,62] More recent studies, however, have shown significant potential for recurrence after conservative treatment, not dissimilar to that of conventional ameloblastoma, with the recommendation being made for more aggressive therapy than has been recommended in the past.[64]

ADENOMATOID ODONTOGENIC TUMOR

The adenomatoid odontogenic tumor (AOT) is a benign, probably hamartomatous, epithelial tumor that occurs in two intraosseous forms (follicular and extrafollicular) as well as a peripheral variant. It has also been known as *adenoameloblastoma*, which is misleading because it behaves clinically in a distinctly different fashion than does ameloblastoma.

Several large clinical and epidemiologic reviews of the adenomatoid odontogenic tumor have been reported.[65-67] The AOT can be subclassified into three variants based on clinical and radiologic findings. Two of these are central or intraosseous variants. The first is the follicular (dentigerous) type in which the tumor is found in association with the crown of an impacted tooth, with the most likely provisional diagnosis being that of a dentigerous cyst. The second and less commonly reported intraosseous variant of the AOT is the extrafollicular type in which there is no association with the crown of an impacted tooth and with the most likely provisional diagnosis being that of a residual, radicular, globulomaxillary, or lateral periodontal cyst, depending upon its location. The third variant of AOT is the peripheral or extraosseous variant, which may appear clinically as a fibroma. Approximately 98% of AOTs are reported as being the intrabony or central type, with the follicular variant accounting for 71%. Although most often asymptomatic, the tumor frequently causes a painless swelling exhibiting slow but progressive growth.

AOTs occur most commonly in the second decade of life. Nearly 70% of patients are younger than 20 years of age and more than 50% of cases occur in the teenage years. Females are involved twice as often as males, and the intraosseous lesions have been noted to occur nearly twice as frequently in the maxilla as in the mandible, with a noticeable predilection for occurrence in the canine and incisor regions. The rare peripheral type is found almost entirely in the anterior maxillary region.

The most common radiographic finding is that of a unilocular radiolucent lesion, which as previously stated may appear radiographically as a dentigerous cyst (Fig. 8-14) or as a residual, radicular, globulomaxillary, or lateral periodontal cyst, depending on its location. Radiopacities of varying size and density are often present. Because these are space-occupying lesions, divergence of roots and displacement of teeth may be noted.

Histologically the AOT is composed of neoplastic odontogenic epithelium with a distinct histologic appearance: an encapsulated proliferation of swirling strands of spindle-shaped or polygonal epithelial cells within which are nodules of ductlike or rosette-like structures composed of a row of definite cuboidal to columnar epithelial cells; these may be empty or may contain variable amounts of an amorphous eosinophilic material, which may become calcified in some areas.

Because these lesions are in almost all cases well encapsulated and show an identical benign biologic behavior, conservative surgical enucleation and curettage is the treatment of choice. There is no propensity for recurrence.

ODONTOGENIC MYXOMA

The odontogenic myxoma is an uncommon benign mesodermal neoplasm of the jaws that is thought to arise from odontogenic ectomesenchyme or undifferentiated mesenchymal cells in the periodontal ligament. In one large review,[68] two thirds of the cases involved the mandible and one third of the cases involved the maxilla, with the molar and premolar region being the most common site of occurrence. Although the majority of cases were diagnosed in the second to fourth decades of life, 33% of the cases were in patients 20 years of age or younger (7% in patients younger than 10 years and 26% in the second decade of life).

Clinically odontogenic myxomas are usually painless, slow-growing lesions that can attain considerable size

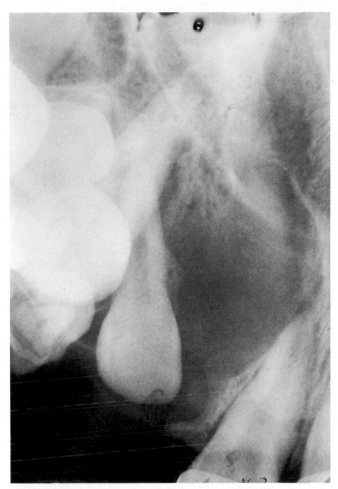

Figure 8-14 Adenomatoid odontogenic tumor in a 12-year-old girl presenting as an expansile radiolucent lesion in the right maxilla associated with the lateral incisor. The lesion was curetted, and the lateral incisor was allowed to erupt and was orthodontically moved into proper alignment. (Courtesy Dr. Dan J. Crocker.)

before manifesting noticeable signs and symptoms such as swelling or mobility and divergence of teeth. Several cases have been reported as occurring in association with impacted or missing teeth, while some cases have been noted to occur in non–tooth-bearing areas, such as the ramus and condyle.

Radiographically odontogenic myxomas may be unilocular or multilocular lesions that may cause expansion, thinning and destruction of the cortical plates of bone, and displacement of teeth. Multilocular lesions often exhibit a mottled, soap bubble or honeycombed appearance. There is no universal agreement as to the relative frequency of presentation as a unilocular versus a multilocular radiographic appearance. In an analysis of 10 cases of odontogenic myxoma in childhood, the most frequent radiographic finding was a unilocular lesion with cortical expansion and tooth displacement.[69] In a review of cases from all age groups, a multilocular appearance was noted in 55% of cases, with a significant correlation between the size of the lesion and its locularity being noted.[68] Perhaps the frequency of unilocular lesions in pediatric cases can be accounted for based on a smaller lesional size in childhood cases with larger lesions more likely being multilocular.[68,69] Because of the variable nature of the radiographic appearance of odontogenic myxomas, the differential diagnosis should include odontogenic lesions such as dentigerous cyst, odontogenic keratocyst, and ameloblastoma, as well as nonodontogenic lesions such as CGCG central hemangioma, traumatic bone cyst, and aneurysmal bone cyst.

Histologically the odontogenic myxoma is made up of stellate to spindle-shaped cells with delicate fibrillar interlacing processes, which produce a loose myxoid appearance. Occasional nests of inactive odontogenic epithelium may be noted, interspersed within this fibromyxoid stroma.

The appropriate treatment for the odontogenic myxoma is still a matter of debate and is certainly dependent on its size and location. The preferred treatment is complete surgical excision, which may prove difficult because of infiltration and expansion of the tumor into bone and the absence of a true capsule. Treatment is complicated by the understandable reluctance to perform wide surgical excision of a benign lesion, especially in a child. Periodic follow-up to check for recurrence is important. In the series of 10 cases of childhood odontogenic myxoma previously discussed, two patients experienced recurrence within the first year after surgery.[69]

AMELOBLASTIC FIBROMA

The ameloblastic fibroma is a true mixed neoplasm of odontogenic origin characterized by the proliferation of both odontogenic epithelium and mesenchymal tissue without the formation of enamel or dentin. It is generally believed to be a less aggressive lesion than the ameloblastoma. The average age of occurrence is approximately 14 years with no obvious sex predilection noted. The lesion occurs in the mandible in approximately 70% of cases, primarily in the molar region. Its initial clinical presentation is most often swelling; however, it is not uncommonly asymptomatic, being found on routine radiographic examination. Radiographically, it may be a unilocular or multilocular radiolucent lesion, usually with well-defined, often sclerotic borders, and may be found in association with unerupted or displaced teeth.

The ameloblastic fibroma has a characteristic histologic appearance, with strands of cuboidal to columnar epithelial cells and islands with peripheral columnar epithelial cells surrounding loosely arranged epithelial cells resembling stellate reticulum, which proliferate along with a primitive-appearing mesenchymal component that resembles the developing dental papilla.

Treatment is by surgical removal that is complete but conservative compared with that advocated for the ameloblastoma. At one time, simple surgical excision was advocated, because there was believed to be little chance for recurrence. Recent evidence, however, indicates that the recurrence rate is higher than originally suspected. In a recent review of published studies with well documented follow-up data, an overall recurrence rate of 33.3% was noted.[70] Hence, somewhat more aggressive

surgical therapy with clinical follow-up is indicated than was previously recommended.

AMELOBLASTIC FIBRO-ODONTOMA

The ameloblastic fibro-odontoma has been defined as "a lesion similar to ameloblastic fibroma, but also showing inductive changes that lead to the formation of both dentine and enamel."[71] The average age of occurrence has been reported as 9 years. The majority of cases are found in the posterior mandible, and the ratio of lesions in this location to those in both the anterior and posterior maxilla is 2.4:1. Described as a painless, slow-growing, and expanding tumor, the lesion is associated with unerupted teeth in 83% of cases, which often leads to its diagnosis. Size may vary from lesions evident only microscopically to a large mass up to 6 cm or more in its greatest dimension.

Histologically the epithelial and mesenchymal components are those of an ameloblastic fibroma, with the formation of osteodentin or dentin-like material and enamel matrix.

It is generally agreed that the ameloblastic fibro-odontoma is a hamartomatous lesion that is a stage preceding the development of a complex odontoma.[71,72] Against this, it has been argued that ameloblastic fibro-odontoma should not be considered a hamartoma because rare cases showing true neoplastic behavior exist and because the existence of a malignant variant has been reported.[73] Conservative surgical enucleation is considered the treatment of choice, and recurrence is unlikely.

ODONTOMA

Odontomas are mixed odontogenic tumors in which both the epithelial and mesenchymal components have undergone functional differentiation to the point that both enamel and dentin are formed. The most common of the odontogenic tumors, odontomas are believed to be hamartomatous rather than neoplastic in nature. The WHO has classified odontomas into two types depending on their degree of morphodifferentiation. The compound odontoma is a lesion in which all the dental tissues are represented in an orderly fashion so that there is at least superficial anatomic resemblance to teeth. In a complex odontoma, on the other hand, although all the dental tissues are represented, they are formed in such a rudimentary fashion that there is little or no morphologic similarity to normal tooth formation (Fig. 8-15).

A review of 149 cases indicated that compound odontomas have a propensity for occurrence in the canine and incisor region, being found more often in the maxilla than in the mandible, whereas complex odontomas show a predilection for occurrence in the posterior jaws.[74] Compound odontomas have been reported as having a mean age of occurrence of 14.8 years compared with 20.3 years of age for complex odontomas, possibly because the odontogenic tissue in the anterior jaws where the compound odontoma predominantly occurs has finished its differentiation earlier than tissues in the posterior part of the jaw.[72]

It has been argued that, because the radiographic and histologic distinction between the compound and complex odontomas is poorly defined and because no appreciable clinical difference separates them, differentiation

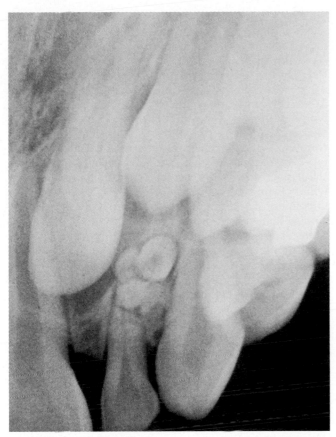

Figure 8-15 Complex composite odontoma delaying eruption of the lateral incisor.

of these two types of odontomas cannot be justified given the obliquity of the diagnostic criteria.[75] Others take exception to this concept, holding the view that complex and compound odontomas are pathogenetically different.[71] Those who take exception argue that complex odontomas are the terminal stage in the series of hamartomatous lesions (termed the *developing complex odontoma line*), including the ameloblastic fibro-dentinoma, the ameloblastic fibro-odontoma, and the "hamartomatous type of ameloblastic fibroma. They argue that ameloblastic fibromas occurring after the age of 20 years represent a benign neoplasm, whereas those occurring during childhood (i.e., during the tooth-development age group) are likely to be nonneoplastic hamartomatous lesions. They believe that the compound odontoma represents a malformation with a high degree of histomorphologic differentiation similar to the process producing supernumerary teeth, "multiple schizodontia," or locally conditioned hyperactivity of the dental lamina.

Although odontomas are usually asymptomatic, they may be the cause of noneruption or impaction of teeth and retained primary teeth (see Fig. 8-15). In one study, for instance, odontomas were found to be in association with an unerupted tooth in 48% of cases and in conjunction with a dentigerous cyst in 28% of cases.[75]

Odontomas are most commonly found on routine radiographic examination, presenting as an irregular radiopaque mass or as small, toothlike structures with the

most frequent presenting symptom being lack of eruption of a permanent tooth or bony expansion or swelling. The recommended treatment for an odontoma is conservative surgical excision, with care taken to remove the surrounding soft tissue. No propensity for recurrence has been noted.

MALIGNANT TUMORS

FIBROMATOSIS AND FIBROSARCOMA IN INFANCY AND CHILDHOOD

Fibromatosis

The fibromatoses represent a heterogenous group of infiltrating fibrous proliferations that have a clinical and biologic behavior between benign fibrous lesions and fibrosarcomas. Often termed *juvenile* or *aggressive* fibromatosis, they are locally aggressive in behavior with a tendency for recurrence, and although they do not metastasize, they can kill by local infiltration and extension into vital structures.

The head and neck region has been reported as a common site of involvement for these lesions, also known as extra-abdominal fibromatoses or desmoid tumors. They most commonly present as a painless mass involving the cheek, tongue, or submandibular region with erosion of bone being a frequent finding in lesions arising in soft tissue adjacent to the jaws.[76] In one large study of fibromatosis occurring in the oral and paraoral region, 74% of cases occurred in the first decade of life.[76]

Histologically fibromatosis is characterized by a proliferation of spindle-shaped or oval bland and uniform cells that are arranged in streaming fascicles with varying amounts of collagen. Cellular pleomorphism and nuclear hyperchromatism are not noted and mitoses are essentially absent.

Fibromatosis occuring in bone has been termed *desmoplastic fibromas* with the mandible being the most common site of involvement.[77] The radiographic findings are variable, ranging from unilocular to multilocular with borders that may vary from ill-defined to well demarcated. Microscopically there is nothing to differentiate desmoplastic fibroma of bone from fibromatosis occurring in the soft tissues. Whereas magnetic resonance imaging may be valuable in surgical planning, computed tomography is best for demonstrating perforation of the cortical plate.[77] Because of its locally aggressive nature, complete surgical excision with a generous margin of normal tissue has been reported as the treatment of choice, with recurrence being dependent on the adequacy of initial treatment.

Fibrosarcoma

Fibrosarcoma is a malignant neoplasm of fibroblastic and myofibroblastic differentiation. Congenital and infantile fibrosarcoma is a relatively rare tumor that usually is manifest in the first year of life, especially in the first 3 months, and almost always before 4 years of age.[78] Compared with fibromatosis, it is generally more cellular in appearance, with increased mitotic activity and radiographically, it may be more destructively expansile.[78] Fibrosarcoma that occurs in children younger than 4 years of age is much less likely to metastasize than it is in adults and has more in common with infantile aggressive fibromatosis than it does with the adult form of the disease. Although recurrence is possible, metastases are rare, and the majority of cases are cured by wide local excision. Adjuvant radiation therapy and chemotherapy are reserved for inoperable, recurrent, or metastatic cases

MALIGNANT LYMPHOMA

Malignant lymphomas are neoplasms of lymphoreticular origin that are divided into two main categories: non-Hodgkin's lymphoma (NHL) and Hodgkin's lymphoma (HL, or Hodgkin's disease). As a group, they are the third most frequent type of cancer in children after leukemia and brain tumors.[79]

Hodgkin's Lymphoma (Hodgkin's Disease)

HL is a malignant neoplasm of lymphoreticular origin distinguished from NHL by diverse but distinctive morphologic features with one common denominator, the presence of the Reed-Sternberg cell, which is widely accepted as the neoplastic cell. Reed-Sternberg cells, which appear to be clonal in origin arising from germinal center B cells, account for only a small percentage of the tumor mass with the majority of tumor composed of a reactive infiltrate of lymphocytes, plasma cells and eosinophils.[79] HL is characterized by a bimodal age distribution with the first peak incidence at approximately 25 years of age and the second peak at approximately 65 years of age. Although the first peak incidence is noted in adolescence and young adulthood, HL may be found even in very young children.

The staging of Hodgkin's disease is anatomically based because of its propensity to spread contiguously from one lymph node group to the next. The Ann Arbor staging classification was initially reported in 1971.[80] In 1989 the Ann Arbor staging was modified at a meeting in Cotswolds, England.[81] The Cotswolds modifications validated the use of computed tomography for identifying intra-abdominal disease, formally introduced bulk of disease into the staging system, and included the concept of unconfirmed complete remission. According to these modifications of the Ann Arbor staging system, stage I HL signifies disease involving one lymph node region (I) or a single extralymphatic organ or site (IE), such as the spleen, thymus, or Waldeyer's tonsillar ring. Stage II signifies involvement of two or more lymph node regions on the same side of the diaphragm (II) or with involvement of an extralymphatic organ or site and one or more lymph node regions on the same side of the diaphragm (IIE). Stage III indicates disease on both sides of the diaphragm (III), which may be accompanied by involvement of the spleen (IIIS) and/or limited contiguous extralymphatic organ or site (IIIE, IIIES). Stage IV indicates the presence of involvement of multiple extralymphatic sites, most often the liver or lungs, bone marrow, or bone with or without lymph node involvement. The absence or presence of symptoms such as unexplained fever with oral temperatures higher than 38°C for 3 or more consecutive days, shaking chills, drenching night sweats, and unexplained weight loss of 10% or more of body weight over a 6-month period are denoted by the suffix A or B, respectively, with B symptoms imparting a worse prognosis within each stage.

HL in the head and neck most commonly presents as a firm, rubbery, asymmetrically enlarged, nontender mass in the cervical lymph node chain. It occurs primarily in lymph nodes, and involvement of the oral cavity or oropharynx, including the Waldeyer's tonsillar ring, is uncommon. HL is classified into four classic histologic subtypes: lymphocyte rich, nodular sclerosing, mixed cellularity, and lymphocyte depletion. The nodular lymphocyte–predominant form, which is relatively uncommon in children, has a distinctive biologic and clinical behavior from the classic subtypes of Hodgkin's disease and hence has been separated from them.[82]

The most important prognostic variable in newly diagnosed cases of HL is the clinical stage, and the strongest predictive factor for patients with relapse after initial treatment is the duration of the initial response. Most treatment programs for limited-stage HL include chemotherapy and involved-field radiation therapy. With advances in therapy, current 5-year recurrence-free survival has been achieved by 95% or more of patients with stage I or II nonbulky disease and absence of systemic B symptoms (mediastinal lymphadenopathy is considered bulky). Five-year survival rates for patients with bulky disease, B symptoms, and/or advanced stage III or IV disease are between 80% and 94%. For patients who have experienced relapse after initial combined-modality therapy and those who experience multiple relapses, hematopoietic stem cell transplantation may offer hope of long-term remission.

Non-Hodgkin's Lymphomas.

The NHLs are a heterogenous group of neoplasms of the lymphoid system that may arise in the head and neck in the lymph nodes (nodal), in extranodal lymphatic areas (Waldeyer's tonsillar ring), or in extranodal, extralymphatic tissue, such as the mandible, salivary glands, pharynx, deep fascial spaces, paranasal sinuses, the orbit, and other areas. Childhood NHL differs from adult NHL in that they are commonly extranodal with the vast majority having an intermediate to high grade pathologic subtype (stage III or IV) at the time of presentation.[83,84] The head and neck is reported as being involved in 30% of cases.[84] Nearly 70% of children who present with NHL are said to have advanced disease or metastatic involvement at the time of diagnosis.[84]

The four major pathologic subtypes of childhood and adolescent non-Hodgkin lymphoma are Burkitt and Burkitt-like lymphoma (40%), lymphoblastic lymphoma (30%), B-large cell lymphoma (20%), and anaplastic large cell lymphoma (10%).[84]

The prognosis for childhood NHL with both limited and advanced stage disease is reported to have improved significantly over the past 2 decades.[84] However, in a study of children with nodal versus extranodal NHL, unlike adults, children whose primary head and neck NHLs were extranodal had a significantly worse treatment outcome than those whose primary tumors were nodal.[85]

Children whose tumors were extranodal and extralymphatic had an even worse outcome than the others, even among children with early stage disease (stage I or II). Owing to the anatomic sites of origin of NHL in childhood, the majority of patients do not present with peripheral lymphadenopathy, which may appear as a firm, nontender swelling, which, when present, may make early detection more likely.

RHABDOMYOSARCOMA

Rhabdomyosarcoma (RMS), a malignant neoplasm of skeletal muscle origin, is the most common soft tissue sarcoma in children, accounting for more than half of all such lesions occurring in childhood. It is one of the small, round blue-cell tumors of childhood, which includes neoplasms such as neuroblastoma, Ewing's sarcoma, and lymphoma. There are two key age ranges for the occurrence of RMS in children: 2 to 6 years of age and adolescence, with the early peak due primarily to occurrences in the head and neck region and genitourinary tract and with the peak during adolescence due to tumors of the testes and adjacent structures.[86]

Three general histologic subtypes of RMS are recognized: embryonal and its botryoid variant, alveolar, and pleomorphic. The embryonal subtype accounts for most cases of RMS in infancy and childhood that occur within the deep soft tissues or along mucosal surfaces.

The most common clinical finding is a mass occurring in any region of the head and neck where striated muscle or its mesenchymal progenitor cells exist. There are three primary sites of involvement for RMS in the head and neck in children: the eyelid and orbit, parameningeal sites, and remaining head and neck sites including the oral cavity.[87] The parameningeal sites include the pterygopalatine and infratemporal fossas, nasal cavity, nasopharynx, paranasal sinuses, and middle ear and mastoid. Although there is not good consensus about site predilection within the oral cavity, the soft palate and tonsillar region, tongue, and cheek seem to be most frequently involved with the gingiva and floor of mouth being unusual locations.[88,89] Typically a rapidly growing, often nonulcerated soft tissue mass, RMS typically metastasizes by hematogenous routes to lungs, bone, and brain but may also disseminate via the lymphatics or direct extension.

RMSs arising in the head and neck region are characterized by a wide variation in survival rate, which is dependent on the site, with orbital lesions having the highest survival rates of any site in the body and parameningeal tumors having a worse prognosis.[90] The high survival rate in patients with orbital lesions is likely because they present with less advanced disease compared with the insidious presentation of parameningeal primaries, which more typically present with advanced stage disease.[90] Even though age, anatomic subsite, and resectability were not shown to correlate with survival, extent of disease including tumor size, invasiveness, nodal metastases, and distant disease at presentation were all significantly associated with mortality.[90] Children 11 years of age or younger with a tumor 5 cm or smaller have ben shown to have the best survival, whereas patients older than 11 years with a tumor larger than 5 cm had the worst survival outcome.[91]

Risk-guided therapy based primarily on the extent of disease using multiagent chemotherapy, surgery, and external-beam radiation therapy has improved survival.

OSTEOGENIC SARCOMA

Osteogenic sarcoma (OS) is an uncommon, highly malignant, primary neoplasm of bone with a soft tissue counterpart with a similar histomorphology. Its peak age of occurrence is the second decade of life, with the modal age of incidence being 16 years for girls and 18 for boys.[92] The most common site of involvement is the distal femur, followed by the proximal tibia and proximal humerus.

Osteogenic sarcoma of the jaws (OSJ) accounts for approximately 6.5% of all cases of OS with the average age of onset being 10 to 20 years later than for skeletal lesions.[93] The mandible seems to be involved more often than the maxilla.[93,94] Swelling with or without pain is the most frequently described early symptom. Paresthesia/anesthesia and loosening of the teeth may be noted. In a clinicopathologic study of 22 cases of OS of the head and neck in a pediatric population ranging from 1 to 18 years (mean age, 12.2 years), the primary symptoms were painless swelling, loss of teeth, headaches, or a mass lesion.[95] The average duration of symptoms was 5.9 months. Nineteen cases (86%) occurred in the mandible, two cases in the sphenoid sinus, and one in the maxilla.

The radiographic findings are typically those of a poorly defined, bone-destructive lesion suggestive of malignancy. Radiographically it may be osteoblastic or osteolytic or may have a mixed radiographic appearance. One study reported that most of the lesions on the maxilla were osteoblastic, whereas most of those on the mandible were osteolytic.[96] A frequently described radiographic feature is a "sun-ray" appearance with delicate, hairlike osteophytes radiating in a sunburst fashion away from the peripheral surface of the lesion. This has been reported to occur in as few as 10 % and as many as 55% of cases.[93,97] An additional radiographic finding in early OSJ is symmetric widening of the periodontal ligament space around one or more of the teeth in the area of the lesion.

Histologically the OS is characterized by the production of tumor osteoid forming a malignant stroma that often appears fibroblastic. These tumors are typically classified histologically into osteoblastic, chondroblastic, or fibroblastic subtypes according to the dominant histologic pattern. There is no agreement, however, as to whether the histologic subtype has any significant bearing on the patient's prognosis.

The primary treatment modality for OSJ should always be radical surgery with the single most important factor in curative therapy being its amenability to radical resection with clear margins.[93] Overall, chemotherapy has not been shown to be as effective in OSJ as in extragnathic sites for two reasons: first, even though almost all patients with OS of the long bones have at least microscopic metastatic disease at the time of diagnosis, the incidence of metastatic disease at the time of diagnosis for OSJ in all age groups is reported to be no higher than 18%[98]; second, OSJs tend to be better differentiated than those involving the long bones, which may be partially responsible for the better prognosis for patients with osteosarcoma of the jaws.[96,98] Even so, it is still recommended that patients with primary osteosarcoma of the jaws should be treated with multiagent chemotherapy in addition to complete surgical excision with free surgical margins being absolutely essential.[99]

EWING'S SARCOMA

After osteosarcoma, the Ewing's sarcoma (ES) family of tumors (ES along with peripheral primitive neuroectodermal tumor [pPNET]) is the second most common primary malignancy of bone in children and adolescents. Ewing's sarcoma of bone and soft tissue, as well as pPNET, are small round-cell tumors, the genetic hallmarks of which are the presence of a translocation of chromosomes 11 and 22, t(11;22)(q24;q12), and in most cases overexpression of the MIC2 gene surface marker (CD99), which differentiates them from the majority of other small round-cell tumors.

The histologic and electron microscopic features of ES and pPNET, as well as expression of antigen of the MIC2 gene, provide the basis for characterizing them as neuroectodermally derived neoplasms.[100,101]

Approximately 4% of primary cases of ES arising in bone arise in the bones of the head and neck, with the skull being the most frequent site of involvement and the mandible being the most commonly involved gnathic bone.[102] A review of 105 cases showed the average age at diagnosis to be 15.9 years with an age range of 2 to 44 years at presentation.[103] There was a slight predilection for occurrence in males, with a male-to-female ratio of 1.5:1. The mandible was involved more than twice as often as the maxilla, with a predilection of 4:1 for occurrence in the posterior aspect of the jaws over other regions.

A histopathologically identical extraskeletal form of ES has been identified.[104] In a series of 130 patients with ES of soft tissue in childhood 18% of cases involved the head and neck. Patients with soft tissue or extraskeletal ES were compared with patients with pPNET.[105] There were no significant differences in patient age, gender, tumor location, or stage at presentation between patients with ES and those with pPNET of the soft tissue.

Localized swelling and pain are the most frequent complaints at the time of presentation, although paresthesia and tooth mobility may also be presenting symptoms. The soft tissue overlying the lesion may be erythematous and warm to the touch, and thus more suggestive of an inflammatory process than a neoplasm (Fig. 8-16). In addition, the patient may have fever, elevated erythrocyte sedimentation rate, increased serum lactic dehydrogenase level, anemia, and leukocytosis.

The radiographic features are those of a diffuse bone-destructive lesion, appearing as an irregular, somewhat mottled, radiolucent lesion that may resemble an osteomyelitis (Fig. 8-17). Although reduplication or lamination of the periosteum has been considered a common radiologic sign of ES of long bones, this has been shown not to be a common feature of this disease in the jaw bones; however, sun-ray spicules of periosteal bone may be seen as previously described for osteogenic sarcoma.[103] Computed tomography and in particular magnetic resonance imaging are invaluable in further

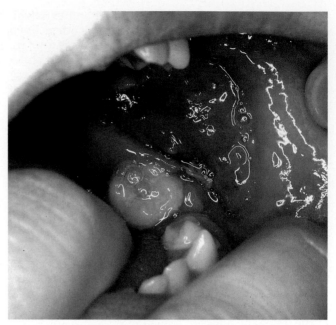

Figure 8-16 Photograph of a 6-year-old boy with Ewing's sarcoma who had a 1-month history of swelling on the left side of his face. Clinically there was swelling with mucosal ulceration in the mucobuccal fold in the first molar area. (Courtesy Drs. Richard L. Miller and William Epstein.)

delineating the extent of disease not readily visible on plain radiographs.[106,107] Histologically, ES appears as sheets of cells with small, dark-staining nuclei and poorly defined cytoplasmic outlines. Mitotic figures are prominent, and necrosis is a common feature. Sheets of cells may be separated by vascular connective tissue septa. The

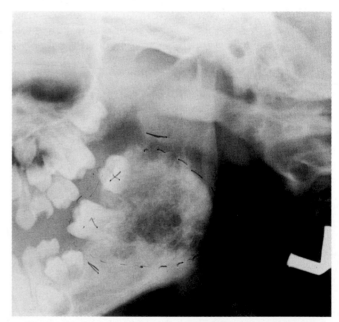

Figure 8-17 Radiograph of the same patient as in Fig. 8-16 with Ewing's sarcoma involving the left angle of the mandible. Notice the mottled radiolucent appearance. (Courtesy Drs. Richard L. Miller and William Epstein.)

presence of intracytoplasmic glycogen and positive results on periodic acid–Schiff staining are essential findings unless there is documented glycogen content on electron microscopy. Detection of MIC2 antigen along with the use of molecular techniques to detect the (11;22)(q24;q12) translocation have generally improved the ability to diagnose these tumors.

In the past, ES as a whole has been associated with an almost uniformly poor prognosis, with nearly all patients having micrometastatic disease at the time of diagnosis. The prognosis for ES in the head and neck, however has been noted to be significantly better than that for ES overall.[102] In a report by the Intergroup Ewing's Sarcoma Study of patients who had been followed in the study for more than 3 years, 80% were alive and well without known progressive recurrent or metastatic disease. Of the 10 patients who had survived 5 years or longer, none had subsequently died, and of the five patients in their study who had died, none had gnathic involvement.

Chemotherapy is the cornerstone of treatment for ES and is usually applied in a neoadjuvant fashion.[107] Therapy consists of systemic multiagent chemotherapy along with local control, which may consist of surgery, radiation therapy, or a combination of the two, depending on the age of the patient, the location of the primary tumor, and the functional consequences of therapy. When surgery is employed, the goal should be complete tumor removal, avoiding marginal resection.[107] Because of the potential for postradiation sarcomas, particularly bone sarcoma in the field of radiation treatment, the importance of local control of the disease with surgery and safe local control with radiation is now emphasized. Patients with clinically detectable metastases at the time of diagnosis and those with relapse after initial therapy have a significantly poorer prognosis.

LANGERHANS CELL HISTIOCYTOSIS (HISTIOCYTOSIS X)

Langerhans cell histiocytosis (LCH) is the current designation replacing the term *histiocytosis X* introduced by Lichtenstein in 1953 as a unifying designation for several previous eponyms, including Letterer-Siwe disease, Hand-Schüller-Christian disease, and eosinophilic granuloma (LCH of bone).[108]

Although clinical forms of LCH were first described at least a century ago, its etiology and pathogenesis remains obscure, with the one common denominator being the Langerhans cell, a bone marrow–derived, antigen- presenting dendritic cell. Langerhans cells reside in the skin, thymus, and mucosal epithelium, including the oropharynx and nasopharynx, esophagus, bronchi, and cervix and are said to be the most potent antigen-presenting cells in the body.[109]

Histologically LCH is characterized by the presence of uniform sheets of large round Langerhans histiocytes, which have been shown to be immature dendritic cells and not a histiocytes at all, with a homogenous pink cytoplasm when stained with hematoxylin and eosin. These Langerhans cell histiocytes are interspersed with variable numbers of eosinophils, lymphocytes, plasma cells, and multinucleated giant cells, particularly in lesions of bone.

Langerhans cells are characterized ultrastructurally by the presence of Langerhans or Birbeck granules, rod-shaped organelles that may have a vesicular portion imparting the so-called tennis racquet appearance under the electron microscope. LCH can now be identified on the basis of immunoreactivity to cell surface markers such as CD-ia and more specifically CD-207 (Langerin), which differentiates it from other dendritic disorders.[110,111] The clinical manifestations of LCH are variable and historically were divided into distinct entities. The term *Letterer-Siwe disease* (now better termed *acute disseminated histiocytosis*) has been used as a moniker for an acute fulminating proliferative disorder involving Langerhans histiocytes that chiefly affects infants and children younger than 3 years of age. It is often characterized initially by the development of a scaly erythematous skin rash initially most prominent on the trunk but progressing to involve the scalp and extremities (Fig. 8-18). This is accompanied by a persistent low-grade fever, anemia, thrombocytopenia, hepatosplenomegaly, and lymphadenopathy.

Bony involvement, indistinguishable from that found in chronic disseminated histiocytosis (Hand-Schüller-Christian disease) and eosinophilic granuloma of bone may be noted (Fig. 8-19). Oral lesions with swelling, pain,

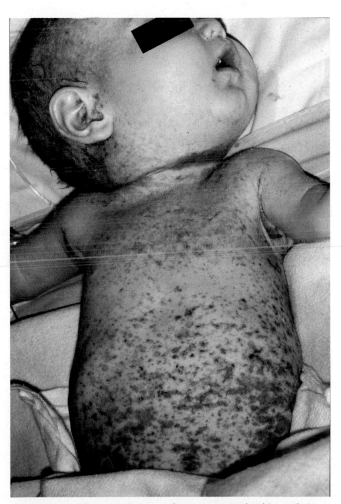

Figure 8-18 Characteristic erythematous scaly skin rash in a 5½-month-old infant with Letterer-Siwe disease.

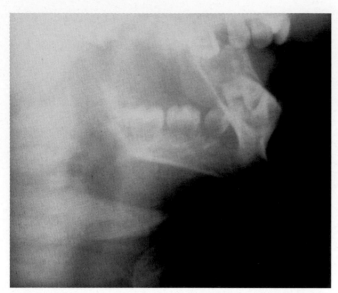

Figure 8-19 Diffuse destruction of maxillary and mandibular alveolar bone around the developing primary teeth in the same patient as in Fig. 8-18. Notice also destruction of the left angle and ramus of the mandible.

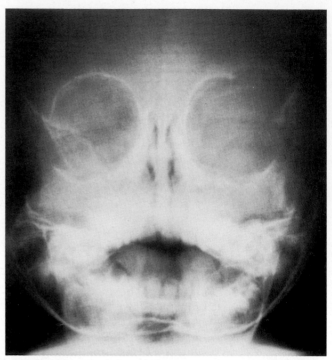

Figure 8-20 Radiograph for a 12-month-old girl with Hand-Schüller-Christian disease. There is an expansile, radiolucent lesion in the right body of the mandible as well as destruction of the greater wing of the sphenoid and supraorbital rim on the left.

ulceration, gingival inflammation and necrosis, and destruction of alveolar bone with premature exfoliation of the teeth may be an early manifestation of this form of the disease. Although multiagent chemotherapy may result in regression of the disease in some cases, patients with this form of the disease have a relatively poor prognosis.

Hand-Schüller-Christian disease (now better termed *chronic disseminated histiocytosis*) has been used to describe the chronic disseminated form of LCH, which is characterized by the development of multifocal eosinophilic granulomas of bone, lymphadenopathy, and visceral involvement, especially hepatosplenomegaly (Fig. 8-20). The classic clinical triad that has often been described for this disease is the occurrence of punched-out–appearing radiolucent defects in membranous bones, exophthalmos, and diabetes insipidus. Chronic otitis media is also a frequent finding. Although usually diagnosed early in the first decade of life, chronic disseminated histiocytosis has been reported to occur as late as the sixth decade.[112]

The treatment varies according to the extent of the disease, with surgical curettage or radiation therapy being used to treat focal disease. Multiagent chemotherapy has been relatively successful in long-term control of disseminated disease.

Eosinophilic granuloma (LCH of bone) is the most common and also least severe form of LCH. It is characterized by single or multiple usually well-defined radiolucent bony lesions, most often accompanied by pain and swelling. Older children and young adults most commonly display this form of the disease. In addition to the mandible and skull, the femur, humerus, ribs, and pelvis are also frequently involved. The maxilla is involved less frequently than the mandible, with the midposterior mandible being the most common site of occurrence. Skin and visceral involvement such as that described for

the acute disseminated and chronic disseminated forms of the disease (Letterer-Siwe disease and Hand-Schüller-Christian disease) are absent. A variety of options exist for patients with this form of the disease. After confirmation of the diagnosis by biopsy, the lesion may be left alone for observation, it may be surgically curetted or excised, intralesional injections of corticosteroids may be given, or low-dose radiotherapy may be used. In one series of 41 lesions in 25 patients, treatment varied from excisional biopsy to curettage and peripheral ostectomy as the only surgical treatment followed by low-dose radiotherapy. Three lesions (7.3%) in three patients (12%) recurred.[113]

REFERENCES

1. Abbey LM, Page DG, Sawyer DR. The clinical and histopathologic features of a series of 464 oral squamous cell papillomas, *Oral Surg* 49:419-428, 1980.
2. Greer RO, Goldman HM. Oral papillomas: clinicopathologic evaluation and retrospective examination for dyskeratosis in 110 lesions, *Oral Surg* 38:435-440, 1974.
3. Praetorius F. HPV-associated diseases of oral mucosa, *Clin Dermatol* 15:399-413, 1997.
4. Syrjänen S. Human papillomavirus infections and oral tumors, *Med Microbiol Immunol* 192(3):123-128; Epub 2003 Jan 18.
5. Naghashfar Z, et al. Identification of genital tract papillomavirus HPV-6 and HPV-16 in warts of the oral cavity, *J Med Virol* 17:313-324, 1985.
6. Zeuss MS, Miller CS, White DK. In situ hybridization analysis of human papillomavirus DNA in oral mucosal lesions, *Oral Surg Oral Med Oral Pathol* 71:714-20, 1991.

7. Jenson AB, et al. Frequency and distribution of papilloma-virus structural antigens in verrucae, multiple papillomas, and condylomata of the oral cavity, *Am J Pathol* 107: 212-218, 1982.

8. Ward KA, et al. Detection of human papilloma virus DNA sequences in oral squamous cell papillomas by the poly-merase chain reaction, *Oral Surg Oral Med Oral Pathol Oral Radiol Endod* 80:63-66, 1995.

9. Eversole LR, Laipis PJ. Oral squamous papillomas: detection of HPV DNA by in situ hybridization, *Oral Surg Oral Med Oral Pathol* 65:545-550, 1988.

10. Angelopoulos AP. Pyogenic granuloma of the oral cavity: statistical analysis of its clinical features, *J Oral Surg* 29: 840-847, 1971.

11. Lawoyin JO, Arotiba JT, Dosumu OO. Oral pyogenic granu-loma: a review of 38 cases from Ibadan, Nigeria, *Br J Oral Maxillofac Surg* 35:185-189, 1997.

12. Cundiff EJ. Peripheral ossifying fibroma: a review of 365 cases, master's thesis, Bloomington, Ind, Indiana University, 1972. Cited in Shafer WG, Hine MK, Levy BM. *Textbook of oral pathology, 4th ed.* Philadelphia, 1983, WB Saunders.

13. Eversole LR, Rovin S. Reactive lesions of the gingival, *J Oral Pathol* 1:30-38, 1972.

14. Cuisia ZE, Brannon RB, Peripheral ossifying fibroma—a clinical evaluation of 134 pediatric cases, *Pediatr Dent* 23(3):245-248, 2001.

15. Gardner DG. The peripheral odontogenic fibroma: an attempt at clarification, *Oral Surg Oral Med Oral Pathol* 54:40-48, 1982.

16. Daley TD, Wysocki GP. Peripheral odontogenic fibroma, *Oral Surg Oral Med Oral Pathol* 78(3):329-336, 1994.

17. Giansanti JS, Waldron CA. Peripheral giant cell granuloma: review of 720 cases, *J Oral Surg* 27:787-791, 1969.

18. Andersen L, Fejerskov O, Philipsen HP. Oral giant cell gran-ulomas: a clinical and histological study of 129 new cases, *Acta Pathol Microbiol Scand* 5(Sec A 81):606-616, 1973.

19. Nedir R, Lombardi T, Samson J. Recurrent peripheral giant cell granuloma associated with cervical resorption, *J Periodontol* 68:381-384, 1997.

20. Hersh JH; American Academy of Pediatrics Committee on Genetics. Health supervision for children with neurofibro-matosis, *Pediatrics* 121(3):633-642, 2008.

21. Lee L, Yan YH, Pharoah MJ. Radiographic features of the mandible in neurofibromatosis: a report of 10 cases and review of the literature, *Oral Surg Oral Med Oral Pathol Oral Radiol Endod* 81:361-367, 1996.

22. Needle MN, et al. Prognostic signs in the surgical manage-ment of plexiform neurofibroma: The Children's Hospital of Philadelphia experience, 1974-1994, *J Pediatr* 131: 678-682, 1997.

23. Robertson RL, et al. Head and neck vascular anomalies of childhood, *Neuroimaging Clin North Am* 9(1):115-132, 1999.

24. Mulliken JB, Glowacki J. Hemangiomas and vascular mal-formation in infants and children: a classification based on endothelial characteristics, *Plast Reconstr Surg* 69(3): 412-422, 1982.

25. Arneja JS, Gosain AK. Vascular malformations, *Plast Recon-str Surg* 122(6):1982-1984, 2008.

26. Lamberg MA, Tasanen A, Jääskeläinen J. Fatality from central hemangioma of the mandible, *J Oral Surg* 37(8): 578-584, 1979.

27. Hancock BJ, et al. Complications of lymphangiomas in children, *J Pediatr Surg* 27(2):220-226, 1992.

28. Ugras W, et al. Immunohistochemical study on histogene-sis of congenital epulis and review of the literature, *Pathol Int* 47:627-632, 1997.

29. Kaiserling E, Ruck P, Xiao JC. Congenital epulis and granu-lar cell tumor: a histologic and immunohistochemical study, *Oral Surg Oral Med Oral Pathol Oral Radiol Endod* 80(6):687-697, 1995.

30. Eversole R, Su L, El Mofty S. Benign fibro-osseous lesions of the craniofacial complex. A review, *Head Neck Pathol* 2:177-202, 2008.

31. Petrikowski CG, et al. Radiographic differentiation of osteo-genic sarcoma, osteomyelitis, and fibrous dysplasia of the jaws, *Oral Surg Oral Med Oral Pathol Oral Radiol Endod* 80:744-750, 1995.

32. Mäkitie AA, Törnwall J, Mäkitie O. Bisphosphonate treat-ment in craniofacial fibrous dysplasia—a case report and review of the literature, *Clin Rheumatol* 27(6):809-812, 2008.

33. Eversole LR, Leider AS, Nelson K. Ossifying fibroma: a clini-copathologic study of sixty-four cases, *Oral Surg Oral Med Oral Pathol* 60:505-511, 1985.

34. Sciubba JJ, Younai F. Ossifying fibroma of the mandible and maxilla: review of 18 cases, *J Oral Pathol Med* 18: 315-321, 1989.

35. Waldron CA. Fibro-osseous lesions of the jaws, *J Oral Surg* 28:58-64, 1970.

36. El-Mofty S. Psammomatoid and trabecular juvenile ossify-ing fibroma of the craniofacial skeleton: two distinct clini-copathologic entities, *Oral Surg Oral Med Oral Pathol Oral Radiol Endod* 93:296-304, 2002.

37. Jaffe HL. Giant-cell reparative granuloma, traumatic bone cyst, and fibrous (fibro-osseous) dysplasia of the jawbones, *Oral Surg Oral Med Oral Pathol* 6(1):159-175, 1953.

38. Kaffe I, et al. Radiologic features of central giant cell granu-loma of the jaws, *Oral Surg Oral Med Oral Pathol Oral Radiol Endod* 81:720-726, 1996.

39. Waldron CA, Shafer WG. The central giant cell reparative granuloma of the jaws: an analysis of 38 cases, *Am J Clin Pathol* 45:437-447, 1966.

40. Auclair PL, et al. A clinical and histomorphologic comparison of the central giant cell granuloma and the giant cell tumor, *Oral Surg Oral Med Oral Pathol* 66: 197-208, 1988.

41. Whitaker SB, Waldron CA. Central giant cell lesions of the jaw. A clinical, radiologic, and histopathologic study, *Oral Surg Oral Med Oral Pathol* 75(2):199-208, 1993.

42. Chuong R, et al. Central giant cell lesions of the jaw: a clinicopathologic study, *Oral Maxillofac Surg* 44(9):708-713, 1986.

43. de Lange J, van den Akker HP, van den Berg H. Central giant cell granuloma of the jaw: a review of the literature with emphasis on therapy options, *Oral Med Oral Pathol Oral Radiol Endod* 104(5):603-615, 2007.

44. Browne RM. The pathogenesis of odontogenic cysts: a review, *J Oral Pathol* 4(1):31-46, 1975.

45. Brannon RB. The odontogenic keratocyst: a clinicopatho-logic study of 312 cases. Part I. Clinical features, *Oral Surg* 42:54-72, 1976.

46. Mourshed F. A roentgenographic study of dentigerous cysts. I. Incidence in a population sample, *Oral Surg Oral Med Oral Pathol* 18:47-53, 1964.

47. Benn A, Altini M. Dentigerous cysts of inflammatory ori-gin. A clinicopathologic study, *Oral Surg Oral Med Oral Pathol Oral Radiol Endod* 81(2):203-209, 1996.

48. Mourshed F. A roentgenographic study of dentigerous cysts. II. Role of roentgenograms in detecting dentigerous cyst in the early stages, *Oral Surg Oral Med Oral Pathol* 18:54-61, 1964.

49. McMillan MD, Smillie AC. Ameloblastomas associated with dentigerous cysts, *Oral Surg* 51:489-496, 1981.

50. Leider AS, Eversole LR, Barkin ME. Cystic ameloblastoma, *Oral Surg* 60:624-630, 1985.

51. Gardner DG, Corio RL. Plexiform unicystic ameloblastoma: a variant of ameloblastoma with a low recurrence rate after enucleation, *Cancer* 53:1730-1735, 1984.

52. Wright JM. The odontogenic keratocyst: orthokeratinized variant, *Oral Surg Oral Med Oral Pathol* 51(6):609-618, 1981.

53. Eyre J, Zakrzewska JM. The conservative management of large odontogenic keratocysts, *Br J Oral Maxillofac Surg* 23:195-203, 1985.

54. Woolgar JA, Rippin JW, Browne RM. A comparative study of the clinical and histological features of recurrent and non-recurrent odontogenic keratocysts, *J Oral Pathol* 16:124-128, 1987.

55. Anand VK, Arrowood JP, Krolls SO. Malignant potential of the odontogenic keratocyst, *Otolaryngol Head Neck Surg* 111:124-249, 1994.

56. Forsell K, Forsell H, Kahnberg KE. Recurrence of keratocysts in a long-term follow-up study, *Int J Oral Surg* 17:25-28, 1988.

57. Meara JG, et al. The odontogenic keratocyst: a 20-year clinicopathologic review, *Laryngoscope* 108:280-283, 1998.

58. Blanas N, et al. Systematic review of the treatment and prognosis of the odontogenic keratocyst, *Oral Surg Oral Med Oral Pathol Oral Radiol Endod* 90:553-558, 2000.

59. Gorlin RJ. Nevoid basal cell carcinoma (Gorlin) syndrome, *Genet Med* 6(6):530-539, 2004.

60. Robinson L, Martinez MG. Unicystic ameloblastoma: a prognostically distinct entity, *Cancer* 40:2278-2285, 1977.

61. Philipsen HP, Reichert PA. Unicystic ameloblastoma. A review of 193 cases from the literature, *Oral Oncol* 34:317-325, 1998.

62. Kahn MA. Ameloblastoma in young persons: a clinicopathologic analysis and etiologic investigation, *Oral Surg Oral Med Oral Pathol* 67:706-715, 1989.

63. Rosenstein T, et al. Cystic ameloblastoma—behavior and treatment of 21 cases, *J Oral Maxillofac Surg* 59:1311-1318, 2001.

64. Ghandhi D, et al. Ameloblastoma: a surgeon's dilemma, *J Oral Maxillofac Surg* 64(7):1010-1014, 2006.

65. Philipsen HP, Reichart PA. Adenomatoid odontogenic tumor: facts and figures, *Oral Oncol* 35:125-131, 1998.

66. Philipsen HP, et al. Adenomatoid odontogenic tumor: biologic profile based on 499 cases, *J Oral Pathol Med* 20:149-158, 1991.

67. Phillipsen HP, et al. An updated clinical and epidemiological profile of the adenomatoid odontogenic tumour: a collaborative retrospective study, *J Oral Pathol Med* 36(7):383-393, 2007.

68. Kaffe I, Naor H, Buchner A. Clinical and radiological features of odontogenic myxoma of the jaws, *Dentomaxillofac Radiol* 26:299-203, 1997.

69. Keszler A, Dominguez FV, Giannunzio G. Myxoma in childhood: an analysis of 10 cases, *J Oral Maxillofac Surg* 53:518-521, 1995.

70. Chen Y, Wang JM, Li TJ. Ameloblastic fibroma: a review of published studies with special reference to its nature and biological behavior, *Oral Oncol* 43(10):960-969, 2007.

71. Philipsen HP, Reichart PA, Praetorius F. Mixed odontogenic tumours and odontomas: considerations on interrelationship. Review of the literature and presentation of 134 new cases of odontomas, *Oral Oncol* 33:86-99, 1997.

72. Slootweg PJ. An analysis of the interrelationship of the mixed odontogenic tumors—ameloblastic fibroma, ameloblastic fibro-odontoma and the odontomas, *Oral Surg* 51:266-276, 1981.

73. Takeda Y. Ameloblastic fibroma and related lesions: current pathologic concept, *Oral Oncol* 35:535-540, 1999.

74. Budnick SD. Complex and compound odontomas, *Oral Surg Oral Med Oral Pathol* 42:501-506, 1976.

75. Kaugars GE, Miller ME, Abbey LM. Odontomas, *Oral Surg Oral Med Oral Pathol* 67:172-176, 1989.

76. Fowler CB, Hartman KS, Brannon RB. Fibromatosis of the oral and paraoral region, *Oral Surg Oral Med Oral Pathol* 77(4):373-386, 1994.

77. Said-Al-Naief N, et al. Desmoplastic fibroma of the jaw: a case report and review of literature, *Oral Surg Oral Med Oral Pathol Oral Radiol Endod* 101(1):82-94, 2006.

78. Fisher C. Fibromatosis and fibrosarcoma in infancy and childhood, *Eur J Cancer* 32A:2094-2100, 1996.

79. Percy CL, Smith MA, Linet M, et al. Lymphomas and reticuloendothelial neoplasms. In Ries LAAG, Smith MA, Gurney JG, et al, eds. *Cancer incidence and survival among children and adolescents: United States SEER Program 1975-1995.* Pub. No. 99-4649. Bethesda, MD, National Cancer Institute, PubSeer program, 1999:35-30.

80. Carbone PP, et al. Report of the Committee on Hodgkin's Disease Staging Classification, *Cancer Res* 31:1 860-1861, 1971.

81. Lister TA, et al. Report of a committee convened to discuss the evaluation and staging of patients with Hodgkin's disease: Cotswolds meeting, *J Clin Oncol* 7:1630-1636, 1989.

82. Franklin J, et al. Lymphocyte predominant Hodgkin's disease: pathology and clinical implication, *Ann Oncol* 9(Suppl 5):39-44, 1998.

83. Harris NL, et al. The World Health Organization classification of neoplasms of the hematopoietic and lymphoid tissues: Report of the Clinical Advisory Committee meeting—Airlie House, Virginia, November, 1997, *Hematol J* 1(1):53-66, 2000.

84. Cairo MS. Raetz E, Perkins SL. Non-Hodgkin lymphoma in children. In: Kufe DW, Pollock RE, Weichselbaum RR, et al, eds. *Cancer medicine E6.* London, 2003, BC Decker Inc.

85. Ribeiro RC, et al. Extranodal primary tumor site indicates poor prognosis in childhood head and neck non-Hodgkin's lymphomas, *Leukemia* 5:615-620, 1991.

86. Miller RW, Calager NA. Fatal rhabdomyosarcoma among children in the United States, 1960-69, *Cancer* 34(6):1897-1900, 1974.

87. Sutow WW, et al. Three-year relapse-free survival rates in childhood rhabdomyosarcoma of the head and neck: report from the Intergroup Rhabdomyosarcoma Study, *Cancer* 1;49(11):2217-2221, 1982.

88. Bras J, Batsakis JC, Luna MA. Rhabdomyosarcoma of the oral soft tissues, *Oral Surg Oral Med Oral Pathol* 64(5):585-596, 1987.

89. Peters E, et al. Rhabdomyosarcoma of the oral and paraoral region, *Cancer* 1:63(5):963-966, 1989.

90. Kraus DH, Saenz NC, Gollamudi S, et al. Pediatric rhabdomyosarcoma of the head and neck, *Am J Surg* 174:556-560, 1997.

91. Simon JH, et al. Prognostic factors in head and neck rhabdomyosarcoma, *Head Neck* 24:468-473, 2002.

92. Meyers PA, Gorlick R. Osteosarcoma, *Pediatr Clin North Am* 44:973-989, 1997.

93. Fernandes R, et al. Osteogenic sarcoma of the jaw: a 10-year experience, *J Oral Maxillofac Surg* 65(7):1286-1291, 2007.

94. Garrington GE, et al. Osteosarcoma of the jaws: analysis of 56 cases, *Cancer* 20:377-391, 1967.

95. Gadwal SR, et al. Primary osteosarcoma of the head and neck in pediatric patients: clinical pathologic study of 22 cases with a review of the literature, *Cancer* 91:598-605, 2001.

96. Clark JL, et al. Osteosarcoma of the jaw, *Cancer* 51:2311-2316, 1983.
97. August M, Magennis P, Dewitt D. Osteogenic sarcoma of the jaws: factors influencing prognosis, *Int J Oral Maxillofac Surg* 26(3):198-204, 1997.
98. Mardinger O, et al. Osteosarcoma of the jaw: The Chaim Shebe Medical Center experience, *Oral Surg Oral Med Oral Pathol Oral Radiol Endod* 91:445-451, 2001.
99. Thiele OC, et al. Interdisciplinary combined treatment of craniofacial osteosarcoma with neoadjuvant and adjuvant chemotherapy and excision of the tumour; a retrospective study, *Br J Oral Maxillofac Surg* 46(7):533-356, 2008.
100. Ambros IM, et al. MIC2 is a specific marker for Ewing's sarcoma and peripheral primitive neuroectodermal tumors. Evidence for a common histogenesis of Ewing's sarcoma and peripheral primitive neuroectodermal tumors from MIC2 expression and specific chromosome aberration, *Cancer* 67(7):1886-1893, 1991.
101. Lombart-Bosch A, et al. Histology, immunohistochemistry, and electron microscopy of small round cell tumors of bone, *Semin Diagn Pathol* 13:153-170, 1996.
102. Siegal GP, et al. Primary Ewing's sarcoma involving the head and neck, *Cancer* 60:2829-2840, 1987.
103. Wood RE, et al. Ewing's tumor of the jaw, *Oral Surg Oral Med Oral Pathol* 69:120-127, 1990.
104. Raney RB, et al. Ewing's sarcoma of soft tissues in childhood: a report from the Intergroup Rhabdomyosarcoma Study, 1972-1991, *J Clin Oncol* 15:574-582, 1997.
105. Siebenrock KA, et al. Comparison of soft tissue Ewing's sarcoma and peripheral neuroectodermal tumor, *Clin Orthop* 329:288-299, 1996.
106. Eggli KD, et al. Ewing's sarcoma, *Radiol Clin North Am* 31:325-337, 1993.
107. Bielack SS, Carrle D. State-of-the-art approach in selective curable tumors: bone sarcoma, *Ann Oncol* 19(Suppl 7): vii 155-160, 2008.
108. Lichtenstein L. Histiocytosis X: integration of eosinophilic granuloma of bone, Letterer-Siwe disease and Schüller-Christian disease as related manifestations of a single nosologic entity, *Arch Pathol* 56:84-102, 1953.
109. Lam KY. Langerhans' cell histiocytosis (histiocytosis X), *Postgrad Med J* 73:391-394, 1997.
110. Valladeau J, et al. Langerin, a novel C-type lectin specific to Langerhans cells, is an endocytic receptor that induces the formation of Birbeck granules, *Immunity* 12(1):71-81, 2000.
111. Hicks J, Flaitz CM. Langerhans cell histiocytosis: current insights in a molecular age with emphasis on clinical oral and maxillofacial pathology practice, *Oral Surg Oral Med Oral Pathol Oral Radiol Endod* 100(Suppl 2): 42-66, 2005.
112. McDonald JS, et al. Histiocytosis X: a clinical presentation, *J Oral Pathol* 9:342-349, 1980.
113. Ardekian L, et al. Clinical and radiographic features of eosinophilic granuloma in the jaws, review of 41 lesions treated by surgery and low-dose radiotherapy, *Oral Surg Oral Med Oral Pathol Oral Radiol Endod* 87:238-242, 1999.

CHAPTER 9

Eruption of the Teeth: Local, Systemic, and Congenital Factors That Influence the Process

▲ Ralph E. McDonald, David R. Avery, and Jeffrey A. Dean

CHAPTER OUTLINE

CHRONOLOGIC DEVELOPMENT AND ERUPTION OF THE TEETH

A variety of developmental defects that are evident after eruption of the primary and permanent teeth can be related to systemic and local factors that influence matrix formation and the calcification process. Thus it is important that the dentist be able to explain to the parents the time factors related to the early stages of tooth calcification both in utero and during infancy.

Lunt and Law made a careful review of the literature on the calcification of the primary teeth.[1] They compared their findings with the values in Table 9-1 showing Logan and Kronfeld's chronology of human dentition, which has been an accepted standard for many years.[2] They offered a revised table that establishes earlier ages than those previously accepted for initial calcification (Table 9-2). A similar review was carried out for the ages at which the primary teeth erupt.[3]

Lunt and Law concluded after reviewing the work of Kraus and Jordan and of Nomata that Table 9-1 should be modified.[4,5] The sequence of calcification of the primary teeth should be changed to central incisor, first molar, lateral incisor, canine, and second molar. They determined that the times of initial calcification of the primary teeth are 2 to 6 weeks earlier than those given in Table 9-1. They also concluded that the maxillary teeth are generally ahead of the mandibular teeth in

development. Exceptions are the second molars, which generally are advanced in the mandible, and the lateral incisors and canines, which at times may be ahead in the mandible.

Lunt and Law also believe that the lateral incisor, first molar, and canine tend to erupt earlier in the maxilla than in the mandible; the Logan and Kronfeld table suggests that eruption in the mandible is generally ahead of that in the maxilla. The ages at which primary teeth erupt are 2 months or more later than suggested in the Logan and Kronfeld table. Finally, Hernandez and colleagues provide confirmation that more recent studies in different white populations have findings similar to these classic studies on eruption chronology.[6]

The time of eruption of both primary and permanent teeth varies greatly. Variations of 6 months on either side of the usual eruption date may be considered normal for a given child. A study by Parner and colleagues compared the well-known general acceleration of the physical development of children over the past century with their own observations of the emergence of permanent teeth.[7] They found that the emergence of permanent teeth has not been subject to a similar acceleration; in fact, the mean age of eruption has increased slightly, but only by a few days per year. They conclude that the age of eruption of the permanent teeth is a much more stable phenomenon than other aspects of physical development of children.

TABLE 9-1

Chronology of the Human Dentition

Tooth	Hard Tissue Formation Begins	Amount Of Enamel Formed At Birth	Enamel Completed	Eruption	Root Completed
Deciduous Dentition					
Maxillary					
Central incisor	4 mo in utero	Five sixths	1½ mo	7½ mo	1½ yr
Lateral incisor	4½ mo in utero	Two thirds	2½ mo	9 mo	2 yr
Cuspid	5 mo in utero	One third	9 mo	18 mo	3¼ yr
First molar	5 mo in utero	Cusps united	6 mo	14 mo	2½ yr
Second molar	6 mo in utero	Cusp tips still isolated	11 mo	24 mo	3 yr
Mandibular					
Central incisor	4½ mo in utero	Three fifths	2½ mo	6 mo	1½ yr
Lateral incisor	4½ mo in utero	Three fifths	3 mo	7 mo	1½ yr
Cuspid	5 mo in utero	One third	9 mo	16 mo	3¼ yr
First molar	5 mo in utero	Cusps united	5½ mo	12 mo	2¼ yr
Second molar	6 mo in utero	Cusp tips still isolated	10 mo	20 mo	3 yr
Permanent Dentition					
Maxillary					
Central incisor	3-4 mo		4-5 yr	7-8 yr	10 yr
Lateral incisor	10-12 mo		4-5 yr	8-9 yr	11 yr
Cuspid	4-5 mo		6-7 yr	11-12 yr	13-15 yr
First bicuspid	1½-1¾ yr		5-6 yr	10-11 yr	12-13 yr
Second bicuspid	2-2¼ yr		6-7 yr	10-12 yr	12-14 yr
First molar	At birth	Sometimes a trace	2½-3 yr	6-7 yr	9-10 yr
Second molar	2½-3 yr		7-8 yr	12-13 yr	14-16 yr
Third molar	7-9 yr		12-16 yr	17-21 yr	18-25 yr
Mandibular					
Central incisor	3-4 mo		4-5 yr	6-7 yr	9 yr
Lateral incisor	3-4 mo		4-5 yr	7-8 yr	10 yr
Cuspid	4-5 mo		6-7 yr	9-10 yr	12-14 yr
First bicuspid	1¾-2 yr		5-6 yr	10-12 yr	12-13 yr
Second bicuspid	2¼-2½ yr		6-7 yr	11-12 yr	13-14 yr
First molar	At birth	Sometimes a trace	2½-3 yr	6-7 yr	9-10 yr
Second molar	2½-3 yr		7-8 yr	11-13 yr	14-15 yr
Third molar	8-10 yr		12-16 yr	17-21 yr	18-25 yr

From Kronfeld R: *Bur* 35:18–25, 1935 (based on research by WHG Logan and R Kronfeld); adapted by Kronfeld R, Schour I: *J Am Dent Assoc* 26: 18-32, 1939; further adapted by McCall JO, Wald SS: *Clinical dental roentgenology: technic and interpretation including roentgen studies of the child and young adult,* Philadelphia, 1940, WB Saunders.

Numerous in vivo animal experiments and human radiographic studies have been done to better understand the process of tooth eruption. Although many theories have been advanced, the factors responsible for the eruption of the teeth are not fully understood. The factors that have been related to the eruption of teeth include elongation of the root, forces exerted by the vascular tissues around and beneath the root, growth of the alveolar bone, growth of dentin, growth and pull of the periodontal membrane, hormonal influences, presence of a viable dental follicle, pressure from the muscular action, and resorption of the alveolar crest.

A series of experiments by Cahill and Marks have established that a viable dental follicle is required for tooth

TABLE 9-2

Modification of the Table "Chronology of the Human Dentition" Suggested by Lunt and Law for the Calcification and Eruption of the Primary Dentition

Tooth	Hard Tissue Formation Begins	Amount Of Enamel Formed At Birth	Enamel Completed	Eruption (±1 Sd)	Root Completed
Deciduous Dentition					
Maxillary					
Central incisor	14 (13-16) wk in utero	Five sixths	1½ mo	10 (8-12) mo	1½ yr
Lateral incisor	16 (14⅔-16½) wk in utero	Two thirds	2½ mo	11 (9-13) mo	2 yr
Canine	17 (15-18) wk in utero	One third	9 mo	19 (16-22) mo	3¼ yr
First molar	15½ (14½-17) wk in utero	Cusps united; occlusal completely calcified plus half to three fourths crown height	6 mo	16 (13-19) mo boys, 16 (14-18) mo girls	2½ yr
Second molar	19 (16-23½) wk in utero	Cusps united; occlusal incompletely calcified; calcified tissue covers one fifth to one fourth crown height	11 mo	29 (25-33) mo	3 yr
Mandibular					
Central incisor	14 (13-16) wk in utero	Three fifths	2½ mo	8 (6-10) mo	1½ yr
Lateral incisor	16 (14⅔-) wk in utero	Three fifths	3 mo	13 (10-16) mo	1½ yr
Canine	17 (16-) wk in utero	One third	9 mo	20 (17-23) mo	3¼ yr
First molar	15½ (14½-17) wk in utero	Cusps united; occlusal completely calcified	5½ mo	16 (14-18) mo	2¼ yr
Second molar	18 (17-19½) wk in utero	Cusps united; occlusal incompletely calcified	10 mo	27 (23-31) mo boys, 27 (24-30) mo girls	3 yr

From Lunt RC, Law DB: *J Am Dent Assoc* 89:8720-879, 1974. *SD,* Standard deviation.

eruption.[8] Further studies by Marks and Cahill resulted in the conclusion that "tooth eruption is a series of metabolic events in alveolar bone characterized by bone resorption and formation on opposite sides of the dental follicle and the tooth does not contribute to this process."[9]

Tooth eruption is influenced by pituitary growth hormone and thyroid hormone and parathyroid hormone-related protein is required for tooth eruption.

Each tooth starts to move toward occlusion at approximately the time of crown completion and the interval from crown completion and the beginning of eruption until the tooth is in full occlusion is approximately 5 years for permanent teeth.

Grøn observed in her study of 874 Boston children that tooth emergence appeared to be more closely associated with the stage of root formation than with the chronologic or skeletal age of the child.[10] By the time of clinical emergence, approximately three fourths of root

formation had occurred. Teeth reach occlusion before the root development is complete.

Demirjian and Levesque presented a large sample of 5437 radiographs from a homogeneous (French-Canadian) population.[11] They used this sample to investigate the sexual differences in the development of permanent mandibular teeth from the early stages of calcification to closure of the apex. The analysis of the developmental curves of individual teeth shows a common pattern, namely, the similarity in timing between the sexes for the early stages of development. For the first stages of crown formation, which they refer to as A, B, and C, there was no difference between boys and girls in the chronology of the dental calcification in the majority of teeth. For the fourth stage, D, which represents the completion of crown development, girls were more advanced than boys by an average of 0.35 year for four teeth. For the stages of root development the mean difference between the sexes for all

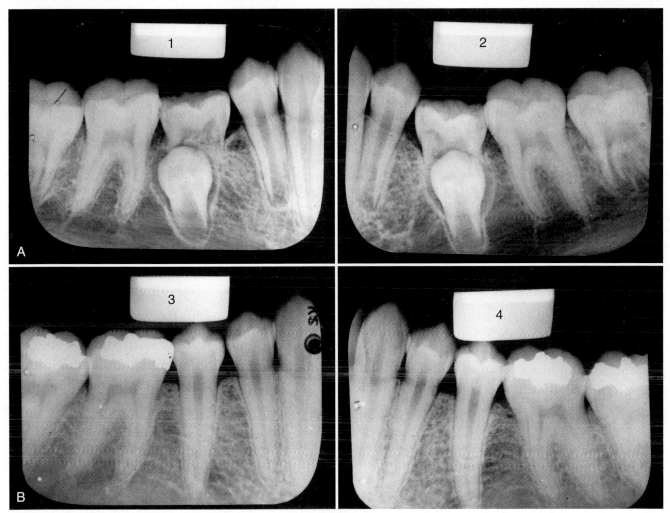

Figure 9-13 A, Bilateral ankylosis of second primary molars. **B,** The ankylosed molars were eventually shed, and the second premolars erupted into good occlusion. Frequently the ankylosed teeth must be removed surgically.

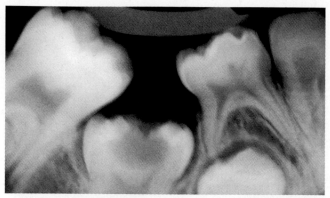

Figure 9-14 Ankylosed second primary molar with a carious lesion in the occlusal surface. This tooth probably became ankylosed soon after root resorption began.

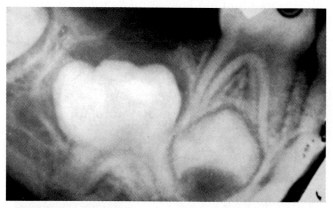

Figure 9-15 An ankylosed, deeply embedded second primary molar. Surgical removal of this tooth is indicated.

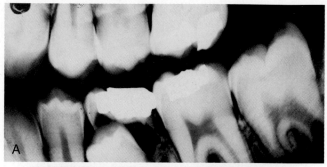

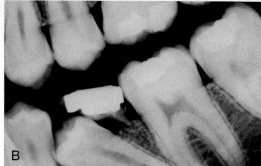

Figure 9-16 A, A small spicule of root of the primary tooth is ankylosed to the alveolar bone. This was overlooked at the time of the routine examination. **B,** One year later the second primary molar is still retained, and the second premolar has moved into a more unfavorable position.

ANKYLOSIS OF PRIMARY MOLARS WITH ABSENCE OF PERMANENT SUCCESSORS

Kurol and Thilander emphasize the importance of the presence of a permanent successor for normal exfoliation of a primary molar. In their longitudinal study, no ankylosed primary molars without permanent successors were found to exfoliate spontaneously. However, very slow root resorption was observed for most of the ankylosed teeth.[51]

The observations of Messer and Cline indicate that failure to carry out timed extraction of severely infraoccluded molars results in reduced alveolar bone support for the premolars.[52] However, Kurol and Olson suggest that infraocclusions and ankylosis of primary molars does not constitute a general risk for future alveolar bone loss mesial to the first permanent molars.[53] In their study of 119 infraoccluded primary molars next to permanent first molars, all but two of the first permanent molars showed a normal alveolar bone level mesially. Therefore the general treatment recommendation to await normal exfoliation and eruption of successors remains valid in their opinion. They suggest that, in patients in whom

there is an abnormality associated with a succedaneous tooth (e.g., agenesis, ectopic eruption), early intervention is most likely required. In situations in which permanent successors of ankylosed primary molars are missing, attempts have been made to establish functional occlusion using stainless steel crowns, overlays, or bonded composite resins on the affected primary molars. Currently, bonded restorations would be the preferred choice. Williams and colleagues reported excellent success with two bonded composite crowns on ankylosed mandibular second primary molars that were well below the occlusal plane.[54] At the time of their report the restorations had been functional for more than 7 years in a young adult patient. This treatment is successful only if maximum eruption of permanent teeth in the arch has occurred. If adjacent teeth are still in a state of active eruption, they will soon bypass the ankylosed tooth (Fig. 9-18).

ANKYLOSED PERMANENT TEETH

The incomplete eruption of a permanent molar may be related to a small area of root ankylosis. The removal of soft tissue and bone covering the occlusal aspect of the crown should be attempted first, and the area should be packed with surgical cement to provide a pathway for the developing permanent tooth (Fig. 9-19). If the permanent tooth is exposed in the oral cavity and at a lower occlusal plane than the adjacent teeth, ankylosis is the probable cause. Biederman as well as Skolnick have described a luxation technique effective in breaking the bony

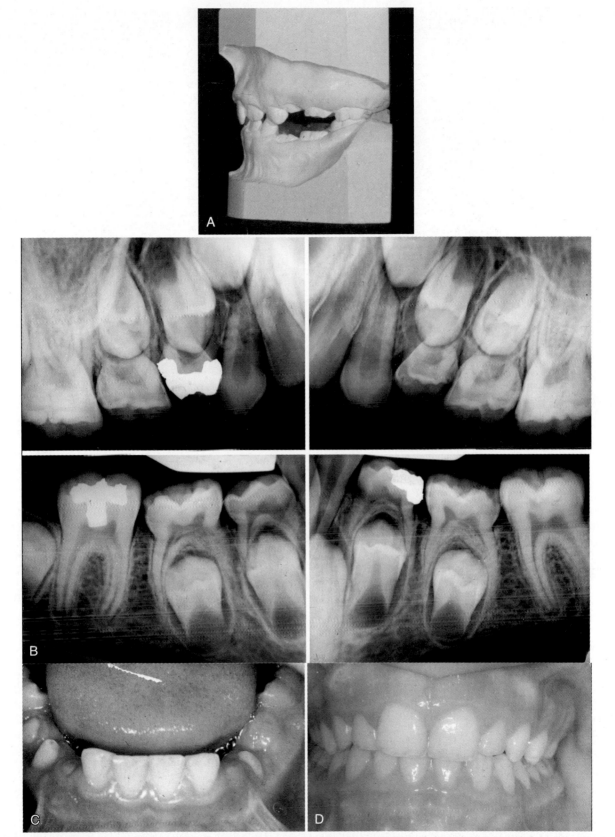

Figure 9-17 A, All eight of the primary molars were ankylosed. Continuing eruption of the adjacent teeth has caused a loss of arch length. **B,** Radiographs aided in the diagnosis of the ankylosed primary molars. The recommended treatment was surgical removal of the ankylosed teeth. **C,** Space maintainers were constructed after removal of the ankylosed teeth and were worn until the permanent teeth erupted. **D,** Ideal occlusion was achieved as a result of early diagnosis and the removal of the ankylosed teeth at the proper time.

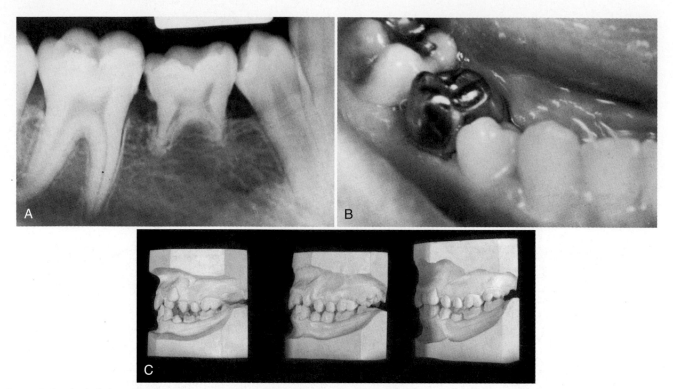

Figure 9-18 A, Ankylosed primary molar without a permanent successor. **B,** Mesiodistal width of the primary molar was reduced to allow the premolar to erupt, and an overlay was constructed to establish occlusion with the opposing teeth. **C,** Models at the left show the original condition. Center models show the occlusion at the time the overlay was placed on the ankylosed tooth. Models at the right show the continued eruption of the adjacent teeth that occurred in the subsequent 18-month period.

ankylosis.[55,56] If the rocking technique is not immediately successful, it should be repeated in 6 months. A delay in treatment may result in a permanently ankylosed molar (Fig. 9-20).

Unerupted permanent teeth may become ankylosed by inostosis of enamel. According to Franklin, the process follows the irritation of the follicular or periodontal tissue resulting from chronic infection.[57] The close association of an infected apex to an unerupted tooth may give rise to the process. In the unerupted tooth, enamel is protected by enamel epithelium. The enamel epithelium may disintegrate as a result of infection (or trauma), the enamel may subsequently be resorbed, and bone or coronal cementum may be deposited in its place. The result is solid fixation of the tooth in its unerupted position (Fig. 9-21).

TRISOMY 21 SYNDROME (DOWN SYNDROME)

Trisomy 21 syndrome (Down syndrome [DS]) is one of the congenital anomalies in which delayed eruption of the teeth frequently occurs. The first primary teeth may not appear until 2 years of age, and the dentition may not be complete until 5 years of age. The eruption often follows an abnormal sequence, and some of the primary teeth may be retained until 15 years of age. A study of 127 males and 128 females with DS by Ondarza and colleagues found that, on average, six primary teeth were delayed in eruption in boys and 11 primary teeth were delayed in girls.[58] A similar study of 116 males and 124 females with DS by Jara and colleagues showed delayed eruption of 13 permanent teeth in boys and eight permanent teeth in girls.[59] These studies seem to confirm that delayed tooth eruption is common but sporadic in children with DS.

Earlier literature refers to DS as *mongolism*, but the use of this term is inappropriate according to Schreiner and it may be insulting to the affected families.[60] DS occurs very early in embryonic development, possibly during the first cell divisions. Anomalies of the eye and external ear are seen, and congenital heart defects are often present. The occurrence of DS is frequently related to maternal age. Benda reported the frequency of DS to be approximately 1.5 per 1000 births for mothers in the 18- to 29-year-old age group.[61] The frequency increases for maternal ages of 30 years and older, reaching 29 per 1000 in the 40-year-old and older age group and a high of 91 per 1000 in the 44-year-old and older age group.

The cause of DS is trisomy 21, that is, the presence of three number 21 chromosomes rather than the normal two (diploid). The diagnosis of DS in a child is not usually difficult to make because of the characteristic facial

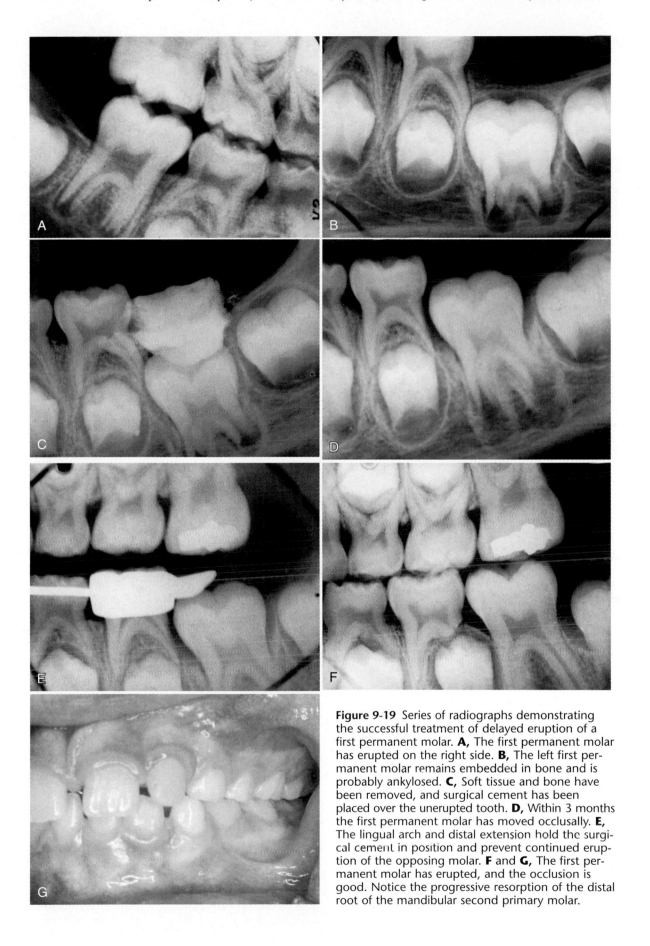

Figure 9-19 Series of radiographs demonstrating the successful treatment of delayed eruption of a first permanent molar. **A,** The first permanent molar has erupted on the right side. **B,** The left first permanent molar remains embedded in bone and is probably ankylosed. **C,** Soft tissue and bone have been removed, and surgical cement has been placed over the unerupted tooth. **D,** Within 3 months the first permanent molar has moved occlusally. **E,** The lingual arch and distal extension hold the surgical cement in position and prevent continued eruption of the opposing molar. **F** and **G,** The first permanent molar has erupted, and the occlusion is good. Notice the progressive resorption of the distal root of the mandibular second primary molar.

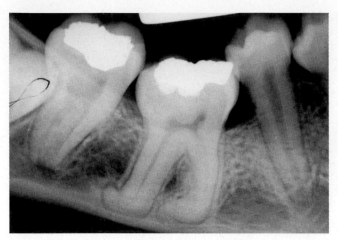

Figure 9-20 Ankylosed first permanent molar.

pattern (Fig. 9-22). The orbits are small, the eyes slope upward, and the bridge of the nose is more depressed than normal. Cohen, in a study of 194 children with DS, reported that 54% demonstrated anomalies in the formation of the external ear, characterized by outstanding "lap" ear with flat or absent helix.[62] Mental retardation is another characteristic finding, with most children in the mild to moderate range of disability (see Table 3-2).

Landau made a cephalometric comparison of children with DS and their normal siblings.[63] Retardation in the growth of the maxillae and mandible was evident in those with DS. Both the maxillae and mandible were positioned anteriorly under the cranial base. The upper facial height was found to be significantly smaller. The midface was also found to be small in the vertical and horizontal dimensions. The smaller jaws contribute to a tendency for protrusion of the tongue and dental crowding, both of which may compromise good occlusion development. The tongue also tends to be larger than normal.

Many children with DS have chronic inflammation of the conjunctiva and a history of repeated respiratory tract infections. The use of antibiotics has reduced the incidence of chronic infection and has resulted in fewer deaths from infection.

Tannenbaum as well as Baer and Benjamin observed that the prevalence and severity of periodontal disease in children with DS are much higher than the norm.[64,65] A high prevalence of necrotizing ulcerative gingivitis was also observed. After a literature review, Cichon and colleagues concluded that individuals with DS have a higher prevalence of periodontal disease than otherwise normal, age-matched control groups and other mentally disabled patients of similar age distribution.[66] Furthermore the reports of exaggerated immunoinflammatory responses of the tissues in DS patients cannot be explained by poor oral hygiene alone and may be the result of impaired cell-mediated and humoral immunities and deficient phagocytic systems. Cichon and colleagues' study of 10 DS patients aged 20 to 31 years demonstrated that the young age of onset, the severe destruction, and the pathogenesis

of disease in the periodontal tissues were consistent with a juvenile periodontitis disease pattern.

Morinushi and associates obtained blood samples and conducted gingival health assessments of 75 individuals with DS aged 2 to 18 years.[67] The extent of gingival inflammation and the antibody titers of the DS subjects suggested that colonization of certain pathogenic organisms for periodontal disease had occurred before 5 years of age. The prevalence and extent of gingivitis was significantly higher than in normal children. The antibody titers also suggested that colonization of additional pathogenic organisms increased with age. The authors believe that there are abnormalities in the systemic defenses that are responsible for the early onset of disease in the DS subjects. Similarly, Carlstedt and colleagues have demonstrated significantly higher oral colonization with *Candida albicans* in DS children compared with an age- and sex-matched control group.[68] They believe that abnormalities of the immune response in DS children are responsible for their greater susceptibility to oral mucosal disease.

Dental caries susceptibility is usually low in those with DS. This finding has been reported by Johnson and associates who noted a much lower dental caries incidence in both the primary and the permanent dentition.[69] Brown and Cunningham found in a study of DS children that 44% were caries-free.[70] Shapira and Stabholz successfully demonstrated caries reduction and improved periodontal health during a 30-month period after initiating a comprehensive preventive oral health program for 20 children with DS.[71]

Although some children with low cognitive ability are unmanageable for dental procedures, most are pleasant, cheerful, affectionate, and well behaved. They often can be managed in the dental office in a conventional manner. The possibility of reduced resistance to infection should be considered in the dental management of the child with DS.

CLEIDOCRANIAL DYSPLASIA

A rare congenital syndrome that has dental significance is cleidocranial dysplasia (CCD), which has also been referred to as *cleidocranial dysostosis, osteodentin dysplasia, mutational dysostosis,* and *Marie-Sainton syndrome.* Transmission of the condition is by either parent to a child of either sex, so that the disorder thus follows a true Mendelian dominant pattern. CCD can also occur sporadically with no apparent hereditary influence and with no predilection for race. The diagnosis is based on the finding of an absence of clavicles, although there may be remnants of the clavicles, as evidenced by the presence of the sternal and acromial ends. The fontanels are large, and radiographs of the head show open sutures, even late in the child's life. The sinuses, particularly the frontal sinus, are usually small.

Richardson and Deussen performed cephalometric analyses of 17 patients with CCD.[72] They found that, on average, the patients exhibited mandibular prognathism caused by increased mandibular lengths and short cranial bases. The maxillae tended to be short vertically but not

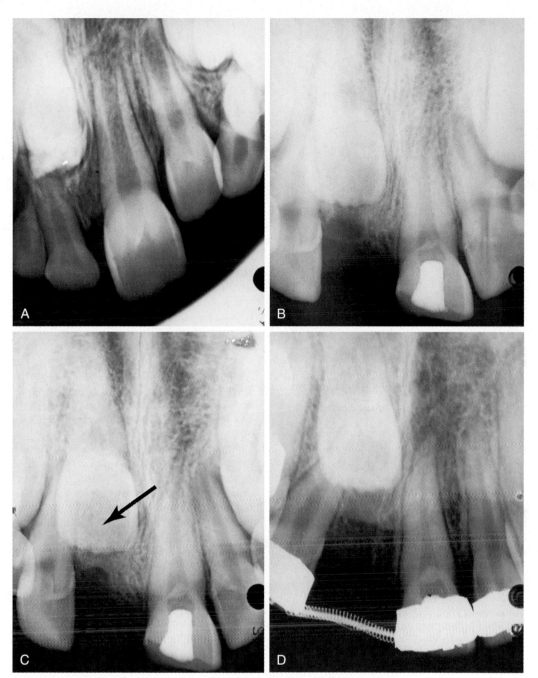

Figure 9-21 Ankylosis by inostosis. **A,** A mesiodens has delayed the eruption of the maxillary right permanent central incisor. **B,** The primary incisors and the mesiodens were removed. During the surgical removal of the mesiodens, there was apparently damage to the enamel epithelium. **C,** There is evidence of resorption of the enamel of the unerupted incisor and ankylosis of the tooth. **D,** The left central incisor crown sustained a fracture and pulp exposure. A calcium hydroxide pulpotomy was successfully performed, which resulted in continued root development.

anteroposteriorly. Somewhat similar findings have been reported by Jensen and Kreiborg in their study of 22 children with CCD.[73]

The development of the dentition is delayed. Complete primary dentition at 15 years of age resulting from delayed resorption of the deciduous teeth and delayed eruption of the permanent teeth is not uncommon

(Fig. 9-23). One of the important distinguishing characteristics is the presence of supernumerary teeth. Some children may have only a few supernumerary teeth in the anterior region of the mouth; others may have a large number of extra teeth throughout the mouth. Even with removal of the primary and supernumerary teeth, eruption of the permanent dentition, without orthodontic

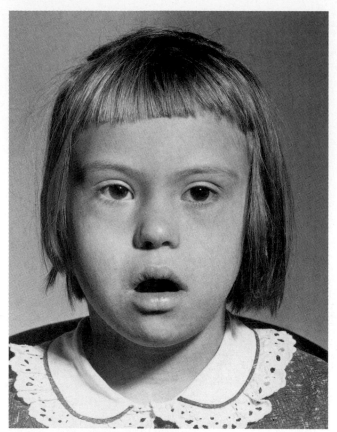

Figure 9-22 Child with Down syndrome, 8 years of age. (Courtesy Dr. Mace Landau.)

intervention, is often delayed and irregular. Other reports by Jensen and Kreiborg, based on their experiences and longitudinal study of 19 patients with CCD, provide information to help clinicians predict the location and time of onset of formation of supernumerary teeth. This information should help the clinician optimally time surgical treatment.[74,75]

Hutton and colleagues have reported the successful dental management of a patient with CCD over a 15-year period.[76] The patient was first seen at 2 years of age. Treatment consisted of timed extractions of primary and supernumerary teeth and conservative uncovering of the permanent teeth. The surgical procedures were planned according to progressive radiographic evidence of the development of the permanent teeth. This management results in a nearly normal but slightly delayed eruption sequence. Orthodontic treatment was begun at 14 years of age, and by 16 years of age the patient displayed acceptable occlusion and normal vertical dimension, root development, and periodontal bone support.

Learning from their experiences with the long-term management of 16 patients with CCD, Becker and colleagues advocate cooperative efforts by clinicians from the disciplines of pediatric dentistry, oral and maxillofacial surgery, and orthodontics and dentofacial orthopedics.[77] The pediatric dentist serves as the coordinator of overall oral health care and disease prevention during an extended treatment regimen that usually

includes two surgical interventions and three stages of orthodontic surgery.

Delayed eruption has also been reported in other forms of osteopetroses.

HYPOTHYROIDISM

Hypothyroidism is another possible cause of delayed eruption. Patients in whom the function of the thyroid gland is extremely deficient have characteristic dental findings.

Congenital Hypothyroidism (Cretinism)

Hypothyroidism occurring at birth and during the period of most rapid growth, if undetected and untreated, causes mental deficiency and dwarfism. This condition was referred to as *cretinism* in earlier medical and dental literature. Congenital hypothyroidism is the result of an absence or underdevelopment of the thyroid gland and insufficient levels of thyroid hormone (Fig. 9-24). Today it is routinely diagnosed and corrected at birth because of mandatory blood screening of newborn infants. An inadequately treated child with congenital hypothyroidism is a small and disproportionate person, with abnormally short arms and legs. The head is disproportionately large, although the trunk shows less deviation from the norm. Obesity is common.

Without adequate hormonal therapy the dentition of the child with congenital hypothyroidism is delayed in all stages, including eruption of the primary teeth, exfoliation of the primary teeth, and eruption of the permanent teeth. The teeth are normal in size but are crowded in jaws that are smaller than normal. The tongue is large and may protrude from the mouth. The abnormal size of the tongue and its position often cause an anterior open bite and flaring of the anterior teeth. The crowding of the teeth, malocclusion, and mouth breathing cause a chronic hyperplastic type of gingivitis.

Although untreated congenital hypothyroidism is rare, even in developing countries, Loevy and colleagues published a case report documenting the condition discovered in a 19-year-old boy.[78] The patient presented with a complete caries-free primary dentition and partially erupted maxillary first permanent molars. All primary teeth showed some abrasion. At a subsequent oral

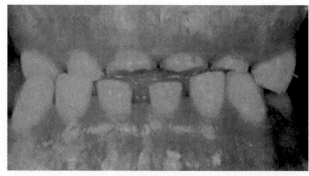

A

Figure 9-23 Cleidocranial dysplasia. **A,** A Primary dentition is still present at 15 years of age.

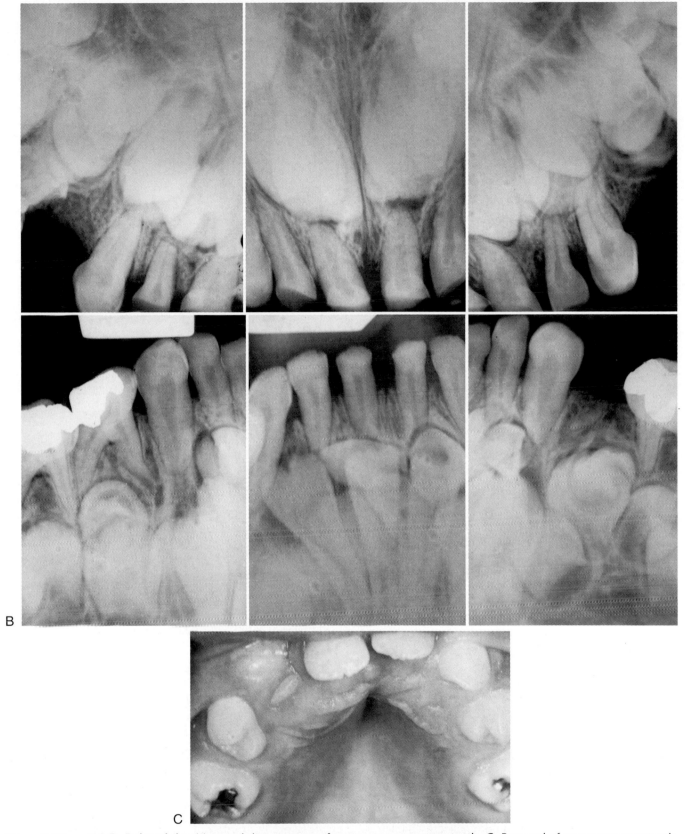

Figure 9-23 cont'd B, Delayed dentition and the presence of many supernumerary teeth. **C,** Removal of supernumerary teeth in the maxillary arch caused irregular and delayed eruption of some of the permanent teeth.

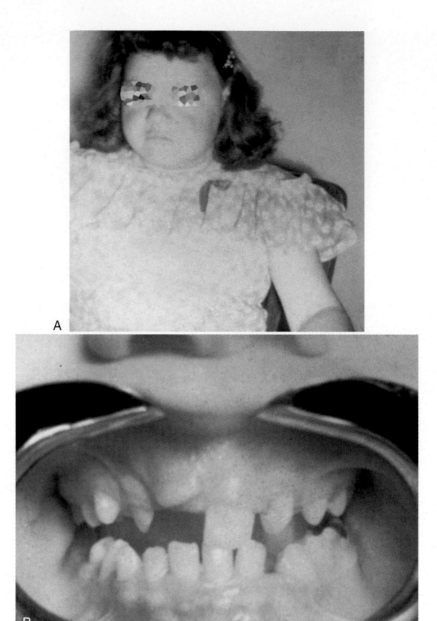

Figure 9-24 A, A 24-year-old patient with congenital hypothyroidism. **B,** Dentition is greatly delayed. With the administration of thyroxine, the eruption of the permanent teeth was accelerated. (Courtesy Dr. David F. Mitchell.)

examination 1 year and 9 months after appropriate l-thyroxine therapy was initiated, several primary teeth had exfoliated, permanent incisors and first molars had erupted, and radiographs showed additional development of other permanent teeth.

Juvenile Hypothyroidism (Acquired Hypothyroidism)

Juvenile hypothyroidism results from a malfunction of the thyroid gland, usually between 6 and 12 years of age. Because the deficiency occurs after the period of rapid growth, the unusual facial and body pattern characteristic of a person with congenital hypothyroidism is not present. However, obesity is evident to a lesser degree. In the untreated case of juvenile hypothyroidism, delayed exfoliation of the primary teeth and delayed eruption of

the permanent teeth are characteristic. A child with a chronologic age of 14 years may have a dentition in a stage of development comparable with that of a child 9 or 10 years of age (Fig. 9-25).

HYPOPITUITARISM

A pronounced deceleration of the growth of the bones and soft tissues of the body will result from a deficiency in secretion of the growth hormone. Pituitary dwarfism is the result of an early hypofunction of the pituitary gland. Again, early diagnosis is routine because of the mandatory blood screening of newborn infants for congenital hypothyroidism.

An individual with pituitary dwarfism is well proportioned but resembles a child of considerably younger chronologic age (Fig. 9-26). The dentition is essentially normal in size.

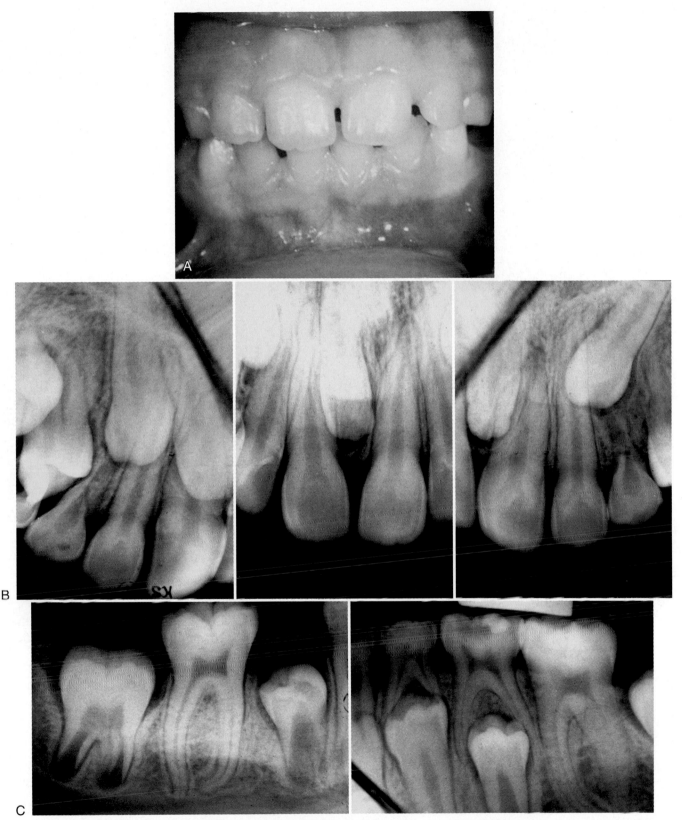

Figure 9-25 A, A 14-year-old girl with juvenile hypothyroidism. **B,** The occlusion was essentially normal but was delayed in its development. **C,** Delayed development of the teeth in juvenile hypothyroidism. The maxillary midline supernumerary tooth is a coincidental finding.

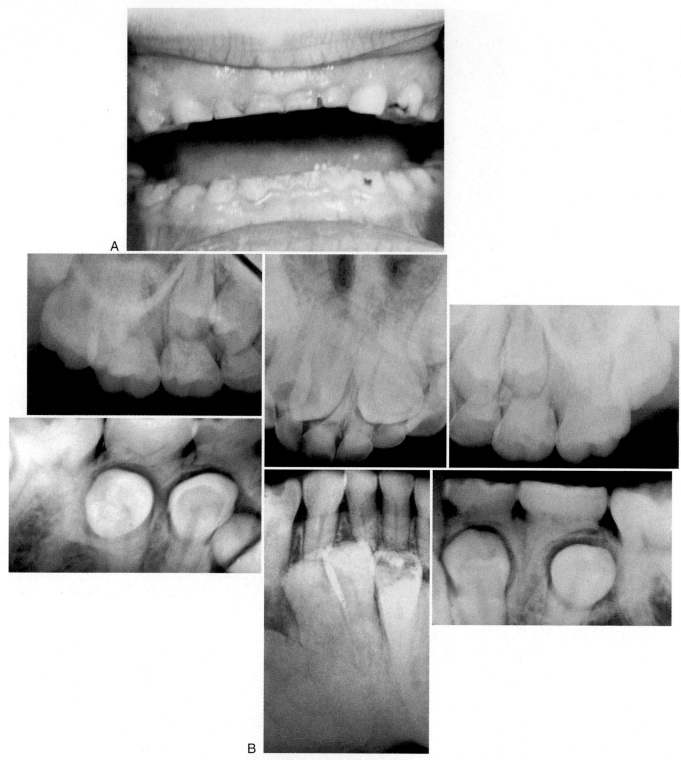

Figure 9-26 A 28-year-old woman diagnosed as having hypopituitary dwarfism. **A,** Complete primary dentition at 28 years of age. The first permanent molars have erupted. **B,** The roots of the primary teeth have not been resorbed to an appreciable degree, although some permanent teeth show complete development.

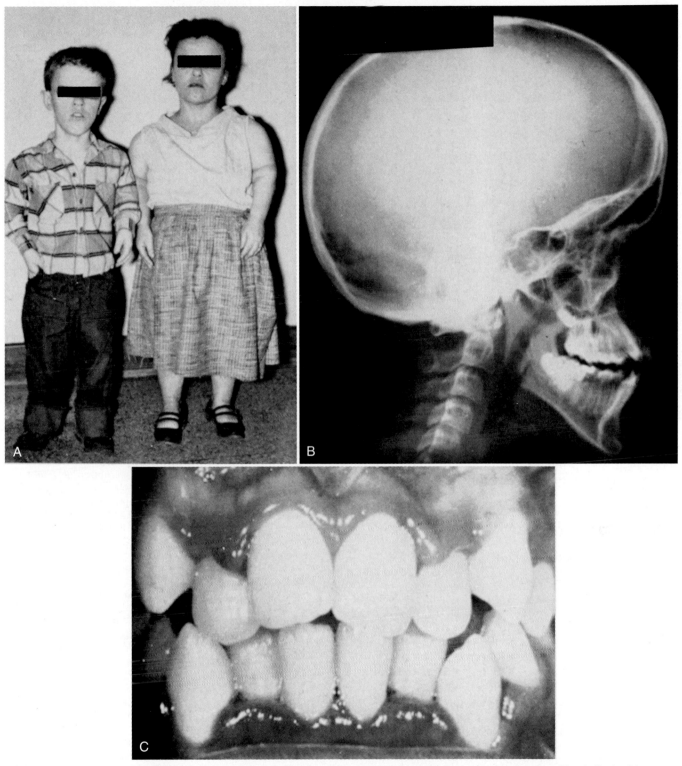

Figure 9-27 A, A 14-year-old boy with achondroplastic dwarfism and his mother. Growth of the extremities is limited in both. **B,** The upper face is greatly underdeveloped. **C,** The arch length is inadequate, and the teeth are crowded. (**A** and **B** courtesy Dr. Ralph E. McDonald. **C** from Shafer W, Hine MK, Levy BM. *A Textbook of Oral Pathology.* Philadelphia, 1958, WB Saunders.)

Delayed eruption of the dentition is characteristic. In severe cases the primary teeth do not undergo resorption but instead may be retained throughout the life of the person. The underlying permanent teeth continue to develop but do not erupt. Extraction of the deciduous teeth is not indicated, since eruption of the permanent teeth cannot be assured. Some degree of cognitive disability often occurs.

ACHONDROPLASTIC DWARFISM

Achondroplastic dwarfism, also diagnosed at birth, demonstrates a few characteristic dental findings. Growth of the extremities is limited because of a lack of calcification in the cartilage of the long bones. Stature improvements have been reported with surgical lengthening of the limbs and also with growth hormone therapy. The head is disproportionately large, although the trunk is normal in size. The fingers may be of almost equal length, and the hands are plump. The fontanels are open at birth. The upper face is underdeveloped, and the bridge of the nose is depressed.

Although the etiology of achondroplastic dwarfism is unknown, it is clearly an autosomal dominant disorder although sporadic spontaneous mutations occur. There is some evidence that the condition is more likely to occur when the ages of the parents differ significantly. In contrast to DS, the increased age of the father may be related to the occurrence of the condition.

Deficient growth in the cranial base is evident in many individuals with achondroplastic dwarfism. The maxilla may be small, with resultant crowding of the teeth and a tendency for open bite. A chronic gingivitis is usually present. However, this condition may be related to the malocclusion and crowding of the teeth. In the patient shown in Fig. 9-27, the development of the dentition was slightly delayed.

OTHER CAUSES

Delayed eruption of the teeth has been linked to other disorders, including fibromatosis gingivae (see Chapter 20), Albright hereditary osteodystrophy, chondroectodermal dysplasia (Ellis-van Creveld syndrome), de Lange syndrome, frontometaphyseal dysplasia, Gardner syndrome, Goltz syndrome, Hunter syndrome, incontinentia pigmenti syndrome (Bloch-Sulzberger syndrome), Maroteaux-Lamy mucopolysaccharidosis, Miller-Dieker syndrome, progeria syndrome (Hutchinson-Gilford syndrome), and familial hypophosphatemia.

Of additional interest is the effect of bisphosphonate therapy on children with osteogenesis imperfecta. Bisphosphonates inhibit the ability of osteoclasts to resorb bone. Indeed, one study demonstrated that children with osteogenesis imperfecta that were treated with bisphosphonates had an associated mean delay of 1.67 years in tooth eruption.[79]

REFERENCES

1. Lunt RC, Law DB. A review of the chronology of calcification of deciduous teeth, *J Am Dent Assoc* 89:599-606, 1974.
2. Logan WHG, Kronfeld R. Development of the human jaws and the surrounding structures from birth to the age of 15 years, *J Am Dent Assoc* 20:379-427, 1933.
3. Lunt RC, Law DB. A review of the chronology of eruption of deciduous teeth, *J Am Dent Assoc* 89:872-879, 1974.
4. Kraus BS, Jordan RE. *The Human Dentition before Birth*, Philadelphia, 1965, Lea & Febiger.
5. Nomata N. Chronological study on the crown formation of the human deciduous dentition, *Bull Tokyo Med Dent Univ* 11:55-76, 1964.
6. Hernandez M, Espasa E, Boj JR. Eruption chronology of the permanent dentition in Spanish children, *J Clin Pediatr Dent* 32:347-350, 2008.
7. Parner E, et al. A longitudinal study of time trends in the eruption of permanent teeth in Danish children, *Arch Oral Biol* 46:425-431, 2001.
8. Cahill DR, Marks SC. Tooth eruption: Evidence for the central role of the dental follicle, *J Oral Pathol* 9:189-200, 1980.
9. Marks SC, Cahill DR. Experimental study in the dog of the non-active role of the tooth in the eruptive process, *Arch Oral Biol* 29:311-322, 1984.
10. Grøn AMP. Prediction of tooth emergency, *J Dent Res* 41:573-585, 1962.
11. Demirjian A, Levesque GY. Sexual differences in dental development and prediction of emergence, *J Dent Res* 59:1110-1122, 1980.
12. Wise GE, et al. Cellular, molecular, and genetic determinants of tooth eruption, *Crit Rev Oral Biol Med* 12(4):323-335, 2002.
13. Kardos TB. The mechanism of tooth eruption, *Br Dent J* 181:91-95, 1997.
14. Marks SC, Schroeder HE. Tooth eruption: Theories and facts, *Anat Rec* 245:374-373, 1996.
15. Posen AL. The effect of premature loss of deciduous molars on premolar eruption, *Angle Orthod* 35:249-252, 1965.
16. Hartsfield J. Premature exfoliation of teeth in childhood and adolescence, *Adv Pediatr* 41:453-470, 1994.
17. Lo RT, Moyers RE. Studies in the etiology and prevention of malocclusion. I. The sequence of eruption of the permanent dentition, *Am J Orthod* 39:460-467, 1953.
18. Carlos JP, Gittelsohn AM. Longitudinal studies of the natural history of caries. I. Eruption patterns of the permanent teeth, *J Dent Res* 44:509-516, 1965.
19. Moyers RE. *Handbook of Orthodontics*, 4th ed. Chicago, 1988, Mosby.
20. Gellin ME. Indications and contraindications for the removal of primary teeth, *Dent Clin North Am* 13:899-911, 1969.
21. Gellin ME, Haley JV. Managing cases of overretention of mandibular primary incisors where their permanent successors erupt lingually, *J Dent Child* 49:118-122, 1982.
22. King DL. Teething revisited, *Pediatr Dent* 16:179-182, 1994.
23. Dally A. The lancet and the gum-lancet: 400 years of teething babies, *Lancet* 348:1710-1711, 1996.
24. Illingworth RS. Teething, *Dev Med Child Neurol* 11:376-377, 1969.

25. Tasanen A. General and local effects of the eruption of deciduous teeth, *Ann Paediatr Fenn* 14(Suppl 29):1-40, 1968.
26. Jaber L, Cohen IJ, Mor A. Fever associated with teething. *Arch Dis Child* 67:233-234, 1992.
27. Macknin M, et al. Symptoms associated with infant teething: A prospective study, *Pediatrics* 105(4):747-752, 2000.
28. Leung AK. Teething, *Am Fam Physician* 39:131-134, 1989.
29. Swann IL. Teething complications: A persisting misconception, *Postgrad Med J* 55:24-25, 1979.
30. Starkey PE, Shafer WG. Eruption sequestra in children, *J Dent Child* 30:84-86, 1963.
31. Watkins JJ. An unusual eruption sequestrum, *Br Dent J* 138:395-396, 1975.
32. Priddy RW, Price C. The so-called eruption sequestrum, *Oral Surg* 58:321-326, 1984.
33. Maki K, Ansai T, Nishida I, Zhang M, Kojima Y, Takehara T, Kimura M: Eruption sequestrum: x-ray microanalysis and microscopic findings, *J Clin Pediatr Dent* 29(3):245-247, 2005.
34. Leung AK. Natal teeth, *Am J Dis Child* 140:249-251, 1986.
35. Kates GA, Needleman HL, Holmes LB. Natal and neonatal teeth: A clinical study, *J Am Dent Assoc* 109:441-443, 1984.
36. Zhu J, King D. Natal and neonatal teeth, *J Dent Child* 62:123-128, 1995.
37. Adekoya-Sofowora CA. Natal and neonatal teeth: A review, *Niger Postgrad Med J* 15(1):38-41, 2008.
38. Spouge JD, Feasby WH. Erupted teeth in the newborn, *Oral Surg* 22:198-208, 1966.
39. Bodenhoff J, Gorlin RJ. Natal and neonatal teeth: Folklore and fact, *Pediatrics* 32:1087-1093, 1963.
40. Nedley MP, Stanley RT, Cohen DM. Extraction of natal and neonatal teeth can leave odontogenic remnants, *Pediatr Dent* 17:457, 1995.
41. Fromm A. Epstein's pearls, Bohn's nodules and inclusion cysts of the oral cavity, *J Dent Child* 34:275-287, 1967.
42. Henderson HZ. Ankylosis of primary molars: A clinical, radiographic, and histologic study, *J Dent Child* 46:117-122, 1979.
43. Alexander SA, et al. Multiple ankylosed teeth, *J Pedod* 4:354-359, 1980.
44. Via WF Jr. Submerged deciduous molars: Familial tendencies, *J Am Dent Assoc* 69:128-129, 1964.
45. Krakowiak FJ. Ankylosed primary molars, *J Dent Child* 45:288-292, 1978.
46. Darling AI, Levers BG. Submerged human deciduous molars and ankylosis, *Arch Oral Biol* 18:1021-1040, 1973.
47. Brown ID. Some further observations on submerging deciduous molars, *Br J Orthod* 8(2):99-107, 1981.
48. Steigman S, Koyoumdjisky-Kaye E, Matrai Y. Submerged deciduous molars and congenital absence of premolars, *J Dent Res* 52:842, 1973.
49. Tsukamoto S, Braham RL. Unerupted second primary molar positioned inferior to the second premolar: Clinical report, *J Dent Child* 53:67-69, 1986.
50. Belanger GK, Strange M, Sexton JR. Early ankylosis of a primary molar with self-correction: Case report, *Pediatr Dent* 8:37-40, 1986.
51. Kurol J, Thilander B. Infraocclusion of primary molars with aplasia of the permanent successor: A longitudinal study, *Angle Orthod* 54:283-294, 1984.
52. Messer LB, Cline JT. Ankylosed primary molars: Results and treatment recommendations from an eight-year longitudinal study, *Pediatr Dent* 2:37-47, 1980.
53. Kurol J, Olson L. Ankylosis of primary molars—a future periodontal threat to first permanent molars? *Eur J Orthod* 13(5):404-409, 1991.
54. Williams HA, Zwemer JD, Hoyt DJ. Treating ankylosed primary teeth in adult patients: A case report, *Quintessence Int* 26:161-166, 1995.
55. Biederman W. Etiology and treatment of tooth ankylosis, *Am J Orthod* 48:670-684, 1962.
56. Skolnick IM. Ankylosis of maxillary permanent first molar, *J Am Dent Assoc* 100:558-560, 1980.
57. Franklin CD. Ankylosis of an unerupted third molar by inostosis of enamel, *Br Dent J* 133:346-347, 1972.
58. Ondarza A, et al. Sequence of eruption of deciduous dentition in a Chilean sample with Down's syndrome, *Arch Oral Biol* 42:401-406, 1997.
59. Jara L, et al. The sequence of eruption of the permanent dentition in a Chilean sample with Down's syndrome, *Arch Oral Biol* 38:85-89, 1993.
60. Schreiner RL. Personal communication, 1992.
61. Benda CE. *The Child with Mongolism.* New York, 1960, Grune & Stratton.
62. Cohen MM. Variability of facial and dental characteristics in trisomy G, *South Med J* 64:51-55, 1971.
63. Landau MJ. A cephalometric comparison of children with Down's syndrome and their normal siblings. Thesis. Indianapolis, Indiana University School of Dentistry, 1966.
64. Tannenbaum KA. The oral aspects of mongolism, *J Public Health Dent* 35:95-108, 1975.
65. Baer PN, Benjamin SD. Periodontal disease in children and adolescents. Philadelphia, 1974, JB Lippincott.
66. Cichon P, Crawford L, Grimm WD. Early-onset periodontitis associated with Down's syndrome: Clinical interventional study, *Ann Periodontol* 3:370-380, 1998.
67. Morinushi T, Lopatin DE, Van Poperin N. The relationship between gingivitis and the serum antibodies to the microbiota associated with periodontal disease in children with Down's syndrome, *J Periodontol* 68:626-631, 1997.
68. Carlstedt K, et al. Oral carriage of *Candida* species in children and adolescents with Down's syndrome, *Int J Paediatr Dent* 6:95-100, 1996.
69. Johnson NP, Young MA, Gallios JA. Dental caries experience of mongoloid children, *Dent Abstr* 6:371, 1961.
70. Brown RH, Cunningham WM. Some manifestations of mongolism, *Oral Surg* 14:664-676, 1961.
71. Shapira J, Stabholz A. A comprehensive 30-month preventive dental health program in a pre-adolescent population with Down's syndrome: A longitudinal study, *Spec Care Dentist* 16:33-37, 1996.
72. Richardson A, Deussen FF. Facial and dental anomalies in cleidocranial dysplasia: A study of 17 cases, *Int J Paediatr Dent* 4:225-231, 1994.
73. Jensen BL, Kreiborg S. Craniofacial growth in cleidocranial dysplasia—a roentgencephalometric study, *J Craniofac Genet Dev Biol* 15:35-42, 1995.
74. Jensen BL, Kreiborg S. Development of the dentition in cleidocranial dysplasia, *J Oral Pathol Med* 19:89-93, 1990.
75. Jensen BL, Kreiborg S. Dental treatment strategies in cleidocranial dysplasia, *Br Dent J* 172:243-247, 1992.

76. Hutton CE, Bixler D, Garner LD. Cleidocranial dysplasia—treatment of dental problems: Report of a case, *J Dent Child* 48:456-462, 1981.

77. Becker A, et al. Cleidocranial dysplasia. Part II. Treatment protocol for the orthodontic and surgical modality, *Am J Orthod Dentofacial Orthop* 111:173-184, 1997.

78. Loevy HT, Aduss H, Rosenthal IM. Tooth eruption and craniofacial development in congenital hypothyroidism: report of case, *J Am Dent Assoc* 115:429-431, 1987.

79. Kamoun-Goldrat A, Ginisty D, Le Merrer M. Effects of bisphosphonates on tooth eruption in children with osteogenesis imperfecta, *Eur J Oral Sci* 116:195–198, 2008.

CHAPTER 10

Dental Caries in the Child and Adolescent

▲ Ralph E. McDonald, David R. Avery, George K. Stookey, Judith R. Chin, and Joan E. Kowolik

CHAPTER OUTLINE

We know that good oral health is an integral component of good general health. Although enjoying good oral health includes more than just having healthy teeth, many children have inadequate oral and general health because of active and uncontrolled dental caries. According to the first-ever United States Surgeon General's report on oral health in America published in May 2000, dental caries is the single most common chronic childhood disease.[1] Dental caries is five times more common than asthma and seven times more common than hay fever. Furthermore, as Edelstein and Douglass noted, dental caries is not self-limiting, like the common cold, nor amenable to treatment with a simple course of antibiotics, like an ear infection.[2] After analyzing the National Health Interview Survey data from 1993 through 1996, Newacheck and colleagues concluded that dental care is the most prevalent unmet health need among American children.[3] Much other available data verify that we learned a great deal during the twentieth century about preventing dental caries, but other variables that contribute to the spread of the disease among many people in the world continue to thwart our efforts to eliminate this major health problem. Although effective methods are known for prevention and management

of the disease, the unmet need for treatment, especially in children, does not seem to be diminishing. Gift has estimated that 51 million school hours per year are lost in the United States because of dental-related illness.[4]

The National Institutes of Health sponsored a Consensus Development Conference on Diagnosis and Management of Dental Caries Throughout Life in March 2001.[5] Thirty-four papers were presented by recognized experts on dental caries. The October 2001 issue of the *Journal of Dental Education* published the entire proceedings of that conference. The complete journal issue provides many good updates on the diagnosis and management of dental caries. A few of the papers from the conference are cited in this chapter.

ETIOLOGY OF DENTAL CARIES

For as long as the science of dentistry has existed, there has been theorizing about the cause of dental caries. Today, all experts on dental caries generally agree that it is an infectious and communicable disease and that multiple factors influence the initiation and progression of the disease. The disease is recognized to require a host (tooth in the oral environment), a dietary substrate, and aciduric bacteria.[6] The saliva (also considered a host component), the substrate, and the bacteria form a biofilm (plaque) that adheres to the tooth surface. Over time the presence of the substrate serves as a nutrient for the bacteria, and the bacteria produce acids that can demineralize the tooth. The flow, dilution, buffering, and remineralizing capacity of saliva are also recognized to be critical factors that affect, and in some ways regulate, the progression and regression of the disease. If the oral environment is balanced and favorable, saliva can contribute to strengthening of the tooth by supplying the components known to help build strong apatite structure. If the oral environment is unfavorable (too much acid is produced too often), an adequate flow of saliva can help dilute and buffer the acid, and thus slow the rate of damage to the tooth or even repair it. The critical pH for dissolution of enamel has been shown to be about 5.5. Once the process reaches dentin, dissolution can occur at a considerably higher pH. In addition, we know of many anatomic, behavioral, dietary, genetic, social, cultural, socioeconomic, and therapeutic variables that can significantly influence the level of caries activity favorably or unfavorably.

We recognize dental caries as a preventable disease. Furthermore we know that the disease typically begins in enamel and progresses slowly in the early stages of the process. Rampant caries is an exception to the typical course and is discussed later. Cavitation of the tooth structure is quite a late stage of the disease. Before cavitation, the progress of the disease may be arrested and/or reversed if a favorable oral environment can be achieved. Even after cavitation occurs, if the pulp is not yet involved and if the cavitated area is open enough to be self-cleansing (plaque-free), the caries process can halt and become an "arrested lesion." Arrested lesions typically exhibit much coronal destruction, but the remaining exposed dentin is hard and usually very dark, there is no evidence of pulpal damage, and the patient has no pain. We also must emphasize that treating a carious tooth by providing a restoration does not cure the disease. If the unfavorable oral environment that caused the cavity persists, so will the disease, and more restorations will be required in time. Treating the oral infection by reducing the number of cariogenic microorganisms and establishing a favorable oral environment to promote predominantly remineralization of tooth structure over time will stop the caries process and cure the disease. Curing the disease currently requires modifications by the patient and/or caretaker and relies on their compliance in making the necessary modifications. Research efforts are ongoing to find a feasible method of achieving caries immunity that would be far less dependent on patient compliance.

Studies by Orland[7] and by Fitzgerald and colleagues[8] demonstrated that dental caries do not occur in the absence of microorganisms. Animals maintained in a germ-free environment did not develop caries even when fed a high-carbohydrate diet. However, dental caries did develop in these animals when they were inoculated with microorganisms from caries-active animals and then fed cariogenic diets.

A number of microorganisms can produce enough acid to demineralize tooth structure, particularly aciduric streptococci, lactobacilli, diphtheroids, yeasts, staphylococci, and certain strains of sarcinae. *Streptococcus mutans* has been implicated as one of the major and most virulent of the caries-producing organisms. Consequently *S. mutans* has been targeted in a large share of research. Loesche conducted an extensive review of the literature regarding the etiology of caries.[9] He concluded that the evidence suggests that *S. mutans*, possibly *Streptococcus sobrinus*, and lactobacilli are human odontopathogens. He stated that aciduricity appears to be the most consistent attribute of *S. mutans* and is associated with its cariogenicity. He also observed that other aciduric species such as *S. sobrinus* may be more important in smooth-surface decay and are perhaps associated with rampant caries. Loesche concluded the review with the suggestion that treatment strategies that interfere with the colonization of *S. mutans* may have a profound effect on the incidence of caries in humans.[9] As caries research proceeds, there seems to be increasing evidence that disease may result from a group of microbial species in the tooth-adhering biofilm. It is not clear which combinations of organisms are most blameworthy.

Wan and colleagues have published a series of three papers that report on 111 infants whom they observed to 2 years of age. They found *S. mutans* colonization in infants as young as 3 months, and more than 50% of the predentate infants were infected by 6 months of age. By 24 months of age, 84% of the children harbored the bacteria.[10-12] Investigations by Davey and Rogers[13] and by Berkowitz and Jones[14] have confirmed that *S. mutans* is transmitted orally from mother to infant, whereas Brown and colleagues[15] have demonstrated a relationship between the numbers of *S. mutans* present in mothers and infants. Research by Kohler and colleagues demonstrated that reducing the numbers of oral *S. mutans* in mothers delayed the colonization of the organisms in the mouths of their children.[16] Their findings also showed that 52% of the children who carried *S. mutans* at 3 years of age had caries, whereas only 3% of the children without demonstrable *S. mutans* had caries at the same age. In 1988, these same investigators reported that, the earlier the colonization of *S. mutans* in the mouths of children, the higher the caries prevalence at 4 years of age.[17] Caufield and colleagues suggested the possibility of a "window of infectivity" between 19 and 33 months of age during which most children acquire the cariogenic organisms.[18] The mother was the most common source of transmission of the bacteria to the child. In a group of 122 children 6 to 24 months of age, Mohan and colleagues found oral mutans streptococci colonization in 20% of the children younger than 14 months of age.[19] In addition, logistic regression models that controlled for both age and number of teeth indicated that children who consumed sweetened beverages in their baby bottle were four times more likely to have mutans streptococci than children who only consumed milk. Although investigations to elucidate how and when mutans streptococci are transmitted to children are continuing, essentially all experts agree that the earlier transmission occurs, the higher the caries risk.

The acids that initially demineralize the enamel have a pH of 5.5 to 5.2 or less and are formed in the plaque material, which has been described as an organic nitrogenous mass of microorganisms firmly attached to the tooth structure. This film, which exists primarily in the susceptible areas of the teeth, has received a great deal of attention. Considerable emphasis is currently being given to plaque and its relationship to oral disease. Methods of chemical plaque control are being investigated. The method that has received the most attention during the past decade is the use of antimicrobial agents whose action is selective against certain types of microorganisms, including *S. mutans*. Chlorhexidine and other agents are available in antimicrobial oral rinse solutions. Another approach involves the use of monomolecular layers on the tooth surface that prevent the adherence of microorganisms. Perhaps by learning how to make enamel resistant to bacterial colonization (plaque formation), both caries and gingival disease can be reduced.

The acids involved in the initiation of the caries process are normal metabolic by-products of the microorganisms and are generated by the metabolism of carbohydrates. Because the outer surface of enamel is far more resistant to demineralization by acid than is the deeper portion of enamel, the greatest amount of demineralization occurs 10 to 15 mm beneath the enamel surface (Fig. 10-1). The continuation of this process results in the formation of an incipient subsurface enamel lesion that is first observed clinically as a so-called white spot. Unless the demineralization is arrested or reversed (remineralization), the subsurface lesion continues to enlarge, with the eventual collapse of the thin surface layer and the formation of a cavitated lesion.

Remineralization of incipient subsurface lesions may occur as long as the surface layer of the enamel remains intact. Saliva, which is supersaturated with calcium and phosphate and has acid-buffering capability, diffuses into plaque, where it neutralizes the microbial acids and repairs the damaged enamel. The time required for remineralization to replace the hydroxyapatite lost during demineralization is determined by the age of the plaque, the nature of the carbohydrate consumed, and the presence or absence of fluoride. For example, it has been suggested that, in the presence of dental plaque that has developed for 12 hours or less, the enamel demineralization resulting from a single exposure to sucrose will be remineralized by saliva within about 10 minutes. In contrast, a period of at least 4 hours is required for saliva to repair the damage to enamel resulting from a similar exposure to sucrose in the presence of dental plaque that is 48 or more hours old. The presence of fluoride has a profound effect on the remineralization process; not only does fluoride greatly enhance the rate of remineralization of enamel by saliva but it also results in the formation of a fluorohydroxyapatite during the process, which increases the resistance of the remineralized enamel to future attack by acids. Fluoride also has antimicrobial effects.

Thus the development of dental caries may be considered as a continuous dynamic process involving repeating periods of demineralization by organic acids of microbial origin and subsequent remineralization by salivary components (or therapeutic agents), but in which the

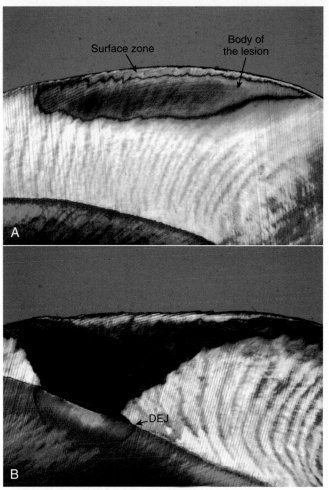

Figure 10-1 Polarized light appearance of natural subsurface caries lesion. **A,** Blue/green line represents surface zone; yellow/brown represents the most demineralized area, the body of the lesion. **B,** More advanced natural subsurface lesion reaching to the dentino-enamel junction (DEJ). (Courtesy Dr. James Wefel.)

overall oral environment is imbalanced toward demineralization. Several factors influence the degree of vulnerability of the tooth.

CARIES PREVALENCE IN PRESCHOOL CHILDREN

Weddell and Klein examined 441 children who ranged in age from 6 to 36 months and resided in a community with water fluoridation.[20] They found dental caries in 4.2% of the children 12 to 17 months of age, 19.8% of those 24 to 29 months of age, and 36.4% of those 30 to 36 months of age. Children in the middle and middle-low socioeconomic groups showed a trend toward higher caries frequencies. Edelstein and Tinanoff found that 30.5% of 200 preschool children had caries detectable by visual or radiographic examination.[21] These children were recruited from a private pediatric dental office and ranged in age from 5 months to 5 years 11 months (mean, 3 years 8 months).

Douglass and colleagues determined the caries prevalence in children 3 to 4 years of age from a fluoridated community in Connecticut who were enrolled in the same Head Start program.[22] They compared the caries prevalence in 517 children enrolled in 1999 with that in 311 children enrolled in 1991. They found a caries prevalence of 38% in the children enrolled in 1999 and 49% in those enrolled in 1991. They noted, however, that the children enrolled in 1999 had a greater severity of maxillary anterior caries. Tang and colleagues performed dental caries examinations on 5171 preschool children recruited from public health assistance programs in Arizona.[23] They found caries in 6.4% of 1-year-olds, nearly 20% of 2-year-olds, 35% of 3-year-olds, and 49% of 4-year-old children in the study.

In general, other reports of caries prevalence among children in various parts of the world show rates that seem to be comparable to those cited here. Another common element of caries prevalence in the United States and throughout the world is that children from families in low socioeconomic groups consistently have greater caries prevalences than their peers from families at a higher socioeconomic level. Vargas and colleagues reported that 27.4% of a sample of 3889 children 2 to 5 years of age had at least one decayed or filled primary tooth.[24] These children were part of a larger sample of individuals included in the third National Health and Nutrition Examination Survey (NHANES III, 1988-1994). This sample of children was 51.4% male and 48.6% female, with an ethnic distribution of 64.1% non-Hispanic white, 16.0% black, 9.5% Mexican American, and 10.4% other ethnicity. The family incomes for these children were distributed into four groups categorized from low to high, and these groups comprised 27.9%, 25.5%, 21.6%, and 24.9% of the sample, respectively.

In a longitudinal evaluation of caries patterns in 317 children followed an average of 7.8 years in private dental practices, Greenwell and colleagues made several noteworthy discoveries.[25] They found that 84% of the children who were caries-free in the primary dentition remained caries-free in the mixed dentition. Children with pit and fissure caries in the primary dentition were more likely to develop smooth-surface caries of primary teeth than the caries-free children. Fifty-seven percent of the children with proximal lesions in primary molars in the primary dentition developed additional primary molar proximal lesions in the mixed dentition. Children with faciolingual decay (nursing caries) were at the highest risk of any group for developing additional carious lesions. These investigators also discovered levels of caries susceptibility in children that can be characterized as caries-free, pit and fissure caries, and proximal molar caries patterns.

CARIES PREVALENCE IN SCHOOL CHILDREN

The report by Vargas and colleagues provides additional representative data for school children as well.[24] Their report revealed that 61% of the sample of children 6 to 12 years of age had at least one decayed or filled primary

tooth. Furthermore, in the sample of 4116 children 6 to 14 years of age, 40% had at least one decayed or filled permanent tooth. Of the 1383 children 15 to 18 years of age, 89.8% had at least one decayed or filled permanent tooth. The ethnic and family income distributions for children in these different age groups were comparable to those outlined in detail for the preschool children. This information, along with that in many other published reports, clearly indicates that managing the disease of dental caries among children remains a formidable task despite the advances made in various preventive programs. Edelstein and Douglass have noted, "The popular statement that half of U.S. school children have never experienced tooth decay fails profoundly to reflect the extremity and severity of this still highly prevalent condition of childhood."[2]

RAMPANT DENTAL CARIES

There is no complete agreement on the definition of rampant caries or on the clinical picture of this condition. It has been generally accepted, however, that the disease referred to as *rampant caries* is, in terms of human history, relatively new. Rampant caries has been defined by Massler as a "suddenly appearing, widespread, rapidly burrowing type of caries, resulting in early involvement of the pulp and affecting those teeth usually regarded as immune to ordinary decay."[26]

There is no evidence that the mechanism of the decay process is different in rampant caries or that it occurs only in teeth that are malformed or inferior in composition. On the contrary, rampant caries can occur suddenly in teeth that were previously sound for many years. The sudden onset of the disease suggests that an overwhelming imbalance of the oral environment has occurred, and some factors in the caries process seem to accelerate it so that it becomes uncontrollable; it is then referred to as *rampant caries*.

When a patient has what is considered an excessive amount of tooth decay, one must determine whether that person actually has a high susceptibility and truly rampant caries of sudden onset or whether the oral condition represents years of neglect and inadequate dental care. Young teenagers seem to be particularly susceptible to rampant caries, although it has been observed in both children and adults of all ages (Fig. 10-2).

There is considerable evidence that emotional disturbances may be a causative factor in some cases of rampant caries. Repressed emotions and fears, dissatisfaction with achievement, rebellion against a home situation, a feeling of inferiority, a traumatic school experience, and continuous general tension and anxiety have been observed in children and adults who have rampant dental caries. Because adolescence is often considered to be a time of difficult adjustment, the increased incidence of rampant caries in this age group lends support to this theory. An emotional disturbance may initiate an unusual craving for sweets or the habit of snacking, which in turn might influence the incidence of dental caries. On the other hand, a noticeable salivary deficiency is not an uncommon finding in

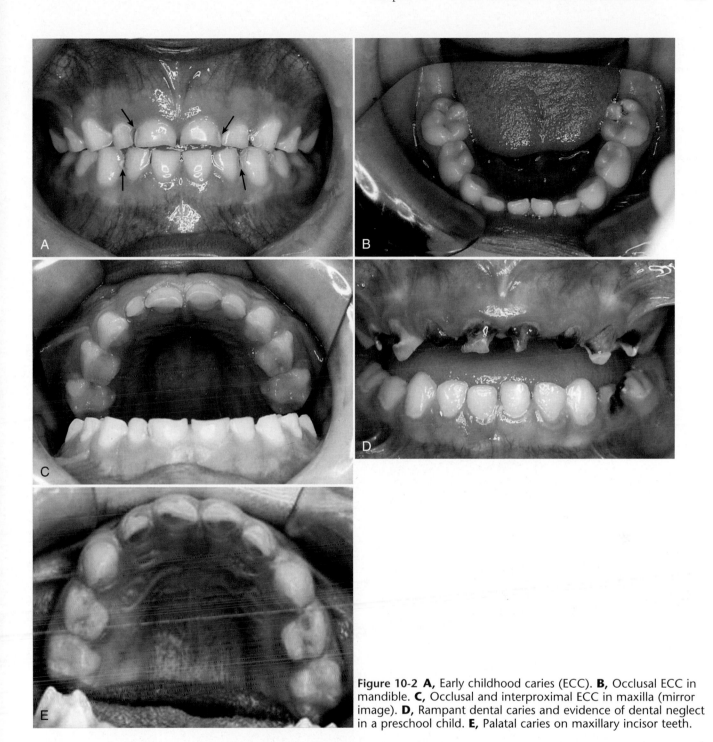

Figure 10-2 A, Early childhood caries (ECC). **B,** Occlusal ECC in mandible. **C,** Occlusal and interproximal ECC in maxilla (mirror image). **D,** Rampant dental caries and evidence of dental neglect in a preschool child. **E,** Palatal caries on maxillary incisor teeth.

tense, nervous, or disturbed persons. Indeed, various forms of stress in both children and adults, as well as various medications (e.g., tranquilizers and sedatives) that are commonly taken to help cope with stress, are associated with decreased salivary flow and decreased caries resistance caused by impaired remineralization. It is well known that radiation therapy to the head and neck often results in significantly diminished salivary function and may place patients at high risk for severe caries development.

EARLY CHILDHOOD CARIES, SEVERE EARLY CHILDHOOD CARIES, NURSING CARIES, BABY BOTTLE TOOTH DECAY

The American Academy of Pediatric Dentistry (AAPD) defines early childhood caries (ECC) as the presence of one or more decayed (noncavitated or cavitated), missing (as a result of caries), or filled tooth surfaces in any primary tooth in a child 71 months of age or younger. The AAPD also specifies that, in children younger than 3 years of age, any sign of smooth-surface caries is indicative of severe early childhood caries (S-ECC).[27]

For many years it has been recognized that, after eruption of the primary teeth begins, excessively frequent bottle feedings and/or prolonged bottle or breast-feeding is often associated with early and rampant caries. The clinical appearance of the teeth in S-ECC in a child 2, 3, or 4 years of age is typical and follows a definite pattern.[28] There is early carious involvement of the maxillary anterior teeth, the maxillary and mandibular first primary molars, and sometimes the mandibular canines (Fig. 10-3). The mandibular incisors are usually unaffected. A discussion with the parents often reveals an inappropriate feeding pattern: the child has been put to bed at afternoon nap time and/or at night with a nursing bottle holding milk or a sugar-containing beverage. The child falls asleep, and the liquid becomes pooled around the teeth (the lower anterior teeth tend to be protected by the tongue). It would seem that the carbohydrate-containing liquid provides an excellent culture medium for acidogenic microorganisms. Salivary flow is also decreased during sleep, and clearance of the liquid from the oral cavity is slowed.

Gardner and colleagues reported four case histories in which the same pattern of caries was observed, and in each child the condition was attributed to a specific breast-feeding habit.[29] In each case the mother explained that human milk was the main source of nutrition. The investigators recommend that from birth the infant should be held while feeding. The child who falls asleep while nursing should be burped and then placed in bed. In addition, the parent should start brushing the child's teeth as soon as they erupt.

The AAPD endorses the policy statement of the American Academy of Pediatrics (AAP) on breast-feeding and the use of human milk.[30] The AAP statement includes the acknowledgment that "breast-feeding ensures the best possible health as well as the best development and psychosocial outcomes for the infant." However, both organizations discourage extended or excessive frequency of feeding times (from the breast or bottle) and encourage appropriate oral hygiene measures for infants and toddlers.

Dilley and colleagues observed a large number of children with prolonged nursing habit caries and concluded that there was no association between the nursing habit

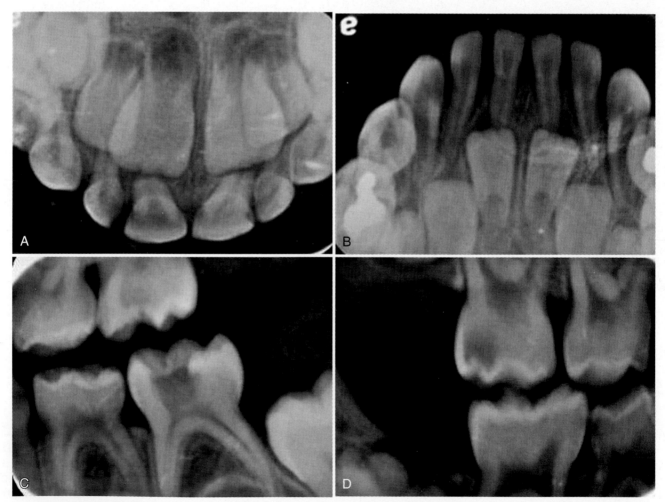

Figure 10-3 Radiographs illustrating early childhood caries. **A,** Maxillary incisors (interproximal). **B,** Mandibular incisors. **C,** Deep caries in mandibular molar. **D,** Maxillary molar distally and on mandibular first molar.

and family background, except that the families were predominantly from lower socioeconomic groups.[31] All subjects demonstrated prolonged breast-feeding or bottle feeding, with milk reported to be the liquid most often used in the bottle. Parents indicated that they did not know when weaning should occur and when oral hygiene should be instituted. The authors also observed nearly symmetric caries patterns.

Hallonsten and colleagues screened 3,000 18-month-old children for dental caries and ongoing breast-feeding.[32] Twelve (19.7%) of the 61 children still being breast-fed had caries, while 51 (1.7%) of the 2,939 children not being breast-fed had caries. The authors found that children who experience prolonged breast-feeding tend to develop unsuitable dietary habits that put them at risk for caries at an early age.

There is considerable scientific evidence from experiments in vitro and in animal models to suggest that some dairy products such as bovine milk and cheese, as well as human breast milk, are not cariogenic and may actually be protective to tooth structure and promote remineralization under certain conditions. Similar experiments show that many infant formulas, with refined food additives, do promote caries. There is much still to learn about caries progression in both the more typical disease and this rampant form. It is prudent to counsel parents to practice good oral hygiene measures for the child and to avoid inappropriate feeding habits that are associated with S-ECC.

S-ECC may be prevented by early counseling of the parents. This is one reason for suggesting that children receive their first dental examination between 6 and 12 months of age when S-ECC is not likely to have developed. In a comprehensive report prepared for the Oral Health Subcommittee of the Healthy Mothers–Healthy Babies Coalition, Ripa states, "Priority needs to be given to a major national educational program directed toward educating the public about nursing caries."[33] The educational program must involve direct contact with pregnant women, parents, and other caregivers in population subgroups with a high prevalence of nursing caries.

ADDITIONAL FACTORS KNOWN TO INFLUENCE DENTAL CARIES

SALIVA

Although saliva was identified in the etiology section earlier as part of the host component and thus a primary part of the caries process, the role of saliva overall is so unique and special that further discussion is warranted here regarding its influence on several aspects of the caries process that may help produce favorable environments to combat the process. Any patient with a salivary deficiency, from any cause, is at higher risk for caries activity.

It is generally accepted that the dental caries process is controlled to a large extent by a natural protective mechanism inherent within the saliva. Many properties of saliva have been investigated to learn their possible role in the caries process. Considerable importance has been

placed on the salivary pH, the acid-neutralizing power, and the calcium, fluoride, and phosphorus content. It has long been suggested that in addition to these properties the rate of flow and the viscosity of saliva may influence the development of caries. The normal salivary flow aids in the solution of food debris on which microorganisms thrive. In addition, the saliva manifests a variety of antibacterial and other anti-infectious properties. All known characteristics of saliva seem somehow relevant to the process of dental caries.

Saliva is secreted by three paired masses of cells—the submaxillary, sublingual, and parotid glands. Small accessory glands are also scattered over the oral mucous membranes. Each of these has its own duct.

The salivary glands are under the control of the autonomic (involuntary) nervous system, receiving fibers from both its parasympathetic and sympathetic divisions. Stimulation of either the parasympathetic (chorda tympani) fibers or the sympathetic fibers to the submaxillary or sublingual gland causes a secretion of saliva. The secretion resulting from parasympathetic stimulation is profuse and watery in most animals. Sympathetic stimulation, however, causes a scanty secretion of a thick, mucinous juice. Stimulation of the parasympathetic fibers to the parotid gland causes a profuse, watery secretion, but stimulation of the sympathetic fibers causes no secretion.

Salivary Deficiency

One of the first descriptions of a severe salivary deficiency with its deleterious effect on the dentition was reported by Hutchinson in 1888.[34] Since that time, many reports have emphasized the importance of a normal flow of saliva in preventing a breakdown of the dentition. A reduction in the salivary flow may be temporary or permanent. When the quantity is only moderately reduced, the oral structures may appear normal. A pronounced reduction or complete absence of saliva, however, results in an acidic environment with rampant caries (Fig. 10-4). In addition to the rapid destruction of the teeth, there may be dryness and cracking of the lips, with fissuring at the corners of the mouth, burning and soreness of the mucous membranes, crusting of the tongue and palate, and sometimes paresthesia of the tongue or mucous membrane.

There are many reasons for a reduction in salivary flow. Acquired salivary dysfunction may be the result of a psychological or emotional disturbance and, again, may be either temporary or permanent. During the acute stages, mumps may cause a temporary reduction in salivary flow. Immune disorders, such as Sjögren syndrome, and genetic conditions, such as hypohidrotic ectodermal dysplasia, often exhibit chronic xerostomia. Many oncology patients receive head and neck or total-body irradiation that also results in salivary gland dysfunction. An interruption in the central pathways of the secretory nerves has been suggested as a cause of salivary failure, but this is usually overshadowed by definite neurologic signs and symptoms. Similarly, a deficiency of vitamin B complex has been reported as a cause of salivary gland dysfunction.

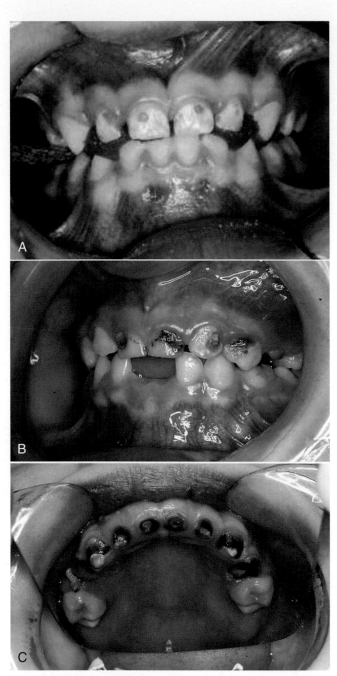

Figure 10-4 Progression of early childhood caries illustrated in three different children. **A,** Restorable with resins. **B,** Restorable with crown forms (possibly). **C,** Nonrestorable.

One study indicated that the minimum effective dose of many of the antihistaminic drugs can reduce salivary flow by as much as 50%.[35] Dryness of the mouth may occur after the use of a variety of tranquilizers and antihistamines. It has likewise been observed that dry mouth and rampant caries may accompany a systemic condition, such as myasthenia gravis. In this disease, the acetylcholine that is necessary for the proper transmission of nerve impulses is destroyed; as a result, the salivary glands do not receive adequate stimulation.

Previous work has shown a great deal of individual variation in the amount of saliva produced by stimulation of the glands. The range is from less than a measurable amount in patients with acquired or congenital dysfunction of the salivary glands to 65 mL during a 15-minute period of stimulation and collection. Patients with deficient salivary flow often have excessive or rampant caries. In contrast, patients with greater than average salivary flow are usually relatively free from dental caries.

Determination of Salivary Flow
If a patient has no known existing conditions that may cause hyposalivation and if the clinician notices a small pool of saliva in the floor of the mouth during oral examination, it is not unreasonable to assume that the patient has adequate salivary quantity and flow. Little information is available about salivary flow rates in children, but Crossner reported that in children 5 to 15 years of age, the rate of mixed whole stimulated saliva increases with age, and boys have consistently higher rates than girls.[36] If inadequate salivary flow is known to exist or is suspected, measurement of salivary flow can provide a baseline useful for comparing with later measurements after implementation of adjunctive therapy.

To evaluate the adequacy of salivary flow, Zunt recommends establishing the unstimulated salivary flow (USF) rate.[37] The USF rate is measured after a period of 1 hour without eating, drinking, chewing gum, or brushing the teeth. Sitting in the "coachman" position, on the edge of the dental chair, the patient passively drools into a funnel inserted into a graduated cylinder for 5 minutes. The eyes should remain open except for blinking during the 5-minute collection period. The head and neck should be bent, and the arms should rest comfortably on the thighs or knees. The volume of saliva collected in the cylinder after 5 minutes is divided by 5 to determine the USF. A USF rate of less than 0.1 mL per minute is diagnostic of salivary gland hypofunction. If the USF rate is less than 0.1 mL per minute, the next step is to measure the stimulated salivary flow (SSF). The patient should chew unflavored paraffin for 45 chews or 1 minute and expectorate into a funnel inserted into a graduated cylinder. The SSF rate should be 1 to 2 mL per minute; less than 0.5 mL per minute is scored as an abnormal rate. A convenient alternative method for measuring USF is the modified Schirmer technique, which uses a calibrated paper test strip to collect saliva in the floor of the mouth.

In patients who are known or suspected to have salivary deficiency, it is not unusual to find a salivary flow ranging from slightly below normal to practically a dry mouth. If there is a deficiency of saliva or a dry mouth, the cause should be sought. Sometimes the cause is readily determinable; sometimes it is obscure. An emotional disturbance should not be overlooked as a cause in a patient of any age. Psychotherapy may be helpful in these cases. If the cause cannot readily be determined, perhaps it should be assumed that the sparse flow is related to inadequacies in the diet, particularly a vitamin deficiency or excessive sugar consumption to the exclusion of needed foods. Monthly quantitative analyses of the saliva should be performed to determine whether dietary improvement is accompanied by an increased flow.

If the salivary glands have not undergone degenerative or metaplastic change and if the nerve pathways between the central nervous system and the salivary glands are still intact, salivary stimulants may be recommended. If dryness of the mouth is attributable to dehydration, increased fluid intake should be recommended. The use of gustatory stimulants (sugar-free candy) or masticatory stimulants (xylitol gum) has been suggested as an adjunct to encourage salivation. Prescription sialagogue medications, also known as secretagogues, such as pilocarpine and cevimeline may be of benefit in improving the salivary flow rate in patients with Sjögren syndrome or with radiation damage to salivary glands. The use of sialagogue medications has not been studied in pediatric populations, but these agents are considered safe for most adult patients and have been used successfully in older children. The use of salivary substitutes has been suggested by Shannon and colleagues as helpful in preventing soft tissue problems associated with dry mouth.[38] Saliva substitutes, as well as fluoride and chlorhexidine rinses, are also reported to enhance remineralization and promote resistance to demineralization of tooth surfaces, and may help prevent radiation-induced caries.

Viscosity of Saliva

It has long been suggested that the viscosity of saliva is related to the rate of dental decay. Both thick, ropy saliva and thin, watery saliva have been blamed for rampant dental caries. Previous work has shown a statistically significant direct relationship between the viscosity of saliva and the number of decayed, missing, and filled teeth.[39] This relationship held true for all members of the observation group, regardless of age. Patients with thick, ropy saliva invariably had poor oral hygiene. The teeth were covered with stain or plaque, and the rate of dental caries ranged from greater than average to rampant.

No evidence exists that viscosity changes with age under normal conditions. This property of the saliva is governed not only by the particular set of glands stimulated but also by the type of nervous stimulation and the amount of mucin (glycoprotein) present.

Children who consume excessive amounts of carbohydrates often have not only a sparse flow but also viscous saliva. Even minimal doses of some antihistaminic drugs will result in a greatly increased viscosity of saliva in some persons.[35]

There are apparently only a limited number of ways to alter the viscosity of saliva. Reduction of refined sugar intake may be effective in some patients.

Although relatively little information specific to salivary function, flow, and viscosity in children is available, an excellent review article by Leone and Oppenheim provides much additional information regarding the relationship between saliva and dental caries.[40]

SOCIOECONOMIC STATUS

The Surgeon General's report of 2000 indicated that one in four American children is born into poverty.[1] The report notes that children and adolescents living in poverty suffer twice as much tooth decay as their more affluent peers and their disease is more likely to go untreated. The report also mentioned that, although continuing reductions of dental caries in permanent teeth have been achieved, caries prevalence in primary teeth has stabilized or possibly increased in some population groups. A Census Bureau report published in March 2003 showed that the poverty rate for children in the United States rose in 2002, whereas it dropped for people 65 years and older.[41] Nearly half of the 35 million people living in poverty were children. These are alarming data calling attention to a huge unmet oral health care need in the United States.

Following the report of the Surgeon General, Edelstein pointed out that, paradoxically, children living in poverty also have the highest rates of dental insurance coverage, largely through the Medicaid program and the State Children's Health Insurance Program.[42] Yet Medicaid-eligible children who have cavities have twice the number of carious teeth and twice the number of visits for pain relief but fewer total dental visits than children in families with higher incomes. He also noted that these disparities continue into adolescence and young adulthood but to a lesser degree. Because practitioners have the opportunity to assess the oral health of poor children individually, they will identify some patients at low risk for dental caries. However, the available data confirm that, from a demographic perspective, economically poor children are at high risk for dental caries.

ANATOMIC CHARACTERISTICS OF THE TEETH

Certain teeth of many patients, particularly permanent teeth, seem vulnerable to dental caries as they emerge and, in caries-active mouths, they may show evidence of the attack almost coincident with their eruption into the oral cavity. Because enamel calcification is incomplete at the time of eruption of the teeth and an additional period of about two years is required for the calcification process to be completed by exposure to saliva, the teeth are especially susceptible to caries formation during the first two years after eruption. Permanent molars often have incompletely coalesced pits and fissures that allow the dental plaque material to be retained at the base of the defect, sometimes in contact with exposed dentin. These defects or anatomic characteristics can readily be seen if the tooth is dried and the debris and plaque removed. In addition to occlusal surfaces, lingual pits on the maxillary permanent molars, buccal pits on the mandibular permanent molars, and lingual pits on the maxillary permanent lateral incisors are vulnerable areas in which the process of dental caries can proceed rapidly.

ARRANGEMENT OF THE TEETH IN THE ARCH

Crowded and irregular teeth are not readily cleansed during the natural masticatory process. It is likewise difficult for the patient to clean the mouth properly with a toothbrush and floss if the teeth are crowded or over-lapped. This condition therefore may contribute to the problem of dental caries.

PRESENCE OF DENTAL APPLIANCES AND RESTORATIONS

Partial dentures, space maintainers, and orthodontic appliances often encourage the retention of food debris and plaque material and have been shown to result in an increase in the bacterial population. Few patients keep their mouths meticulously clean, and even those who make an attempt may be hampered by the presence of dental appliances that retain plaque material between brushings. Patients who have had moderate dental caries activity in the past might be expected to have increased caries activity after the placement of appliances in the mouth unless they practice unusually good oral hygiene.

Rosenbloom and Tinanoff evaluated the *S. mutans* level of patients before, during, and after orthodontic treatment.[43] *S. mutans* levels were significantly elevated during active treatment. When samples were taken 6 to 15 weeks into the retention phase of treatment, however, the microbial levels were found to have decreased significantly to levels comparable to those of untreated children.

Dentists have known for many years that the tooth structure at the interface with restorative material is especially vulnerable to recurrent caries. Clinical studies suggest that dentists and their patients should not expect successful restorative treatment to reduce a patient's risk for future development of carious lesions. Tinanoff and colleagues found higher numbers of salivary *S. mutans* in patients after they received restorative treatment.[44] Wright and colleagues observed significant reductions in the number of mutans streptococci and lactobacilli immediately after restoration; however, mutans streptococci returned to prerestoration levels in many of their subjects.[45] Gregory and colleagues observed that postoperative counts of salivary streptococci essentially equaled the preoperative counts after all restorative work had been completed in their patients.[46] Effective prevention programs are required to protect the patient from additional caries and to better justify the investment in restorative care.

HEREDITARY FACTORS

Although parents of children with excessive or rampant caries tend to blame the condition on hereditary factors or tendencies, and some scientific evidence, as reviewed in Chapter 6, acknowledges certain genetic influences on the caries process, most authors agree that genetic influences on dental caries are relatively minor in comparison with the overall effect of environmental factors. The fact that children acquire their dietary habits, oral hygiene habits, and oral microflora from their parents makes dental caries more an environmental than a hereditary disease. Although several hereditary factors identified in Chapter 6 may be influential in promoting or preventing dental caries activity, available effective preventive therapies along with proper dietary and plaque control measures can override the hereditary factors that contribute to caries development.

EARLY DETECTION OF DISEASE ACTIVITY

Traditionally, dentists have relied upon a visual-tactile-radiographic procedure for the detection of dental caries. This procedure involves the visual identification of demineralized areas (typically white spots) or suspicious pits or fissures and the use of the dental explorer to determine the presence of a loss of continuity or breaks in the enamel and assess the softness or resilience of the enamel. Carious lesions located on interproximal tooth surfaces have generally been detected with the use of bite-wing radiographs. These procedures have been used routinely in virtually every dental office in the United States for the past 50 years.

Because the reversal of the caries process depends on an intact surface layer of the lesion and the typical use of the dental explorer to probe the suspicious areas often results in the rupture of the surface layer covering early lesions, the use of the dental explorer to probe enamel is no longer recommended. The recommended use of the dental explorer is to judiciously remove plaque and debris to permit visual inspection of pits and fissures.

Tactile probing procedures are no longer used for caries detection in most European countries and this protocol has now been adopted by many U.S. dental schools. The primary concerns that led to the discontinuation of the probing procedure were (1) the insertion of the probe into the suspected lesion inevitably disrupts the surface layer covering very early lesions, thereby eliminating the possibility for remineralizing the decalcified area; (2) the probing of lesions and suspected lesions results in the transport of cariogenic bacteria from one area to another; and (3) frank lesions requiring restoration are generally apparent visually without the need for probing. The clinical caries detection procedures commonly used in Europe have been described by several clinical investigators.[47-51]

Carious lesions are detected visually on the basis of their location (decalcification can only occur in areas where dental plaque may accumulate regularly) and the presence of enamel opacities with or without staining. The state of activity is determined by the visual appearance of an opacity, the color of the area (i.e., presence of brown or green stain), and the roughness of the enamel surface as assessed by dragging the explorer across the surface. The only use of the dental explorer as a probe is to remove plaque or debris from tooth surfaces.

While this visual examination procedure for clinically detecting dental caries maintains the integrity of the enamel surface over the demineralized area and the possibility for the remineralization of the area, there remain some practical limitations to this caries detection procedure. The detection process requires the visual detection of demineralized areas as so-called white spots with or without additional pigmentation, which presents two significant limitations. First, these areas, particularly if they are relatively small, may be overlooked during the visual examination due to reflections or inadequate drying of the tooth surfaces. Second, by the time these areas may be detected visually as white spots, the demineralization will have progressed through at least one third of the outer portion of the enamel. Decalcifications of this magnitude require longer time periods and a greater number of treatments to completely remineralize. Lesions detected on radiographs have generally progressed to the initial involvement of dentin. The increased desire of dental professionals and patients for more conservative restorative procedures as well as the implementation of measures to control and reverse the caries process led to significant efforts to develop technologies for the early detection of dental caries. Dental scientists have explored other measures to assist with the detection of the caries at an earlier stage of the formation process, which resulted in the development and evaluation of a variety of instruments.[51]

INFRARED LASER FLUORESCENCE (DIAGNOdent)

An instrument designed to facilitate the detection of dental caries, DIAGNOdent (Kaltenbach & Voigt GmbH & Co., Biberach/Riss, Germany) (Fig. 10-5), has recently become available in several countries. This instrument was developed for the detection and quantification of dental caries of occlusal and smooth surfaces. It uses a diode laser light source and a fiberoptic cable that transmits the light to a handheld probe with a fiberoptic eye in the tip. The light is absorbed and induces infrared fluorescence by organic and inorganic material. The emitted fluorescence is collected at the probe tip, transmitted through ascending fibers, and processed and presented on a display window as an integer between 0 and 99. Increased fluorescence reflects carious tooth substance. What material is responsible for the fluorescence is still under investigation, but it appears to be bacterial metabolites, particularly the porphyrins.

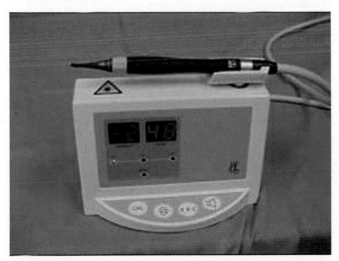

Figure 10-5 Infrared laser fluorescence diagnostic machine (DIAGNOdent, Kaltenbach & Voigt GmbH & Co., Biberach/Riss, Germany).

An appreciable number of in vitro studies and a few in vivo (clinical) studies of the performance of this instrument have been reported in the past five years. The results of the various in vitro studies have indicated that the DIAGNOdent instrument is capable of detecting relatively advanced carious lesions, and DIAGNOdent readings show a very good correlation with histologic evidence of caries but not with the depth of the lesions into dentin. However, the results of the in vitro studies have also indicated that the readings are influenced by several variables, including the degree of dehydration of the lesion, the presence of dental plaque, and the presence of various types of stain in occlusal fissures.

The results of clinical investigations have shown significant differences in readings between different DIAGNOdent instruments with regard to extent of occlusal caries, which raises questions regarding the selection of a value of 20 or 25 to indicate the presence of caries. For a given instrument, intraoperator reliability was generally good and interoperator reliability typically ranged from good to very good. Furthermore, DIAGNOdent readings increased linearly with clinical histologic measurements. The instrument was reported to be able to distinguish with good sensitivity between sound tooth structure and deeper carious lesions extending into dentin. The instrument is very good at indicating the presence of deeper lesions into dentin that may not be apparent yet on radiographs but is unable to reliably indicate the depth of a dentinal lesion.

Instrument readings higher than 20 or 25 suggest the presence of caries, and higher readings generally reflect more extensive lesion progression, although there does not appear to be a linear relation between the readings and the extent of the lesions. Prudent use of the instrument can identify early lesions that should be considered for preventive rather than restorative treatment.

INFRARED AND RED FLUORESCENCE (Midwest Caries ID)

Recently an instrument was introduced that reflected a further improvement in the use of infrared-induced fluorescence involving the combination of infrared and red fluorescence (Fig. 10-6). This instrument (Midwest Caries ID) uses both infrared (880 nm) and red (660 nm) light provided by light-emitting diodes in a handheld probe that is designed for use on all tooth surfaces. The inclusion of the red light permits observations related to light-scattering properties associated with the loss of tooth structure. As noted earlier, the infrared light induces fluorescence from bacterial porphyrins and related exogenous materials that may be present in pits and fissures, dental plaque, or cavitated carious lesions. Originally developed in Canada and introduced in 2006, there is little evidence-based information available in the dental literature. Preliminary data suggest that the added presence of red light to the system improves the accuracy for caries detection. In particular, the combination instrument appears to be more useful for detecting so-called hidden occlusal caries. However, there is no indication that either the

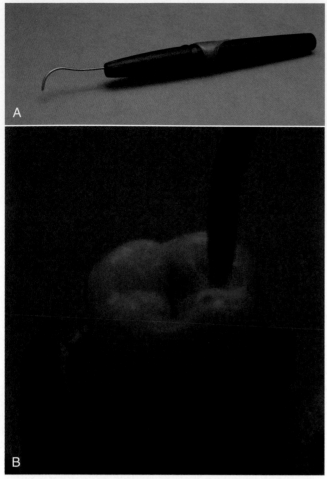

Figure 10-6 Infrared and fluorescence (Midwest Caries ID). **A,** Handheld probe. **B,** Handheld probe being used on molar tooth.

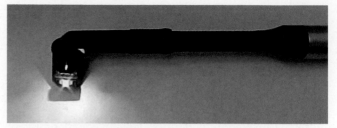

Figure 10-7 Digital imaging fiberoptic transillumination handheld probe (DIFOTI).

the use of FOTI with visual and radiographic examinations, and a recent investigation indicated that dental practitioners were able to detect more proximal lesions with FOTI than with a visual examination with or without the use of radiographs.

Digital Imaging Fiber Optic Trans-Illumination (DIFOTI) (Electro-Optical Sciences, Inc., Irvington, NY 10533) is a further advancement of this technology in which the visually observed images are captured using a digital charge-coupled device (CCD) camera and sent to a computer for analysis using dedicated algorithms. This instrument has become commercially available relatively recently, and very few investigations of its capabilities and limitations have been reported. The results of an in vitro study involving the imaging of extracted teeth indicated that the instrument had greater sensitivity for the detection of caries on all tooth surfaces than did radiologic imaging. However, a more recent in vitro study in which artificial lesions developed over 14 weeks underwent intermittent imaging and radiography at 2-week intervals indicated that the DIFOTI system, unlike radiography, was not able to determine the depth of lesions. Although at least one clinical investigation of this instrument is in progress, there are currently no published reports of the clinical use of the instrument demonstrating its usefulness in practice. Nevertheless, based on prior reports of the use of FOTI, it is reasonable to expect that DIFOTI should be at least as good as radiography for detection of caries on interproximal tooth surfaces.

QUANTITATIVE LIGHT FLUORESCENCE

Without question the most extensively investigated technique available for the early detection of dental caries is quantitative light fluorescence (QLF) (Fig. 10-8). This methodology began with the observation in 1978, by a dental scientist in Sweden, that the use of a laser light of selected wavelength markedly enhanced the visibility of early noncavitated lesions. Subsequent investigations by this group confirmed the value of this approach for the early detection of caries clinically. Further studies established a relationship between the loss of fluorescent intensity and increasing mineral loss from the lesions compared with sound enamel. Numerous additional in vitro and in situ studies confirmed this important correlation between the amount of observed fluorescence and the mineral content of the lesions, and

DIAGNOdent nor this instrument is capable of detecting noncavitated "lesions" confined to the outer half of enamel. Nevertheless, the instrument may be considered as a useful adjunct to the visual examination for the diagnosis of dental caries that are considered visually suspicious.

DIGITAL IMAGING FIBEROPTIC TRANSILLUMINATION

Conventional clinical caries examinations routinely use transillumination to identify lesions located on the interproximal surfaces of the anterior teeth (Fig. 10-7). For at least 30 years, a fiberoptic transillumination (FOTI) instrument has been available for clinical use. It provides an intense light beam that is transmitted through a fiberoptic cable to a specially designed probe to permit the use of transillumination on the proximal surfaces of posterior teeth. Repeated improvements have been made in the instrument so that it may be used on occlusal as well as proximal tooth surfaces, and the instrument is commonly used, often in place of radiographs, in private practices in Europe. Numerous studies have compared changes in the enamel, the QLF method has continued to undergo further development with respect to both software and hardware. A number of clinical investigations of this newer system have been conducted and have convincingly demonstrated the ability of the QLF instrument to detect early carious lesions and to accurately monitor either lesion progression or regression. The first of these studies monitored the changes in white spot lesions in orthodontic patients following the removal of the appliances and the institution of improved oral hygiene and use of a fluoride dentifrice; the remineralization of the lesions was impressively demonstrated within a few weeks. Another study of school-aged children showed that the QLF instrument detected 5 to 10 times more early lesions than conventional detection methods, was particularly useful for examination of occlusal pits and fissures, and gave reproducible results. A clinical study of white spot lesions in caries-active children in Sweden demonstrated significant remineralization of the lesions within 6 months after treatments with a fluoride varnish. An additional clinical study by this group involving multiple examiners demonstrated the reproducibility of clinical QLF measurements. A team of Japanese scientists conducted a clinical trial using QLF to monitor changes in white spot lesions of children brushing with a fluoride dentifrice and reported a significant decrease in the size of the lesions within 3 months of the 1-year test period. From these clinical studies, it is apparent that QLF enhances the early detection of dental caries and is uniquely useful in monitoring the progression or regression of lesions.

Numerous investigations have demonstrated the practical usefulness of QLF for the early detection of dental caries on occlusal and smooth tooth surfaces as well as for the quantification of lesion changes related to treatment procedures and environmental factors such as oral hygiene. The only significant limitation to this instrument is its inability to detect or monitor interproximal lesions.

Applications

Caries detection is entering a new era with new technologies capable of detecting lesions at an earlier stage of development and quantifying the impact of noninvasive professional fluoride treatments such as fluoride varnishes. DIAGNOdent appears to be most useful in confirming the presence of caries in suspicious occlusal pits and fissures and detecting deep dentinal lesions of the occlusal surface (so-called hidden caries). DIFOTI, pending further study, may have greatest usefulness as a potential replacement for bite-wing radiography in the detection of caries on interproximal surfaces. QLF has been shown to be most useful for the early detection of dental caries on occlusal, buccal, and lingual surfaces and for the quantification of changes in early lesions associated with various preventive treatments. Such early identification will provide evidence to guide the dental professional in implementing various measures for the reversal and control of these lesions.

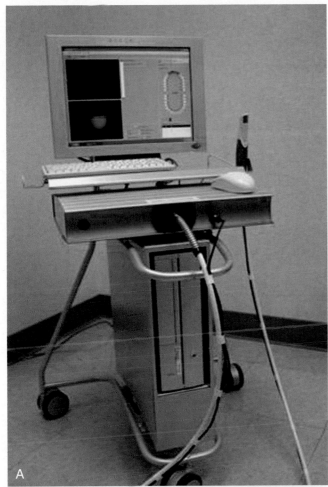

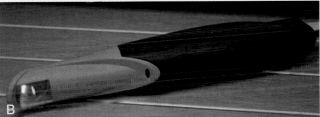

Figure 10-8 Quantitative light fluorescence. (QLF). **A**, QLF machine. **B**, QLF handheld probe.

made possible the development of a system that could truly assess changes in either the progression or regression of carious lesions.

To facilitate clinical investigations, as well as the use of the device in clinical practice, a small portable system (Omnii Oral Pharmaceuticals, West Palm Beach, FL 33409) was developed in which the laser source was replaced by a regular light source and filter system. The light illuminating the tooth is transported through a liquid-filled light guide. The fluorescent filtered images are captured using a color CCD camera and a frame grabber. Data are collected, stored, and analyzed by custom software. Since the first attempts at in vivo quantification of mineral

PREDICTION OF PATIENTS' RISK FOR FUTURE DISEASE (RISK ASSESSMENT)

In contemporary health care practices, caries-risk assessment is now recognized as a useful component in providing appropriate care for children and adolescents. The AAPD has adopted a policy statement on caries risk assessment and a caries risk assessment tool (CAT). The CAT is illustrated in Table 10-1. The policy statement, almost in its entirety except for references, follows[53]:

Purpose

The American Academy of Pediatric Dentistry (AAPD) recognizes that caries-risk assessment is an essential element of contemporary clinical care for infants, children, and adolescents.

Background

While assessment of caries risk undoubtedly will benefit from emerging science and technologies, the AAPD believes that sufficient evidence exists to support the

Table **10-1**

American Academy of Pediatric Dentistry Caries-risk Assessment Tool

RISK FACTORS TO CONSIDER	RISK INDICATORS		
(For each item below, circle the most accurate response found to the right under "Risk Indicators")	**High**	**Moderate**	**Low**
Part 1- History (determined by interviewing the parent/primary caregiver)			
Child has special health care needs, especially any that impact motor coordination or cooperation[A]	Yes		No
Child has condition that impairs saliva (dry mouth)[B]	Yes		No
Child's use of dental home (frequency of routine dental visits)	None	Irregular	Regular
Child has decay	Yes		No
Time lapsed since child's last cavity	<12 mo	12 to 24 mo	>24 months
Child wears braces or orthodontic/oral appliances[C]	Yes		No
Child's parent and/or sibling(s) have decay	Yes		No
Socioeconomic status of child's parent[D]	Low	Mid-level	High
Daily between-meal exposures to sugars/cavity-producing foods (includes on demand use of bottle/sippy cup containing liquid other than water; consumption of juice, carbonated beverages, or sports drinks; use of sweetened medications)[E]	>3	1 to 2	Mealtime only
Child's exposure to fluoride[F,G]	Does not use fluoridated toothpaste; drinking water is not fluoridated; and is not taking fluoride supplements	Uses fluoridated toothpaste; usually does not drink fluoridated water; and does not take fluoride supplements	Uses fluoridated toothpaste; drinks fluoridated water; or takes fluoride supplements
Times per day that child's teeth/gums are brushed	<1	1	2-3
Part 2- Clinical Evaluation (determined by examining the child's mouth)			
Visible plaque (white, sticky buildup)	Present		Absent
Gingivitis (red, puffy gums)[H]	Present		Absent
Areas of enamel demineralization (chalky white-spots on teeth)	More than 1	1	None
Enamel defects, deep pits/fissures[I]	Present		Absent

Table **10-1**			
American Academy of Pediatric Dentistry Caries-risk Assessment Tool—cont'd			
RISK FACTORS TO CONSIDER	**RISK INDICATORS**		
(For each item below, circle the most accurate response found to the right under "Risk Indicators")	**High**	**Moderate**	**Low**
Part 3- Supplemental Professional Assessment (Optional)^J			
Radiographic enamel caries	Present		Absent
Levels of *mutans* streptococci or lactobacilli	High	Moderate	Low

Each child's overall assessed risk for developing decay is based on the highest level of risk indicator circled above (ie, a single risk indicator in any area of the "high risk" category classifies a child as being "high risk").

Adapted from American Academy on Pediatric Dentistry Council on Clinical Affairs. Policy on use of a caries-risk assessment tool (CAT) for infants, children, and adolescents, *Pediatr Dent* 30(Suppl):29-33, 2008.

^AChildren with special health care needs are those who have a physical, developmental, mental, sensory, behavioral, cognitive, or emotional impairment or limiting condition that requires medical management, health care intervention, and/or use of specialized services. The condition may be developmental or acquired and may cause limitations in performing daily self-maintenance activities or substantial limitations in a major life activity. Health care for special needs patients is beyond that considered routine and requires specialized knowledge, increased awareness and attention, and accommodation.

^BAlternation in salivary flow can be the result of congenital or acquired conditions, surgery, radiation, medication, or age-related changes in salivary function. Any condition, treatment, or process known or reported to alter saliva flow should be considered an indication of risk unless proven otherwise.

^COrthodontic appliances include both fixed and removable appliances, space maintainers, and other devices that remain in the mouth continuously or for prolonged time intervals and which may trap food and plaque, prevent oral hygiene, compromise access of tooth surfaces to fluoride, or otherwise create an environment supporting caries initiation.

^DNational surveys have demonstrated that children in low-income and moderate-income households are more likely to have caries and more decayed or filled primary teeth than children from more affluent households. Also, within income levels, minority children are more likely to have caries. Thus, socioeconomic status should be viewed as an initial indicator of risk that may be offset by the absence of other risk indicators.

^EExamples of sources of simple sugars include carbonated beverages, cookies, cake, candy, cereal, potato chips, French fries, corn chips, pretzels, breads, juices, and fruits. Clinicians using caries-risk assessment should investigate individual exposures to sugars known to be involved in caries initiation.

^FOptimal systemic and topical fluoride exposure is based on use of a fluoride dentifrice and American Dental Association/American Academy of Pediatrics guidelines for exposure from fluoride drinking water and/or supplementation.

^GUnsupervised use of toothpaste and at-home topical fluoride products are not recommended for children unable to expectorate predictably.

^HAlthough microbial organisms responsible for gingivitis may be different than those primarily implicated in caries, the presence of gingivitis is an indicator of poor or infrequent oral hygiene practices and has been associated with caries progression.

^ITooth anatomy and hypoplastic defects (eg, poorly formed enamel, developmental pits) may predispose a child to develop caries.

^JAdvanced technologies such as radiographic assessment and microbiologic testing are not essential for using this tool.

creation of a framework for classifying caries risk in infants, children, and adolescents based on a set of physical, environmental, and general health factors.

The table [Table 10-1] represents a first step toward incorporating available evidence into a concise, practical tool to assist both dental and nondental health care providers in assessing levels of risk for caries development in infants, children, and adolescents. The AAPD intends this to be a dynamic instrument that will be evaluated and revised periodically as new evidence warrants.

Clinicians using this tool should:

1. Be able to visualize adequately a child's teeth and mouth and have access to a reliable historian for nonclinical data elements.
2. Assess all three components of caries risk—clinical conditions, environmental characteristics, and general health conditions.
3. Be familiar with footnotes that clarify use of individual factors in this instrument.
4. Understand that each child's ultimate risk classification is determined by the highest risk category where a risk indicator exists (i.e., the presence of a single risk indicator in any area of the "high-risk" category is sufficient to classify a child as being at "high risk"; the presence of at least one "moderate-risk" indicator and no "high-risk" indicators results in a "moderate-risk" classification; and a child designated as "low risk" would have no "moderate-risk" or "high-risk" indicators).

Users of the AAPD caries-risk assessment tool (CAT) must understand the following caveats:

1. CAT provides a means of classifying dental caries risk at a point in time and, therefore, should be applied periodically to assess changes in an individual's risk status.

2. CAT is intended to be used when clinical guidelines call for caries-risk assessment. Decisions regarding clinical management of caries, however, are left to qualified dentists (ideally, the dentist responsible for the child's "dental home").
3. CAT can be used by both dental and nondental personnel. It does *not* render a diagnosis. However, clinicians using CAT must be familiar with the clinical presentation of dental caries and factors related to caries initiation and progression.
4. Since clinicians with various levels of skill working in a variety of settings will use this instrument, advanced technologies such as radiographic assessment and microbiologic testing (darker shaded areas in Table 10-1) have been included but are not essential for using this tool.

Policy Statement

The AAPD:

1. Encourages both dental and nondental health care providers to use CAT in the care of infants, children, and adolescents.
2. Encourages dentists to use advanced technologies such as radiographic assessment and microbiologic testing with CAT when assessing an individual's caries risk.
3. Recognizes the need to evaluate CAT periodically and revise the tool as new science and technologies warrant.

Zero and colleagues presented an extensive review of the literature to determine the predictive validity of available multivariate caries risk assessment strategies for children and adults.[54] They concluded the following:

- The predictive validities of the models reviewed depended strongly on the caries prevalence and characteristics of the population for which they were designed.
- Many models included similar categories of risk indicators but provided very different outcomes depending on the study population.
- In many instances, the use of a single risk indicator gave results that were equally as good as those obtained using a combination of indicators.
- No combination of risk indicators was consistently considered a good predictor when applied to different populations, across different age groups. In general, however, the best indicators of caries risk were easily obtained from dental charts and did not require additional testing.
- Previous caries experience was an important predictor for primary, permanent, and root surface caries in most models tested.
- Most of the research in this area has been done in children, for both primary and permanent teeth.

It is obvious from their report that the caries risk assessment process is very much a work in progress. Further refinements will continue for some time in the future.

Of course, accurate caries risk assessments of patients can guide clinicians and health care facilities toward better allocation of their time and resources for their high-risk patients. As our accuracy and efficiency in identifying patients with active disease or high potential to develop disease improves, and as parents, patients, and health care insurance plans accept this newer approach to care, the standard "6-month recall visit" for children may change to a more customized plan for individual patients or groups of patients. Children who are at low risk for caries and who do not present with other oral conditions that need frequent monitoring may not require oral health care visits as often as those at high risk (with or without active disease), whereas compliant high-risk patients may, at times, require frequent visits and multiple forms of caries control therapies in addition to their voluntary modification of caries-promoting dietary and behavioral habits.

CONTROL OF DENTAL CARIES

Many practical measures for the control of dental caries are applicable to private practice. Most practitioners have tried control measures with varying degrees of success. One cannot emphasize too strongly, however, that no single measure for the control of dental caries will be entirely satisfactory. All possible preventive measures and approaches must be considered in the hope of successfully controlling and preventing the caries process.

Pediatric dentists who see patients on a referral basis may hear a parent remark, "My child has so many cavities that my dentist doesn't know where to start." Although it is true that the problem may at first seem overwhelming, a systematic, understanding approach often results in a gratifying response. An outline of procedures for the control of active or rampant caries in cooperative and communicative patients follows. With this approach and with patient cooperation, the problem can usually be explained and brought under control. The successful management of active dental caries, however, depends on the parents' or patient's interest in maintaining the patient's teeth and their cooperation in a customized and specific caries control program.

CONTROL OF ALL ACTIVE CARIOUS LESIONS

When rampant caries occurs, the first steps are to initiate treatment of all carious lesions to stop or at least slow the progression of the disease and to identify the most important causes of the existing condition. Next, and even simultaneously, if possible, the practitioner begins working with the parents and/or the patient to achieve the appropriate behavioral modifications required to prevent recurrence. The problem may then be approached in a systematic manner. Invariably modifications in oral hygiene procedures and dietary habits are necessary. Often, achieving patient compliance with the recommended modifications is the greatest challenge of all.

If the initial restorative treatment is to be done in one appointment under general anesthesia or in one or two appointments with sedation, then control of the existing lesions will be definitive at that time. If the restorative care is to be performed over several visits in the outpatient setting, gross caries excavation as an initial approach in the control of rampant dental caries has several advantages. The removal of the superficial caries and the filling of the cavity with a glass ionomer material or zinc oxide–eugenol cement (IRM, Intermediate Restorative Material, LD Caulk Co., Milford, DE, 19963) will at least temporarily arrest the caries process and prevent its rapid progression to the dental pulp. Gross caries removal can usually be accomplished easily in one appointment. If there are many extensive carious lesions, however, a second appointment may be necessary.

An alternative approach for some compliant children (with compliant parents) old enough to rinse and expectorate and for compliant adolescents is to initiate intensive and multiple antimicrobial and topical fluoride therapies in conjunction with the necessary behavioral lifestyle modifications and then to proceed systematically with restorations and other indicated therapies.

REDUCTION IN THE INTAKE OF FREELY FERMENTABLE CARBOHYDRATES

Excellent studies have shown a relationship between diet and dental caries. As a result of these studies, considerable emphasis has been given to this phase of the caries control program. There is also much evidence to confirm that between-meal snacking and the frequency of eating and drinking are related to dental caries incidence.

Gustafsson and colleagues conducted a well-controlled study of dental caries, now considered a classic, and observed that a group of patients whose diet was high in fat, low in carbohydrates, and practically free of sugar had low caries activity.[55] When refined sugar was added to the diet in the form of a mealtime supplement, there was still little or no caries activity. However, when caramels were given between meals, a statistically significant increase in the number of new carious lesions occurred. It was concluded from these studies that dental caries activity could be increased by the consumption of sugar if the sugar was in a form easily retained on the tooth surface. The more frequently this form of sugar was consumed between meals, the greater was the tendency for an increase in dental caries.

Weiss and Trithart reported additional evidence for the relationship between the incidence of dental caries and between-meal eating habits.[56] In a group of preschool children, it was found that most between-meal snacks were of high sugar content or were high in adhesiveness. The children who did not eat between meals had 3.3 decayed, extracted, or filled primary teeth (deft), whereas those who ate four or more items between meals had a deft rate of 9.8.

As mentioned earlier, sweetened liquids provided to young children in nursing bottles can have enormous cariogenic potential. Likewise, carbonated soft drinks and other sweetened drinks are popular with older children and adolescents and are readily available. Frequent ingestion of these drinks is another form of snacking that can promote and accelerate caries progression.

Investigations by Schachtele and Jensen[57] as well as by Park and colleagues[58] have indicated that the acidity of plaque located in interproximal areas, which generally have less exposure to saliva, may remain below the critical pH for periods in excess of 2 hours after carbohydrate ingestion. Because foods containing sugars in solution as well as retentive sugars are included in the diet analysis,

20 minutes may be considered as the minimal time each exposure permits acid concentrations to be available in the bacterial plaque.

The following can be used in explaining the dental caries process to a parent or child:

$$\text{Fermentable carbohydrate} + \text{Oral bacteria}$$
$$\text{within plaque} \rightarrow \text{Acid within plaque}$$

$$\text{Acid} + \text{Susceptible tooth} \rightarrow \text{Tooth decay}$$

REDUCTION OF DENTAL PLAQUE (AND MICROORGANISMS) WITH GOOD ORAL HYGIENE PROCEDURES

Chapter 11 discusses the importance of good oral hygiene in more detail, but it must be mentioned here as a critically important component of any caries control program. Berenie and colleagues studied the relationship between frequency of toothbrushing, oral hygiene, gingival health, and caries in 384 children, 9 to 13 years of age, who resided in a fluoride-deficient western New York community.[59] Of the children studied, 37% brushed their teeth once a day, 37% brushed twice a day, and 13% brushed less than once a day. The remaining children in the group, approximately 13%, brushed their teeth three or more times each day. A trend toward decreased scores for decayed, missing, or filled permanent teeth (DMFT) and decayed, missing, or filled permanent tooth surfaces (DMFS) accompanied increased daily brushing. The increased frequency of daily toothbrushing had its most significant positive effect on the level of oral hygiene.

Beal and colleagues studied the caries incidence and gingival health of children who were 11 to 12 years old at the start of the study.[60] The children's dental cleanliness was evaluated at yearly examinations for a 3-year period. The children whose dental cleanliness was consistently good had lower caries increments than those whose dental cleanliness was consistently bad. Horowitz and colleagues have demonstrated the benefits of a school-based plaque removal program in a 3-year study of children in grades 5 to 8.[61] At the end of the study, the adjusted mean DMFS scores were 13% lower in the supervised plaque removal group than in the control group. The difference between groups was accounted for entirely by a 26% difference in affected mesial and distal surfaces, a figure that approached statistical significance ($P = .07$). Similarly, Tsamtsouris and colleagues demonstrated that supervised toothbrushing with instruction produces significantly and consistently lower plaque scores, even in preschool children, than were achieved through a control test of the same children when they were neither supervised nor instructed.[62] The investigators concluded that constant reinforcement is necessary to maintain effective plaque control in preschool children.

Wright and colleagues conducted a clinical study to evaluate the effect of frequent interdental flossing on the incidence of proximal dental caries.[63] School children from a fluoride-deficient area were studied after clinical and radiographic examinations were performed. Based on the observations of this study, the authors concluded that frequent interdental flossing resulted in a 50% reduction in the incidence of proximal caries in primary teeth during a 20-month period. The longer the period of interdental flossing, the greater the benefit; however, there was little residual effect after flossing was discontinued.

USE OF FLUORIDES AND TOPICAL ANTIMICROBIAL AGENTS

Without doubt, the repeated use of fluorides is of critical importance for the control and prevention of dental caries in both children and adults. Numerous controlled clinical investigations have consistently demonstrated the cariostatic properties of fluoride provided in a variety of manners. These studies have also shown that the maximal benefit from fluoride is achieved only through the use of multiple delivery systems.

Existing evidence indicates that the cariostatic activity of fluoride involves several different mechanisms. The ingestion of fluoride results in its incorporation into the dentin and enamel of unerupted teeth; this makes the teeth more resistant to acid attack after eruption into the oral cavity. In addition, ingested fluoride is secreted into saliva. Although it is present in low concentrations, the fluoride is accumulated in plaque, where it decreases microbial acid production and enhances the remineralization of the underlying enamel. Fluoride from saliva is also incorporated into the enamel of newly erupted teeth, thereby enhancing enamel calcification (frequently called *enamel maturation*), which decreases caries susceptibility. As a topically applied therapeutic agent, fluoride is effective in preventing future lesion development, in arresting or at least slowing the progression of active cavitated lesions, and in remineralizing active incipient lesions. Topical fluoride also has some antimicrobial properties.

The exposure of the teeth to fluoride through professional application of fluoride solutions, gels, foams, and varnishes plus exposure from dentifrices and other fluoride preparations used at home engages almost all of the foregoing mechanisms except the preeruptive incorporation into enamel. Although it is difficult to separate the benefits of the different mechanisms of action of fluoride, research has suggested that the predominant mechanism is the impact of fluoride on the remineralization of demineralized enamel. Numerous studies have shown that the presence of fluoride greatly enhances the rate of remineralization of demineralized enamel and dentin. Moreover, tooth structure remineralized in the presence of fluoride contains increased concentrations of fluorohydroxyapatite, which makes the remineralized tissue more resistant to future attack by acids than was the original structure. In view of fluoride's multiple mechanisms of action, it is not surprising that treatment with fluoride through multiple delivery systems has additive benefits. This supports the recommendation that frequent exposure to fluoride is beneficial for maximal caries prevention and control.

Communal Water Fluoridation

Research studies and observations in private practice continue to support the contention that fluoridation of the communal water supply is the most effective method of reducing the dental caries problem in the general population.

In 1998, Stookey noted that approximately half of the population of the United States enjoys the benefits of fluoridated communal water supplies.[64] Cohen has cited observations in Philadelphia, the first city with a population over 1 million to fluoridate its water supply.[65] The reduction in DMFT has averaged 75% at 6 years of age, 54.5% at 8 years, 42.6% at 12 years, and 46.7% at 14 years. A 50% reduction in the decay rate has been noted in the primary teeth.

Murray and Rugg-Gunn reviewed 94 studies conducted in 20 countries to help clarify varying reports on the benefits to primary teeth of communal water fluoridation.[66] A thorough review of the data clearly showed that water fluoridation provides protection for primary teeth against dental caries but to a somewhat lesser degree than for permanent teeth. The caries reduction benefits to primary teeth ranged between 40% and 50%, whereas the range for permanent teeth was between 50% and 60%.

Carmichael and colleagues[67] and Rock and colleagues[68] have reported data in separate studies comparing the caries incidence in children living in two fluoridated communities with that in children living in two nonfluoridated communities in England. The role of fluoridation in reducing dental caries is obvious in both studies. The study by Carmichael and colleagues also demonstrated that children in lower social classes gain an even greater caries prevention benefit than children in higher social classes. The reason is that, as a group, the children in the lower social classes have a higher prevalence of proximal carious lesions, and proximal tooth surfaces derive the greatest benefit from fluoridation.

The protection afforded by the ingestion of fluoridated water persists throughout the lifetime of the person. Several studies have shown that the continuous ingestion of fluoridated water during adulthood decreases the prevalence of dental caries by about the same magnitude observed in children.[69,70] In addition, Stamm and Banting have reported a 56% decrease in the prevalence of root-surface caries in adults who lived continuously in a fluoridated community.[71]

The posteruptive benefits associated with the ingestion of fluoridated water also have been demonstrated. The posteruptive ingestion of fluoridated water can result in decreases in caries prevalence as great as 30%.[72,73] Similarly, Hardwick and colleagues have reported a 27% reduction in caries prevalence after 4 years of ingestion of fluoridated water by teenagers who were 12 years of age when fluoridation was initiated.[74] These observations are consistent with the multiple mechanisms of action of fluoride cited earlier and support the significant contribution of the exposure of the teeth to fluoride even in the very low concentrations present in fluoridated drinking water.

More recent studies concerning the reduced prevalence of dental caries associated with the presence of fluoride in communal water supplies have demonstrated appreciably lesser benefits, typically ranging between 18% and 30%.[75-77] This decrease in attributable benefit is due to the so-called halo effect associated with the preparation of numerous foods and beverages in fluoridated communities and their consumption in nonfluoridated communities. Recent reports have attempted to quantify this halo effect by measuring the fluoride intake of children residing in communities that do not have a fluoridated communal water supply and have shown that fluoride ingestion is nearly 70% that of residents of optimally fluoridated communities.[78-80] Thus it is not surprising that only modest differences in caries prevalence rates are noted between children residing in fluoridated and nonfluoridated communities.

When fluoridation is discontinued in a community, an crease in the dental caries incidence follows. Way has ported that, after a 2-year lapse of drinking fluoride-free water in Galesburg, Illinois, children experienced as much as a 38% increase in tooth decay.[81] Lemke and colleagues have reported that in Antigo, Wisconsin, a city of 9600, tooth decay rose 92% among kindergarten children, 183% among second-graders, and 100% among fourth-graders when fluoridation was discontinued.[82]

Attwood and Blinkhorn reported on the dental health of school children in Stranraer, Scotland, five years after fluoridation of their water supply had ended.[83] They found that, among children 5 years of age, the dmft score had increased to 3.08 compared with 2.48 among the same age group five years earlier. After five years of no fluoridation, the scores for decayed, missing, or filled primary teeth (dmft) and DMFT were quite similar to the scores of children from another city in the same region (Annan, Scotland) that had never had fluoridated water. Most of the 44% difference in dmft scores and the 50% difference in DMFT scores that previously favored the Stranraer children were lost five years after the fluoride had been removed from their water. The authors point out that, although there is a general decline in dental caries because of the almost universal use of fluoride toothpaste (the Annan children also had lower dmft and DMFT scores at the end of the study), fluoridation of water has a significantly beneficial added effect.

Eichenbaum and colleagues reported interesting information related to the long-term impact of communal fluoridation on the private practice of pediatric dentistry.[84] A survey conducted from 1948 to 1950 showed that 86% of the pediatric patients in a private pediatric dental practice needed restorative treatment, and nearly half of these children required pulp therapy. The results of this survey encouraged the city health officials to implement dental health education and preventive programs that included communal water fluoridation. A survey of the same practice almost 30 years later (1977 to 1979) revealed a dramatic change in the restorative needs of the children. The majority of children needed no restorations, and the number of teeth with pulp involvement was negligible.

In 1986, Smith estimated that the average annual cost of fluoridating communal water supplies is approximately $0.25 per person.[85] Gish pointed out in 1979 that the annual cost varies with the size of the community and may range from approximately $1.50 per person in very small communities to as low as $0.10 per person in larger metropolitan areas.[86] These estimates are still valid, with just

upward adjustment for inflation. Communal water fluoridation remains by far the most cost-effective caries prevention measure available.

Horowitz and colleagues have reported findings that have relevance for the millions of Americans who are deprived of the benefits of community water fluoridation because they live in areas not served by central water supplies.[87] The water supply of a rural school was fluoridated for 12 years at a level of 5 ppm, which is 4.5 times the optimum level for community fluoridation in the area. In the final survey, children who had attended the school continuously during the study had 39% fewer DMFTs than did their counterparts who had not attended the school continuously. Late-erupting teeth (canines, premolars, and second molars) demonstrated twice as much caries protection as early-erupting teeth (incisors and first molars). In both categories of teeth, the greatest benefits were observed on proximal surfaces, with as much as 69% fewer caries for late-erupting teeth.

Considerable research related to the effect of school water fluoridation on dental caries has been conducted using even higher concentrations of fluoride. Heifetz and colleagues completed another 12-year study in Seagrove, North Carolina, where school water is fluoridated at the level of 6.3 ppm, or approximately seven times the optimum recommended for community water fluoridation.[88] Observations after 12 years show only a slight improvement in DMFS reduction compared with the earlier 12-year study using 5 ppm (or 4.5 times the optimum). The researchers concluded that there is little justification for recommending the higher fluoride level for school water fluoridation programs.

When these investigations were conducted, it was thought that school water fluoridation would provide a mechanism for children in rural, nonfluoridated areas to receive the public health benefits of fluoride. At its peak, school water fluoridation programs were in operation in 13 states, serving about 170,000 children in 470 schools. However, numerous problems associated with equipment maintenance and monitoring coupled with the recently recognized impact of increased amounts of fluoride in the food chain (i.e., the halo effect) has led the Centers for Disease Control and Prevention (CDC) to discontinue promoting these programs in the United States. In 2001, the Task Force on Community Preventive Services of the CDC strongly recommended community water fluoridation and school-based or school-linked pit and fissure sealant delivery programs for prevention and control of dental caries.[89] However, the task force found insufficient evidence of effectiveness for the remaining interventions reviewed, including school water fluoridation.

Fluoride-Containing Dentifrices
Extensive research initiated in the early 1950s ultimately resulted in the identification of the first fluoride-containing dentifrice (Crest, Proctor & Gamble, Cincinnati, Ohio) capable of decreasing the incidence of dental caries. This dentifrice contained stannous fluoride (SnF_2) in combination with calcium pyrophosphate as the cleaning and polishing system and in 1964 was accepted as the first therapeutic dentifrice by the Council on Dental

Therapeutics of the American Dental Association (ADA) based on more than 20 clinical trials. The significance of this original development has been profound; in fact, a review by Jenkins concluded that the general decline in caries prevalence in Great Britain and other developed countries appears to be attributable in large part to the widespread use of effective fluoride-containing dentifrices.[90]

Caretakers should be counseled so they know that no more than a small, pea-sized amount of fluoridated toothpaste should be used when they brush the teeth of young children (Fig. 10-9).

For nearly 3 decades after the completion of the first successful clinical trial in 1954, this stannous fluoride dentifrice served as a standard of reference for the development of additional fluoride dentifrices as well as for efforts to identify even more effective compositions. An extensive review of the literature by Stookey in 1985 indicated that more than 140 clinical trials of fluoride dentifrices had been reported.[91] These investigations identified several fluoride dentifrice systems with demonstrated cariostatic activity and verified the commercial availability of many such systems. In the United States, 55 dentifrice formulations from 13 manufacturers have received the Seal of Approval of the ADA. These ADA-accepted dentifrices now comprise approximately 90% of all dentifrices sold in the United States. Fluoride dentifrices similarly represent 85% to 90% of the dentifrice sales in Great Britain as well as several in other countries.

Before 1981, attempts to identify a fluoride dentifrice system significantly more effective than the original stannous fluoride formulation were unsuccessful. However, in 1981 the results of two clinical studies demonstrated the superiority of a sodium fluoride composition.[92,93] A clinical study of 3 years' duration was conducted by Beiswanger and colleagues[92] to determine the effect of a sodium fluoride–silica abrasive dentifrice on dental caries. The dentifrice, containing 0.243% sodium fluoride, was compared with stannous fluoride in a study group of 1824 school children 6 to 14 years of age in Indiana cities where water supplies were fluoride deficient (containing less than 0.35 ppm fluoride). After three years, the group

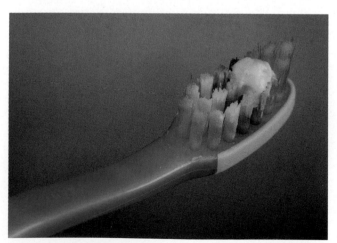

Figure 10-9 Toothbrush with pea-sized amount of toothpaste.

brushing with the sodium fluoride dentifrice had significantly lower DMFT and DMFS increments than the group brushing with the stannous fluoride dentifrice. Two independent examiners found that the reductions were 14.8% and 10.5% for DMFT and 16.4% and 13.1% for DMFS. These results are consistent with those reported by Zacherl in which the sodium fluoride dentifrice resulted in a 40.7% decrease in DMFS compared with a 23.4% decrease observed with the stannous fluoride dentifrice.[93] Similarly, studies conducted by Gerdin[94] and by Edlund and Koch[95] indicated that the use of sodium fluoride dentifrices by children resulted in significantly fewer caries than the use of dentifrices containing sodium monofluorophosphate. The results of these studies and several similar reports led Stookey to conclude in 1985 that the use of sodium fluoride in a highly compatible formulation resulted in greater cariostatic activity than the use of other fluoride dentifrice systems available at that time.[91]

Topical Fluorides in the Dental Office

The periodic professional topical application of more concentrated fluoride solutions, gels, foams, or varnishes has been repeatedly demonstrated to result in a significant reduction in the incidence of dental caries in both children and adults as well as the arrestment of incipient lesions. As a result, professional topical fluoride applications are routinely recommended for all children and adolescents. Even in the absence of dental caries activity, topical fluoride applications to children are recommended as a means of raising the fluoride content of the enamel of newly erupted teeth and thereby increasing the resistance of these teeth to caries formation.

Historically the periodic topical application of fluoride was first demonstrated to be effective for the prevention of dental caries in the early 1940s. Since that time, many hundreds of publications have provided additional data to confirm the efficacy of professionally applied topical fluoride treatments for caries prevention.

A 4-minute treatment time has been typically recommended for professionally applied topical fluoride solutions, gels, or foams. Recently some manufacturers recommend only a 1-minute application. It is known that most of the fluoride uptake in the enamel occurs during the first minute after application. However, measurable benefits do continue to accrue for approximately 4 minutes if the topical preparation remains in contact with the teeth. We continue to recommend the 4-minute application whenever possible. If gel or foam is applied with a tray technique, use of an ample amount will force the substance into the proximal areas. The trays should be about one third to one half full for gel and full (level with the edge) for foam (Fig. 10-10A). Usually both upper and lower trays are inserted at once to complete the topical fluoride treatment in one 4-minute application. Some trays are supplied as a connected double set. The patient sits in an upright position with head tipped slightly forward to allow excess saliva and fluoride to flow toward the lips (see Fig. 10-10B). Patients who follow instructions well may be provided with the high-velocity evacuator tip to help control the drooling themselves, or they may be given a plastic "drool bag" that enables them to tip the

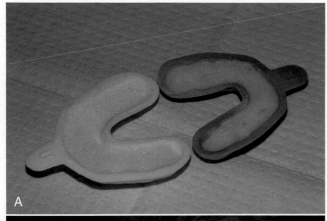

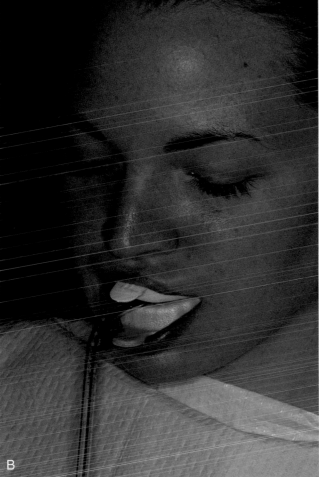

Figure 10-10 A, Sufficient topical fluoride foam is placed in the upper and lower trays so that each tray is half filled. **B,** The teeth are dried and the trays are inserted in the patient's mouth to provide a complete-mouth topical fluoride treatment in a single 4-minute application. The evacuator tip is positioned to remove the excess saliva and foam as the liquids flow toward the lips.

head forward even more and catch the drooled liquid in the bag, which is later discarded. The dentist or appropriate office staff should supervise the treatment and provide assistance as needed. If necessary the auxiliary may manipulate the evacuator tip or help hold the patient's

head forward and the trays in place over the drool bag. Patients requiring assistance also often need positive reinforcement during the procedure. Extra caution and special application techniques are required when topical solutions, gels, or foams are placed in the mouths of young children (around 4 years old and younger). The agent is usually brushed on to the teeth in small amounts and the excess is wiped away with gauze.

The results of independent clinical trials have seriously questioned the need for dental prophylaxis before the topical application of acidulated phosphate fluoride (APF). Ripa and colleagues compared the caries incidence during a 3-year period in children given semiannual topical applications of APF after different cleaning procedures.[96] Before each fluoride treatment, the children either received conventional prophylaxis using a nonfluoride prophylactic paste, performed supervised toothbrushing and flossing, or rinsed their mouths with water. Caries increments after three years were essentially identical in all the treatment groups, a finding that indicates that the manner of cleaning the teeth before the APF treatment may not influence the cariostatic activity of the fluoride applications. Similarly designed clinical trials were conducted by Houpt and colleagues[97] and by Katz and colleagues[98]; in both instances the results were comparable to those observed by Ripa and colleagues.[96] An additional study by Bijella and colleagues likewise demonstrated that the presence or absence of a prophylactic procedure did not alter the efficacy of a topical APF application.[99] Collectively these studies indicate that prophylaxis before an APF topical application may be an optional procedure with regard to caries reduction.

Beginning with reports by Ekstrand and colleagues[100] and by LeCompte and Whitford,[101] several investigators have expressed concern regarding the amount of fluoride swallowed by children during a topical fluoride application. These reports indicated that, depending on the manner of application, 15 to 31 mg of fluoride may be swallowed during the treatment. Stookey and colleagues explored the feasibility of permitting patients to rinse after a topical fluoride application as a means of reducing fluoride ingestion.[102] However, they observed that rinsing with water after a topical fluoride application significantly decreased fluoride deposition in incipient carious lesions. A report by LeCompte and Doyle indicated that one could drastically reduce the amount of fluoride ingested during topical fluoride application to about 1.6 mg by using only the necessary amount of fluoride gel, having the patient seated in an upright position, using high-velocity saliva evacuation during the treatment, and asking the patient to expectorate thoroughly for 1 minute after completion of the treatment.[103] Thus the latter procedures are recommended to minimize fluoride ingestion during the application, particularly in younger children, and the patient should be encouraged not to eat, drink, or rinse for 30 minutes after the treatment to maximize fluoride uptake in enamel.

Fluoride-containing varnishes have been widely used in Europe and other parts of the world for approximately 40 years but were not available in the United States until 1994. The first fluoride varnish was introduced in Europe in 1964 and contained 5.0% sodium fluoride (or 2.26%

fluoride). A second product was introduced in Europe in 1975 and contained 0.9% silane fluoride (or 0.1% fluoride). Much more research has been conducted using the sodium fluoride system, and it is the most widely accepted.

Petersson,[104] Horowitz and Ismail,[105] and Petersson and colleagues[106] have reviewed the numerous controlled clinical trials of fluoride varnishes and concluded that these materials are equally as effective as professional topical fluoride applications for the prevention of dental caries in children. Seppa and colleagues investigated the effect of the sodium fluoride varnish in children with a high past caries experience and found that this measure resulted in numerically fewer new caries lesions than was achieved with semiannual applications of an APF gel during a 3-year study period.[107] These investigators also noted that the data for use of this varnish satisfied the criteria of the ADA for the claim of being "at least as good as" professionally applied topical fluoride gels. Helfenstein and Steiner performed a statistical meta-analysis of the data from a number of clinical trials and found that use of the sodium fluoride varnish resulted in an overall reduction in caries of 38% in the permanent teeth.[108]

The sodium fluoride varnish (Fig. 10-11) is particularly recommended for use in preschool-age children because of its ease of application and equal efficacy to APF systems.[64] Before application of the varnish, the teeth may receive prophylaxis or are brushed with a dentifrice to remove plaque and oral debris. The varnish is then applied with a soft brush, with reapplications recommended at 3- to 6-month intervals depending on caries risk assessment. A more intensive annual treatment regimen consisting of three applications within a 10-day period has been investigated, and this regimen was observed to be as effective as applications every four months.[109-111] Furthermore, single annual applications have been found to be without clinical benefit. Varnish may have a light yellow color but it is lost from the tooth surfaces within 24 to 48 hours. Some varnishes are clear or have a white color. Because less than a milliliter of varnish is used for a professional treatment in preschool-aged children, the amount of fluoride that will ultimately be ingested when the varnish is lost from the tooth surfaces is less than 3 mg. Thus there are no practical concerns regarding safety, and this procedure is frequently recommended for use in young children in place of the traditional topical fluoride gel application.

Topical Fluorides for the General Anesthesia Patient

The application of fluoride to the teeth of children receiving dental care under a general anesthetic, after the placement of restorations, is certainly recommended. Thorough prophylaxis should precede the placement of the rubber dam for a quadrant of restorations. The fluoride should be applied after the restorative work has been completed for that quadrant but before removal of the rubber dam.

Home Fluoride Mouth Rinses and Gels

The use of dilute oral fluoride rinses and/or gels as an additional dental caries control measure has become another helpful adjunct. Children younger than 4 years of

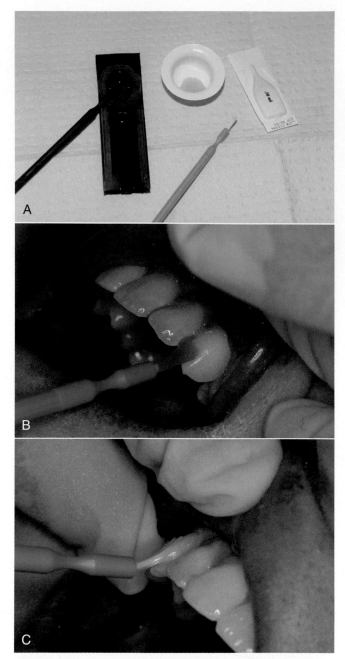

Figure 10-11 A, Fluoride varnishes. **B,** Application of colored fluoride varnish. **C,** Application of white fluoride varnish.

age may not have full control over their swallowing reflexes; therefore caution should be exercised in recommending these products for home use for this age group. However, some small children can expectorate rinses quite reliably under proper supervision, or the parent can brush on the gel and wipe away the excess. In nonfluoridated areas it may be appropriate to have the child swallow the rinse after "swishing" it to gain the systemic fluoride effect as well. Some rinses (acidulated or aqueous solutions that do not contain alcohol) are prepared to provide the necessary supplemental systemic dose of fluoride if the child does not drink fluoridated water. However, current Food and Drug Administration (FDA) regulations specify that fluoride rinses not be recommended for children younger than 6 years of age unless they are intended for use as a systemic fluoride supplement.

Radike and colleagues observed school children who rinsed their mouths once each school day for two school years with a stannous fluoride mouth rinse containing 250 ppm fluoride (about 0.1% stannous fluoride).[112] There was a significant reduction in dental caries at the end of the first and second school years. Two independent examiners found caries reductions of 33% and 43% in DMFS scores. The anticaries benefit from the stannous fluoride mouth rinse was especially encouraging because the children already were receiving the optimum benefit of water fluoridation.

APF mouthwashes in concentrations of either 100 or 200 ppm fluoride ion used twice daily have been shown by Finn and colleagues to be effective.[113] They reported that during a 26-month period the APF rinses containing relatively small amounts of fluoride were effective in reducing dental caries.

Miller made a preliminary report on results of the National Caries Program sponsored by the National Institute of Dental Research.[114] A nationwide school-based fluoride mouth rinse program that included 85,000 children in 17 states and Guam produced encouraging results. The school children rinsed their mouths for 60 seconds once weekly with 5 mL of a 0.2% neutral sodium fluoride solution. Children in the 7-, 11-, and 13-year-old groups experienced a reduction in dental decay. There was also evidence of caries decrease in the primary teeth.

Leske and colleagues[115,116] have reported on results of a fluoride rinsing program that was begun in 1975 in the Three Village Central School District of Long Island, New York. The program was one of 17 demonstration projects sponsored by the National Institute of Dental Research, which initially enrolled approximately 4500 elementary school children (kindergarten through the sixth grade), who rinsed once a week with a 0.2% neutral sodium fluoride solution under the supervision of homeroom teachers. The prevalence of caries in the children who participated in the rinse program for 2 to 4 years was 20.4% DMFT and 24.4% DMFS lower than that of children who had never rinsed. The reduction in proximal caries was 49.6%. The reductions in occlusal and buccolingual caries were 21.0% and 18.8%, respectively. The examination of exfoliated teeth also indicated that fluoride rinsing may produce a residual benefit. The later report on children who had participated in the program for seven years demonstrated caries prevalence reductions of 55.7% DMFT and 60.9% DMFS, with 85.4% reduction of proximal surface caries.

Extensive field research has been conducted on the use of fluoride mouth rinses. Most studies incorporate the use of a 0.2% sodium fluoride rinse once weekly or a 0.05% sodium fluoride rinse once daily. As does the work previously summarized, these other studies show unquestionable caries prevention benefits of the regular use of self-administered fluoride rinses when properly supervised. These benefits accrue to primary and permanent teeth, and seem to be helpful both in fluoridated areas

and in areas with nonfluoridated water. The studies of Heifetz[117] and of Ripa and Leske[118] are cited in the references listed at the end of this chapter as good examples of clinical research with fluoride rinses. Based on numerous studies indicating the efficacy of fluoride rinses, some rinses were approved by the FDA in 1974 and by the ADA Council on Dental Therapeutics in 1975. Studies supporting the use of the dilute gels are not as numerous as those for the rinses, but some gels have also subsequently been approved.

Dietary Fluoride Supplements

A review of the literature on the value of fluorides administered during pregnancy fails to disclose any valid evidence to support such use even in nonfluoridated areas. In 1966, the FDA banned the manufacturers of fluoride supplements from marketing products bearing the claim that dental caries would be prevented in the offspring of women who used such products during pregnancy. The FDA took this action because of the insufficiency of clinical evidence to substantiate such a claim. There was no question of safety. Although some medical and dental practitioners have continued to prescribe dietary fluoride supplements for pregnant women since the FDA's advertising ban, generally there is unanimity among most research experts and public health officials that fluoride ingestion by gravid women does not benefit the teeth of their offspring, at least not the permanent teeth.

Participants in a symposium concerning the use of prenatal fluorides agreed that transfer of fluoride does occur from the mother to the fetus through the placenta.[119] Only in recent years has such a transfer been generally acknowledged. How much fluoride is transferred from the blood of the mother to the blood of the fetus, however, remains uncertain. Nevertheless, the members of the symposium generally agreed that some benefit of caries prevention accrues to the primary teeth when the fetus is subjected to fluoride. There was considerable doubt about the benefit to the permanent teeth. The symposium discussions seemed to lead to the conclusion that additional well-controlled research efforts are needed to define more clearly the possible benefits of prenatal fluoride administration. Some research into this issue continues, as does the controversy.

A study by Katz and Muhler suggested that the effect of fluoride on primary teeth is mainly postnatal.[120] In a study to determine the effect of waterborne fluoride on dental caries in primary teeth, 890 children from 4 to 7 years of age were examined in one Indiana city having a communal water supply with only 0.05 ppm fluoride and in three cities having a supply with a concentration of 1 ppm fluoride. Children living in the cities with fluoridated water had between 35% and 65% fewer dental caries in their primary teeth than those living in the fluoride-deficient city. Comparisons of dental caries incidence in the primary teeth of children living in the same city who were exposed either prenatally or postnatally or exclusively postnatally showed no difference between the groups.

Hennon and colleagues conducted a clinical study that included 815 children between 18 and 39 months of age residing in three fluoride-deficient Indiana communities.[121] The children received chewable tablets containing vitamins, vitamins plus fluoride, or fluoride alone (1 mg as sodium fluoride) and were examined for dental caries initially and at 6-month intervals. The findings during the first 2 years of the 5½-year study indicated a significant reduction of about 37% in the incidence of dental caries after 6 months in the children ingesting either the fluoride or vitamin-fluoride supplements.[122] This degree of protection increased to about 55% and 63%, respectively, after the children had used the supplement for 1 and 2 years. The important finding was the significant reduction in the incidence of dental caries after use of the tablets for only 6 months. This observation indicates a highly effective topical benefit of chewing the tablets, because most of the primary teeth had already erupted when the study began.

The natural fluoride content of the water should first be determined. If the natural fluoride content is 0.6 ppm or higher, supplements should not be administered. If the fluoride content is below 0.6 ppm, the administration of fluoride supplements should be considered only after a review of all other types of fluoride sources and use have been considered as indicated in Table 10-2.

A number of studies report the caries-preventive effects of adding fluoride to a variety of foods and beverages. Fluoride has been used as a caries-preventive additive in salt, milk, and even sugar. Some suppliers now offer controlled concentrations of fluoride in bottled water. Numerous reports show that these products can have measurable and favorable results when used as intended. Such products are designed for use by specific and targeted population groups. These products have not yet had widespread popularity, although there is growing interest in this concept and public acceptance seems to be growing for fluoridated bottled water for children who either do not have or do not use community fluoridated water.

Combinations of Fluoride Therapies

There is considerable evidence to suggest that using combinations of therapeutic fluoride agents often produces additive anticariogenic effects. The evidence also indicates that the earlier fluoride therapy is initiated in children, the more effective the caries control will be. However, one must use caution in prescribing multiple

therapies in very young children to avoid excessive fluoride ingestion.

Fluoride is the most effective caries prevention agent commercially available today. Except in a patient who has a fluoride allergy (very rare), it is considered completely safe when properly used. The ingestion of high concentrations can lead to nausea, vomiting, dental fluorosis (mottling), or, in extreme cases, even death, especially in children. Extreme care must be used to safeguard the agents from inappropriate or inadvertent ingestion. It is imperative that the dental profession have full awareness of the hazards accompanying its use and yet be prepared to use it to the patient's maximum advantage through careful consideration of each patient's individual situation.

Chlorhexidine and Thymol

As an oral antimicrobial, chlorhexidine has been used in oral rinses, dentifrices, chewing gum, varnish, and gel. In the United States it is used most often in the form of a prescription oral rinse. Many children object to the taste of these products, but they have been shown to be effective against microorganisms causing both caries and periodontal disease. Thymol has also been included with chlorhexidine in some varnish preparations. To date, these products have not shown superior caries prevention results when compared with multiple fluoride therapies, and they may require more frequent application to be effective. However, they should provide an additive effect and may be used in combination with fluoride, particularly in high-risk patients. In the rare situation in which a provider is trying to control or prevent caries in a patient with fluoride allergy, they could be very important therapies.

Povidone-Iodine

Considerable data exist from laboratory and animal studies to confirm the dramatic suppression of mutans streptococci by iodine. Several studies reconfirm this observation in humans as well. Lopez and colleagues published two human studies demonstrating that topical application of povidone-iodine at 2-month intervals in dentate infants is effective in preventing S-ECC in children at high risk for the disease.[123,124] The authors called for more and larger in-depth clinical trials. If such trials prove as successful as these initial reports, they might lead to widespread implementation of an effective defense against this devastating disease for which minimal parental compliance is required.

Xylitol

Xylitol is a low-calorie sweetener that inhibits the growth of *S. mutans*. Numerous studies seem to confirm its anticariogenic capability. Xylitol has been tested as an additive to a variety of foods and to dentifrice. However, the vast majority of published data come from studies in which xylitol was incorporated into chewing gum. Makinen has reported numerous studies on the topic, most of them performed with many different coworkers in different parts of the world. In 2000, he published a concise summary titled "The Rocky Road of Xylitol to Its Clinical Application."[125] The available data not only show that xylitol chewing gum reduces caries activity but

---

Table **10-2**

Dietary Fluoride Supplementation Schedule

Age	Less Than 0.3 ppm Fluoride	0.3 to 0.6 ppm Fluoride	More Than 0.6 ppm Fluoride
Birth to 6 mo	0	0	0
6 mo to 3 yr	0.25 mg	0	0
3 yr to 6 yr	0.50 mg	0.25 mg	0
6 yr up to at least 16 yr	1 mg	0.50	0

From American Academy of Pediatric Dentistry. Guideline on fluoride therapy. Pediatr Dent 2001;24(Suppl 7):66. [Special issue: Reference manual 2002-2003.]

also provide evidence that it decreases the transmission of *S. mutans* from gum-chewing mothers to their children. The use of xylitol chewing gum seems to be gaining popularity as another caries prevention strategy. It should be readily accepted by many children.

RESTORATIVE DENTISTRY IN THE CONTROL PROGRAM

Excellent restorative dentistry is also valuable in the dental caries control program. For patients who do not comply with nonrestorative caries control recommendations (e.g., use of fluorides and/or antimicrobials, appropriate diet, and plaque control), the restorative care will be more aggressive than it would otherwise need to be. Further discussion of appropriate selection of restorative materials and procedures is in Chapters 16, 17, and 18.

PIT AND FISSURE SEALANTS

For many years, attempts have been made to eliminate pit and fissure caries. In 1923, Hyatt recommended that all pits and fissures be opened with a bur and filled with amalgam.[126] Attempts have been made to prevent pit and fissure caries by applying a variety of different chemical solutions, including silver nitrate and potassium ferrocyanide with zinc chloride, and by covering the depressions with various types of dental cement. None of these methods proved successful over time.

Pit and fissure sealants have been used successfully by many dentists. Many recent clinical studies have shown that the placement of pit and fissure sealants is an effective caries-preventive measure; the subject is covered in detail in Chapter 17.

CARIES VACCINE

A vaccine to prevent the disease of dental caries has been an anticipated scientific breakthrough since at least the early 1940s. Most recent research efforts assume that *S. mutans* is the principal etiologic organism of dental caries, and the development of a method of immunization specifically targeted at neutralizing *S. mutans* has been a major thrust of caries vaccine research. Bowen reported that monkeys remained caries-free for more than six years after the animals received intraoral injections of killed *S. mutans*, even though the monkeys were fed highly cariogenic diets and had severe malocclusion that would predispose them to caries.[127]

Most current research is being directed toward a greater understanding of the immune system and specifically of immune responses to mutans streptococci. The route of administration of the vaccine is usually mucosal absorption by intraoral or intranasal tissues. For more information, refer to the review article by Michalek and colleagues.[128]

DENTAL CARIES ACTIVITY TESTS

For the larger part of a century, dental scientists have been trying to develop a convenient method of measuring quantitatively the degree of dental caries activity in individual patients. Techniques requiring laboratory procedures to determine oral bacterial counts or their aciduric potential have been developed and used. More recently, convenient paper test strips to gauge salivary microbial density in patients have been tested. No truly convenient and efficient test method has yet been developed that has sufficient accuracy to be a reliable caries activity indicator. Research continues in this area because having an accurate, convenient, and efficient test to measure early caries activity and its level of potential, especially in young children, would be a very useful diagnostic tool for private practitioners and public health assistance providers.

DENTIST'S ROLE IN THE CARIES CONTROL PROGRAM

The success of a dental caries control program depends to a great extent on the interest and cooperation of the patient and the patient's caretakers. Rampant caries should not be viewed as a hopeless problem. Diagnostic, therapeutic, and preventive measures are available to control it. In the clinical management of rampant caries, the dentist's role consists of seeking and eliminating the cause to the extent possible. This includes trying to correct inappropriate habits or deficiency states that may be contributing factors, restoring the salvageable teeth to good form and function, and, finally, making use of all available therapeutic preventive and control measures in an established, ongoing manner.

Successful management of all active dental caries problems also requires careful and complete dental and medical history taking, the use of currently accepted diagnostic aids, initiation of a comprehensive preventive program, the application of sound principles of restorative dentistry, and establishment of regular recall schedule for maintenance and reemphasis of the preventive procedures. The recall appointment should be set at each visit based on the clinician's judgment of the patient's risk for future disease at that time.

REFERENCES

1. US Department of Health and Human Services. Oral health in America: A report of the Surgeon General. Rockville, MD, US Department of Health and Human Services, National Institute of Dental and Craniofacial Research, National Institutes of Health, 2000.
2. Edelstein BL, Douglass CW. Dispelling the myth that 50 percent of U.S. schoolchildren have never had a cavity, *Public Health Rep* 110:522-530, 1995.
3. Newacheck PW, et al. The unmet health needs of America's children, *Pediatrics* 105:989-997, 2000.
4. Gift HC. Oral health outcomes research—challenges and opportunities. In Slade GD. Measuring Oral Health and Quality of Life. Chapel Hill, University of North Carolina Department of Dental Ecology, 1997.
5. NIH Consensus Development Conference on Diagnosis and Management of Dental Caries Throughout Life, March 26-28, 2001, conference papers, *J Dent Educ* 65:935-1179, 2001.
6. Keyes P, Fitzgerald RJ. Dental caries in the Syrian hamster, *Arch Oral Biol* 7:267-77, 1962.
7. Orland FJ. Bacteriology of dental caries: formal discussion, *J Dent Res* 43:1045-1047, 1964.
8. Fitzgerald RJ, Jordan HV, Archard HL. Dental caries in gnotobiotic rats infected with a variety of *Lactobacillus acidophilus, Arch Oral Biol* 11:473-476, 1966.
9. Loesche WJ. Role of *Streptococcus mutans* in human dental decay, *Microbiol Rev* 50:353-380, 1986.

10. Wan AK, et al. Association of *Streptococcus mutans* infection and oral developmental nodules in pre-dentate infants, *J Dent Res* 80:1945-1948, 2001.

11. Wan AK, et al. Oral colonization of *Streptococcus mutans* in six-month-old predentate infants, *J Dent Res* 80: 2060-2065, 2001.

12. Wan AK, et al. A longitudinal study of *Streptococcus mutans* colonization in infants after tooth eruption, *J Dent Res* 82:504-508, 2003.

13. Davey AL, Rogers AH. Multiple types of the bacterium *Streptococcus mutans* in the human mouth and their intra-family transmission, *Arch Oral Biol* 29:453-460, 1984.

14. Berkowitz RJ, Jones P. Mouth-to-mouth transmission of the bacterium *Streptococcus mutans* between mother and child, *Arch Oral Biol* 30:377-379, 1985.

15. Brown JP, Junner C, Liew V. A study of *Streptococcus mutans* levels in both infants with bottle caries and their mothers, *Aust Dent J* 30:96-98, 1985.

16. Kohler B, Andreen I, Jonsson B. The effect of caries-preventive measures in mothers on dental caries and the presence of the bacteria *Streptococcus mutans* and lactobacilli in their children, *Arch Oral Biol* 29:879-883, 1984.

17. Kohler B, Andreen I, Jonsson B. The earlier the colonization by mutans streptococci, the higher the caries prevalence at 4 years of age, *Oral Microbiol Immunol* 3:14-17, 1988.

18. Caufield PW, Cutter GR, Dasanayake AP. Initial acquisition of mutans streptococci by infants: evidence for a discrete window of infectivity, *J Dent Res* 72:37-45, 1993.

19. Mohan A, et al. The relationship between bottle usage/content, age, and number of teeth with mutans streptococci colonization in 6–24-month-old children, *Commun Dent Oral Epidemiol* 26:12-20, 1998.

20. Weddell JA, Klein AI. Socioeconomic correlation of oral disease in six- to thirty-six-month children, *Pediatr Dent* 3:306-311, 1981.

21. Edelstein B, Tinanoff N. Screening preschool children for dental caries using a microbial test, *Pediatr Dent* 11: 129-132, 1989.

22. Douglass JM, et al. Dental caries experience in a Connecticut Head Start program in 1991 and 1999, *Pediatr Dent* 24:309-314, 2002.

23. Tang JM, et al. Dental caries prevalence and treatment levels in Arizona preschool children, *Public Health Rep* 112:319-331, 1997.

24. Vargas CM, Crall JJ, Schneider DA. Sociodemographic distribution of pediatric dental caries: NHANES III, 1988-1994, *J Am Dent Assoc* 129:1229-1238, 1998.

25. Greenwell AL, et al. Longitudinal evaluation of caries patterns from the primary to the mixed dentition, *Pediatr Dent* 12:278-282, 1990.

26. Massler JN. Teen-age caries, *J Dent Child* 12:57-64, 1945.

27. American Academy of Pediatric Dentistry. Policy on early childhood caries (ECC): Unique challenges and treatment options, *Pediatr Dent* 30(Suppl 7):44-46, 2008. [Special issue: Reference manual 2008-2009.]

28. American Academy of Pediatric Dentistry: Policy on early childhood caries (ECC): Classifications, consequences and preventive strategies, *Pediatr Dent* 30(Suppl 7):40-43, 2008. [Special issue: reference manual 2008-2009.]

29. Gardner DE, Norwood JR, Eisenson JE. At-will breast feeding and dental caries: four case reports, *J Dent Child* 44: 186-191, 1977.

30. American Academy of Pediatric Dentistry. Policy on dietary recommendations for infants, children, and adolescents, *Pediatr Dent* 30(Suppl 7):L47-L48, 2008. [Special issue: reference manual 2008-2009.]

31. Dilley GJ, Dilley DH, Machen JB. Prolonged nursing habit: a profile of parents and their families, *J Dent Child* 47: 102-108, 1980.

32. Hallonsten AL, et al. Dental caries and prolonged breast-feeding in 18-month-old Swedish children, *Int J Paediatr Dent* 5:149-155, 1995.

33. Ripa LW. Nursing caries: a comprehensive review, *Pediatr Dent* 10:268-282, 1988.

34. Hutchinson J. A case of dry mouth, *Trans Clin Soc Lond* 21:180-181, 1888.

35. McDonald RE. The effect of antihistaminic drugs on salivary flow and viscosity, *J Dent Res* 32:224-226, 1953.

36. Crossner CG. Salivary flow rate in children and adolescents, *Swed Dent J* 8:271-276, 1984.

37. Zunt SL. Evaluation of the dry mouth patient, *Alpha Omegan* 4:203-209, 2008.

38. Shannon IL, McCrary BR, Starcke EN. A saliva substitute for use by xerostomic patients undergoing radiotherapy of the head and neck, *Oral Surg* 44:656-666, 1977.

39. McDonald RE. Human saliva: a study of the rate of flow and viscosity and its relationship to dental caries, thesis. Indianapolis, Indiana University School of Dentistry, 1951.

40. Leone CW, Oppenheim FG. Physical and chemical aspects of saliva as indicators of risk for dental caries in humans, *J Dent Educ* 65:1054-1062, 2001.

41. US Census Bureau. Poverty in the United States: 2002, Washington, DC, US Department of Commerce, Economics and Statistics Administration, US Census Bureau, March 10, 2003.

42. Edelstein BL. Disparities in oral health and access to care: Findings of national surveys, *Ambul Pediatr* 2(Suppl): 141-147, 2002.

43. Rosenbloom RG, Tinanoff N. Salivary *Streptococcus mutans* levels in patients before, during and after orthodontic treatment, *Am J Orthod Dentofacial Orthop* 100:35-37, 1991.

44. Tinanoff N, Siegrist B, Lang NP. Safety and antibacterial properties of controlled release SnF2, *J Oral Rehabil* 13: 73-81, 1986.

45. Wright JT, et al. Effect of conventional dental restorative treatment on bacteria in saliva, *Commun Dent Oral Epidemiol* 20:138-143, 1992.

46. Gregory RL, El-Rahman AMA, Avery DR. Effect of restorative treatment on mutans streptococci and IgA antibodies, *Pediatr Dent* 20:273-277, 1998.

47. Pitts NB. Clinical diagnosis of dental caries. A European perspective, *J Dent Educ* 65:973-980, 2001.

48. Pitts NB. Modern concepts of caries measurement, *J Dent Res* 83:43-47, 2004.

49. Pitts NB. Are we ready to move from operative to non-operative/preventive treatment of dental caries in clinical practice? *Caries Res* 38:294-304, 2004.

50. Ekstrand KR. Improving clinical visual detection—potential for caries clinical trials, *J Dent Res* 83:C67-C71, 2004. [Special issue.]

51. Nyvad B, Machiulskiene V, Baelum V. The Nyvad criteria for assessment of caries lesion activity. In Stookey GK, ed. *Clinical Models Workshop: Remin-Demin, Precavitation, Caries.* Indianapolis, Proceedings of the 7th Indiana Conference, 2005.

52. Stookey GK, Gonzales-Cabezas C. Emerging methods of caries diagnosis, *J Dent Educ* 65:1001-1006, 2001.

53. American Academy of Pediatric Dentistry. Policy on use of a caries-risk assessment tool (CAT) for infants, children, and adolescents, *Pediatr Dent* 30(Suppl 7):29-33, 2008. [Special issue: Reference manual 2007-2008.]

54. Zero D, Fontana M, Lennon AM. Clinical applications and outcomes of using indicators of risk in caries management, *J Dent Educ* 65:1126-1132, 2001.
55. Gustafsson BE, et al. The Vipeholm dental caries studies: The effect of different levels of carbohydrate intake on caries activity in 436 individuals observed for five years (Sweden), *Acta Odontol Scand* 11:232-364, 1954.
56. Weiss RL, Trithart AH. Between-meal eating habits and dental caries experience in preschool children, *Am J Public Health* 50:1097-1104, 1960.
57. Schachtele CG, Jensen ME. Comparison of methods for monitoring changes in the pH of human dental plaque, *J Dent Res* 61:1117-1125, 1982.
58. Park KK, Ashmore RW, Stookey GK. Prolonged response period for indwelling plaque pH studies, *J Dent Res* 65:282, 1986. (abstract 1014; special issue).
59. Berenie J, Ripa LW, Leske G. The relationship of frequency of toothbrushing, oral hygiene, gingival health, and caries experience in schoolchildren, *J Public Health Dent* 33: 160-171, 1973.
60. Beal JF, et al. The relationship between dental cleanliness, dental caries incidence and gingival health, *Br Dent J* 146:111-114, 1979.
61. Horowitz AM, et al. Effects of supervised daily plaque removal by children after 3 years, *Commun Dent Oral Epidemiol* 8:171-176, 1980.
62. Tsamtsouris A, White GE, Clark ER. The effect of instruction and supervised toothbrushing on the reduction of dental plaque in kindergarten children, *J Dent Child* 46: 204-209, 1979.
63. Wright GZ, Banting DW, Feasby WH. The Dorchester dental flossing study: final report, *Clin Prev Dent* 1(3):23-26, 1979.
64. Stookey GK. Caries prevention, *J Dent Educ* 62:803-811, 1998.
65. Cohen A. Fluoridation in Philadelphia, *Dent Abst* 11:552, 1966.
66. Murray JJ, Rugg-Gunn AJ. A review of the effectiveness of artificial water fluoridation throughout the world. Paper presented at ORCA XXVI Congress, 1979 (abstract 65).
67. Carmichael CL, et al. The effect of fluoridation upon the relationship between caries experience and social class in 5-year-old children in Newcastle and Northumberland, *Br Dent J* 149:163-167, 1980.
68. Rock WP, Gordon PH, Bradnock G. Dental caries experience in Birmingham and Wolverhampton schoolchildren following the fluoridation of Birmingham water in 1964, *Br Dent J* 150:61-66, 1981.
69. Russell AL, Elvolve E. Domestic water and dental caries VIII. A study of the fluoride-dental caries relationship in an adult population, *Public Health Rep* 66:1389-1401, 1951.
70. Englander HR, Reuss RC, Kesel RG. Dental caries in adults who consume fluoridated versus fluoride-deficient water, *J Am Dent Assoc* 68:14-19, 1964.
71. Stamm JW, Banting DW. Adult root caries survey of two similar communities with contrasting natural water fluoride level, *J Am Dent Assoc* 120:143-149, 1990.
72. Arnold FA, et al. Effect of fluoridated public water supplies on dental caries prevalence. Tenth year of the Grand Rapids-Muskegon study, *Bull Am Assoc Public Health Dent* 17:32-38, 1957.
73. Hayes RL, Littleton NW, White CL. Posteruptive effects of fluoridation on first permanent molars of children in Grand Rapids, Mich, *Dent Abst* 2:615, 1987.
74. Hardwick JL, Teasdale J, Bloodworth G. Caries increments over 4 years in children aged 12 at the start of water fluoridation, *Br Dent J* 153:217-222, 1982.
75. Brunelle JA, Carlos JP. Recent trends in dental caries in U.S. children and the effect of water fluoridation, *J Dent Res* 69:723-727, 1990.
76. Clark DC, et al. Effects of lifelong consumption of fluoridated water or use of fluoride supplements on dental caries experience, *Commun Dent Oral Epidemiol* 23:20-24, 1995.
77. Newbrun E. Effectiveness of water fluoridation, *J Public Health Dent* 49:279-289, 1989.
78. Griffin SO, et al. Quantifying the halo effect of water fluoridation, *J Dent Res* 77:699 (abstract 540; special issue B).
79. Jackson RD, et al. Fluoride levels of biological samples collected from adolescents, *J Dent Res* 77:143, 1998. (abstract 303; special issue A).
80. Jackson RD, et al. The fluoride content of foods and beverages from negligibly and optimally fluoridated communities. *Commun Dent Oral Epidemiol* 30:382-391, 2002.
81. Way RM. The effect on dental caries of a change from a naturally fluoridated to a fluoride-free communal water, *J Dent Child* 31:151-157, 1964.
82. Lemke CW, Doherty JM, Arra MC. Controlled fluoridation: the dental effects of discontinuation in Antigo, Wis, *J Am Dent Assoc* 80:782-786, 1970.
83. Attwood D, Blinkhorn AS. Dental health in schoolchildren 5 years after water fluoridation ceased in south-west Scotland, *Int Dent J* 41:43-48, 1991.
84. Eichenbaum IW, Dunn NA, Tinanoff N. Impact of fluoridation in a private pedodontic practice: thirty years later, *J Dent Child* 48:211-214, 1981.
85. Smith CE. Personal communication, 1986.
86. Gish CW. The dollar and cents of prevention, *J Indiana Dent Assoc* 58(2):12-14, 1979.
87. Horowitz HS, Heifetz SB, Law FE. Effect of school water fluoridation on dental caries: final results in Elk Lake, Pa., after 12 years, *J Am Dent Assoc* 84:832-838, 1972.
88. Heifetz SB, Horowitz HS, Brunelle JA. Effect of school water fluoridation on dental caries: results in Seagrove, NC, after 12 years, *J Am Dent Assoc* 106:334-337, 1983.
89. Centers for Disease Control and Prevention. Promoting oral health: interventions for preventing dental caries, oral and pharyngeal cancers, and sports-related craniofacial injuries. A report on the recommendations of the task force on community preventive services, *MMWR Recomm Rep* 50 (RR-21):1-13, 2001.
90. Jenkins GN. Recent changes in dental caries, *Br Med J* 291:1297-1298, 1985.
91. Stookey GK. Are all fluoride dentifrices the same? In Wei SHY, ed. *Clinical uses of fluorides.* Philadelphia, 1985, Lea & Febiger.
92. Beiswanger BB, Gish CW, Mallatt ME. A three year study of the effect of a sodium fluoride-silica abrasive dentifrice on dental caries, *Pharmacol Ther Dent* 106:9-16, 1981.
93. Zacherl WA. A three-year clinical caries evaluation of a sodium fluoride-silica abrasive dentifrice, *Pharmacol Ther Dent* 6:1-7, 1981.
94. Gerdin PO. Studies in dentifrices. VI. The inhibitory effect of some grinding and non-grinding fluoride dentifrices on dental caries, *Swed Dent J* 65:521-532, 1972.
95. Edlund D, Koch G. Effect on caries of daily supervised toothbrushing with sodium monofluorophosphate and sodium fluoride dentifrices, *Scand J Dent Res* 85:41-45, 1977.
96. Ripa LW, et al. Effect of prior toothcleaning on bi-annual professional acidulated phosphate fluoride topical fluoride gel-tray treatments: results after three years, *Caries Res* 18:457-464, 1984.

97. Houpt M, Koenigsberg S, Shey Z. The effect of prior tooth-cleaning on the efficacy of topical fluoride treatment: two-year results, *Clin Prev Dent* 5(4):8-10, 1983.

98. Katz RV, et al. Topical fluoride and prophylaxis: a 30-month clinical trial, *J Dent Res* 63:256, 1984. (abstract 771; special issue).

99. Bijella MFTB, et al. Comparison of dental prophylaxis and toothbrushing prior to topical APF applications, *Commun Dent Oral Epidemiol* 13:208-211, 1985.

100. Ekstrand J, et al. Pharmacokinetics of fluoride gels in children and adults, *Caries Res* 15:213-220, 1981.

101. LeCompte EJ, Whitford GM. Pharmacokinetics of fluoride from APF gels and fluoride tablets in children, *J Dent Res* 61:469-472, 1982.

102. Stookey GK, et al. The effect of rinsing with water immediately after a professional fluoride gel application on fluoride uptake in demineralized enamel: an in vivo study, *Pediatr Dent* 8:153-157, 1986.

103. LeCompte EJ, Doyle TE. Effects of sectioning devices on oral fluoride retention, *J Am Dent Assoc* 110:357-360, 1986.

104. Petersson LG. Fluoride mouthrinses and fluoride varnishes, *Caries Res* 27(Suppl 1):35-42, 1993.

105. Horowitz HS, Ismail AI. Topical fluorides in caries prevention. In Fejerskov O, Ekstrand J, Burt BA, eds. *Fluoride in dentistry,* 2nd ed. Copenhagen, 1996, Munksgaard.

106. Petersson LG, et al. Fluoride varnish for community based caries prevention in children. Geneva, 1997, World Health Organization, WHO/NCD/ORH/FV/97.1

107. Seppa L, et al. Fluoride varnish versus acidulated phosphate fluoride gel: a 3-year clinical trial, *Caries Res* 27:327-330, 1995.

108. Helfenstein U, Steiner M. Fluoride varnishes (Duraphat): a meta-analysis, *Commun Dent Oral Epidemiol* 22:1-5, 1994.

109. Petersson LG, et al. Caries-inhibiting effect of different modes of Duraphat varnish reapplication: a three-year radiographic study, *Caries Res* 25:70-73, 1991.

110. Petersson LG, Westerberg I. Intensive fluoride varnish program in Swedish adolescents: economic assessment of a 7-year follow-up study on proximal caries incidence, *Caries Res* 28:59-63, 1994.

111. Skold L, et al. Four-year study of caries inhibition of intensive Duraphat application in 11–15-year-old children, *Commun Dent Oral Epidemiol* 22:9-12, 1994.

112. Radike AW, et al. Clinical evaluation of stannous fluoride as an anticaries mouth rinse, *J Am Dent Assoc* 86:404-408, 1973.

113. Finn SB, et al. The clinical cariostatic effectiveness of two concentrations of acidulated phosphate-fluoride mouthwash, *J Am Dent Assoc* 90:398-402, 1975.

114. Miller AJ. National caries program. National Institutes of Health, American Academy of Pedodontics meeting, Miami Beach, Fla, 1977.

115. Leske GS, et al. Post-treatment benefits from participating in a school-based fluoride mouthrinsing program, *J Public Health Dent* 41:103-108, 1981.

116. Leske GS, Ripa LW, Green E. Posttreatment benefits in a school-based fluoride mouthrinsing program: final results after 7 years of rinsing by all participants, *Clin Prev Dent* 8:19-23, 1986.

117. Heifetz SB. Evaluation of the comparative effectiveness of fluoride mouthrinsing, fluoride tablets, and both procedures in combination: interim findings after two years, *Pediatr Dent* 9:121-125, 1987.

118. Ripa LW, Leske G. Effect on the primary dentition of mouthrinsing with a 0.2 percent neutral NaF solution: results from a demonstration program after four school years, *Pediatr Dent* 3:311-315, 1981.

119. Symposium: Perspectives on the use of prenatal fluorides, *J Dent Child* 48:100-133, 1981.

120. Katz S, Muhler JC. Prenatal and postnatal fluoride and dental caries experience in deciduous teeth, *J Am Dent Assoc* 76:305-311, 1968.

121. Hennon DK, Stookey GK, Muhler JC. The clinical anticariogenic effectiveness of supplementary fluoride-vitamin preparation: results at the end of three years, *J Dent Child* 33:3-12, 1966.

122. Hennon DK, Stookey GK, Muhler JC. The clinical anticariogenic effectiveness of supplementary fluoride-vitamin preparations: results at the end of five and a half years, *Pharmacol Ther Dent* 1(1):1-6, 1970.

123. Lopez L, et al. Topical antimicrobial therapy in the prevention of early childhood caries, *Pediatr Dent* 21:9-11, 1999.

124. Lopez L, et al. Topical antimicrobial therapy in the prevention of early childhood caries: a follow-up report, *Pediatr Dent* 24:204-206, 2002.

125. Makinen KK. The rocky road of xylitol to its clinical application, *J Dent Res* 79:1352-1355, 2000.

126. Hyatt TP. Prophylactic odontotomy: the cutting into the tooth for the prevention of disease, *Dent Cosmos* 65:234-241, 1923.

127. Bowen WH. Relevance of caries vaccine investigations in rodents, primates, and humans: critical assessment, *Immunology* 11-20, 1976. (abstract; special suppl).

128. Michalek SM, Katz J, Childers NK. A vaccine against dental caries: An overview, *Biodrugs* 15:501-508, 2001.

CHAPTER 11

Mechanical and Chemotherapeutic Home Oral Hygiene

▲ **Jeffrey A. Dean** and **Christopher V. Hughes**

CHAPTER OUTLINE

*A*s the technological level of health care increases, it is important not to lose sight of the basics of patient care. In dentistry, this means establishing and maintaining effective preventive habits in our patients. No matter how sophisticated our dental techniques and procedures have become, preventive dentistry is the foundation on which all oral health care must be built. In 1960, McDonald discussed how pediatric medicine had changed in the previous 30 years (since 1930) from 90% treatment and 10% prevention to just the reverse.[1] He stated that preventive measures for dentistry were available and remained to be applied, as they had been in pediatrics. With this preventive philosophy, dentistry, particularly dentistry for children, has come a long way toward reaching this ratio of 90% prevention to 10% treatment.

At the core of this preventive foundation is home oral hygiene and plaque control. The area of oral hygiene has undergone recent developments that have turned a mundane subject into a field of surprising growth and research. Modern biology has made new inroads in the area of plaque control and will continue to exert a strong influence on how we look at oral hygiene and plaque in the future. The traditional focus of oral hygiene has been and will continue to be the control of the two most prevalent oral diseases: caries and periodontal disease. Although plaque control is essential to oral hygiene, unlike with periodontal disease, no clear relationship exists between plaque control and the prevention of caries. As discussed in Chapter 10, the complex etiology of decay centers on the following factors: tooth susceptibility, bacterial plaque, refined carbohydrates, and time. Many other variables, such as oral sugar clearance, salivary flow, and pH and immune factors, add to the complexity of this process. This may help explain the difficulty in demonstrating a relationship between oral hygiene practices and caries prevention.

Despite this ambiguity, plaque control remains an essential element for oral health. Although Marsh has shown that the natural oral microflora confers several benefits on the host, in the absence of oral hygiene, dental plaque accumulates, which leads to shifts in bacterial populations away from those associated with health.[2] Treatment should therefore be designed to control rather than to eliminate dental plaque.

Not only have there been advances in biology, but the public's consciousness regarding home oral hygiene also has been raised to new levels by the advertising of home health care products. The oral care market in the United States was estimated to reach nearly $8 billion in 2007. Health and cosmetic awareness by patients is possibly at an all-time high; they are willing to pay for the best in health products.

This chapter addresses the broad area of home oral hygiene for the child and adolescent, from the biology of plaque development to plaque removal techniques and patient motivation. Dental health care professionals need to make home oral hygiene the core of their preventive foundation.

MICROBIAL ASPECTS OF ORAL HYGIENE AND PLAQUE FORMATION

Although Miller proposed in the late nineteenth century that microorganisms play a role in dental disease,[3] definitive evidence of the microbial etiology of dental caries and periodontal diseases did not appear until three fourths of a century later with the work of Keyes[4] and of Löe and colleagues.[5] Since these seminal studies were performed, the major focus of dental research has been to define the specific microorganisms in dental plaque that mediate these diseases. Although great progress has been made in identifying these pathogens, our primary tools in preventing dental diseases remain mechanical removal of plaque and promotion of the remineralization of the tooth surface. Therefore the following brief review of the timing, mechanisms, and biology of plaque formation provides a scientific rationale for any clinical program of oral hygiene and prevention.

The development of anaerobic culturing techniques and, more recently, genetic techniques that allow for the detection of uncultivable species have identified more than 700 bacterial species and numerous distinct bacterial habitats in the mouth. Interestingly, only a limited number of species are found in high numbers in dental plaque.[6-8] These species are uniquely suited to this habitat. The formation of plaque on the tooth surface is characterized by progression from a limited number of pioneer species (mainly streptococci and other gram-positive organisms) to the complex flora of mature dental plaque. This maturation involves initial adherence of bacteria to the salivary pellicle and subsequent formation of a complex multispecies biofilm. Most oral bacteria have evolved specific adherence mechanisms that enable them to colonize the tooth surface. In addition, bacteria undergo a number of phenotypic changes as they initiate the formation of a biofilm. The molecular mechanisms that underlie these processes have been intensively studied. Kolenbrander and Kuramitsu have provided recent reviews of these areas.[8-10] Although their reports offer the possibility of new methods of plaque control, mechanical plaque removal with supplementation by chemotherapeutic agents currently offers the most practical method of controlling plaque.

Not only do microbial changes occur as plaque matures on the tooth surface, but mature dental plaques associated with oral diseases appear to differ from those associated with oral health. Many studies have demonstrated that, in dental caries, the pathogenicity of plaque is related to the numbers of *Streptococcus mutans* and related species present.[11] In contrast, the plaques associated with gingival inflammation are characterized by a predominance of gram-negative bacteria rather than the predominantly gram-positive flora found in oral health. This transition seems to coincide with inflammatory changes that occur at the gingival margin. Plaque control efforts should be directed toward two goals: (1) limiting the numbers of mutans streptococci in dental plaques for prevention of caries by mechanical elimination of supragingival plaque and limitation of dietary sucrose, and (2) maintaining the predominantly gram-positive flora associated with gingival health by mechanical removal of plaque from the subgingival area on a regular basis. The use of chemotherapeutic agents, particularly chlorhexidine, can also play a role in maintenance of gingival health. The incorporation of these methods into the daily routines of patients and their parents is perhaps the greatest challenge facing the dentist.

MECHANICAL METHODS OF PLAQUE CONTROL

Mechanical methods of plaque control are the most widely accepted techniques for plaque removal. Toothbrushing and flossing are the essential elements of these mechanical methods; adjuncts include disclosing agents, oral irrigators, and tongue scrapers.

MANUAL TOOTHBRUSH

The toothbrush is the most common method for removing plaque from the oral cavity. A number of variables enter into the design and fabrication of toothbrushes. These include the bristle material; length, diameter, and total number of fibers; length of brush head; trim design of brush head; number and arrangement of bristle tufts; angulation of brush head to handle; and handle design. In addition, many features, such as the use of neon colors or familiar cartoon caricatures, are designed to attract the attention of potential purchasers (Fig. 11-1).

Today, most commercially available toothbrushes are manufactured with synthetic (nylon) bristles. Park and colleagues identify the bristle and head of the toothbrush as the most important part of the toothbrush, noting that the length of most bristles is 11 mm.[12] Toothbrushes are classified as soft, medium, or hard based on the diameter of these bristles. The diameter ranges for these classifications are 0.16 to 0.22 mm for soft, 0.23 to 0.29 mm for medium, and 0.30 mm and greater for hard. In addition to the bristle diameter, the bristle end has been studied to determine the most beneficial type for plaque control. Of the three types of bristle ends (Fig. 11-2A to C), coarse-cut, enlarged bulbous, and round, the round end is the bristle type of choice because it is associated with a lower incidence of gingival tissue irritation. However, even the coarse-cut bristles round off eventually with normal use (see Fig. 11-2D).

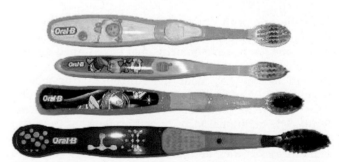

Figure 11-1 Features such as neon colors or cartoon characters on toothbrushes are designed to attract the attention of purchasers.

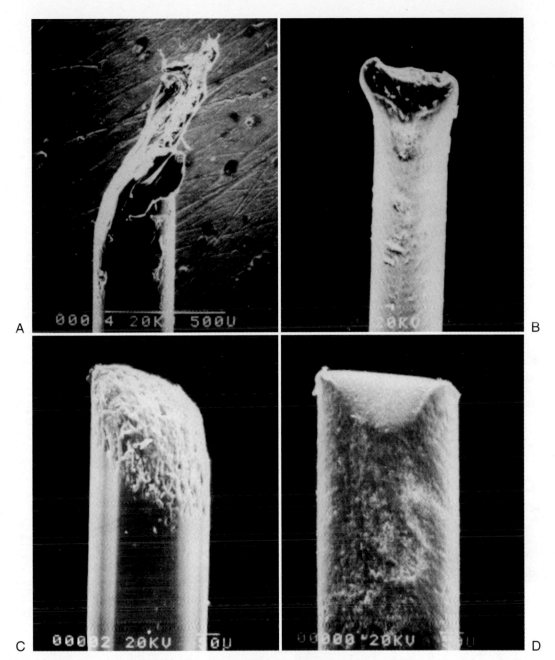

Figure 11-2 Scanning electron micrographs of toothbrush bristles manufactured by different processes. **A,** Coarse-cut bristle end, probably the result of an incomplete single-blade cut. **B,** Slightly enlarged, bulbous nylon bristle end, resulting from a double-blade or scissors cut. **C,** Tapered or round-end nylon toothbrush bristle produced by heat or a mechanical polishing process. **D,** Scrubbing, mechanical action of a toothbrush wear machine has nicely rounded off this bristle removed from a brush that was originally coarse-cut. (From Park KK, Matis BA, Christen AG. Choosing an effective toothbrush, *Clin Prev Dent* 7[4]:5-10, 1985.)

The soft brush is preferable for most uses in pediatric dentistry because of the decreased likelihood of gingival tissue trauma and increased interproximal cleaning ability. In evaluating the best toothbrush head and handle for children, Updyke concludes that it is best to use a toothbrush with a smaller head and a thicker handle than an adult-size toothbrush to better access the oral cavity and facilitate the child's grip of the handle.[13] However, no single toothbrush design has been scientifically proven

to be superior for removal of plaque. Multiple variables influence a toothbrush's ability to remove plaque; therefore the practitioner should make recommendations only after assessing a patient's individual needs.

Wear rates of toothbrush bristles and their subsequent ability to remove plaque raise another concern. Dean suggests that toothbrushes remain effective well after patients identify a brush as being worn out.[14] The cleansing effectiveness of toothbrushes is maintained until pronounced toothbrush wear has occurred. This implies that patients are much more likely to dispose of a brush well before its clinical usefulness actually ends than to continue to use a toothbrush that no longer cleans effectively. In this regard, one manufacturer claims that their commercial toothbrush (Oral-B Indicator, Oral-B Laboratories, Inc., Belmont, Calif) indicates when the brush should be replaced by means of centrally located tufts of bristles dyed with food colorant. When the blue band fades to halfway down the bristle, it is time to replace the brush (Fig. 11-3). The company states that on average this occurs after 3 months but that the time varies depending on the individual's brushing habits.

Parents frequently ask how often they should change a child's toothbrush. It is best to replace the toothbrush when it appears well worn. This can present some problems for parents, because some children, especially toddlers, chew their brushes when brushing, which rapidly gives the bristles a well-worn appearance.

FLOSS

Although toothbrushing is the most widely used method of mechanical plaque control, toothbrushing alone cannot adequately remove plaque from all tooth surfaces. In particular, it is not efficient in removing interproximal plaque, which means that interproximal cleaning beyond

brushing is necessary. Indeed, Corby and colleagues found that after a 2-week study period of 12- to 21-year-old well-matched twins, tooth and tongue brushing plus flossing significantly decreased the abundance of microbial species associated with periodontal disease and dental caries.[15] Many devices have been suggested for interproximal removal of plaque, such as interdental brushes, floss holders and floss, and end tuft brush (Fig. 11-4). According to Mauriello and associates, there appears to be no substantial difference between these devices in their ability to remove plaque and their tendency to produce gingival inflammation effects when they are used properly; however, floss is the standard device to which other devices are most often compared.[16] The other devices are more often recommended in certain unique circumstances, for example, the interdental brush may be recommended for orthodontic patients. Unfortunately, regular flossing does not occur daily in most households. Chen and Rubinson demonstrated that daily flossing was practiced by only 20% of mothers, 12% of fathers, and 6% of children within families.[17] In addition, 28% of mothers, 45% of fathers, and 48% of children never floss their teeth. This low compliance rate, particularly in children, is a problem requiring our attention as practitioners.

Several different types of floss are available: flavored and unflavored, waxed and unwaxed, and thin, tape, and meshwork (Super Floss, Oral-B Laboratories, Inc., Belmont, Calif) (Fig. 11-5). Almost all commercially available floss is made of nylon, although floss made of Teflon material (polytetrafluoroethylene) (Glide, W.L. Gore and Associates, Inc., Flagstaff, Ariz) is also available. The manufacturer claims that, because the material has a lower coefficient of friction than nylon, this floss does not shred, slides easily between tight contacts, and minimizes snapping of the floss.

Based on the work of Bass, unwaxed nylon-filament floss has generally been considered the floss of choice because of the ease of passing the floss between tight contacts, the lack of a wax residue, the squeaking sound produced by moving the floss over a clean tooth, and the

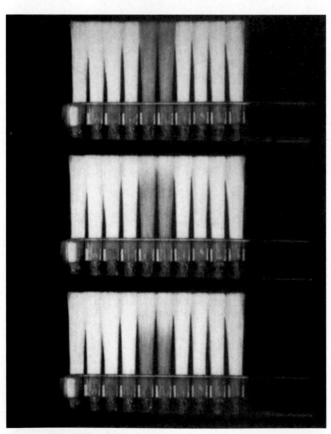

Figure 11-3 Blue dye in the center bristle tufts of this toothbrush fades down from the end with use. When the dye reaches the half-way point (bottom), the manufacturer suggests replacing the toothbrush.

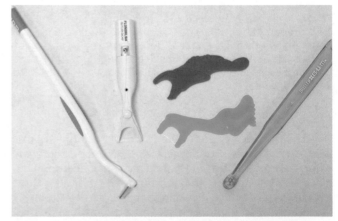

Figure 11-4 Several different methods for interproximal cleaning. Left to right, Interdental brush, Y-shaped floss holder, disposable floss holders, and end tuft brush.

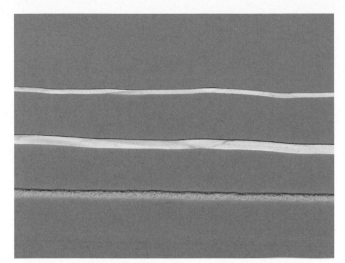

Figure 11-5 Dental floss. Thin (*top*), tape (*middle*), and meshwork (*bottom*).

fiber spread, which results in increased surface contact and greater plaque removal.[18]

However, more recent work indicates clearly that individual patient needs and preferences should be taken into account before floss selection recommendations are made. Carr and colleagues tested four different types of floss: waxed, unwaxed, woven, and shred resistant.[19] They studied the reductions in interproximal plaque scores for 24 dental hygiene students. Statistical analysis revealed no significant differences between floss types in cleaning efficacy, comfort of use, or ease of use.

With these results kept in mind, it may help when making floss recommendations to parents for their children to consider both the parent's and the child's preferences and individual needs. From the perspective of patient acceptance, flavored waxed floss may be most effective. In addition, many parents complain that their fingers are too large for their child's mouth. Floss-holding devices (see Fig. 11-4) are an excellent alternative for parents when this complaint is voiced or when the dexterity of the parent or child prevents handholding of floss. For orthodontic patients, the use of Super Floss or a floss threader (Fig. 11-6) helps in negotiating the floss under the archwires to allow for interproximal cleaning. For

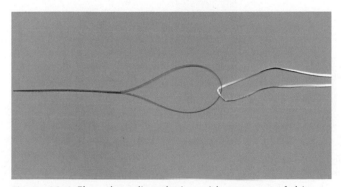

Figure 11-6 Floss-threading device with segment of thin floss attached.

orthodontic patients, flossing is a tedious process but is nonetheless essential to maintenance of oral health.

POWERED MECHANICAL PLAQUE REMOVAL

The use of powered or electric toothbrushes has received considerable attention since the 1960s. The rationale for using powered brushes is that many patients remove plaque poorly because they lack adequate manual dexterity to manipulate the brush. The powered brushes should decrease the need for dexterity by automatically including some movement of the toothbrush head. However, initial studies into the plaque removal effectiveness of powered toothbrushes failed to demonstrate greater efficacy for powered than for manual toothbrushes. Although improvement was seen initially, over time the level of cleaning achieved with power toothbrushes declined to the same level obtained using manual toothbrushes. Kerlinger refers to this as the *Hawthorne effect*: almost any change or experimental manipulation will induce an improvement in behavior, apparently because of a novelty effect.[20] The introduction of powered toothbrushes caused an initial increase in use, and therefore plaque and gingivitis were controlled. Over time, however, the results were comparable to those achieved with manual toothbrushes.

Use of the latest power toothbrushes, such as the Sonicare (Philips Oral Healthcare, Inc., Snoqualmie, Wash) or the Braun Oral-B Kids' Power Toothbrush (D10) (Oral-B Laboratories, Inc., Belmont, Calif), however, may prove to be more beneficial than use of other toothbrushes.

The Sonicare uses sonic technology in the form of acoustic energy to improve removal ability of traditional toothbrush bristles. The brush has an electromagnetic device that drives the bristles' motions at 261 Hz, or 31,320 brush strokes per minute. Ho and Niederman found that the Sonicare toothbrush was significantly more effective than the manual toothbrush in reducing the plaque index, gingival index, percentage of sites that bled on probing, pocket depth, and total gram-negative bacteria in a subgingival plaque sample.[21] Nowak and colleagues have demonstrated a 40% improvement in the debris index component of the Simplified Oral Hygiene Index in children aged 4 to 9 years who were using the Braun Oral-B Kids' Power Toothbrush (D10).[22] Studies by Grossman and Proskin[23] and by Jongenelis and Wiedemann[24] also compared the effectiveness of electric versus manual toothbrushes when the toothbrushes were specifically designed for children. Both studies concluded that the powered toothbrushes removed significantly more plaque than the manual toothbrushes for children. Finally, Heanue and associates performed a meta-analysis showing that power toothbrushes with a rotation-oscillation action design removed more plaque and reduced gingivitis more effectively than manual brushes in both the short and the long term.[25] No other powered toothbrush designs were consistently superior to manual toothbrushes.

The Toothbrush Acceptance Program Guidelines of the American Dental Association (ADA) Council on Scientific Affairs list several requirements for powered toothbrushes that are not imposed on manual toothbrushes.[26] Among these are evidence that the product can be used under unsupervised conditions by the average layperson to provide a 15% statistically significant reduction over baseline in gingivitis and a statistically significant reduction in plaque.

Also noteworthy is the development of the Braun Oral-B Interclean. (Braun GmbH, Kronberg, Germany). This electrically powered cleaning device requires only single-handed usage while its filament rotates to undergo an elliptical movement, disrupting plaque attached to adjacent and proximate teeth. Gordon and colleagues compared the effect of Interclean use and manual flossing over a 4-week period on level of interproximal plaque, gingivitis, and papillary bleeding in 52 healthy volunteers.[27] The results demonstrated no statistically significant difference between manual flossing and use of the electric interdental cleaning device. Results from the personal preference phase of the study demonstrated that significantly more subjects preferred the interdental cleaning device (69.5%) to floss (24.5%). This new type of interdental cleaning device may be particularly helpful for adolescent orthodontic patients

DENTIFRICES

Dentifrices serve multiple functions in oral hygiene through the inclusion of a variety of agents. They act as plaque- and stain-removing agents through the use of abrasives and surfactants. Pleasant flavors and colors encourage their use. They have tartar control properties because of the addition of pyrophosphates. Finally, dentifrices have anticaries and desensitization properties through the action of fluoride and other agents. A child's dentifrice should contain fluoride, rank low in abrasiveness, and carry the ADA seal of acceptance. In 2009, 51 different fluoride-containing dentifrices were listed as accepted dental therapeutic products by the Council on Scientific Affairs. Many of the 51 dentifrices are specifically designed and flavored to catch the attention of children.

These formulations are useful because a child is more likely to practice oral hygiene procedures if the tools to be used are pleasing. Although the caries-preventive efficacy of fluoride toothpastes in children has been well documented, the impact of dentifrices on the total fluoride intake in children must be considered. Adair and associates confirmed that children tend to use larger amounts of dentifrice, brush for a longer period, and rinse and expectorate less when using a children's dentifrice than when using an adult dentifrice.[28] Levy and Zarei-M studied toothbrushing habits and quantities of toothpaste used on toothbrushes in children from birth through 6 years of age. Fig. 11-7 shows their results.[29] This study did not quantify the amount of toothpaste, and therefore of fluoride, ingested from the use of this much toothpaste on the brush. However, the investigators suggest that ingestion was likely a substantial source of systemic fluoride for these children during the years when a risk of dental fluorosis is present. It is interesting to note that many toothpaste advertisements show children with large amounts of toothpaste on their brushes. Clearly, this is not the perception dentists want the public to have when regarding the use of fluoridated toothpastes in young children.

Simard and colleagues concluded from their study of 12- to 24-month-old children that 20% of the children ingested more than 0.25 mg of fluoride per day by toothbrushing alone.[30] They suggest the following to reduce the chance of dental fluorosis in children secondary to toothpaste ingestion. Manufacturers should market a low-fluoride dentifrice for infants or reduce the diameter of the tube orifice. Parents should be advised to delay the use of fluoride dentifrice until the child is older than 36 months and to use small, pea-sized quantities of toothpaste. Pediatricians should take into consideration all sources of fluoride before prescribing supplements. In the wake of these recommendations, one manufacturer

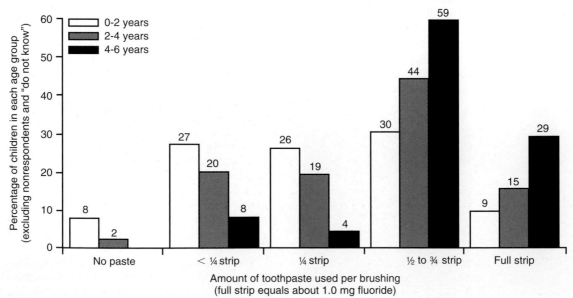

Figure 11-7 Quantity of toothpaste used by children from birth to 6 years of age. (From Levy SM, Zarei-M Z. Evaluation of fluoride exposures in children. J Dent Child 1991;58:467-473.)

has developed a dentifrice for children called Baby Orajel Tooth and Gum Cleanser (Del Pharmaceuticals, Inc., Plainview, NY). The manufacturer states that it is non-abrasive, nonfoaming, without fluoride, safe for infants, and ideal for babies aged 4 months to 3 years. It contains a mild surfactant and simethicone, is sugar-free, and comes in vanilla and fruit flavors.

DISCLOSING AGENTS

To increase the patient's ability to remove plaque, several agents have been developed to allow for patient visualization of plaque. These include iodine, gentian violet, erythrosin, basic fuchsin, fast green, food dyes, fluorescein, and a two-tone disclosing agent. Use of these agents is particularly helpful in teaching children toothbrushing techniques and educating them on the rationale for oral hygiene. FDC red No. 28 is a plaque-disclosing agent commonly used either as a liquid to be dabbed onto the teeth with a cotton swab or in the form of a chewable tablet (Fig. 11-8). Unfortunately, this dye stains the oral soft tissues and dental pellicle, as well as plaque, leaving an objectionable pink discoloration that lasts up to several hours after use. Most younger children do not appear to be bothered by the discoloration, but as children approach adolescence it can become a problem. Fluorescein disclosing agents were developed to address this problem because fluorescein is not visible under normal light. Their use does, however, require special equipment.

In a study by Lim and colleagues, four different techniques were compared for clinically detecting plaque in patients using different dietary regimens.[31] Subjects ranging in age from 18 to 27 years had their plaque levels assessed using a caries probe, a plaque-detection probe, erythrosin, and a two-tone disclosing agent at 3, 6, and 18 hours after thorough cleaning of their teeth. Thirty-eight patients were assigned to a sucrose-restricted (SR) diet in the first part of the study, and 32 patients were assigned to a sucrose-supplemented (SS) diet in the second part of the study. At 3 hours, plaque was detectable on more than 12% of sites in those consuming the SR diet and up to 23% in those on the SS diet. After 18 hours, the proportion of plaque-covered surfaces had increased to between 52% (SR diet) and 73% (SS diet). For minimal amounts of plaque, the disclosing solutions were found to be the most sensitive assessment techniques. For moderate and abundant plaque deposits, however, the probe techniques were more sensitive.

The clinical significance of these data is that, in measuring a patient's oral hygiene abilities, one must assess plaque deposits immediately after the patient has cleaned his or her teeth. Otherwise, allowances must be made for factors such as the time elapsed since the teeth were

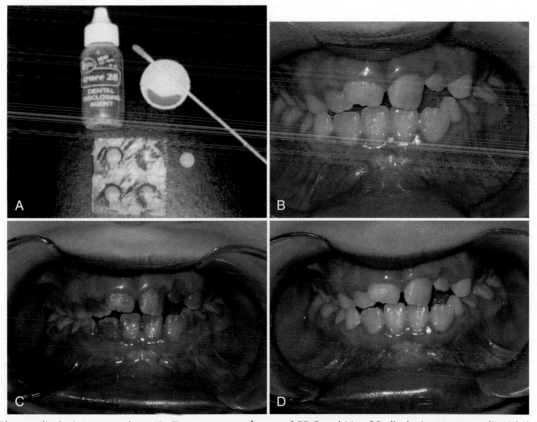

Figure 11-8 Plaque-disclosing procedure. **A,** Two common forms of FDC red No. 28 disclosing agent: a liquid that is dabbed on with a cotton swab and a chewable tablet. **B,** Mixed dentition in a patient before oral hygiene and disclosing. **C,** Patient before oral hygiene but after disclosing. **D,** Patient after oral hygiene and disclosing.

cleaned and the patient's diet. If a patient is seen several hours after the teeth have been cleaned, the quality of plaque control may be deemed unsatisfactory regardless of the quality of the patient's performance. Disclosing agents also have some antimicrobial activity, according to Baab and colleagues.[32] Although short-term quantitative inhibition of plaque growth has not been observed clinically, long-term home use of disclosing agents may contribute to qualitative differences in plaque composition. Further studies are needed to measure the long-term in vivo effect of these agents.

OTHER ADJUNCTS FOR PLAQUE CONTROL

Several other devices, such as oral irrigators and tongue scrapers, have been suggested for routine oral hygiene. Oral irrigators use pulsed water or chemotherapeutic agents to dislodge plaque from the dentition. Tongue scrapers, which are flat, flexible plastic sticks, are used to remove bacterial and food deposits that accumulate within the rough dorsal surface of the tongue. In addition, gauze or special dental washcloths are useful in infants to massage the gums and to remove plaque on newly erupted teeth. Although these adjuncts add to our basic hygiene tools, toothbrushes and floss remain the most effective means of mechanical plaque removal. Professional recommendation of these adjuncts should be to suggest them as supplements to and not substitutes for the basic tools and should take into consideration the patient's and caregiver's individual needs, abilities, and preferences.

TECHNIQUES

As with toothbrush design, several different types of toothbrushing techniques for children have been advocated over the years. The more predominant techniques are the roll method, the Charters method, the horizontal scrubbing method, and the modified Stillman method. Anaise, in his study of the effectiveness of these four techniques in children 11 to 14 years of age, describes them as follows[33]:

Roll Method
The brush is placed in the vestibule, the bristle ends directed apically, with the sides of the bristles touching the gingival tissue. The patient exerts lateral pressure with the sides of the bristles, and the brush is moved occlusally. The brush is placed again high in the vestibule, and the rolling motion is repeated. The lingual surfaces are brushed in the same manner, with two teeth brushed simultaneously.

Charters Method
The ends of the bristles are placed in contact with the enamel of the teeth and the gingiva, with the bristles pointed at about a 45-degree angle toward the plane of occlusion. A lateral and downward pressure is then placed on the brush, and the brush is vibrated gently back and forth a millimeter or so.

Horizontal Scrubbing Method
The brush is placed horizontally on buccal and lingual surfaces and moved back and forth with a scrubbing motion.

Modified Stillman Method
The modified Stillman method combines a vibratory action of the bristles with a stroke movement of the brush in the long axis of the teeth. The brush is placed at the mucogingival line, with the bristles pointed away from the crown, and moved with a stroking motion along the gingiva and the tooth surface. The handle is rotated toward the crown and vibrated as the brush is moved.

Anaise concluded that the horizontal scrubbing method exhibited a more significant plaque-removing effect than the roll, Charters, and modified Stillman methods.[33] This finding supports the work done by McClure[34] and by Sangnes and colleagues.[35]

In a study by Rugg-Gunn and Macgregor, uninstructed videotaped toothbrushing behavior in three age groups (5, 11, and 18 to 22 years) was analyzed.[36] The following conclusions were drawn:

- In the three age groups, the proportions of the areas that were brushed were 25% 5-year-old group, 50% in the 11-year-old group, and 67% in the 18- to 22-year-old group.
- More time was spent brushing the lower than the upper teeth.
- The contralateral side (the left side in right-handed persons) was brushed more than the ipsilateral side in children, but equally in adults.
- Less than 10% of the time was spent brushing lingual areas.
- The most popular brushing strokes were the horizontal stroke in children and the vertical stroke in adults; the roll and circular strokes were seldom used.
- Eighty-four percent of subjects used more than one type of stroke.

The horizontal scrub technique removes as much or more plaque than the other techniques, regardless of how old the child is and whether the brushing is performed by the parent or the child. In addition, it is the technique most naturally adopted by children. Therefore, in most situations the horizontal scrubbing method can be recommended for brushing children's teeth, regardless of the brushing method.[37] By following a systematic approach, as shown in Fig. 11-9, the child or parent can help ensure that all areas of the mouth are cleaned. Notice also on this figure the positioning of the brush head on the lingual surfaces of the anterior teeth and on the distal aspect of the most posterior tooth in each quadrant.

For flossing, the following technique is recommended (Fig. 11-10):
1. A 46- to 61-cm (18- to 24-inch) length of floss is obtained, and the ends are wrapped around the patient's or parent's middle fingers. Floss should be long enough to allow the thumbs to touch each other when the hands are laid flat.
2. The thumbs and index fingers are used to guide the floss as it is gently sawed between the two teeth to be cleaned. Care must be taken not to snap the floss down through the interproximal contacts to avoid gingival trauma.
3. The floss is then manipulated into a C shape around each tooth individually and moved in a cervical-occlusal reciprocating motion until the plaque is

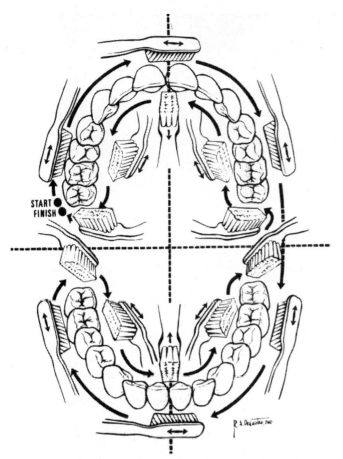

Figure 11-9 Systematic approach to brushing the teeth begins with the buccal aspects of the teeth in the maxillary right quadrant and follows the arrows. Bristles are held at a 45-degree angle to the long axis of the teeth and are directed to the gum line. Short back-and-forth strokes are used, allowing bristles to remain in the same place. The handle of the brush is placed parallel to the biting surfaces except when brushing the lingual aspects of the anterior teeth and the posterior aspects of the last tooth in each quadrant, when a heel-toe direction of brushing is used. (Courtesy Dr. Paul Starkey.)

removed. In between cleaning each pair of teeth the floss is repositioned on the fingers so that fresh, unsoiled floss is used at each new location.

Learning a flossing technique is difficult and takes some practice. Some children and their parents prefer to make a loop of floss. Tying the two ends of the floss together, instead of wrapping it around their fingers, assists them in holding and controlling the floss. However, Rodrigues and colleagues demonstrated that, even when the looped floss technique is used, a training program is required for children 6½ to 7½ years of age to accomplish significant reduction in proximal surface dental plaque indices.[38]

VISUAL-MOTOR SKILL MASTERY

Several attempts have been made to develop specific recommendations for when children can begin performing oral hygiene procedures themselves with adequate effectiveness. Terhune stated that the variables of age,

gender, and eye-hand coordination could not precisely predict when particular children were ready to learn an effective dental flossing technique.[39] However, all 8- to 11-year-old children in his study learned how to use dental floss effectively within 10 days. Mescher and associates found that hand function was an age-related factor in children's ability to perform sulcular toothbrushing, but that hand function test scores were not accurate predictors of an individual's toothbrushing ability.[40]

Preisch, however, did find a significant relationship between developmental age and oral hygiene scores using a visual-motor integration developmental test.[41] With the use of this test, significant correlations have been shown between the ability of children to copy geometric forms and their academic achievement and motor skill level. Higher levels of thinking and behavior require integration among sensory inputs and motor action. A child can have well-developed visual and motor skills but may be unable to coordinate the two. Although both chronologic and developmental ages were found to be predictors of plaque removal ability, only developmental age demonstrated statistically significant predictive power. Because of the complexity of this test, however, we are left without a practical method for making recommendations to parents as to when their child can begin brushing on their own. As Preisch laments, many dentists use anecdotal accounts and tell parents to supervise their children's brushing until the children can color within the lines, tie their own shoelaces, or cut through a tough piece of meat.[41] However, this may still be our best practical recommendation.

TIME CONSIDERATIONS

Another of the important questions regarding home oral health care involves time considerations in oral hygiene practices. How often should patients brush and floss their teeth and for how long? In discussing frequency of oral hygiene procedures, Löe suggests that oral cleanliness should be regarded as a defined state in which all surfaces of all teeth are plaque-free.[42] He states that it may not be surprising to find that complete removal of plaque once daily or every second day, or possibly even once every third day, is more valuable in preventing dental disease than performing two or three inadequate brushings per day. Indeed, Lang and colleagues observed that completion of effective oral hygiene procedures at intervals of up to 48 hours is compatible with gingival health.[43] Studies addressing the relation between the frequency of hygiene procedures and caries experience in children have yielded inconclusive results.

In addition to optimal brushing frequency, the most efficacious length of brushing time has been investigated. In a study by Hodges and colleagues, 84 children aged 5 to 15 years brushed their teeth with a fluoridated dentifrice for 30, 60, 120, and 180 seconds.[44] The results of the study suggest that, statistically, a 1-minute brushing period provides the greatest plaque removal benefit of all time periods tested.

The following recommendations are made based on the preceding information. In children, thorough oral hygiene procedures should be performed at least once

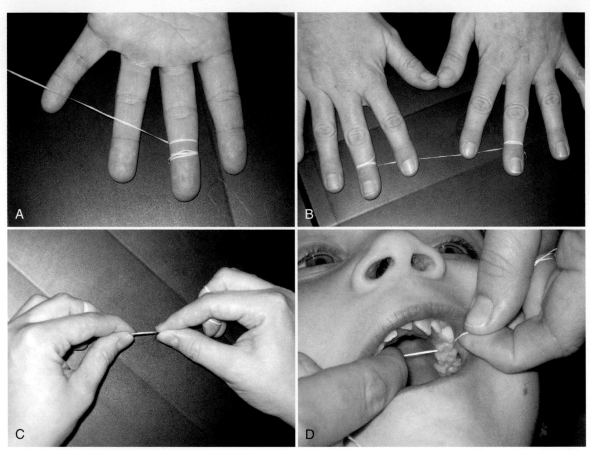

Figure 11-10 Flossing technique. **A,** The length of floss is wrapped around the middle fingers of each hand. **B,** Enough floss should be left between the middle fingers to allow the thumbs to touch when the hands are laid flat. **C,** The index fingers and thumbs are used to manipulate the floss. **D,** The floss is carefully placed in a C shape between the interproximal contacts and gently sawed up and down until each tooth surface is clean.

daily, preferably twice, with parental supervision. Teeth should be brushed for at least 1 minute with a fluoridated dentifrice; flossing and other plaque removal activities are added to this time. If oral hygiene is accomplished only once per day, it should be the last thing the child does before bedtime at night. Because the flow of saliva and its buffering capacity are reduced during sleep, it is advantageous to remove plaque before bedtime. In addition, the development in children of a learned behavior performed at a specific time of day, each and every day, will be helpful throughout childhood and into adulthood.

CHEMOTHERAPEUTIC PLAQUE CONTROL

Although the use of mechanical therapy for plaque control can provide excellent results, it is clear that many patients are unable, unwilling, or untrained to practice routine effective mechanotherapy. In addition, certain patients with dental diseases (e.g., periodontitis) or medical diseases (e.g., immunocompromised conditions) require additional assistance beyond mechanotherapy to maintain a normal state of oral health. Because of this, chemotherapeutic agents have been developed as adjuncts in plaque control.

Van der Ouderaa has stated that the ideal chemotherapeutic plaque control agent should have the following characteristics[45]:
- Specificity only for the pathogenic bacteria
- Substantivity, the ability to attach to and be retained by oral surfaces and then be released over time without loss of potency
- Chemical stability during storage
- Absence of adverse reactions, such as staining or mucosal interactions
- Toxicologic safety
- Ecologic safety so as not to adversely alter the microbiotic flora
- Ease of use

No agent has yet been developed that has all of these characteristics.

There are several main routes of administration of antiplaque agents designed for home use. They are mouthwashes, dentifrices, gels, irrigators, floss, chewing gum, lozenges, and capsules. All of these are designed for local, supragingival admin tration, except the irrigator and capsule delivery methods. The irrigators can provide both supragingival and subgingival delivery. The capsules are designed for systemic distribution.

Box 11-1

Chemotherapeutic Plaque Control Agents

ANTISEPTIC AGENTS
Positively Charged Organic Molecules:
Quaternary ammonium compounds—cetylpyridinium chloride
Pyrimidines—hexedine
Bis-biguanides—chlorhexidine, alexidine
Noncharged Phenolic Agents: Listerine (thymol, eucalyptol, menthol, and methylsalicylate), triclosan, phenol, and thymol
Oxygenating Agents: Peroxides and perborate
Bis-Pyridines: Octenidine
Halogens: Iodine, iodophors, and fluorides
Heavy Metal Salts: Silver, mercury, zinc, copper, and tin

ANTIBIOTICS
Niddamycin, kanamycin sulfate, tetracycline hydrochloride, and vancomycin hydrochloride

ENZYMES
Mucinases, pancreatin, fungal enzymes, and protease

PLAQUE-MODIFYING AGENTS
Urea peroxide

SUGAR SUBSTITUTES
Xylitol, mannitol

PLAQUE ATTACHMENT INTERFERENCE AGENTS
Sodium polyvinylphosphonic acid, perfluoroalkyl

Both van der Ouderaa[45] and Mandel[46] have provided excellent reviews of the various chemotherapeutic agents and their uses. Box 11-1 is adapted from those reviews. Space does not allow a complete discussion of the agents listed in this box; however, a few pertinent subjects are addressed.

ANTISEPTIC AGENTS

The antiseptic agents used in chemotherapeutic plaque control have been shown to exhibit little or no oral or systemic toxicity in the concentrations used. Virtually no drug resistance is induced, and in most instances these agents have a broad antimicrobial spectrum. Chlorhexidine, a positively charged organic antiseptic agent, has received considerable attention and study because of its ability to reduce plaque and gingivitis scores. It has strong substantivity, binding well to many sites in the oral cavity and maintaining an ongoing antibacterial presence. Chlorhexidine binds with anionic glycoproteins and phosphoproteins on the buccal, palatal, and labial mucosa and the tooth-borne pellicle. Its antibacterial effects include binding well to bacterial cell membranes, increasing their permeability, initiating leakage, and precipitating intracellular components.

Grossman and colleagues conducted a 6-month clinical trial in which 430 adults rinsed twice daily with either 0.12% chlorhexidine or a placebo.[47] Gingivitis and plaque

scores were lower in the chlorhexidine group (34% to 41%) than in the placebo group (61%). Several studies have demonstrated the use and efficacy of chlorhexidine therapy in children as young as 8 years of age. Studies have examined its use in the form of a rinse, a spray, a varnish, and a chlorhexidine gel used in flossing.

Lang and associates investigated the effects of supervised rinsing with chlorhexidine in 158 schoolchildren, aged 10 to 12 years.[48] The children were divided into four groups. Group A rinsed with a 0.2% solution of chlorhexidine digluconate (CHX) six times weekly. Group B rinsed with 0.2% CHX two times weekly. Group C rinsed with a 0.1% CHX solution six times weekly. Group D rinsed six times weekly with a placebo solution. All rinsing was performed under supervision, and no effort was made to change the children's oral hygiene habits. Fig. 11-11 shows the results of the study. All three experimental groups, A, B, and C, exhibited statistically significant reductions in the gingival index compared with the control group (group D). The investigators concluded that gingivitis can be controlled successfully in children by regular rinsing with a chlorhexidine solution over an extended period.

Chlorhexidine spray has stimulated interest regarding its use in disabled populations because of its effectiveness and ease of administration. Burtner and colleagues demonstrated a 35% reduction in plaque levels with use of the spray compared with placebo use in a study of 16 institutionalized adult males with severe and profound mental retardation.[49] Chikte and colleagues conducted a 9-week, double-blind, randomized crossover clinical trial involving 52 institutionalized mentally disabled individuals 10 to 26 years of age. By the end of the trial, plaque and gingival indices had been reduced by 48% and 52%, respectively, in the group treated with a stannous fluoride

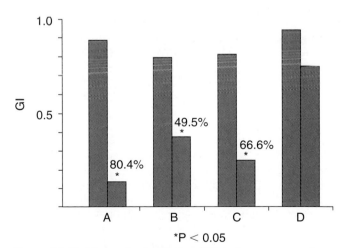

Figure 11-11 Mean gingival index (GI) in four groups of schoolchildren rinsing with chlorhexidine digluconate (CHX) or placebo solution for 6 months under supervision. Clear bars, Before treatment; screened bars, after treatment. Group A: 0.2% CHX six times weekly; group B: 0.2% CHX two times weekly; group C: 0.1% CHX six times weekly; group D: placebo six times weekly. (From Lang NP, et al. Effects of supervised chlorhexidine mouthrinses in children. J Periodontal Res 1982;17:101-111.)

spray.[50] In the group treated with chlorhexidine spray, reductions in plaque and gingival indices were 75% and 78%, respectively.

In addition to its use in institutionalized patients with mental retardation, chlorhexidine has been studied for its use in immunocompromised patients. Ferretti and colleagues found that the prophylactic use of chlorhexidine mouthrinse produced reductions in gingivitis and mucositis and oral microbial burden in patients undergoing bone marrow transplantation.[51] Raether and associates, however, studying a similar patient population, found no significant difference between the group receiving chlorhexidine and that given a placebo, in terms of number of oral ulcerations, development of bacteremia, and length of hospital stay.[52] Despite these findings, they suggested the use of a chlorhexidine mouthrinse as an antiplaque and antigingivitis agent in bone marrow transplant patients to augment their oral hygiene. Finally, chlorhexidine varnish has been shown by Fennis-le and associates[53] and by Petersson and colleagues[54] to suppress the level of mutans streptococci. However, recent clinical studies have failed to demonstrate a transfer of this effect into a decrease in caries on either smooth enamel surfaces or occlusal pits and fissures.[55] Additional work is needed to conclusively demonstrate the value of chlorhexidine varnishes in reducing dental caries.

The use of positively charged antiplaque agents has been hampered by adverse reactions such as staining of teeth, impaired taste sensation, and increased supragingival calculus formation. Different attempts have been made to decrease these side effects, such as alteration of dietary habits, increase in mechanical plaque removal efforts, and use of hydrogen peroxide solutions in conjunction with the antiseptic agent. Continued research is needed to find methods to limit these adverse reactions.

The most widely known noncharged phenolic antiseptic agent is Listerine (Pfizer Warner Lambert Division, Morris Plains, NJ). It has demonstrated a long history of efficacy and was among the original antiseptic agents studied by W. D. Miller in 1890.[3] In addition, it was the first over-the-counter mouthrinse to be accepted by the Council of Dental Therapeutics for its help in controlling plaque and gingivitis.[26] Despite its long history of use, studies by Clark and colleagues[56] and by Brownstone and associates[57] have shown chlorhexidine to be significantly more effective than Listerine in reducing plaque and gingivitis indices. Listerine tends to give patients a burning sensation, and it has a bitter taste. Lang and Brecx have summarized the changes in plaque index, gingival index, and discoloration index scores resulting from the use of four well-known chemotherapeutic plaque control agents (Fig. 11-12).[58] The effects of two daily 10-mL rinses with either 0.12% chlorhexidine digluconate, the quaternary ammonium compound cetylpyridinium chloride, the phenolic compound Listerine, or the plant alkaloid sanguinarine were compared with those of rinses with a placebo. All rinses were supervised by registered dental hygienists during these 21-day studies. The subjects were divided into five groups of eight individuals each and were instructed to refrain from oral hygiene during the 21 days. Although the sanguinarine, Listerine, and cetylpyridinium

chloride inhibited plaque formation to some extent, they did not prevent gingivitis significantly more than the placebo. The chlorhexidine, however, maintained the preexperimental gingival index scores throughout the 21 days. Unfortunately, all of the antiseptics demonstrated higher discoloration index scores than the placebo. As can be seen in Fig. 11-12C, chlorhexidine had the second highest discoloration score of the four agents. Not surprisingly, studies have shown improvement in plaque and gingivitis when antiseptic rinses are used in conjunction with dentifrices when compared with dentifrice use alone.[59,60]

Listerine has one of the highest alcohol contents of any mouthwash, approximately 25%. The alcohol content of some mouthwashes has been the cause of some concern. Although the development of oral and pharyngeal cancer with long-term mouthwash use has been investigated, alcohol intoxication is more relevant to pediatric dentistry. In addition, the relationship of alcohol-containing mouthwashes to oral carcinomas is equivocal. Alcohol intoxication of children and adolescents from mouthwashes is a concern because of the products' availability. Most parents do not recognize the potential harm from these rinses. Selbst and associates reported the case of a 4-year-old boy who died after consuming approximately 12 oz of a 10% alcohol mouthwash.[61] They urge for stronger legislation that would restrict the level of alcohol in substances that might be available to children and for continued education of practitioners and parents regarding the potential lethality of most mouthwashes so that accidental ingestions are prevented. One consumer advocacy group states that it is inconsistent for cough and cold products with 12% alcohol to have child-resistant tops whereas some mouthwashes with an even higher alcohol content have designer shot-glass tops. The ADA Council on Dental Therapeutics requires any mouthrinses that carry the ADA seal of acceptance and contain more than 5% ethyl alcohol to be packaged in bottles with child-resistant caps.

Chitosans are another cationic antimicrobial finding their way into oral health care. They are derived from the shells of shrimp and other crustaceans and appear to reduce biofilm viability.[62]

A few comments regarding the use of fluoride as a halogen antiseptic plaque control agent are appropriate here, although its use in dentistry is discussed in other portions of the text. The fluoride ion inhibits carbohydrate use of oral organisms by blocking enzymes involved in the glycolytic pathway; however, at preventive-use levels it probably does not alter the plaque ecosystem. As mentioned earlier, stannous fluoride can produce reductions in plaque and gingivitis scores approaching those of chlorhexidine, but this effect is caused by the tin content of this salt, not the fluoride content. It is interesting to note that two antiseptic agents, chlorhexidine and triclosan, have been incorporated into dentifrice formulations.

ENZYMES, PLAQUE-MODIFYING AGENTS, AND PLAQUE ATTACHMENT INTERFERENCE AGENTS

Enzyme systems intended to alter plaque architecture and adherence, as well as enzymes designed to generate antibacterial products, have been investigated. However,

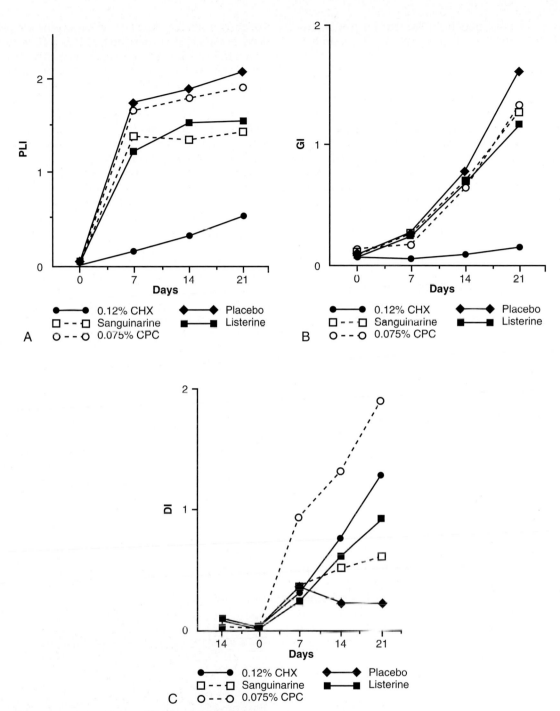

Figure 11-12 Mean indices in five groups of eight individuals refraining from oral hygiene for 21 days rinsing with either 0.12% chlorhexidine digluconate (CHX), 0.075% cetylpyridinium chloride (CPC), Listerine, sanguinarine, or placebo. **A,** Mean plaque index (PLI). **B,** Mean gingival index (GI). **C,** Mean discoloration index (DI). (From Lang NP, Brecx MC. Chlorhexidine digluconate: An agent for chemical plaque control and prevention of gingival inflammation. J Periodontal Res 1986;16[Suppl 21]:74-89.)

problems associated with the long-term stability of enzyme molecules in environments with potentially high concentrations of alcohol or surfactants have yet to be addressed. The use of urea peroxide as a plaque-modifying agent has been investigated because of its increased stability over hydrogen peroxide and the protein denaturation effect of urea. Only limited success has been demonstrated.

The use of agents designed to interfere with the initial adherence of bacteria to the salivary pellicle or the subsequent accumulation by growth and interbacterial adherence seems encouraging. Delmopinol, derived from orpholinoethanol, exerts its affects by binding to salivary proteins and altering the cohesiveness and adhesiveness properties of the films formed.

Although these areas may hold promise for future chemotherapeutic control of plaque, additional research is needed.

SUGAR SUBSTITUTES

The use of sugar substitutes such as xylitol, mannitol, sucralose, and aspartame has been advocated. Although Park and colleagues have shown that sugar substitutes can have a positive influence on plaque pH, the intrinsic antiplaque activity is much lower than that of other plaque control agents.[63] These agents have been suggested for use in chewing gum to decrease plaque accumulation and pH. Advocating the use of chewing gum as a preventive technique is not without controversy, however. Hoerman and colleagues demonstrated that in a no-oral-hygiene environment, plaque accumulation was lower when gum with sucrose or sorbitol was chewed than when gum was not chewed.[64] In addition, Isokangas and associates carried out a 2-year study of 11- and 12-year-old children with moderate and decreasing caries prevalence.[65] They demonstrated that the combination of xylitol gum chewing and fluoride use resulted in a significantly lower incidence of caries than fluoride use alone. Continued research into the use of sugar substitutes as plaque control agents is needed.

In closing this section, one final comment is in order. Because of conflicting results published on the effectiveness of the commercially available prebrushing rinse containing sodium benzoate, it is not included in the list of chemotherapeutic plaque control agents. In addition, it is not accepted by the ADA. O'Mullane suggests that the positive results found for this prebrushing rinse may stem purely from the advantage of rinsing with water before brushing.[66] Indeed, an in vitro study by Jakober and Perritt supports this idea.[67] They demonstrated that brushing with hot water (40°C to 43°C) was more efficient at removing simulated plaque on ceramic tiles than brushing alone or brushing with toothpaste. They also showed that flowing hot water was more effective at removing the simulated plaque than flowing cold water (30°C to 35°C). The idea of using water to help remove plaque is not new. The "swish-and-swallow" method of removing material from the mouth immediately after eating in circumstances where brushing is impractical has been advocated for a long time. Ciancio recommends that, when a product is selected for a patient, consideration be given to necessity, efficacy, adverse effects, and cost effectiveness.[68]

AGE-SPECIFIC HOME ORAL HYGIENE INSTRUCTIONS

The appropriateness and effectiveness of home oral hygiene procedures change throughout childhood. Specific age-related home oral hygiene recommendations are described in the following sections. It is necessary to involve the parent at some level of the oral hygiene procedure for each of the age categories.

PRENATAL COUNSELING

The best time to begin counseling parents and establishing a child's dental preventive program is actually before the birth of the child. It is beneficial to begin at this time

for numerous reasons. For an expectant couple, particularly if the child is their first, this is a time in their lives when they are most receptive to preventive health recommendations. These parents-to-be become acutely aware of their child's dependence on them for all of the child's nurturing and health care needs. Parents have a strong instinct to provide the best that they can for the child. Counseling them on their own hygiene habits and the effect they can have on their children as role models will aid in improving both the parents' and child's oral health. Discussing pregnancy gingivitis with the mother-to-be and dispelling some of the myths about childbirth and dental health can be beneficial. In addition, a review of infant dental care is useful for the expectant parents.

INFANTS (0 TO 1 YEAR OLD)

It is important that a few basic home oral hygiene procedures for the child begin during the first year of life. There is general agreement that plaque removal activities should begin on eruption of the first primary teeth. Some practitioners recommend cleaning and massaging of the gums before this to help in establishing a healthy oral flora and to aid in teething. This early cleaning must be done totally by the parent. It can be accomplished by wrapping a moistened gauze square or washcloth around the finger and gently massaging the teeth and gingival tissues. The child can be positioned in numerous ways during this procedure, but cradling the child with one arm while massaging the teeth with the hand of the other may be the simplest and provides the infant with a strong sense of security (Fig. 11-13). This procedure should be performed once daily. Generally, other plaque removal techniques are not necessary. The introduction of a moistened, soft-bristled, child- or infant-sized toothbrush during this age is advisable only if the parent feels comfortable using the brush. The use of a dentifrice is neither necessary nor advised as the foaming action of the paste tends to be objectionable to the infant. Because fluoride

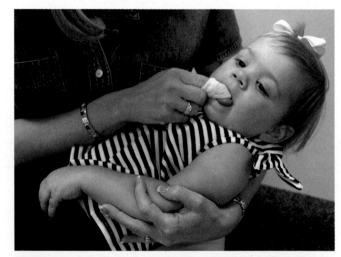

Figure 11-13 Arm-cradled position of child for effective cleansing of the oral cavity. This figure shows the use of a gauze square for wiping the child's dentition and gingival tissues.

ingestion is possible, however, as mentioned earlier, use of a nonfluoridated tooth and gum cleanser may be beneficial.

The child's first visit to the dentist should take place during this period. The American Academy of Pediatric Dentistry recommends that parents or caregivers establish a dental home for infants by 12 months of age.[69] When the child has special dental needs, such as medical problems or trauma, this visit can be sooner. Several objectives are accomplished at this visit. Certainly, instruction of the parents in the use of the oral hygiene practices mentioned herein is necessary. In addition, an infant dental examination and fluoride status review should be accomplished, dietary issues related to nursing and bottle caries as well as other health concerns should be addressed, anticipatory guidance should be provided, and caries risk assessment should be accomplished. These subjects are discussed in more detail in other sections of this text. These first dental visits are also a time for the child to become familiar with the dental environment and the dental staff and the dentist, which makes any future dental treatment less anxiety provoking.

TODDLERS (1 TO 3 YEARS OLD)

During toddlerhood, the toothbrush should be introduced into the plaque removal procedure if this was not accomplished previously. Because of the inability of children in this age group to expectorate and because of the potential for fluoride ingestion, careful and minimal (a "smear" of toothpaste on the brush) introduction of fluoridated dentifrice can be used in 2- and 3-year-olds. Most children enjoy imitating their parents and will readily practice toothbrushing. Adequate plaque removal is not usually accomplished by the child alone, however. Although the child should be encouraged to begin rudimentary brushing, the parent remains the primary caregiver in these hygiene procedures. The use of additional instruments for plaque control is generally unnecessary, although flossing may be needed if any interproximal contacts are closed. The use of a flossing aid may also be indicated.

Positioning of the child and parent is again important. Although most children enjoy brushing their own teeth, many are resistant to allowing anyone else to do the brushing. Several positions can be used by the parent, but the lap-to-lap position, as shown in Fig. 11-14, allows one adult to control the child's body movements while the other adult brushes the teeth. Notice how the child's arms and legs are controlled with the hands and elbows of the adult responsible for body movements. The parents should be encouraged to make this a special time for the child and to praise the child as much as possible. For single-parent households, a one-adult position often becomes necessary. In this situation the parent sits on the floor with his or her legs stretched out in front and the child is positioned between the legs. The child's head is placed between the thighs of the parent, with the child's arms and legs carefully controlled by the legs of the parent. This position is a little awkward, but for a young child resistant to oral hygiene, it does allow these procedures to be accomplished.

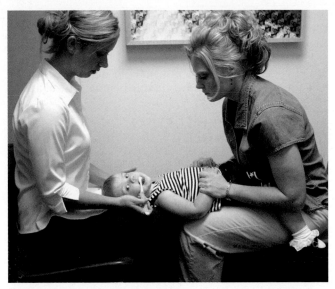

Figure 11-14 Lap-to-lap position of child. Two adults sit with knees touching, using their laps as a table on which to rest the child. The adult on the right holds the child's legs and arms while the adult on the left performs the oral hygiene procedures.

PRESCHOOLERS (3 TO 6 YEARS OLD)

Although children in the preschool age range begin to demonstrate significant improvements in their ability to manipulate the toothbrush, it is still the responsibility of the parent to be the primary provider of oral hygiene procedures. All too often, parents of these children feel that the child has adequately achieved the skills necessary to clean the teeth. It is important to stress to the parents that they must continue to brush their child's teeth. Although fluoride ingestion remains a concern for this age group, during this time, most children develop the skills to expectorate toothpaste adequately. Until this occurs, it is important for parents to use only a pea-sized amount of toothpaste on the child's brush. In addition, it is during this age that flossing is most likely to begin. As mentioned previously, if the interproximal contacts are closed, the parent must begin flossing procedures. In the primary dentition, the posterior contacts may be the only areas where flossing is needed. The closure of the spaces between the primary molars tends to occur somewhere near the start of this age range. If any interproximal area has tooth-to-tooth contact, however, daily flossing of that area becomes necessary.

Proper positioning of the child continues to be useful for this age group in performing oral hygiene. One method advocated is that in which the parent stands behind the child and both face the same direction. The child rests his or her head back into the parent's nondominant arm. With the hand of this arm the cheeks can be retracted, and the other hand is used to brush. This position is also appropriate for flossing. To brush their child's teeth, many parents use a frontal approach, which is awkward and provides little head support. This positioning technique should be discouraged.

It is also during this stage that fluoride gels and rinses for home use may be introduced. Because of the risk of ingestion, however, these agents should be employed in small quantities and their use should be limited to those patients demonstrating a moderate to high risk of caries. The use of other chemotherapeutic plaque control agents is generally not recommended.

SCHOOL-AGED CHILDREN (6 TO 12 YEARS OLD)

The 6- to 12-year stage is marked by acceptance of increasing responsibilities by the children. The need to assume responsibility for homework and household chores tends to occur during this time. In addition, the child can begin to assume more responsibility for oral hygiene. Parental involvement is still needed. However, instead of performing the oral hygiene, parents can switch to active supervision. By the second half of this stage, most children can provide their basic oral hygiene (brushing and flossing). Parents may find they only need to brush or floss their child's teeth in certain difficult-to-reach areas of the mouth or if there is a compliance problem. Parents do need to actively inspect their child's teeth for cleanliness on a regular basis. One helpful adjunct is the use of a disclosing agent. After the child has brushed, flossed, and used the disclosing agent on his or her teeth, the parent can easily visualize any remaining plaque and assist the child in removing it.

By this age, ingestion of fluoridated materials, such as dentifrices, gels, or rinses, is not as pronounced a concern because these children are able to expectorate well. Certainly the use of fluoridated dentifrices is essential; however, fluoridated gels and rinses can be reserved for those children at risk for caries. In addition, the use of chlorhexidine or Listerine can be introduced to those at risk for periodontal disease and caries, although some children who might benefit from these chemotherapeutic agents will find their use objectionable.

Because early treatment of malocclusions has increased, this age group has undergone more of this treatment and experienced its accompanying increased risk for caries and periodontal disease. Special attention to oral hygiene is necessary for these patients. Increased frequency and adequacy of brushing and flossing becomes necessary. Although fluoridated dentifrices provide cost-efficient fluoride exposure, the use of fluoridated gels or rinses is strongly encouraged. In addition, as with other patients at risk for caries and periodontal disease, the use of chemotherapeutic agents and adjuncts such as oral irrigators is recommended. Feil and colleagues published an interesting study on the intentional use if the Hawthorne effect to improve oral hygiene compliance in orthodontic patients.[70] Forty orthodontic adolescent patients with histories of poor oral hygiene were assigned to one of two groups. The experimental subjects were presented with a situation that stimulated participation in an experiment, whereas the control subjects had no knowledge of study participation. Although there were no statistically significant differences between the control and the experimental group at baseline, the experimental group showed significantly lower plaque scores at 3 months and again at 6 months. The experimental subjects had significantly improved oral hygiene, which suggests that the Hawthorne effect (participating in an "experimental study") caused the adolescent patients to pay more attention to oral hygiene and therefore to do a better job.

ADOLESCENTS (12 TO 19 YEARS OLD)

Although the adolescent patient usually has developed the skills for adequate oral hygiene procedures, compliance is a major problem during this age period. Griffen and Goepferd point out that motivating an adolescent to assume responsibility for personal oral hygiene may be complicated by reactions of rebellion against external authority and some incapacity to appreciate long-term consequences.[71] Macgregor and Balding's survey of 4075 children 14 years old suggests a positive relationship between self-esteem and toothbrushing behavior and motivation for mouth care in adolescents.[72] Because self-esteem declines between the ages of 11 and 14 and then shows a gradual improvement into adulthood, it is not hard to understand why plaque control in these patients declines. In addition, poor dietary habits and pubertal hormonal changes increase adolescents' risk for caries and gingival inflammation.

Therefore, it is important for practitioners and parents to continually help and guide adolescents as they progress through this difficult stage. Stressing their increased responsibility as young adults without appearing authoritarian can aid them in accepting their new role. The parents must be ready to adapt to their child's changing personality and to continue to reinforce the need for oral health care and hygiene. Increasing adolescents' knowledge regarding plaque control and oral diseases, as well as appealing to their appearance, may also help in motivating these patients.

IN-OFFICE ORAL HYGIENE PROGRAMS

Preventive dentistry is the foundation on which all oral health care must be built. In establishing this foundation for their patients, practitioners must first look at themselves and their office environment. Each practice must establish a preventive philosophy that is evident throughout the patient's encounter with the dental office. This means that the dentist, the staff, and the practice systems and design must reflect this concept. All staff members must have a personal understanding and appreciation of the importance of this basic concept. This must be evident from their own personal hygiene and in their routine interactions with patients.

After this introspective look and adjustment, the practitioner can turn to the patient directly. Ong discusses several basic concepts for developing a plaque control program in the dental office.[73] Gathering information from the child and parent is necessary for the practitioner to understand what their concerns are and to let them know that he or she understands these concerns. By discussing the patient's and parents' needs, and listening to and observing their reactions, the practitioner can gauge their readiness to begin the plaque control program. Dental education of the parent and child should be accomplished next with tailoring to the patient's individual problem. Describing exactly why oral hygiene is important in the patient's particular case can help with motivation. The information should be delivered in simple terms and with enthusiasm and conviction. It also needs to be conveyed to the child in age-appropriate language.

When specific age-appropriate oral hygiene instructions are given, it is important to be positive and reassuring, not critical. Use phrases like "Let me show you how to improve," rather than saying, "You're doing it all wrong." Be gentle but firm, and enlist the parent and patient's help in the treatment plan and therapy. Setting goals and complimenting achievements will assist in keeping the parent and patient's attitudes positive. It is very useful to be open to parental and patient feedback regarding their priorities and progress. As with many long-term commitments, cyclic participation can be expected and accepted to a certain extent. However, the parents and patient must know the consequences of neglect. Finally, establishment of a regular maintenance schedule is imperative. Along with prophylaxis, reinstruction and remotivation in the plaque control program is a necessary element for success. Recare intervals should be personalized to the individual patient's needs, with consideration of factors such as caries and periodontal disease risk; restorative, orthodontic, and prosthetic concerns; and individual patient and parental dental education and skill levels. It is the responsibility of every dental practitioner to make oral hygiene and prevention the core of his or her practice. By listening to, educating, adapting to, and motivating our patients and their parents, we can make our preventive practices successful and enjoyable.

REFERENCES

1. McDonald RE. Pediatrics allied with pedodontics, *Pediatr Herald* 1(5):1, 1960.
2. Marsh PD. The significance of maintaining the stability of the natural microflora of the mouth, *Br Dent J* 171(6):174-177, 1991.
3. Miller WD. *Microorganisms of the human mouth.* Philadelphia, 1890, SS White Dental Manufacturing.
4. Keyes PH. The infectious and transmissible nature of experimental dental caries, *Arch Oral Biol* 1:304-320, 1960.
5. Löe H, Theilade E, Jensen SB. Experimental gingivitis in man, *J Periodontol* 35:177-187, 1965.
6. Moore WE. Microbiology of periodontal disease, *J Periodontal Res* 22:335-341, 1987.
7. Aas JA, et al. Defining the normal bacterial flora of the oral cavity, *J Clin Microbiol* 43:5721-5732, 2005.
8. Kuramitsu HK, et al. Interspecies interactions with oral microbial communities, *Microbiol Mol Biol Rev* 71:653-670, 2007.
9. Kolenbrander PE. Oral microbial communities: biofilms, interactions, and genetic systems, *Annu Rev Microbiol* 54:413-437, 2000.
10. Kolenbrander PE, et al. Bacterial interactions and successions during plaque development, *Periodontology* 2000 42:47-79, 2006.
11. Balakrishnan M, Simmonds RS, Tagg JR. Dental caries is a preventable infectious disease, *Aust Dent J* 45(4):235-245, 2000.
12. Park KK, Matis BA, Christen AG. Choosing an effective toothbrush, *Clin Prev Dent* 7(4):5-10, 1985.
13. Updyke JR. A new handle for a child's toothbrush, *J Dent Child* 46:123-125, 1979.
14. Dean DH. Toothbrushes with graduated wear: correlation with in vitro cleansing performance, *Clin Prev Dent* 213(4):25-30, 1991.
15. Corby PM, et al. Treatment outcomes of dental flossing in twins: Molecular analysis of the interproximal microflora, *J Periodontal* 79(8):1426-1433, 2008.
16. Mauriello AM, et al. Effectiveness of three interproximal cleaning devices, *Clin Prev Dent* 9(3):18-22, 1987.
17. Chen MS, Rubinson L. Preventive dental behavior in families: A national survey, *J Am Dent Assoc* 105:43-46, 1982.
18. Bass CC. An effective method of personal oral hygiene. Part II, *J La State Med Soc* 106:100, 1954.
19. Carr MP, et al. Education of floss types for interproximal plaque removal, *Am J Dent* 13(4):212-214, 2000.
20. Kerlinger FN. *Foundations of behavioral research, educational and psychological injury.* New York, 1965, Holt, Rinehart and Winston.
21. Ho HP, Niederman R. Effectiveness of the Sonicare toothbrush on reduction of plaque, gingivitis, probing pocket depth and subgingival bacteria in adolescent orthodontic patients, *J Clin Dent* 8:15-19, 1997.
22. Nowak AJ, et al. A practice based study of a children's power toothbrush: efficiency and acceptance, *Compendium* 23(Suppl 2):25-32, 2002.
23. Grossman E, Proskin H. A comparison of the efficacy and safety of an electric and a manual children's toothbrush. *J Am Dent Assoc* 128:469-474, 1997.
24. Jongenelis AP, Wiedemann W. A comparison of plaque removal effectiveness of an electric versus a manual toothbrush in children, *J Dent Child* 64:176-182, 1997.
25. Heanue M, et al. Manual versus powered toothbrushing for oral health (Cochrane Review). The Cochrane Library, Issue 1, 2003.
26. American Dental Association, Council on Scientific Affairs. Toothbrushes Acceptance Program Guidelines, Chicago, 2006, American Dental Association.
27. Gordon JM, Frascella JA, Reardon RC. A clinical study of the safety and efficacy of a novel electric interdental cleaning device, *J Clin Dent* 7:70-73, 1996.
28. Adair SM, Picitelli WP, McKnight-Hanes C. Comparison of the use of a child and an adult dentifrice by a sample of preschool children, *Pediatr Dent* 19:99-103, 1997.
29. Levy SM, Zarei-M Z. Evaluation of fluoride exposures in children, *J Dent Child* 58:467-473, 1991.
30. Simard PL, et al. Ingestion of fluoride from dentifrices by children aged 12 to 24 months, *Clin Pediatr* 30:614-617, 1991.
31. Lim LP, et al. A comparison of four techniques for clinical detection of early plaque formed during different dietary regimes, *J Clin Periodontol* 13:658-665, 1986.
32. Baab DA, Broadwell AH, Williams BL. A comparison of anti-microbial activity of four disclosant dyes, *J Dent Res* 62:837-841, 1983.
33. Anaise JZ. The toothbrush in plaque removal, *J Dent Child* 42:186-189, 1975.
34. McClure DB. A comparison of toothbrushing technics for the preschool child, *J Dent Child* 33:205-210, 1966.
35. Sangnes G, Zachrisson B, Gjermo P. Effectiveness of vertical and horizontal brushing techniques in plaque removal, *J Dent Child* 39:94-97, 1972.
36. Rugg-Gunn AJ, Macgregor ID. A survey of toothbrushing behavior in children and young adults, *J Periodontal Res* 13:382-389, 1978.
37. Starkey P. Instructions to parents for brushing the child's teeth, *J Dent Child* 28:42-47, 1961.

38. Rodrigues CR, et al. The effect of training on the ability of children to use dental floss, *J Dent Child* 63:39-41, 1996.

39. Terhune JA. Predicting the readiness of elementary school children to learn an effective dental flossing technique, *J Am Dent Assoc* 86:1332-1336, 1973.

40. Mescher KD, Brine P, Biller I. Ability of elementary school children to perform sulcular toothbrushing as related to their hand function ability, *Pediatr Dent* 2:31-36, 1980.

41. Preisch JW. The relationship between visual motor integration and oral hygiene in children. Master's thesis. Bloomington, Indiana, Indiana University, 1984.

42. Löe H. How frequently must patients carry out effective oral hygiene procedures in order to maintain gingival health? *J Periodontol* 42:312-313, 1971.

43. Lang NP, et al. Toothbrushing frequency as it relates to plaque development and gingival health, *J Periodontol* 44:396-405, 1973.

44. Hodges CA, Bianco JG, Cancro LP. The removal of dental plaque under timed intervals of toothbrushing, *J Dent Res* 60:425, 1981 (abstract 460)

45. van der Ouderaa FJ. Anti-plaque agents: rationale and prospects for prevention of gingivitis and periodontal disease, *J Clin Periodontol* 18:447-454, 1991.

46. Mandel ID. Chemotherapeutic agents for controlling plaque and gingivitis, *J Clin Periodontol* 15:488-498, 1988.

47. Grossman E, et al. Six-month study of the effects of a chlorhexidine mouthrinse on gingivitis in adults, *J Periodontal Res* 16(Suppl 21):33-43, 1986.

48. Lang NP, et al. Effects of supervised chlorhexidine mouthrinses in children, *J Periodontal Res* 17:101-111, 1982.

49. Burtner AP, et al. Effects of chlorhexidine spray on plaque and gingival health in institutionalized persons with mental retardation, *Spec Care Dentist* 11(3):97-100, 1991.

50. Chikte UM, et al. Evaluation of stannous fluoride and chlorhexidine sprays on plaque and gingivitis in handicapped children, *J Clin Periodontol* 18:281-286, 1991.

51. Ferretti GA, et al. Control of oral mucositis and candidiasis in marrow transplantation: a prospective, double-blind trial of chlorhexidine gluconate oral rinse, *Bone Marrow Transplant* 3:483-493, 1988.

52. Raether D, et al. Effectiveness of oral chlorhexidine for reducing stomatitis in a pediatric bone marrow transplant population, *Pediatr Dent* 11:37-42, 1989.

53. Fennis-le YL, et al. Effect of 6-month application of chlorhexidine varnish on evidence of occlusal caries in permanent molars: a three-year study, *J Dent* 26:233-238, 1998.

54. Petersson LG, et al. Effect of semi-annual applications of a chlorhexidine/fluoride varnish mixture on approximal caries incidence in schoolchildren: a three-year radiographic study, *Eur J Oral Sci* 106:623-627, 1998.

55. Autio-Gold J. The role of chlorhexidine in caries prevention, *Oper Dent* 33(6):710-716, 2008.

56. Clark MJ, et al. The effect of 3 mouthrinses on plaque and gingivitis development, *J Clin Periodontol* 19:19-23, 1992.

57. Brownstone BM, et al. Efficacy of Listerine, Meridol, and chlorhexidine mouthrinses as supplements to regular tooth-cleaning measures, *J Clin Periodontol* 19:202-207, 1992.

58. Lang NP, Brecx MC. Chlorhexidine digluconate: an agent for chemical plaque control and prevention of gingival inflammation, *J Periodontal Res* 16(Suppl 21):74-89, 1986.

59. Sharma N, et al. Adjunctive benefit of an essential oil-containing mouthrinse in reducing plaque and gingivitis in patients who brush and floss regularly: a six-month study, *J Am Dent Assoc* 135(4):496-504, 2004.

60. White DJ, Barker ML, Klukowska M. In vivo antiplaque efficacy of combined antimicrobial dentifrice and rinse hygiene regimens, *Am J Dent* 21(3):189-196, 2008.

61. Selbst AM, DeMaio JG, Boenning D. Mouthwash poisoning, *Clin Pediatr* 24:162-163, 1985.

62. Busscher HJ, et al. Influence of a chitosan on oral bacterial adhesion and growth in vitro, *Eur J Oral Sci* 116(5):493-495, 2008.

63. Park K, et al. Comparison of plaque pH response from a variety of sweeteners. J Dent Res 1992;71(AADR Abstract):269.

64. Hoerman KC, et al. Effect of gum chewing on plaque accumulation, *J Clin Dent* 2(1):17-21, 1990.

65. Isokangas P, et al. Xylitol chewing gum in caries prevention: a field study in children, *J Am Dent Assoc* 117:315-320, 1988.

66. O'Mullane D. New agents in the chemical control of plaque and gingivitis: reaction paper, *J Dent Res* 71: 1455-1456, 1992.

67. Jakober RL, Perritt AM. Comparative evaluation of test parameters in plaque removal: a preliminary report, *Clin Prev Dent* 13(2):29-31, 1991.

68. Ciancio SG. Agents for the management of plaque and gingivitis, *J Dent Res* 71:1450-1454, 1992.

69. American Academy of Pediatric Dentistry. *Guideline on Infant Oral Health Care, Reference Manual*. Chicago, 2004, Author.

70. Feil PH, et al. Intentional use of the Hawthorne effect to improve oral hygiene compliance in orthodontic patients, *J Dent Educ* 66(10):1129-1135, 2002.

71. Griffen AL, Goepferd SJ. Preventive oral health care for the infant, child, and adolescent, *Pediatr Clin North Am* 38(5):1209-1226, 1991.

72. Macgregor ID, Balding JW. Self-esteem as a predictor of toothbrushing behavior in young adolescents, *J Clin Periodontol* 18:312-316, 1991.

73. Ong G. Practical strategies for a plaque-control program, *Clin Prev Dent* 13(3):8-11, 1991.

SUGGESTED READINGS

Brightman LJ, et al. The effects of a 0.12% chlorhexidine gluconate mouthrinse on orthodontic patients aged 11 through 17 with established gingivitis, *Am J Orthod Dentofacial Orthop* 100:324-329, 1991.

Coontz EJ. The effectiveness of a new oral hygiene device on plaque removal, *Quintessence Int* 7:739-742, 1983.

de la Rosa M, Sturzenberger OP, Moore DJ. The use of chlorhexidine in the management of gingivitis in children, *J Periodontol* 59:387-389, 1988.

Glass RT. The infected toothbrush, the infected denture, and transmission of disease: a review, *Compendium* 8:592-598, 1992.

Hancock E, Nowell D. Preventive strategies and supportive treatment, *Periodontology* 2000 25:59-76, 2001.

Kallio PJ. Health promotion and behavioral approaches in the prevention of periodontal disease in children and adolescents, *Periodontology 2000* 26:135-145, 2001.

Kimmelman BB, Tassman GC. Research in designs of children's toothbrushes, *J Dent Child* 27:60-64, 1960.

Loesche WJ. Role of *Streptococcus mutans* in human dental decay, *Microbiol Rev* 50:353-380, 1986.

Pinkham JR. Oral hygiene in children: relationship to age and brushing time, *J Prev Dent* 2(2):28-31, 1975.

Sandham HJ, Nadeau L, Phillips, HI. The effect of chlorhexidine varnish treatment on salivary mutans streptococcal levels in child orthodontic patients, *J Dent Res* 71:32-35, 1992.

Whittaker CJ, Klier CM, Kolenbrander PE. Mechanisms of adhesion by oral bacteria, *Annu Rev Microbiol* 50:513-552, 1996.

CHAPTER 12

Nutritional Considerations for the Pediatric Dental Patient

▲ Laura Romito and James L. McDonald, Jr.

CHAPTER OUTLINE

When the leading causes of death in the United States are tabulated (Table 12-1), the list is headed by heart disease and cancer, with stroke a distant third. However, when evaluating the underlying causes of these diseases, three major lifestyle factors can be identified: tobacco use, a sedentary lifestyle, and inappropriate dietary choices. It has become increasingly apparent that what we eat (and do not eat) is an important factor influencing both the quantity and quality of our lives. The basis of our dietary choices, and thus our nutritional status, is established early in life. It follows that food choices and dietary patterns initiated in childhood can affect our health and well-being at every stage of life. There are many ways in which health professionals can promote the health of their patients. One major way is to educate them regarding the importance of following sound nutritional principles. This chapter focuses on those nutritional factors that have the greatest potential to influence the systemic and oral health of the pediatric dental patient.

It was recognized several decades ago that our health is profoundly affected by our dietary choices; since then, an evolution has occurred in efforts to promote healthy food choices in the United States. In 1977, the Senate Select Committee on Nutrition and Human Needs first published the Dietary Goals for the United States. This was followed in 1979 by *Healthy People: The Surgeon General's Report on Health Promotion and Disease Prevention* and in 1988 with *The Surgeon General's Report on Nutrition and Health*. This latter document concluded that, of the 10 leading causes of death in the United States, half were related to poor dietary choices. In 1990, the U.S. Department of Health and Human Services released *Healthy People 2000*, which outlined goals, including those concerning nutrition, for increasing life span, reducing health disparities, and achieving better access to preventive services for all Americans over the following decade. In January 2000, *Healthy People 2010* was released. Its overall nutritional focus is to promote health and to reduce chronic disease associated with diet and weight. Chapter 19 of this report discusses a number of these objectives, many of which are related to pediatric nutrition and are summarized in Table 12-2. The table includes both the initial target level for each objective and the progress made toward reaching each of these targets after a mid-decade review. Other nutrition-related objectives for children include reducing sodium consumption, increasing calcium intake, and reducing iron-deficiency anemia. The Midcourse Review noted that none of the objectives related to nutrition and overweight met or exceeded their targets. However, objectives concerning food security (19-18) and iron deficiency (19-12) made progress toward their targets. No significant progress was noted on some objectives, whereas others, such as prevalence of overweight and obesity among children and adolescents, actually moved further away from their targets.

The *Healthy People 2020* document, which is intended to build on the objectives and goals set in *Healthy People 2010*, is currently being developed. The *Healthy People 2020* objectives will be released in January 2010 along

Table 12-1

Leading Causes of Death in the United States (Final 2005 Data)

Cause	Number of Deaths
Heart disease	652,091
Cancer	559,312
Stroke	143,579
Chronic lower respiratory disease	130,933
Accidents	117,809
Diabetes	75,119
Alzheimer's disease	71,599
Influenza/pneumonia	63,001
Nephritis, nephritic syndrome, and nephrosis	43,901
Septicemia	34,136

From US Department of Health and Human Services, Centers for Disease Control and Prevention. Natl Vital Stat Rep 2008;56(10).

with guidance for achieving new 10-year targets that reflect assessments of major health risks, public health priorities, and emerging technologies affecting disease prevention and health preparedness in the United States.[1]

The Dietary Guidelines for Americans (the ABCs) promulgated by the U.S. Department of Agriculture (USDA) support the objectives in *Healthy People 2010* and include the following recommendations:

- Aim for fitness.
- Aim for a healthy weight.
- Be physically active each day.
- Build a healthy base.
- Let the Food Guide Pyramid guide your food choices.
- Choose a variety of grains daily, especially whole grains.
- Choose a variety of fruits and vegetables daily.
- Keep food safe to eat.
- Choose sensibly.
- Choose a diet low in saturated fat and cholesterol and moderate in fat.
- Choose beverages and foods so as to moderate your intake of sugars.
- Choose and prepare foods with less salt.
- If you drink alcoholic beverages, do so in moderation.

MYPYRAMID FOOD GUIDANCE SYSTEM

The MyPyramid Food Guidance System is a pictorial representation of the USDA's Daily Food and Physical Activity recommendations. Released in 2005, MyPyramid replaced the nation's previously well-known nutrition education tool, the Food Guide Pyramid (1992). In MyPyramid, daily physical activity is represented by the stairs on the left side of the pyramid. Food groups are represented by the vertical bands, which comprise the body of the pyramid. Bandwidth indicates portion size; the wider the band, the more foods from that group should be consumed. Examples of portions, or serving sizes, are further delineated for each food group. However, in most cases, the serving sizes used in MyPyramid are considerably smaller than the exaggerated portion sizes that many Americans have become accustomed to. In MyPyramid, foods are organized into five major groups and one miscellaneous category. The latter

Table 12-2

Healthy People 2010 Selected Nutritional Goals

Number	Objective	Current	Target
19-3	Reduce the proportion of children and adolescents who are overweight or obese	11%	5%
19-4	Reduce growth restriction among low-income children under 5 years of age	8%	5%
19-5	Increase the proportion of persons aged 2 and older who consume at least two daily servings of fruit	28%	75%
19-6	Increase the proportion of persons aged 2 and older who consume at least three daily servings of vegetables, with at least one third being dark green or deep yellow vegetables	3%	50%
19-7	Increase the proportion of persons aged 2 and older who consume at least six daily servings of grain products, with at least three being whole grains	7%	50%
19-8	Increase the proportion of persons aged 2 and older who consume less than 10% of calories from saturated fat	35%	75%
19-9	Increase the proportion of persons aged 2 and older who consume no more than 30% of calories from fat	33%	75%
19-15	Increase the proportion of children and adolescents age 6-19 whose intake of meals and snacks at schools contributes proportionally to good overall dietary quality	*	*

*No target established.

category includes fats, oils, and sweets, all of which should be consumed sparingly. An individualized nutrition plan based on personal factors such as age, gender, and physical activity, can be developed using the online tools, such as the MyPyramid Menu Planner and the MyPyramid Tracker (http://www.MyPyramid.gov). This website, which contains a host of useful nutrition information for the public and health professionals, also offers a number of food guidance pyramids for special populations, such as pregnant women, vegetarians, and children. The child-friendly version of MyPyramid, called MyPyramid for Kids, is designed to educate children ages 6 to 11 years old about nutrition and to assist them in making appropriate dietary choices (Fig. 12-1).

DIETARY PATTERNS

Myriad national surveys measuring nutritional status and dietary patterns of children and adolescents were conducted from the 1970s through the 1990s. These studies revealed some intriguing trends regarding caloric intake, beverage consumption, dining out, portion sizes, meal patterns and frequency, and school meal participation. Over the past quarter century, the total caloric intake of American children has increased and the dietary patterns of children are reflective of changes seen in the U.S. diet overall.[2] In comparing food intake trends among children ages 6 to 11 years old, over approximately a 20-year period from 1977 through 1998, Enns and colleagues reported increases in consumption of soft drinks, grain products as a whole, grain mixtures (crackers, popcorn, pretzels, corn chips), fried potatoes, noncitrus juices and nectars, cheese, candy, and fruit drinks and ades.[3] Decreases were noted in the intake of milk in general, and whole milk, various vegetables and legumes, beef, pork, and eggs. For any given pyramid group, less than one half of the children consumed the recommended number of servings, and their intakes of discretionary fat and added sugar were much higher than recommended.

Similar findings were reported by Cullen and colleagues, who evaluated the intake of soft drinks, fruit-flavored beverages, and fruits and vegetables by children in grades 4 through 6.[4] Lower parental education level was associated with higher consumption of soft drinks and sweetened beverages, and students who had a high consumption of sweetened beverages reported low fruit and high calorie intakes. Troiano and associates have also reported that beverages contribute 20% to 24% of energy intake among youth aged 2 to 19 years and that soft drinks provide 8% of energy intake among adolescents.[5]

However, recent studies have been inconsistent as to whether the increase in soft drinks and other sweetened beverages has increased obesity risk in children. For example, O'Connor and colleagues found no correlation between body mass index (BMI) of preschool children and their consumption of such beverages. They also found that, although nearly 83% of preschoolers consumed milk, consumption was at levels below recommended amounts. Only 8.3% of the children drank low-fat milk, which is recommended by Dietary Guidelines for Americans for children older than 2 years of age.[6]

Additional trends include an increase in eating out as well as expanded portion sizes in the U.S. marketplace. In examining the changes in dietary intake patterns between 1977 and 1996, Guthrie and colleagues reported that food prepared away from home increased from 18% to 32% of total calories consumed.[7] Both meals and snacks prepared away from home contained more calories per eating event. Food eaten outside the home was also higher in both total and saturated fat on a percentage basis, and contained less dietary fiber, calcium, and iron per calorie. In 2001, Gillis and Bar-Or compared dietary patterns of obese and non-obese youth aged 4 to 16 years in relation to meals eaten away from home. They found a significant correlation between obesity and increased frequency of eating out.[8] Further complicating the situation is that most marketplace portions of foods exceed standard serving sizes by at least a factor of 2 (e.g., bagels and sodas) and sometimes by a factor of 8 (e.g., cookies).[9] Fast-food chains offer larger sizes of hamburgers, sodas, and French fries. The current serving sizes are often two to five times larger than the size originally marketed. These changes in dietary patterns parallel the progressive increase in obesity rates seen in the United States. Based on this information, eating away from home is associated with a compromised quality of nutritional intake and may increase risk for chronic diseases.

Meal patterns and meal frequency have also changed in the last few decades. Breakfast consumption, which has been shown to be important to cognition, school performance, and attendance, has declined significantly in U.S. children and adolescents. Although it is estimated that 10% to 30% of youth skip breakfast, of those who do consume breakfast, about equal numbers eat at home as at school.[10,11] More youth are participating in school meals, such as the School Breakfast Program (SBP) and the National School Lunch Program (NSLP). In 2006, for example, more than 30 million youth in the United States participated in the NSLP daily. These federally funded programs evolved as efforts to assist children in low-income households.

Children from households with incomes at or below the poverty level are eligible for free meals; those with higher incomes may be eligible for reduced price meals.[12] Because school meal programs can have a significant impact on children's health, their ability to meet nutritional quality standards is important. As such, the Physicians Committee for Responsible Medicine (PCRM) evaluates meals served in the NSLP every year and documents changes, improvements, or the lack thereof in the foods offered by schools. They have found that compliance with established nutrition standards varies considerably among school districts countrywide. Many schools continue to offer less than healthful choices, such as hot dogs, cheeseburgers, and other foods high in fat and cholesterol. However, since the PCRM began issuing its "report card" style evaluations of school lunches in 2001, there has been a concerted effort at all levels to improve the nutritional quality of the meals provided by these programs. A 2007 study of NSLP participants in three high schools found that when the program promoted a broad selection of both healthy and less healthy choices,

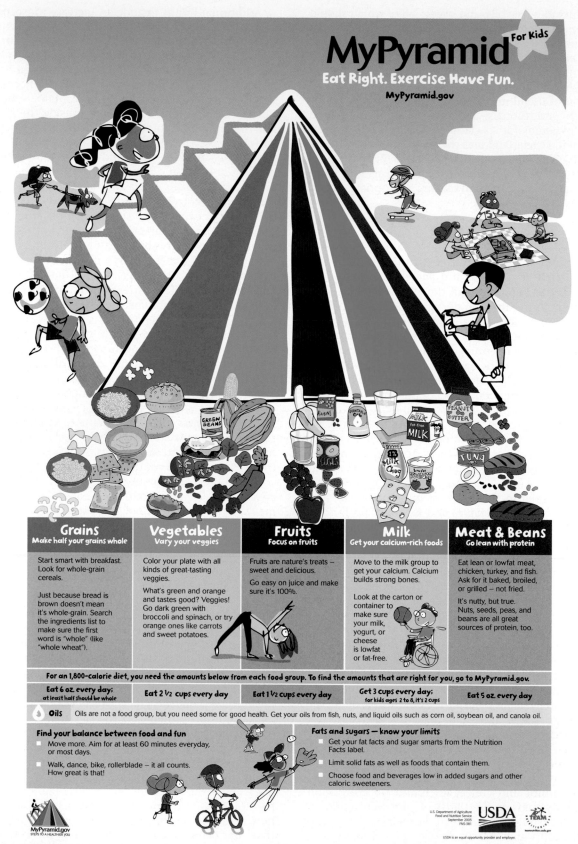

Figure 12-1 USDA MyPyramid for Kids. (From the United States Department of Agriculture; http://www.usda.org.)

consumption of nutritious foods increased; however, consumption of foods with minimal nutritional value increased even more. The investigators concluded that the sale of less nutritious foods should be closely regulated.[13]

Cullen and colleagues examined the effect of the implementation of a public nutrition policy in Texas on the lunches of middle school children. Improvements in dietary intake after the policy change led investigators to conclude that statewide nutrition policy changes can have a positive impact on school lunch programs.[14] Despite the quality issues surrounding the national school meal programs, the American Dietetic Association reported that children who participated in the School Breakfast Program had higher intakes of many vitamins and minerals compared to those who consumed breakfast at home or skip breakfast entirely.[15,16]

Meal frequency, primarily via snacking, has also increased significantly among U.S. children. Jahns and colleagues examined the prevalence of snacking from 1977 to 1996 in individuals 2 to 18 years of age. They found that snacking, which now accounts for a significant portion of total calories and macronutrients consumed relative to 30 years ago, increased amongst all age groups. Compared with that of regular meals, the nutritional content of snacks decreased in calcium and increased in energy density and fat calories.[17] Sebastian and associates assessed the impact of snacking on nutrient intake and the ability to meet MyPyramid recommendations in a population of 12- to 19-year-olds. Results demonstrated that, as snacking frequency increased, total energy increased, primarily due to the amount of refined carbohydrates. One third of all oil was consumed in snacks; chips were a major contributor. Snacking improved intakes of vitamins C, A, and E, and increased fruit consumption, which improved the likelihood of meeting fruit recommendations. Less healthful outcomes were increased intakes of discretionary calories and added sugars, primarily via soft drinks, via fruit drinks and ades.[18] Some snacks can be purchased at school, for example, from vending machines; these offerings usually contain little nutritional value and are highly cariogenic. The widespread use of vending contracts that permit the targeted marketing of soft drinks and other nonnutritious foods to children and teens has come under scrutiny in recent years by many health organizations, including the American Dental Association.

MALNUTRITION AND FOOD INSECURITY

Malnutrition includes undernutrition (inadequate intake of nutrients that potentially leads to deficiency diseases) and overnutrition (excessive dietary intake of energy, fat, or cholesterol that predisposes individuals to chronic diseases). While the latter excessive consumption pattern may be quantitatively more relevant to overall mortality and morbidity rates in contemporary U.S. society than are nutrient deficiencies, malnutrition from dietary insufficiency has not been eradicated.

Chronic malnutrition as measured by low weight for age and low growth rates has decreased; some of this decline has been attributed to better nutrition. Today, the proportion of mothers receiving early prenatal care is at a record high. Data released in 2004 by the U.S. Department of Health and Human Services reported that as of 2002, the rate at which infants die before their first birthday was 7 deaths per 1000 live births. Even so, the U.S. infant mortality rate continues to rank among the highest of the industrialized nations. In addition, African-American babies have a mortality rate that is more than double that of white children.

It is estimated that more than 13 million children in the United States are living below the poverty level, and some estimates indicate that approximately 10% suffer to some degree from clinical malnutrition.[19] Knol and colleagues evaluated the dietary patterns of low-income children 2 to 3 years of age and 4 to 8 years of age and found that the predominant eating patterns in both groups were not indicative of a balanced diet as described by national recommendations. Rather, the diets mimicked those of older adults with high intakes of added sugars and discretionary fats as a percentage of daily calories.[20] Thus children of low socioeconomic status are at risk for the long-term consequences of malnutrition.

The concept of food security evolved in the 1990s to better define and measure access to foods by individuals and households. Food security implies the ready availability of adequate and safe foods, whereas food insecurity is having "limited or uncertain availability of nutritionally adequate and safe foods or limited or uncertain ability to acquire acceptable foods in socially acceptable ways." Hunger refers to the "uneasy or painful sensation caused by lack of food." Thus while food insecurity is a household level social and economic condition, hunger is an individual-level physiological condition that may be a consequence of food insecurity. Likewise, malnutrition is a potential, but not inevitable, result of food insecurity.[21-23]

Data on the food security of US households is obtained by the USDA from federally sponsored national surveys. The food security status of each household is categorized according to the following labels:

High food security: Households had no problems, or anxiety about, consistently accessing adequate food.

Marginal food security: Households had problems at times, or anxiety about, accessing adequate food, but the quality, variety, and quantity of their food intake were not substantially reduced.

Low food security: Households reduced the quality, variety, and desirability of their diets, but the quantity of food intake and normal eating patterns were not substantially disrupted.

Very low food security: At times during the year, eating patterns of one or more household members were disrupted and food intake reduced because the household lacked money and other resources for food.

The USDA reported that in 2006, 89.1% of U.S. households were food secure; however, 6.9 % of households reported low and 4% reported very low food security. Thus although nearly 11% of U.S. households are affected, this represents a decrease from the 16.1% of households reported to be food insecure in 2001.[24]

Prevalence of food insecurity was greater in metropolitan areas, southern and southwestern states, poor households, households with children headed by a single woman, and African-American and Hispanic households. In 2006, 35.5 million people, including 12.6 million children, lived in food-insecure households.[25]

Because food insecure households are eligible to receive assistance from federally funded programs such as the Food Stamp Program, research has been ongoing to understand the impact these programs have on food insecurity and nutrition. In addition, studies seek to clarify the relationships between food insecurity and nutritional status, health risks, and reduced quality of life, especially in children. Rose and Oliveira found that in adult women and older adults, food insecurity was associated with reduced intake of calories and nutrients; however, household food insufficiency was not significantly associated with low intakes among preschoolers.[26] Likewise, a USDA Economic Research Service report noted that even in conditions of very low food insecurity, children are usually shielded from substantial reductions in food. It is believed that this occurs as a result of the adults sacrificing their own food intake for that of the children in the household.[24] Nevertheless, research has linked food insecurity with increased developmental risk and poor health outcomes; however, an explanation for the so-called "obesity paradox" remains elusive.[27,28] This phenomenon, which describes an association between hunger and obesity, was first proposed by Dietz in 1995.[29] One hypothesis for this finding of some studies is that individuals overeat when food is available to compensate for times when food is scarce. The scientific literature is inconsistent in finding a clear association between food insecurity and overweight in children and adolescents.[30-33] Clearly, more research is needed in this area to improve understanding of these relationships.

PEDIATRIC UNDERNUTRITION

Infants and young children whose weight curve has fallen 20% below the ideal weight for their height from a previously established growth rate are described as *failure to thrive*. Typically, in mild chronic undernutrition, weight loss with normal height and head circumference is observed. If the situation becomes chronic, growth will slow, and head circumference and height will be below age- and gender-related standards. Severe lack of caloric intake results in a wasting condition known as *marasmus*. Consumption of adequate calories without sufficient protein can produce kwashiorkor, a condition often characterized by the onset of infections and edema. There are numerous causes of pediatric undernutrition; however, the most common is inadequate dietary intake. Some cases may be secondary to poor socioeconomic status, lack of knowledge, perceived allergies/food intolerances, or neglect and abuse. Iron and zinc are two micronutrients commonly found to be at marginal levels in youth with poor nutrition. In addition, other nutrients such as vitamin D, calcium, and vitamin B_{12} are difficult to obtain at recommended levels in child and adolescent cases of undernutrition.[34]

IRON

As a component of blood hemoglobin and muscle myoglobin, iron fulfills its primary role in the body, which is to provide cells with a constant supply of oxygen. In addition, iron functions as cofactor for many enzymatic reactions in the body and is important to proper functioning of the immune system. Although the prevalence of iron deficiency has declined in recent years, it remains an important pediatric public health problem in the United States. Many of the adverse consequences of iron deficiency are associated with its most severe form, iron-deficiency anemia.[35-37] However, iron deficiency without anemia is associated with poor cognition and lower scholastic achievement in children and adolescents.[38,39] Typically, the high iron needs for growth, when combined with a low dietary intake, produce a low iron status in children. Iron deficiency early in life appears related to behavioral problems in infants who score significantly lower on various tests measuring intellectual and motor functioning. It has long been recognized that toddlers and adolescent females are among the most susceptible groups.[40] An assessment of iron deficiency prevalence in U.S. children 1 to 3 years of age during the period 1976-2002 showed no significant changes, with overall prevalence ranging from 8% to 10%. Iron deficiency prevalence decreased from 22% to 9% in toddlers in low-income households, but remained at 7% in toddlers from households above the poverty level. During this 26-year period, iron deficiency prevalence in African-American toddlers decreased from 16% to 6%, but remained unchanged in both Hispanic and white children at 13% and 6%, respectively.[41] Prolonged bottle feeding of up to 48 months of age was positively correlated with increased prevalence of iron deficiency and may account for the higher prevalence seen in Hispanic toddlers.[42]

Compared with normal weight or underweight peers, iron deficiency prevalence was significantly higher in overweight toddlers.[41] Similar findings have been reported in older children and adolescents. Possible explanations for the association between overweight and iron deficiency include high-calorie, low-iron diets, altered iron metabolism, genetic influences, and physical inactivity, which would lead to decreased myoglobin breakdown and therefore decreased blood iron. Also, overweight girls may grow faster and mature earlier than normal weight peers, making it more difficult to meet their iron requirements.[43] To prevent iron deficiency, vulnerable populations should be encouraged to eat iron-rich foods and breast-feed or use iron-fortified formula for infants. Iron is found primarily in meat, poultry, and fish. However, other foods such as beans, lentils, fortified cereal grain products, and certain vegetables can also contribute to dietary intake of iron.

Clinical signs of iron-deficiency anemia may include weakness, fatigue, pallor, and numbness and tingling of the extremities. Common oral manifestations are glossitis and fissures at the corners of the mouth (angular cheilitis). The papillae of the tongue may be atrophied, which gives the tongue a smooth, shiny, red appearance. In addition, pallor of the oral mucosa or lips may be observed. Affected individuals may also be at increased risk for fungal infections, such as candidiasis.

ZINC

Zinc is crucial to proper growth and development, sexual maturation, immune function, and wound healing. Zinc plays a role in taste and smell acuity as well as in facilitating the activity of vitamin A. Zinc deficiency may result from low dietary intakes, low bioavailability, and/or interaction with other nutrients, or through disease processes.

Iron and zinc share common food sources, so individuals at risk for iron deficiency may also be at risk for zinc deficiency.

Briefel and colleagues assessed zinc intakes from food and supplements in the U.S. population between 1988 and 1994 using National Health and Nutrition Examination Survey (NHANES III) data. Results indicated that in children younger than 10 years, boys and girls had similar zinc intakes, but in children older than age 10 years, boys' intakes exceeded that of the girls. Eighty-one percent of 1- to 3-year-olds and 48% of 4- to 6-year-olds had inadequate zinc intake, defined as less than 77% of the 1989 Recommended Dietary Allowance. In addition, roughly 61% of adolescent girls had inadequate intake compared with 38% of adolescent boys.[44]

In a 2002 feeding study of infants and toddlers ages 4 to 24 months, vitamin and mineral intakes of children taking supplements were compared with intakes of children not consuming supplements. Investigators noted that excessive intake (i.e., above the Tolerable Upper Intake level) was found in both groups for several nutrients including zinc, leading them to conclude that healthy infants and toddlers can achieve the recommended intake levels from food alone.[45] Similarly, Arsenault and Brown found that the zinc intake of U.S. preschool children increased appreciably from 1994 to 1998. In 1998, zinc intake exceeded the new Dietary Reference Intakes for zinc in 99% of children 5 years of age and younger. In this study, milk and fortified ready-to-eat breakfast cereals were the highest contributors of zinc for children aged 1 to 2 and 4 to 5 years, respectively.[46] These studies suggest that, as a result of the new dietary recommendations for zinc, increases in the consumption of zinc-fortified foods, and supplement use, excess zinc intakes may be more commonplace than zinc inadequacy in the youngest populations of U.S. children. Further research is needed to monitor patterns of zinc intake in children and adolescents as well any adverse health effects produced by these changes.

Zinc is present in foods that are high in protein, such as beef, eggs, poultry, and legumes, as well as in whole grains, fortified, ready-to-eat cereals, and dark green and yellow vegetables. However, like iron, zinc from plant food sources is not as well absorbed as that found in animal foods.

Clinically, one of the first manifestations of zinc deficiency in children is stunted growth. Other signs and symptoms include abnormal immune responses, decreased reproductive development and function, and skeletal abnormalities. Oral manifestations include impaired wound healing, alterations of the oral epithelium, xerostomia, reduced or altered sense of taste or smell, and reduced appetite. During tooth formation, children with zinc deficiency may be at increased risk for dental caries. In addition, because of its impact on immune function, zinc deficiency may increase the risk of oral infections such as periodontal disease and candidiasis.

CALCIUM

Calcium is essential for proper nerve and muscle activity, blood clotting, transport of ions across cell membranes and mineralization of the skeleton and dentition. Individuals at risk for inadequate calcium intake include those who dislike milk and other food sources of calcium, as well as those with milk allergies, lactose intolerance, and malabsorptive disorders. Inadequate calcium intake over time can increase the risk of bone demineralization and osteoporosis.

Osteoporosis is a bone disease of older individuals and is most commonly diagnosed in postmenopausal women. It is characterized by a reduction in the quantity of skeletal tissue and thus is often considered to be a geriatric disorder. Education for its prevention, however, is legitimately within the domain of pediatricians and pediatric dentists. Childhood and adolescence are crucial times for development of the skeletal system, and the dietary requirement for calcium peaks during the teenage years. The Food and Nutrition Board of the Institute of Medicine recommends an intake of 1300 mg per day of calcium during adolescence. This equals roughly the amount of calcium present in 4⅓ cups of milk, so this is not a particularly easy recommendation to meet.

Achieving a high peak bone mass is the first line of defense against osteoporosis. Low calcium intake, particularly in combination with low levels of physical activity, may compromise the attainment of optimal peak bone mass. This is a particularly important consideration for adolescent girls, because almost half of the adult skeletal mass is formed during the second decade of life and calcium accumulation normally triples during the pubertal growth spurt.[47] Unfortunately, this is the very age group that is at highest risk for low calcium intakes. Only 30% of adolescent girls reach 75% of the recommended daily allowance for calcium, and calcium intake appears to be declining among 6- to 11-year-olds.[48] This problem may be alleviated by educating youth to select more calcium-rich foods (e.g., cheese, yogurt, fortified breakfast cereals, fortified orange juice concentrates) or to consider using calcium supplements. Calcium carbonate has a good absorption rate and has been characterized as a relatively inexpensive supplement containing a high percentage level of calcium.[49] The concept that dental alveolar bone height loss is associated with osteoporosis is supported by research; therefore strategies for reducing osteoporosis risk also may help retard alveolar bone loss. Dental professionals can help improve both the oral and systemic health of their pediatric patients long term by guiding them in meeting calcium intake recommendations.[50]

VITAMIN D

Adequate stores of vitamin D are crucial for proper skeletal and dental development. Vitamin D increases calcium absorption from the gastrointestinal tract; when vitamin D concentrations are inadequate, calcium absorption decreases. Vitamin D acts in concert with parathyroid hormone to maintain tight control of blood calcium levels. A slight decrease in blood calcium concentration stimulates secretion of parathyroid hormone, which mobilizes calcium and phosphorus from the skeleton to reestablish calcium homeostasis in the blood. Vitamin D may play a role in immune function; in addition, lack of the vitamin may contribute to a number of diseases including hypertension, multiple sclerosis, and cancer.[51]

Although hypovitaminosis D is not well defined in children, recent studies suggest suboptimal vitamin D status is common in otherwise healthy young children. Weng and colleagues found that in a large sample of youth ages 6 to 21 years in the northeastern United States, more than half the children had low serum vitamin D concentrations; prevalence was increased with older age, and in the winter months, especially in African-American children.[52] In a study of nearly 400 healthy Massachusetts infants and toddlers, 12.1% of the subjects had suboptimal serum levels of vitamin D and 1/3 of these children exhibited radiographic evidence of bone demineralization. Predictors of vitamin D deficiency included breast-feeding without supplementation in infants and low milk intake among the toddlers.[53] Cushman and colleagues evaluated the effects of subclinical vitamin D deficiency on bone mineral density (BMD) and bone turnover in healthy adolescent boys and girls. Even though no relation between BMD and vitamin D status was observed in boys, the 12- to 15-year-old girls with high vitamin D status had significantly greater bone density, lower serum parathyroid hormone, and lower bone turnover markers than girls with low vitamin D status.[54] Furthermore, a review of the scientific literature indicates that suboptimal levels of vitamin D are widespread in U.S. youth.[55]

The major source of vitamin D is exposure to sunlight. Ultraviolet rays from the sun trigger vitamin D synthesis from its precursor, 7-dehydrocholesterol, in the skin. Only a few foods are natural sources of the vitamin, including fatty fish such as salmon, mackerel, and herring, as well as fish oil, including cod liver oil. In the United States, although some juices, bread, yogurt, and cheese are now fortified with vitamin D, fortified milk is still generally regarded as the primary dietary source of the vitamin.[56]

Because vitamin D is an essential nutrient for proper skeletal development growth, children who receive too little can develop the bone disease rickets. Rickets is characterized by bone deformities, poor muscle development, spinal curvature, and bowed legs. The latter manifestation occurs because the skeleton cannot support the body weight of the child. In addition, enlarged joints and delayed closing of the skull bones may be present. The presence of rickets during tooth development may result in enamel and dentin hypoplasia, incomplete development, or delayed tooth eruption.[57]

During the first half of the twentieth century, thousands of cases of nutritional rickets were reported in the United States, particularly in the northern climates during the winter months when exposure to sunlight was minimal. This disease was virtually eradicated once vitamin D began to be added to milk. In recent years, however, somewhat of a resurgence of rickets has occurred, particularly in African-American breast-fed babies. There appear to be two major reasons for this resurgence. First is the increase in breast-feeding. Breast-feeding is the preferred method of infant nutrition, but by itself does not supply adequate amounts of vitamin D. Second, endogenously produced vitamin D via effective sun exposure has decreased; it can vary with time exposed, amount of skin exposed, air pollution, cloud cover, time of day, latitude, season, sunscreen use, and skin pigmentation. Compared with individuals with a lighter complexion, those with heavily pigmented skin are less efficient in synthesizing vitamin D from sunlight. In addition, some African-Americans are unable to efficiently digest the lactose in milk, which leads to a significant reduction in milk intake and consequently in vitamin D levels. The increase in reported cases of nutritional rickets prompted the American Academy of Pediatrics to issue new guidelines in 2003 recommending supplemental vitamin D for all breast-fed infants. However, the recommendation has not been universally adopted by pediatricians, which leaves concerns about the continued risks of vitamin D–dependent rickets in U.S. children.[58-61]

VITAMIN B$_{12}$

Vitamin B$_{12}$ is one of the B-complex vitamins, and contains cobalt in the molecule; thus it is the only vitamin that contains a mineral. Vitamin B$_{12}$ is essential for the synthesis of red blood cells and for myelin synthesis in the nervous system. This vitamin is not thought to be present in plant foods, and as a result, strict vegetarians are considered to be at risk for a dietary deficiency of this vitamin. During 2001, neurologic impairment resulting from a vitamin B$_{12}$ deficiency was reported in two children breast-fed by mothers who followed vegetarian diets (consumption of limited food of animal origin).[62] In one of these cases, the diagnosis was made at 15 months, and vitamin B$_{12}$ therapy was initiated. At age 28 months, the child's developmental skill levels ranged from 9 months for fine motor skills to 18 months for gross motor skills. Her expressive language was at a 10-month level. Health care providers should be alert to the possibility of B$_{12}$ deficiency under these circumstances. Patients following vegetarian diets should ensure an adequate intake of vitamin B$_{12}$. The only reliable unfortified sources of this vitamin are animal products, including meat, dairy products, and eggs. Plant foods fortified with this vitamin, such as some cereals, meat analogues, soy or rice beverages, and nutritional yeast, can be reliable and regular sources.

Chronic vitamin B$_{12}$ deficiency can result in the condition known as pernicious anemia, which is characterized by large, immature blood cells. Additional signs and symptoms of vitamin B$_{12}$ deficiency include pallor, dizziness, fatigue, weight loss, confusion, hypotension, and peripheral nerve degeneration. Oral manifestations of vitamin B$_{12}$ deficiency include oral soreness and atrophic glossitis.[57]

PEDIATRIC OVERNUTRITION

For most children and adolescents in the United States, compromised health brought on by malnutrition is much more likely to be related to overconsumption of food rather than to underconsumption. The eating environment in contemporary America has been characterized as consisting of convenient, relatively inexpensive, highly palatable foods served in large portions.[63] Adherence to this type of eating pattern from childhood through adult life contributes to obesity and to numerous diseases, including diabetes, hypertension, coronary heart disease, and certain types of cancer. Those diseases that become evident during adulthood but have their origins in childhood and adolescence provide the health care professional with a potential avenue for preventive medicine. Atherosclerotic heart disease is such a case. Modifiable risk factors can be identified and addressed in the pediatric population, with the goal of preventing or ameliorating heart disease in later life. Thus prevention of coronary heart disease is a pediatric health issue, as is prevention of the other diseases mentioned earlier.

OVERWEIGHT AND OBESITY

Data from a variety of sources strongly indicate that we are in the midst of an obesity epidemic among children, adolescents, and adults in the United States. Simply stated, obesity results from a chronic imbalance between energy intake and energy expenditure. However, its increasing incidence is related to a complex array of genetic, environmental, psychosocial, biological, and economic factors. Although obesity is defined as the excessive accumulation of fat in the body, it is typically diagnosed based on body mass index (BMI). The BMI is calculated by dividing the individual's weight in kilograms by the square of the height in meters. By plotting the BMI on age- and gender-appropriate growth charts, overweight individuals can be identified as those between the 85th and 95th percentile for age and gender (http://www.cdc.gov/growthcharts). A major focus of the nationwide health promotion and disease prevention agenda in Healthy People 2010 is to reduce the proportion of children and adolescents who are overweight or obese. Unfortunately, a large disparity is found between the existing prevalence rates of obesity and the prevalence rate goals targeted in Healthy People 2010.[64] The prevalence of overweight among children ages 6 to 11 more than doubled in the past 20 years, rising from 7% in 1980 to 18.8% in 2004. The rate among adolescents more than tripled, increasing from 5% to 17.1%.[65]

There are many consequences of obesity, both short term and long term. An estimated 61% of overweight youth have at least one additional risk factor for heart disease such as high cholesterol or high blood pressure. Overweight children are at greater risk for bone and joint problems, as well as obstructive sleep apnea, which has been observed in as many as one in six obese children. The latter condition can lead to daytime somnolence, neurocognitive abnormalities, and impaired learning.

Aside from the obvious health risks associated with obesity in childhood and adolescence, there are also significant psychological and quality-of-life issues to be considered. Ackard and associates reported that objective overeating with loss of control in adolescents was associated with lower scores on measures of body satisfaction and self-esteem and higher scores on a measure of depressive mood.[66] Overeating was also associated with suicide risk. Thus objective overeating among adolescents is linked to a number of adverse behaviors and negative psychological experiences. It remains to be determined whether objective overeating is an early warning sign of psychological distress or rather a potential consequence of compromised psychological health.

Schwimmer and colleagues compared the health-related quality of life of obese children and adolescents with that of both their healthy non-obese counterparts and a cohort of children and adolescents with cancer.[67] Quality-of-life ratings of severely obese children and adolescents were lower than those of healthy children and adolescents and similar to those of children and adolescents with cancer. An impaired self-image and perception of low quality of life in this population is not surprising, because obesity is one of the most stigmatizing and least socially acceptable conditions in childhood. These and similar findings emphasize how critical it is for health professionals, teachers, and parents to be aware not only of the medical risks of obesity in children but also of the potential psychological significance of this condition.

Because obese children tend to become obese adults, the potential impact of childhood obesity on the health care system is enormous. It has been suggested that the increased medical care costs associated with obesity may be greater than those associated with smoking and drinking alcohol.[68] As overweight young people age, they are at increased risk for heart disease, type 2 diabetes mellitus, stroke, several types of cancer, and osteoarthritis. The current epidemic of type 2 diabetes in children and adolescents is associated with obesity and a persistently elevated BMI. A recent study found that 25% of obese children (aged 4 to 10 years) were glucose intolerant.[69] Glucose intolerance is a precursor to diabetes.

Severe obesity has long been thought to reduce life expectancy. A recent report states that 20-year-old white men with BMI greater than 45 (extreme obesity) are estimated to lose 13 years of life because of their obesity.[70] Despite several decades of various public health efforts to educate the population regarding the dangers of obesity, the trend toward progressively increasing body weight has not abated.

The epidemiologic approach highlights a web of factors that can contribute to the obesity epidemic in U.S. children and adolescents. It includes factors at the individual, family, community, and societal levels. These include changing meal environments, increased TV viewing, food availability, decreased parental leisure time, suburban changes that discourage walking, increased concern for neighborhood safety, increased advertising and availability of fast, high-fat, calorie-dense food, changes in parental work patterns, increased need for child care, and increased utilization of work-saving machines (e.g., cars, computers). Because the problem is multifactorial, solutions could target a number of factors. An extensive review of the literature by Wofford clearly identified the preschool years as a critical time to intervene in obesity prevention. Parental involvement and the role of health care practitioners in emphasizing recommendations were vital to successful interventions. In addition, prevention strategies should focus on building positive, healthy behaviors because these have better long-term results than strategies that focus on limiting behaviors.[71]

Physical activity is a major determinant of both morbidity and mortality. It has been identified as a national priority area for promoting the health of the U.S. population. However, many children and adolescents do not meet the recommendations for physical activity. This fact is particularly sobering because the adolescent years are thought to be the period during which adult health-related behaviors such as dietary and physical activity patterns begin to develop. Thus childhood may be a critical time for promoting physical activity. In 2005, the Centers for Disease Control and Prevention (CDC) reported that 27.8% of high school girls and 43.8% of high school boys participated in at least 60 minutes of physical activity per day. Only 29% of girls and 37.1% of boys attended a physical education class 5 days a week during school.[72]

Walking for transportation is part of an active lifestyle associated with decreased risk of chronic diseases and an increased sense of well-being; however, time spent walking has declined in U.S. children. One of the objectives of Healthy People 2010 (#22-14b) is to increase among children and adolescents the proportion of trips to school made by walking from 31% to 50%. In 1969, approximately half of all U.S. schoolchildren walked or biked to and from school; of those living within 1 mile of school, 87% walked or biked to school. By 2004, fewer than 15% of children used an active mode of transportation. In 2004, the CDC reported the results of a ConsumerStyles survey of parents that cited distance to school as the most common barrier to walking to school; traffic-related dangers was the next most cited.[73] The reduction in total physical activity that occurs from mid to late adolescence appears to be related more to a reduction in the number of activities in which adolescents choose to participate than in a decline in the time spent on each activity.[74] This finding supports other evidence that physical activity declines during adolescence.

It is recommended that children and adolescents participate in at least 60 minutes of moderately intense physical activity most days of the week, preferably daily, according to Dietary Guidelines for Americans, 2005. For youth, regular physical activity has beneficial effects on weight, muscular strength, cardiorespiratory fitness, bone mass, blood pressure, anxiety, and self-esteem. The approximate energy expenditure of various physical activities is shown in Table 12-3. Walking programs are increasingly being promoted for youth in selected school systems. Many of these programs are using pedometers to register the number of steps being taken. These small units, which clip onto waistbands, resemble tiny pagers and are reasonably accurate in counting all the steps taken over a given period of time. For some programs, the goal is to reach 12,000 steps per day, but for all the programs, a general objective is to motivate the person wearing the pedometer to progressively increase the step count over time and perhaps to maintain a minimally acceptable level of steps per day.

Research shows that the prevalence of obesity is lowest among children watching 1 or fewer hours of television a

Table 12-3

Approximate Energy Expenditure of Various Types of Exercise

Type of Exercise	Calories Used Per 30 Minutes*
Raking leaves	100
Walking (15-minute miles)	200
Playing singles tennis	210
Stationary cycling	300
Stair climbing	300
Jogging (10-minute miles)	330
Shoveling snow	350
Rowing	350

*Values will be higher for larger individuals, lower for smaller individuals.
Data from National Institute of Sports Medicine.

day and highest among those watching 4 or more hours of television a day.[75] Not only will sedentary children expend less energy, but they will also invariably be increasing their consumption of high-fat, high-sugar, high-calorie snack foods during these sedentary periods. Research from more than a decade ago indicates that food (typically sweet snacks) is consumed or referred to three to five times per half-hour on prime-time programming.[76] Also, the majority of commercials shown during children's programming promote foods with low nutritional value, including candy, soft drinks, sugared cereals, and potato chips, as well as other high-salt, high-fat snacks.[77]

EATING DISORDERS

Physical appearance is of prime importance for most teenagers, and for some adolescent girls in particular, getting "thin enough" can become an obsession. Estimates are that 5 million Americans suffer from eating disorders and that 5% of female and 1% of male Americans have anorexia nervosa, bulimia nervosa, or binge eating disorder. Because women and men are often secretive about their eating disorders, existing epidemiologic studies may underestimate the true prevalence of these conditions.[78] Some personality traits, such as perfectionism and concern with weight and shape, may cluster in families of women with eating disorders. Perfectionism may be an environmentally transmitted or genetically mediated trait that is transferred to offspring.[79]

Disordered eating is a term that includes a full spectrum of unhealthy eating behaviors from inappropriate dieting to clinical eating disorders.[80] The mass media is viewed by many as a major contributor in influencing disordered eating behaviors in young people through its presentation of often unattainable physical images and emphasis on the "thin ideal." Analyses of body measurements of 500 models listed on modeling agency websites and of *Playboy* centerfolds from 1985 to 1997 showed that nearly all the centerfolds and three fourths of the models had BMIs of 17.5 or below, a figure that meets the American Psychological Association's criterion for anorexia nervosa.[81] Although boys may be increasingly influenced by the portrayals of muscular men in the media, most research has focused on the effects of media portrayals on girls' eating and dietary habits. Teenaged girls are most at risk for developing eating disorders as they struggle with bodies that are getting larger in a culture that simultaneously attempts to sell them junk food and tells them that they should be thin. A study by Field found that more than 10% of adolescent girls and 3% of boys binge eat or purge at least once a week. Risk factors for these disordered eating behaviors included frequent dieting, concerns about weight, and in girls younger than 14 years, maternal history of an eating disorder.[82]

Research has shown that childhood overweight is a risk factor for disordered eating, and both are risk factors for full-syndrome eating disorders. Shape and weight concerns appear to be elevated in overweight children and teenagers, especially in white girls. Up to 79% of overweight youth report unhealthy weight control behaviors and up to 17% report extreme weight control behaviors such as self-induced vomiting or laxative or diuretic abuse.[83]

A national survey by Neumark-Sztainer of 6728 adolescents reported approximately 24% of the population was overweight and nearly half of the girls had been on a diet at some time, compared with 20% of the boys. Disordered eating behaviors were reported by 13% of girls and 7% of boys. These behaviors were positively correlated with overweight, low self-esteem, depression, suicidal ideation, and alcohol and drug use. In girls, tobacco use was directly associated with both dieting and disordered eating behaviors.[84] Considering the high prevalence of weight-related concerns among young people in the United States, it would be prudent to aim appropriate interventions at all youth.

ANOREXIA NERVOSA

Preoccupation with appearance and body weight during adolescence may lead to anorexia nervosa, a condition of self-induced starvation. Anorexia may be of the restrictive type, in which food intake is severely limited or the binge eating/purging type, in which individuals engage in self-induced vomiting or the misuse of laxatives, diuretics, or enemas. This illness, which is much less common in males and is also less common than bulimia nervosa, is characterized by self-imposed weight loss, amenorrhea, and a distorted attitude toward eating and body weight. In some instances this behavior is used as a means of establishing a sense of identity and control. Anorexia nervosa has captured the interest of psychoanalysts, behavior therapists, family therapists, nutritionists, and endocrinologists alike because of the interplay between the powerful psychological and physiologic components of the disease. Anorexia nervosa rarely begins before puberty and probably is manifest across a wide range of severity levels. Affected individuals often lack the ability to recognize that their emaciated bodies are too thin. Despite their advanced state of wasting, they may continue to believe that they are overweight. The four diagnostic criteria for anorexia nervosa are the following[85,86]:

• Refusal to maintain a body weight equal to or greater than 85% of that expected for the patient's age and height.
• An intense fear of gaining weight or becoming fat, even though the individual is underweight.
• A distorted view of one's body weight, size, or shape; the emaciated anorexic individual actually feels fat.
• In postmenarchal women and girls, the absence of at least three consecutive menstrual cycles.

A wide range of complications, including many of the consequences of starvation, is possible in anorexia nervosa. Fat depletion is the most obvious physical consequence. Qualitative deficiencies in the diet may lead to anemia, hypoproteinemia, and sometimes vitamin deficiencies. Serious electrolyte imbalances, notably hypokalemia, can occur when vomiting or laxative or diuretic abuse is practiced. Anorexia may be accompanied by enlargement of the parotid glands, edema of the legs, increased facial hair, and reductions in blood pressure and pulse rate. Nutritional deficiencies may lead to glossitis, gingivitis, a reduction in the amount and pH of the saliva, and an increase in dental caries susceptibility. Dental erosion may be evident on the palatal aspect of anterior and posterior teeth (perimolysis) secondary to the use of sports drinks, caffeinated/carbonated drinks, wine, vinegar and lemon juice used to quell sensations of hunger. Anorexics who engage in self-induced vomiting may exhibit epithelial erosion, gingivitis, and dental erosion on the palatal surfaces of the maxillary anterior teeth.[86]

Long-term studies have demonstrated diverse outcomes ranging from full recovery to chronicity and death. Outpatient treatment is preferred for most individuals. If the illness is severe and family and environmental circumstances are too damaging or if there is little response to outpatient treatment, then hospitalization is indicated. Fluoxetine hydrochloride appears to help control the obsessive-compulsive behavior involved in both anorexia nervosa and bulimia. This drug raises the brain levels of serotonin, and as a consequence the urge to binge and the preoccupation with food appears to lessen.

BULIMIA

Another eating disorder, bulimia nervosa, is characterized by binge eating and invariably by self-induced vomiting. It also is more prevalent in young women and is more common than is anorexia nervosa. It usually begins during late adolescence or early adult life. Its prevalence among males is probably vastly underestimated because of underreporting. The American Psychiatric Association diagnostic criteria for bulimia nervosa are the following[85]:

• Consumption of an unusually large amount of food in a discrete time period (within 2 hours)
• A perceived lack of control over eating during an episode
• Compensatory behavior to rid the body of excess calories and prevent weight gain
• The occurrence of binge eating and compensatory behaviors at least twice a week for 3 months
• A persistent concern with body shape and size

Although it is more medically benign than anorexia nervosa, bulimia nervosa is associated with significant health consequences. Approximately half of patients with this disorder have fluid and electrolyte abnormalities. Hypokalemia develops in a small percentage. Enlargement of the parotid glands, esophagitis, and gastric necrosis may also occur. Because of the exposure of the tooth surfaces to the highly acidic regurgitated gastric contents, enamel erosion is common among bulimia nervosa patients. The degree of enamel damage can be extensive. Although unanimity of opinion does not exist, the suggestion has been made that toothbrushing after vomiting actually promotes enamel loss and that, instead, patients should be instructed to rinse with an alkaline solution such as sodium bicarbonate dissolved in water. Other suggestions include use of liquid sugar-free antacids, water, or milk. Fluoride treatment should be considered because of its potential for remineralizing previously demineralized areas of the dentition. Daily rinses with 0.5% sodium fluoride and administration of a 1.1% neutral fluoride gel in custom trays can be recommended.

Most bulimic patients can be treated effectively as outpatients. Although antidepressant medications may be helpful in some cases, a multidisciplinary approach to treatment is often indicated. There is some evidence that individuals who eat dinner with their families regularly score significantly lower on the bulimia risk scale.[87] Family meals may serve a protective function against disordered eating as well as other problems by acting as a forum for working through various issues.

BINGE EATING DISORDER

Although binge eating disorder has not yet achieved official diagnostic recognition, it is defined by the consumption of excessive amounts of food along with the sensation of loss of control. The following are the *Diagnostic and Statistical Manual, Fourth Edition, Text Revision* criteria for this disorder[88]:

- Recurrent episodes of binge eating are characterized by eating in a discrete period of time more food than most people would eat in similar circumstances and having a sense of lack of control over eating during the episode.
- Binge eating episodes are associated with three or more of the following:
  - Eating much more rapidly than normal
  - Eating until feeling uncomfortably full
  - Eating large amounts of food when not feeling hungry
  - Eating alone from embarrassment of the amount consumed
  - Feeling disgusted, depressed, or guilty after overeating
  - Feeling marked distress regarding binge eating
  - Binge eating at least 2 days per week for 6 months, on average
- Binge eating is not associated with regular use of inappropriate compensatory behavior.

Binge eating disorder patients may be treated as outpatients in a multidisciplinary manner. In overweight patients with binge eating disorder, the goals include achieving a sustainable weight loss and abstaining from binge eating. Pharmacotherapy using antidepressants and selective serotonin reuptake inhibitors has been employed. Other classes of medications such as antiobesity drugs and anticonvulsants have also been studied and have shown some success. Psychotherapy in the form of cognitive-behavioral therapy has been a popular approach and other modalities such as exercise, self-help, and virtual reality therapy have also been tried as adjunctive therapies for binge eating disorder. Furthermore, some studies indicate there may be a benefit to combined behavioral therapy and pharmacotherapy in treating binge eating disorder; however, more research is needed to better understand the long-term effects of these treatments.[89,90] As health care professionals deal with eating disorders in their patients, they recognize that primary prevention combined with early detection and treatment clearly helps reduce morbidity and mortality in affected youth.[91]

NUTRITIONAL CONSIDERATIONS FROM INFANCY THROUGH ADOLESCENCE

During postnatal life, childhood exposure to environmental factors, primarily via dietary intake, will slowly begin to condition adult susceptibility to diseases both positively and negatively.[92] Dietary factors include calories, saturated fat, sodium, calcium, and antioxidants, among others. Although dietary intervention for disease prevention is possible in adult life, it is difficult and the beneficial results are sometimes limited. A better option is to promote intake of a diet with high nutritional quality early in life; this can reduce risk factors and potentially accomplish major reductions in the incidence of several chronic diseases of adulthood.

INFANT AND TODDLER (0 TO 3 YEARS OLD)

Except for prenatal existence, the period of most rapid growth in humans occurs during the first 6 months of life. Thus energy and nutrient requirements are high during this time. A full-term infant is capable of digesting and absorbing protein, fats, and simple carbohydrates. Proteins are essential for optimal infant growth; rates of protein synthesis and turnover are very high in infants relative to their body weight. Fats are the main dietary source of energy and essential fatty acids for infants and can account for up to 50% of the calories in breast milk. Fats are required for absorption of the fat-soluble vitamins and proper development of the central nervous system. The primary carbohydrate in both human milk and cow's milk formulas is lactose, or milk sugar. Starch presents some digestive challenges, however, because amylase, the starch-splitting enzyme, is not produced in significant quantities until approximately the age of 3 months. Moreover, the immature kidneys of an infant cannot concentrate waste efficiently. As a result, the infant must excrete relatively more water than does an adult to eliminate a comparable amount of waste. When dealing with infants, one must always be on guard against dehydration, which has potentially serious consequences.

Liquid or semiliquid foods are the choice until the teeth begin to erupt. Breast-feeding continues to be the best overall method of infant feeding, and breast milk could well be the infant's only food source for the first 4 to 6 months. Observational studies in affluent populations generally show no difference in weight or length gain between exclusively breast-fed and partially breast-fed infants during the first 4 to 6 months of life. Thereafter, milk can be supplemented with various pureed foods, either homemade or commercially prepared. Breast milk complemented by the infant's own internal stores will meet most of the nutrient needs until the first 6 months have elapsed. Supplements of nutrients such as vitamin D, iron, and fluoride should be considered after consulting with the child's pediatrician and pediatric dentist. Evidence suggests that low tissue levels of iron adversely affect brain and intellectual development and performance. Whether breast-fed infants should receive iron supplements is still the subject of debate. Although infants who are exclusively breast-fed appear to be iron sufficient at 6 months of age, some breast-fed infants who do not receive iron supplements are in negative iron balance between the ages of 3 and 6 months. Therefore it may be desirable to begin iron supplementation (often with ferrous sulfate) for the breast-fed infant at about 4 months of age. If the baby is formula fed, the makeup of the formula determines what additional supplementation is indicated. If an iron-fortified formula is not used, iron supplements again may be recommended after 4 months of age. The use of infant fluoride supplements to maximize caries resistance is discussed elsewhere in this text. The pediatrician and pediatric dentist may be consulted regarding specific situations and local circumstances.

There is no nutritional need for introducing solid foods to infants before 6 months of age.[93] Earlier use may contribute to the development of allergies or increased risk of obesity. New foods should be introduced singly to permit detection of allergies. For the first 6 months of life, the optimal single food for the infant is human milk or alternative formula when indicated. Some concerns have been expressed over inclusion of egg yolk when solid foods begin to be added to the weanling diet because of the potential for elevation of blood cholesterol levels. However, a recent study indicates that egg yolk may be safely introduced into the weanling diet with no elevation in plasma cholesterol level or increase in the prevalence of egg allergies.[94]

Regular unmodified cow's milk is not considered suitable for infants. It is an insufficient source of vitamin C and iron. Moreover, it may cause gastrointestinal bleeding, and its solute load is too heavy for the infant's renal system to handle. Low-fat milks should not be used by infants because of their insufficient energy provision and their lack of essential fatty acids. In addition, health food beverages are not appropriate for infants. Cases of severe nutrient deficiencies resulting in kwashiorkor and rickets have been reported from regular consumption of nonfortified, rice, and soy-based health food milk alternatives.[95]

When the infant becomes a toddler and the rapid growth rate of the first year declines, parents are frequently concerned about a noticeable reduction in appetite. This is normal. Although fewer calories may be needed for growth at this stage, the dietary needs for protein and minerals to promote muscle and skeletal development remain high. Thus a variety of foods should be offered in smaller amounts several times a day to provide these key nutrients. Attractive, brightly colored foods seem to be particularly appealing to children. During the first 2 years of life, 40% to 50% of energy intakes should come from fat, for example, by the consumption of whole milk. However, children older than 2 years should be gradually switched to a diet containing roughly 30% of total calories from fat, with no more than 10% of the calories from either saturated fats or polyunsaturated fats. Carbohydrates should comprise 55% to 60% of calorie requirements, with no more than 10% from simple sugars in toddlers older than 2 years of age. In addition, the recommended daily grams of dietary fiber should be equal to 5 plus the child's age in years.[34]

PRESCHOOLER (3 TO 6 YEARS OLD)

Physical growth occurs in spurts between 3 and 6 years of age. The child is not growing as rapidly as in the first years of life. Thus fewer calories are required but relatively high protein and mineral needs remain. A variety of foods should be offered but in lesser amounts. Parents sometimes provide adult-sized food servings to a child who may be only one-fifth the size of an adult. Care must be taken not to turn mealtimes into major struggles for control over what to eat, how much to eat, and when to eat.

Although it is important to keep the total fat, saturated fat, and cholesterol at recommended levels in the diet, care must be taken not to overdo this approach. With insufficient intake of calories and nutrients, the child cannot grow and develop to full potential. The child of this age should be helped to lose their "baby fat" by increasing physical activity rather than by severely restricting calories. Providing wholesome, nutritious, low-sugar snacks can promote adequate intake of essential nutrients without adding excessive calories or promoting dental caries.

SCHOOL-AGED CHILD (6 TO 12 YEARS OLD)

The 6- to 12-year stage is generally accompanied by a reduced rate of growth, which results in a decline in food requirements per unit of body weight. As a result, there is some need to be more discriminating in food selection, with emphasis on high nutrient density (foods having a high ratio of nutrients to calories). Vegetables are generally among the least-favored foods in this age group, but children usually like fruits, which provide many of the same nutrients. In this age group, regular eating patterns should be established; at the same time, consumption of nutritious snacks should be stressed and the use of foods, particularly sweets, as rewards should be minimized. Children should be encouraged to eat breakfast. This long-standing advice seems consistent with scientific literature. In a study of fourth through sixth graders in a school with a universal school breakfast program, Reddan and colleagues found that the majority of students believed that eating breakfast provides benefits of increased energy and ability to pay attention in school.[96] Barriers to eating breakfast cited by students were not having time and not being hungry in the morning. A focus on eating foods with high nutrient value and maintaining sufficient physical activity levels is important throughout this age range, because overweight and obesity often develop during these years.

ADOLESCENT (12 TO 18 YEARS OLD)

The nutritional requirements of adolescents are influenced primarily by the onset of puberty and the final growth spurt of childhood. This profound increase in growth rate is accompanied by increased needs for energy, protein, vitamins, and minerals. In general, girls consume far less food than do boys and must meet their needs for individual nutrients within a smaller range of caloric intakes. As a result, adolescent females are at high risk for nutritional inadequacies. In addition, girls often encounter significant social and peer pressure to restrict food intake for weight-control purposes. A multitude of fad weight-loss diets and disordered eating behaviors may be experimented with at this time. Some adolescent girls also turn to cigarette smoking to help control their body weight. The nutritional status of adolescent girls remains of concern because of low dietary intakes and attendant marginal iron, calcium, and folic acid status. Generally, as girls progress through adolescence, their average intake of vitamins and minerals and calories declines, while their nutritional requirements actually increase.

Particularly among adolescent female athletes in sports that emphasize leanness, research indicates that reported energy and nutrient intakes are generally well below recommended levels and lower than those of typical teenage girls.[97] This condition has been referred to as *female athlete triad* by the American College of Sports Medicine (ACSM) since 1992. The syndrome, which is characterized by disordered eating behaviors, amenorrhea and osteoporosis, has been observed in elite athletes, recreational athletes, and nonathletic, highly active females. Whether inadvertently or intentionally, some females do not ingest enough calories to adequately fuel themselves for their body's needs; it is thought that the amenorrhea results from lack of energy relative to the demands of the active lifestyle. Disordered menstrual cycles can lead to low estrogen levels and bone loss; studies have shown decreased bone mineral density in some young female athletes. However, it is worthy to consider that the need for education and screening should be balanced with the importance of promoting regular vigorous physical activity among adolescent girls.[98-100]

Teenagers, particularly boys, receive a greater proportion of their total energy intake from snacks than do other population groups. Although these snack items may have significant nutritional value, more often than not they are high in fat and sugar and thus contribute relatively low quantities of essential nutrients relative to their caloric content. The result may be the establishment of lifetime eating patterns that promote future risk of heart disease, obesity, hypertension, and cancer.

Table 12-4 summarizes some major gender differences in adolescent nutrition issues.

Table 12-4

Gender Differences in Adolescent Nutritional Issues

Females	Males
Lower energy needs	Higher energy needs
Thinness considered important	Strength considered important
Concern about peak bone mass	Less concern about bone mass
Higher risk for eating disorders	Lower risk for eating disorders
Higher risk for nutritional deficiencies	Lower risk for deficiencies

ADOLESCENT PREGNANCY

During adolescence, many young people become sexually active, and this often results in unplanned pregnancy; more than 400,000 babies are born to teenage mothers in the United States every year. In 2004, more than 10% of all U.S. births were to adolescent girls. However, after peaking in 1990, the teen birth rate has steadily declined each year. Between 1991 and 2004, the teen birth rate decreased by one third; even so, about 4 % of teenage girls delivered a baby.[101] Despite the continuous declines, the U.S. teenage pregnancy rate is still among the highest of industrialized nations.

The pregnant adolescent represents a population with unique nutritional needs. As stated earlier, even in a nonpregnant state, adolescent females often have difficulty meeting their nutritional requirements; pregnancy compounds this burden. The competition between maternal and fetal needs puts both the teen mother and the infant as risk. Due to a variety of physiological, socioeconomic, and behavioral factors, pregnant teens are at risk for adverse outcomes including preterm delivery, anemia, excessive postpartum weight gain, and delivery of a low-birth-weight baby. Two modifiable risk factors that should be addressed with this population are adequate nutritional intake and appropriate gestational weight gain. Enhanced prenatal care designed to address the unique psychosocial and nutritional needs of adolescents, health education classes, home visits, and nutritional prescriptions are interventions that have improved the outcomes of adolescent pregnancy.[102] Pregnant adolescents can develop a personalized guide for meeting their nutritional needs by using the MyPyramid Food Guidance System designed for them, Pregnancy and Breastfeeding (http://www.mypyramid.gov/mypyramidmoms/index.html).

Because gestational weight influences fetal growth and predicts birthweight, gaining a sufficient amount of weight during pregnancy may reduce infant morbidity and mortality. In 1990, the Institute of Medicine (IOM) released recommendations stating that adolescents age 16 years and younger should gain weight at the upper end of the recommendations, because they deliver more low birthweight babies than older women with the same weight gain. For pregnant teens older than 16 years, the IOM recommended a weight gain similar to that for adult women. However, some studies indicate that pregnant adolescents, especially those with high pre-pregnancy BMI and rapid pregnancy weight gain, experience weight retention after childbirth, which can be long lasting. As such, these individuals are at risk for obesity. There is no clear consensus on the long-term impact of the IOM recommendations on infant and maternal health. Thus more research is needed to better understand the effects of gestational weight gain in adolescents in order to prevent overweight and obesity in this population.[103]

TOBACCO, ALCOHOL, AND ILLICIT DRUG USE IN YOUTH

The pre-teen and teenage years are typically a period of search for identity, independence, and peer acceptance. Enmeshed within this search are a myriad of personal choices to be made, including decisions concerning the use of tobacco, alcohol, and illicit drugs. If the choice is made to use these substances, the individual should recognize that they all have a significant negative impact on health and fitness. Aside from the dangers of establishing a lifetime addiction and increasing the risk of numerous diseases, the use of tobacco, alcohol, and other drugs has a significant negative impact on the nutrient status of the affected individual.

Nicotine is the psychoactive substance in tobacco products. Based on the fact that 90% of tobacco users become addicted to nicotine, it may be considered one of the most addictive substances known. Cigarette smoking affects nutrition in numerous ways. Studies have shown that smokers have a lower intake than nonsmokers of numerous essential nutrients, including vitamins C and A, beta-carotene, folic acid, and dietary fiber. Moreover, several of these nutrients have been associated with a reduced risk of lung cancer, a disease for which cigarette smokers are at high risk. Therefore, the typical smoker is receiving less of the very nutrients most needed. Evidence also exists that smokers metabolize vitamin C more rapidly than do nonsmokers. The result is that smokers require approximately twice as much vitamin C as do nonsmokers to maintain similar blood levels. Smoking also influences both hunger and body weight, tending to postpone feelings of hunger and to reduce weight. Even though smokers as a group weigh less than nonsmokers, there are strong indications that smoking is associated with greater fat accumulations in the central portion of the body (a higher waist-to-hip ratio).

Tobacco use in youth has long been considered to be a gateway to the subsequent introduction and use of other drugs. For example, in a study of 20,000 children and adolescents, those who were pack-a-day smokers were more likely to drink alcohol, were seven times more likely to use smokeless tobacco, and were 10 to 30 times more likely to use illicit drugs than were nonsmokers.[104] Moreover, there was a strong dose-dependent relationship between smoking behavior and binge drinking, as well as between smoking and the use of alcohol and illicit drugs.

Alcohol is a very popular substance among many of the nation's youth and is not difficult to obtain for the vast majority of them. Some adolescents, as well as adults, use alcohol as an inappropriate way to cope with boredom, negative feelings, and the stresses of life. Nutritionally speaking, alcohol is a relatively high-energy substance (7 kcal/g versus 4 kcal/g for carbohydrates) that is devoid of any significant nutritional value. Alcohol use displaces the intake of essential nutrients. With long-term, excessive use, it adversely affects the absorption, transport, and metabolism of nutrients, which sometimes leads to serious nutritional inadequacies. In addition, many alcoholic beverages contain fermentable carbohydrates and as such, may increase risk of dental caries.

The long-term use of other drugs, such as methamphetamine, cocaine, and heroin, often produces numerous adverse physiologic effects, many of which compromise the nutritional state of the user and may result in multiple nutritional problems. Chronic abuse of these drugs may lead to eating disorders, in part because of chronic loss of appetite produced by the drugs. Often, during the "highs" produced by drugs, the individual loses interest in food, eating, and nutrient intake. The nutritional quality of the diet suffers under these circumstances and the individual is at risk for malnutrition. In the last decade, the use of methamphetamine by adolescents, especially in the Midwestern states, has increased. Chronic abuse of the drug is associated with xerostomia, frequent and excessive intake of sugared carbonated beverages, and poor oral hygiene; rampant dental caries is often the result.[105]

REFERENCES

1. Centers for Disease Control: CDC helps launch 2020 collaboration. CDC in the News, Available at: http://www.cdc.gov/news/2008/03/HealthyPeople2020.html. Accessed June 6, 2008.
2. ADA Reports. Position of the American Dietetic Association: Dietary guidance for healthy children ages 2-11 years, *J Am Diet Assoc* 104:660-667, 2004.
3. Enns CW, et al. Trends in food and nutrient intakes by children in the United States, *Fam Econ Nutr Rev* 14(2): 56-68, 2002.
4. Cullen KW, et al. Intake of soft drinks, fruit-flavored beverages, and fruits and vegetables by children in grades 4 through 6, *Am J Public Health* 92(9):1475-1478, 2002.
5. Troiano RP, et al. Energy and fat intakes of children and adolescents in the United States: data from the National Health and Nutrition Examination Surveys, *Am J Clin Nutr* 72(Suppl 5):1343S-1353S, 2000.
6. O'Connor TM, et al. Beverage intake among preschool children and its effect on weight status, *Pediatrics* 118(4):1010-1018, 2006.
7. Guthrie J, et al. Role of food prepared away from home in the American diet, 1977-78 versus 1994-96: changes and consequences, *J Nutr Educ Behav* 34:140-150, 2002.
8. Gillis LJ, Bar-Or O. Food away from home, sugar-sweetened drink consumption and juvenile obesity, *J Am Coll Nutr* 22(6):539-545, 2003.
9. Young L, Nestle M. Expanding portion sizes in the U.S. marketplace: implications for nutrition counseling, *J Am Diet Assoc* 103(2):231-234, 2003.

10. Nicklas T, et al. Nutrient contribution of the breakfast meal classified by source in 10-year-old children: home versus school, *School Food Serv Rev* 17:125-132, 1993.

11. Rampersaud GC, et al. Breakfast habits, nutritional status, body weight and academic performance in children and adolescents, *J Am Diet Assoc* 105(5):743-762, 2005.

12. USDA: Food and Nutrition Service National School Lunch Program (NSLP) 2007. Available at: http://www.fns.usda.gov/cga/FactSheets/NSLP_Quick_Facts.pdf . Accessed June 2008.

13. Snelling AM, et al. The national school lunch and competitive food offerings and purchasing behaviors of high school students, *J Sch Health* 77(10):701-705, 2007.

14. Cullen KW, et al. Improvements in middle school student dietary intake after implementation of the Texas Public School Nutrition Policy, *Am J Public Health* 98(1):111-117, 2008. [Epub Nov. 29, 2007]

15. ADA Reports. Position of the American Dietetic Association: Dietary guidance for healthy children ages 2-11 years, *J Am Diet Assoc* 104:660-667, 2004.

16. Nicklas TA, et al. Breakfast consumption affects adequacy of total daily intake in children, *J Am Diet Assoc* 93:886-891, 1993.

17. Jahns L, et al. The increasing prevalence of snacking among US children between 1977 to 1996, *J Pediatr* 138: 493-498, 2001.

18. Sebastian S, et al. Effect of snacking frequency on adolescents' intakes and meeting national recommendations, *J Adolesc Health* 42:503-511, 2008.

19. Karp R. Malnutrition among children in the United States: The impact of poverty. In Shils M, et al, eds. *Modern nutrition in health and disease.* Philadelphia, 1999, Lippincott Williams & Wilkins.

20. Knol LL, Haughton B, Fitzhugh EC. Dietary patterns of young, low-income US children, *J Am Diet Assoc* 105(11):1765-1773, 2005.

21. Holben D. The concept and definition of hunger and its relationship to food insecurity. Available at: http://www7.nationalacademies.org/cnstat/Concept_and_Definition_of_Hunger_Paper.pdf. Accessed June 20, 2008.

22. USDA ERS Briefing Rooms. Food security in the United States: Measuring household food security. Available at: http://www.ers.usda.gov/Briefing/FoodSecurity/measurement.htm. Accessed June 24, 2008.

23. Andersen SA. Core indicators of nutritional state for difficult to sample populations, *J Nutr* 20:1557S-1600S, 1990.

24. Nord M. USDA food assistance research brief: food insecurity in households with children. Food Assistance and Nutrition Research Report Number 34-13, July 2003. Available at: http://www.ers.usda.gov/publications/fanrr34/fanrr34-13/. Accessed June 6, 2008.

25. USDA ERS Briefing Rooms. Food security in the United States: Conditions and trends, Available at: http://www.ers.usda.gov/Briefing/FoodSecurity/trends.htm. Accessed June 24, 2008

26. Rose D, Oliveira V. Nutrient intakes of individuals from food-insufficient households in the United States, *Am J Pub Health* 87(12):1956-1961, 1997.

27. Cook JT, et al. Food insecurity is associated with adverse health outcomes among human infants and toddlers, *J Nutr* 134(6):1432-1438, 2004.

28. Rose-Jacobs R, et al. Household food insecurity: associations with at-risk infant and toddler development, *Pediatrics* 121(1):65-72, 2008.

29. Dietz WH. Does hunger cause obesity? *Pediatrics* 95(5): 766-767, 1995.

30. Casey PH, et al. The association of child and household food insecurity with childhood overweight status, *Pediatrics* 118(5):e1406-e1413, 2006.

31. Guilliford MC, et al. Food insecurity, weight control practices and body mass index in adolescents, *Public Health Nutr* 9(5):570-574, 2006.

32. Alaimo K, et al. Low family income and food insufficiency in relation to overweight in US children: is there a paradox? *Arch Pediatr Adolesc Med* 155(10):1161-1167, 2001.

33. Gundersen C, et al. Child-specific food insecurity and overweight are not associated in a sample of 10-15 year-old low-income youth, *J Nutr* 138(2):371-378, 2008.

34. Krebs N, et al. Normal childhood nutrition abd its disorders. In Hay W et al, eds. *Current Pediatric Diagnosis and Treatment,* 17th ed. New York, 2003, Lange/McGraw-Hill.

35. Haas JD, Brownlie T. Iron deficiency and reduced work capacity: a critical review of the research to determine a causal relationship, *J Nutr* 131:676S-688S, 2001.

36. Rasmussen KM. Is there a causal relationship between iron deficiency or iron-deficiency anemia and weight at birth, length of gestation and perinatal mortality? *J Nutr* 131:590S-601S, 2001.

37. Iron deficiency—United States, 1999-2000, *MMWR Morb Mortal Wkly Rep* 51(40):897-899, 2002.

38. Grantham-McGregor S, Ani C. A review of studies on the effect of iron deficiency on cognitive development in children, *J Nutr* 131:649S-666S, 2001.

39. Halterman JS, et al. Iron deficiency and cognitive achievement among school-aged children and adolescents in the United States, *Pediatrics* 107(6):1381-1386, 2001.

40. Looker AC, et al. Prevalence of iron deficiency in the United States, *JAMA* 277(12):973-976, 1997.

41. Brotanek JM, et al. Secular trends in the prevalence of iron deficiency among US toddlers, 1976-2002, *Arch Pediatr Adolesc Med* 162(4):374-381, 2008.

42. Brotanek JM, et al. Iron deficiency, prolonged bottle-feeding, and racial/ethnic disparities in young children, *Arch Pediatr Adolesc Med* 159(11):1038-1042, 2005.

43. Nead K, et al. Overweight children and adolescents: a risk group for iron deficiency, *Pediatrics* 114(1):104-108, 2004.

44. Briefel R, et al. Zinc intake of the US population: findings from the third national health and nutrition examination survey, 1988-1994, *J Nutr* 130:1367S-1373S, 2000.

45. Briefel R, et al. Feeding infants and toddlers study: do vitamin and mineral supplements contribute to nutrient adequacy or excess among US infants and toddlers? *J Am Diet Assoc* 106(Suppl 1):S52-S65, 2006.

46. Arsenault JE, Brown KH. Zinc intake of US preschool children exceeds new dietary reference intakes, *Am J Clin Nutr* 78(5):1011-1017, 2003.

47. Kreipe RE. Bones of today, bones of tomorrow, *Am J Dis Child* 146:22-25, 1992.

48. Committee on Nutrition, American Academy of Pediatrics: Policy statement on calcium requirements of infants, children, and adolescents (RE9904), *Pediatrics* 104(5):1152-1157, 1999.

49. Keller J, et al. The consumer cost of calcium from food and supplements, *J Am Diet Assoc* 102:1669-1671, 2002.

50. Kaye EK. Bone health and oral health, *J Sch Health* 77(10): 701-705, 2007.

51. Holick MF. Vitamin D: importance in prevention of cancers, type 1 diabetes, heart disease and osteoporosis, *Am J Clin Nutr* 79:362-371, 2004.

52. Weng F, et al. Risk factors for low serum 25-hydroxyvitamin D concentrations in otherwise healthy children and adolescents, *Am J Clin Nutr* 86:150-158, 2007.

53. Gordon CM, et al. Prevalence of vitamin D deficiency among healthy infants and toddlers, *Arch Pediatr Adolesc Med* 162(6):505-512, 2008.

54. Cushman K, et al. Low vitamin D status adversely affects bone health parameters in adolescents, *Am J Clin Nutr* 87:1039-1044, 2008.

55. Rovner AJ, O'Brien KO. Hypovitaminosis D among healthy children in the United States: a review of the current evidence, *Arch Pediatr Adolesc Med* 162(6):513-519, 2008.

56. Holick M, Chen TC. Vitamin D deficiency: a worldwide problem with health consequences, *Am J Clin Nutr* 87(Suppl):1080-1086, 2008.

57. Palmer C. Vitamins today. In Palmer C. *Diet and nutrition in oral health,* 2nd ed. Saddle River, NJ, 2007, Prentice Hall.

58. Pugliese M, et al. Nutritional rickets in suburbia, *J Am Coll Nutr* 17(6):637-641, 1998.

59. Weisberg P, et al. Nutritional rickets among children in the United States: review of cases reported between 1986 and 2003, *Am J Clin Nutr* 80(Suppl):1697-1705, 2004.

60. Taylor J. Defining vitamin D deficiency in infants and toddlers, *Arch Pediatr Med* 162(6):583-584, 2008.

61. Gartner L, Greer F. Prevention of rickets and vitamin D deficiency: new guidelines for vitamin D intake, *Pediatrics* 3(4):908-909, 2003.

62. Neurologic impairment in children associated with maternal dietary deficiency of cobalamin—Georgia, 2001, *MMWR Morb Mortal Wkly Rep* 52(4):61-64, 2003.

63. Rolls B, et al. Portion size of food affects energy intake in normal-weight and overweight men and women, *Am J Clin Nutr* 76:1207-1213, 2002.

64. Neumark-Sztainer D, et al. Overweight status and eating patterns among adolescents: where do youths stand in comparison with the Healthy People 2010 objectives? *Am J Public Health* 92(5):844-851, 2002.

65. Centers for Disease Control and Prevention. Child overweight. Available at: http://www.cdc.gov/HealthyYouth/overweight/index.htm. Accessed June 28, 2008

66. Ackard DM, et al. Overeating among adolescents: prevalence and associations with weight-related characteristics and psychological health, *Pediatrics* 111(1):67-74, 2003.

67. Schwimmer JB, et al. Health-related quality of life of severely obese children and adolescents, *JAMA* 289(14):1813-1819, 2003.

68. Sturm R. The effects of obesity, smoking, and drinking on medical problems and costs: obesity outranks both smoking and drinking in its deleterious effects on health and health costs, *Health Aff (Millwood)* 21:245-253, 2002.

69. Sinha R, et al. Prevalence of impaired glucose tolerance among children and adolescents with marked obesity [erratum in *N Engl J Med* 346(22):1756, 2002.] *N Engl J Med* 346(11):802-810, 2002.

70. Fontaine K, et al. Years of life lost due to obesity, *JAMA* 289:187-193, 2003.

71. Wofford L. Systematic review of childhood obesity prevention, *J Pediatr Nurs* 23(1):5-19, 2008.

72. Centers for Disease Control and Prevention. Youth risk behavior surveillance, United States, 2005, *MMWR Morb Mortal Wkly Rep* 55(SS-5):1-108, 2006. Available at: http://www.cdc.gov/HealthyYouth/PhysicalActivity. Accessed June 6, 2008

73. Centers for Disease Control and Prevention. Barriers to children walking to or from school-United States, 2004, *MMWR Morb Mortal Wkly Rep* 54(38):949-952, 2005.

74. Aaron DJ, et al. Longitudinal study of the number and choice of leisure time physical activities from mid to late adolescence: implications for school curricula and community recreation programs, *Arch Pediatr Adolesc Med* 156(11):1075-1080, 2002.

75. Crespo CJ, et al. Television watching, energy intake, and obesity in U.S. children: results from the third National Health and Nutrition Examination Survey, 1988-1994, *Arch Pediatr Adolesc Med* 155(3):360-365, 2001.

76. Story M, Faulkner P. The prime time diet: a content analysis of eating and food messages in television content and commercials, *Am J Public Health* 80:738-740, 1990.

77. Taras HL, Gage M. Advertised foods on children's television, *Arch Pediatr Adolesc Med* 149:649-652, 1995.

78. Faine MP. Recognition and management of eating disorders in the dental office, *Dent Clin North Am* 47(2):395-410, 2003.

79. Woodside D, et al. Personality, perfectionism, and attitudes toward eating in parents of individuals with eating disorders, *Int J Eat Disord* 31:290-299, 2002.

80. Sherman RT, Thompson RA. The female athlete triad, *J Sch Nurs* 20(4):197-202, 2004.

81. Brown JK, Witherspoon EM. The mass media and American adolescents' health, *J Adolesc Health* 31(Suppl 6):153-170, 2002.

82. Field EM, et al. Family, peer, and media predictors of becoming eating disordered, *Arch Pediatr Adolesc Med* 162:574-579, 2008.

83. Goldschmidt A, et al. Disordered eating attitudes and behaviors in overweight youth, *Obesity* 16(2):257-264, 2008.

84. Neumark-Sztainer D, Hannan P. Weight related behaviors among adolescent girls and boys, *Arch Pediatr Adolesc Med* 154:569-577, 2000.

85. American Psychiatric Association. *Diagnostic and statistical manual for mental disorders,* 4th ed. Washington, DC, 2000, American Psychiatric Association.

86. Lo Muzio L, et al. Eating disorders: a threat for women's health. Oral manifestations in a comprehensive review, *Minerva Stomatologica* 56(5):281-292, 2007.

87. Ackard D, Neumark-Sztainer D. Family mealtime while growing up: associations with symptoms of bulimia nervosa, *Eat Disord* 9:239, 2001.

88. Bulik C, et al. Diagnosis and management of binge eating disorder, *World Psychiatry* 6:142-148, 2007.

89. Brewerton T. Binge eating disorder: recognition, diagnosis, and treatment. Medscape Psychiatry & Mental Health eJournal 2(3), 1997. Available at: http://www.medscape.com/viewarticle/431260. Accessed June 28, 2008.

90. Pull C. Binge eating disorder, *Curr Opin Psychiatry* 17(1):43-48, 2004.

91. Rome ES, et al. Children and adolescents with eating disorders: the state of the art, *Pediatrics* 111(1):e98-e108, 2003.

92. Caballero B. Early nutrition and risk of disease in the adult, *Public Health Nutr* 4(6a):1335-1336, 2001.

93. WHO Working Group on the Growth Reference Protocol and WHO Task Force on Methods for the Natural Regulation of Fertility: growth of healthy infants and the timing, type and frequency of complementary foods, *Am J Clin Nutr* 76:620-627, 2002.

94. Makrides M, et al. Nutritional effect of including egg yolk in the weaning diet of breast-fed and formula-fed infants: a randomized controlled trial, *Am J Clin Nutr* 75:1084-1092, 2002.

95. Carvalho NF, et al. Severe nutritional deficiencies in toddlers resulting from health food milk alternatives, *Pediatrics* 107(4):E46, 2001.

96. Reddan J, et al. Children's perceived benefits and barriers in relation to eating breakfast in schools with or without Universal School Breakfast, *J Nutr Educ Behav* 34(1):47-52, 2002.

97. Beals K. Eating behaviors, nutritional status, and menstrual function in elite female adolescent volleyball players, *J Am Diet Assoc* 102(9):1293-1296, 2002.

98. Gabel K. Special nutritional concerns for the female athlete. *Curr Sports Med Rep* 5:187-191, 2006.

99. Sherman R, Thompson R. The female athlete triad, *J School Nurs* 20(4):197-202, 2004.

100. DiPietro L, Stachenfeld NS. The myth of the female athlete triad, *Br J Sports Med* 40:490-493, 2006.

101. Martin JA, et al. Births: Final data for 2004. National Vital Statistics Reports 2006;55(1).

102. Nielsen J, et al. Interventions to improve diet and weight gain among pregnant adolescents and recommendations for future research, *J Am Diet Assoc* 106:1825-1840, 2006.

103. Groth S. Adolescent gestational weight gain, *MCN Am J Matern Child Nursing* 31(2):101-105, 2006.

104. Waldman HB. Do your pediatric patients drink alcohol? Are they heavy or binge drinkers? *J Dent Child* 65:194-197, 1998.

105. Goodchild JH, Donaldson M. Methamphetamine abuse in dentistry: a review of the literature and presentation of a clinical case, *Quintessence Int* 38(7):583-590, 2007.

SUGGESTED READINGS

US Department of Health and Human Services, Centers for Disease Control and Prevention, *Natl Vital Stat Rep* 56(16), 2006.

CHAPTER 13

Local Anesthesia and Pain Control for the Child and Adolescent

▲ Ralph E. McDonald, David R. Avery, Jeffrey A. Dean, and James E. Jones

CHAPTER OUTLINE

It is generally agreed that one of the most important aspects of child behavior guidance is the control of pain. If children experience pain during restorative or surgical procedures, their future as dental patients may be damaged. Therefore it is important at each visit to reduce discomfort to a minimum and to control painful situations. There are many pharmacologic pain control strategies to help children cope with these situations, both preoperatively and postoperatively. Most of these strategies involve the use of local anesthetics or analgesics.

Because there is usually some discomfort associated with the procedure, use of a local anesthetic is generally indicated when operative work is to be performed on the permanent teeth, and the same is true of cavity preparations in primary teeth. Dental procedures can be carried out more effectively if the child is comfortable and free of pain. The local anesthetic can prevent discomfort that may be associated with placing a rubber dam clamp, ligating teeth, and cutting tooth structure. Even the youngest child treated in the dental office normally presents no contraindications for the use of a local anesthetic.

Investigators have found that injection is the dental procedure that produces the greatest negative response in children. Responses become increasingly negative over a series of four or five injections. Venham and Quatrocelli[1] have reported that a series of dental visits sensitized children to the stressful injection procedure while reducing their apprehension toward relatively nonstressful procedures. Thus dentists should anticipate the need for continued efforts to help the child cope with dental injections.

TOPICAL ANESTHETICS

Topical anesthetics reduce the slight discomfort that may be associated with the insertion of the needle before the injection of the local anesthetic. Some topical anesthetics, however, present a disadvantage if they have a disagreeable taste to the child. Also, the additional time required to apply them may allow the child to become apprehensive concerning the approaching procedure.

Topical anesthetics are available in gel, liquid, ointment, and pressurized spray forms. However, the pleasant-tasting and quick-acting liquid, gel, or ointment preparations seem to be preferred by most dentists. These agents are applied to the oral mucous membranes with a cotton-tipped applicator. A variety of anesthetic agents have been used in topical anesthetic preparations, including ethyl aminobenzoate, butacaine sulfate, cocaine, dyclonine, lidocaine, and tetracaine.

Ethyl aminobenzoate (benzocaine) liquid, ointment, or gel preparations are probably best suited for topical anesthesia in dentistry. They offer a more rapid onset and longer duration of anesthesia than other topical agents. They are not known to produce systemic toxicity as oral topical anesthetics, but a few localized allergic reactions have been reported from prolonged or repeated use. Examples of commercially available products are Hurricaine (Beutlich L.P. Pharmaceuticals, Inc., Chicago, Ill), Topicale (Premier Dental Products, Inc., Plymouth Meeting, Pa), and Gingicaine (Gingi-Pak, Inc., Camarillo, Calif). All three products are available in gel form. Gingicaine is also available in liquid and spray forms, and Hurricaine is available as a liquid. Topicale is available in ointment form.

The mucosa at the site of the intended needle insertion is dried with gauze, and a small amount of the topical anesthetic agent is applied to the tissue with a cotton swab. Topical anesthesia should be produced in approximately 30 seconds.

During the application of the topical anesthetic, the dentist should prepare the child for the injection. The explanation should not necessarily be a detailed description but simply an indication that the tooth is going to be put to sleep so that the treatment can proceed without discomfort.

A more recently developed product for achieving topical anesthesia is known as DentiPatch (Noven Pharmaceuticals, Inc., Miami, Fla), a lidocaine transoral delivery system. This system seems to be designed primarily for situations in which superficial oral tissue anesthesia is desired for several minutes rather than the shorter time required for local anesthetic injections. The use of this product has not yet been shown to be convenient or efficacious in young children.

JET INJECTION

The jet injection instrument is based on the principle that small quantities of liquids forced through very small openings under high pressure can penetrate mucous membrane or skin without causing excessive tissue trauma. One jet injection device, the Syrijet Mark II (iMizzy, Inc., Cherry Hill, NJ) holds a standard 1.8-mL cartridge of local anesthetic solution. It can be adjusted to expel 0.05 to 0.2 mL of solution under 2000 psi pressure.

Jet injection produces surface anesthesia instantly and is used by some dentists instead of topical anesthetics. The method is quick and essentially painless, although the abruptness of the injection may produce momentary anxiety. This technique is also useful for obtaining gingival anesthesia before a rubber dam clamp is placed for isolation procedures that otherwise do not require local anesthetic. Similarly, soft tissue anesthesia may be obtained before band adaptation of partially erupted molars or for the removal of a very loose (soft tissue–retained) primary tooth. O'Toole has reported that the Syrijet may be used instead of needle injections for nasopalatine, anterior palatine, and long buccal nerve blocks.[2]

A more recently developed jet injection device reported by Duckworth and colleagues delivers a dose of

dry powdered anesthetic to the oral mucosa.[3] In this study, an initial trial with 14 adult subjects, successful topical analgesia without tissue damage was reported. More clinical trials are required before substantial claims can be made regarding how efficacious the technique is and whether its routine use for topical anesthesia is warranted.

LOCAL ANESTHESIA BY CONVENTIONAL INJECTION

Wittrock and Fischer[4] and later Trapp and Davies[5] demonstrated that human blood can be readily aspirated with the smaller-gauge needles. Trapp and Davies reported positive aspiration through 23-, 25-, 27-, and 30-gauge needles without a clinically significant difference in resistance to flow. Malamed recommends the use of larger-gauge needles (i.e., 25 gauge) for injection into highly vascular areas or areas where needle deflection through soft tissue may be a factor.[6] Regardless of the size of the needle used, it is generally agreed that the anesthetic solution should be injected slowly and that the dentist should watch the patient closely for any evidence of an unexpected reaction.

The injections that are most commonly used in the treatment of children are described in the following sections.

ANESTHETIZATION OF MANDIBULAR TEETH AND SOFT TISSUE

INFERIOR ALVEOLAR NERVE BLOCK (CONVENTIONAL MANDIBULAR BLOCK)

When deep operative or surgical procedures are undertaken for the mandibular primary or permanent teeth, the inferior alveolar nerve must be blocked. The supraperiosteal injection technique may sometimes be useful in anesthetizing primary incisors, but it is not as reliable for complete anesthesia of the mandibular primary or permanent molars.

Olsen reported that the mandibular foramen is situated at a level lower than the occlusal plane of the primary teeth of the pediatric patient.[7] Therefore the injection must be made slightly lower and more posteriorly than for an adult patient. An accepted technique is one in which the thumb is laid on the occlusal surface of the molars, with the tip of the thumb resting on the internal oblique ridge and the ball of the thumb resting in the retromolar fossa. Firm support during the injection procedure can be given when the ball of the middle finger is resting on the posterior border of the mandible. The barrel of the syringe should be directed on a plane between the two primary molars on the opposite side of the arch. It is advisable to inject a small amount of the solution as soon as the tissue is penetrated and to continue to inject minute quantities as the needle is directed toward the mandibular foramen.

The depth of insertion averages about 15 mm but varies with the size of the mandible and its changing proportions depending on the age of the patient. Approximately

1 mL of the solution should be deposited around the inferior alveolar nerve (Figs. 13-1 and 13-2).

LINGUAL NERVE BLOCK

One can block the lingual nerve by bringing the syringe to the opposite side with the injection of a small quantity of the solution as the needle is withdrawn. If small amounts of anesthetic are injected during insertion and withdrawal of the needle for the inferior alveolar nerve block, the lingual nerve will invariably be anesthetized as well.

LONG BUCCAL NERVE BLOCK

For the removal of mandibular permanent molars or sometimes for the placement of a rubber dam clamp on these teeth, it is necessary to anesthetize the long buccal nerve. A small quantity of the solution may be deposited in the mucobuccal fold at a point distal and buccal to the indicated tooth (Fig. 13-3).

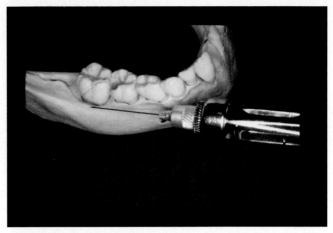

Figure 13-3 In anesthetizing the long buccal nerve, a small quantity of the solution may be deposited in the mucobuccal fold adjacent to the first permanent molar.

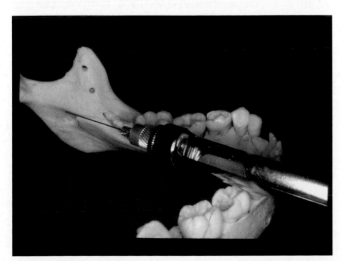

Figure 13-1 The mandible is supported by the thumb and middle finger, while the needle is directed toward the inferior alveolar nerve.

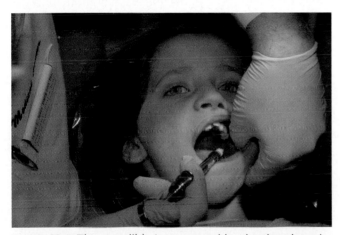

Figure 13-2 Anesthetic solution is deposited around the inferior alveolar nerve.

All facial mandibular gingival tissue on the side that has been injected will be anesthetized for operative procedures, with the possible exception of the tissue facial to the central and lateral incisors, which may receive innervation from overlapping nerve fibers from the opposite side.

INFILTRATION ANESTHESIA FOR MANDIBULAR PRIMARY MOLARS

Wright and colleagues have studied the effectiveness of injecting local anesthetic solution in the mucobuccal fold between the roots of primary mandibular molars.[8] Based on observational data, little or no pain was experienced by 65% of the children during cavity preparation. It was also noted that children who demonstrate comfort at the time of injection are likely to exhibit no pain during successive procedures.

Oulis and associates[9] reported very similar studies comparing the effectiveness of mandibular infiltration anesthesia to mandibular block anesthesia in children 3 to 9 years of age for restorative pulpotomy and extraction therapies in primary mandibular molars. Eighty-nine and 80 children, respectively, were included in their studies. Oulis and associates found that the two anesthesia techniques were equally effective for restorative procedures, but the mandibular infiltration technique was less effective than mandibular block for extraction and pulpotomy.[9] In 1976 a new local anesthetic, articaine, was introduced in Europe and by 1983 it was in use in Canada. It was not available in the United States until 2000, by which time the preservative had been removed from the formulation, and it received Food and Drug Administration (FDA) approval. Articaine (Septocaine), manufactured by Septodont (http://www.septodontusa.com) underwent several research studies to test reliability and effectiveness, and became readily available and widely used. Articaine is unique among local anesthetics because it contains a thiophene group as well as both ester and amide groups. Articaine is an amide anesthetic (it has an amide intermediate chain) that is metabolized in the liver. The associated ester group also allows plasma metabolism via pseudocholinesterase, which purportedly increases the rate of breakdown and reduces toxicity. This difference in metabolism gives articaine the advantage of having a 30-minute half-life; lidocaine, for example, has a 90-minute half-life.[10-14]

Sharaf[15] demonstrated that behavior in young children can be adversely affected by the painful mandibular block. It is well known that articaine has a high bone penetrating ability, which suggests that it may be more successful as a locally injected infiltration. From these reports, one may infer that mandibular infiltration anesthesia may produce adequate anesthesia in mandibular deciduous molars for most restorative procedures.

INFILTRATION FOR MANDIBULAR INCISORS

The terminal ends of the inferior alveolar nerves cross over the mandibular midline slightly and provide conjoined innervation of the mandibular incisors. A single inferior alveolar nerve block may not be adequate for operative or surgical procedures on the incisors, even on the side of the block anesthesia. The labial cortical bone overlying the mandibular incisors is usually thin enough for supraperiosteal anesthesia techniques to be effective.

If only superficial caries excavation of mandibular incisors is needed or if the removal of a partially exfoliated primary incisor is planned, infiltration anesthesia alone may be adequate. Incisor infiltration is most useful as an adjunct to an inferior alveolar nerve block when total anesthesia of the quadrant is desired. In this case the infiltration injection is made close to the midline on the side of the block anesthesia, but the solution is deposited labial to the incisors on the opposite side of the midline. For example, if block anesthesia is used for the mandibular right quadrant, anesthetic solution is infiltrated over the left mandibular incisors by insertion of the needle just to the right of the midline diagonally toward the left incisors.

MANDIBULAR CONDUCTION ANESTHESIA (GOW-GATES MANDIBULAR BLOCK TECHNIQUE)

In 1973, Gow-Gates introduced a new method of obtaining mandibular anesthesia, which he referred to as *mandibular conduction anesthesia*.[16] This approach uses external anatomic landmarks to align the needle so that anesthetic solution is deposited at the base of the neck of the mandibular condyle. This technique is a nerve block procedure that anesthetizes virtually the entire distribution of the fifth cranial nerve in the mandibular area, including the inferior alveolar, lingual, buccal, mental, incisive, auriculotemporal, and mylohyoid nerves. Thus with a single injection the entire right or left half of the mandibular teeth and soft tissues can be anesthetized, except possibly the mandibular incisors, which may receive partial innervation from the incisive nerves of the opposite side. Gow-Gates suggested that, once the technique is learned properly, it rarely fails to produce good mandibular anesthesia.[16] He had used the technique in practice more than 50,000 times. The technique has become increasingly popular and is often referred to as the *Gow-Gates technique*.

The external landmarks to help align the needle for this injection are the tragus of the ear and the corner of the mouth. The needle is inserted just medial to the tendon of the temporal muscle and considerably superior to the insertion point for conventional mandibular block anesthesia. The needle is also inclined upward and parallel to a line from the corner of the patient's mouth to the lower border of the tragus (intertragic notch). The needle and the barrel of the syringe should be directed toward the injection site from the corner of the mouth on the opposite side (Fig. 13-4).

ANESTHETIZATION OF MAXILLARY PRIMARY AND PERMANENT INCISORS AND CANINES

SUPRAPERIOSTEAL TECHNIQUE (LOCAL INFILTRATION)

Local infiltration (supraperiosteal technique) is used to anesthetize the primary anterior teeth. The injection should be made closer to the gingival margin than in the patient with permanent teeth, and the solution should be deposited close to the bone. After the needle tip has penetrated the soft tissue at the mucobuccal fold, it needs little advancement before the solution is deposited (2 mm at most) because the apices of the maxillary primary anterior teeth are essentially at the level of the mucobuccal fold. Some dentists prefer to pull the upper lip down over the needle tip to penetrate the tissue rather than advancing the needle upward. This approach works quite well for the maxillary anterior region (Figs. 13-5 to 13-7).

In the anesthetizing of the permanent central incisor teeth, the puncture site is at the mucobuccal fold, so that the solution may be deposited slowly and slightly above and close to the apex of the tooth. Because nerve fibers may be extending from the opposite side, it may be necessary to deposit a small amount of the anesthetic solution adjacent to the apex of the other central incisor to obtain adequate anesthesia in either primary or permanent teeth. If a rubber dam is to be applied, it is advisable to inject a drop or two of anesthetic solution into the

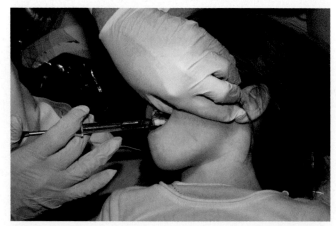

Figure 13-4 Barrel of the syringe is aligned with a line from the corner of the mouth to the intertragic notch.

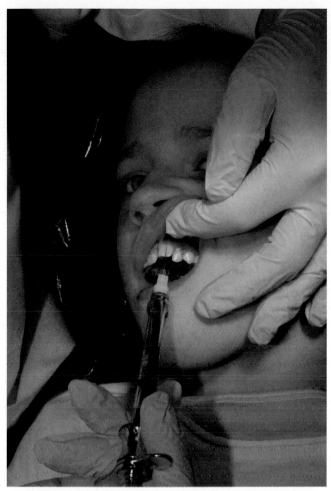

Figure 13-5 Anesthetizing a central incisor. The supraperiosteal injection should be close to the bone and adjacent to the apex of the tooth.

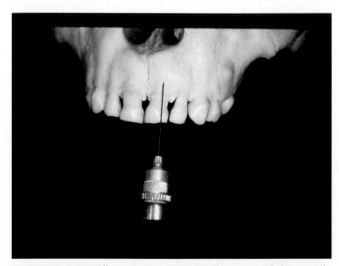

Figure 13-6 Needle point is opposite the apex of the maxillary primary incisor.

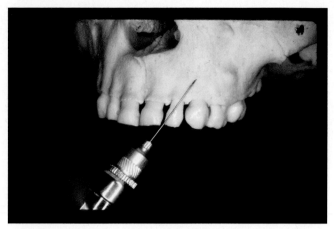

Figure 13-7 Position of the needle for anesthetizing a maxillary primary canine.

lingual free marginal tissue to prevent the discomfort associated with the placement of the rubber dam clamp and ligatures.

Before extraction of the incisors or canines in either the primary or permanent dentition, it is necessary to anesthetize the palatal soft tissues. The nasopalatine injection provides adequate anesthesia for the palatal tissues of all four incisors and at least partial anesthesia of the canine areas. Nerve fibers from the greater (anterior) palatine nerve usually extend to the canine area as well. If only a single anterior tooth is to be removed, adequate palatal anesthesia may also be obtained when anesthetic solution is deposited in the attached palatal gingiva adjacent to the tooth to be removed. If it is observed that the patient does not have profound anesthesia of anterior teeth during the operative procedures with the supraperiosteal technique, a nasopalatine injection is advisable.

ANESTHETIZATION OF MAXILLARY PRIMARY MOLARS AND PREMOLARS

Traditionally, dentists have been taught that the middle superior alveolar nerve supplies the maxillary primary molars, the premolars, and the mesiobuccal root of the first permanent molar. There is no doubt that the middle superior alveolar nerve is at least partially responsible for the innervation of these teeth. However, Jorgensen and Hayden have demonstrated plexus formation of the middle and posterior superior alveolar nerves in the primary molar area on child cadaver dissections.[17] The role of the posterior superior alveolar nerve in innervating the primary molar area has not previously received adequate attention. In addition, Jorgensen and Hayden have demonstrated maxillary bone thickness approaching 1 cm overlying the buccal roots of the first permanent and second primary molars in the skulls of children.[17]

The bone overlying the first primary molar is thin, and this tooth can be adequately anesthetized by injection of anesthetic solution opposite the apices of the roots (Figs. 13-8 and 13-9). However, the thick zygomatic process overlies the buccal roots of the second primary and first permanent molars in the primary and early mixed

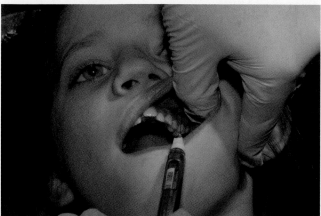

Figure 13-8 Injection of the anesthetic solution to anesthetize the maxillary second primary molar for operative procedures.

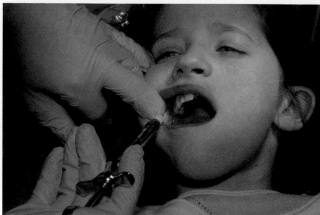

Figure 13-10 Posterior superior alveolar injection for maxillary permanent molars and second primary molar.

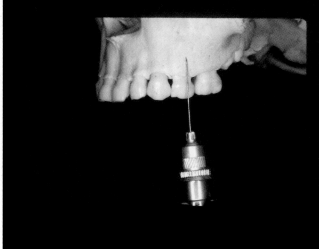

Figure 13-9 Anesthetic solution is injected opposite the apices of the buccal roots of the first primary molar.

dentition. This thickness of bone renders the supraperiosteal injection at the apices of the roots of the second primary molar much less effective; the injection should be supplemented with a second injection superior to the maxillary tuberosity area to block the posterior superior alveolar nerve as has been traditionally taught for permanent molars (Fig. 13-10). This supplemental injection helps compensate for the additional bone thickness and the posterior middle superior alveolar nerve plexus in the area of the second primary molar, which compromise the anesthesia obtained by injection at the apices only.

To anesthetize the maxillary first or second premolar, a single injection is made at the mucobuccal fold to allow the solution to be deposited slightly above the apex of the tooth. Because of the horizontal and vertical growth of the maxilla that has occurred by the time the premolars erupt, the buccal cortical bone overlying their roots is thin enough to permit good anesthesia with this method. The injection should be made slowly, and the solution

should be deposited close to the bone; these recommendations hold true for all supraperiosteal and block anesthesia techniques in dentistry.

Before operative procedures for maxillary primary molars and maxillary premolars, the appropriate injection techniques for the buccal tissues, as described, should be performed. If the rubber dam clamp impinges on the palatal tissue, injection of a drop or two of the anesthetic solution into the free marginal tissue lingual to the clamped tooth alleviates the discomfort and is less painful than the true greater (anterior) palatine injection. The greater palatine injection is indicated if maxillary primary molars or premolars are to be extracted or if palatal tissue surgery is planned.

ANESTHETIZATION OF MAXILLARY PERMANENT MOLARS

To anesthetize the maxillary first or second permanent molars, the dentist instructs the child to partially close the mouth to allow the cheek and lips to be stretched laterally. The tip of the dentist's left forefinger (for a right-handed dentist) will rest in a concavity in the mucobuccal fold and is rotated to allow the fingernail to be adjacent to the mucosa. The ball of the finger is in contact with the posterior surface of the zygomatic process. Bennett suggests that the finger be on a plane at right angles to the occlusal surfaces of the maxillary teeth and at a 45-degree angle to the patient's sagittal plane.[18] The index finger should point in the direction of the needle during the injection. The puncture point is in the mucobuccal fold above and distal to the distobuccal root of the first permanent molar. If the second molar has erupted, the injection should be made above the second molar. The needle is advanced upward and distally, depositing the solution over the apices of the teeth. The needle is inserted for a distance of approximately ¾ inch (2 cm) in a posterior and upward direction; it should be positioned close to the bone, with the bevel toward the bone (see Fig. 13-10).

To complete the anesthesia of the first permanent molar for operative procedures, the supraperiosteal injection is made by insertion of the needle in the mucobuccal fold and deposition of the solution at the apex of the mesio-buccal root of the molar.

ANESTHETIZATION OF THE PALATAL TISSUES

Anesthesia of the palatal tissues can be one of the more exquisitely painful procedures performed in dentistry. Ramirez and colleagues discuss methods for achieving profound anesthesia with minimal pain in the palatal and lingual aspects.[19] After buccal infiltration, they suggest interdental (interpapillary) infiltration, with slow injection of the anesthetic solution as the needle is penetrating the papilla. The interdental infiltration allows diffusion of the anesthetic to the palatal aspect via the craterlike area of the interproximal oral mucosa joining the lingual and buccal interdental papillae, known as the *col.* Blanching of the area is indicative of sufficient anesthesia of the superficial soft tissues; however, additional palatal infiltration may be given as needed.

NASOPALATINE NERVE BLOCK

Blocking the nasopalatine nerve anesthetizes the palatal tissues of the six anterior teeth. If the needle is carried into the canal, it is possible to anesthetize the six anterior teeth completely. However, this technique is painful and is not routinely used before operative procedures. If the patient experiences incomplete anesthesia after supraperiosteal injection above the apices of the anterior teeth on the labial side, it may be necessary to resort to the nasopalatine injection. The path of insertion of the needle is alongside the incisive papilla, just posterior to the central incisors. The needle is directed upward into the incisive canal (Fig. 13-11). The discomfort associated with the injection can be reduced by deposition of the anesthetic solution in advance of the needle. When anesthesia of the canine area is required, it may be necessary to inject a small amount of anesthetic

solution into the gingival tissue adjacent to the lingual aspect of the canine to anesthetize overlapping branches of the greater palatine nerve.

GREATER (ANTERIOR) PALATINE INJECTION

The greater palatine injection anesthetizes the mucoperiosteum of the palate from the tuberosity to the canine region and from the median line to the gingival crest on the injected side. This injection is used with the middle or posterior alveolar nerve block before surgical procedures. The innervation of the soft tissues of the posterior two thirds of the palate is derived from the greater and lesser palatine nerves.

Before the injection is made, it is helpful to bisect an imaginary line drawn from the gingival border of the most posterior molar that has erupted to the midline. Approaching from the opposite side of the mouth, the dentist makes the injection along this imaginary line and distal to the last tooth (Figs. 13-12 and 13-13). In the child in whom only the primary dentition has erupted, the injection should be made approximately 10 mm posterior to the distal surface of the second primary molar. It

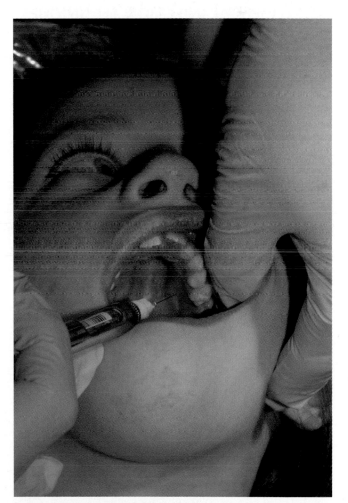

Figure 13-12 Greater palatine injection is used in conjunction with the middle or posterior alveolar nerve block before removal of a maxillary primary molar.

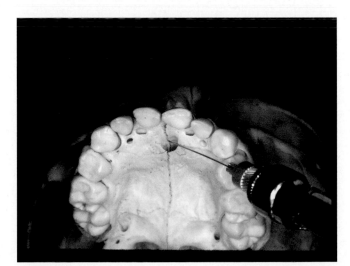

Figure 13-11 The needle is directed upward into the incisive canal when anesthetizing the nasopalatine nerve.

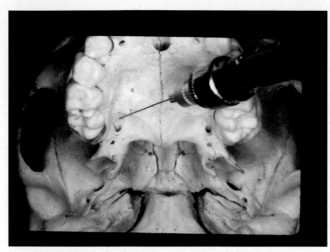

Figure 13-13 The needle is inserted approximately 10 mm posterior to the distal surface of the second primary molar.

is not necessary to enter the greater palatine foramen. A few drops of the solution should be injected slowly at the point where the nerve emerges from the foramen.

SUPPLEMENTAL INJECTION TECHNIQUES

INFRAORBITAL NERVE BLOCK AND MENTAL NERVE BLOCK

The infraorbital nerve block and the mental nerve block are two additional local anesthetic techniques used by many dentists. The infraorbital nerve block anesthetizes the branches of the anterior and middle superior alveolar nerves. It also affects innervation of the soft tissues below the eye, half of the nose, and the oral musculature of the upper lip on the injected side of the face. This leaves the child with a feeling of numbness above the mouth similar to that below the mouth when an inferior alveolar nerve is blocked. In addition, there is temporary partial oral paralysis. These effects do not contraindicate use of the technique when it is truly needed. However, we find its use difficult to justify in routine operative and extraction procedures for teeth innervated by the anterior and middle superior alveolar nerves, because the supraperiosteal techniques are more localized and just as effective. The infraorbital block technique is preferred when impacted teeth (especially canines or first premolars) or large cysts are to be removed, when moderate inflammation or infection contraindicates use of the supraperiosteal injection site, or when longer duration or a greater area of anesthesia is needed.

The mental nerve block leaves the patient with essentially the same feelings of numbness as the inferior alveolar nerve block. Blocking the mental nerve anesthetizes all mandibular teeth in the quadrant except the permanent molars. Thus the mental nerve block makes it possible to perform routine operative procedures on all primary teeth without discomfort to the patient. However, we believe that the inferior alveolar nerve block should be favored unless there is a specific contraindication to its use at the inferior alveolar nerve injection site.

The mental nerve block is no more comfortable for the patient, and the technique puts the syringe in clear view of the patient, whereas the inferior alveolar nerve block may be performed with the syringe out of the child's direct vision.

Refer to the textbooks by Jorgensen and Hayden[17] and by Malamed[6] for more detailed information concerning the infraorbital block, the mental block, and other local anesthetic techniques.

PERIODONTAL LIGAMENT INJECTION (INTRALIGAMENTARY INJECTION)

The periodontal ligament injection has been used for many years as an adjunctive method of obtaining more complete anesthesia when supraperiosteal or block techniques failed to provide adequate anesthesia. This technique has also gained credibility as a good method of obtaining primary anesthesia for one or two teeth.

The technique is simple, requires only small quantities of anesthetic solution, and produces anesthesia almost instantly. The needle is placed in the gingival sulcus, usually on the mesial surface, and advanced along the root surface until resistance is met. Then approximately 0.2 mL of anesthetic is deposited into the periodontal ligament. For multirooted teeth, injections are made both mesially and distally. Considerable pressure is necessary to express the anesthetic solution.

A conventional dental syringe may be used for this technique. However, the great pressure required to express the anesthetic makes it desirable to use a syringe with a closed barrel to offer protection in the unlikely event that the anesthetic cartridge breaks. Some syringes are equipped with a metal or Teflon sleeve that encloses the cartridge and provides the necessary protection in case of breakage.

Syringes designed specifically for the periodontal ligament injection technique have been developed. One syringe, the Peri-Press (University Dental Implements, Fanwood, NJ), is designed with a lever-action "trigger" that enables the dentist to deliver the necessary injection pressure conveniently. The Peri-Press syringe has a solid metal barrel and is calibrated to deliver 0.14 mL of anesthetic solution each time the trigger is completely activated.

There are some possible psychological disadvantages to use of the periodontal ligament injection technique, especially for the inexperienced pediatric patient. The technique provides the patient with an opportunity to see the syringe and to watch the administration of the anesthetic. This may not be a significant problem for the experienced, well-adjusted dental patient, but it may contribute to the anxiety reaction of the new or anxiety-prone patient. In addition, the very design of the Peri-Press (which resembles a handgun) probably has some adverse psychological effects.

There are two types of syringes designed specifically for intraligamentary injections. One is gunlike and the other is penlike. They both have the additional disadvantage of being quite expensive compared to a good, conventional aspirating syringes. The penlike syringe would be preferred in pediatric dentistry, but it is even more expensive than the gunlike instrument.

Nevertheless, the periodontal ligament injection technique seems to offer a valuable adjunctive method of achieving dental anesthesia.

Malamed has reported a clinical study in which impressive results were obtained for certain procedures when the periodontal ligament injection technique was used.[20] The sample size was small for some procedures, and he pointed out that additional research was warranted. However, seven periodontal procedures (curettage and root planing) were performed with 100% effective anesthesia, and two teeth were extracted with 100% effective anesthesia (injections were administered to the mesial, distal, buccal, and lingual areas for these procedures). Seventy-one routine restorative procedures were performed under periodontal ligament anesthesia, with 91.5% effectiveness. The technique proved 66.6% effective for crown preparation procedures on 12 teeth, and for eight endodontic procedures adequate anesthetization was achieved only 50% of the time. Several different anesthetics were used, with and without vasoconstrictors, yet there seemed to be little difference in success rates or duration of pulpal anesthesia with the various agents. Because of the confined space and the limited blood circulation at the injection site for the periodontal ligament technique, the use of vasoconstrictors as an additive to the anesthetic solution may not be warranted. In fact, vasoconstrictors might conceivably contribute to ischemia of the periodontal ligament, which could at least add to localized postoperative discomfort or possibly cause more serious damage to the periodontal ligament. Walton and Abbott have also reported a clinical evaluation of the technique that showed a 92% success rate.[21]

The periodontal ligament injection offers the following advantages for either primary or adjunctive anesthesia:

1. It provides reliable pain control rapidly and easily.
2. It provides pulpal anesthesia for 30 to 45 minutes, long enough for many single-tooth procedures without an extended period of postoperative anesthesia.
3. It is no more uncomfortable than other local anesthesia techniques.
4. It is completely painless if used adjunctively.
5. It requires very small quantities of anesthetic solution.
6. It does not require aspiration before injection.
7. It may be performed without removal of the rubber dam.
8. It may be useful in patients with bleeding disorders that contraindicate use of other injections.
9. It may be useful in young or disabled patients in whom the possibility of postoperative trauma to the lips or tongue is a concern.

INTRAOSSEOUS INJECTION, INTERSEPTAL INJECTION, AND INTRAPULPAL INJECTION

Intraosseous, interseptal, and intrapulpal injection techniques have been known for many years, but they have recently received renewed attention. The intrapulpal injection is an adjunctive anesthesia technique designed to obtain profound pulpal anesthesia during direct pulp therapy when other local anesthesia attempts have failed. The intrapulpal injection often provides the desired anesthesia, but the technique has the disadvantage of being painful initially, although the onset of anesthesia is usually rapid.

Intraosseous injection techniques (of which the interseptal injection is one type) require the deposition of local anesthetic solution in the porous alveolar bone. One may do this by forcing a needle through the cortical plate and into the cancellous alveolar bone, or a small, round bur may be used to make an access in the bone for the needle. A small, reinforced intraosseous needle may be used to penetrate the cortical plate more easily. This procedure is not particularly difficult in children because they have less dense cortical bone than adults. The intraosseous techniques have been advocated for both primary anesthesia and adjunctive anesthesia when other local injections have failed to produce adequate anesthesia. These techniques have been reported by Lilienthal to produce profound anesthesia.[22] They do not seem to offer any advantages over the periodontal ligament injection except when use of the latter is contraindicated by infection in the periodontal ligament space.

COMPUTER-CONTROLLED LOCAL ANESTHETIC DELIVERY SYSTEM (WAND)

Reports by Friedman and Hochman[23] and by Krochak and Friedman[24] emphasize the advantages of a computer-controlled local anesthetic delivery system known as the Wand (Milestone Scientific, Livingston, NJ). The system includes a conventional local anesthetic needle and a disposable wandlike syringe held by a pen grasp when used for oral local anesthetic injections. A microprocessor with a foot control regulates the delivery of anesthetic solution through the syringe at a precision-metered flow rate, constant pressure, and controlled volume. The system includes an aspiration cycle for use when necessary. Block, infiltration, palatal, and periodontal ligament injections are all reported to be more comfortable for the patient with the Wand than with conventional injection techniques. In a randomized clinical trial comparing the Wand with the traditional anesthetic delivery system, Allen and associates demonstrated that use of the Wand led to significantly fewer disruptive behaviors ($P < 0.1$) in preschool-aged children.[25] None of the preschool-aged children exposed to the Wand required restraint during the initial interval while nearly half of the children receiving a traditional injection required some type of immediate restraint.

COMPLICATIONS AFTER A LOCAL ANESTHETIC

ANESTHETIC TOXICITY

Systemic toxic reactions from the anesthetics are rarely observed in adults. However, young children are more likely to experience toxic reactions because of their lower body weight. Young children are also often sedated with pharmacologic agents before the treatment. The potential for toxic reactions increases when local anesthetics are used in conjunction with sedation medications. Aubuchon found a direct lineal relationship between the number of cartridges of local anesthetic administered and the frequency of severe reactions.[26] It is most important for dentists who treat children to be acutely aware of the maximum recommended dosages of the anesthetic agents they use, because allowable dosages are based on the patient's weight (Table 13-1). For example, the toxic dose of lidocaine would be attained if hardly more than 1½ cartridges (3 mL) of 2% lidocaine with 1:100,000 epinephrine were injected at one time in a patient weighing 14 kg (30 lb). Yet 5½ cartridges of the same anesthetic agent would be required to reach the toxic level in an adolescent patient weighing 46 kg (100 lb).

Because there is the possibility of toxic reaction to local anesthetic in some children, Wilson and colleagues have studied and reported on the clinical effectiveness of 1% and 2% lidocaine.[27] They found that 1% and 2% lidocaine were equally effective when performing minor procedures on primary molars.[27] The 1% lidocaine had a slightly lower effectiveness for major procedures, including pulpotomies and extractions.

TRAUMA TO SOFT TISSUE

Parents of children who receive regional local anesthesia in the dental office should be warned that the soft tissue in the area will be without sensation for a period of 1 hour or more. These children should be observed carefully so that they will not purposely or inadvertently bite the tissue. Children who receive an inferior alveolar injection for routine operative procedures may bite the lip, tongue, or inner surface of the cheek. Sometimes a parent calls the dentist's office an hour or two after a dental appointment to report an injury to the child's oral mucous membrane. The parent may wonder if the accident occurred during the dental appointment; in all probability the child has chewed the area, and the result 24 hours later is an ulceration, often termed a *traumatic ulcer* (Fig. 13-14). Complications after a self-inflicted injury of this type are rare. However, the child should be seen in 24 hours, and a warm saline mouth rinse is helpful in keeping the area clean.

In a prospective study, College and colleagues evaluated unilateral versus bilateral mandibular nerve block anesthesia with regard to postoperative soft tissue trauma and

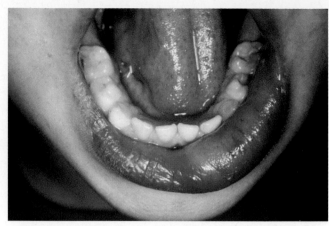

Figure 13-14 Child who has chewed his lip after an inferior alveolar nerve block for operative procedures.

other complications in a pediatric population.[28] Their results showed that after unilateral and bilateral blocks, 13% of patients experienced postoperative soft tissue trauma, with the younger patients (younger than 4 years of age) experiencing more than twice as many problems as the older patients (older than 12 years of age). Interestingly, the study showed that, in the group younger than age 4, patients receiving the unilateral nerve blocks had a statistically significantly higher incidence of trauma than the patients receiving the bilateral nerve blocks (35% versus 5%). Although the use of bilateral mandibular nerve blocks has been discouraged in the past, College and colleagues concluded that there is no contraindication to the use of bilateral mandibular block anesthesia in pediatric patients.

ELECTRONIC DENTAL ANESTHESIA

Although an excellent record of effective and safe local anesthesia has been achieved in dentistry and medicine by injection, it is common knowledge that many children and adults have acquired a significant aversion to any form of therapy requiring injection with a needle. This

Table **13-1**

Maximum Recommended Doses of Local Anesthetics

Dose	Proprietary Name	Percent of Local Anesthetic	Vasoconstrictor	Duration of Anesthetic	Maximum Recommended Dose (Malamed)
Lidocaine	Xylocaine	2	Epinephrine 1:100,000	Pulpal: 60 min Soft tissue: 3-5 hr	4.4 mg/kg
Mepivacaine	Carbocaine	3	—	Pulpal: 20-40 min Soft Tissue: 2-3 hr	4.4 mg/kg
Prilocaine	Citanest Forte	4	Epinephrine 1:200,000	Pulpal: 60-90 min Soft Tissue: 3-8 hr	6.0 mg/kg
Articaine	Septocaine	4	Epinephrine 1:100,000	Pulpal: 60-75 min Soft Tissue: 180-360 min	7 mg/kg

Adapted from Malamed SF. Handbook of Local Anesthesia, 4th ed. St. Louis, Mosby, 1997.

aversion has prompted the investment of much time, energy, and resources in the search for effective and practical local anesthesia techniques that do not require the use of needles. During the late twentieth century, renewed interest in electronic dental anesthesia (EDA) as a viable alternative to conventional local injections occurred. At least six clinical studies have been completed to evaluate the efficacy of EDA in children.[29-34] In general, these studies show that EDA can produce sufficient oral local anesthesia and analgesia to comfortably allow many invasive dental procedures in children. However, the procedures cannot be performed as efficiently, and the effectiveness of anesthesia is not consistently as reliable as with conventional techniques. Further research on EDA and the refinement of EDA delivery systems are required before EDA can be recommended as a superior substitute for conventional procedures.

REVERSAL OF DENTAL ANESTHESIA

With the granting of marketing approval by the FDA in May 2008, OraVerse (Novalar Pharmaceuticals, Inc., San Diego, Calif; http://www.novalar.com) (phentolamine mesylate) became the first pharmaceutical agent indicated for the reversal of soft tissue anesthesia, that is, anesthesia of the lip and tongue, and the associated functional deficits resulting from an intraoral submucosal injection of a local anesthetic containing a vasoconstrictor.

In randomized, double-blind, controlled phase 3 studies, following the administration of local anesthetics and completion of the dental procedure, patients were given either OraVerse or the control treatment. OraVerse reduced the median time to recovery of normal sensation in the lower lip (as measured by standardized lip tapping procedures) by 85 minutes compared with the control. OraVerse reduced the median time to recovery of normal sensation in the upper lip by 83 minutes. Within 1 hour after administration

of OraVerse, 41% of the patients reported normal lower lip sensation compared with 7% in the control group, and 59% of patients in the OraVerse group reported normal upper lip sensation compared with 12% in the control group. Similar results in additional pediatric subjects (ages 6 to 11 years of age) have been recently reported.[35]

In all OraVerse clinical trials, there were no serious adverse events reported. The most common adverse reaction was transient injection site pain. Although tachycardia and cardiac arrhythmia may occur with the parenteral use of alpha-adrenergic blocking agents, such events are uncommon after submucosal administration of OraVerse. OraVerse is not recommended for use in children younger than 6 years of age or who weigh less than 15 kg (33 lb).

ANALGESICS

In addition to local administration of anesthetics to aid in pain control, occasionally systemic administration of analgesics is necessary to help control pain. These analgesics may be needed in instances of moderate to severe pain associated with trauma or infectious processes such as abscessed teeth, or they may be administered preoperatively or postoperatively in association with a dental procedure that may cause pain for the child. The rationale for preoperative administration of analgesics draws on the theory that giving the drug before the procedure provides effective analgesia because it precedes the inflammatory response and subsequent pain incurred during the operative procedure. This theory is not without controversy, however, and there are conflicting reports within the literature as to the efficacy of this technique.

Tate and Acs suggest that the selection and dosages of analgesics vary because of the change in body weight and composition that occur throughout childhood.[30] The first choice in most cases is the least potent analgesic with the fewest side effects. Table 13-2, adapted from Tate and Acs,

Table 13-2

Medications and Dosages for Oral Pediatric Postoperative Pain Management

Medication	Availability	Dosage	40-lb child	80-lb child
Acetaminophen	Elixir: 160 mg/5 mL Tablets: 325 mg Chewable: 160 mg	10-15 mg/kg/dose given at 4-6 hr intervals	160 mg = 1 tsp 160 mg = 1 chewable	325 mg = 1 tablet 320 mg = 2 chewables
Ibuprofen	Suspension: 100 mg/5 mL Tablets: 200, 300, 400, 600, 800 mg	4-10 mg/kg/dose given at 6- to 8-hr intervals	100 mg = 1 tsp	200 mg = 2 tsp 200 mg = 1 tablet
Tramadol	Tablets: 50, 100 mg	1-2 mg/kg/dose given at 4- to 6-hr intervals-maximum 100 mg	25 mg = ½ tablet	50 mg = 1 tablet
Codeine and acetaminophen	Suspension: 12 mg/5 mL	0.5-1.0 mg codeine/kg/dose given at 4- to 6-hr intervals	12 mg = 1 tsp	24 mg = 2 tsp
Meperidine	Syrup: 50 mg/5 mL Tablets: 50 mg, 100 mg	1-2 mg/kg/dose given at 4- to 6-hr intervals	25 mg = ½ tsp	50 mg = 1 tsp

Adapted from Tate AR, Acs G. Dental postoperative pain management in children. Dent Clin North Am 2002;46:707-717.

shows common pediatric pain management agents and their appropriate dosage schedules.[36] Tate and Acs suggest that only rarely does the recommended dosage of acetaminophen or nonsteroidal anti-inflammatory drugs fail to control the dental pain. In the rare cases in which acetaminophen or nonsteroidal anti-inflammatory drugs are not sufficient to manage the pain, the combination of codeine and acetaminophen provides the needed pain relief. Finally, in cases of severe pain in which codeine and acetaminophen are not effective, meperidine may be indicated.

REFERENCES

1. Venham L, Quatrocelli S. The young child's response to repeated dental procedures, *J Dent Res* 56:734-738, 1977.
2. O'Toole TJ. Administration of local anesthesia. In Snawder KD. *Handbook of clinical pedodontics.* St. Louis, 1980, Mosby.
3. Duckworth GM, et al. Oral PowderJect: a novel system for administering local anaesthesia to the oral mucosa, *Br Dent J* 185:536-539, 1998.
4. Wittrock JW, Fischer WE. The aspiration of blood through small-gauge needles, *J Am Dent Assoc* 76:79-81, 1968.
5. Trapp LD, Davies RO. Aspiration as a function of hypodermic needle internal diameter in the in vivo human upper limb, *Anesth Prog* 27:49-51, 1980.
6. Malamed SF. *Handbook of local anesthesia,* 5th ed. St. Louis, 2004, Elsevier Mosby.
7. Olsen NH. Anesthesia for the child patient, *J Am Dent Assoc* 53:548-555, 1956.
8. Wright GZ, et al. The effectiveness of infiltration anesthesia in the mandibular molar region, *Pediatr Dent* 13:278-283, 1991.
9. Oulis CJ, Vadiakas GP, Vasilopoulou A. The effectiveness of mandibular infiltration compared to mandibular block anesthesia in treating primary molars in children, *Pediatr Dent* 18:301-305, 1996.
10. Oertel R, Rahn R, Kirch W. Clinical pharmacokinetics of articaine, *Clin Pharmacokinet* 33(6):417-426, 1997.
11. Ortel R, et al. The concentration of local anesthetics in the dental alveolus. Comparative studies of lidocaine and articaine in the mandible and maxilla, *Schweiz Monatsschr Zahnmed* 104(8):952-955, 1994.
12. Vree TB, Gielen MJ. Clinical pharmacology and the use of articaine for local regional anaesthesia, *Best Pract Res Clin Anaesthesiol* 19(2):293-308, 2005.
13. Claffey E, et al. Anesthetic efficacy of articaine for inferior alveolar nerve blocks in patients with irreversible pulpitis, *J Endodont* 30(8):568-571, 2004.
14. Kanaa MD, et al. Articaine and lidocaine mandibular buccal infiltration anesthesia: a prospective randomized double blind cross-over study, *J Endodontics* 32(4):296-298, 2006.
15. Sharaf AA. Evaluation of mandibular infiltration versus block anesthesia in pediatric dentistry, *J Dent Child* 64:276-281, 1997.
16. Gow-Gates GAE. Mandibular conduction anesthesia: a new technique using extraoral landmarks, *Oral Surg* 36:321-328, 1973.
17. Jorgensen NB, Hayden J Jr. *Sedation, local and general anesthesia in dentistry,* 3rd ed. Philadelphia, 1980, Lea & Febiger.
18. Bennett CR. *Monheim's local anesthesia and pain control in dental practice,* 7th ed. St. Louis, 1984, Mosby.
19. Ramirez K, et al. Painless pediatric local anesthesia, *Gen Dent* 49(2):174-176, 2001.
20. Malamed SF. The periodontal ligament (PDL) injection: an alternative to inferior alveolar nerve block, *Oral Surg* 53:117-121, 1982.
21. Walton RE, Abbott BJ. Periodontal ligament injection: a clinical evaluation, *J Am Dent Assoc* 103:571-575, 1981.
22. Lilienthal B. A clinical appraisal of intraosseous dental anesthesia, *Oral Surg* 39:692-697, 1975.
23. Friedman MJ, Hochman MN. A 21st century computerized injection system for local pain control, *Compend Contin Educ Dent* 18:995-1000, 1002-1004, 1997.
24. Krochak M, Friedman N. Using a precision-metered injection system to minimize dental injection anxiety, *Compend Contin Educ Dent* 19:137-143, 146-150, 1998.
25. Allen KD, et al. Comparison of a computerized anesthesia device with a traditional syringe in preschool children, *Pediatr Dent* 24(4):315-320, 2002.
26. Aubuchon RW. Sedation liabilities in pedodontics, *Pediatr Dent* 4:171-180, 1982.
27. Wilson TG, et al. Clinical effectiveness of 1 and 2% lidocaine in young pediatric dental patients, *Pediatr Dent* 12:353-359, 1990.
28. College C, et al. Bilateral unilateral mandibular block anesthesia in a pediatric population, *Pediatr Dent* 22(6):453-457, 2000.
29. Baghdadi ZD. Evaluation of audio analgesia for restorative case in children treated using electronic dental anesthesia, *J Clin Pediatr Dent* 25:9-12, 2000.
30. Cho SY, et al. Effectiveness of electronic dental anesthesia for restorative care in children, *Pediatr Dent* 20:105-111, 1998.
31. Harvey M, Elliott M. Transcutaneous electrical nerve stimulation (TENS) for pain management during cavity preparations in pediatric patients, *J Dent Child* 62:49-51, 1995.
32. Modaresi A, et al. A partial double-blind, placebo-controlled study of electronic dental anaesthesia in children, *Int J Paediatr Dent* 6:245-251, 1996.
33. te Duits, et al. The effectiveness of electronic dental anesthesia in children, *Pediatr Dent* 15:191-196, 1993.
34. Toppi GR. The use of cell demodulated electronic targeted anesthesia to control dental operative pain in pediatric patients, thesis. Indianapolis, Indiana University School of Dentistry, 1999.
35. Tavares M, et al. Reversal of soft-tissue local anesthesia with phentolamine mesylate in pediatric patients, *JADA* 139:1095-1104, 2008.
36. Tate AR, Acs G. Dental postoperative pain management in children, *Dent Clin North Am* 46(4):707-117, 2002.

SUGGESTED READINGS

Berde CB, Sethna NF. Drug therapy: analgesics for the treatment of pain in children, *N Engl J Med* 347(14):1094-1103, 2002.
Blanton PL, Jeske AH. The key to profound local anesthesia: neuroanatomy, *J Am Dent Assoc* 134:753-760, 2003.

CHAPTER 14

Pharmacologic Management of Patient Behavior

▲ Murray Dock

FUNDAMENTAL CONCEPTS

To perform the highest quality dental care for the pediatric patient, the practitioner may need to use pharmacologic means to obtain a quiescent, cooperative patient. Techniques that use drugs to induce a cooperative yet conscious state in an otherwise anxious or uncooperative child are most commonly referred to as *techniques of sedation.* Levels of sedation are defined as follows (American Academy of Pediatric Dentistry [AAPD] guidelines):

Minimal sedation. A drug-induced state during which patients respond normally to verbal commands. Although cognitive function and coordination may be impaired, ventilatory function and cardiovascular function are unaffected.

Moderate sedation. A drug-induced depression of consciousness during which patients respond purposefully to verbal commands. For older patients, this level of sedation implies an interactive state; for younger patients, age-appropriate behavior (e.g., crying) occurs and is expected. No intervention is required to maintain a patent airway, and spontaneous ventilation is adequate. Cardiovascular function is usually maintained.

Deep sedation. A drug-induced depression of consciousness during which patients cannot be easily aroused but respond purposefully after repeated verbal or painful stimulation. The ability to independently maintain ventilatory function may be impaired. Patients may require assistance in maintaining a patent airway, and spontaneous ventilation may be inadequate. There

may be partial or complete loss of protective airway reflexes.

The goals of sedation for the pediatric patient are (1) to guard the patient's safety and welfare, (2) to minimize physical discomfort and pain; (3) to control anxiety, minimize psychological trauma, and maximize the potential for amnesia; (4) to control behavior or movement so as to allow the safe completion of the procedure; and (5) to return the patient to a physiologic state in which safe discharge, as determined by recognized criteria, is possible. In-office sedation techniques used by pediatric dentists produce a minimally depressed state or level of consciousness in which the patient retains the ability to maintain a patent airway independently and continuously, and is able to respond appropriately to physical stimulation or verbal commands. This means that the patient can in some way purposefully acknowledge a request to move or open the eyes, or react to an uncomfortable applied stimulus. All reflexes are essentially intact. If the patient is incapable of response by virtue of being very young or severely disabled, one should exercise care not to depress the patient to a point where such a determination is difficult to make. The techniques and drugs used to produce this state should possess a margin of safety of ample width to preclude unintended loss of consciousness.

In contrast to this awake state, deep sedation and general anesthesia are defined as conditions of the patient characterized by an incomplete, partial, or total loss of protective reflexes. In addition, there may be a partial or complete loss of the ability to independently and continuously maintain a patent airway. Cardiovascular function may also be impaired. Under these circumstances, the patient is noninteractive and does not respond purposefully to physical stimulation or verbal command.

Occasionally the sedated patient will drift into normal sleep. When this occurs, it becomes the practitioner's responsibility to be assured that what is being observed is a normal sleep state by frequently arousing the patient. This may be frustrating, because the objective is to produce a patient who is totally cooperative and the sleeping patient is just that.

Often, deep sedation and general anesthesia are differentiated; however, for the purposes of describing what is required to manage the patient in this condition in terms of training, monitoring, facilities, and personnel, the two conditions are treated as a single physiologic state of the patient. The requirements for management of the unconscious patient are much more stringent and address a greater concern for the safety of the patient.

A caution for the practitioner should be to avoid thinking of the patient's state in terms of the techniques employed rather than the level of consciousness. Historically, many sedation techniques have been defined by the route of administration. It is not the technique of administration but the drugs or agents employed that produce the effect observed in the patient. For example, one can produce an unconscious or fully anesthetized patient using the oral route. The concept of rescue is essential to safe sedation. Practitioners of sedation must have the skills to rescue the patient from a deeper level than that intended for the procedure (AAPD guidelines).

Several requisites should be satisfied when the use of sedation for pediatric dental patients is considered. They are the following:

1. The practitioner should possess a thorough knowledge of the agent or agents to be used and should be formally trained in the proper method of their administration. When sedating pediatric patients, practitioners must adhere to the guidelines published by the American Dental Association as well as the joint guidelines of the American Academy of Pediatric Dentistry (AAPD) and the American Academy of Pediatrics (AAP) for the management of pediatric patients during and after sedation for diagnostic and therapeutic procedures.[1,2] It is unwise and no longer acceptable to learn sedation by experimenting in one's own practice setting.

2. There should be a carefully planned and documented rationale for the use of sedation for each patient. The decision should be made based on a careful analysis of the behavioral profile of the patient, the nature and extent of the treatment required, the risk-to-benefit ratio with regard to the physical status of the patient, the capability of the family to meet the demands of an extensive treatment plan, and the economic feasibility of alternative choices.

3. The patient should be carefully evaluated to ensure that no condition exists that might alter the expected response to the sedative agent or technique and pose added risk to the patient.

4. There should be a well-documented informed consent. No sedation technique should be attempted unless the parent or guardian has participated in a thorough consultation on the alternatives to sedation and foreseeable risks, knows what is expected in the postsedation period, and willingly agrees to proceed.

5. The office facilities should be such that a comfortable experience can be assured. There should be no physical barriers or lack of proper equipment to complicate the management of any emergency that might arise. Personnel should be thoroughly trained in techniques of monitoring a sedated patient. Practitioners should be certified in either Advanced Cardiac Life Support (ACLS) or Pediatric Advanced Life Support (PALS). These personnel should be trained and frequently rehearsed in patient resuscitation.

6. Mobile emergency medical services should be readily available. The capabilities of these facilities and their personnel should be appraised and their response time to the office known before reliance on them is considered a part of the emergency protocol.

ANATOMIC AND PHYSIOLOGIC DIFFERENCES

When a regimen of sedation for the pediatric patient is prepared, it is important to consider the differences between the adult patient and one in the pediatric age group. The sedation of children is different from the sedation of adults. Differences in size, weight, and age as a measure of maturation of systems are obvious. Less obvious, but equally important, are the differences in basal metabolic rate between the adult and pediatric patient. Basal metabolic activity is greater in children, which ultimately affects not only drug response but also important physiologic parameters as well. Because oxygen demand is greater but the alveolar system is less mature, the respiratory rate is far higher in children than in adults (Table 14-1). This is an important consideration when drugs that depress the respiratory system are administered.

Airway management requires different consideration in the pediatric patient because of anatomic variations. The narrow nasal passages and glottis, combined with

Table 14-1
Vital Signs at Various Ages

Age (yr)	Heart Rate (beats/min)	Blood Pressure (mm Hg)	Respiratory Rate (breaths/min)
1 to 3	70 to 110	90 to 105/55 to 70	20 to 30
3 to 6	65 to 110	95 to 110/60 to 75	20 to 25
6 to 12	60 to 95	100 to 120/60 to 75	14 to 22
12	55 to 85	110 to 135/65 to 85	12 to 18

Adapted from Behrman RE, et al. Nelson Textbook of Pediatrics, 17th ed. Philadelphia, Elsevier Science, 2004.

hypertrophic tonsils and adenoids, enlarged tongue, and greater secretions, produce a much greater risk of airway obstruction. The airway of all patients should be examined before sedation (Fig. 14-1). Patients with tonsillar tissue that occupies more than 50% of the pharyngeal space are at increased risk for respiratory obstruction, and alternative treatment options should be considered.[3] Children demonstrate a reduced tolerance to respiratory obstruction. Thus sudden apnea is a greater concern in the pediatric age group. Because the thorax is smaller, with less expansion capability, children have less functional reserve. Consequently they are more prone to

rapid desaturation on obstruction or respiratory depression. For this reason children with sleep apnea are not good candidates for sedation.

Cardiovascular parameters are different for children. The heart rate is faster and blood pressure is lower than in the adult. Children are more susceptible to bradycardia, decreased cardiac output, and hypotension. Unlike in the adult population, heart rate is the primary determinate of blood pressure in children. Compensatory mechanisms to maintain adequate blood pressure when the heart rate is depressed are not as well developed in children. Thus a decrease in heart rate leads to a corresponding decrease in

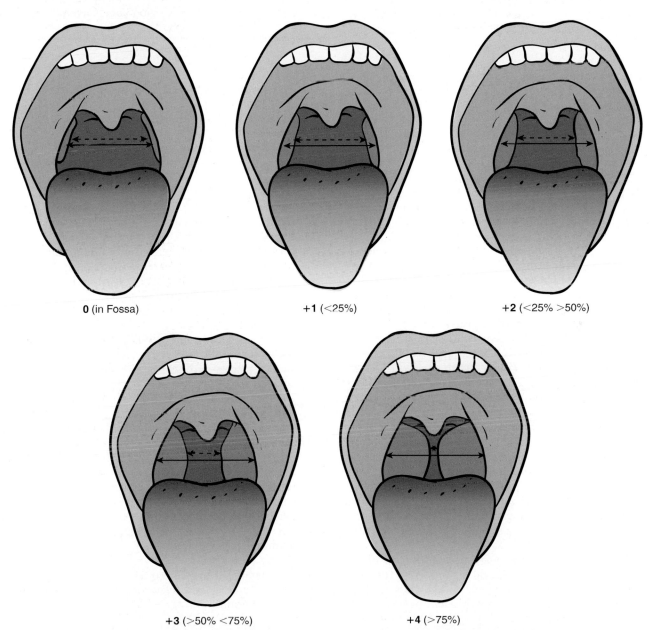

Figure 14-1 Standardized system for evaluation of tonsillar size. Classification of tonsil size should be completed for all patients before sedation. Patients classified as +3 or greater (having more than 50% of the pharyngeal area occupied by tonsils) are at increased risk for developing airway obstruction. (From Brodsky L. Modern assessment of tonsils and adenoids. Pediatr Clin North Am 1989;36:1551-1569; and Cote CJ, et al. A practice of Anesthesia for Infants and Children. Philadelphia, WB Saunders, 1993:313-314.)

blood pressure and tissue oxygenation. This concept must be well appreciated when giving drugs that depress the heart rate in the pediatric age population.

The effect and duration of action of drugs is much more variable in children. For agents that are more lipophilic, retention may be prolonged, especially in children who are obese. For some patients, drug metabolism may be increased. Because of better peripheral perfusion in children, the onset of intramuscularly administered drugs may be more rapid.

The anatomic and physiologic differences between children at different age levels and adults lead one to the conclusion that dosage is not simply an application of a formula for derivation of a percentage of the adult dosage of any agent. Drug dosages for children should be carefully individualized for each patient following established guidelines.

PATIENT SELECTION AND PREPARATION

INDICATIONS

Because sedation embodies a group of techniques designed to alter patient behavior, the practitioner should have a rationale for making the choice as to which patients will most likely benefit from their use. The indiscriminate application of these techniques to all patients must be avoided. Several behavioral or anxiety-assessment profiles have been developed that can be of great help to the practitioner as the various techniques are introduced into a practice.[4,5] As one gains experience, this decision becomes more one of clinical judgment and intuition as to which approach produces the most successful results for specific types of patients for that individual practitioner. No one technique or agent, or combination of agents, should be expected to be successful every time. There are also degrees of success, and total immobilization and near unconsciousness of a patient should not necessarily be equated with the most successful sedation. One should choose the agent and technique that best fits the patient type as well as the nature of what needs to be accomplished.

A thorough medical history is required to determine whether a patient is suitable for sedative procedures. This, along with a recent physical examination, constitute a risk assessment or physiologic status evaluation. This health evaluation should be used to place the patient in one of the categories set forth by the American Society of Anesthesiologists (http://www.asahq.org/clinical/physicalstatus.htm) and should be documented in the record (Box 14-1).

Patients who are in ASA I are frequently considered appropriate candidates for minimal, moderate, or deep sedation. Some children assigned to ASA class II or III may actually benefit from this approach, but this must be determined in consultation with the child's physician. Generally, patients categorized into classes III and IV, children with special needs, and those with anatomic airway abnormalities or extreme tonsillar hypertrophy are better managed in a hospital setting. (AAPD guidelines).

Box 14-1

American Society of Anesthesiologists' Physical Status Classification System

Class I	A normal healthy patient
Class II	A patient with mild systemic disease (e.g., controlled reactive airway disease)
Class III	A patient with severe systemic disease (e.g., a child who is actively wheezing)
Class IV	A patient with severe systemic disease (e.g., a child with status asthmaticus)
Class V	A moribund patient who is not expected to survive without operation (e.g., a patient with severe cardiomyopathy requiring heart transplantation)

The medical history should include information regarding the following:
1. Allergies and previous allergic or adverse drug reactions.
2. Current medications, including dosage, time, route, and site of administration for prescription, over-the-counter, herbal, or illicit drugs. Many drugs, including herbal agents (e.g., St. John's Wort, Echinacea, kava, valerian), may alter drug pharmacokinetics, prolonging the effect of sedative agents.
3. Diseases or abnormalities in the patient, including pregnancy status of adolescents and neurologic impairment that might increase the potential for airway obstruction, such as a history of snoring or obstructive sleep apnea (AAPD).
4. Previous hospitalizations, including the date, purpose, and hospital course.
5. History of general anesthesia or sedation and any associated complication.
6. Family history of diseases and sedation or anesthetic complications.
7. Review of body systems.
8. Age in years and months and weight in kilograms.

The physical evaluation should include the following:
1. Vital signs, including heart, respiratory rates, blood pressure, and temperature. If determination of baseline vital signs is prevented by the patient's physical resistance or emotional condition, the reason(s) should be documented.
2. Evaluation of airway patency to include tonsillar size (see Fig 14-1) and any anatomic abnormality (e.g., mandibular hypoplasia) that may increase the risk of airway obstruction.
3. ASA classification (see Box 14-1).
4. Name, address, and telephone number of the child's medical home.

INFORMED CONSENT

The parent or legal guardian must be agreeable to the use of sedation for the child. These individuals are entitled to receive complete information regarding the reasonably foreseeable risks and the benefits associated with the

---

**CONSENT FOR THE USE OF SEDATION OR GENERAL ANESTHESIA
FOR
PEDIATRIC DENTAL TREATMENT**

I _____, as the legally responsible parent or guardian of _____, give my consent to the use of local anesthetics, sedative drugs, or general anesthetic agents that Dr(s). _____ may deem necessary on the child's examination chart, as previously explained to me, and any other procedure deemed necessary or advisable as a cor-ollary to the planned treatment for _____, except for: (if none, so state) _____.

I have been informed and understand that occasionally there are complications of the treatment, drugs, or anesthetic agents, including but not limited to: numbness, infection, swelling, bleeding, discoloration, nausea, vomiting, allergic reactions, brain damage, stroke, or heart at-tack. I further understand and accept that complications may require hospitalization and may even result in death.

Dr(s). _____ discussed with me, to my satisfaction, these compli-cations. I acknowledge the receipt of and understand the preoperative and postoperative instruc-tions. The treatment and sedation or anesthesia procedures have been explained to me, to my satisfaction, along with possible alternative methods and their advantages and disadvantages, risks, consequences, and probable effectiveness of each, as well as the prognosis if no treatment is provided.

I have read this consent and understand, to my satisfaction, the procedures to be performed and accept the possible risks.

Legally responsible parent or guardian: _____ Date: _____

Address: _____

Witness: _____

I certify that I explained the above procedures to the parent or guardian before requesting his or her signature.

_____ Date: _____
Signature of dentist

Figure 14-2 Example of form for informed consent. (Courtesy of Dr. Kenneth C. Troutman.)

particular technique and agents being used, as well as any alternative methods available. Therefore the explanation should be in clear, concise terms that are familiar to them (Fig. 14-2). The consent form can be on or part of a sedation record with space provided for the signatures of all parties.

Because sedation is not considered a routine part of every dental visit, this consent should be separate and distinct from permission to treat the patient.

INSTRUCTIONS TO PARENTS

Information in written form should be reviewed with the person caring for the child and given to this person along with the notice of the scheduled appointment (Fig. 14-3). This information should include a 24-hour contact number for the practitioner.

Dietary instructions should be as follows (AAPD guidelines):

1. Clear liquids: water, fruit juices without pulp, carbonated beverages, clear tea, black coffee up to 2 hours before the procedure.
2. Breast milk up to 4 hours before the procedure.
3. Infant formula up to 6 hours before the procedure.
4. Nonhuman milk up to 6 hours before the procedure.
5. A light meal up to 6 hours before the procedure. A light meal typically consists of toast and clear liquids. Meals that include fried or fatty foods or meat may prolong gastric emptying times and should be avoided.
6. It is permissible for routine necessary medications to be taken with a sip of water on the day of the procedure.

INSTRUCTIONS TO FOLLOW BEFORE YOUR CHILD'S SEDATION

EATING AND DRINKING
1. No milk or solid foods 6 hours before the sedation appointment.
2. Clear liquids such as water, clear juices, gelatin, Popsicles, or broth, may be given up to 3 hours before the appointment.
3. Let everyone in the home know the above information, because siblings or others living in the home often unknowingly feed the child.

ACTIVITY
1. Plan the child's sleep and awakening times to encourage the usual amount of sleep the day before the sedation appointment.
2. Please arrive on time for your scheduled appointment. This is a long appointment, and you may be here for several hours.
3. The legal guardian must accompany the child to the sedation appointment.
4. A second responsible adult must join you and your child at the time of discharge. This enables one adult to drive the car while the second adult focuses attention on your child after the treatment is completed. The child should be carefully secured in a car seat belt during transportation.
5. Make sure your child uses the restroom before the sedation.

ACTIVITY AFTER THE SEDATION
1. Your child may take a long nap. He/she may sleep from 3 to 8 hours and may be drowsy and irritable for up to 24 hours after sedation. When your child is asleep, you should be able to awaken him/her easily.
2. Your child may be unsteady when walking or crawling and will need support to protect him/her from injury. An Adult must be with the child at all times until the child has returned to his/her usual state of alertness and coordination.
3. Closely supervise any activity for the remainder of the day.

CHANGE IN HEALTH
It is important that you notify the office of the development of a cold, cough, fever, or any illness within 14 days before the sedation appointment. For your child's safety, the sedation may need to be rescheduled.

Figure 14-3 Example of presedation instructions to the parent or caregiver.

The reasons for these recommendations are twofold. First, emesis during or immediately after a sedative procedure is a potential complication that can result in aspiration of stomach contents leading to laryngospasm or severe airway obstruction. Aspiration may even present difficulties later in the form of aspiration pneumonia. At the very least, it creates an unfavorable disruption of the office routine. Second, because most sedative agents are administered by the oral route, drug uptake is maximized when the stomach is empty.

The parent or guardian should also be advised that he or she will be expected to remain in the area of the office during the sedation appointment. With regard to transportation, the instructions should request that a second person accompany the parent so that the person caring for the child may be free to attend to the child's needs during the trip home.

The caregiver should be advised that, on arriving home, the child may sleep for several hours and may be drowsy and irritable for up to 24 hours after the sedation.

It is important to stress the need for frequent observation if the child is sleeping, to ensure an open airway. Activity should be restricted to quieter pursuits and be closely supervised for the remainder of the day.

Following treatment, the child should first be offered clear liquids and may advance to solid foods as tolerated. Once solids are tolerated, there are no dietary restrictions other than those imposed as a result of the dental procedure performed. Nausea and vomiting may occur, especially when narcotics have been used, which may thus prolong the delay before beginning solid food intake. In this event, special attention should be paid to the fluid intake to ensure adequate hydration.

Knowledge on the part of the parent of what to expect is the most reliable way to ensure a calm, comfortable, and uncomplicated postsedation period. Therefore these instructions and recommendations should be in written form and should be reviewed again with the person responsible for the patient and given to this person at the time of discharge from the office (Fig. 14-4).

CARE OF YOUR CHILD AFTER SEDATION

Today your child had dental treatment under conscious sedation.

He/she received the following medicine(s) for sedation:

☐ Chloral hydrate   ☐ Meperidine (Demerol)   ☐ Hydroxyzine (Vistaril)
☐ Diazepam (Valium) ☐ Midazolam   ☐ Other_____

Children repond to sedation in their own way, but the following guidelines will help you know what to expect at home:

GOING HOME
1. Your child will not be able to walk well, so we suggest that you carry your child or use wheelchair to transport your child to the car.
2. Young children must be restrained in a car safety seat and older children must be restrained with a seat belt during transportation.

ACTIVITY
1. Your child may take a long nap. He/she may sleep from 3 to 8 hours and may be drowsy and irritable for up to 24 hours after sedation. When your child is asleep, you should be able to awaken him/her easily.
2. Your child may be unsteady when walking or crawling and will need support to protect him/her from injury. An ADULT must be with the child at all times until the child has returned to his/her usual state of alertness and coordination.
3. Your child should not perform any potentially dangerous activities, such as riding a bike, playing outside, handling sharp objects, working with tools, or climbing stairs until he/she is back to his/her usual alertness and coordination for at least 1 hour.
4. We advise you to keep your child home from school or daycare after treatment and possibly the next day if your child is still drowsy or unable to walk well. Your child should return to his/her usual state of alertness and coordination within 24 hours.

EATING AND DRINKING INSTRUCTIONS
Begin by giving clear liquids such as clear juices, water, gelatin, Popsicles, or broth. If your child does not vomit after 30 minutes, you may continue with solid foods.

REASONS TO CALL THE DOCTOR
1. You are unable to arouse your child.
2. Your child is unable to eat or drink.
3. Your child experiences excessive vomiting or pain.
4. Your child develops a rash.

FOR THESE OR ANY OTHER CONCERNS about your child's sedation, please contact our office at_____.

Figure 14-4 Example of postsedation instructions to the parent or caregiver.

DOCUMENTATION

Meticulous and accurate documentation of the sedation experience is imperative. In the event of an adverse reaction, the best insurance is an accurate, clear, continuous, documented account of what occurred before, during, and after the encounter.

Preprocedural records should document (1) proper adherence to food and liquid intake restrictions; (2) the preoperative health evaluation, including the patient's health history and a complete physical assessment along with the patient's current weight, age, and baseline vital signs; (3) name and address of the physician who usually cares for the child; (4) a note as to why the particular method of management was chosen; (5) the presence of informed consent; and (6) the delivery of instructions to the caregiver.

Before the sedation, a "time out" should be performed to confirm the patient's name, the procedure to be performed, and the site of the procedure; this should be documented in the record (AAPD #43).

Intraoperatively the appropriate vital signs should be recorded as they are assessed (Table 14-2). Timed notations regarding the patient's appearance should be

Table 14-2

Template of Definitions and Characteristics for Levels of Sedation and General Anesthesia

	Minimal sedation	Moderate Sedation	Deep Sedation
Responsiveness	Responds normally to verbal commands; uninterrupted interactive ability; totally awake.	Responds purposefully to verbal commands or following light tactile stimulation.	Cannot be easily aroused but responds purposefully after repeated verbal or painful stimulation.
Personnel required	2	2 In addition to the practitioner, the support personnel shall be capable of pediatric basic life support. May assist in patient-related tasks of short duration.	3 In addition to the practitioner and assistant, there shall be one individual whose only responsibility is to observe the patient's vital signs, airway patency, and adequacy of ventilation, and to either administer drugs or direct their administration.[1] Individual must be PALS certified.
Monitoring equipment	Clinical observation*	Pulse oximeter, BP.	Pulse oximeter, BP, ECG, and defibrillator. Precordial stethoscope and capnography encouraged.[†]
Monitoring information during procedure	Intermittent assessment of level of sedation	Continuous monitoring of oxygen saturation; heart rate; intermittent recording of respiratory rate and blood pressure.	Continuous monitoring every 5 minutes of BP, respiratory rate, oxygen saturation, and heart rate.

*Clinical observation should accompany any level of sedation and general anesthesia.
†"Encouraged" should be interpreted as not a necessity but as an adjunct in assessing patient status.
BP, Blood pressure; ECG, electrocardiography; PALS, Pediatric Advanced Life Support.
Adapted from American Academy of Pediatric Dentistry. Guidelines on the elective use of conscious sedation, deep sedation and general anesthesia in pediatric dental patients. Pediatr Dent 2003;24(7):74-80.

included. The type of drug, the dose given, and the route, site, and time of administration should be clearly indicated. If a prescription is used, either a copy of the prescription or a note as to what was prescribed should also be a part of the permanent record.

After completion of treatment, the patient should be continuously observed in an appropriately equipped recovery area. The patient should remain under direct observation until respiratory and cardiovascular stability have been ensured. The patient should not be discharged until the presedation level of consciousness or a level as close as possible for that child has been achieved (Box 14-2). At the time of discharge, the condition of the patient should be noted.

SEDATION TECHNIQUES

A variety of methods are available for producing sedation or alteration of mood in the pediatric patient. These systemic procedures are based on the thoughtful use of various drugs that produce sedation as one of their principal effects, as well as the use of differing routes of administration. Sedative drugs may be administered by inhalation or by oral, rectal, submucosal, intramuscular, or intravenous routes. The use of combinations of drugs and specific selection of routes of administration to maximize

effect and increase safety, as well as maximize patient acceptability, are common. Inhalation of a nitrous oxide–oxygen mixture is often coupled with administration of an agent by any of the other routes.

Prescription medications intended to accomplish procedural sedation must not be administered without the

Box 14-2

Discharge Criteria

1. Cardiovascular function is satisfactory and stable.
2. Airway patency is uncompromised and satisfactory.
3. Patient is easily arousable and protective reflexes are intact.
4. State of hydration is adequate.
5. Patient can talk, if applicable.
6. Patient can sit unaided, if applicable.
7. Patient can ambulate, if applicable, with minimal assistance.
8. If the child is very young or disabled, incapable of the usually expected responses, the presedation level of responsiveness or the level as close as possible for that child has been achieved.
9. Responsible individual is available.

benefit of direct supervision by trained personnel. It is no longer acceptable to administer any sedative drug outside of the treatment facility (e.g., given at home by the parent or caregiver). Administration of sedating medications at home poses an unacceptable risk, particularly for infants and preschool-aged children traveling in car-safety seats. (AAPD guidelines).

The selection of technique is often made as a matter of clinical judgment. It is a question of successfully matching a method to a specific objective.

The primary goal of these techniques is to produce a quiescent patient to ensure the best quality of care. Another goal might be to accomplish a more complex or lengthy treatment plan in a shorter period by lengthening appointment times and thereby reducing the number of repeat visits required. Children presenting with a dental injury or acute pain may require sedation for completion of treatment as well as postoperative analgesia. In fact, the reduction in anxiety may reduce the amount of analgesia required. Sedation may also allow for more comfortable and acceptable treatment for physically impaired or cognitively disabled patients. Often these patients may benefit from parenteral sedation. Although the presence of a compromising medical condition is generally a contraindication to sedation, some patients in this category may in fact benefit from its use.[6] This would, of course, include patients for whom stress reduction would reduce the likelihood of complications. These children should be managed in close cooperation with the physicians who regularly cares for them.

NITROUS OXIDE AND OXYGEN SEDATION

Eighty-five percent of pediatric dentists use nitrous oxide and oxygen for sedation of patients. This makes it the most frequently used sedative agent.

Nitrous oxide is a slightly sweet-smelling, colorless, inert gas. It is compressed in cylinders as a liquid that vaporizes on release. This is an endothermic reaction that pulls heat from the cylinder and environment; consequently the cylinder becomes cool or even cold when in use. The gas is nonflammable but will support combustion.

The objectives of nitrous oxide sedation include (AAPD guidelines):
- Reducing or eliminate anxiety
- Reducing untoward movement and reaction to dental treatment
- Enhancing communication and patient cooperation
- Raising the pain threshold
- Increase tolerance for longer appointments
- Aiding in treatment of the mentally/physically disabled or medically compromised patient
- Reducing gagging
- Potentiating the effect of sedatives

Disadvantages of nitrous oxide–oxygen inhalation may include (AAPD guidelines):
- Lack of potency
- Dependence on psychological reassurance
- Interference of the nasal hood with injection to anterior maxillary region
- Need for patient to be able to breathe through the nose
- Nitrous oxide pollution and potential occupational exposure health hazards

Pharmacokinetics

Nitrous oxide is slightly heavier than air, with a specific gravity of 1.53, and has a blood to gas partition coefficient of 0.47. Because of its low solubility in blood, it has a very rapid onset and recovery time. Nitrous oxide will become saturated in blood within 3 to 5 minutes following administration and is physically dissolved in the serum fraction of the blood. There is no biotransformation, and the gas is rapidly excreted by the lungs when the concentration gradient is reversed. Very small amounts may be found in excreted body fluids and intestinal gas.

A phenomenon termed diffusion hypoxia may occur as the sedation is reversed at the termination of the procedure. The nitrous oxide escapes into the alveoli with such rapidity that the oxygen present becomes diluted; thus the oxygen–carbon dioxide exchange is disrupted and a period of hypoxia is created. However, this phenomenon is reported not to occur in healthy pediatric patients.[7] Nonetheless, to minimize this effect, the patient should be oxygenated for 3 to 5 minutes after a sedation procedure, if for no other reason than to allow for proper nasal hood evacuation of the exhaled gas.

Pharmacodynamics

Nitrous oxide produces nonspecific central nervous system (CNS) depression. Although it is classed with inhalational general anesthetics, it produces limited analgesia, and thus surgical anesthesia is unlikely unless concentrations producing anoxia are reached. Nitrous oxide is the weakest of all inhalation agents, with a minimum alveolar concentration of 105. The minimum alveolar concentration of an inhalation agent is a measure of its potency. It is the concentration required to produce immobility in 50% of patients. At concentrations between 30% and 50%, nitrous oxide will produce a relaxed, somnolent patient who may appear dissociated and easily susceptible to suggestion. Amnesia may occur in some patients, but there is little alteration of learning or memory. At concentrations greater than 60%, patients may experience discoordination, ataxia, giddiness, and increased sleepiness. The concentration of nitrous oxide should not routinely exceed 50%. One of the advantages of nitrous oxide is that it can easily be titrated up for stimulating procedures (e.g., injections) and titrated down during easier periods of the procedure (e.g., restorations).

Nitrous oxide reduces hypoxic-driven ventilation and has minimal effect on the hypercapnic respiratory drive. When used as a single agent, nitrous oxide will not cause hypoxemia. It should be avoided, however, in patients who rely significantly on hypoxia-driven ventilation, in whom exposure to high levels of oxygen can result in respiratory depression. When combined with other agents that depress respiration, nitrous oxide decreases the body's normal response to low oxygen tension. These effects are usually negligible, however, because of the high concentration of oxygen administered with the combination. Nitrous oxide slightly increases the respiratory minute volume. As the patient becomes more relaxed from the effects of nitrous oxide, the respiratory rate may decrease slightly. The gas is nonirritating to the respiratory tract and can be given to patients with asthma without fear of bronchospasm. Problems can arise, however, from the added respiratory effects when it is given in combination with narcotics or other CNS depressants.

Cardiac output is decreased and peripheral vascular resistance is increased when nitrous oxide is used. This is generally of insignificant degree and is a consideration only in patients with severe cardiac disease. The respiratory and cardiac effects may be secondary to the high concentration of oxygen administered in conjunction with nitrous oxide.

Adverse Effects and Toxicity

Nitrous oxide–oxygen has an excellent safety record with few adverse effects. Nausea and vomiting are the most common adverse effects occurring in 1% to 10% of patients. The incidence increases significantly with concentrations in excess of 50%, with lengthy procedures, with rapid fluctuations in concentrations, and with rapid induction and reversal. Fasting is not required for nitrous oxide–oxygen sedation; however, in certain situations, patients may be advised to consume only a light meal within 2 hours of the appointment.

Nitrous oxide will become entrapped in gas-filled spaces such as the middle ear, sinuses, and gastrointestinal tract. Middle ear pressure will increase significantly, and although it is of little significance in a patient with normal patency of eustachian tubes, it can induce pain in patients with acute otitis media. Consequently, use of nitrous oxide should be avoided in patients with acute otitis media.

Other contraindications include severe behavioral problems and emotional illness, uncooperativeness, fear of "gas," claustrophobia, maxillofacial deformities that prevent nasal hood placement, nasal obstruction (e.g., upper respiratory infection, nasal polyps, deviated septum), chronic obstructive pulmonary disease, pregnancy, and situations in which high oxygenation is inadvisable (e.g., bleomycin therapy).

In clinical use for sedation at proper concentrations of medical-quality nitrous oxide and oxygen, the gas has no toxic effects. The greatest concern regarding toxicity centers on exposure of dental personnel to high ambient air levels of the gas for periods of time during its use for patient sedation. Chronic exposure to nitrous oxide, including recreational abuse, can over time produce neurotoxicity, impotence, and renal and liver toxicity. The rate of spontaneous abortion is known to be higher in operating room personnel and in the spouses of operating room personnel.[8] In addition, individuals exposed over long term may experience a decrease in fertility.[9] An increase in hepatic disease was found in dentists and dental personnel exposed to high levels of nitrous oxide for periods longer than 3 hours per week. Therefore, leakage from open systems, such as those used in the dental office, should be reduced as much as possible. This can be accomplished by limiting the amount of mouth breathing

by the patient and using an efficient scavenging system. The installation of laminar air-flow systems might also be considered in new office constructions when it is known that considerable amounts of nitrous oxide will be in use. In addition, the office as well as office personnel should be periodically monitored for exposure to unscavenged nitrous oxide. A variety of units are available that use infrared spectrophotometry to measure ambient levels. These machines can detect levels as low as 1 ppm and are particularly useful for uncovering leaks around tanks and flowmeters. A less costly and more practical approach is the use of dosimetry badges that are worn by office personnel when using nitrous oxide. These units are generally worn for an 8-hour period and report exposure as time-weighted averages. Exposure-limiting methods are listed in Box 14-3.

Box 14-3
Controlling Ambient Nitrous Oxide Levels

VENTILATION
Operatories must have good cross ventilation. Exhaust vents should preferably be located in the ceiling as close to the head of the chair as possible.
Nitrous oxide exhaust must be vented to the outside.
Room air exchanges of 10 or more per hour are recommended.

WORK PRACTICES
Inspect equipment each day to ensure that all connectors are tight and that tubing and bags are free of holes and cracks.
Always use a scavenger system when administering nitrous oxide and oxygen. Adjust the scavenger flow rate to 45 L/min.
Select an appropriately sized mask to ensure a sealed but comfortable fit.
Instruct patients to refrain from mouth breathing and talking during the procedure.
Adjust the nitrous oxide and oxygen flow rate to keep the bag from overfilling. The bag should collapse and expand as the patient breathes.
After administration, flush the patient and system by administering 100% oxygen to the patient for at least 5 minutes.

MAINTENANCE
Schedule periodic inspections of all aspects of the system every 3 months, paying particular attention to areas of potential leaks.
Document results of inspections as well as all corrective actions taken.
Ensure that repairs and modifications are performed only by authorized dealers.
Consider periodic personal sampling of dental personnel with a dosimeter.

Adapted from American Dental Association Council on Scientific Affairs, Council on Dental Practice, *J Am Dent Assoc* 128:364-365, 1997; and Howard WR. *J Am Dent Assoc* 128:356-360, 1977. (See Suggested Readings for full references.)

Equipment

Several manufacturers produce machines for the safe delivery of nitrous oxide–oxygen mixtures for use in conscious sedation in the dental office. The machine should be of the continuous-flow design, with flowmeters capable of accurate regulation and capable of delivering 100% oxygen. A fail-safe mechanism that provides automatic shutdown if oxygen falls below 30% and audible and visual alarms that are activated by oxygen failure are important design features. If equipment is used capable of delivering less than 30% oxygen, an in-line oxygen analyzer must be used. There should be a flush lever for easy and immediate flushing of the system with 100% oxygen.

Mobile, self-contained units are available, as are those operating from a central supply. A major safety consideration with either type is the presence of a good pin-indexed yoke system to absolutely prevent crossover of the cylinder hookup. One should be continuously aware of the danger of crossed lines or cylinders. Such crossover becomes possible when office renovations are done and when fittings wear with age and use.

An efficient scavenger system is an important component of any hose-mask system. The double-mask type is the most efficient type of scavenger (Fig. 14-5). These systems exhaust into the vacuum waste system, which should be vented to the outside to prevent dispersal of gases to other areas of the office or building. Nasal hoods should be of good design and should be available in pediatric and adult sizes to ensure adequate fit, which further reduces leakage (Fig. 14-6).

Technique

After a thorough inspection of the equipment, the mask should be introduced to the patient with an explanation delivered at the appropriate level of understanding, and then the mask should be carefully placed over the nose. Traditional behavior guidance techniques should be employed as the effectiveness of nitrous oxide–oxygen sedation is largely dependent on psychological reassurance. The delivery tubes are tightened behind the chair back in a comfortable position. The bag is filled with 100% oxygen and delivered to the patient for 1 or 2 minutes at an appropriate flow rate, typically between 4 and 6 L/min. With an appropriate flow rate, slight movement of the mixing bag should be apparent with each inhalation and exhalation. With too high a flow rate, the bag will be over-inflated, movement will not be seen with each breath, and leakage will occur from around the mask. In this instance, the flow rate should be adjusted downward. Too low a flow rate will deplete the bag of mixed gases. Once the proper flow rate is achieved, the nitrous oxide can be introduced by slowly increasing the concentration at increments of 10% to 20% to achieve the desired level. The operator should encourage the patient to breathe through

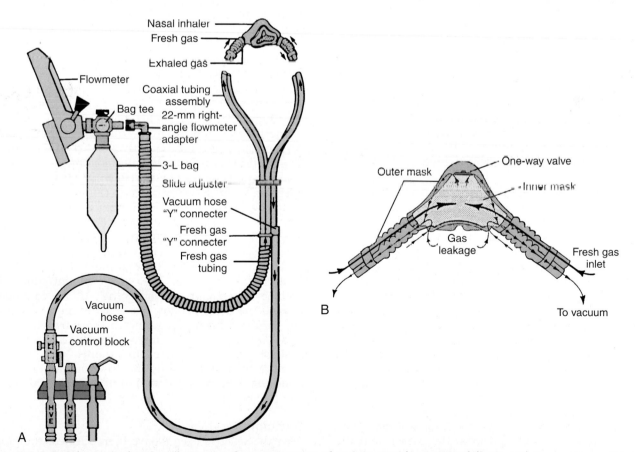

Figure 14-5 A, Schematic drawing illustrating the components of a nitrous oxide–oxygen delivery and scavenging system. **B,** Components of the system's nasal hood. (Courtesy of Porter Instrument Co., Hatfield, Pa.)

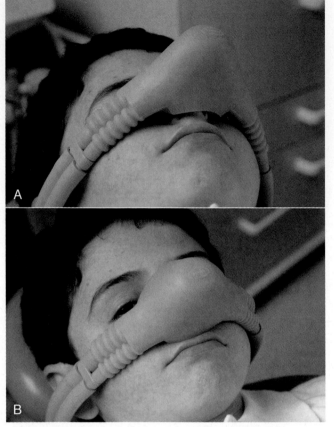

Figure 14-6 A, Poorly fitting mask with leakage under nares. **B,** Well-fitting mask. (A and B, Mask from Olympic Medical Corp., Seattle, Wash.)

the nose with the mouth closed. The sensations should be explained as they begin to be felt. They are best described as a floating, giddy feeling with tingling of the digits. The eyes will take on a distant gaze with sagging eyelids. When this state is reached, the local anesthetic may be given. Once this is completed, the concentration can be reduced to 30% nitrous oxide and 70% oxygen or lower. The rate can then be maintained and the patient monitored, so that the contemplated procedure carried out. As the need arises, the concentration can be titrated in either direction depending upon the procedure being performed and the response of the patient. The dentist should communicate with the patient throughout the procedure, paying particular attention to the maintenance of an open, relaxed airway. The level of nitrous oxide may be periodically reduced to determine the minimum level required for that patient. This should be recorded for future reference. An emesis basin should be readily available; if vomiting does occur, the patient's head should be rotated to the side. However, the laryngeal reflex is not obtunded with nitrous oxide, so aspiration of vomitus is unlikely.[10]

Recovery can be achieved quickly by reverse titration. Once the sedation is reversed, the patient should be allowed to breathe 100% oxygen for 3 to 5 minutes. Oxygenation purges residual gas from the patient and the nitrous oxide system. The patient should be allowed to remain in the sitting position for a brief period to ensure

against dizziness upon standing. The patient is then ready for discharge. Even though psychomotor effects return to normal within 5 to 15 minutes, it is not advisable to allow teenage patients to drive themselves home.

Monitoring
Clinical observation and intermittent assessment of the level of sedation must occur throughout the procedure. This must include the patient's responsiveness, color, and assessment of respiratory rate and rhythm.

Documentation
Informed consent along with the indication for the use of nitrous oxide/oxygen must be documented in the record. In addition, the percent of nitrous oxide used, flow rate, duration of the procedure, and posttreatment oxygenation must be documented.

ORAL SEDATION

By far the most universally accepted and easiest method of drug administration is the oral route. From the patient's point of view, this is certainly true, particularly in pediatrics, because there is no discomfort. That is not to say that all patients will readily accept orally administered drugs. The taste may be quite objectionable, especially in very young children. This can usually be overcome when the drug is mixed with a palatable liquid (e.g., flavoring drops). It has been suggested that, for children who object, a syringe be used to squirt the solution into the oral cavity. Caution is advised, however, because there are reported cases of aspiration of the drug with too forceful an effort.[11] Although complications can and do arise when drugs are administered by the oral route, their frequency and severity are usually reduced.

The oral route of administration is the most variable. The method is dependent on absorption through the gastrointestinal mucosa. This means that the condition of the stomach and intestines, the absorption characteristics of the drug, and the bioavailability of the drug are all considerations. Drugs administered by mouth vary in peak and consistency of effect. Reversal of any unwanted effect is also difficult. The operator cannot titrate the drug to achieve optimal effect with moment-to-moment control as with other methods. Recovery time may be prolonged, because the drug is slowly metabolized.

Many practitioners attempt to overcome the problems of length of onset by having the parent administer medications at home. This, however, introduces the problem of reliability as well as the inability to properly monitor a sedated patient. This practice must be avoided and is unacceptable according to the most recent AAP and AAPD sedation guidelines. A suitable area should be available in the office so that trained personnel can monitor the patient during the onset of sedation as well as during the recovery period until discharge criteria are met (see Box 14-2).

Technique
After the sedative agents have been selected, the proper dose of medication is calculated for the child. It is important to keep in mind the maximum recommended dose of

each agent. Once the sedative is administered, the patient should be kept in an area of the office that allows for continuous monitoring. When the desired effect is observed (usually after a period of 30 to 60 minutes), the patient is transferred to the chair. For small children or children who may become physically combative, placing the patient in a reclining restraint, such as a Papoose Board* (Fig. 14-7A) is advisable. The arms, legs, and midbody should be secured; however, the chest and diaphragm must not be

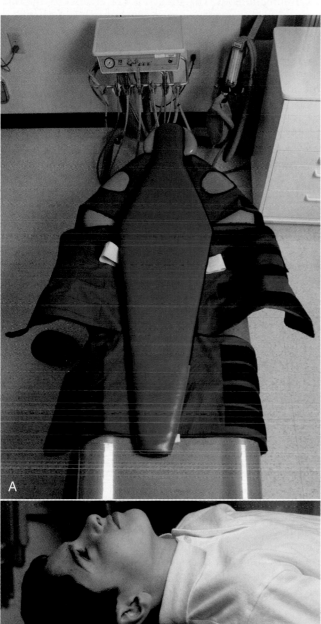

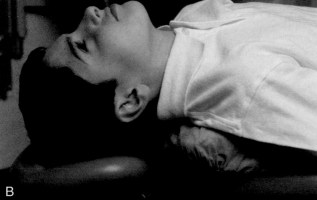

Figure 14-7 A, Papoose Board. **B,** Shoulder Roll Placement. The shoulder roll functions to keep the head rolled up and back, which allows for a more patent airway.

restrained to avoid obstruction of respiratory muscles. A shoulder roll should be placed to keep the head slightly rolled up and back, to allow for a more patent airway (see Fig. 14-7B). Nitrous oxide and oxygen may be started at this time for added effect, as well as for oxygenation. If the patient is not adequately sedated to the point that treatment can be accomplished, the attempt should be aborted and considered a sedation failure. The patient should be given a reappointment for another attempt, in which either the dose or the technique is altered or another form of management considered (e.g., deep sedation or general anesthesia). Increments of medication should not be administered to avoid the risk of an overdose caused by variable and unpredictable absorption. Titration is dangerous and should be reserved for intravenous techniques that do not rely on variable absorption.

The patient should be monitored carefully during the procedure to ensure responsiveness (see Table 14-2). Discharge to the parent should occur only after minimal discharge criteria have been met (see Box 14-2). Full oral and written instructions on postsedation care should be carefully reviewed with the caregiver and the written information given to that person for easy reference at home (see Fig. 14-4).

Oral sedation may be achieved by using a combination of drugs. This is done either to achieve a combined effect or, more often, to reduce the amount required of drugs with a greater potential for problems at higher dosages.

INTRAMUSCULAR SEDATION

Parenteral administration of drugs for sedation requires additional training and skill. For intramuscular injections, some attention must be paid to the anatomy of the injection site and the different pharmacologic effects to be expected. For obvious reasons, the injection method is usually not preferred over the oral route by the pediatric patient, especially those in the younger age group.

Occasions may arise, however, when it is advantageous for the dentist to choose this method. An example would be the sedation of patient who refuses to take medication orally or for some reason cannot do so. The situation is one in which the patient can be momentarily restrained for the administration.

Oral and intramuscular sedation share common problems. A prolonged time is still required to reach peak effect, although it is shorter than with the oral route, and variability and unpredictability are seen in onset and effect. Another problem is the total lack of reversibility. Except in the case of the narcotics or benzodiazepines, whose effects can be reversed, once the drug is deposited in the muscle mass, the operator must be prepared to deal with unexpected problems for the extent of the effect. The opportunity for idiosyncratic reaction is also greater.

Anatomic Considerations

Injection-site selection is a very important aspect of the intramuscular drug administration. The primary considerations are the presence of adequate tissue for deposition of the drug volume and reduction of the risk of injury from needle penetration. Use of the vastus lateralis muscle on the anterior thigh is the safest for small children.

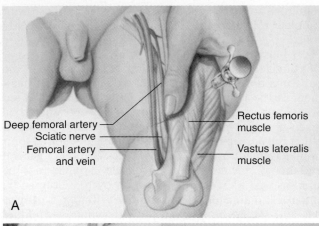

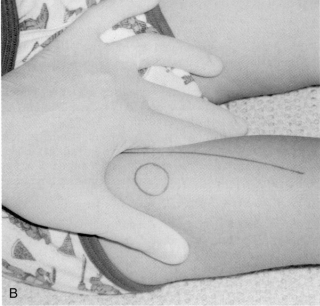

Deep femoral artery
Sciatic nerve
Femoral artery
and vein

Rectus femoris
muscle

Vastus lateralis
muscle

A

B

Figure 14-8 A, Anatomy of the anterior thigh of a child. **B**, Demonstration of patient injection site. (**A** Courtesy Wyeth Laboratories, Philadelphia, Pa.; **B** Courtesy Dr. David R. Avery.)

This is a rectangular area over the anterior lateral aspect of the thigh (Fig. 14-8). The upper outer quadrant of the gluteus maximus muscle and the middle of the posterior lateral aspect of the deltoid muscle are other acceptable sites as long as muscle development is adequate.

Once the medication has been injected, if the desired effect is not achieved in a reasonably expected time of 20 to 30 minutes, either the treatment should be performed under existing circumstances or the patient should be given a reappointment at which either an increased dose or an alternative method of achieving cooperation is used. As with oral administration, titration to a desired level of sedation by injection of incremental amounts of medication is dangerous and must be avoided.

SUBMUCOSAL SEDATION

Submucosal sedation involves the deposition of the drug beneath the mucosa. Its use is almost exclusively the province of dentistry. Although the effectiveness of oral local anesthetics is best if they are placed subperiosteally, most infiltrations are in fact submucosal injections. As is the case with local anesthetics, care must be taken that sedatives are not injected into any of the muscles of the face and jaw lest the absorption and effect of the drug be unduly and unexpectedly prolonged. The site usually chosen for injection is the buccal vestibule, particularly in the area of the maxillary primary molar or canine teeth.

The term *submucosal* is often used interchangeably with subcutaneous. This usage may be erroneous, because research has shown the serum level of a drug to rise very quickly after injection into the vessel-rich areas just described. The response time probably should be considered to be somewhere between those of the intramuscular and the intravenous administration of a drug. This fact makes the method suitable for the pediatric patient for whom quick administration and onset is desirable. Caution should be exercised, however, to select a drug that is not irritating to tissue. The information provided with the drug will indicate its suitability for tissue injection. This is a parenteral route of administration, and adherence to all of the necessary precautions and requirements must be ensured.

Technique

The technique requires only a syringe suitably sized for the volume of drug affixed with a 27- or 30-gauge, ½-inch needle. A tuberculin syringe is recommended for volumes less than 1 mL. Some patient restraint is usually required. Placement of a small quantity of local anesthesia without vasoconstrictor in the area of injection is preferred if the drug being used is known to be painful on injection. The local anesthetic required for pain control of the procedure should not be given in the same area after the injection of the sedative drug, because the action of the vasoconstrictor will slow the uptake of the sedative drug. Also, the physiochemical properties of the sedative agent may interfere with the effectiveness of the local anesthetic agent.

The drugs most commonly administered by the submucosal technique are the narcotics meperidine and fentanyl, however, in recent years, this technique has fallen out of favor.

INTRAVENOUS SEDATION

Sedation levels in which the patient remains conscious are readily achievable through the use of intravenous techniques. In the hands of properly trained professionals, this method can be the easiest, most efficient, and safest next to sedation by inhalation. Controversy has existed for several years over what constitutes adequate training in the use of this modality. The individual state boards are resolving this controversy by writing requirements in terms of didactic and clinical hours required to be certified by the board to use intravenous sedation. Generally, these requirements are following those set forth by the ADA Guidelines for the Use of Conscious Sedation, Deep Sedation, and General Anesthesia for Dentists.[1]

The use of intravenous conscious sedation in pediatric dentistry is somewhat restricted to certain types and ages of patients. Venipuncture is difficult to accomplish in the very young or the combatant child. Such difficulty is attributable to smaller vein size and availability together with the need to restrain the patient. Consequently, the technique is often more suitable for the apprehensive preteen and adolescent patient.

The attribute that makes intravenous sedation desirable for some patients also makes it undesirable for others in the hands of the untrained practitioner. In very young children, the incidence of untoward effects is increased. The onset of action of the drug or drugs used is approximately 20 to 25 seconds, which is the most rapid among all techniques. Thus the opportunity to render the patient unconscious unintentionally is much greater. A practitioner with limited training in management of the airway or of the unconscious patient should never consistently crowd this line between consciousness and unconsciousness.

The possibility of phlebitis is also a disadvantage, particularly with drugs insoluble in water. Hematoma at the site of venipuncture is a complication. There is also an increased need to monitor the patient more closely on a continuous basis, and this usually means the use of an assistant who has had extensive training in the monitoring of sedated patients. In fact, current sedation guidelines require the presence of a third person for the sole purpose of monitoring.

With the intravenous method of sedation, one must also consider that, although the onset of effect is rapid, the reversal of effect is not.

Techniques

There are basically two techniques for using intravenous sedation. The first employs a single drug, usually a benzodiazepine, whereas the second requires a sophisticated combination of several drugs, usually including a narcotic. The single-drug technique is probably the most adaptable to pediatric practice. Unless extensive training opportunities exist, the multiple-drug method should not be considered.

COMBINATIONS OF METHODS AND AGENTS

It is often advantageous to consider combining methods and agents to produce a state of balanced conscious sedation. A goal of combining agents should be to establish a balance between sedation, analgesia, and amnesia, all while minimizing adverse effects and maintaining physiologic homeostasis. When agents are combined, often one drug will be potentiated by another. Their combination thus enables the operator to reduce the dosage of a stronger drug, such as a narcotic, and thus reduce the possibility or degree of an adverse effect, such as severe respiratory depression. Another goal in combining agents might be to quiet the behavior of the patient for the introduction of a method requiring more patient cooperation, such as placement of an intravenous line.

Sedation is usually most effective when combined with the use of local anesthesia. Sedation techniques are not pain-control techniques, and the sedative effects are often overridden when intraoperative pain is experienced by the patient. To overcome this circumstance with the use of sedative agents alone requires the use of very high doses or the addition of a narcotic to the regimen; this produces a deeper level of sedation than might be required and increases the possibility of adverse effects. Sedation techniques should not be used simply to escape the need to inject a local anesthetic. Local anesthetic agents are CNS depressants and effects are additive. Occasionally a drug with a known capacity to improve postoperative comfort also may be used, particularly if surgical procedures are required.

Inhalation sedation is the next most frequently combined technique. Nitrous oxide and oxygen can be combined with all other methods of sedation. Not only does this combination provide increased sedation, but it also increases the availability of oxygen for the patient. In fact, inhalation sedation is so often used in combination that one should be reminded that nitrous oxide is also a CNS depressant and should be the first agent to be reduced or reversed when the sedation level becomes deeper than desired.

The orally administered sedatives are the next most commonly employed in combination. Most frequently combined include sedative hypnotics, narcotics, and antihistamines. A great deal of care must be taken when combining oral agents to avoid deepening the patient's state to deep sedation or general anesthesia. It is important to appreciate that oral agents are potent and that combinations are capable of deepening the patient's sedation to the point that protective reflexes may be lost.

Oral premedication of the patient with minor tranquilizers in advance of the use of inhalation or parenteral sedation methods is common. This technique works especially well to calm the patient for a smoother beginning of a sedative appointment. When parenteral agents are used, unless the result of admixture is definitely known, it is not good practice to mix the agents before administration to the patient, because they may be incompatible in mixed solution. Combining drugs complicates their use because of their additive, synergistic, or potentiating effects. This makes recognition of the causative agent of the untoward effect and subsequent efficient management very difficult. The combination of methods or agents should be viewed as a balancing technique and should be manipulated to produce a maximum result with minimum risk of complication.

Multiple-drug use is also common with intravenous methods of sedation. All the previous cautions pertain in these situations as well. Because of the great potential for swiftly occurring, serious adverse reactions, these multiple-drug intravenous techniques should never be used by anyone who is not specifically trained in their use.

Regardless of the method of administration, the combining of agents should be approached with great caution because of the possibility of additive effects. Individual drug doses should be reduced by 20% to 50% when the drugs are given in combination.

FACILITIES AND EQUIPMENT

The primary requisite for successful sedative management of the pediatric patient is a comfortable, quiet environment. All necessary supplies and equipment should be readily available to ensure a minimum amount of disturbance once the procedure is under way. Although not necessary, a comfortable, single-patient, quiet room is helpful. The facility should also be equipped with adequate suction, monitoring devices, and a positive-pressure oxygen delivery system that is capable of sustaining greater than 90% oxygen at a flow of 10 L/min for at least 60 minutes (650-L E cylinder). When a self-inflating bag-valve-mask device is used for delivering positive-pressure oxygen, a 15-L/min flow is recommended. A functional suction apparatus with appropriate suction catheters and a sphygmomanometer with cuffs of appropriate size for pediatric patients must be immediately available. All equipment must be adaptable to children of all ages and sizes.[2]

As previously stated, all inhalation sedation equipment must have the capability for immediate delivery of 100% oxygen with a minimum delivery of 30%. The apparatus must have a fail-safe system that accomplishes complete shutdown when the oxygen supply drops below the 30% level. If nitrous oxide–oxygen delivery equipment capable of delivering more than 70% nitrous oxide and less than 30% oxygen is used, an in-line oxygen analyzer must be used. This system must be checked and calibrated annually.

Emergency drugs and equipment needed to resuscitate a nonbreathing, unconscious patient must be close at hand and kept up to date and functional (Box 14-4). Portability is essential so that a patient can be supported during transfer to a medical facility if necessary. The best way to provide a portable, reliable oxygen system is with an E-sized (650-L) cylinder to which a self-inflating bag and mask, commonly called an Ambu bag, can be attached (Fig. 14-9). With this apparatus, oxygen from the cylinder mixed with room air can be delivered to the patient. The device is equipped with a valve to prevent rebreathing and can be used alone to supply room air to the patient during movement from one area to another.

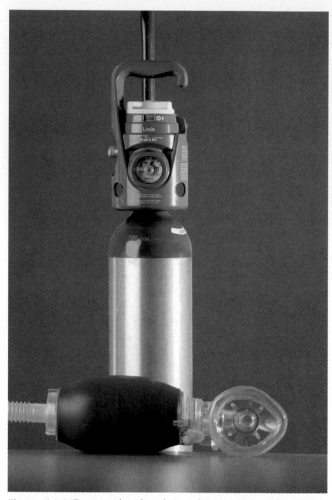

Figure 14-9 Bag-mask-valve device for assisting respiration.

Establishing an open airway and administering oxygen should be the first thought in any emergency-related to sedation. These situations almost always are respiratory in nature at the outset. If respiratory problems are ignored, other systemic problems will rapidly ensue. Quick action is the means to preventing deterioration of adverse reactions.

COMMON AGENTS

GASES

As previously mentioned, only two gases are used in sedation techniques—nitrous oxide and oxygen. The pharmacology of nitrous oxide is discussed in the section on inhalation sedation and need not be repeated here. Oxygen requires no discussion, because its sole purpose is to avoid anoxia, which is produced when nitrous oxide is used alone.

ANTIHISTAMINES

Hydroxyzine
Hydroxyzine is an antihistamine with mild sedative and antiemetic properties. In normal doses, it has no cardiovascular or respiratory depressant effects. It is rapidly absorbed from the gastrointestinal tract with clinical effect

---

Box 14-4

Emergency Drugs That May Be Needed to Rescue a Sedated Patient (AAPD Guidelines)

Albuterol for inhalation
Ammonia spirits
Atropine
Diazepam
Diphenhydramine
Epinephrine (1:1000, 1:10,000)
Flumazenil
Fosphenytoin
Glucose (25% or 50%)
Lidocaine
Lorazepam
Methylprednisolone
Naloxone
Oxygen
Racemic epinephrine
Rocuronium
Sodium bicarbonate
Succinylcholine

seen in 15 to 30 minutes, peak levels occur at 2 hours, and mean half-life is 3 hours. Administration is preferably by the oral route. Intramuscular injections must be deep in a large muscle mass. The drug should not be injected subcutaneously or intravenously because of potential tissue necrosis and hemolysis.

Adverse reactions: Extreme drowsiness, dry mouth, hypersensitivity

Dosage: Oral—1 to 2 mg/kg; intramuscular—1.1 mg/kg

Supplied: Tablets—10, 25, 50, and 100 mg; syrup—10 mg/5 mL; injectable—25 or 50 mg/mL

Promethazine (Phenergan)

Promethazine is a phenothiazine with sedative and antihistaminic properties. It is well absorbed after oral ingestion. Onset is within 15 to 60 minutes, with a peak at 1 to 2 hours and a duration of 4 to 6 hours. Phenothiazines should be used with caution in children with a history of asthma, sleep apnea, or family history of sudden infant death syndrome. Phenothiazines lower the seizure threshold and should be avoided in seizure-prone patients.

Interactions: Potentiates other CNS depressants

Adverse reactions: Dry mouth, blurred vision, thickening of bronchial secretions, mild hypotension, extrapyramidal effects

Dosage: Oral/intramuscular—0.5 to 1.1 mg/kg; subcutaneous—not recommended; maximum recommended single dose—25 mg

Supplied: Tablets—12.5, 25, and 50 mg; syrup—6.25 and 25 mg/mL; injectable—25- and 50-mg/mL ampules

Diphenhydramine (Benadryl)

Diphenhydramine is an antihistamine with sedative properties. It is rapidly absorbed through the gastrointestinal tract, with maximum effect in 1 hour and a duration of 4 to 6 hours. It is metabolized by the liver and completely excreted in 24 hours. Diphenhydramine produces a mild sedative effect but has additive effects with other CNS depressants.

Adverse reactions: Disturbed coordination, epigastric distress, and thickening of bronchial secretions

Dosage: Oral, intramuscular, or intravenous—1.0 to 1.5 mg/kg; maximum single dose is 50 mg

Supplied: Capsules—25 and 50 mg; elixir—12.5 mg/5 mL; injectable—50 mg/mL

BENZODIAZEPINES

Diazepam (Valium)

Diazepam is a benzodiazepine that is lipid soluble and water insoluble. It is rapidly absorbed from the gastrointestinal tract, reaching peak levels at 2 hours. Biotransformation of the drug occurs quite slowly and it has a half-life of 20 to 50 hours. The drug has three active metabolites, one of which is also lipophilic with a half-life of 96 hours. These metabolites are more anxiolytic than sedative.

After intravenous administration, diazepam is redistributed within 30 to 45 minutes, and the patient seems not to be sedated but rather seems to be free from anxiety. The patient should not be considered recovered from the drug. It has simply been redistributed. In fact, stored drug can be redistributed to the CNS by a fatty meal consumed some time later, and the patient will suddenly feel resedated. This is referred to as the *rebound effect*.

Diazepam has strong anticonvulsant activity and provides some prophylaxis against this adverse reaction of other drugs during the operative procedure.

Diazepam can be administered orally, rectally, or parenterally. If the intravenous route is selected, use of a large vein and slow administration is recommended because of the drug's propensity to cause irritation of the vein, with resultant thrombophlebitis. In addition, rapid administration may result in apnea.

Ataxia and prolonged CNS effects are the only common adverse reactions that can be anticipated when diazepam is used for minimal or moderate sedation.

Dosage: Oral or rectal—0.2 to 0.5 mg/kg to a maximum single dose of 10 mg; intravenous—0.25 mg/kg

Supplied: Tablets—2, 5, and 10 mg; suspension—5 mg/mL

Midazolam

A significant advantage of midazolam over diazepam is its high water solubility. Consequently, the possibility of thrombophlebitis is reduced to a minimum. Midazolam is packaged in an acidic solution at a pH of 3.3, a state in which the drug is water soluble. Once the drug enters the blood, which has a pH of 7.4, the chemical structure changes to an active form with high lipid solubility. In fact, its lipid solubility is among the highest of all benzodiazepines.

After intravenous administration, sedation occurs in 3 to 5 minutes. Recovery occurs in 2 hours but is variable and may require up to 6 hours for complete return to baseline values. There is no rebound phenomenon from metabolites. Midazolam can also be given effectively intramuscularly.

Midazolam is effective when given orally and is available as a syrup. Approximately 50% to 65% of the oral dose will go through first-pass hepatic metabolism. Onset of action when given orally is between 20 and 30 minutes with an elimination half life of 1 to 4 hours, which provides approximately 30 minutes of working time. Oral administration is indicated primarily for anxious patients requiring relatively short dental procedures. As a single agent, it should not be used to control combative behavior.

Midazolam may produce respiratory depression with higher doses. There is also a dose-related risk of apnea, which is believed to be influenced by the rapidity with which the drug is administered.[12] Apnea is more likely to occur when midazolam is used with narcotics.[13] Hypotension also occurs more frequently with this combination. Doses should be adjusted downward when midazolam is used with any other CNS depressant, especially narcotics. These effects are not usually seen if the drug is appropriately titrated.

Compared with diazepam, midazolam produces better anxiolysis and amnesia. Between 75% and 90% of patients experience retrograde amnesia for up to 4 hours when given midazolam. Midazolam is three to four times more potent than diazepam and has twice the affinity for the benzodiazepam receptor.

Dosage: Oral—0.25 to 1.0 mg/kg to a maximum single dose of 20 mg; intramuscular—0.1 to 0.15 mg/kg to a maximum dose of 10 mg; intravenous—slow titration; see manufacturer's recommended dosage guidelines

Supplied: Syrup—2 mg/mL; injectable—1- and 5-mg/mL vials

BENZODIAZEPINE ANTAGONIST

Flumazenil (Romazicon)

Flumazenil is a benzodiazepine receptor antagonist. The drug selectively inhibits the CNS effects of the benzodiazepines by a competitive, high-affinity interaction with benzodiazepine receptors. It has no antagonistic properties against the opioids. When carefully titrated, flumazenil has been shown to be effective in reversing the sedative effects but not necessarily the amnesic or anxiolytic qualities of benzodiazepines.

Flumazenil is well tolerated in patients having no dependence on or increased tolerance to benzodiazepines. In patients with benzodiazepine dependency, withdrawal symptoms occur when flumazenil is given. Induced seizure activity occurs in patients receiving benzodiazepines for control of convulsive disorders when flumazenil is used. The drug is recommended for intravenous use only. For reversal of sedation, the initial dose should be 0.01 mg/kg (up to 0.2 mg) given over 15 seconds. If the desired level of consciousness does not occur after waiting an additional 45 seconds, another dose of 0.01 mg/kg (up to 0.2 mg) should be administered and dosing repeated at 60-second intervals to a maximum total dose of 0.05 mg/kg or 1 mg, whichever is lower. Most patients respond to doses in the range of 0.6 to 1.0 mg. A series of injections is preferable to a single bolus to titrate to a desired end point and thus manage the problem with the minimally effective amount of drug. Onset of reversal is usually seen within 1 to 2 minutes. The duration and degree of reversal are related to dose and plasma concentration of the sedating benzodiazepine, as well as that of the antagonist given. This, coupled with the fact that the duration of effect is shorter for flumazenil than for most benzodiazepines, means that resedation can occur. Patients should be carefully monitored for resedation and respiratory depression throughout the period of reversal. The longer the period of sedation, the longer the period required for monitoring and surveillance for resedation. If resedation occurs, repeated doses of flumazenil at no less than 20-minute intervals may be used.

Dosage: Intravenous—as described

Supplied: 5- and 10-ml multiple-use vials containing 0.1 mg/mL in boxes of 10

SEDATIVE HYPNOTICS

Barbiturates

Barbiturates can produce all levels of CNS depression, ranging from mild sedation to general anesthesia and deep coma. Their use has fallen out of favor, however, with the availability of sedatives and hypnotics with fewer adverse effects. Consequently, barbiturates are of very limited value for pediatric patients.

Chloral Hydrate

Chloral hydrate is an extremely well known and widely used drug for pediatric sedation. It has an onset of action of 30 to 60 minutes when given orally. It has a duration of action between 4 and 8 hours and a half-life of 8 to 11 hours as a result of the formation of active metabolites. The primary metabolite of choral hydrate is trichloroethanol, which is responsible for most of the CNS effects that occur.

Chloral hydrate is irritating to gastric mucosa and unless diluted in a flavored vehicle will frequently cause nausea and vomiting. Children given chloral hydrate often enter a period of disinhibition resulting in excitement and irritability before becoming sedated. The drug causes prolonged drowsiness or sleep and respiratory depression. In large doses it produces general anesthesia. Large doses also depress the myocardium and can sensitize the myocardium to the effects of catecholamines resulting in arrhythmias, and thus should be avoided in patients with cardiac disease.[14,15] The lethal dose of chloral hydrate is stated to be 10 g in adults, yet ingestion of 4 g has caused death.

Because the drug does not reliably produce sedation of a degree to permit operative procedures at lower doses, the tendency is to push the dosage higher to achieve the necessary sedation. With such a wide range of reported toxicity, this drug may be an unwise choice for many pediatric patients. It is recommended that young children receive not more than 1 g as a total dose. Risks are increased when chloral hydrate is combined with nitrous oxide, narcotics, or local anesthetic agents. At higher doses and in combination with other agents, loss of a patent airway is a common problem.[16]

Dosage: Must be individualized for each patient recommended: 25 to 50 mg/kg to a maximum of 1 g

Supplied: Oral capsules—500 mg; oral solution—250 and 500 mg/5 mL; rectal suppositories—324 and 648 mg

NARCOTICS

Narcotics are the "heavy artillery" of pediatric sedation. They are not employed with any great consideration for their analgesic properties. They do produce sedation and euphoria to a greater degree in children than in adults. Local anesthesia is still required for intraoperative pain control. Local anesthetics are also CNS depressants.

A significant drug-drug and drug-physiologic interaction can occur when narcotics or other drugs that depress respiration are combined with local anesthetics. In usual doses, local anesthetics are CNS depressants and will provide additive depression when combined with other CNS depressants. In addition, when drugs that depress respiration are used (particularly narcotics), varying degrees of hypercarbia can occur, with a resultant decrease in serum pH. As the respiratory depression continues to deepen, respiratory and metabolic acidosis result in an increase in the availability of lidocaine to the CNS. This occurs as a result of less serum protein binding of lidocaine along with central vasodilation and an increase in blood flow to the CNS in an acidotic state. Consequently the threshold for CNS lidocaine toxicity is lowered. Lidocaine toxicity results in CNS excitation and seizures and ultimately coma and death. As a result, the maximum dosage of local anesthetic must be reduced when used in combination with a CNS and/or respiratory depressant. This very important and significant interaction is often overlooked and is the cause of many of the adverse incidents reported in pediatric sedation. The maximum local anesthetic dose in children may allow for the use of only one or two dental cartridges, which is quite different than for adult patients.

Combination with other sedative drugs, including nitrous oxide–oxygen, reduces the need for larger doses of narcotics and thus reduces the potential for unwanted effects from these potent drugs. A practitioner employing narcotics should be thoroughly familiar with their actions and interactions and should have had some supervised experience in their use as well as in management of the airway and patient resuscitation procedures.

Meperidine (Demerol)

Meperidine is a synthetic opiate agonist. It is water soluble but is incompatible with many other drugs in solution. Meperidine may be administered orally or by subcutaneous, intramuscular, or intravenous injection. It is least effective by mouth. It is bitter and requires taste masking by a flavoring agent. By the oral route, peak effect occurs in 1 hour and lasts about 4 hours. Parenteral administration shortens the time of onset and duration. High doses that lead to an accumulation of normeperidine, a primary metabolite of meperidine, have resulted in seizures. Meperidine should be used with extreme caution in patients likely to accumulate or be sensitive to this metabolite (e.g., patients with hepatic or renal disease, or history of seizures).

Dosage: Oral, subcutaneous, or intramuscular—1.0 to 2.2 mg/kg, not to exceed 100 mg when given alone or 50 mg when in combination with other CNS depressants

Supplied: Oral tablets—50 and 100 mg; oral syrup—50 mg/5 mL; parenteral solution—25, 50, 75, and 100 mg/mL

Fentanyl (Sublimaze)

Fentanyl is a synthetic opiate agonist in the same chemical class as meperidine. It is a potent narcotic analgesic. A dose of 0.1 mg is approximately equivalent to 10 mg of morphine or 75 mg of meperidine. Fentanyl has a rapid action, and after a submucosal or intramuscular injection the onset occurs in 7 to 15 minutes; duration of effects is 1 to 2 hours. The drug is metabolized by the liver and is excreted in the urine.

Respiratory depression is the same as with other narcotics. Respiratory rate decreases but returns to near normal rapidly. Tidal volume, however, remains depressed. The response to carbon dioxide can be depressed for extended periods, long after the analgesic effect has disappeared. It is believed that this characteristic is attributable to redistribution of the drug. When fentanyl is used, one should be attentive to and competent in airway management. When higher doses are administered rapidly intravenously,

rigidity of skeletal muscle has been reported. Apnea has also occurred under these circumstances. This effect can be reversed by administration of naloxone along with a skeletal muscle relaxant and/or managed by assisted or controlled ventilation. Bradycardia has been reported. Atropine can be used to normalize heart rate.

Fentanyl produces little histamine release and has much less emetic effect than morphine or meperidine.

Fentanyl can be administered by the intramuscular, intravenous, or submucosal route. When it is used with other CNS depressants, the dose should be reduced. The drug works well with orally administered diazepam and nitrous oxide–oxygen. It is not recommended for use in children younger than 2 years of age.

Dosage: 0.002 to 0.004 mg/kg

Supplied: 0.05 mg/mL in 2- and 5-mL ampules

NARCOTIC ANTAGONIST

Naloxone (Narcan)

A semisynthetic opiate antagonist used for the sole purpose of reversing the effects of narcotic drugs. Naloxone is a pure antagonist, with no agonist activity even in large doses. It acts in 2 to 5 minutes after subcutaneous or intramuscular injection and 1 to 2 minutes intravenously. After intravenous administration the duration of reversal is about 45 minutes; it is slightly longer when the drug is administered intramuscularly or subcutaneously. This is an important difference, because the duration of effect of the opiate is in all likelihood longer than that of the antagonist. Consequently, patients undergoing reversal of sedation with naloxone should be kept under continual surveillance until it has been determined that the narcotic will not produce a rebound effect. The time period will vary depending on the duration of action of the narcotic. Repeated doses of naloxone may be necessary to establish patient stability. If the decision has been made to administer an antagonist, other resuscitative measures must be available and must be used as necessary. Naloxone administration should never take precedence over basic resuscitative measures. There is no evidence to support the contention that naloxone will reverse respiratory depression but not the sedative action of the opiate.

Adverse reactions include nausea, vomiting, sweating, hypotension, hypertension, ventricular tachycardia and fibrillation, and pulmonary edema. None of these effects, however, has been reported with its use in pediatric conscious sedation.

Dosage: Intravenous, subcutaneous, intramuscular—initial dose: 0.01 mg/kg; subsequent doses: 0.1 mg/kg (2 mg maximum) every 2 to 3 minutes

Supplied: Parenteral solution—0.02, 0.4, 1.0 mg/kg

MONITORING

For successful monitoring of the vital physiologic parameters of a patient receiving treatment with the aid of sedation, baseline values taken preoperatively at a time when the patient is calm are extremely helpful. Admittedly this is not possible in all circumstances, but the attempt should be made to establish these values.

INTRAOPERATIVE MONITORING

Intraoperative monitoring must include an assessment of oxygenation, ventilation, and circulation. The depth of sedation dictates the degree and frequency of monitoring required (see Table 14-2).[2]

As the treatment progresses, the state of consciousness should be evaluated frequently by verbal communication with the patient. How often this is done is related directly to the level of sedation at any one time. As the patient becomes quieter with deeper levels of sedation, more vigilance to all physiologic parameters is required. If the patient is responding to questions and commands, the patient is conscious by definition. For those patients incapable of communication, either because of age or disability, some means of evoking a response should be used. For the very lightly sedated patient capable of verbal response, this may be the extent of the monitoring required.

Another area of assessment is the patient's appearance. The oral mucosa, the nail beds, and the complexion of the skin provide indications of perfusion of the patient. This should be done at intervals throughout the procedure and documented in the record. If restraining devices that cover the patient are used, a hand or foot should be exposed. These devices should be carefully applied to the sedated patient to ensure that there is no restriction of the chest.

The heart and respiratory rates can be continuously monitored by means of a stethoscope with a custom-fitted earpiece. The bell of the instrument is taped over the trachea in the suprasternal notch. This piece of equipment is referred to as a *precordial* or, more accurately, a *pretracheal* stethoscope (Fig. 14-10).

In addition to the rate, the quality of heart and breath sounds should be assessed and recorded. The patient should have a strong, regular pulse and an airway without noisy movement of air.

The excursion of the chest is important also, because the rate of respiration can remain steady while the depth becomes increasingly shallow. Shallow respiration is a reduction in tidal volume, and the exchange of oxygen is correspondingly reduced.

For deeper levels of sedation, such as with the use of narcotics, it is desirable to monitor blood pressure at frequent intervals. Again, the frequency is determined by the depth of the sedation (see Table 14-2). However, physiologic deterioration occurs long before changes in blood pressure are detected.

Although it is acceptable to measure physiologic parameters using the basic methods of auscultation and an aneroid sphygmomanometer with a manually inflated cuff, numerous electronic, automatic, continuous-monitoring devices are available. These range from the uncomplicated and reasonably priced to the elaborate and expensive. In all instances, the cuff should be of the appropriate size for the patient (Fig. 14-11). Pulse monitors are available that attach to the finger or earlobe and produce both visual and audible signals. There are variable-cycled blood pressure monitors with automatically inflating cuffs (Fig. 14-12). These are monitors in which both blood presure and pulse

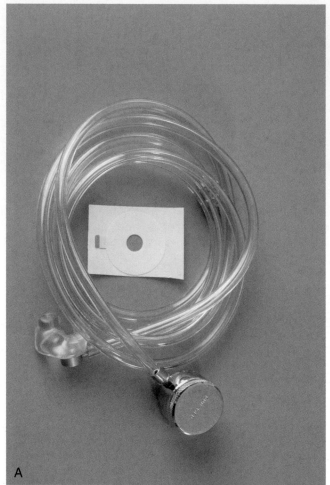

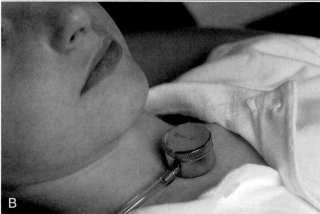

Figure 14-10 A, Pretracheal stethoscope with fitted earpiece. Double-stick disks. **B,** Placement of pretracheal stethoscope. (**A** Courtesy 3M Corporation, St. Paul, Minn.)

rate are continuously assessed together and automatically recorded on a paper strip. The device carries adjustable visual and audible alarms.

One of the most valuable pieces of electronic monitoring equipment is the pulse oximeter (Fig. 14-13). This device continuously assesses arterial hemoglobin oxygen saturation and pulse rate, with values updated with every heartbeat. An oxisensor is attached noninvasively to a

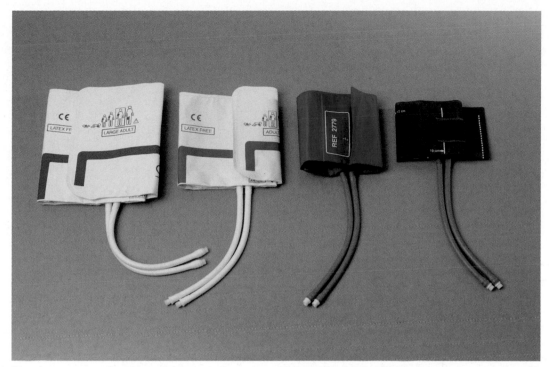

Figure 14-11 Blood pressure cuffs are available in various sizes. The width of the cuff should cover approximately two thirds of the upper arm.

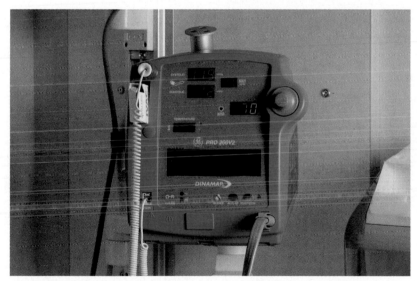

Figure 14-12 Automated vital signs monitor. (Courtesy Dinamap by Critikon, Inc., Tampa, Fla.)

digit on the hand or foot or to the earlobe and consists of a light-emitting diode and light-detecting diode (Fig. 14-14). The light-emitting diode emits both red and infrared wavelengths of light, and the light-detecting diode detects light transmitted through the tissue. Red wavelengths are absorbed primarily by oxygenated hemoglobin, whereas infrared wavelengths are absorbed primarily by deoxygenated hemoglobin. The device's processor then calculates the percent of oxygenation of hemoglobin and the results are conveyed both audibly

and visually. A delay of more than a minute occurs before respiratory compromise is reflected in oxygen saturation levels as determined by pulse oximetry.

There is a correlation between the percent oxygen saturation of hemoglobin (Sao_2) and oxygen tension in arterial blood (Pao_2) that must be appreciated when interpreting oxygen saturation. The relationship between the two parameters is plotted on the oxyhemoglobin dissociation curve (Fig. 14-15). It is the unbound oxygen dissolved in blood that produces the tension (Pao_2)

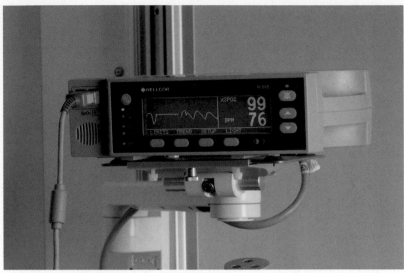

Figure 14-13 Pulse oximeter. (Courtesy Nellcor, Pleasanton, Calif.)

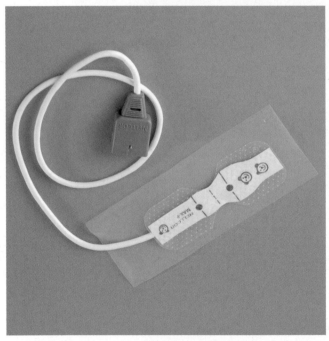

Figure 14-14 Two types of optical sensors. Sensors with adhesive tabs are less likely to dislodge in pediatric patients than are clip-on sensors.

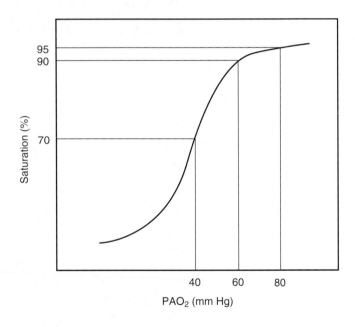

Figure 14-15 Oxyhemoglobin dissociation curve, which shows the saturation of hemoglobin with oxygen (Sao_2) relative to the oxygen tension (Pao_2). Hypoxemia is defined as Pao_2 below 80 mm Hg (95% Sao_2). (From Dionne R, Phero, J, Becker D. *Management of pain and anxiety in the dental office.* Philadelphia, 2002, WB Saunders.)

required to drive oxygen into tissues. Hypoxemia occurs when oxygen saturation drops to 95%, corresponding to an oxygen tension of 80 mm Hg. Once the arterial saturation levels drop to 90% (Pao_2 = 60 mm Hg), the patient will begin to desaturate rapidly, and the cells of vital organs will begin to be deprived of oxygen. The patient's oxygen saturation level should be as close to 100% as possible during the sedation. A number of conditions can lead to false oximeter readings, including (1) failure to place diodes directly opposite each other, (2) interference from ambient light, (3) placement of diodes on the same limb as a blood pressure cuff, (4) fingernail polish on the

digit to which the sensor is attached, (5) cold limbs, (6) profound tissue pigmentation, (7) reuse of disposable oxisensors, and (8) motion artifact. Sensor displacement is the most common cause for false readings in children and can be minimized by using a sensor with adhesive tabs rather than a clip-on sensor. Securing the sensor with additional tape and using a toe rather than a finger may also help minimize displacement. The new generation of pulse oximeters is less susceptible to motion artifacts and may be more useful than older oximeters that do not contain the updated software (AAPD guidelines).

Knowing the peripheral oxygen saturation from moment to moment is important to detect sudden deterioration of the patient's physiologic status during sedation. Hypoxia is almost always the primary complication with these techniques of patient management. Oxygen saturation measures oxygenation, the transport of oxygen to metabolically active tissues. It does not, however, reflect ventilation—the movement of gases from the atmosphere to alveoli. Thus oxygenation represents only half of the results of ventilation. Ventilation must be evaluated independently from oxygenation.[17] Methods used to monitor ventilation include visual monitoring for chest wall movement, listening for breath sounds with a precordial stethoscope, determination of respiratory rate, and capnography. Capnography is considered the gold standard for monitoring ventilatory status and reveals respiratory compromise within 15 seconds. The use of expired carbon dioxide monitoring devices is encouraged for sedated children, particularly in situations where other methods of assessing the adequacy of ventilation are limited . Several manufacturers have produced nasal cannulae that allow simultaneous delivery of oxygen and measurement of expired carbon dioxide values. These devices have a high degree of false-positive alarms; however, they are very accurate in detecting complete airway obstruction or apnea (AAPD guidelines).

The capnography monitor (Fig. 14-16A) detects both the presence and the quality of ventilation by analyzing the concentration of carbon dioxide in the exhaled gasses through differential infrared absorption. The end-tidal carbon dioxide concentration is the concentration of carbon dioxide measured at the terminal portion of the exhalation curve (see Fig. 14-16B).[18] The sampling line is placed either in the nostril or in close approximation to the nose or mouth and allows for suctioning of a sample of exhaled air into the unit. There are limitations to the accuracy of readings that must be kept in mind, especially when the device is used in children. Head movement, mouth breathing, crying, and tube blockage by mucous all result in inaccurate readings. Technology is being developed to overcome these obstacles. Capnography is rapidly becoming the most important monitoring instrument when patient sedation is used.

The availability of appropriately trained personnel to evaluate the patient and interpret monitoring results is just as important as using the correct monitoring devices. In addition to the operating practitioner, an individual trained to monitor appropriate physiologic parameters must be present during sedation, must be trained in basic life support, and must be familiar with the office emergency cart or kit.

POSTOPERATIVE MONITORING

Before any patient receiving conscious sedation is discharged, all vital signs must be stable. The child must be reasonably alert, able to talk, ambulating with minimal assistance, and sitting unaided. Some patients may benefit from a longer period of less-intense observation. The child should be able to remain awake for at least 20 minutes, unstimulated, before discharge (AAPD guidelines #100). For the very young or disabled patient who might be

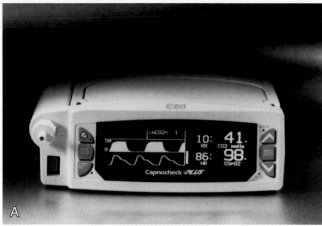

Normal capnogram

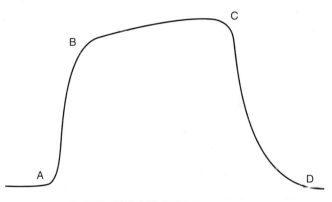

A: Exhalation begins
B-C: Plateau = outflow of alveolar gas
D: End-tidal CO_2

Figure 14-16 Capnography. **A,** The monitor produces a waveform by the continuous analysis of expired gas for carbon dioxide. **B,** The presence of a waveform implies exhalation of gases from the lungs. The end-tidal carbon dioxide concentration (point C) corresponds to the concentration of alveolar gas, which correlates closely with the arterial partial pressure of carbon dioxide. (**A** Courtesy Capnocheck by Pryon Inc., Beaverton, Ore. **B** From Anderson J, Vann W. Respiratory monitoring during pediatric sedation: pulse oximetry and capnography, *Pediatr Dent* 10:94-101, 1988.)

incapable of the usually expected responses, a level of awareness that is as close to the usual state for that person must be achieved before discharge (see Box 14-2).

These patients should be monitored at frequent and regular intervals, and the condition of these children should be fully documented before they are discharged to the care of the parent or guardian.

RISK MANAGEMENT

To minimize the risk of adverse events occurring during the treatment of a patient under sedation, the practitioner should consider the following recommendations set forth in a policy statement of the ADA:

• Use only drugs and techniques that are thoroughly understood with regard to indications, contraindications, adverse reactions and their management, drug interactions, and proper dosage for the desired effect.

- Limit the use of these modalities to patients who require them because of factors such as the extent and type of operative procedure, psychological need, or medical status.
- Conduct comprehensive preoperative evaluation of each patient, including recording of a complete medical history and determination of current physical and psychological status, age, and preference for and past experience with sedation and anesthesia.
- Conduct continuous physiologic and visual monitoring of the patient from onset through recovery.
- Have available appropriate emergency drugs, equipment, and facilities and maintain proficiency in their use.
- Keep fully documented records of drugs used, dosages, vital signs monitored, adverse reactions, and any emergency procedures employed.
- Use sufficient support personnel who are properly trained for the functions they are assigned to perform.
- Treat high-risk patients in a hospital or similar setting equipped to provide for their care.

REFERENCES

1. American Dental Association. Guidelines for Teaching Pain Control and Sedation to Dentists and Dental Students. Chicago, ADA, 2007.
2. American Academy of Pediatric Dentistry. Guideline on for Monitoring and Management of Pediatric Patients During and After Sedation for Diagnostic and Therapeutic Procedures, *Pediatr Dent* 29(7):134-143, 2008.
3. Cote CJ, et al. A Practice of Anesthesia for Infants and Children. Philadelphia, 1993, WB Saunders, pp 313-314.
4. Venham LL, et al. Interval rating scales for children's dental anxiety and uncooperative behavior, *Pediatr Dent* 2:195-202, 1980.
5. Frankl SN, et al. Should the parent remain with the child in the dental operatory? *J Dent Children* 29:150-163, 1962.
6. National Institutes of Health. Consensus development conference statement on anesthesia and sedation in the dental office, *J Am Dent Assoc* 111:90-94, 1985.
7. Dunn-Russell T, et al. Oxygen saturation and diffusion hypoxia in children following nitrous oxide sedation, *Pediatr Dent* 15(2):88-92, 1993.
8. Cohen EN, et al. A survey of anesthetic health hazards among dentists: report of ad hoc committee on the effects of trace anesthetic agents on the health of operating room personnel, *J Am Dent Assoc* 90:1291-1296, 1975.
9. Kugel G, et al. Effect of nitrous oxide on the concentrations of opioid peptides, substance P, and LHRH in the brain and B-endorphin in the pituitary, *Anesth Prog* 38:206-211, 1991.
10. Allen GD, et al. The efficacy of the laryngeal reflex in conscious sedation, *J Am Dent Assoc* 96:901-903, 1977.
11. Granoff DM, et al. Cardiorespiratory arrest following aspiration of chloral hydrate, *Am J Dis Child* 122:170-171, 1971.
12. Reeves JG, et al. Midazolam: pharmacology and uses, *Anesthesiology* 62:310-324, 1985.
13. Kanto J, et al. Effect of different kinds of premedication on the induction properties of midazolam, *Br J Anaesth* 54:507-511, 1982.
14. Bowyer K, Glasser SP. Chloral hydrate overdose and cardiac arrhythmias, *Chest* 77:232-235, 1980.
15. Brown AM, Cade JF. Cardiac arrhythmias after chloral hydrate overdose, *Med J Aust* 1:28-29, 1980.
16. Moore PA, et al. Sedation in pediatric dentistry: a practical assessment procedure, *J Am Dent Assoc* 109:564-569, 1984.
17. Dionne R, et al. Management of Pain and Anxiety in the Dental Office. Philadelphia, 2002, WB Saunders.
18. Anderson J, Vann W. Respiratory monitoring during pediatric sedation: pulse oximetry and capnography, *Pediatr Dent* 10(2):94-101, 1988.

SUGGESTED READINGS

Agurell S, Berlin A, Ferngren H. Plasma levels of diazepam after parenteral and rectal administration in children, *Epilepsia* 16:277-283, 1975.

American Academy of Pediatric Dentistry, Guideline on Appropriate Use of Nitrous Oxide for Pediatric Dental Patients, *Pediatr Dent* 29(7) 131-133, 2008

American Dental Association. Guidelines for Teaching Pain Control and Sedation to Dentists and Dental Students, October 2007

American Dental Association. Report of Council on Scientific Affairs, Council on Dental Practice: nitrous oxide in the dental office, *J Am Dent Assoc* 128:364-365, 1997.

Brodsky L. Modern assessment of tonsils and adenoids, *Pediatr Clin North Am* 36:1551-1569, 1989.

Caudill WA et al. Absorption rates of alpha-prodine from the buccal and intravenous routes, *Pediatr Dent* 4:168-170, 1982.

Chrysikopoulou A, et al. Effectiveness of two nitrous oxide scavenging nasal hoods during routine pediatric dental treatment, *Pediatr Dent*, 28:3, 242-247, 2006

Fayans E. Pediatric oral premedication: changes in the patterns of administration and safety, *Compendium* 10:568, 570, 572, 574, 1989.

Fishbaugh D, et al. Relationship of tonsil size on an airway blockage maneuver in children during sedation, *Pediatr Dent* 19(4): 227-281, 1997.

Flaitz CM, Nowak AJ. Evaluation of the sedative effect of rectally administered diazepam for the young dental patient, *Pediatr Dent* 7:292-296, 1985.

Houpt MI, Limb R, Livingston R. Clinical effects of nitrous oxide conscious sedation in children, *Pediatr Dent* 26:1, 29-36, 2004

Howard WR. Nitrous oxide in the dental environment: assessing the risk, reducing the exposure, *J Am Dent Assoc* 128: 356-360, 1997.

Knudson FU. Plasma diazepam in infants after rectal administration in solution and by suppository, *Acta Pediatr Scand* 66:563, 1977.

Lundgren S, Rosenquist JB. Comparison of sedation, amnesia, and patient comfort produced by intravenous and rectal diazepam, *J Oral Maxillofac Surg* 42:646-650, 1984.

Malamed SF. Sedation: a guide to patient management, ed 4, St Louis, 2003, Mosby.

Trapp LD. Pharmacologic management of pain and anxiety. In Stewart RE et al, editors: *Pediatric dentistry: scientific foundation and clinical practice*, St Louis, 1982, Mosby.

CHAPTER 15

Hospital Dental Services for Children and the Use of General Anesthesia

▲ James A. Weddell and James E. Jones

CHAPTER OUTLINE

*D*entists can provide essential services to patients within an operating room setting in addition to providing consultative and emergency services. Staff membership is necessary. National commissions such as the Joint Commission (formerly the Joint Commission on Accreditation of Healthcare Organizations [JCAHO]) issue the standards for hospital governance for all hospital services.

In recent years, with the increasing number of general practice residencies and postdoctoral specialty programs, the qualified dentist finds that hospital staff privileges are a necessity. Active involvement in hospital dentistry has added a rewarding component to the practice of many dentists. Many hospitals have incorporated not only dental specialties but also general dental services, providing a comprehensive health care facility in which to serve the community.

OBTAINING HOSPITAL STAFF PRIVILEGES

Requirements for obtaining hospital staff privileges vary among institutions. The dentist must fulfill the following three basic requirements to become a hospital staff member:

1. The applicant must have graduated from an accredited dental school.
2. The applicant must be licensed to practice dentistry in the state in which the facility is located.
3. The applicant must have high moral and ethical standards.

Additional requirements may have to be met to obtain staff privileges. Many hospitals ask staff members to sign a "Delineation of Privileges" form indicating the procedures that staff members are qualified to perform and that are accepted by the governing body of the hospital. In addition, the applicant must show proof of professional liability insurance, and membership in the American Dental Association is desirable.

In a children's hospital, dentists might be required to have adequate advanced training to treat and manage children in the hospital. The requirements may include a dental residency of 1 to 4 years in a teaching hospital in which the dentist (1) gains experience in recording and evaluating the medical history and current medical status of children; (2) receives instruction in physical examination techniques and in recognition of conditions that may influence dental treatment decisions; (3) learns to initiate appropriate medical consultations when a problem arises during treatment; (4) learns the procedure for admitting, monitoring, and discharging children; and (5) develops proficiency in operating room protocol. A rotation in which the dental resident was actively involved in administering general anesthetics to children is highly desirable. Current certification in basic cardiopulmonary resuscitation should be maintained by all members of the hospital's professional staff, including dentists.

As active members of the hospital staff, dentists should be aware of the hospital's bylaws, rules, regulations, and meetings. A copy of the bylaws should be obtained for easy reference. Fully understanding the responsibilities of staff membership will enable dentists to treat their patients within the established protocol of the institution. Most important, dentists should endeavor to provide the highest quality care within the specialty area for which they are trained. The American Academy of Pediatric Dentistry encourages the participation of pediatric dentistry practitioners on hospital medical-dental staffs, recognizes the American Dental Association as a corporate member of the Joint Commission, and encourages hospital member pediatric dentists to maintain strict adherence to the rules and regulations of the policies of the hospital medical staff.

INDICATIONS FOR GENERAL ANESTHESIA IN THE TREATMENT OF CHILDREN

The use of general anesthesia for dental care in children is sometimes necessary to provide safe, efficient, and effective care. Depending on the patient, this will be done in an ambulatory care setting or inpatient hospital setting. It should be only one component of the dentist's overall treatment regimen. Oral hygiene and preventive care must be implemented at the onset of treatment with parents or guardians and patients to eliminate the cause of the dental problem.

The safety of the patient and practitioner, as well as the need to diagnose and treat, must justify the use of general anesthesia. All available management techniques, including acceptable restraints and sedation, should be considered before the decision is made to use a general anesthetic. Crespi and Friedman cite several authors who agree in recommending that at least one or two attempts be made using conventional behavior management techniques or conscious sedation before general anesthesia is considered.[1]

Parental or guardian written consent must be obtained before the use of general anesthesia. Documentation regarding dental treatment needs, unmanageability in the dental setting, and contributory medical problems must be included in the patient's hospital record. Records must be clearly written so others are able to read and understand them. Review organizations examine dental admissions for proper documentation in the hospital chart for insurance payment and quality assurance purposes.

Patients for whom general anesthesia has been the management technique of choice include the following:
1. Patients unable to cooperate with a certain physical, mental, or medically compromising disability
2. Patients with dental restorative or surgical needs for whom local anesthesia is ineffective because of acute infection, anatomic variations, or allergy
3. The extremely uncooperative, fearful, anxious, physically resistant, or uncommunicative child or adolescent with substantial dental needs for whom there is no expectation that the behavior will soon improve.
4. Patients who have sustained extensive orofacial or dental trauma and/or require significant surgical procedures
5. Patients requiring immediate comprehensive oral or dental needs
6. Patients requiring dental care for whom the use of general anesthesia may protect the developing psyche and/or reduce medical risks

If the benefits of the procedure outweigh the risk of anesthesia, there are few if any contraindications to general

anesthesia. However, when a concern about the medical condition exists, an anesthesia consult would be desirable. Patients for whom general anesthesia is usually contraindicated include those with a medical contraindication to general anesthesia and healthy and cooperative patients with minimal dental needs.

PSYCHOLOGIC EFFECTS OF HOSPITALIZATION ON CHILDREN

Hospitalization is a frequent source of anxiety for children. According to King and Nielson, 20% to 50% of children demonstrate some degree of behavioral change after hospitalization.[2] Separation of the child from the parent appears to be a significant factor in post-hospitalization anxiety, although other causes are also documented. Allowing the parent to stay with the child during the hospitalization, and especially to be present when the child leaves for and returns from surgery, can reduce anxiety for the child and parent alike.

According to Camm and colleagues, postoperative behavioral changes reported by mothers in a limited sample of children who received dental treatment with general anesthesia in a hospital were similar to those observed in children who received treatment under conscious sedation in a dental clinic.[3] Mothers of children receiving dental treatment with general anesthesia in a hospital setting were found to experience more stress during the procedure. Ways to decrease these stresses include the following: providing a prior tour of the operating room facility, informing the parents of the status of the child during the procedure, and letting them know that "everything is all right." Seventy-five percent of the children receiving general anesthesia exhibited some type of behavioral change. Positive changes included less fuss about eating, fewer temper tantrums, and better appetite. Negative changes included biting the fingernails, becoming upset when left alone, being more cautious or avoiding new things, staying with the parent more, needing more attention, and being afraid of the dark. Ways to minimize negative changes include (1) involving the child in the operating room tour, (2) allowing the child to bring along a favorite doll or toy, (3) giving preinduction sedation, (4) providing a nonthreatening environment, (5) giving postprocedure sedation as needed, and (6) allowing parents to rejoin their children as early as possible in the recovery area.

To limit the severity and duration of psychologic disturbances, the dentist should strive to reduce parental apprehension concerning the operative procedure. Because children often sense apprehension in their parents, effectively reducing the parents' anxiety will put the child more at ease. Thoroughly explaining the procedure, describing the normal postanesthetic side effects, and familiarizing the child and parents with the hospital can reduce postoperative anxiety.

Peretz and colleagues concluded that children treated for early childhood caries under general anesthesia or under conscious sedation at a very young age behaved similarly or better in a follow-up examination approximately 14 months after treatment than at their pretreatment visit, as measured by the Frankl scale and by the "sitting pattern."[4]

Fuhrer and colleagues found children were more likely to exhibit positive behavior at their 6-month recall appointment following dental treatment for childhood caries under general anesthesia versus those treated under oral conscious sedation.[5]

OUTPATIENT VERSUS INPATIENT SURGERY

During the past 30 years, the popularity of outpatient anesthesia and surgery has continually increased. Currently more than 70% of all pediatric surgical and diagnostic procedures are performed on an outpatient basis. The criteria for and advantages of ambulatory general anesthesia procedures are well recognized. The increasing cost of inpatient hospital care, advances in anesthetic management, and quality assessment of patient care have led to changes in preoperative and postoperative management of many surgical procedures done under general anesthesia that were previously assumed to be possible only on an inpatient basis. Ambulatory care is more expeditious, better tolerated both by family and hospital teams, and less traumatic for the patient. Development of freestanding ambulatory care surgical centers (i.e., same-day surgery centers) and hospital ambulatory surgical care areas has cut health care costs for consumers and third-party providers. The advances in perioperative anesthesia care are related to the wider availability of more highly qualified anesthesia care providers (board-certified anesthesiologists with subspecialty training) and the availability of modern, safer short-acting anesthetic and adjuvant drugs and monitoring equipment. A number of studies have reported a significant decrease in anesthesia-related morbidity and mortality in children over the past 2 decades.

Good patient selection is an important criterion of a successful outpatient surgery program. A young child or adolescent who requires a general anesthetic and is free of any significant medical disorders (i.e., is categorized as class I or II on the American Society of Anesthesiologists (ASA) physical status classification—see Box 14-1) can be considered a candidate for outpatient surgery. Certain patients with well-controlled chronic systemic diseases such as asthma, diabetes, and congenital heart disease can also be considered for outpatient anesthesia following prior consultation with an anesthesiologist.

When the outpatient surgery is planned, the child undergoes a complete preoperative evaluation, including a comprehensive medical history and physical examination, anesthesia assessment, and limited hematologic evaluation. Many medical facilities allow this preadmission preparation to be performed outside of the medical outpatient treatment facility. Biery and associates suggest that routine laboratory tests, such as urinalysis and complete blood count with indices and electrolyte levels, are not cost effective nor are they necessary for patients categorized as ASA class I in whom the prior complete medical history and physical examination was unremarkable.[6]

As an outpatient, the child should be brought by the parents to the hospital at least 1½ hours before the dental surgery. The nursing staff will verify that all preoperative instructions have been followed and that the appropriate laboratory tests have been performed. Several hours after the procedure is completed, the patient is released to the parent or guardian. Postoperative instructions are given, and a follow-up appointment is scheduled.

The dentist will be more responsible for team communication, physical assessment, management, and postoperative evaluation for outpatient procedures under general anesthesia than for inpatient procedures. Ferretti reported that pediatric outpatient general anesthesia patients must have reliable parents or guardians to qualify for treatment.[7] For example, the parents must have transportation available to return the child to the hospital in case postoperative complications develop at home.

The child should be treated as an inpatient if a medical condition exists that requires close follow-up, if the child lives outside the general area of the hospital, or if the parents demonstrate questionable ability to comply with preoperative or postoperative instructions. In many instances, medically or developmentally disabled patients with multiple problems requiring lengthy dental treatment are not good candidates for ambulatory care using general anesthesia. However, even some of these patients can be managed in an ambulatory setting when they are properly assessed and when no postoperative complications are anticipated.

MEDICAL HISTORY AND PHYSICAL EXAMINATION

Once the decision has been made that a general anesthetic would be preferable for a pediatric patient, the dentist should evaluate the child's medical history, the current medical status, and the possibility of complications resulting from the procedure. This risk assessment process is discussed in Chapter 14, and the patient-classification categories are shown in Box 14-1. The parents should be told of any potential complications, and their informed consent must be obtained (Fig. 15-1).

Intraoperative medical complications of dental patients with and without disabilities undergoing general anesthesia have been reported at 0% to 1.4%. In a survey of 200 pediatric dental general anesthesia cases, Enger and Mourino indicated that the most common postoperative complications following general anesthesia in children younger than the age of 5 years were vomiting, fever, and sore throat.[8] Treatment of complications consisted of administration of antiemetic medications for nausea with vomiting, ice chips for sore throat, and acetaminophen (Tylenol) for fever postoperatively. Bradley and Lynch found that no significant long-term complications resulting from anesthesia or operative procedures were observed in 100 disabled and nondisabled patients.[9]

The Joint Commission requires that all patients admitted to a hospital or treated under general anesthesia as an outpatient have a physical examination performed by a physician or qualified dentist. The child's physician must therefore be consulted for the completion of a comprehensive

---

35258
CH-1096
(FEB 02)

ᛝ Clarian Health
Methodist·IU·Riley

CONSENT FOR PROCEDURE

By signing this form, I agree that _____ , M.D., his or her associates, members of the Clarian medical staff and appropriately licensed personnel of Clarian Health may perform the following operations or procedure. I understand that Clarian Health provides educational training for health care professionals and agree that residents and students may assist in my care.

☐ Inpatient   ☐ Outpatient

Procedure: **Any necessary dental treatment under general anesthesia, including x-rays, prophylaxis, periodontal therapy, restorations, extractions, pulpal therapy, space maintainers, fluoride treatment and photographs.**

Exceptions, if any: _____ **None** _____ (If none, write "none")

- I acknowledge that I have had an opportunity to discuss with _____ M.D., my condition, the planned operation or procedure, its purpose and nature, reasonable alternatives, possible consequences of remaining untreated, risks, benefits and possible consequences.

- The procedure stated above is the one planned by my physician at this time. I realize my physician is not able to anticipate or explain all the possible risks and complications which could occur. I agree that additional procedures may be performed if my physician believes they become necessary during this procedure.

- I understand there are no guarantees that this procedure will be successful and that an undesirable result does not necessarily mean that an error was made.

- During this procedure I also consent to have any anesthetics given to me that the anesthesiologist or the physician performing the procedure believe are needed. I realize that there are medical risks associated with the anesthesia.

- If I am scheduled to receive blood or blood products, my physician has advised me of the risk and alternative therapies available. If it becomes medically necessary for me to receive blood or blood products, I agree to be transfused and accept the related risks.

- I agree to the disposal of any tissue, organ or body part removed during surgery. Provided that I am not identified, I agree that any material removed during surgery may be used for research purposes.

- I give my permission for pictures to be taken for educational purposes as long as my identity is not made known.

PHYSICIAN'S NOTE: Please list the most common and serious risks, benefits, reasonable alternatives and complications of the intended procedure(s) you discussed with the patient.

Common		Uncommon	Rare
Sore throat	Pain	Aspiration	Heart and lung complications
Nausea and vomiting	Swelling	Idiosyncratic drug reaction	Cardiac depression and arrest
Bleeding	Iatrogenic trauma	Dental trauma	Life-threatening events are statistically remote
	Sleepiness		
	Separation anxiety		

ADDITIONAL NOTES (*Optional*):

_____

Signed: _____ , M.D.

WITNESS TO SIGNATURE:

_____

Patient's Name: _____

Date: _____

Patient's Signature (see reverse side)

Time: _____ AM PM

Relationship or authority if not signed by the Patient

┌── PHYSICIAN USE ONLY/DAY OF PROCEDURE ──

☐ I have verified the correct surgical/procedural site prior to incision.

Signed: _____ , M.D.   Date: _____

Medical Record Copy	**CONSENT FOR PROCEDURE**	**M-1**

B-CLIN. NOTES	E-LAB	G-X-RAY	K-DIAGNOSTIC	M-SURGERY	Q-THERAPY	T-ORDERS	W-NURSING	Y-MISC.

Figure 15-1 Sample of form similar to one that may be used to obtain parental consent for dental treatment of a child under general anesthesia.

SIGNATURES REQUIRED

1. If the patient is an adult (age 18 or over) – signature of patient; or, if the patient is incompetent, the guardian's signature.

2. Minor patient (under age 18) – if emancipated (providing own support and living apart from the parents) patient's signature.

   If married, signatures of patient and spouse are required.

   Otherwise, signature of parent or guardian is required.

3. In an emergency threatening the life or well-being of the patient, and if signatures as required above are not available, there should be an entry in the chart documenting the emergency nature of theprocedure and the need for prompt action, attested by the signatures of two physicians. Also, the signature of the closest adult relative should be obtained, if available.

Figure 15-1 cont'd

medical history and physical examination (Box 15-1). If the physician is not a member of the hospital staff, a staff physician should complete the medical history and physical examination before admission. The dentist should perform a thorough intraoral examination and submit a record of the findings together with a summary of the child's dental history and the reason for admission (Box 15-2). The hospital must be notified to reserve an appropriate surgical suite and a bed for the child. Two weeks before admission or an outpatient dental surgery appointment, a letter containing general instructions concerning the procedure, results of the dental examination, and pertinent dates and times should be mailed to the parents.

A dental procedure may be canceled before the administration of general anesthesia, due to patient illness; productive cough, rhinitis, or wheezing; failure to comply with preoperative instructions such as abstention from eating or drinking; or risks related to coexisting diseases.

ADMISSION TO THE HOSPITAL

The "inpatients" for elective surgery are no longer admitted to the hospital the night before but on the day of surgery as an "AM admit." In this instance the child may come to the hospital the same day as the operative procedure and stay postoperatively until the next morning.

Box 15-1

Components of the Pediatric Medical History and Physical Examination for Admission to the Hospital

A. Pediatric history
  1. Identification: age, sex, racial-ethnic profile
  2. Informant and estimate of reliability
  3. Problem leading to admittance
  4. History of present illness: date of onset, chronologic description of illness, presence or absence of previous similar episodes, treatment given prior to admittance
  5. Medical survey
     a. Immunization against diphtheria, pertussis, tetanus, polio, measles, mumps, rubella
     b. Previous hospitalizations, operations, major illnesses, or injuries
     c. Allergies, including allergies to food and drugs
     d. Dietary history (younger than 2 years of age)
     e. Current medications
  6. Developmental status
     a. Infants younger than 2 years: statement regarding motor and language development
     b. Preschool children: general statement regarding development
     c. Children in school: statement regarding school performance
  7. Family history

B. Physical examination
  1. Vital signs: Temperature, pulse, respiration, blood pressure if older than 12 months of age
  2. Measurements: weight, height or length, head circumference if younger than 12 months of age
  3. General observations: nutrition, color, distress
  4. Head: description of fontanel if present
  5. Eyes: pupils, extraocular movements
  6. Ears: tympanic membranes
  7. Nose: patency, secretions
  8. Mouth: teeth, pharynx, and tonsils
  9. Neck: masses
  10. Lungs: auscultation
  11. Cardiovascular system: heart sounds, rate, rhythm, murmurs; femoral pulses
  12. Abdomen: masses, viscera
  13. Genitalia
     a. Male testes
     b. Female introitus
  14. Skin: eruption
  15. Lymph nodes
  16. Skeleton: joints, spine
  17. Nervous system: state of consciousness, gait (if walking)
  18. Summary list of problems on tentative diagnosis

Box 15-2

Components of the Dental History and Intraoral Examination to Be Completed Before Hospitalization

1. Past dental history
2. Head and neck physical examination
   a. General
   b. Head
   c. Neck
   d. Face
   e. Lateral facial profile
3. Intraoral examination
   a. Lips
   b. Tongue
   c. Floor of mouth
   d. Buccal mucosa
   e. Hard and soft palate
   f. Oropharynx
   g. Periodontium
4. Teeth
   a. Caries
   b. Eruption sequence
   c. Occlusion molar, cuspid, overbite, overjet, and midline
5. Oral habits
6. Behavior
7. Recommendations

The parents must complete the necessary forms for admission to the hospital. The dentist must write the child's admission orders, which give the nursing staff the preliminary information needed and outline the basic care procedures for the child (Fig. 15-2). The nursing staff will explain standard hospital procedures to the parents and make any recommendations needed to foster a comfortable experience for the patient.

During this time, the child will be visited by the anesthesiologist involved in the anticipated procedure. The anesthesiologist will assess the child's present state of health and review the past and present hospital records, focusing on prior exposures to general anesthetics and any complications that may have occurred. The anesthesiologist will explain the procedures involved during his or her part of the procedure and answer any questions that the child or parent might have. The decision regarding how long to keep the child off solid foods and liquids before the procedure is also determined by the anesthesiologist and may vary for younger patients to prevent hypoglycemia (Fig. 15-3).

Before surgery, the dentist can answer any questions the parents or the child might have. The dentist should also evaluate the preoperative laboratory data so that appropriate consultations can be initiated if any abnormal values are found. The dentist should record an admitting note in the medical chart to provide the supporting staff with a concise record of the child's medical history, current medical and oral status, diagnosis, and proposed treatment (Box 15-3). Abbreviations can be used when information is recorded in the medical chart (Box 15-4).

Thirty minutes before the dental procedure, the dentist and the staff should be in the operating room area.

OPERATING ROOM PROTOCOL

All persons involved in the care of patients in the operating room must follow Occupational Safety and Health Administration (OSHA) guidelines. They must wear appropriate attire designed to prevent contamination of the surgical suite, hallways, and recovery room. This generally consists of a shirt, pants or skirt, and coverings for the face, head, and feet. A hood is used to cover all unshaven facial hair. Eyeglasses, goggles, or a face shield must be used to protect the surgeon's eyes, and a mask must cover the mouth and nose.

The dentist and staff should be familiar with the standard scrub technique for sterile procedures. Neither the medical nor the dental literature documents that a sterile technique is more advantageous than a modified sterile, or clean, technique for restorative dental procedures. Therefore intraoral dental procedures are generally considered clean procedures rather than sterile procedures. However, the dentist should wear sterile gloves. A sterile gown is worn at the discretion of the dentist. The barrier technique should be followed to prevent cross-contamination between patients in the hospital.

PROPERTIES OF INHALATION GENERAL ANESTHETICS

All inhalation anesthetic agents produce anesthesia by depressing specific areas of the brain. The magnitude of depression is proportional to the partial pressure of the inhalation agents reaching specific sites in the central nervous system (CNS) after entering through the lungs and being distributed by the circulation to the tissues. The resulting physiologic signs of CNS depression produced by general anesthetic agents have been described by Guedel and modified by Roberts as stages of anesthesia with ether (Fig. 15-4).[10,11] Guedel's classification of the stages of anesthesia is largely of historical interest, however. The modern inhaled anesthetics are extremely potent. Induction of anesthesia occurs quickly, and passage through the stages of anesthesia is quite rapid.

Techniques of inhalation anesthesia vary with the type of equipment used (i.e., reservoir bag, directional valves), chemical absorption of expired carbon dioxide, and rebreathing of expired gases. The techniques range from insufflation to open or nonbreathing systems, semiopen systems, semiclosed systems, and closed systems. The semiclosed system is most often used in modern anesthesia. Exhaled gases mingle with fresh gas and are rebreathed after all the carbon dioxide is removed by a chemical absorber. Inhaled gases are humidified and a reservoir bag or ventilator allows assisted respiration. Reduced loss of body heat and water vapor, increased economy of flow, and decreased environmental contamination are advantages of the low-flow semiclosed system.

INDIANA UNIVERSITY

SCHOOL OF DENTISTRY
University Pediatric Dentistry Associates
IUPUI

July 7, 2009

Mr. and Mrs. Smith
75 Mulberry Lane
Indianapolis, Indiana University

Dear Mr. and Mrs. Smith:

Re: William Smith

After evaluating William and discussing with you the extent of his dental disease, it has been decided to accomplish all necessary dental care in the hospital. A medical history and physical examination must be completed by your physician, Dr. Charles Brown, prior to William's admission to the hospital. It has been scheduled for him at 9:00 a.m. on August 9, 2009 at Dr. Brown's office. You should also bring your child to the hospital at 10:00 a.m. on August 10, 2009 for admission.

You are encouraged to remain with your child overnight if possible. Your child may bring his favorite toy or book. If any cold symptoms (runny nose or congestion) should develop before the scheduled admission, please contact our office immediately. It is better to postpone the general anesthesia procedure if your child has a cold.

If you have any further questions concerning this procedure, please contact our office.

Sincerely,

John J. Doe

John J. Doe, D.D.S.

JJD;db

Department of Pediatric Dentistry   702 Barnhill Drive   Room 4205   Indianapolis, IN 46202-5200   (317) 274-9604   fax (317) 278-0760
Indiana University–Purdue University Indianapolis

Figure 15-2 Sample letter sent to parents two weeks before their child's admission to the hospital.

CLARIAN HEALTH
Preoperative Care Center
Riley Day Surgery

NPO Guidelines - Policy

All patients will receive specific instructions regarding preanesthetic dietary limitations during the preoperative phone call. These instructions will be appropriate and specific for the age of the patient and the time for which the procedure is scheduled. Patients with a history of neurological impairment, gastroesophageal reflux or delayed gastric emptying time may require a longer NPO period. Before giving instruction to these patients an anesthesiologist must be consulted.

Over one year of age			
Time of surgery	**Light meal**	**Clear liquids**	**Nothing by mouth**
0730	Until 2400	2400-0430	After 0430
0800	Until 2400	2400-0500	After 0500
0830	Until 2400	2400-0530	After 0530
0900	Until 2400	2400-0600	After 0600
0930	Until 2400	2400-0630	After 0630
1000	Until 2400	2400-0700	After 0700
1030	Until 2400	2400-0730	After 0730
1100	Until 2400	2400-0800	After 0800
1130	Until 2400	2400-0830	After 0830
1200	Until 2400	2400-0900	After 0900
1230	Until 2400	2400-0930	After 0930
1300	Until 2400	2400-1000	After 1000
1330	Until 2400	2400-1030	After 1030
1400	Until 0600	0600-1100	After 1100
1430	Until 0630	0630-1130	After 1130
1500	Until 0700	0700-1200	After 1200
1530	Until 0730	0730-1230	After 1230
1600	Until 0800	0800-1300	After 1300
1630	Until 0830	0830-1330	After 1330
1700	Until 0900	1930-1400	After 1400
1730	Until 0930	0930-1430	After 1430

- Clear liquids are those you can see through such as water, Gatorade, Kool-Aid, apple or white grape juice, carbonated drinks, etc. They do not include mild, gelatin, ALL other fruit juices, formula, or cereal.
- Light meals include items that can be easily digested such as soup, ice cream, toast, cereal, and crackers. They do not include steak, potatoes, pizza, eggs, bacon, sausage, or other heavy breakfast food.
- Meals that include fried or fatty foods of meat may prolong gastric emptying time. Both the amount and type of foods ingested must be considered when determining an appropriate fasting period. Following the guidelines does not guarantee a complete gastric emptying has occurred.

Revised 9/2008
Gopal Krishna, MD
Department of Anesthesia
Riley Hospital for Children

Figure 15-3 Nothing by mouth (nil per os [NPO]), times according to age.

An anesthetic's potency is defined as the concentration of the agent required to inhibit response to a standard surgical stimulus. The potency is expressed in terms of the minimal alveolar concentration (MAC) value for the agent. The MAC of a given agent will abolish the response to stimulus in 50% of patients. Expressed as a number, MAC values are additive when different agents are used in combination. MAC is useful, in that it provides an estimate of the anesthetic requirement for each patient. Fine adjustment of anesthetic administration can then be made by monitoring the patient's physiologic responses (e.g., heart rate, blood pressure, and respiratory rate). MAC values and some other properties of inhalation anesthetics are listed in Table 15-1.

Commonly used inhalation anesthetics in children include nitrous oxide, isoflurane, desflurane, and sevoflurane. In children, because they dislike needles, anesthesia is commonly induced by inhalation of a halogenated

Box 15-3

Components of Dentist's Admitting Note on the Medical History-Physical- Progress Note Form

1. Name, age, sex, race, chief complaint, and rationale for admission
2. History of the present illness
3. Past medical history
4. Present medications (list all with dosages and times given)
5. Results of current laboratory tests
6. Documentation of informed consent and physical examination
7. Impression of case (intraoral examination, diagnosis, and prognosis)
8. Plan for treatment
9. Dentist's signature

volatile anesthetic via a face mask. Due to the pleasant odor, for decades, halothane enjoyed widespread popularity as an induction agent in children. Sevoflurane became available in 1995 and in comparison to halothane has a lower blood/gas partition coefficient (producing more rapid induction and emergence) and is associated with less myocardial depression and fewer and less significant respiratory problems when used for inhalational induction. Like halothane, it has a pleasant odor. As a result, sevoflurane has become the agent of choice for inhalational induction. For maintenance of anesthesia, sevoflurane, isoflurane, and desflurane are all acceptable.

ANESTHETIC PREPARATION OF THE CHILD

TIME OUT PROTOCOL

After donning operating room attire, the dentist should report to the surgical suite and inform the anesthesiologist of any special requests concerning the procedure

Box 15-4

Abbreviations Commonly Used in the Hospital

a.c.	Before meals (ante cibos)	HEENT	Head, eyes, ears, nose, and throat
ad lib.	At liberty or at pleasure	Hg	Mercury
anom	Anomalies	Hx	History
AP	Anteroposterior	HPI	History of present illness
aq.	Aqueous, water	h.s.	Just before sleep (hora somni)
BP	Blood pressure	I & D	Incision and drainage
BRP	Bathroom privileges	IM	Intramuscular
BUN	Blood urea nitrogen	I & O	Intake and output
bx	Biopsy	IV	Intravenous
c	With (cum)	kg	Kilogram
C	Celsius (formerly centigrade)	Mand	Mandible
Caps.	Capsule	Max	Maxilla
CBC	Complete blood count	M	Molar, in moles
CC	Chief complaint	MCH	Mean corpuscular hemoglobin
CNS	Central nervous system	MCHC	Mean corpuscular hemoglobin
cong	Congenital		concentration
CP	Cerebral palsy	MCV	Mean corpuscular volume
CV	Cardiovascular	Med	Medication
d/c	Discontinue	norm	Normal
Dent	Dental	neg	Negative
Diff	Differential blood count	N2O	Nitrous oxide
disch	Discharge	NPO	Nothing by mouth (nil per os)
D5W	5% dextrose in water	NSA	No significant abnormality
Dx	Diagnosis	n/v	Nausea and vomiting
ECG	Electrocardiogram (also EKG)	op	Operation
Elix	Elixir	OPD	Outpatient department
ER	Emergency room	OR	Operating room
FHx	Family history	PA	Posteroanterior
FUO	Fever of unknown origin	p.c.	After meals (post cibos)
Fx	Fracture	PE (or Px)	Physical examination
GA	General anesthesia or (gen an)	Ped	Pediatric
ging	Gingiva	PH	Past history
Hr	Hour	PMH	Past medical history
Hct	Hematocrit	p.o.	By mouth (per os)

Continued

Box 15-4

Abbreviations Commonly Used in the Hospital—cont'd

postop	Postoperative	Subq	Subcutaneous
preop	Preoperative	SH	Social history
prep	Prepare	Hep	hepatitis
prn	As required (pro re nata)	S/P	Status post
pro Time	Prothrombin time	Stat	At once (statim)
Pt	Patient	rect	Rectal
PT	Physical therapy	surg	Surgery
PTT	Partial thromboplastin time	Sx	Signs and symptoms
Px	Physical examination	tbsp	Tablespoon
q	Every (quaque)	TPR	Temperature, pulse, and respiration
qs	Sufficient quantity (quantum sufficiat)	Tx	Treatment
R/O	Rule out	UA	Urinalysis
ROS	Review of symptoms	WBC	White blood count
RR	Respiratory rate	WD	Well developed
RR	Recovery room	W/F	White female
RSR	Regular sinus rhythm	W/M	White male
Rx	treatment (or prescription)	WN	Well nourished
s	Without (sine)	WNL	Within normal limits
SBE	Subacute bacterial endocarditis	w/o	Without

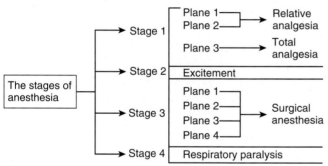

Figure 15-4 Stages of anesthesia observed with ether. (Adapted from Roberts GJ. Relative analgesia in clinical practice. In Coplans MD, Green RA, eds. *Anaesthesia and sedation in dentistry,* vol 12. Amsterdam, 1983, Elsevier Science.)

Table 15-1

Physical and Chemical Properties of Commonly Used Inhalation Anesthetics

	Vapor Pressure (mm Hg at 20°C)	Blood Gas Partition Coefficient at 37°C	Minimum Alveolar Concentration in Adults
Nitrous oxide	—	0.47	104
Isoflurane	238	1.43	1.15
Sevoflurane	157	0.63	2.1
Desflurane	664	0.42	6.0

Courtesy Dr. Gopal Krishna.

before the induction of anesthesia. When the patient enters the operating room, the mandatory "time out protocol" initiated by the circulating nurse identifies the patient, allergies, planned medications and proposed treatment to the dentist and anesthesiologist before induction for the child's safety (Fig. 15-5). Nasotracheal intubation is preferred to ensure good access to the oral cavity. Oral tracheal intubation is not contraindicated, however, and can be used in a dental case with minimal restorative needs. The anesthesiologist should be careful to avoid complications during induction (i.e., laryngospasm, tooth avulsion or aspiration, traumatic intubation, compromised airway, malignant hyperthermia).

The anesthesiologist is responsible for starting intravenous fluids (IV), securing the necessary monitoring equipment, performing the intubation, and stabilizing the endotracheal tube. The anesthesiologist will select the type of IV fluid and calculate the estimated fluid replacement and fluid deficit volumes, and perform a physical assessment of dehydration. The monitoring equipment should include (1) an automatic sphygmomanometer, (2) electrocardiographic leads, (3) a temperature-monitoring device, (4) a pulse oximeter, and (5) a capnography device. The anesthesiologist must confirm that the child is in a stable condition for anesthesia and that the equipment is functioning properly (Fig. 15-6).

Special care is taken to protect the child's eyes (Fig. 15-7). In addition, a shoulder roll is placed, padding is added to the patient's pressure points, the endotracheal tube and head are stabilized, heating or cooling blankets are used as needed, and the safety belt is secured. The dentist has the table positioned to conduct dental procedures, and the anesthesiologist administers any preoperative IV medications requested.

Before scrubbing, the dentist should obtain any necessary preoperative radiographic studies. All persons

49993
CH-6817 (MAR 09)
Page 1 of 1

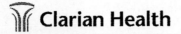

UNIVERSAL PROTOCOL CHECKLIST
To be completed by Licensed Professional

A. 1) Before Patient is in the Procedure Room

- ☐ Patient identity *(2 patient identifiers)*
- ☐ Procedure, location, allergies
- ☐ Consents complete
- ☐ H&P complete with up-date
- ☐ DVT Prophylaxis is addressed if ordered
- ☐ Anesthesia assessment is completed
- ☐ Site marked with "YES" if appropriate

Completed by: _____ Date/Time: _____

2) Before Patient is in the Procedure Room

- ☐ Correct diagnostic and radiology tests are available
- ☐ Blood availability addressed
- ☐ Correct devices and equipment including implants are available

Completed by: _____ Date/Time: _____

B. Upon Arrival to the Procedural Room – *complete prior to procedure or if at bedside*

- ☐ Patient identity *(2 patient identifiers)*
- ☐ Procedure to be performed
- ☐ Allergies
- ☐ The responsible proceduralist *(per policy)* is available
- ☐ Verbal acknowledgment from all members of the team present

Completed by: _____ Date/Time: _____

C. To Be Completed Immediately Prior to Incision/Start of Procedure

- ☐ Patient identity *(2 patient identifiers)*
- ☐ Procedure to be performed
- ☐ Consent is accurate and signed
- ☐ Position is correct, site marking visible
- ☐ Antibiotic type and time if appropriate
- ☐ Special precautions due to patient history discussed if applicable
- ☐ Irrigation present if needed
- ☐ All images correctly displayed
- ☐ Verbal acknowledgment from all essential members of the Procedure team

Completed by: _____ Date/Time: _____

D. Before Patient Leaves the Procedure Room

- ☐ Consent(s) checked – all procedures have been done
- ☐ All Specimens are identified and correctly labeled   ☐ No Specimens
- ☐ All foreign bodies not intended for implantation are removed
- ☐ Verbal acknowledgment from all members of the Procedure team
- ☐ Counts addressed

Completed by: _____ Date/Time: _____

UNIVERSAL PROTOCOL
CHECKLIST (Page 1 of 1)

M-22

Figure 15-5 Universal protocol checklist.

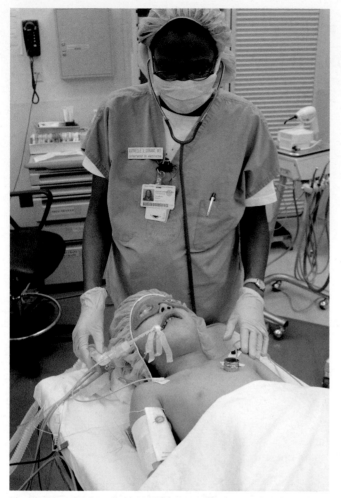

Figure 15-6 Patient is in a stable anesthetic condition and ready for the dental procedure. Notice the position of the precordial stethoscope, blood pressure cuff, and nasotracheal tube.

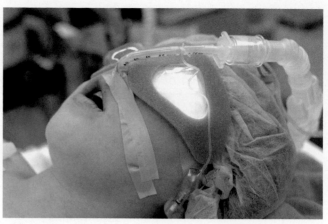

Figure 15-7 Special eye guard protects the patient's eyes during the procedure

involved in the radiologic procedure should wear protective lead apparel. Radiographs of excellent quality can be made while a patient is under general anesthesia without exposing the patient or staff to unnecessary radiation (Fig. 15-8). Digital radiographs are advantageous because radiation exposure is decreased and image feedback is immediate.

PERIORAL CLEANING, DRAPING, AND PLACEMENT OF PHARYNGEAL THROAT PACK

Before the dental procedure is begun, the perioral area is cleansed with three sterile 4- × 4-inch gauze pads. The first gauze pad is saturated with a bacteriostatic cleansing agent, the second with sterile water, and the third with alcohol (Fig. 15-9). This procedure is not intended to sterilize the area but only to remove gross debris (Fig. 15-10). A surgical sheet is then positioned over the remainder of

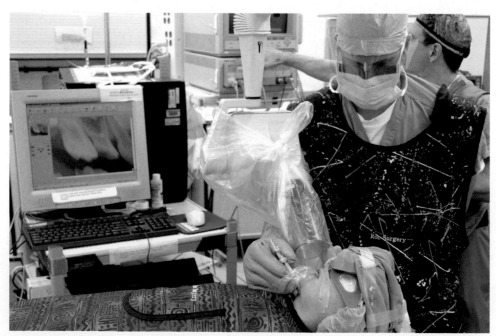

Figure 15-8 Obtaining diagnostic radiographs. Notice the use of protective lead gloves, gown, and apron.

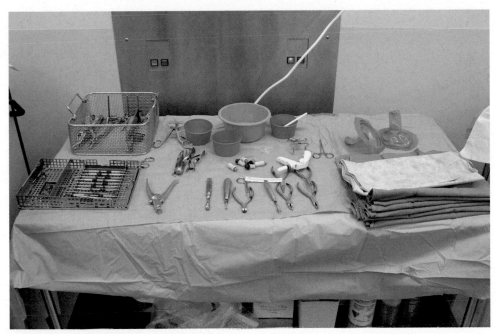

Figure 15-9 Materials required for perioral cleaning. From upper left: pharyngeal throat pack, towel clamps, patient drapes, bacteriostatic cleaning agent, sterile water, and alcohol.

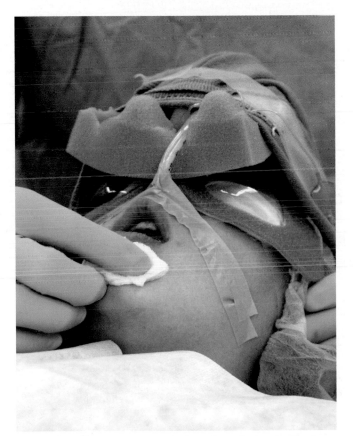

Figure 15-10 Special care must be taken during perioral cleaning to prevent materials from entering the oral cavity.

the child's body. This helps maintain body temperature and provides a clean field during the procedure. The head is draped with three towels arranged to form a triangular access space for the mouth. The towels are secured in place with towel clamps or hemostats. The mouth should

be fully exposed (Fig. 15-11). The anesthesiologist may request that part of the nasotracheal tube remain exposed so that all connections can be easily monitored. The assistants then place all supporting carts and stands around the table in positions that the dentist finds comfortable and efficient (Fig. 15-12).

The patient's mouth is opened with the aid of a molt mouth prop. Care should be taken not to impinge on the lips or tongue with the prop (Fig. 15-13). The mouth is thoroughly aspirated. The pharyngopalatine area is sealed off with a strip of moist 3-inch sterile gauze approximately 12 to 18 inches long (Fig. 15-14). Written documentation of throat pack placement and removal is required on the physical history form of the medical chart. This packing reduces the escape of anesthetic agents and prevents any material from entering the pharynx. The gauze should be tightly packed around the tube, so that a good seal is ensured. Once the pack is in place, a thorough intraoral examination is performed, followed by dental prophylaxis. The dentist should then evaluate any new radiographic studies that have been obtained and formulate a final treatment plan.

RESTORATIVE DENTISTRY IN THE OPERATING ROOM

Instruments used for restorative dental procedures in the operating room are the same as those for procedures in the dental operatory. Local anesthesia may be used to minimize pain and bleeding. The use of quadrant isolation with a rubber dam is preferred (Fig. 15-15). After the completion of the procedures for each quadrant, a topical fluoride treatment should be applied before the removal of the rubber dam. Written documentation of blood loss and hydration in the medical chart is required.

Restorative dental care under general anesthesia allows excellent patient compliance and easy achievement of a

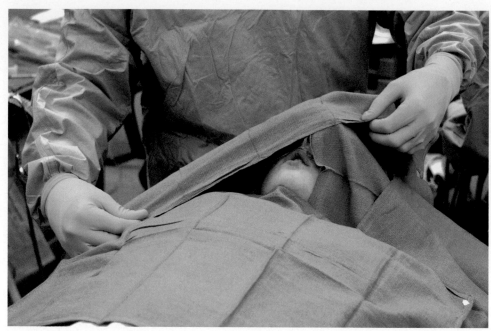

Figure 15-11 Placement of the surgical sheet and triangular draping of the oral cavity area. The nasotracheal tube is exposed to allow easy monitoring of its connections.

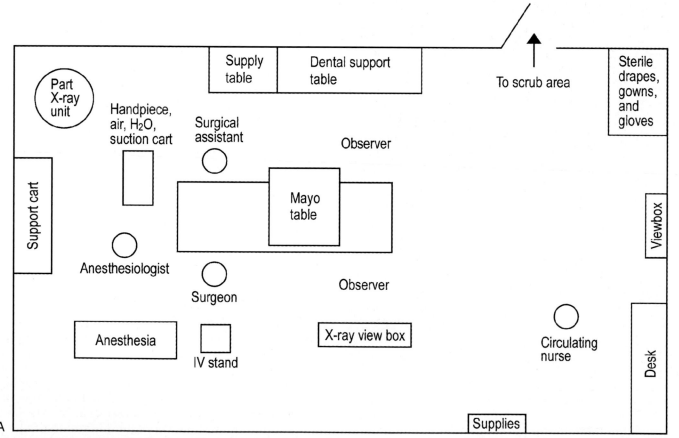

A

Figure 15-12 A, Schematic drawing of one example of the positioning of personnel and equipment in the operating room. IV, intravenous.

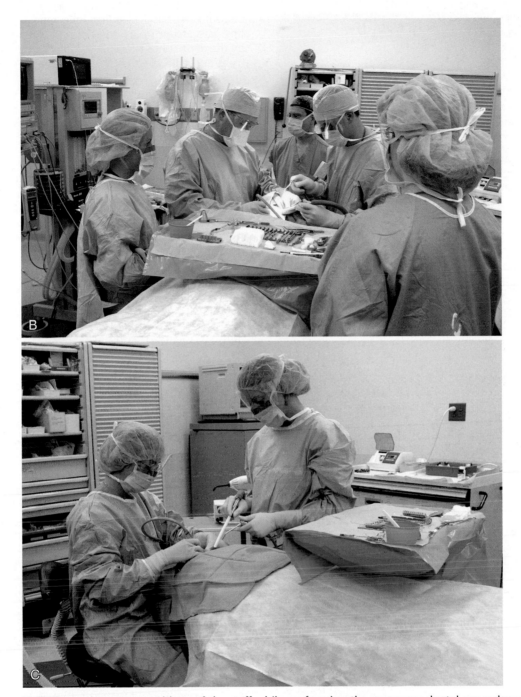

Figure 15-12 cont'd B, Operating room positions of the staff while performing the necessary dental procedures. From left: Dental assistant, dental surgeon, anesthesiologist, assistant dental surgeon, and circulating nurse. **C,** Sitting position operating room. From left: Dental surgeon, dental assistant (anesthesiologist is out of the picture to the left).

well-lighted field, and therefore increases the quality and quantity of dental care while decreasing the anxiety level for the clinician and patient during dental treatment. Spiro and Burns found that they were able to treat seven teeth per hour in children under general anesthesia compared with only three teeth per hour in children of similar age in a clinic setting.[12] Eidelman and associates reported that the quality of restorative treatment performed was better under general anesthesia than under conscious sedation.[13]

The dentist should place restorations that will provide the greatest longevity with the least amount of maintenance, for example, full-coverage stainless steel crowns rather than large amalgam restorations on posterior primary teeth. In a 3-year study of comprehensive dental cases treated under general anesthesia, O'Sullivan and Curzon found stainless steel crowns to be significantly more successful (3% failure rate) than an amalgam or composite restoration (29% failure rate).[14] A 6-month retrospective study by Tate and colleagues to assess the failure

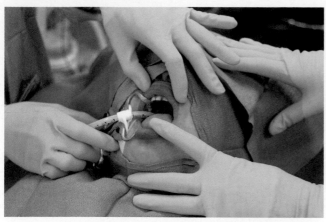

Figure 15-13 Positioning of a mouth prop. Special care is taken not to impinge on the lips or tongue with the prop.

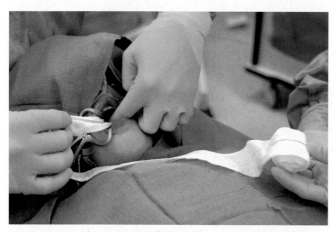

Figure 15-14 Placement of the pharyngeal throat pack.

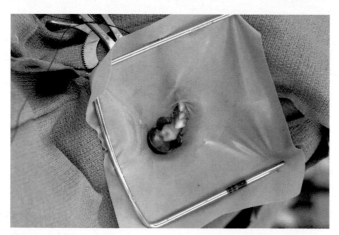

Figure 15-15 Rubber dam isolation of the maxillary left quadrant.

rates of dental restorative procedures performed under general anesthesia by pediatric dental residents found stainless steel crowns to be best (8%), followed by amalgam (21%) and composite (30%); composite strip crowns (51%) had the lowest successful restorative treatment rate.[15]

Intraoperative anesthesia complications (e.g., dislodged or obstructed endotracheal tube, IV infiltrates or disconnects, nasal bleeding or edema of the tongue and lips, and arrhythmias) rarely occur. Care should be taken by the dentist not to displace the endotracheal tube. Priority is given by the dentist to the anesthesiologist to treat any adverse event quickly, even to the point of stopping treatment and removing rubber dams to allow access.

COMPLETION OF THE PROCEDURE

END TIME OUT PROTOCOL

The anesthesiologist should be notified 10 minutes before the completion of the procedure so that the child can begin to be aroused and preparations can be made for extubation. The recovery room personnel are notified that the child will soon be arriving so that they can begin preparations. On completion of the dental procedure, the oral cavity is thoroughly débrided and the throat pack is removed carefully to prevent aspiration of any materials that might be lodged against it. The "end time out protocol" is called by the circulating nurse to identify any patient safety concerns (see Fig. 15-5). The dentist verbalizes a needle and sponge count and removal of the throat pack to the nurse. At this time, the anesthesiologist assumes responsibility for the child. The dentist should remain in the operating room during the extubation process to assist the anesthesiologist if necessary. When the child is transported to the recovery room, the dentist should accompany the anesthesiologist and provide assistance during the transportation.

POSTANESTHESIA CARE UNIT

When the child arrives in the postanesthesia care unit or recovery room, the dentist should inform the nursing staff of the procedures accomplished and of any special requests or instructions. If teeth have been removed, the nurse should be specifically instructed how and where to apply gauze packs for hemostasis. The nurses and other medical staff are available to deal with immediately postoperative complications if they occur (i.e., fever, nausea, vomiting, croup, hypoxia, bleeding, and laryngospasm). After the dentist has confirmed that the airway is patent and the vital signs are stable, and after the anesthesiologist is confident the child is recovering well, the dentist should meet with the parents or guardian to provide a brief report of the child's condition and a review of the treatment. The parents or guardian of inpatients should be informed of the approximate time the child will be transported to the ward. The parents or guardian of outpatients should be informed of the time to meet the child in the recovery area. Prescriptions may be written for pain control agents (i.e., acetaminophen with codeine, or ibuprofen suspension) antibiotics (i.e., amoxicillin, clindamycin), or antiemetics for nausea (i.e., prochlorperazine, ondansetron [Zofran]).

POSTOPERATIVE CARE

Postoperative orders and the operative note for the staff should be completed by the dentist and recorded in the medical chart while the child is in the postanesthesia care unit (Fig. 15-16 and Box 15-5). Transfer orders may be

Outpatient Orders

1. PACU care per protocol.
2. Discontinue IV when released from PACU.
3. Begin clear liquids in Day Surgery.
4. Acetaminophen_____mg. (10-15 mg./kg/ standard dose)
5. Call Dental House officer at _____if questions.
6. Release from Day surgery when discharge criteria are met.
7. Return appointment.
8. Call if problems arise.

Office number_____
Pager number_____
Signature_____

A

Inpatient Orders

1. Admit to_____ to Dr. _____ Service.
2. Allergies
3. Vital signs q2h x 2, then q4h x 2, then q8h
4. Continuous pulse oximetry x 24h
5. Head of bed elevated 30 degrees
6. Protective stabilization, if needed.
7. Encourage oral fluids
8. Advance to soft diet as tolerates.
9. Medications: list all meds, dosage, times given
10. Pain medication: Acetaminophen_____mg po q4h prn pain (typical dose 10-15 mg/kg)
11. Nausea medication (if indicated): Ondansetron_____mg po or IV prn nausea (0.1-0.2 mg/kg, adult dose 4-8 mg)
12. IV fluids: D5 1/2 NS + 20 meq KCL at _____(typical maintenance fluid rate = 4 ml/kg for patients < 10kg, 40 + 2 ml/kg for patients 10-20 kg, and 60 + 1 ml/kg for patients > 30 kg)
13. Antibiotics (if indicated): Amoxicillin_____mg if not allergic to penicillins, Clindamycin_____mg, if allergic to penicillins.
14. Apnea monitor, if indicated.
15. For oral swelling — apply ice pack to area for 30 minutes.
16. Check for oral bleeding q15 min x 1 hr. If needed, apply moist 4x4 sterile gauze to area with pressure.
17. Call if needed.

Office number _____
Pager number _____
Signature _____

B

Transfer Medical Orders

1. Transfer to pediatric medical service: Dr. _____MD_____ pager number_____
2. Vital signs per PACU protocol.
3. Change intravenous fluids per pediatric medical service.
4. Encourage clear liquids.
5. Advance to soft diet as tolerated.
6. Monitor for oral hemorrhage for 24 hours. Apply moist strile gauze and pressure, if necessary. Call Dentist for excessive hemorrhage or swelling.
7. Medications per pediatric medical service.
8. Continue additional medications per prescription: i.e. mild pain — acetaminophen or ibuprofen suspension; moderate pain — acetaminophen with codeine elixir, antibiotic — amoxicillin; allergy clindamycin nausea — ondansetron
9. Give and eview appropriate home care instructions, and return appointment with family prior to discharge.
10. For dental questions contact: Dr. _____Dentist_____ Pager number_____

_____
Dentist Signature

C

Figure 15-16 Components of the dentist's postoperative orders for a patient. **A,** Inpatient orders. **B,** Outpatient orders. **C,** Transfer medical orders.

Box 15-5

Components of the Dentist's Operative Note

1. Title of dental procedure
2. Type of intubation and anesthesia used
3. Teeth restored
4. Teeth extracted
5. Other procedures completed
6. Dental prophylaxis and topical fluoride used
7. Summary (e.g., length of procedure, how the child tolerated the procedure, blood loss, complications)
8. Prognosis
9. Dentist's signature

used for individuals requiring more specialized care than the pediatric dentist usually provides (see Fig. 15-16C). The operative report should be dictated as soon after the completion of the procedure as possible (Box 15-6).

If the child was treated as an outpatient, once the child is awake and alert, displays appropriate behavior, maintains his or her own airway, has stable vital signs, has no uncontrolled bleeding or pain, is voiding, and has no retention of liquids, a decision is made to release the child rather than keep the child overnight for further evaluation. If the child is to be kept for 23-hour observation (inpatient), an appropriate note is recorded in the medical chart and a discharge summary is dictated (Box 15-7) after the child is released. Postoperative instructions and

Box 15-6
Components of the Dentist's Operative Report

1. Doctor's name and assistants' names
2. Patient's name and hospital number
3. Preoperative diagnosis
4. Postoperative diagnosis
5. Title of the operative procedure
6. Preparation for anesthesia (preoperative medications, type of intubation, and anesthetic agents used)
7. Surgical procedure
   a. Radiographs taken
   b. Description of scrub, draping procedure, and throat pack
   c. Number of teeth restored and type of restorations
   d. Number of teeth receiving pulp therapy
   e. Teeth extracted (name each)
   f. Gingival therapy procedures
   g. Band(s) for appliance(s) and impression(s)
   h. Dental prophylaxis and fluoride applied
   i. Type and amount of intraoperative fluids used
   j. Other information (if indicated)
8. Estimated blood loss and hemostasis
9. Condition of the patient at the conclusion of the surgical procedure (complications incurred if indicated)
10. Condition of the patient on arrival in the recovery room
11. Prognosis

Box 15-7
Components of the Dentist's Discharge Summary Statement

1. Patient's name and hospital number
2. Date of admission
3. Date of discharge
4. Date of dictation
5. Preoperative diagnosis
6. Postoperative diagnosis
7. Age, race, and sex of patient
8. Reason for admission and treatment using general anesthetic
9. Results of preoperative history and physical examination (medical and dental) and present medications
10. Name of the physician completing the history and physical examination
11. Complete description of the surgical procedure (see Box 15-6)
12. Patient's tolerance in the recovery room and ward
13. Condition of patient on discharge
14. Individual to whom patient is discharged
15. Home care instructions given to parents and medications prescribed (dosage and times to be given)
16. Patient's next appointment
17. Copies of discharge summary sent to patient's physician and referring dentist or physician

necessary prescriptions are given to the parents or guardian, and an observation appointment for the child is arranged before the discharge. The dentist must be available that evening (a contact number must be given) in the event the parents or guardian need assistance in caring for the child after returning home. These instructions and prescriptions help the patient deal with common complications after discharge, such as fever, nausea, vomiting, pain, and bleeding.

Effective communication is essential at this time to reaffirm the parents' or guardian's cooperation in performing oral health care and in keeping follow-up observation appointments and recall appointments. Enger and Mourino reported that only 57% of dental patients undergoing a treatment in the operating room returned for 6-month recall visits.[8] They suggest that procedures requiring monitoring (i.e., space maintenance) be postponed if the patient's return is unlikely.

A study by Almeida et al of future caries susceptibility in children with early childhood caries following dental treatment under general anesthesia found that, despite implementation of increased preventative measures for these children, they were still highly predisposed to greater caries incidence in later years.[16] The researchers concluded that more aggressive preventive therapies may be required in children who experience early childhood caries.

There are several categories of dental problems in children that cannot be handled well in the office setting and are best managed in the hospital or outpatient surgery center. The ability to treat children in the hospital environment and to provide comprehensive dental care using a general anesthetic for such children is a valuable part of the dentist's treatment regimen. Granting hospital staff privileges to qualified dentists has become routine at many hospitals seeking to provide comprehensive health care for the community. The dentist who uses the hospital or outpatient surgery center in the care of patients often finds it to be a rewarding component of practice.

REFERENCES

1. Crespi P, Friedman RB. Hospitalization for the pediatric dental patient: an update on admission indications and third party review, *N Y State Dent J* 52(2):40-43, 1986.
2. King KJ, Nielson RR. Dental treatment in the hospital utilizing general anesthesia. In Nowak AJ, ed. *Dentistry for the handicapped patient.* St Louis, 1976, Mosby.
3. Camm JH, et al. Behavioral changes of children undergoing dental treatment using sedation versus general anesthesia, *Pediatr Dent* 9(2):111-117, 1987.
4. Peretz B, et al. Children with baby bottle tooth decay treated under general anesthesia or sedation: behavior in a follow-up visit, *J Clin Pediatr Dent* 24(2):97-101, 2000.
5. Fuhrer CT, et al. Effect on behavior of dental treatment rendered under conscious sedation and general anesthesia in pediatric patients, *Pediatr Dent* (in press)
6. Biery KA, Shamaskin RG, Campbell RL. Analysis of preoperative laboratory values prior to outpatient dental anesthesia, *Anesth Prog* 34:58-60, 1987.
7. Ferretti GA. Guidelines for outpatient general anesthesia to provide comprehensive dental treatment, *Dent Clin North Am* 28(1):107-120, 1984.

8. Enger DJ, Mourino AP. A survey of 200 pediatric dental general anesthesia cases, *J Dent Child* 52(1):36-41, 1985.
9. Bradley GS, Lynch S. Safety of hospital dental treatment for the high-risk patient, *Spec Care Dentist* 4(6):253-260, 1984.
10. Guedel AE. Inhalation Anesthesia. New York, 1937, Macmillan.
11. Roberts GJ. Relative analgesia in clinical practice. In Coplans MD, Green RA, eds. *Anaesthesia and sedation in dentistry, vol 12. Amsterdam,* 1983, Elsevier Science.
12. Spiro SR, Burns J. Current concepts of premedication and anesthesiological management for the pediatric dental patient who is hospitalized for dento-oral rehabilitation, *J Hosp Dent Pract* 14(1):35-39, 1980.
13. Eidelman E, Faibis S, Peretz B. A comparison of restorations for children with early childhood caries treated under general anesthesia or conscious sedation, *Pediatr Dent* 22:33-37, 2000.
14. O'Sullivan EA, Curzon MEJ. The efficacy of comprehensive dental care for children under general anesthesia, *Br Dent J* 171:56-58, 1991.
15. Tate AR, et al. Failure rates of restorative procedures following dental rehabilitation under general anesthesia, *Pediatr Dent* 24(1):69-71, 2002.
16. Almeida A, et al. Future caries susceptibility in children with early childhood caries following treatment under general anesthesia, *Pediatr Dent* 22(4):1-5, 2000.

SUGGESTED READINGS

American Academy of Pediatric Dentistry. Special issue: Reference manual 2007-2008, *Pediatr Dent* 29(7 suppl):66-68, 121-122, 2007.

Bohaty B, Spencer P. Trends in dental treatment rendered under general anesthesia, 1978 to 1990, *Pediatr Dent* 16(3):222-224, 1992.

Coplans MD, Green RA. Anaesthesia and sedation in dentistry, vol 12, Amsterdam, 1983, Elsevier Science.

Diner MH, Marcous P, Legault V. Intraoral radiographic techniques for the anaesthetized patient, *J Int Assoc Dent Child* 20(1):17-21, 1990.

Dripps RD, Eckenhoff JE, Vandam LD. *Introduction to anesthesia: the principles of safe practice,* ed 6, Philadelphia, 1988, WB Saunders.

Gotowka T, Bailit HL. Quality assurance systems for hospital outpatient dental programs: background, *Spec Care Dentist* 1:211-217, 1981.

Hill CM, Morris PJ. General anesthesia and sedation in dentistry, Bristol, England, 1983, John Wright & Sons.

Persliden B, Magnusson BO. Medical complications of dental treatment under general anesthesia in children, *Swed Dent J* 4(4):155-159, 1980.

Sheehy E, Hirayama K, Tsamtsouris A. A survey of parents whose children had full-mouth rehabilitation under general anesthesia regarding subsequent preventive dental care, *Pediatr Dent* 16(5):362-364, 1994.

Trapp LD. Special considerations in pedodontic anesthesia, *Dent Clin North Am* 31(1):131-138, 1987.

Vermeulen M, Vinckeir F, Vandenbroucke J. Dental general anesthesia: clinical characteristics of 933 patients, *J Dent Child* 52:36-41, 1991.

Wenner JII, Greene VW, King JL. Monitoring microbial aerosols in an operating room during restorative dentistry, *J Dent Child* 43:25-29, 1977.

CHAPTER 16

Dental Materials

▲ B. Keith Moore

CHAPTER OUTLINE

*A*lthough the past 30 years have seen a marked reduction in the dental caries rate in children, restorative dentistry remains an important part of pediatric dentistry. Recurrent caries remains a major diagnosis indicating necessity for replacement of existing restorations. Development continues on improved restorative materials and manipulation techniques for restorative dentistry for the general population. As these become available to the pediatric dentist they may displace materials that have been used for many years. Much current effort addresses the growing awareness, expectations, and concerns of the dental consumer. Aesthetics has become a major consideration in choice of materials and procedures. Concern is also increasing about the biocompatibility of materials from the standpoint of the patient and the environment. Research has resulted in an ever-increasing body of knowledge related to the behavior of dental materials and an avalanche of new products. These developments place a continuing responsibility on the dentist, who must critically analyze the literature and the claims of manufacturers to determine which materials and techniques will provide optimal service to the patient. For intelligent and best choices to be made, an appreciation of the clinical significance of the chemical, physical, and biologic properties of dental materials is essential.

The oral cavity is a formidable obstacle to maintenance of the integrity of tooth structure and the materials used in its restoration or replacement. Biting stress on the cusp of a molar tooth may be as high as 207 MPa (30,000 psi). The pH of saliva, dental plaque, foods, and beverages fluctuates daily from very acid to alkaline. The temperature of a meal may vary as much as 150° F (66° C). The warm, moist oral cavity contains a variety of enzymes and debris, providing optimum conditions for the accumulation of surface deposits that can degrade restorations and tooth structure. For these and other reasons, restorative materials are readily subject to fracture, solubility, dimensional change, and discoloration. If these problems are to be minimized, a dental material must possess certain minimum chemical and physical properties. Furthermore, those properties must be maintained during the manipulation and placement of the restoration and for its projected lifetime in service.

The American Dental Association (ADA)/American National Standards Institute Specification Program has contributed greatly to providing the dentist with high-quality dental materials that have been carefully developed to resist the rigors of the oral cavity. Many commonly used restorative materials are encompassed by this certification program.

The website of the ADA (http://www.ADA.org) should be consulted for listings of materials that meet the ADA specifications. From that list the dentist should be able to select a brand that provides the desired manipulative characteristics.

In a like manner to the ADA, the Fédération Dentaire Internationale has been instrumental in the development of international specifications under the auspices of the International Standards Organization (ISO). The dental materials market has become international. The Medical Devices Amendments of 1976 to the Food and Drug Act gave the U.S. Food and Drug Administration (FDA) regulatory authority to protect the public from hazardous or ineffective medical and dental devices. Some dental products with claims for therapeutic effects (e.g., fluoride products) are considered drugs, but most dental materials used professionally are considered devices and are subject to regulation by the FDA Bureau of Medical Devices. Also included are over-the-counter dental products sold to the public, such as floss and denture adhesives.

In addition to the issue of the safety of dental materials and devices for the patient, other safety issues have been raised in recent years that have dramatically influenced the practice of dentistry. Concern about the transmission of infectious disease during dental procedures has led state and federal agencies to develop rigorous standards for infection control. These standards have placed new demands on dental materials, devices, and equipment. Today, most of these must be capable of being subjected to disinfection procedures and, in some cases sterilization, without loss of properties. Delivery systems for materials have been significantly influenced. Most materials are now packaged for unit-dose delivery at chairside, which makes infection control much easier than when bulk containers of materials are used.

The second safety issue to come to the forefront is the safety of individuals working in the dental office. Federal and state occupational safety and health administrations (OSHAs) are responsible for developing and enforcing standards to ensure safety in the workplace. Dental offices that employ any person besides the dentist fall within the regulatory scope of these agencies. Many of the dental materials commonly used in restorative dentistry are considered to present an occupational hazard. One of the federal OSHA regulations requires the dentist to have on file a Material Safety Data Sheet for every material—from impression materials to the cleaning fluids used in the office. All employees must be informed about the nature of any hazardous materials to which they may be exposed and must receive training in the safe handling of these materials. Information to assist the dentist/employer is available from sources such as the ADA Regulatory Compliance Manual, first published in 1989 and continuously updated as new regulations are developed.

Environmental concerns also have affected the practice of dentistry. State and federal environmental protection agencies are giving scrutiny to all waste discharged from the dental office, whether solid, liquid, or gas. Disposal of hazardous materials, such as toxins or biohazards, is regulated and the level of such regulation can be expected to grow. In most cases the generator of waste material remains legally responsible even if another party has been paid to dispose of it.

All of the concerns mentioned can seriously affect the practice of dentistry and require on the part of the dentist an increasing body of knowledge about dental materials and a constant vigilance to stay current with developing regulations.

MICROLEAKAGE AND BIOLOGIC CONSIDERATIONS

Possibly the greatest deterrent to the development of an "ideal" restorative material is the leakage that occurs along the restoration-tooth interface. There is as yet no truly adhesive dental material. No restorative dental material exactly duplicates the physical properties of tooth structure. Changes in temperature and mechanical stress can result in the development of gaps at the tooth-material junction. Moreover, no matter how proficient the dentist may be, no restoration exactly fits the prepared space in the tooth. Overwhelming evidence shows that all restorative materials permit ingress of deleterious agents, such as acid, food debris, and microorganisms, between the walls of the prepared cavity and the restoration. A certain incidence of the clinical failure of materials can be associated with this phenomenon. Microleakage may be the precursor of secondary caries, marginal deterioration, postoperative sensitivity, and pulp pathology. With restorations, microleakage often results in unsightly marginal discoloration and necessitates replacement of the restoration. Microleakage poses a particular problem for teeth in the pediatric patient because the floor of the cavity preparation may be close to the pulp. The added insult to the pulp caused by the seepage of irritants that penetrate around the restoration and through the thin layer of dentin, or a microscopic pulpal exposure, may produce irreversible pulp damage.

One method of bonding substances together is entirely mechanical. A liquid adhesive is used that will flow into irregularities in the surfaces being bonded and then solidify. In dentistry, acid etching is commonly used to accomplish bonding of a restorative resin to enamel by the formation of resin tags into the etched enamel.

For true adhesion to occur, bonding must take place at a molecular level and must involve a chemical interaction between the molecules of the adhesive and the adherend. The only dental materials currently in use that have the potential for true adhesion to tooth structure and an established clinical record for success are based on polyacrylic and other polyalkenoic acids. These materials are the polycarboxylate and glass ionomer cements (GICs).

With the advancements that have been made in surface chemistry and the development of adhesives for all types of unusual applications, the dentist may ask why other adhesive dental materials have not been developed. Availability of a truly adhesive restorative material would greatly alter many phases of dental practice. The need for the typical cavity preparation would no longer be a prime consideration because adhesion would eliminate the need for mechanical retention by the cavity preparation. It would no longer be necessary to use auxiliary aids, such as cavity varnishes and etching techniques, to minimize the microleakage around direct filling restorations. The compromised tooth could actually be reinforced by the restorative material, which would reduce the need for full occlusal coverage to protect the tooth.

However, tooth structure possesses numerous undesirable characteristics as a substrate for bonding of an adhesive. It is rough, inhomogeneous in composition, covered with a tenacious layer of surface debris, and wet. These factors discourage adhesion. Furthermore, the reactivity (surface energy) of enamel is low, and therefore the surface does not easily attract other molecules to it.

It has been shown that topical fluoride applications reduce even further the surface energy of enamel. Although this may be beneficial because it can reduce plaque accumulation and hence caries, it also interferes with the wetting of the tooth surface by a liquid adhesive.

On the other hand, the surface energy of most restorative materials, particularly metallic ones, is higher than that of normal intact tooth structure. Therefore, debris accumulates on the surface of restorations more than on the adjoining enamel. This could, in part, account for the surprisingly high incidence of secondary caries associated with most restorative materials, except for those that release fluoride ion. Debris accumulation can promote marginal deterioration by the loss of tooth structure or restorative material at the interface. Such deterioration would normally increase microleakage.

CAVITY VARNISHES

Cavity varnishes have been used empirically for many years as a liner for cavity preparations. When varnish is painted onto the cavity preparation, the solvent evaporates and leaves a thin resin film. The varnish may reduce microleakage when it is used with certain restorative materials. Cavity varnish may reduce initial microleakage around amalgam. Because varnish films are very thin and do not adhere to tooth structure, some clinicians have replaced cavity varnish with one of the dental adhesives currently marketed. In theory, if such a material adheres to dentin and enamel, any leakage should occur between the amalgam and the adhesive. The results of laboratory studies provide limited support for this theory, although a controlled clinical study by Mahler and colleagues showed no reduction in postoperative sensitivity with the use of dentin adhesives as liners for amalgam restorations. Application of cavity varnish before applying a dental adhesive negates any potential for adhesion or sealing on the part of the adhesive system.

CEMENT BASES

The function of the cement base is to promote recovery of the injured pulp and to protect it against further insult. The base serves as a thermal insulator and replaces missing dentin when it is used under the metallic restoration. The base must be of sufficient thickness to provide effective thermal insulation. A minimum of approximately 0.5 mm is required for this purpose.

A base must be able to support the condensation of the restorative material placed over it. If the strength of the base is inadequate, it may fracture during condensation and permit amalgam to penetrate and come into contact with the dentin floor, which thereby compromises the thermal protection afforded by the base. Zinc phosphate, hard-setting calcium hydroxide, zinc oxide–eugenol, and GICs have sufficient strength to serve effectively. In certain cases, such as a class II preparation that involves the restoration of an angle or of a deep depression, it may be necessary to cover a calcium hydroxide base with a layer of stronger zinc phosphate or GIC.

AMALGAM

Controversy regarding the safety of the dental amalgam restoration has existed since the material was introduced to the profession more than 150 years ago. Periodically this controversy surfaces in the news media and becomes a matter for public, as well as professional, debate. As a result, the dentist who uses dental amalgam can expect questions to be raised by patients and their guardians and can expect requests for replacement of intact amalgam restorations with other materials.

Amalgam is no longer the most commonly used material for restoring posterior carious lesions. Tooth-colored restorative materials, such as composite resins and resin-modified glass ionomers, are increasingly being used. The popularity of dental amalgam likely will continue to decline as these other materials demonstrate their longevity and their suitability as general amalgam replacements in the permanent dentition.

The unique clinical success of amalgam during 150 years of use has been associated with many characteristics. It is likely that its excellent clinical service, even under adverse conditions, is attributable to the tendency for its microleakage to decrease as the restoration ages in the oral cavity. Although amalgam does not bond to tooth structure and the margins of an amalgam restoration may appear open, the restoration-tooth interface immediately below the exposed margin becomes filled with relatively insoluble corrosion products that inhibit leakage. Amalgam is unique from this standpoint. The microleakage around other restorative materials usually increases with time. Amalgam is the least technique sensitive of all current direct restorative materials. One of the factors slowing the acceptance of posterior composite resin restorations has been the very exacting clinical technique and time required for placement. Another unique property of amalgam as a direct filling material is its lack of dimensional change during hardening. The ADA specification for dental amalgam limits maximum acceptable dimensional change to ±0.2%. If this is compared with a typical value of 2% or higher for the polymerization shrinkage of a resin matrix composite material, the potential impact on microleakage is obvious.

Nevertheless, failures of amalgam restorations are observed. These may occur in the form of recurrent caries, fracture (either gross or severe marginal breakdown), dimensional change, or involvement of the pulp or periodontal membrane. More significant than the type of failure is its cause. Two factors that lead to such clinical failures are improper design of the prepared cavity and faulty manipulation. In other words, the deterioration of amalgam restorations often can be associated with neglect in observing the fundamental principles of cavity design or abuse in preparing and inserting the material. One other factor also is involved, and that is the choice of the alloy used.

SELECTION OF THE ALLOY

Several criteria are involved in the selection of an amalgam alloy. The first criterion is that the alloy should meet the requirements of the ADA Specification No. 1 or the corresponding ISO specification for dental amalgam alloys.

The manipulative characteristics of dental amalgam are extremely important and a matter of subjective preference. Rate of hardening, smoothness of the mix, and ease of condensation and finishing vary with the alloy. For example, the resistance felt with lathe-cut amalgams during condensation is entirely different from that with spherical amalgams. The alloy selected must be one with which the dentist feels comfortable, because the operator variable is a major factor influencing the clinical lifetime of the restoration. Use of alloys and techniques that encourage standardization in the manipulation and placement of the amalgam enhances the quality of the service rendered. Coincident with this is the delivery system provided by the manufacturer—its convenience, expediency, and ability to reduce human variables.

Obviously the physical properties should be reviewed in the light of claims made for the superiority of one alloy over competing products. Ideally such a list of properties should be accompanied by documented clinical performance in the form of well-controlled clinical studies. Although the cost of the alloy is a factor, this criterion should not be overemphasized when balanced against the alloy's ability to render maximum clinical service. The dentist should always consider the fractional costs of any material to the overall total charges for a dental procedure when making price comparisons between brands, particularly when comparing a brand with documented clinical performance against a generic brand of material.

Dental amalgam alloys generally are available as either small filings called lathe-cut alloys or spherical particles called spherical alloys. Spherical alloys tend to amalgamate readily. Therefore amalgamation can be accomplished with smaller amounts of mercury than required for lathe-cut alloys, and the material gains strength more rapidly. Also, the condensation pressure and technique employed by the dentist in placing the restoration are somewhat less critical in achieving the same properties of the amalgam. This is an advantage in difficult clinical situations in which optimal access for condensation is limited. Spherical amalgam alloys have a somewhat different feel during condensation and require less condensation pressure than lathe-cut alloys. The dentist and auxiliary should familiarize themselves with the handling characteristics of a new alloy before clinical restorations are placed.

HIGH-COPPER ALLOYS

The original dental amalgam alloys were alloys of silver and tin with a maximum of 6% copper. When significantly more copper is available, improved laboratory properties and clinical performance have been demonstrated. This improvement has been attributed to the displacement of the tin-mercury reaction product with a copper-tin phase during the amalgamation reaction. Alloys that contain enough copper to eliminate the formation of the tin-mercury phase (11% to 30%) are called high-copper amalgam alloys. The first such alloy of this type was an admixed system. Small spherical particles of a silver-copper alloy were added to filings of a conventional silver-tin alloy. High-copper alloys also can be made using single composition particles. Each of these alloy particles has the same chemical composition, usually silver, copper, and tin. Amalgams made from high-copper alloys have low creep. Creep is the tendency of a material to deform continuously under a constant applied stress. This property has been associated with the marginal breakdown (ditching) commonly noted with amalgam restoration. Although the ADA specification for dental amalgam permits a maximum of 3% creep, creep of a modern high-copper amalgam alloy should not exceed 1%.

Choice of amalgam alloy today should be limited to high-copper alloy systems.

Regardless of the alloy used, manipulation plays a vital role in controlling the properties and the clinical performance of the restoration.

MERCURY/ALLOY RATIO

Most of the properties of amalgam restorations have been shown to depend on the relative amount of mercury contained in the finished restoration (the residual mercury). One of the variables that control the final mercury content is the amount of mercury used to mix the amalgam.

Although dental amalgam alloy still may be available in the form of powder or preweighed compressed pellets and bulk mercury can be dispensed by volume, most of the amalgam alloy sold today is in the form of prefilled, disposable mixing capsules containing the proper amounts of alloy and mercury. This delivery system should be used for several reasons. The alloy/mercury ratio is accurately preproportioned. The need for disinfection procedures is minimized because the capsule system is discarded after use. Most importantly, exposure of dental personnel and environmental contamination by mercury vapor is minimized. These prefilled capsules are usually available for different size mixes, often called single- or double-spill capsules.

TRITURATION

The second manipulative variable that controls the residual mercury content is trituration. Trituration time can significantly influence both consistency and working time of the mixed amalgam. These in turn relate to the ability to bring excess mercury to the surface during condensation. The correct trituration time varies depending on the composition of the alloy, the mercury/alloy ratio, the size of mix, and other factors. The best practice is to acquire an appreciation for the appearance of a proper mix and then to adjust the trituration time accordingly. The most serious error in amalgamation generally is undertrituration. An undertriturated mix appears dry and sandy and does not cohere into a single mass. Such an amalgam will set too rapidly, which results in a high residual mercury content, reduced strength, and the increased likelihood of fracture or marginal breakdown. Properly mixed amalgam is a shiny, coherent mass that can be readily removed from the capsule.

MECHANICAL AMALGAMATORS

When first introduced, mechanical amalgamators for dental amalgam operated at a single speed that was usually below 3000 cpm. High-copper alloys in prefilled, self-activating capsules are designed for shorter trituration times at higher trituration speeds. Failure to activate these capsules reliably results in undertrituration and is a common problem with the use of older single-speed amalgamators. Because amalgamators also deteriorate with time, replacement of an older unit with a new high-speed amalgamator is desirable. A unit that allows multiple speeds of operation should be selected, because numerous other products such as dental cements are now marketed in capsules to be mixed in a dental amalgamator. The trituration times suggested by the amalgam alloy supplier are starting points. Amalgamators may vary in operating speed even within the same brand, and a unit's performance may vary with line voltage or the number of times it is used in rapid succession. Trituration speed, as well as time, significantly influences the rate at which some amalgams harden(Fig. 16-1).

CONDENSATION

The purpose of condensation is to adapt the amalgam to the walls of the cavity preparation as closely as possible, to minimize the formation of internal voids, and to express excess mercury from the amalgam. Within reasonable limits, the greater the condensation pressure, the lower the amount of residual mercury left in the restoration and the greater the strength of the restoration. The selection of the condenser and the technique of "building" the amalgam should be designed to achieve those

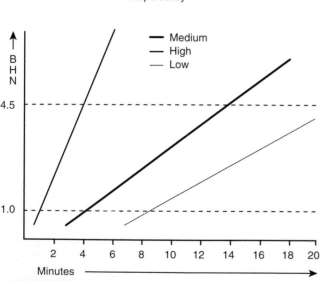

Dispersalloy

— Medium
— High
— Low

Figure 16-1 The influence of amalgamator speed (low-medium-high) on the hardening rate of a high-copper amalgam alloy as measured by the Brinell Hardness test (BHN). BHN = 1.0 indicates the working time, and BHN = 4.5 indicates the carving time. (Redrawn from Brackett W. Master's thesis. Indianapolis, Indiana University School of Dentistry, 1986.)

objectives, as described in detail in textbooks of operative dentistry, and should be tailored to the handling characteristics of the type of amalgam alloy chosen.

MOISTURE

Moisture contamination of an amalgam restoration can promote failure. If zinc is present in the alloy, it will react with water, and hydrogen gas will be formed. As this gas builds up within the amalgam, a significant delayed expansion can occur and may cause protrusion of the amalgam from the cavity preparation, which enhances the possibility of fracture at the margins.

Such moisture contamination can result from failure to maintain a dry field during the placement of the restoration. Exposure to saliva after the amalgam has been completely condensed is not harmful. It is only moisture incorporated within the amalgam as it is being prepared or inserted that must be avoided.

Zinc-free alloys are available, and their physical properties are generally comparable to those of their counterparts that contain zinc. A zinc-free, high-copper alloy should be used when the dentist operates in a field where moisture control is difficult.

MARGINAL BREAKDOWN AND BULK FRACTURE

Because dental amalgam is a brittle material, a commonly observed type of amalgam failure is the restoration in which the marginal areas have become severely chipped. The exact mechanisms that produce this breakdown of the amalgam or the adjoining tooth structure are not established, but it is likely that the deterioration is precipitated by manipulation and technique of finishing rather than by dimensional changes during setting.

If the restoration is improperly finished by the dentist, a thin ledge of amalgam may be left that extends slightly over the enamel at the margins. These thin edges of such a brittle material cannot support the forces of mastication. In time they fracture, leaving an opening at the margins.

Bulk fracture of amalgam is much less common with high-copper amalgam alloys. Those cases that do occur likely have one of two causes. Poor cavity design resulting in an insufficient bulk of material across the isthmus can lead to failure of even a high-strength alloy, as illustrated in Fig. 16-2. The other reason for bulk fracture is premature loading of the restoration. Unlike a resin matrix composite, amalgam gains strength slowly over the first 24 hours. Premature loading can result in minute fractures that are not apparent for weeks or even months. The use of a rapid-setting amalgam with a high 1-hour compressive strength should be considered when treating a pediatric patient in whom compliance with instructions to refrain from biting down hard on the freshly placed amalgam is in question.

BONDED AMALGAM RESTORATIONS

Because dental amalgam does not adhere to tooth structure, it must be retained mechanically by the design of the cavity preparation and/or mechanical devices such as pins. The placement of an amalgam does not strengthen

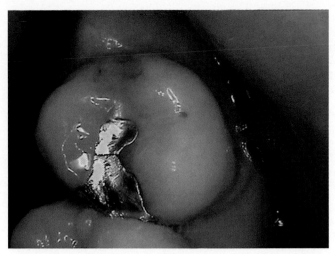

Figure 16-2 Bulk fracture of an amalgam restoration. Such failure may occur from improper cavity design or premature occlusal loading. (Photo courtesy of Dr. Jeffrey Platt)

the compromised remaining tooth structure and subsequent fracture may occur, particularly in molar teeth with relatively large mesiodistocclusal amalgam restorations. The use of dental adhesive systems, as described in detail in the section related to resin composites, as lining materials for amalgam to create a "bonded amalgam restoration" has been suggested. Several products are marketed specifically for this purpose. In general, they are chemically activated dentin-bonding systems over which the amalgam is condensed before the resin adhesive has hardened. This results in an intermixing of the unset resin and the plastic amalgam at the interface and forms a mechanical bond as both materials harden. It is important to distinguish this application from the use of a dental adhesive to seal the dentin surface and reduce early microleakage as previously discussed. When dental adhesives are used to seal the dentin surface, the adhesive should be polymerized before the amalgam is placed. Bond strengths reported in laboratory studies between amalgam and dentin are lower than the maximum reported for resin composite bonded to dentin. In vitro studies also show that teeth restored with bonded amalgams are more resistant to fracture than those in which amalgam is placed without a bonding adhesive.

These are relatively short-term laboratory studies. Even though longer-term clinical data are available, little is known about the potential influence of embedding the resin into the bulk of the amalgam on the long-term properties of the restoration. At the present time, amalgam bonding should be considered only as an adjunct for conventional, accepted practices of cavity preparation and mechanical retention of amalgam.

MERCURY TOXICITY

The amalgam restoration is possible only because of the unique characteristics of mercury. Mixing this liquid metal with the alloy powder provides a plastic mass that can be inserted into the tooth and then hardens rapidly to a structure that resists the rigors of the oral environment.

As the restoration hardens, mercury reacts with silver and tin to form stable, intermetallic compounds. Most of the public controversy about the safety of dental amalgam has focused on the hazards associated with elemental mercury and some of its organic compounds. Many substances commonly regarded as quite safe contain extremely dangerous elemental ingredients. No one would ever consider human ingestion of elemental sodium or chlorine, but ordinary table salt, which is the compound sodium chloride, is an important dietary substance. From the time of the earliest use of amalgam, it has been asked whether mercury in a dental restoration can produce local or systemic toxic effects in humans. It is periodically conjectured that mercury toxicity from dental restorations is the cause for numerous illnesses of unknown etiology.

The possibility of toxic reactions by the patient to traces of mercury penetrating the tooth or sensitization from mercury dissolving from the surface of the amalgam is remote, however. The danger has been evaluated in numerous studies. The patient's encounter with mercury vapor during insertion of the restoration is brief, and the total amount of mercury vapor is too small to be injurious. Furthermore, the amount of mercury released from the amalgam in service is small compared with other sources of mercury from air, water, and food. Metallic mercury in the human digestive track is apparently not converted to lethal organo-mercury compounds and is excreted by the body.

Both the National Institutes of Health and the FDA have examined the evidence for risk of dental restorative materials to the patient. The conclusion was that, except for the very small fraction of the population with a true allergic reaction to mercury or other constituents of amalgam, the dental amalgam restoration remains a safe and effective treatment. No evidence was found that related the presence of amalgam restorations to disorders such as arthritis, multiple sclerosis, or other diseases in which amalgam has been implicated. It should be noted that no currently available restorative material is completely risk free and that patients should be informed of the relative risks associated with all dental treatment alternatives.

The question about the replacement of existing serviceable amalgams with other materials remains one of professional judgment. Both the ADA and some state dental licensing boards have found that a dentist who recommends replacement of amalgam restorations with other materials on the claim that this will improve the physical health of the patient may be acting unethically and may be subject to sanctions by licensing bodies and to suits for civil damages. Patients who feel that they have medical problems related to the presence of any dental restorative material should be referred to a physician for diagnosis and treatment recommendations.

What about dental office personnel? Restorative dentists and their office personnel potentially are exposed daily to mercury, even in offices in which amalgam restorations are not being placed. Although metallic mercury can be absorbed through the skin or by ingestion, the primary risk to dental personnel is from inhalation. A potential hazard exists for dentist and staff from long-term inhalation of mercury vapor in the dental clinic, although the few actual incidents reported have been related to poor technique in handling mercury. The maximum level considered safe for occupational exposure is 50 mg of mercury per cubic meter of air averaged over a standard 8-hour workday. Mercury at room temperature has a vapor pressure almost 400 times the maximum level considered safe. This vapor has no color, odor, or taste and cannot be readily detected by simple means at the level of maximum safe exposure. Because liquid mercury is almost 14 times more dense than water, a small spill can be significant. Eliminating the use of bulk mercury by employing prefilled, disposable capsules should significantly reduce exposure to mercury vapor.

The dental operatory should be well ventilated. All mercury waste and amalgam scrap removed during placement or removal of amalgam restorations should be collected and stored in well-sealed containers. When amalgam is cut, water spray and high-speed evacuation should be used. More detailed recommendations can be obtained from the Regulatory Compliance Manual published by the ADA. The risk to dental personnel from mercury exposure cannot be ignored. However, adherence to simple hygienic procedures will ensure a safe working environment.

Waste materials containing mercury or amalgam scrap should be disposed of responsibly in accordance with the regulations of the local Environmental Protection Agency. These materials should not be incinerated or subjected to heat sterilization. Biologically contaminated wastes containing mercury, including extracted teeth, should be cold-sterilized with a chemical agent before disposal. The most significant threat to the continued use of dental amalgam will likely be from government regulations on environmental waste discharge. In Japan, use of amalgam has been discontinued because it is not feasible for a dental office using amalgam to meet restrictions on mercury discharge into sewers. Amalgam-mercury separators on dental clinic wastewater discharge lines are now required in several countries in Europe. Local and state authorities should be consulted about limitations on discharge of mercury into wastewater from a dental practice.

CEMENTS

Dental cements have several functions in restorative dentistry. One is to serve as a luting agent to fill the space between a restoration fabricated outside the mouth and the tooth structure. By flowing into irregularities in both materials and then hardening, the cement provides mechanical retention as previously discussed. A second function is to serve as a filling material for either permanent or temporary restorations. Cements are also used as bases for other restorative materials as previously described.

Silicate cement was an early tooth-colored filling material. Although it is no longer used, its ability to reduce development of secondary caries has made it a model for the development of caries-resisting dental materials. Recurrent or secondary caries was seldom encountered around silicate cement restorations even when gross disintegration had occurred. Most other restorative materials have not shown such an ability to resist recurrent

caries, which is today the most common cause for replacement of restorations.

This beneficial characteristic is attributed to the presence of fluoride in silicate cement powder, which typically contains approximately 15% fluoride. After placement of the silicate restoration, fluoride ion is released and reacts with the adjoining tooth structure in much the same manner as does topically applied fluoride. The enamel solubility is reduced, which builds up its resistance to acid attack and caries. Because there is evidence that the fluoride ions are released slowly throughout the life of the restoration, the protective mechanism is undoubtedly a continuous one.

LUTING CEMENTS

Several types of cement may be used as luting agents. Each has inherent advantages and disadvantages. Thus the selection of a particular type of cement is governed by the individual situation presented by the patient.

ZINC PHOSPHATE CEMENT

Formerly, zinc phosphate cement was the most widely used luting agent. Composed essentially of phosphoric acid liquid that is mixed with zinc oxide powder, the cement has excellent handling characteristics such as setting time, fluidity, and film thickness. Furthermore, this type of cement has a long history of successful application for permanent cementation. It does not have an anticariogenic effect, does not adhere to tooth structure, and does demonstrate a moderate degree of intraoral solubility.

Because of the phosphoric acid liquid, zinc phosphate cement is an irritant, and proper pulp protection is recommended. When experience indicates that sensitivity and pulp response are likely to be problems, use of a cement that is more biologically compatible, such as a polycarboxylate cement, is recommended.

POLYCARBOXYLATE CEMENT

Polycarboxylate cement is one of the few dental materials that demonstrate true adhesion to tooth structure. The powder is primarily zinc oxide, and the liquid is polyacrylic acid or a copolymer of that acid. Although the final pH of the set cement is comparable to that of zinc phosphate cement, its biologic properties are excellent. For this reason, polycarboxylate cement is useful as a base or as a luting agent, particularly when the cavity preparation is close to the pulp. In addition, as the cement sets against the tooth structure, a chemical bond is formed between the cement liquid and the calcium in the hydroxyapatite in enamel and dentin.

When the cement is used as a luting agent, several manipulative factors influence the wetting of the tooth by the cement and thereby retention of the restoration. After cavity preparation, the enamel and dentin surfaces are covered with a thin layer of tenacious debris, referred to as the *smear layer*. Also the preparation may be covered by a thin film of material, such as zinc oxide–eugenol, if a provisional restoration was placed. Unless this contamination is removed, it may inhibit adhesive bonding of the setting cement to the tooth. One means of cleaning the surface is a 10- to 15-second swabbing with 10% polyacrylic acid.

As with all types of cement, the liquid should not be dispensed until just before the mix is to be made. To slow down the setting reaction and provide longer working time, a chilled mixing slab may be used. The powder and liquid should be mixed rapidly, and the mix should be completed within 30 seconds.

The recommended powder/liquid ratio should be used. If the mix is too thick, insufficient acid is present to produce bonding to the tooth. If excess liquid is used, the intraoral solubility increases significantly. When properly prepared, the mix has a glossy appearance and can be extruded into a thin film. It is important that minimal time elapsed between completion of the mix and placement of the cement; the mix must not have lost its glossy appearance.

When polycarboxylate cement is used with cast restorations, the inside surface of the casting must be cleaned thoroughly. After the casting is cleaned in a pickling bath, the interior should be treated with an air abrasive or a fine stone. Polycarboxylate cement will not wet a chemically dirty surface. In time, leakage and loss of retention may occur along the cement restoration interface.

Although polycarboxylate cement demonstrates adhesion to tooth structure, it has a relatively low tensile strength, no significant fluoride release, and modest intraoral solubility. Good practices of tooth preparation should be used to insure retention of the restoration.

GLASS IONOMER CEMENT

Another type of cement that is based on polyacrylic acid is GIC. Because of its biologic kindness, fluoride release, and potential for adherence to the calcium in the tooth (as with the polycarboxylate system), GIC is used as a restorative material (type II) for treatment of the eroded area, as a luting agent (type I), and as a base and liner material (type III).

Like zinc polycarboxylate cement, the glass ionomer liquid is polyacrylic acid or other alkenoic acids, such as itaconic or maleic, with tartaric acid added to improve handling properties. The acid has the potential for bonding to calcium in the manner described for polycarboxylate. This chemical bond provides retention of the cement to the tooth.

The powder is a fluoro-aluminosilicate glass similar to silicate cement powder and displays fluoride release patterns similar to that of silicate cement. Data from glass ionomer restoration of class V erosion lesions for periods of more than 7 years indicates that GIC shows resistance to secondary caries. One can immediately see the attraction of the GIC system: it has a potential for adherence to tooth structure and possesses anticariogenic potential.

The material is supplied as a powder and liquid and is commonly preproportioned in a disposable capsule to be mixed in an amalgamator. With type I GIC, the liquid acid may be freeze-dried and combined in the powder. When this powder is mixed with water, the acid reconstitutes, which results in the same setting reaction. The freeze-dried products have better shelf life and somewhat

lower viscosity, which are important characteristics for luting cements.

The mix can be made either on a disposable, moisture-resistant paper pad or on a glass slab. A plastic spatula is preferred to a metal one to minimize contamination of the mix from abraded metal. As with polycarboxylate cement, the polyacrylic acid–based liquid is not dispensed until just before the start of the mix. The GICs are mixed in a manner like that used for polycarboxylate cements: large increments of the powder are rapidly incorporated into the liquid, and the mix should be completed within 40 seconds. The working time is short, usually no more than 3 minutes from the start of the mix. In no instance should the material be used if the mix has lost its gloss or a skin has formed on the surface.

After setting, the material is more brittle than a polycarboxylate cement. It can be trimmed and finished in much the same manner as zinc phosphate cement. Before the patient is dismissed, all the accessible margins should be covered with the varnish or protective resin supplied by the manufacturer. This protects the cement from oral fluids and dehydration during the next few hours as the setting reaction continues.

Instances of postoperative sensitivity have been reported when GIC is used as a luting agent, particularly in deep preparations with minimal remaining dentin. This is possibly attributable to the low initial pH of the cement and its relatively slow set. To guard against potential irritation, in very deep areas calcium hydroxide should be placed. The cut dentin surface can be cleaned mechanically with pumice, but the smear layer should not be removed. After cleaning, the dentin should be rinsed and dried but not desiccated. A slightly damp surface appears to help minimize sensitivity and does not interfere with the setting reaction.

Glass ionomer luting cements have mechanical properties similar to those of zinc phosphate cements and lower intraoral solubility. Because of their potential for fluoride release and adhesion to tooth structure, they are becoming the most commonly employed luting cements for metallic restorations.

In addition to its use as a luting agent for cast restorations, GIC has been employed for bonding orthodontic brackets to acid-etched enamel. GIC has lower cohesive strength than do the resin orthodontic adhesives, but the fluoride release from the GIC should minimize the white spotting and decalcification sometimes seen around orthodontic brackets or bands. If orthodontic bands are employed on posterior teeth, the GIC is the luting agent of choice.

RESIN-MODIFIED GLASS IONOMER CEMENTS

The most recent addition to the cement field is the resin-modified GIC. These cements are also sometimes referred to as *hybrid glass ionomers* or in the case of type II and III cements as *light-cured glass ionomers*. Disadvantages of conventional glass ionomers include short working time, slow development of ultimate properties, sensitivity to both moisture exposure and dehydration during setting, and lower cohesive strength compared with resin cements. These problems have been addressed by the development of resin- modified GIC. Resin monomers or a co-monomer of acrylic acid and a methacrylate such as hydroxyethyl methacrylate are added to the glass ionomer formulation. The resin component hardens immediately on exposure to the light, which results in an initial set of the cement. The material then continues to undergo the acid-base GIC setting reaction that occurs more slowly than that of a conventional GIC, resulting in a much longer working time for the light-cured glass ionomer. The rapid set after light exposure yields a material that is much less sensitive to dehydration or moisture. Type I resin-modified GIC luting cements are also available; in this case the resin component is either chemically activated or dual (chemical and light) activated. Resin-modified GIC type II restorative materials appear to exhibit the advantages of conventional GIC and have received rapid acceptance. The use of resin-modified GIC luting cements is less well established. Fracture of all-ceramic crowns cemented with some resin-modified GIC has been reported, which prompts concern about their use with ceramic restorations.

ZINC OXIDE–EUGENOL

The acid-base reaction between zinc oxide and eugenol results in a cement that can be used as both a luting and restorative material. Because of its low strength and high oral solubility, zinc oxide–eugenol is not recommended as a permanent luting cement. However, because of its exceptionally kind biologic behavior, it is often used as a base material, as a temporary luting cement, and as a temporary restorative material. Eugenol is an inhibitor for additional polymerizing resins and can interfere with subsequent use of resin cements, restorative materials, and even impression materials.

RESIN CEMENTS

Resin luting cements are derived from the composite resin systems used for restorative materials. They may be viewed as lightly filled composites. The resin matrix systems used are the same as those employed for restorative resins. Although these materials are not new to dentistry, they are becoming more extensively employed. Their first major clinical application was in direct bonding of orthodontic attachments to acid-etched enamel, for which they quickly became the materials of choice. Similar formulations were developed into pit and fissure sealants, which are discussed in Chapter 17. The resin-bonded bridge such as the "Maryland" bridge is another application in which resin cements came to the forefront. The demand for dentistry has resulted in extensive use of both resin and ceramic veneers. Here, too, resin cements are the cements of choice. Finally, new technology for fabricating all-ceramic crowns and inlays has greatly increased the use of these restorations, which are normally cemented with resin cements. Resin cements have high strength, low film thickness, and very low oral solubility, and can be bonded to etched enamel, ceramics, resins,

and etched or treated metal surfaces. With the advent of dentin adhesives, resin cements provide the possibility of bonded, indirect restorations.

Resin cements are usually available in different shades for color matching beneath translucent restorations, and opaque cements are made for masking metal substructure or discolored tooth structure. The first resin cements were two-component, chemically activated curing systems. Visible light–activated, single-component systems are now available and are popular when used with translucent restorative materials. Dual-activated materials, which are both chemical and light activated, are recommended for use beneath thick restorations and in locations where geometry may limit access to the curing light.

TEMPORARY AND PERMANENT RESTORATIONS

The temporary restoration should possess good biologic characteristics, have minimal solubility, and be rigid, strong, and resistant to abrasion. The relative importance of each of these properties depends on the degree of permanence desired. For example, in the carious mouth it is often desirable to remove some or all of the caries immediately and place temporary restorations. These restorations subsequently are replaced with more permanent restorative materials. In such situations it may be necessary for the temporary restoration to serve for several months or longer. Strength and resistance to abrasion and dissolution are of paramount importance in these cases. Usually, temporary restorations need to remain in place only for days. In the latter instance more emphasis may be placed on the biologic properties when a material is selected.

Because of its excellent tissue tolerance and ability to minimize initial microleakage, zinc oxide–eugenol cement has been commonly used for holding or intermediate restorations. The strength, rigidity, and resistance to abrasion of the conventional zinc oxide–eugenol mixture have been improved by the addition of polymers and by the surface treatment of the zinc oxide powder.

Type II GICs or the newer resin-modified GICs also are useful as long-term, temporary restoratives, for example, in restoring eroded areas in patients when exposed areas of cementum and dentin are present. Because of its desirable biologic and adhesive characteristics, the GIC can be used to restore these lesions without the need for a retentive cavity preparation. If conventional GICs are employed as restorative materials, they must be protected from exposure to moisture in the early stages of setting and from dehydration for a very long time, likely the entire time the restoration will serve. In general, a resin-modified glass ionomer is a better choice for reasons given previously.

GIC formulations that include fillers to improve their mechanical properties are marketed. In one product particles of amalgam alloy are mixed with the GIC powder; another uses a cermet—silver sintered onto the GIC glass powder. Although use of these materials for core buildup and for very conservative class I and class II restorations in primary dentition has been advocated, the improvements in mechanical properties of these "reinforced"

GICs are modest. Whether their mechanical properties, such as fracture toughness, are adequate to resist masticatory stress is questionable. Again, the resin-modified glass ionomer is probably a better choice.

RESTORATIVE RESINS

CONVENTIONAL COMPOSITES

The term *composite material* refers to a combination of at least two chemically different materials with a distinct interface separating the components. When properly constructed, such a combination of materials provides properties that could not be obtained with any of the components alone. (Examples of natural composites are bone, tooth enamel, and wood.) In a resin composite dental restorative material, an inorganic filler has been added to a resin matrix in such a way that the properties of the matrix have been improved.

A number of parameters have a pronounced influence on the properties that are obtained by the addition of inorganic fillers to a resin matrix. The characteristics of the dispersed phase in terms of its shape, size, orientation, concentration, and distribution are very important. Likewise, the composition of the continuous phase, the resin matrix, is equally significant.

The resin matrix of many currently available composite materials is bisphenol A–glycidyldimethacrylate (bis-GMA) or urethane dimethacrylate resin. Triethylene glycol dimethacrylate, a lower-viscosity resin, is usually added as a diluent. Among the materials used for macro fillers are ground particles of fused silica, crystalline quartz, and soft glasses such as barium, strontium, and zirconium silicate glass. These particles, which make up 70% to 80% of the material by weight, resist deformation of the soft resin matrix. The high filler content and the chemistry of the resin matrix substantially reduce the coefficient of thermal expansion compared with an unfilled acrylic resin. The filler also reduces the polymerization shrinkage and increases the hardness.

The filler and the resin matrix must be chemically bonded together with a coupling agent on the surface of the filler. If this is not done, the particles may be easily dislodged, water sorption at the filler-matrix interface may take place, and stress transfer between matrix and filler may not occur. The filler particles are coated with a reactive silane product. Despite use of this coupling system, the filler particles do become dislodged during cutting and finishing and under abrasive action such as tooth brushing or occlusal contact. This abrasive action likely affects the softer resin matrix, which becomes worn away and exposes the filler particles. When enough of the filler particle is exposed, it will break free of the resin. This process leaves a continual rough surface (Fig. 16-3). Because the composites are 70% to 80% filled, this surface roughness is clinically noticeable.

Based on clinical experience, there has been a definite preference for use of smaller filler particles. In the early resin composites it was common for the particle size to approach 100 mm; now the coarsest particles would not exceed 30 mm. The average mean particle size of

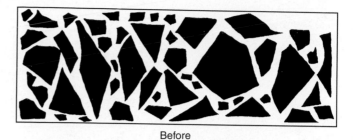

Before

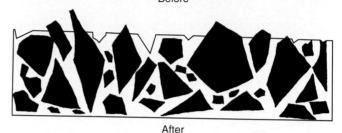

After

Figure 16-3 Schematic drawing of a conventional composite resin with macrofiller (*black areas*) before and after finishing or wear. (Redrawn from Phillips RW. Science of Dental Materials, 9th ed. Philadelphia, WB Saunders, 1991.)

the fillers in conventional composites is in the 8- to 12-mm range, and the trend is to reduce the filler size even further.

MICROFILLED COMPOSITES

Efforts to improve the surface smoothness and polish ability of composite resins led to the development of the microfilled composite. These composites are based on the use of an extremely small silica filler particle, whose size is 0.02 to 0.04 mm, and hence are called microfine, microfilled, or polishable resins. The particles may be dispensed directly into the paste, but the amount that can be added in this manner is very limited. Addition of amounts in excess of 20% results in a paste too viscous for the dentist to use. Matrix resin monomer can be heavily filled with microfine silica and polymerized in the manufacturing process. The resulting composite is ground to filler particle sizes comparable to those of the inorganic filler in conventional composite. This "organic" filler with additional colloidal silica is then added to the resin monomer to form the composite resin paste. The structure of such a resin is illustrated in Fig. 16-4.

The appealing characteristic of these microfilled resins is their ability to be finished to an extremely smooth surface, which was a major problem with the conventional composites. When microfilled resins are finished, the polymerized resin filler particles cut at the same rate as the matrix and a much smoother surface results, as shown in Fig. 16-4. Even if some of the very small silica particles are dislodged, the surface irregularities cannot be detected by the eye.

Because of the small silica particle size, the filler has a very large surface area, and the total amount of filler that can be incorporated is reduced to about 50% by weight compared with a filler loading of 70% to 80% for conventional composites. Thus the microfilled composite has a higher resin matrix content. As a result, such resins are

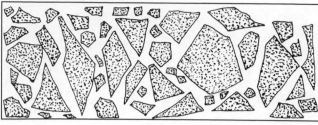

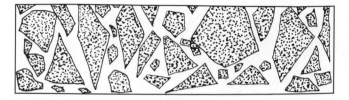

Figure 16-4 Structure of a microfilled resin showing microfiller *(dots)* and prepolymerized macrofiller particles before and after finishing. (Redrawn from Phillips RW. Science of Dental Materials, 9th ed. Philadelphia, WB Saunders, 1991.)

softer and have a slightly higher coefficient of thermal expansion, a higher water absorption, more polymerization shrinkage, and somewhat lower mechanical properties. Because of this tradeoff in properties, microfilled resins should be used where esthetics is the principal consideration and where undue stress will not be placed on the restoration, such as in class III or class V restorations. When the restoration is subject to stress, such as the incisal margin of a class IV restoration, a composite having better physical properties is preferred. The development of hybrid and small-particle composites has significantly reduced the use of microfilled composites.

SMALL-PARTICLE AND HYBRID COMPOSITES

The conventional macrofilled composite is no longer in common use. Filler sizes have been continually reduced to approach the surface smoothness of the microfilled resin but retain the filler levels and physical properties of the conventional composite. Small-particle composites have an average filler size of 1 to 5 mm, with a broad distribution of sizes. This permits higher filler loading than in the conventional composites and results in the best combination of physical properties of all the currently available composites. Small-particle composites are recommended for stress-bearing applications such as class IV and class II restorations. Their surface finish is inferior to that of a microfill resin but much better than that of a conventional composite.

Hybrid composites are the most recent step toward smaller particle size. They contain radiopaque glass particles with an average size of 0.6 to 1.0 mm in addition to 10% to 20% colloidal silica. The total filler level, 70% to 80%, is lower than in a small-particle composite but higher than in a microfill resin. Because these combine two types of fillers, the result is called a *hybrid composite*.

Although the surface of hybrid resins is not as smooth as that of microfilled resins, these resins find extensive anterior use if they are carefully polished. Also, one of the primary motivations in the development of these hybrid materials was to find a material that could compare favorably with dental amalgam in wear resistance in class I and II restorations. The use of composites in such situations is discussed in the section on posterior composite restorations. The most recent trend in resin composites has been the marketing of so-called universal or all-purpose restorative materials for use in either anterior or posterior applications.

LIGHT-CURED COMPOSITES

Originally, composite resins were chemically activated, which required the mechanical mixing of two pastes to initiate the chemical reaction. Light-cured or light-activated composites have largely supplanted the chemically activated composites. Light-activated resins do not differ significantly in composition from the chemically activated resins except for the polymerization activation mechanism. However, light curing provides an advantage in working time and other handling characteristics. The dentist has complete control over the working time and is not confined to the rather short working time of the chemically activated systems. This is particularly beneficial when large restorations such as class IV restorations are placed.

Most currently available visible light–cured resins contain the photosensitive initiator camphoroquinone, which absorbs visible light at wavelengths between 450 and 500 nm (blue light) and forms free radicals that activate an amine accelerator.

Visible light activation units are simple and relatively inexpensive, and their output remains fairly constant throughout the life of the bulb. Visible light is capable of polymerizing a reasonable thickness of resin (2 mm). It also will cure the resin through a layer of enamel, a particular advantage in class III restorations. Although protective glasses are recommended to shield the operator's eyes from the glare of the intense blue light, visible-spectrum curing lights do not pose a significant safety risk.

One major disadvantage of light-cured composites must be emphasized. Polymerization will only occur if the resin is exposed to light of sufficient intensity for an adequate length of time. The top surface of a restoration that is nearly in direct contact with the light source will always be cured if the light and resin are serviceable. However, the curing of the portion of the restoration farthest removed from the light is less certain. Normally this portion of the restoration is not accessible for any kind of probing to test its hardness. If the cure is incomplete on the bottom side of the resin compared with the top surface, the physical properties will be reduced and a color shift may occur in time. Likewise, unpolymerized monomer may increase the potential for pulpal irritation. Microleakage is another likely scenario. To ensure maximum polymerization, the end of the light source should be within 1 mm of the surface of the resin. The curing time should be at least 40 seconds, and the depth of resin to be cured should not exceed 2.5 mm. Larger restorations and dark shades of resin require an incremental placement technique. Dual-activated resins are available that combine both light and chemical activation. In situations in which light access to parts of the restoration is problematic, a dual-activated material may be preferred.

When visible light curing systems first were introduced into dentistry, considerable emphasis was placed on the claim that the light output of the visible light curing unit remained constant with use, unlike the previously employed ultraviolet light units. Unfortunately, this statement is only partially true. Numerous factors do influence the light output of a visible light curing unit such as power line variations, aging of the filters, aging of the lamp, damage to the light-conducting pipe or optic fiber, and resin buildup on the end of the light tip. The curing light should be tested regularly to ensure adequate light intensity. Inexpensive meters are available for this purpose and should be used regularly. Many of the newer visible light activation units have built-in meters to verify adequate light intensity. If such a device is not available, a simple usage test should be performed. Place a mass of light-curing resin that is about the thickness of a nickel over a Mylar matrix strip on a sheet of white paper. Cover this mass with a Mylar matrix strip. Holding the curing light within 1 mm of the top surface, cure the resin for the length of time normally used. Remove the matrix strips and probe both the top and bottom resin surfaces with an explorer. There should be no noticeable difference in hardness or scratch resistance. Dark shades of composite resin may require longer curing times or curing of a thinner layer according to the manufacturer's instructions. If a comparable cure on both top and bottom cannot be achieved, the combination of resin and curing light is unsatisfactory for clinical use.

The original visible light activation units employed a quartz-tungsten-halogen lamp (QTH) as a light source. This light is filtered to retain the wavelengths between 400 and 500 nm (blue light). In an effort to accomplish more rapid polymerization of a greater thickness of resin, other light sources have been marketed. These include plasma arc lamps and lasers. These are significantly more expensive than the QTH units, and there is evidence that more rapid polymerization may increase polymerization shrinkage stresses at the tooth-resin interface. A more recent addition to activation units uses blue light-emitting diodes (LED). More than 95% of the electrical energy delivered to a QTH light becomes heat and light of wavelengths longer than 500 nm. LEDs are nearly 100% efficient at generating light over a relatively narrow wavelength band (460 to 480 nm). This makes it possible to construct self- contained, rechargeable, battery-powered activation lights. These lights generate much less heat than QTH units. Unlike QTH lamps, an LED should maintain a constant output throughout its lifetime.

The total power delivered in the 400- to 500-nm band from LED lights was initially much lower than that of QTH units. Recently marketed LED lights have significantly improved power output and the useful light intensity for some LED units exceeds that of the best QTH units. Some evidence exists that suggests that compared with QTH lights, the LED light does not result in as great a depth of cure with the same exposure time for all resin composites. Light-activated resin composites that use

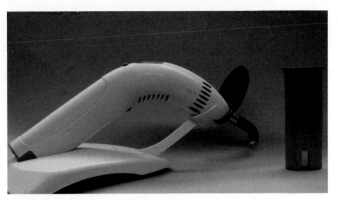

Figure 16-5 Rechargeable battery-powered light-emitting diode–type visible light activation unit.

photoinitiators other than camphoroquinone may not be effectively activated by the narrow bandwidth of light emitted by LED units. The main advantage of the LED lights appears to be convenience, because they do not require a fixed power cord to a base unit (Fig. 16-5).

POSTERIOR COMPOSITE RESTORATION

Composite resins were originally used for anterior or non–stress-bearing locations such as class III, class V, and class IV restorations. Since the introduction of resin composites, however, attempts have been made to use them as alternatives to dental amalgam for class I and II restorations. These attempts with conventional macrofilled composite failed because of unacceptable wear on the occlusal surface. Only in the case of conservative restorations in primary dentition was any success observed. A major goal of composite resin research has been to develop properties adequate to allow their use as an alternative to dental amalgam.

The improved strength, hardness, and modulus of elasticity of some of the newer composite resins, with their low thermal conductivity and superior esthetics, indicate that they may serve as alternatives for amalgam in the restoration of occlusal and proximal surfaces in posterior teeth (class I and class II restorations). Extensive clinical testing has been done to compare the performance of these new resins with that of amalgam. There now exists resin composites, mostly of the small-particle type, with documented clinical wear of less than 20 microns per year over a 5-year period. These materials qualify for full acceptance under the ADA acceptance program for posterior composite resins. In a patient who has a known sensitivity to dental amalgam, use of a composite chosen from the ADA list of accepted materials should be considered. The patient and guardian should be cautioned that the profession does not have long-term data to suggest that such restorations will perform as well as amalgam over long periods (5 to 10 years or longer), and the wear and occlusal relationships of the restorations should be monitored.

The dentist needs to be aware of an additional factor when choosing resin composites for posterior occlusal service. Whereas dental amalgam is one of the least technique-sensitive direct restorative materials and one whose microleakage decreases with time, composite resins are the opposite. The microleakage problem with anterior composite restorations was significantly reduced by the development of the acid-etched enamel bonding technique that is discussed later. Unfortunately, posterior class II restorations often have gingival margins in dentin or cementum. As mentioned, exposure to light of adequate intensity is essential to cure a light-cured composite. This is usually straightforward in an anterior or class V restoration. However, the class II restoration presents a proximal surface with poor, if any, direct access to the curing light. Various solutions have been suggested, including the use of light-conducting interproximal wedges. Careful incremental buildup is probably the best general procedure.

Another problem with posterior restorations is related to the curing shrinkage pattern. Most composite resins exhibit linear shrinkage of 2% or more during curing. The light-cured composite hardens first on the surface immediately adjacent to the curing light tip. As a consequence, the shrinkage is directed toward the curing light and away from the floor of the preparation or the gingival margin. This places the largest stresses from curing shrinkage on the sections of resin that are least well cured and whose bond to tooth structure may be the poorest. Increased microleakage may be the result. Recent developments have resulted in marketing of new resin matrix systems with very low polymerization shrinkage. Laboratory data show that these materials minimize polymerization stresses at the resin interface. Long-term clinical data, however, is not available for these new materials.

Resin composites are also compromised by moisture contamination during placement, and effective isolation of the operative field is essential.

Operative techniques reduce these effects, as described in Chapter 18, but the dentist must understand the basic phenomena to appreciate the importance of the rather detailed and meticulous techniques recommended for placement of posterior composite restorations. Unless the practitioner is able and willing to take the time to place posterior composites properly, the restorations are likely to fail prematurely. The dentist must be compensated for this service in keeping with the time required for placement and should carefully explain to the patient the advantages and disadvantages of the treatment alternatives along with their costs. Placement of bonded resin restorations in posterior permanent teeth of young patients is problematic if those restorations have an expected clinical lifetime of 5 years or less. Each time a bonded restoration is replaced, additional tooth structure will be lost. Repeated replacement of resin composites over the lifetime of a patient is not only costly but may eventually compromise the tooth.

Because the dentist may frequently be faced with a request for placement of resin composites rather than amalgam restorations, knowledge about the safety of these materials is important. A resin monomer often used in restorative resin composites is bis-GMA. This monomer is the reaction product of bisphenol A and a dimethacrylate. Commercial bisphenol A often contains impurities that are chemically similar to synthetic estrogen. Concerns have been raised about the potential for promoting certain types of malignancies. Complete conversion of resin monomers into polymers does not occur in dental restorative materials. Degree of conversion of 60% to 70% is typical. Although bisphenol A is commonly employed in many commercial polymers, certain areas including the State of California have promulgated severe restrictions on its use in food or drink containers and in particular in resin baby bottles. Components used in the light activation of polymerization initiation are very reactive. Traces of these components remain after the resin has hardened. Moreover, enzymes in saliva and in oral tissues may promote degradation of dental resins, which could release reactive species. It is important that the dental consumer, who may be the parent of a pediatric patient, be aware of the risks and benefits of the dental materials used in a proposed treatment plan.

The clinical application of pit and fissure sealants is discussed in a separate chapter; however, some comments about these materials are relevant to the discussion of light-activated resin composites. Clinicians often tend to assume that the film thickness of a sealant is so thin that if the surface is hard, the material is properly polymerized. Cross sections through extracted molar teeth show that thicknesses exceeding 2 mm are common in occlusal pits. Deep developmental grooves may have exposed dentin at the bottom and if the bottom of the sealant is not adequately polymerized, the dentin is in contact with reactive components of the resin. The geometry of the occlusal surface may result in reduced light intensity because of the distance of the tip from the occlusal groves. Use of a large-diameter curing tip further reduces the intensity. Opaque sealants are popular, but the opacity also reduces the light transmitted to the bottom of the sealant. Adequate polymerization is a function of the energy delivered to the entire mass of the resin. Energy is the product of light intensity and the activation time.

RESIN INLAYS

The resin inlay restoration addresses some of the shortcomings of composite resins, particularly the difficulties with placement and light curing discussed previously. The indirect inlay restoration is fabricated in the laboratory on a die poured from an impression of the prepared tooth like a wax pattern for a cast restoration. An alternative for the resin inlay is a direct technique. A separating medium is applied to the prepared tooth, and the resin is condensed and light-cured. It is then removed from the mouth and subjected to additional curing procedures. Either technique allows better access for light-curing the composite, and the finished restoration can be subjected to additional curing under intense light, heat, and pressure or some combination of these. In theory, the properties of the resulting composite are maximized, and the presence of unreacted monomer is minimized. More importantly, the polymerization shrinkage occurs outside the mouth. The finished inlay is cemented in the mouth using a resin cement. The stresses at the tooth-restoration interface should be much lower than in a direct-placement resin restoration.

Although laboratory data support some of the claims made for these inlays, long-term clinical data are not yet available. The resin inlay systems have not achieved wide popularity in the United States, although they are commonly used in Europe. Resin inlay restorations are more time consuming and expensive than direct resin restorations. Their appropriateness as alternatives to dental amalgam or cast restorations needs long-term clinical investigation.

ACID-ETCHING TECHNIQUE

Marginal leakage is probably a more acute problem with resins than it is with any other restorative material. As has been noted, the amalgam restoration tends to counteract the microleakage phenomenon by the formation of corrosion products along the tooth-restoration interface. Other restorative materials may provide a mechanism for resisting secondary caries attributable to microleakage, such as the fluoride released from GIC. With the presently available direct restorative resins, however, there is no inherent resistance to the dangers of marginal penetration of deleterious agents. Thus the resin restoration presents a challenge to the dentist to attain good initial adaptation of the material to the tooth surface and maintain it under oral conditions.

One of the most satisfactory methods for mechanical bonding of resin to enamel is the use of the acid-etch technique. The enamel is etched with a solution of phosphoric acid (usually about 35%) for approximately 15 to 20 seconds. Both liquid and gel etching agents are available; placement is more readily controlled with the gel.

The next critical step in the technique is the use of a water rinse to remove the debris produced during etching. If this debris is not flushed off the enamel surface, the resin will not wet the etched surface. A minimum wash time of 30 seconds is usually recommended. Before the resin is placed, the etched surface must then be dried for at least 15 seconds.

Any film of moisture on this cleaned surface will inhibit resin penetration into the etched enamel. If the surface is accidentally contaminated by saliva, the saliva film cannot be completely removed by washing. Rather, the surface should be re-etched for 10 seconds, washed, and dried.

An etched enamel surface is shown in Fig. 16-6A. The acid cleans the enamel to provide better wetting of the resin and creates pores into which the resin flows to produce "tags" that greatly increase retention (see Fig. 16-6B). The resulting bond should reduce the possibility of marginal stain, which is the invariable result of microleakage. In addition to providing a seal between the resin and tooth, the acid-etch technique results in mechanical retention. Resin bond strengths to etched enamel range from 16 to 22 MPa.

BONDING AGENTS

As an adjunct to the acid-etch technique, manufacturers formerly supplied enamel-bonding agents. The bonding agent consisted of bis-GMA resin matrix material diluted with a low-viscosity methacrylate monomer. After acid etching of the enamel, the bonding agent was applied. The composite resin was then immediately inserted, and it in turn bonded to the intermediate layer of resin-bonding agent. The resulting bond to tooth structure was strictly mechanical.

The success of the acid-etch, enamel-bond technique led to attempts to do the same for bonding to dentin. Early efforts to etch dentin and apply enamel-bonding agents were not successful. The structure of dentin is far more complex, and it has a lower concentration of inorganic material; because of its microstructural organization, the regular etch patterns seen with enamel are not produced. Due to the organic component of dentin and to the permeability that results from the dentinal tubules, the dentin surface has low surface energy and is constantly wet. This presents the ultimate challenge for adhesion. For the past 20 years, research has focused on the development of agents that will bond adhesively to dentin. This has led to the introduction of dentin-bonding agents, which are either chemically activated or light cured. They are applied to the dentin before placement of the composite.

The chemistry of the different products is complex and varied. Some rely on mechanical retention whereas the claim is that others form chemical bonds to the organic or inorganic portions of the dentin. Such claims are not generally supported by direct evidence of chemical bonding. Instead, bond strengths to dentin are measured and reported. These vary from a few megapascals to values comparable to those for etched enamel. Often the bond strengths measured in vitro decrease markedly with time, exposure to water, and thermocycling.

Probably no area of dental materials has seen as much activity as that of dentin bonding in the past 15 years. Many of the products currently marketed have been available for less than 2 years, and their development has been a continuing process. By the time short-term clinical data are available, these products often have been replaced by a new generation of bonding systems.

The dentin-bonding systems that first exhibited good bond strengths involved removal of the dentin smear layer and decalcification of the outer layer of intact dentin with an acid. A hydrophilic primer component carried by a volatile solvent that displaces water was then applied. Resin components in the primer penetrate the decalcified dentin and react with and modify the remaining dentin structure, which results in creation of a so-called hybrid layer between the intact dentin and the resin adhesive. High in vitro bond strengths are generally reported for these systems along with good short-term clinical performance. Unlike with enamel bonding, it is important that the etched dentin surface not be desiccated before application of the primer when systems with hydrophilic primers are used. Current advances have focused on the development of delivery systems that simplify the steps involved in using dentin-bonding systems. Acidic primers that are self-etching have been introduced. These simultaneously demineralize and penetrate the smear layer and underlying dentin. Other systems combine the primer and the resin adhesive into one component.

The most recently introduced systems mix together the acidic primer and resin adhesive before they are placed on the tooth surface. Even though these newer systems use fewer separate components, their application

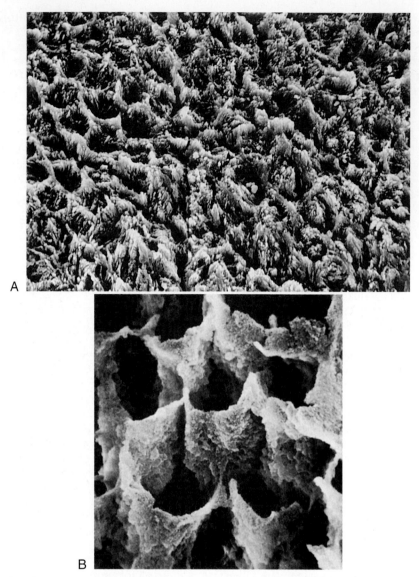

Figure 16-6 Effects of acid etching. **A,** Scanning electron micrograph of enamel surface etched with phosphoric acid. **B,** Scanning electron micrograph of resin tags formed by penetration of resin into etched enamel surface (×5000). (**A** and **B** from Anusavice KJ. Phillips' Science of Dental Materials, 11th ed. St. Louis, WB Saunders, 2003; courtesy of K-J Söderholm.)

still requires that several steps be performed with great attention to detail. Use of these materials remains extremely technique sensitive.

Little if any convincing evidence exists that any of the dentin-bonding agents currently marketed form significant chemical bonds to dentin. More likely the bonding mechanism is micromechanical. The status of these agents remains controversial, particularly with regard to their long-term stability in the oral cavity. Until these matters are resolved, one should not deviate too far from accepted restorative procedures. One should assume that the dentin adhesive will not eliminate the need for the use of traditional methods for retention of the resin restoration, such as acid etching of the enamel and retentive cavity preparations in dentin or cementum.

Recent laboratory data have shown incompatibility between some of the newer dental bonding systems and restorative resins or resin cements that are activated by chemical or dual means. Many of the resins used for crown buildup as core materials fall into these categories. It appears that the use of acidic primers may interfere with the chemical activation of these resin materials unless a separate resin adhesive is placed over the primer and light activated before the core material or cement is placed.

Most of the bonding agents currently marketed are sold as universal bonding agents to be used with both dentin and enamel. Bond strengths reported for etched enamel usually equal those for the original enamel-bonding agents that have largely disappeared. Regardless of whether an auxiliary resin-bonding agent is used, adequate etching of the enamel is an important step in securing mechanical bonding of any restorative resin to enamel. Some of the systems that use self-etching primers or acids other than phosphoric acid do not routinely yield enamel-bond strengths as high as expected with conventional acid etching. Questions exist about the effectiveness of dental bonding systems employing self-etching primers when these are used in place of phosphoric acid treatment for bonding orthodontic appliances and pit and fissure sealing. Conventional phosphoric acid etchants can be used to ensure etching of the enamel margins of a cavity preparation.

In the context of dental bonding, one should not ignore the polyacrylic acid systems. GIC has been recommended for use as a dentin-bonding agent in the so-called sandwich technique. Fast-setting GICs are available for use as cavity-lining materials (type III GIC and light-cured GIC). The enamel is not covered with the GIC but rather acid etched in the conventional manner. Then a resin-bonding agent is applied and a composite resin placed. The ionomer bonds adhesively to the tooth whereas the bonding agent bonds mechanically to the ionomer and the enamel. This adds yet another dimension to dentin-bonding technology, particularly for the class II restoration.

Dental resins are no more or less irritating to the pulp than are several other commonly used restorative materials. Whenever the cavity preparation is deep, the same precautions should be taken with resins as with other restorative materials.

SUGGESTED READINGS

General

Anusavice KJ. *Phillips' science of dental materials,* ed 11, Philadelphia, 2003, WB Saunders.

Baum L, Phillips RW, Lund MR: *Textbook of operative dentistry,* ed 3, Philadelphia, 1995, WB Saunders.

Medical devices; dental device classification; final rule and withdrawal of proposed rules, Federal Register, p. 30082, Aug 12, 1987.

O'Brien WJ. *Dental materials and their selection,* ed 3, Chicago, 2002, Quintessence Publishing.

Phillips RW: Changing trends of dental restorative materials, *Dent Clin North Am* 33:285-291, 1989.

Adhesion

Brauer GM: Adhesion and adhesives. In von Fraunhofer J, editor: *Scientific aspects of dental materials,* London, 1975, Butterworths.

Buonocore MG. *The use of adhesives in dentistry,* Springfield, Ill, 1975, Charles C. Thomas.

Garcia-Godoy F, Donly KJ. Dentin/enamel adhesives in pediatric dentistry, *Pediatr Dent* 24:462-464, 2002.

Gerdolle DA, Mortier E, Droz D. Microleakage and polymerization shrinkage of various polymer restorative materials, *J Dent Child* 75:125-133, 2008.

Mitra SB. Adhesion to dentin and physical properties of a light cured glass ionomer liner/base, *J Dent Res* 70:72-74, 1991.

Wilson AD. Adhesion of glass ionomer cements. In Allen KW, editor: Aspects of adhesion, London, 1975, Transcriptor Books.

Amalgam

Anusavice KJ. Quality evaluation of dental restorations: Criteria for placement and replacement, Chicago, 1989, Quintessence Publishing.

Browning WD, Johnson WW, Gregory PN. Clinical performance of bonded amalgam restorations at 42 months, *J Am Dent Assoc* 131:607-611, 2000.

Klausner LH, Green TG, Charbeneau GT. Placement and replacement of amalgam restorations: A challenge for the profession, *Oper Dent* 12:105-112, 1987.

Kulapongs KJ, Moore BK, Cochran MA. Microleakage of resin-lined amalgams using confocal microscopy and fluorescent markers, *J Dent Res* 77:243, special issue A, abst 1100, 1998.

Letzel H et al. A controlled clinical study of amalgam restorations: Survival, failures, and causes of failure, *Dent Mater* 5:115-121, 1989.

Mahler DB et al. One-year clinical evaluation of bonded amalgam restorations, *J Am Dent Assoc* 127:345-349, 1996.

Marshall GW, Marshall SJ, Letzel H. Mercury content of amalgam restorations, *Gen Dent* 37:473-477, 1989.

Mjor IA. Problems and benefits associated with restorative materials: Side-effects and long-term costs, *Adv Dent Res* 6:7-16, 1992.

Osborne JW, Summitt JB, Roberts HW. The use of dental amalgam in pediatric dentistry: Review of the literature, *Pediatr Dent* 24:439-447, 2002.

Rogers KD. Status of scrap (recyclable) dental amalgams as environmental health hazards or toxic substances, *J Am Dent Assoc* 119:159-166, 1989.

Sutow EJ, Jones DW, Hall GC: Correlation of dental amalgam crevice corrosion with clinical ratings, *J Dent Res* 68:82-88, 1989.

Tangsgoolwatana J et al. Microleakage evaluation of bonded amalgam restorations: Confocal microscopy versus radioisotope, *Quintessence Int* 28:467-477, 1997.

Cements

Berg JH. Glass ionomer cements, *Pediatr Dent* 24:430-438, 2002.

Croll TP. Light-hardened luting cement for orthodontic bands and appliances, *Pediatr Dent* 21:121-123, 1999.

Croll TP, Killian C. Glass ionomer resin restoration of primary molar with adjacent class II carious lesions, *Quintessence Int* 24: 723-727, 1993.

Croll TP et al. Clinical performance of resin-modified glass ionomer cement restorations in primary teeth. A retrospective evaluation, *J Am Dent Assoc* 132:1110-1116, 2001.

Hunt PR, editor. Glass ionomers: The next generation. A summary of the current situation, *J Esthet Dent* 6:192-194, 1994.

McLean JW. Limitations of posterior composite resins and extending their use with glass ionomer cements, *Quintessence Int* 18:517-529, 1987.

Mount GJ. *An atlas of glass ionomer cements: A clinician's guide,* ed 3, London, 2002, Martin Dunitz.

Phillips RW. Glass ionomers: Impact on restorative dentistry, *J Am Dent Assoc* 120:19 (theme issue, guest editor), 1990.

Phillips RW et al. In vivo disintegration of luting agents, *J Am Dent Assoc* 114:489-492, 1987.

Swartz ML, Phillips RW, Clark HE. Long-term F release from glass ionomer cements, *J Dent Res* 63:158-160, 1984.

Smith DC, Norman RD, Swartz ML. Dental cements: Current status and future prospects. In Reese JA, Valega TM, editors: *Restorative dental materials: an overview,* London, 1985, Quintessence Publishing.

Smith DC, Ruse ND. Acidity of glass ionomer cements during setting and its relation to pulp sensitivity, *J Am Dent Assoc* 112:654-657, 1986.

Taleghani M, Leinfelder KF. Evaluation of a new glass ionomer cement with silver as a core buildup under a cast restoration, *Quintessence Int* 19:19-24, 1988.

Wilson AD, McLean JW. *Glass-ionomer cements,* Chicago, 1988, Quintessence Publishing.

Composites

Albers H. Tooth colored restoratives: principles and techniques, ed 9, Hamilton, Ont, 2002, BC Decker.

Baum L, Phillips RW, Lund MR. *Textbook of operative dentistry,* ed 3, Philadelphia, 1995, WB Saunders.

Donly KJ, Garcia-Godoy F. The use of resin-based composite in children, *Pediatr Dent* 24:480-488, 2002.

Lambrechts P, Braem M, Vanherle G. Evaluation of clinical performance for posterior composite resins and dentin adhesives, *Oper Dent* 12:53-78, 1987.

Lutz F, Phillips RW. A classification and evaluation of composite resin systems, *J Prosthet Dent* 50:480-488, 1983.

Moore BK et al, *Oper Dent* 33:408-12, 2008.

Platt JA, Clark H, Moore BK. Curing of pit and fissure sealants using Light Emittimg Diode curing units. *Oper Dent* 30:764-71, 2005.

Roulet JF. The problems associated with substituting composite resins for amalgam: a status report on posterior composites, *J Dent* 16:101-113, 1988.

Bonding agents

Asmussen E, Munksgaard EC. Bonding of restorative resins to dentine: status of dentine adhesives and impact on cavity design and filling techniques, *Int Dent J* 38:97-104, 1988.

Bowen RL et al. Adhesive bonding of composites, *J Am Coll Dent* 56(2):10-13, 1989.

Douglas WH. Clinical status of dentine bonding agents, *J Dent* 17:209-215, 1989.

Gwinnett AJ. Quantitative contribution of resin infiltration/hybridization to dentin bonding, *Am J Dent* 6:7-9, 1993.

Kanca J 3rd. Wet bonding: effect of drying time and distance, *Am J Dent* 9:273-276, 1996.

Suh B. One-step: the fifth generation dentin adhesive. Proceedings of a symposium on the fifth generation of dentin adhesives, sec 6:1-6, 1995.

Tsai YH et al. Comparative study: bond strength and microleakage with dentin bond systems, *Oper Dent* 15:53-60, 1990.

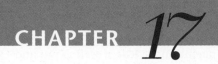
Pit and Fissure Sealants and Preventive Resin Restorations

▲ **Brian J. Sanders, Robert J. Feigal,** and **David R. Avery**

CHAPTER OUTLINE

*I*n 1955, Buonocore described the technique of acid etching as a simple method of increasing the adhesion of self-curing methyl methacrylate resin materials to dental enamel.[1] He used 85% phosphoric acid to etch enamel for 30 seconds. This produces a roughened surface at a microscopic level, which allows mechanical bonding of low-viscosity resin materials.

The first materials used experimentally as sealants were based on cyanoacrylates but were not marketed. By 1965, Bowen had developed the bis-GMA resin, which is the chemical reaction product of bisphenol A and glycidyl methacrylate.[2] This is the base resin to most of the current commercial sealants. Urethane dimethacrylate and other dimethacrylates are alternative resins used in sealant materials.

For the chemically cured sealants, a tertiary amine (activator) in one component is mixed with another component containing benzoyl peroxide, and their reaction produces free radicals, which initiates polymerization of the sealant material.

The other sealant materials are activated by an external energy source. The early light-activated sealants were polymerized by the action of ultraviolet rays (which are no longer used) on a benzoin methyl ether or higher-alkyl benzoin ethers to activate the peroxide curing system. The visible light–curing sealants have diketones and aromatic ketones, which are sensitive to visible light in the wavelength region of 470 nm (blue region). Some sealants contain filler, usually silicon dioxide microfill or even quartz.

Sealant materials may be transparent or opaque. Opaque materials are available in tooth color or white. Transparent sealants are clear, pink, or amber. The clear and tooth-colored sealants are esthetic but are difficult to detect at recall examinations. Recent advances in sealant technology include light-activated coloring agents that allow for color change during and/or after polymerization. These compositional changes do not affect the sealant, but only offer some arguable benefit in the recognition of sealed surfaces.

The cariostatic properties of sealants are attributed to the physical obstruction of the pits and grooves. This prevents colonization of the pits and fissures with new bacteria and also prevents the penetration of fermentable carbohydrates to any bacteria remaining in the pits and fissures, so that the remaining bacteria cannot produce acid in cariogenic concentration.

CLINICAL TRIALS

Many clinical studies have reported on the success of pit and fissure sealants with respect to caries reduction. As the longevity of the sealant increases, the retention rate becomes a determinant of its effectiveness as a caries-preventive measure.

In 1983, a National Institutes of Health Consensus Panel considered the available information on pit and fissure sealants and concluded that "the placement of sealants is a highly effective means of preventing pit and fissure caries.... Expanding the use of sealants would substantially reduce the occurrence of dental caries in the population beyond that already achieved by fluorides and other preventive resources."[3]

In 1991, Simonsen reported on a random sample of participants in a sealant study recalled after 15 years.[4] He reported that, in the group with sealant, 69% of the surfaces were sound 15 years after a single sealant application, whereas 31% were carious or restored. In the group without sealant, matched by age, gender, and residence, 17% of the surfaces were sound, whereas 83% were carious or restored. He also estimated that a pit and fissure surface on a permanent first molar is 7.5 times more likely to be carious or restored after 15 years if it is not sealed with a single application of pit and fissure sealant.

The use of glass ionomer as a sealant material has the advantage of continuous fluoride release, and its preventive effect may continue with the visible loss of the material. Glass ionomer may be useful as a sealant material in deeply fissured primary molars that are difficult to isolate due to the child's precooperative behavior and in partially erupted permanent molars that the clinician believes are at risk for developing decay. In such cases, glass ionomer materials must be considered a provisional sealant to be reevaluated and probably replaced with resin-based sealants when better isolation is possible. Because questions exist regarding the strength and retention of glass ionomer, further long-term research is necessary before it is recommended as a routine pit and fissure sealant material.

A 1996 survey of Indiana dentists[5] found that 91% of them were placing sealants on permanent teeth, whereas in 1985 a similar study[6] had found that only 73.5% were placing sealants on permanent teeth. This increased use of sealants may be related to increased practitioner comfort with the materials, because a direct correlation was found between sealant use and year of graduation from dental school. The increase may also be related to a decreased concern over the possibility of caries developing under the sealant.

Several studies have reported decreased viable bacterial counts in occlusal fissures that have been sealed. Handleman and colleagues placed an ultraviolet-radiation–polymerized sealant on pits and fissures of teeth with incipient caries.[7] They reported a 2000-fold decrease in the number of cultivable microorganisms in the carious dentin samples of the sealed teeth compared with unsealed control teeth at the end of 2 years.

Going and colleagues obtained bacteriologic samples from teeth that had been sealed with an ultraviolet-radiation–polymerized sealant for 5 years.[8] They found an apparent 89% reversal from a caries-active to a caries-free state in the sealed teeth.

Jeronimus and associates placed three different pit and fissure sealants on molars with incipient, moderate, and deep carious lesions.[9] Samples of carious dentin were removed immediately after and 2, 3, and 4 weeks after placement of the sealants and bacteriologic cultures were made. They reported usually positive culture results in teeth where the sealant was lost. Although their short-term study indicated that incipient carious lesions may not be of prime concern when sealants are applied, they cautioned against the use of sealants over deeper lesions because of the potential for advancement of caries when sealants over these lesions are lost. One must keep in mind that their deep-lesion group consisted of teeth with caries that had advanced pulpally greater than half the distance from the dentinoenamel junction.

Studies have shown definitively that deficient sealants are not effective in caries prevention and that loss of sealants leads to immediate risk of caries attack from undercover surfaces. Sealants require regular maintenance and repair or replacement to assure success in caries prevention over the long term.

Going declared that, given the results of many well-documented studies, practitioners' fear of sealing pits and fissures with incipient caries is not warranted.[10] He pointed out that sufficient studies of scientific merit reported negative or low bacterial concentrations after sealant had been in place for several years.

Wendt and Koch annually followed 758 sealed occlusal surfaces in first permanent molars for 1 to 10 years.[11] At the end of their study, evaluation of the surfaces that had been sealed 10 years previously revealed that only 6% showed caries or restorations. Romcke and associates annually monitored 8340 sealants placed on high-risk (for caries) first permanent molars during a 10-year period.[12] Maintenance resealing was performed as indicated during the annual evaluations. One year after the sealants were placed, 6% required resealing; thereafter 2% to 4% required resealing annually. After 8 to 10 years, 85% of the sealed surfaces remained caries free.

Retrospective studies based on billing data from large third-party databases reveal that sealant use is still surprisingly low, even in populations for which sealants are a covered benefit.[13,14] In addition, these studies show that the effectiveness of sealants in preventing the need for future restorative care on the sealed surfaces declines after the first 3 years following sealant treatment. These data argue again for the importance of vigilant recall and upkeep of sealants after placement.

Another concern is the placement of sealants immediately after topical fluoride application. Clinical and in vitro studies have shown that topical fluoride does not interfere with the bonding between sealant and enamel.[15,16]

RATIONALE FOR USE OF SEALANTS

The 2008, Evidence Based Clinical Recommendations for the Use of Pit and Fissure Sealants report by the American Dental Association on Scientific Affairs concluded that sealants are effective in caries prevention and can prevent the progression of early noncavitated carious lesions.[17]

The American Academy of Pediatric Dentistry's Pediatric Restorative Dentistry Consensus Conference[18] confirmed support for sealant use and published these recommendations:

1. Bonded resin sealants, placed by appropriately trained dental personnel, are safe, effective, and underused in preventing pit and fissure caries on at-risk surfaces. Effectiveness is increased with good technique and appropriate follow-up and resealing as necessary.
2. Sealant benefit is increased by placement on surfaces judged to be at high risk or surfaces that already exhibit incipient carious lesions. Placing sealant over minimal-enamel caries has been shown to be effective at inhibiting lesion progression. As with all dental treatment, appropriate follow-up care is recommended.
3. The best evaluation of risk is made by an experienced clinician using indicators of tooth morphology, clinical diagnostics, past caries history, past fluoride history, and present oral hygiene.
4. Caries risk, and therefore potential sealant benefit, may exist in any tooth with a pit or fissure, at any age,

including primary teeth of children and permanent teeth of children and adults.

5. Sealant placement methods should include careful cleaning of the pits and fissures without removal of any appreciable enamel. Some circumstances may indicate use of a minimal-enameloplasty technique.

6. Placement of a low-viscosity, hydrophilic material-bonding layer as part of or under the actual sealant has been shown to enhance the long-term retention and effectiveness.

7. Glass ionomer materials have been shown to be ineffective as pit and fissure sealants but can be used as transitional sealants.

8. The profession must be alert to new preventive methods effective against pit and fissure caries. These may include changes in dental materials or technology.

SELECTION OF TEETH FOR SEALING

To gain the greatest benefit, the clinician should determine the caries risk; thus, the term risk-based sealant treatment has come into use. In risk-based sealant treatment, the practitioner takes into account prior caries experience, fluoride history, oral hygiene, and fissure anatomy in determining when sealant should be applied.

Good professional judgment should be used in the selection of teeth and patients. The use of pit and fissure sealants is contraindicated when rampant caries or interproximal lesions are present. Occlusal surfaces that are already carious with involvement of dentin require restoration.

All caries-susceptible surfaces should be carefully evaluated, because caries is unlikely in well-coalesced pits and fissures. In this case, sealants might be unnecessary or, at least, not cost effective. Finally, although sealant application is relatively simple, the meticulous technique requires patient cooperation and should be postponed for uncooperative patients until the procedures can be properly executed.

SEALANT TECHNIQUE

After selection, the tooth is washed and dried and the deep pits and fissures are reevaluated (Fig. 17-1A). If caries is present, restoration or a combination of restoration and sealing may be indicated (see later).

Marking centric stops with articulating paper provides information so that excess sealant does not interfere with the occlusion. This is not necessary when the tooth has just erupted but is helpful in a well-established occlusion.

CLEANING

Adequate retention of the sealant requires that the pit and fissures be clean and free of excess moisture (see Fig. 17-1B, C). Acid etching completely removes the enamel pellicle, and a dental prophylaxis (even with a dental explorer) does not increase the retention of sealants. From a practical standpoint, in cases of poor oral hygiene, fissure cleansing with a rotating dry bristle brush may be beneficial.

Pope and colleagues found that the use of a quarter round bur produced the greatest penetration of the sealant into etched enamel in laboratory studies.[19] The use of an aluminum oxide air abrasion system allows sealant penetration greater than that achievable by use of pumice or a dry bristle brush alone. It is not known if the increased depth of sealant penetration will result in greater sealant retention. When pumice or aluminum oxide is used, particulate matter is left in the deep recesses of the pits, the impact of which has not been determined.

Hatibovic-Kofman and colleagues measured the microleakage of sealants placed in three groups of extracted teeth.[20] The teeth received conventional (etch), quarter round bur, or air abrasion surface preparation. Teeth prepared with the bur exhibited the least microleakage. The amount of microleakage in the conventional and air abrasion groups was about equal. No clinical studies exist to substantiate the value of using a bur to clean fissure surfaces before sealant placement.

The routine procedure of fissure eradication is probably not necessary. In fact, inappropriate or aggressive use of fissure opening or enameloplasty often removes the last of the enamel overlying dentin at the bottoms of fissures, which leaves the tooth more susceptible to future caries in case of sealant loss. Good sealant methodology and proper sealant volume is probably more beneficial than enameloplasty.

ISOLATION

The tooth (or quadrant of teeth) to be sealed is first isolated. Rubber dam isolation is ideal but may not be feasible in certain circumstances. Cotton rolls, absorbent shields, and high-volume evacuation with compressed air may also be used effectively.

Eidelman and associates reported comparable retention results with the use of rubber dam and the use of cotton rolls for the isolation of teeth to be sealed.[21] Matis reported 96% retention of sealants with rubber dam isolation and 91% retention with cotton roll isolation at 12 months in young adults.[22] These values are not statistically different, however, which indicates that retention rates are probably not related to isolation technique, as long as the insertion technique is sound.

ETCHING

Microporosities in the enamel surface are created by the acid-etching technique. This permits a low-viscosity resin to be applied that penetrates the roughened surface and produces a mechanical lock of resin tags when cured.

Various phosphoric acid solutions have been evaluated for the etching procedure. Zidan and Hill tested the amount of surface loss of enamel after 60 seconds of etching with different phosphoric acid concentrations ranging from 0.5% to 80%.[23] They reported that the maximum loss of enamel was produced by the 35% concentrations, whereas the bond strengths were not significantly different after etching with 2%, 5%, and 35% concentrations. Generally, 30% to 50% acid solutions or gels are recommended.

The etchant in solution should be placed on the enamel with either a brush, small sponge, cotton pellet,

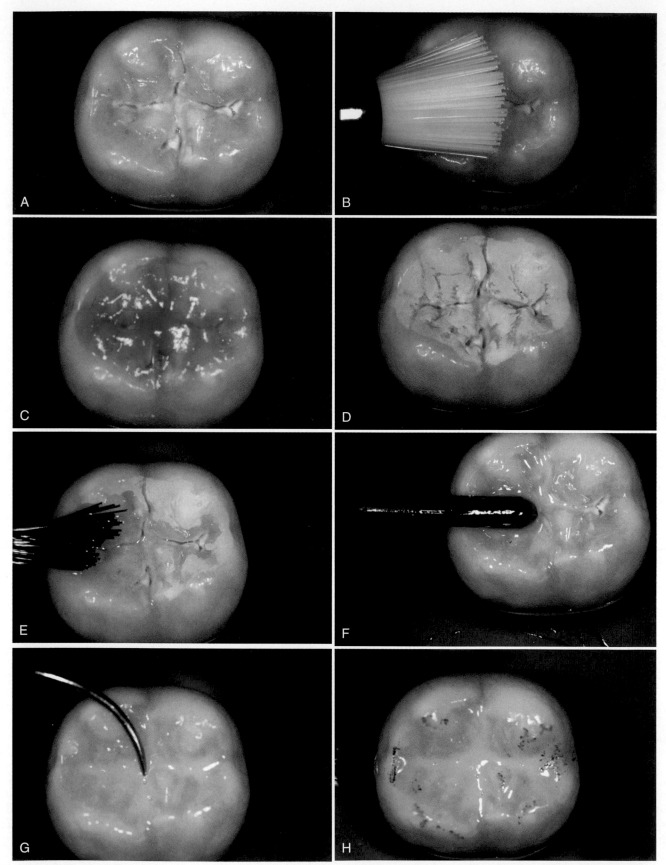

Figure 17-1. A, An occlusal view of a molar with susceptible pits and fissures. **B,** The tooth is cleaned with a rotary brush. **C,** The tooth is etched. **D,** The tooth appears frosty after etching, washing, and drying. **E,** The bonding agent is placed on the tooth. **F,** The sealant is applied to the tooth. **G,** The sealant is checked for polymerization voids and excess. **H,** The occlusion is adjusted as necessary.

or applicator provided by the manufacturer. The etchant should be placed widely across the surface to be sealed so that there is no chance that resin placement and polymerization will occur over an unetched enamel area. If a solution is used, one should gently agitate and replenish it, making an effort to avoid rubbing and breaking the enamel rods.

Occasionally a viscous gel etchant may show a "skipping" effect, which occurs when the etchant does not completely and uniformly wet the entire enamel surface, and unetched areas are evident after washing and drying. If this occurs, retching is necessary.

Generally, a 20-second etching time is recommended. Enamel rich with fluorhydroxyapatite may be resistant to etching and may need to be exposed for longer periods. Primary teeth may also sometimes be resistant to etching and may require a longer etching time. Redford and colleagues reported no increase in bond strength with 120-second etching on primary teeth compared with 15-, 30-, or 60-second etching times.[24] Their in vitro study showed that the etch depth increased between 60 and 120 seconds, but there was no corresponding increase in bond strength.

Some advocate preparing enamel for sealant application with an aluminum oxide air abrasion system or a laser system approved for hard-tissue procedures. To date, studies indicate that additional acid etching is needed after each of these techniques to allow adequate resin bonding to enamel.

WASHING

Most manufacturers' instructions advocate a thorough washing and drying of the etched tooth surface but do not specify a time interval. Phillips advocated a 40-second washing time.[25] Norling has advocated 20 seconds.[26]

The etched enamel is dried using a compressed air stream that is free of oil contaminants. The dry etched enamel should exhibit the characteristic frosty appearance (see Fig. 17-1D).

Feigal and colleagues found that the use of a dentin-bonding agent increased sealant retention in teeth even when salivary contamination occurred.[27] Choi and colleagues have reported corresponding findings in vitro on moisture-contaminated bovine enamel.[28] In a later extensive review article, Feigal recommended routine placement of bonding agents before all sealant applications.[29]

Although the recommendation is still to avoid moisture contamination whenever possible during sealant application, the use of a dentin-bonding agent as part of the technique appears to be warranted (see Fig. 17-1E). Furthermore, the use of a dentin-bonding agent is definitely recommended in clinical situations that do not lend themselves to strict isolation, for example, when newly erupted teeth are sealed or when patient cooperation is not ideal. The use of a dentin-bonding agent is also advantageous on the buccal surfaces of molars, which traditionally have shown a lower retention rate than the occlusal surfaces of teeth.[30] When used, the bonding agent must be thoroughly air-dried across the surface to be sealed to avoid a thick layer of adhesive residue.

APPLICATION OF SEALANT

Chemically Cured Sealant
The manufacturer's instructions should be followed. Precise mixing without vigorous agitation can help prevent the formation of air bubbles.

The addition of the catalyst to the base immediately begins the polymerization of the material, and this should be kept in mind so that no time is lost in carrying the material to the etched and dried tooth. Working time is limited with a chemically cured sealant.

Visible Light–Cured Sealant
The curing of a light-polymerized sealant is not completed without the exposure of the material to the curing light, but the operating light and ambient light can also affect the material over a period of time, and so material should be dispensed only when it is time to place it on the tooth. The working time is longer than with chemically cured sealant. The method of placement varies with the different applicators provided by the manufacturers. The sealant is applied to the prepared surface in moderation and then gently teased with a brush or probe into the pits and grooves (see Fig. 17-1F, G). With careful application, incorporation of air bubbles is avoided. Care should also be taken to avoid applying large amounts of the sealant material.

If a light-curing material is used, the intensity of the light should be considered. If a large surface area requires polymerization, place the light directly over each area of the occlusal surface for the recommended time.

With light-cured sealants there is less chance of incorporating air bubbles, because no mixing of materials is required. After the material has been cured and while the treated teeth are still isolated, the unpolymerized surface layer should be removed by washing and drying the surface to avoid an unpleasant taste.

CHECK OF OCCLUSAL INTERFERENCES

Articulating paper should be used to check for occlusal interferences and the occlusion adjusted if necessary (see Fig. 17-1H). All centric stops should be on enamel.

If a filled sealant has been used, it is essential to adjust the occlusion before the patient is dismissed.

Other excess sealant that may have flowed over the marginal ridge or toward the cervical area should also be removed. If the tooth is isolated with a rubber dam, the excess should be removed before detaching the rubber dam. A small round bur at slow speed will remove the excess effectively. If etchant has been well localized, excess sealant may be removed with a sharp instrument from unetched tooth enamel without removing sealant from the etched groove areas.

REEVALUATION

It is important to recognize that sealed teeth should be observed clinically at periodic recall visits to determine the effectiveness of the sealant. Periodic recall and reapplication of sealants is necessary, because it is estimated that between 5% and 10% of sealants need to be repaired or replaced yearly. If a sealant is partially or completely lost, any discolored or defective old sealant should be removed and the tooth reevaluated. A new sealant can be applied using the method previously described.

PREVENTIVE RESIN RESTORATION (SEALED COMPOSITE RESIN RESTORATION)

The preventive resin restoration is an alternative procedure for restoring young permanent teeth that require only minimal tooth preparation for caries removal but also have adjacent susceptible fissures.

Simonsen and Stallard described the technique of removing only the carious tooth structure in small class I cavities.[31] A resin restoration was then placed, and the adjacent pits and fissures were sealed at the same time.

Henderson and Setcos described the sequence of the preventive resin restoration that is particularly applicable for young patients with recently erupted teeth and minimally carious pits and fissures.[32] They pointed out that this preparation requires a meticulous technique that involves more time than the traditional occlusal amalgam restoration. This type of restoration was advocated for carefully selected non–stress-bearing areas to minimize anatomic wear.

Occlusal surfaces often have small carious pits. For minimal caries, restorations are not likely to be subjected to substantial stresses that might lead to wear of resin materials. Figure 17-2 shows diagrams illustrating the principles of the sealant-composite combination. In this case a small carious lesion has penetrated to the dentin. In general, bite-wing radiographs should indicate no interproximal caries.

A clinical series showing the sequence for this conservative preparation and restoration is portrayed in Figure 17-3. Caries is identified by careful visual examination of a dry occlusal tooth surface using a sharp explorer, a mirror, and a light (see Fig. 17-3A). Articulating paper marks on the tooth would indicate the points of occlusal contact.

The tooth is anesthetized if necessary, isolated, and reexamined to determine the extent of the caries process. A No. 329 bur, aluminum oxide air abrasion, or a laser system approved for hard tissue can be used to gain access to the depth of the lesion and to complete caries removal (see Fig. 17-3B). The preparation, which should not extend to the occlusal contact marks, is washed, dried, and examined.

The cavity and the enamel beside the susceptible grooves are etched (see Fig. 17-3C). A gel or liquid form of 37% phosphoric acid is commonly used for 20 seconds. Surface preparation with aluminum oxide air abrasion or a laser system approved for hard tissue may not substitute for acid etching. If these cleaning methods are used, etchant must still be applied to provide adequate resin-bonding enamel. The lingual groove of maxillary molars and the buccal groove of mandibular molars are also commonly etched and sealed. The tooth is thoroughly washed for approximately 30 to 40 seconds and completely dried.

A thin layer of bonding agent is applied to the cavity (see Fig. 17-3D). A stream of air must be used to thin the

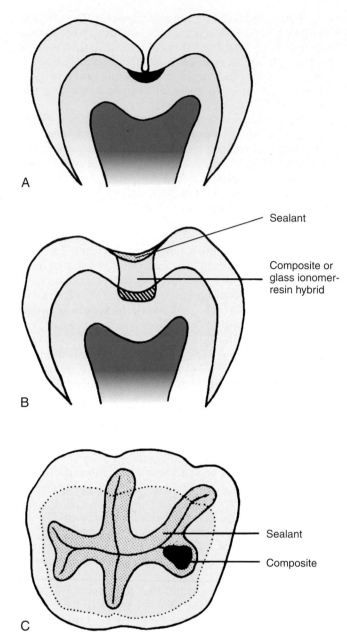

Figure 17-2. Diagrams illustrating the sealed composite resin restoration. **A,** A cross section showing caries extending to the dentin. **B,** A cross section through a preparation with a glass ionomer or composite restoration and a sealant. **C,** An occlusal view of the outline of a small restoration where a pit and fissure sealant provides the extension-for-prevention principle of cavity preparation.

bonding agent and to prevent pooling of bonding agent in the cavity.

The cavities are filled with a light-curing composite or resin-modified glass ionomer, which may be cured at this time (see Fig. 17-3E). A light-curing sealant is placed over the remaining susceptible areas and brushed into the pits and grooves (see Fig. 17-3F). The materials are polymerized with visible light in accordance with the manufacturer's instructions.

The rubber dam is removed, and the occlusal contacts are checked. A small-particle diamond rotary instrument

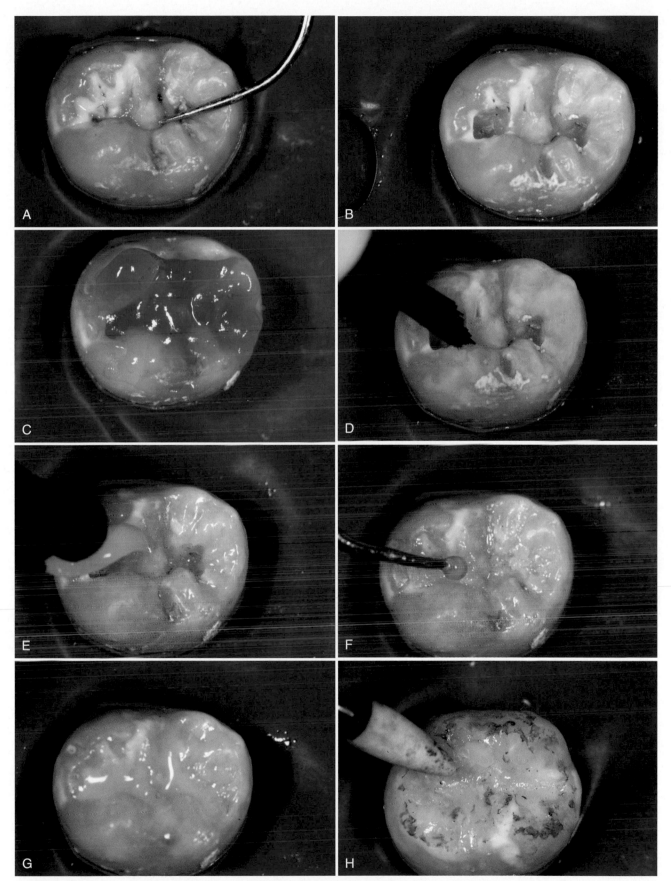

Figure 17-3. A, An occlusal caries identified with susceptible pits and grooves. **B,** Caries is removed into dentin. **C,** The tooth is etched. **D,** The bonding agent is placed. **E,** Composite resin is placed. **F,** Sealant is placed over resin. **G,** Polymerized preventive resin restoration. **H,** The occlusion is adjusted.

can be used to remove excess sealant and ensure centric stops on enamel (see Fig. 17-3G, H).

A meticulous technique is used in the selection, preparation, and restoration of small pit and fissure caries using the preventive resin restoration.

The bonded restoration with sealant overlay has proven long-term effectiveness. The restorations have equivalent or better success than amalgam restorations. Once again, however, success is dependent upon keeping the sealant intact.

The use of flowable composite systems is also gaining in popularity because they are easy to apply and because evidence shows that less microleakage occurs with these systems than when teeth are restored with condensable composite resins, such as sealant materials that have slightly more filler than filled sealants. Therefore the practical results of sealing with a flowable or a filled sealant should not differ.

There is no single perfect conservative restoration. Each dentist must decide, on an individual basis, the appropriate type of procedure. The restoration described can be very effective in carefully selected cases.

Walker and associates reported on preventive resin restorations placed in patients 6 to 18 years of age and observed for up to 6.5 years.[33] Of the 5185 restorations, 83% did not require further intervention. Those requiring intervention included 37% that needed sealant alone and 21% that required treatment because of the development of an interproximal lesion. Houpt and associates reported complete retention of 54% of their preventive resin restorations, partial loss of sealant in 25%, and complete loss of sealant in 20% after 9 years.[34] Caries occurred in 25% of the teeth that had sealant loss, and 88% of the restored surfaces remained caries-free 9 years after treatment. These researchers concluded that preventive restorations produce excellent long-term results. Conservative cavity preparation with sealing for prevention is a successful approach for treating selected decayed teeth.

REFERENCES

1. Buonocore MG. A simple method of increasing the adhesion of acrylic filling materials to enamel surfaces, *J Dent Res* 34:849-853, 1955.
2. Bowen RL. Method of preparing a monomer having phenoxy and methacrylate groups linked by hydroxyl glycerol groups. US Patent No 3, 194, 783, July 1965.
3. Dental sealants in the prevention of tooth decay. Proceedings of the National Institutes of Health Consensus Development Conference, *J Dent Educ* 48:4-131, 1984.
4. Simonsen RJ. Retention and effectiveness of dental sealant after 15 years, *J Am Dent Assoc* 122:34-42, 1991.
5. Sanders BJ, Smith CE. The use of sealants by Indiana dentists, *J Indiana Dent Assoc* 76:11-14, 1997.
6. Henderson HZ, et al. The use of pit and fissure sealants by Indiana dentists, *J Indiana Dent Assoc* 64(5):35-38, 1985.
7. Handleman SL, et al. Two-year report of sealant effect on bacteria in dental caries, *J Am Dent Assoc* 93:967-970, 1976.
8. Going RE, et al. The viability of micro-organisms in carious lesions five years after covering with a fissure sealant, *J Am Dent Assoc* 97:455-462, 1978.
9. Jeronimus DJ, et al. Reduced viability of microorganisms under sealants, *J Dent Child* 42:275-280, 1975.
10. Going RE. Sealant effect on incipient caries, enamel maturation and future caries susceptibility, *J Dent Educ* 48(Suppl 2):35-41, 1984.
11. Wendt L, Koch G. Fissure sealant in permanent first molars after 10 years, *Swed Dent J* 12:181-185, 1988.
12. Romcke RG, et al. Retention and maintenance of fissure sealants over 10 years, *J Can Dent Assoc* 56:235-237, 1990.
13. Dennison JB, et al. Effectiveness of sealant treatment over five years in an insured population, *J Am Dent Assoc* 131:597-605, 2000.
14. Robison VA, et al. A longitudinal study of school children's experience in the North Carolina dental Medicaid program, 1984 through 1992, *Am J Public Health* 88:1669-1673, 1998.
15. Koh SH, et al. Effects of topical fluoride treatment on tensile bond strength of pit and fissure sealants, *Gen Dent* 46:278-280, 1998.
16. Warren DP, et al. Effect of topical fluoride on retention of pit and fissure sealants, *J Dent Hyg* 75:21-24, 2001.
17. Beauchamp J, et al. Evidence based clinical recommendations for the use of pit and fissure sealants, *J Am Dent Assoc* 139:257-268, 2008.
18. Papers from the Pediatric Restorative Dentistry Consensus Conference. San Antonio, Texas, April 15-16, 2002, *Pediatr Dent* 24(5):374-516, 2002.
19. Pope BD, et al. Effectiveness of occlusal fissure cleansing methods and sealant micromorphology, *J Dent Child* 63:175-180, 1996.
20. Hatibovic-Kofman S, et al. Microleakage of sealants after conventional, bur, and air-abrasion preparation of pits and fissures, *Pediatr Dent* 20:173-176, 1998.
21. Eidelman E, et al. The retention of fissure sealants: rubber dam or cotton rolls in a private practice, *J Dent Child* 50:259-261, 1983.
22. Matis BA. Pit and fissure sealants in young adults: an evaluation of placement time and retention rate using two isolation techniques. Master's thesis. Indianapolis, Indiana University School of Dentistry, 1983.
23. Zidan O, Hill G. Phosphoric acid concentration: enamel surface loss and bonding strength, *J Prosthet Dent,* 55: 388-391, 1986.
24. Redford DA, et al. The effect of different etching times on the sealant bond strength, etch depth, and pattern in primary teeth, *Pediatr Dent* 8:111-115, 1986.
25. Phillips RW. Personal communication, 1986.
26. Norling BK. Bonding. In Anusavice KJ, ed. *Phillips' science of dental materials,* 11th ed. St. Louis, 2003, Saunders.
27. Feigal RJ, et al. Retaining sealants on salivary contaminated enamel, *J Am Dent Assoc* 124:88-96, 1993.
28. Choi JW, et al. The efficacy of primer on sealant shear bond strength, *Pediatr Dent* 19:286-288, 1997.
29. Feigal RJ. Sealants and preventive restorations: review of effectiveness and clinical changes for improvement, *Pediatr Dent* 20:85-92, 1998.
30. Feigal RJ, et al. Improved sealant retention with bonding agents: a clinical study of two-bottle and single-bottle systems, *J Dent Res* 79:1850-1856, 2000.
31. Simonsen RJ, Stallard RE. Sealant-restorations utilizing a diluted filled composite resin: one year results, *Quintessence Int* 8(6):77-84, 1977.
32. Henderson HZ, Setcos JC. The sealed composite resin restoration, *J Dent Child* 52:300-302, 1985.
33. Walker J, et al. The effectiveness of preventive resin restorations in pediatric patients, *J Dent Child* 63:338-340, 1996.
34. Houpt M, et al. The preventive resin (composite resin/sealant) restoration: nine-year results, *Quintessence Int* 25:155-159, 1994.

SUGGESTED READINGS

Azarpazhooh A, Main P: Pit and fissure sealants in the prevention of dental caries in children and adolescents: a systemic review, *JCDA* 74:171-177, 2008.

Brown LJ et al. Dental caries and sealant usage in US children 1988-1991, *J Am Dent Assoc* 127:335-343, 1996.

Feigal RJ. The use of pit and fissure sealants, *Pediatr Dent* 24:415-422, 2002.

Mertz-Fairhurst EJ et al. Ultraconservative and cariostatic sealed restorations: results at year 10, *J Am Dent Assoc* 129:55-66, 1998.

Selwitz RH et al. The prevalence of dental sealants in the US population: findings from NHANES III, 1988-1991, *J Dent Res* 75(special issue):652-660, 1996.

Waggoner WF, Siegal M. Pit and fissure sealant application: updating the technique, *J Am Dent Assoc* 1:351-361, 1996.

Walker J, Floyd K, Jakobsen J. The effectiveness of sealants in pediatric patients, *J Dent Child* 63:268-270, 1996.

CHAPTER 18

Restorative Dentistry

▲ **Ralph E. McDonald, David R. Avery,** and **Jeffrey A. Dean**

CHAPTER OUTLINE

*A*dvances in preventive dentistry and their application in the private dental office, the widespread acceptance of communal fluoridation, and greater emphasis on dental health education have dramatically changed the nature of dental practice. Today the dentist devotes more time to preventive procedures and less time to the routine restoration of carious teeth.

Nevertheless, the restoration of carious lesions in primary and young permanent teeth continues to be among the important services that pediatric dentists and general practitioners provide for the children in their practices. Patients and fellow practitioners often judge dentists on the effectiveness of their preventive programs and the skill with which they perform routine operative procedures.

The *Reference Manual* of the American Academy of Pediatric Dentistry (AAPD) includes a Guideline on Pediatric Restorative Dentistry (revised in 1998 and in 2001) that states in part[1]:

Restorative treatment is based upon the results of an appropriate clinical examination and is ideally part of a comprehensive treatment plan. The treatment plan shall take into consideration:
1. The developmental status of the dentition
2. A caries-risk assessment
3. Patient's oral hygiene
4. Anticipated parental compliance and likelihood of timely recall
5. Patient's ability to cooperate for treatment

The restorative treatment plan must be prepared in conjunction with an individually tailored preventive program. Restoration of primary teeth differs significantly from restoration of permanent teeth, due in part to the differences in tooth morphology.

In 2002, the AAPD, with financial assistance from the American Society of Dentistry for Children, held a pediatric restorative dentistry consensus conference in San Antonio, Texas. Sixteen literature review and position papers were presented at the conference and numerous consensus statements about appropriate pediatric restorative materials and procedures were developed. The papers and consensus statements are compiled in the September/October 2002 issue 24 of *Pediatric Dentistry*.

STATUS OF COMMON RESTORATIVE MATERIALS

Recent advances in the development of improved biomaterials for dental restorations have been rapid, and they continue to occur at a fast pace. This fact creates a significant challenge for dentists striving to remain at the cutting edge of dental technology. The more common restorative materials used in pediatric dentistry are composite and other resin systems, glass ionomers, silver amalgam alloys, and stainless steel alloys. Porcelain and cast metal alloy materials are also used in pediatric restorative dentistry but less frequently than those listed in the previous sentence.

Composite resins, glass ionomers, or some combination of the two are being used progressively more and silver amalgam progressively less in pediatric restorative dentistry. Many pediatric dentistry practices do not use silver amalgam at all; instead, some form of composite resin and/or glass ionomer is used. These materials have bonding capability. Glass ionomers may be considered pharmacologically therapeutic because they release fluoride over time; they also have minimal shrinkage during setting. Composite resins possess durability and superior esthetic qualities. When managed properly, both materials are capable of providing superior marginal sealing at the tooth–restorative material interface. The manufacturers of these materials have also combined them in an effort to join the primary advantages of each type of material. Berg has suggested that we think of these materials and their combinations on a continuum, with glass ionomer on the left, composite resin on the right, and the combined materials somewhere in between depending on the relative amounts of each material in the mix. Two major categories on the continuum are described as "resin-modified glass ionomer" (or "hybrid ionomer" or "light-cured glass ionomer") and "compomers" (or "polyacid-modified composite resin" or "glass ionomer-modified composite resin"). A fifth formulation has been added on the right side of the continuum in the form of "flowable composite resin." Berg points out that knowing the particular strengths and weaknesses of each type of material on the continuum will enhance the clinician's ability to make the best choices for each individual restorative situation.[2] Use of any of these restorative materials generally requires more effort and time than corresponding conventional amalgam restorations.

Despite its declining use, silver amalgam remains one of the most durable and cost-effective restorative materials. Success in using this filling material depends on adherence to certain principles of cavity preparation that do not always apply when materials on the glass ionomer–composite resin continuum are used. Some renewed interest in silver amalgam has occurred because of the development of "bonded amalgams." Bonded amalgams are silver amalgam restorations that have been condensed into etched cavity preparations lined with a dentin-bonding agent and some material on the glass ionomer–composite resin continuum. Bonded amalgams require considerable extra effort and expense to place compared with conventional amalgam restorations. The improvements in tooth support and marginal integrity gained with these restorations have been demonstrated in many studies. Some longer-term studies, however, suggest that the advantages of bonded amalgams may be transient and relatively short-lived, possibly 1 year or less.[3,4] In general, the use of bonded amalgams seems difficult to justify for the routine restoration of primary teeth because traditional silver amalgam should provide comparable quality more efficiently and cost effectively in most situations.

Stainless steel alloy is another commonly used pediatric restorative material. It is used extensively for full coronal coverage restorations of primary teeth. Stainless steel crowns have undoubtedly preserved the function of many primary teeth that otherwise would have been unrestorable. In addition, stainless steel crowns are often used to restore all posterior teeth in young patients with high risk for caries who exhibit multiple proximal lesions that could otherwise be restored with silver amalgam or esthetic materials. Crowns are used instead simply because they better protect all posterior tooth surfaces from developing additional caries and because the posterior crown restoration has proven to be the most durable and cost effective in the primary dentition. Anterior, as well as posterior, stainless steel crowns may have labial and/or occlusal resin or porcelain veneers to enhance esthetics.

MAINTENANCE OF A CLEAN FIELD

The maintenance of a clean operating field during cavity preparation and placement of the restorative material helps ensure efficient operation and development of a serviceable restoration that will maintain the tooth and the integrity of the developing occlusion.

The rubber dam aids in the maintenance of a clean field. It is generally agreed that the use of the rubber dam offers the following advantages:

1. *Saves time.* The dentist who has not routinely used the rubber dam needs only to follow the routine presented later in this chapter or a modification of it for a reasonable period to be convinced that operating time can be appreciably reduced. The time spent in placing the rubber dam is negligible, as long as the dentist works out a definite routine and uses a chairside assistant. Heise reported an average time of 1 minute and 48 seconds to isolate an average of 2.8 teeth with the rubber dam in 302 cases.[5] These applications of the rubber dam, placed with the aid of a capable dental assistant, were for routine operative dentistry procedures. The minimum time recorded for placing a rubber dam was 15 seconds (single-tooth isolation), and the maximum time was 6 minutes. Many of the applications ranged from 25 to 50 seconds. Heise also observed that approximately 10 seconds is required to remove the rubber dam. The time required for the placement of the rubber dam will invariably be made up and additional time saved through the elimination of rinsing and spitting by the pediatric patient.

2. *Aids management.* A few explanatory words and reference to the rubber dam as a "raincoat" for the tooth or as a "Halloween mask" helps allay the child's anxiety. It has been found through experience that apprehensive or otherwise uncooperative children can often be controlled more easily with a rubber dam in place. Because the rubber dam efficiently controls the tongue and the lips, the dentist has greater freedom to complete the operative procedures.

3. *Controls saliva.* Control of saliva is an extremely important consideration when one is completing

an ideal cavity preparation for primary teeth. The margin of error is appreciably reduced when a cavity is prepared in a primary tooth that has a large pulp and extensive carious involvement. Small pulp exposures may be more easily detected when the tooth is well isolated. It is equally important to observe the true extent of the exposure and the degree and type of hemorrhage from the pulp tissue. Thus the rubber dam aids the dentist in evaluating teeth that are being considered for vital pulp therapy.

4. *Provides protection.* The use of the rubber dam prevents foreign objects from coming into contact with oral structures. When filling material, debris, or medicaments are dropped into the mouth, salivary flow is stimulated and interferes with the operative or restorative procedure. A rubber dam also prevents the small child in a reclining position from swallowing or aspirating foreign objects and materials.

5. *Helps the dentist educate parents.* Parents are always interested in the treatment that has been accomplished for their child. While the rubber dam is in place, the dentist can conveniently show parents the completed work after an operative procedure. The rubber dam creates the feeling that the dentist has complete control of the situation and that a conscientious effort has been made to provide the highest type of service.

ARMAMENTARIUM FOR RUBBER DAM PLACEMENT

The armamentarium consists of 5- × 5-inch sheets of medium latex, a rubber dam punch, clamp forceps, a selection of clamps, a flat-blade instrument, dental floss, and a rubber dam frame. If one visualizes an approximately 1¼-inch square in the center of a sheet of rubber dam, each corner of the square indicates where the punch holes for the clamp-bearing tooth in each of the four quadrants of the mouth are to be made (Fig. 18-1). As experience is gained in applying the dam, the dentist and assistant will soon learn the proper location for punching the holes. If the holes are punched too far apart, the dam will not readily fit between the contact areas. In addition, the greater bulk of material between the teeth will greatly increase the possibility that the rubber will become a barrier to proximal surface preparation. Conversely, if the holes are punched too close together, salivary leakage will contaminate the operating field. In general, the holes should be punched the same distance apart as the holes on the cutting table of the rubber dam punch.

The large punch hole is used for the clamp-bearing tooth and for most permanent molars. The medium-sized punch hole generally is used for the premolars and primary molars. The second smallest hole is used for maxillary permanent incisors, whereas the smallest hole is adequate for the primary incisors and lower permanent incisors.

SELECTION OF A CLAMP

The operator will soon develop a personal preference for which clamps to use to secure the dam in isolating different areas in the mouth. Unless the clamp is firmly anchored to the tooth, the tension of the stretched rubber

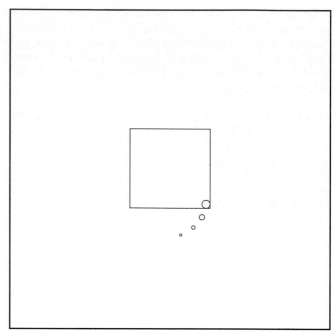

Figure 18-1 The corners of the square represent points where punch holes should be made for the clamp-bearing tooth.

will easily dislodge it. Therefore the proper selection of a clamp is of utmost importance. It is recommended that the clamp be tried on the tooth before the rubber dam is placed to ascertain that the clamp can be securely seated and will not be easily dislodged by the probing tongue, lip, or cheek musculature. An 18-inch length of dental floss should be doubled and securely fastened to the bow of the clamp. The floss will facilitate retrieval in the unlikely event that the clamp slips and falls toward the pharynx (Fig. 18-2).

The following procedure is recommended for rubber dam application (Fig. 18-3). The previously selected and

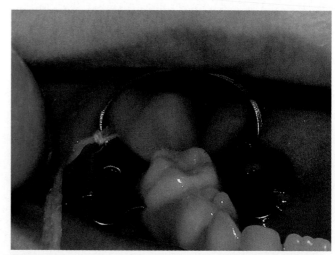

Figure 18-2 An Ivory No. 3 clamp has been trial-fitted to the second primary molar. The clamp will be removed and placed in the rubber dam.

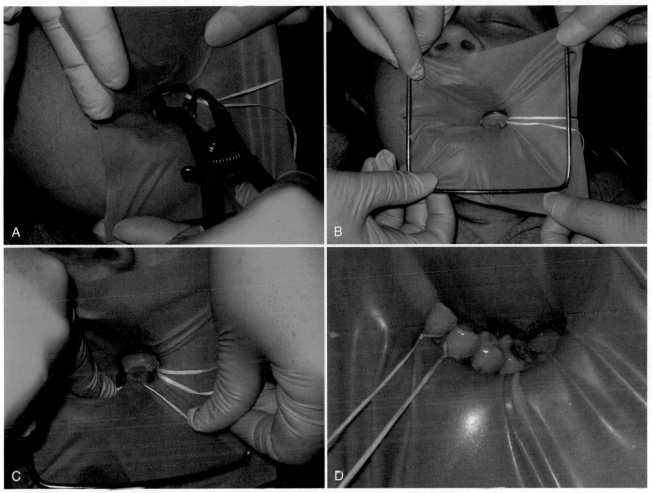

Figure 18-3 A, The dental assistant holds the top and lower right corners of the rubber dam as the dentist holds the lower left corner and carries the clamp to the tooth. **B,** The assistant and dentist attach the corners of the rubber dam to the frame. **C,** Dental floss is used to carry the rubber dam between the teeth. **D,** The teeth are isolated and ready for the operative procedure. **(A, B,** and **C** Courtesy of Dr. Richard Troyer.)

ligated clamp is placed in the rubber dam. The dentist grasps the clamp forceps with the clamp engaged. The assistant, seated to the left of the patient (the dentist is right-handed in this example), grasps the upper corners of the dam with the right hand and the lower left corner between the left thumb and index finger. The dam is moved toward the patient's face as the dentist carries the clamp to the tooth while holding the lower right portion of the dam. After securing the clamp on the tooth, the dentist transfers the clamp forceps to the assistant, who receives it while continuing to hold the upper corners of the dam with the right hand. The dentist then places the frame over the rubber dam. Together the assistant and dentist attach the corners of the dam to the frame. The flat blade of a plastic instrument or a right-angle explorer may be used to remove the rubber dam material from the wings of the clamp and to complete the seal around the clamped tooth. If necessary, light finger pressure may seat the clamp securely by moving it cervically on the tooth. If additional teeth are to be isolated, the rubber is stretched over them, and the excess rubber between the punched holes is placed between the contact areas with

the aid of dental floss. The most anterior tooth and others if necessary are ligated to aid in the retention of the dam and the prevention of cervical leakage. The free ends of the floss are allowed to remain, because they may aid in the further retraction of the gingival tissue or the patient's lip during the operative procedure. At the end of the operative procedure, the length of floss will also aid in removing the ligature.

When a quadrant of restorations in the primary dentition is planned and no pulp therapy is anticipated, Croll recommends the "slit-dam method."[6] One long opening is made in the dam, and the entire quadrant is isolated without interseptal dam material between the teeth.

It is unwise to include more teeth in the rubber dam than are necessary to isolate the working area adequately. If the first or second permanent molar is the only tooth in the quadrant that is carious and if it requires only an occlusal preparation, it is often desirable to punch only one hole in the dam and to isolate the single tooth (Fig. 18-4). This procedure will require only seconds and will save many minutes.

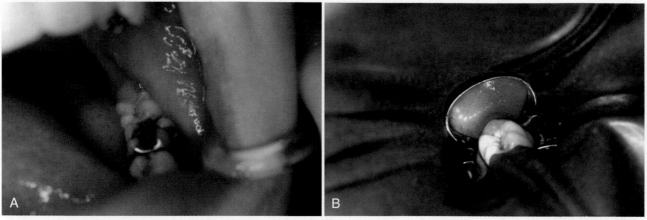

Figure 18-4 A, The second permanent molar requires an occlusal restoration. It is not necessary to isolate more than a single tooth. **B,** A No. 200 clamp has been selected to hold the rubber dam in place. The rubber dam has retracted the tissue that extended over the distal marginal ridge.

MORPHOLOGIC CONSIDERATIONS

The crowns of the primary teeth are smaller but more bulbous than the corresponding permanent teeth, and the molars are bell-shaped, with a definite constriction in the cervical region. The characteristic sharp lingual inclination occlusally of the facial surfaces results in the formation of a distinct faciogingival ridge that ends abruptly at the cementoenamel junction. The sharp constriction at the neck of the primary molar necessitates special care in the formation of the gingival floor during class II cavity preparation. The buccal and lingual surfaces of the molars converging sharply occlusally form a narrow occlusal surface or food table; this is especially true of the first primary molar.

The pulpal outline of the primary teeth follows the dentoenamel junction more closely than that of the permanent teeth. The pulpal horns are longer and more pointed than the cusps would indicate. The dentin also has less bulk or thickness, and so the pulp is proportionately larger than that of the permanent teeth. The enamel of the primary teeth is thin but of uniform thickness. The enamel surface tends to be parallel to the dentinoenamel junction.

BASIC PRINCIPLES IN THE PREPARATION OF CAVITIES IN PRIMARY TEETH

Traditional cavity preparations for class I and class II lesions include areas that have carious involvement and, in addition, those areas that retain food and plaque material and may be considered areas of potential carious involvement. A flat pulpal floor is generally advocated. However, a sharp angle between the pulpal floor and the axial wall of a two-surface preparation should be avoided. Rounded angles throughout the preparation will result in less concentration of stresses and will permit better adaptation of the restorative material into the extremities of the preparation.

Although the traditional class I cavity preparation and restoration may occasionally be the most practical treatment for a tooth in certain circumstances, such treatment is currently obsolete for most class I lesions. The traditional treatment has been replaced, for the most part, by conservative caries excavation and restoration using a combination of bonding restorative and sealant materials (see Chapter 17).

Likewise, the traditional class II cavity preparation and restoration, although not yet considered obsolete, is currently used less frequently as steadily improving restorative materials with therapeutic and bonding capability are developed. In the traditional class II cavity preparation for amalgam, the buccal and lingual extensions should be carried to self-cleansing areas. The cavity design should have greater buccal and lingual extension at the cervical area of the preparation to clear contact with the adjacent tooth. This divergent pattern is necessary because of the broad, flat contact areas of the primary molars and because of the distinct buccal bulge in the gingival third. Ideally, the width of the preparation at the isthmus should be approximately one-third the intercuspal dimension (Fig. 18-5). The axiopulpal line angle

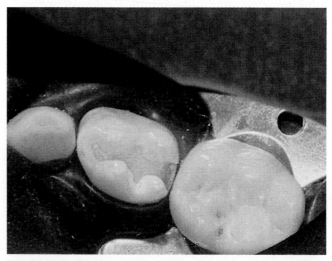

Figure 18-5 Conservative but adequate extension of a traditional class II cavity preparation in a mandibular first primary molar.

should be beveled or grooved to reduce the concentration of stresses and to provide greater bulk of material in this area, which is vulnerable to fracture.

Because many occlusal fractures of amalgam restorations are caused by sharp opposing cusps, it is advisable to identify these potentially damaging cusps with articulating paper before cavity preparation. The slight reduction and rounding of a sharp opposing cusp will reduce the number of such fractures.

CAVITY PREPARATION IN PRIMARY TEETH

The steps in the preparation of a cavity in a primary tooth are not difficult but do require precise operator control. Many authorities advocate the use of small, rounded-end carbide burs in the high-speed handpiece to establish the cavity outline and perform the gross preparation. For efficiency and convenience, all necessary high-speed instrumentation for a given preparation may be completed with a single bur in most situations. Therefore the dentist should select the bur that is best designed to accomplish all the high-speed cutting required for the procedure being planned. Fig. 18-6 illustrates four high-speed carbide burs designed to cut efficiently and yet allow conservative cavity preparations with rounded line angles and point angles. Alternatively, cavity preparations may be made with aluminum oxide air abrasion systems or with laser systems approved for hard-tissue procedures, when indications allow.

INCIPIENT CLASS I CAVITY IN A VERY YOUNG CHILD

During the routine examination of a child younger than 2 years of age, the dentist may occasionally discover a small but definite carious lesion in the central fossa of one or two first primary molars, with all other teeth being sound. Thus restorative needs are present but minimal.

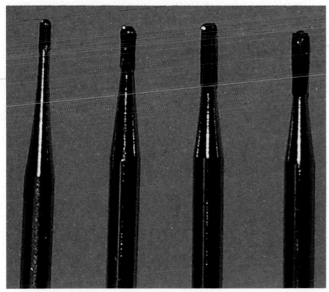

Figure 18-6 Rounded-end, high-speed carbide burs No. 329, No. 330, No. 245, and No. 256, which may be used for cutting cavity preparations.

Because of the child's psychological immaturity and because it is usually impossible to establish effective communication with the child, the parent should hold the child on his or her lap in the dental chair. This helps the child feel more secure and provides a better opportunity to restrain the child's movement during the operative procedure. The small-cavity preparation may be made without the aid of a rubber dam or local anesthetic. A No. 329 or No. 330 bur is used to open the decayed area and extend the cavosurface margin only to the extent of the carious lesion. If the patient is resistant (usually), completing the preparation with an air abrasion or laser system would be inconvenient. The preparation can be completed in just a few seconds. Restoring the tooth with amalgam or a resin-modified glass ionomer arrests the decay and at least temporarily prevents further tooth destruction without a lengthy or involved dental appointment for the child. If the child is cooperative, a preventive resin restoration, preceded by application of a dentin-bonding agent, may be used.

PIT OR FISSURE CLASS I CAVITY

The preparation and restoration of a pit or fissure class I cavity are discussed in the section on preventive resin restoration in Chapter 17.

DEEP-SEATED CLASS I CAVITY

If an amalgam restoration is planned, the first step in the preparation of an extensive class I cavity is to plane back the enamel that overhangs the extensive carious lesion. Then the cavity preparation should be extended throughout the remaining grooves and anatomic occlusal defects. The carious dentin should next be removed with large, round burs or spoon excavators. If a carious exposure is not encountered, the cavity walls should be finished as previously described. With deep carious lesions and near pulp exposures, the depth of the cavity should be covered with a biocompatible base material to provide adequate thermal protection for the pulp.

If a composite resin and/or glass ionomer restoration is planned, any disease-free pits and grooves may be sealed as part of the bonded restoration. The restorative material also provides thermal insulation to the pulp.

CLASS II CAVITY

Proximal lesions in a preschool child indicate excessive caries activity; a preventive and restorative program should be undertaken immediately.

Small Lesions

Very small incipient proximal lesions may be chemically restored with topical fluoride therapy provided by the dentist, along with the judicious use of fluoride products designed for topical application at home. If this treatment regimen is accompanied by improved diet and improved oral hygiene, some incipient proximal lesions may remineralize or remain in an arrested state indefinitely. However, the parents should be informed of the incipient lesions and emphasis should be placed on the need to continue practicing the recommended procedures and to bring the child back for periodic examinations. If the parents and the patient do not follow the instructions properly, subsequent bitewing radiographs will reveal growth of the lesion, and restorative procedures should be initiated before the defects become extensive carious lesions.

As bonded restorations have improved, especially those restorations capable of fluoride release, more conservative cavity preparation designs have also been advocated. In otherwise sound teeth free of susceptible pits and fissures, accessing small class II carious lesions via small openings in the marginal ridges or in the facial surfaces of the teeth is becoming a popular technique (Fig. 18-7). Gaining access to the lesion with openings only large enough to allow caries excavation is the goal. Caries is removed by pendulous motions of small burs or by tilting of the air abrasion tip laterally and pulpally at the initial opening. This technique is particularly useful in cooperative patients with one or two affected primary molars who are judged to be at relatively low risk for additional caries activity. Suwatviroj and colleagues have shown in vitro that various tooth-colored restorations placed in box-only preparations did not differ in fracture resistance from those placed in dovetail preparations.[7] However, resin-modified glass ionomer restorations placed in box-only preparations were more likely to show adhesive failure than those placed in dovetail preparations.

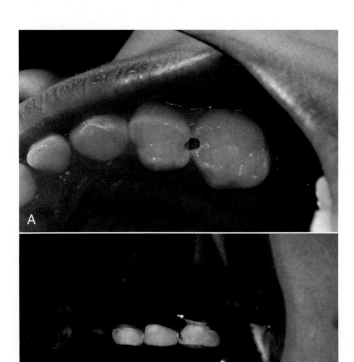

Figure 18-7 Approximating conservative preparations to remove small class II carious lesions in primary molars. **A,** Marginal ridge access. **B,** Facial surface access.

Other researchers, Croll[8] as well as Vaikuntam,[9] have also advocated conservative preparations and restorations with fluoride-releasing restorative materials. Our experience has shown that local anesthesia is usually unnecessary to make the preparation. When performing this short procedure in cooperative patients, rubber dam isolation is often optional, especially on maxillary teeth. Use of resin-modified glass ionomer materials results in excellent restorations for this conservative procedure (Fig. 18-8).

Marks and associates,[10] as well as Welbury[11] and colleagues (who also restored class I preparations), have reported satisfactory results using conservative class II preparations and compomers to restore primary molars in studies of 36 and 42 months' duration, respectively. In a 3-year study, Hubel and Mejare reported the successful performance of conservative class II resin-modified glass ionomer restorations in primary molars.[12]

Lesions with Greater Dentin Involvement

The first step in the traditional preparation of a class II cavity in a primary tooth for an amalgam or an esthetic restoration involves opening the marginal ridge area. Extreme care must be taken when breaking through the marginal ridge to prevent damage to the adjacent proximal surface.

Amalgam

The gingival seat and proximal walls should break contact with the adjacent tooth. The angle formed by the axial wall and the buccal and lingual walls of the proximal box should approach a right angle. The buccal and lingual walls necessarily diverge toward the cervical region, following the general contour of the tooth (Fig. 18-9). The occlusal extension of the preparation should include any caries-susceptible pits and fissures. If the occlusal surface is sound and not caries susceptible, then a minimal occlusal dovetail is still often needed to enhance the cavity retention form. If carious material remains after the preparation outline is established, it should next be removed. The appropriate liner or intermediate base, if indicated, and a snug-fitting matrix should be placed before the insertion of the amalgam.

Esthetic Materials

Because of the improvements in the properties of composite resins, many dentists use them routinely for posterior restorations. More recently the use of glass ionomer restoratives (or other materials on the glass ionomer–composite resin continuum) has also been advocated. The preparation and restoration may be similar to that described earlier for amalgam when significant caries exists on both the occlusal and proximal surfaces (Fig. 18-10). However, little or no occlusal preparation may be required when the occlusal pits and fissures are caries susceptible but sound or incipient. Then the proximal restoration may be combined with application of an occlusal sealant (with or without enameloplasty). Whenever composite restorative materials are employed, enamel beveling, etching, and application of bonding agents are recommended.

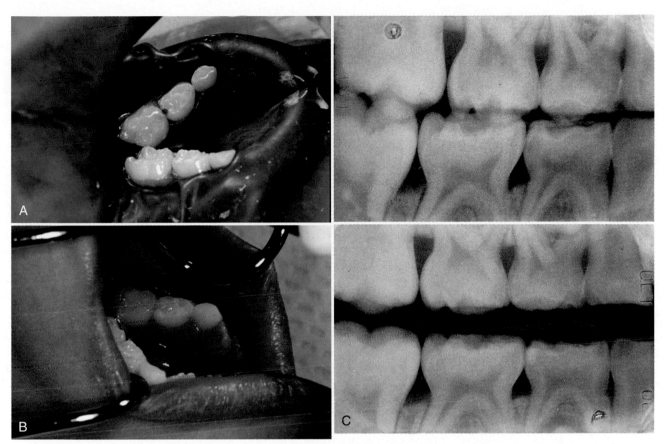

Figure 18-8 A, Conservative class II preparation. **B,** Resin-modified glass ionomer restoration. **C,** Preoperative radiograph (top) and 17-month postoperative film.

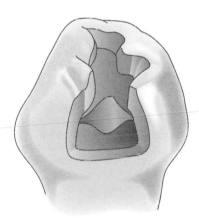

Figure 18-9 Traditional class II cavity preparation for a primary molar. The preparation includes diverging proximal walls and a beveled and grooved axiopulpal line angle.

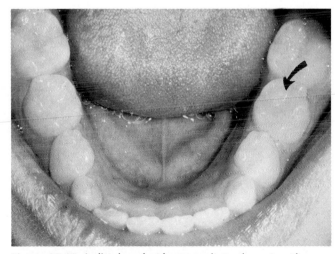

Figure 18-10 A distal occlusal composite resin restoration was placed in the lower left second primary molar 6 months before the photograph.

Clinical trials of restoration of primary molars reported by Paquette and colleagues[13] and by Oldenburg and associates[14] revealed that traditional preparations modified only by beveling of enamel margins and restored with bonded composite resins yielded highly successful results during 12- and 24-month observation periods. Tonn and

Ryge also reported acceptable 2-year results for primary molars restored with bonded composite resins in traditional cavity preparations modified only by beveling of enamel margins.[15]

Dilley and colleagues have demonstrated that the placement and finishing of posterior composite restorations are significantly more time consuming than those for comparable amalgam restorations.[16] In addition to increasing the cost of care, the extra time required for treatment may complicate patient management for some young patients.

Donly and associates have reported successful results for class II resin-modified glass ionomer restorations in primary molars after 3 years of observation.[17] In an interesting study by dos Santos and colleagues, class I and II preparations in primary molars were restored with either a resin modified glass ionomer, polyacid modified composite or composite. After 24 months, no statistical differences were found between the materials, although not too surprisingly, the class I restorations showed higher survival rates than the class II restorations.[18] The dentist's sound professional judgment is the key to selecting the restoration that will best serve the patient in each situation.

CLASS III CAVITY

Carious lesions on the proximal surfaces of anterior primary teeth sometimes occur in children whose teeth are in contact and in children who have evidence of arch inadequacy or crowding. Carious involvement of the anterior primary teeth, however, may be interpreted as evidence of excessive caries activity requiring a comprehensive preventive program.

If the carious lesion has not advanced appreciably into the dentin and removal of the caries will not involve or weaken the incisal angle, a small conventional class III cavity may be prepared and the tooth may be restored with the dentist's choice of bonding materials (Fig. 18-11).

Mandibular primary incisors with small proximal carious lesions may not require conventional restorations at all. Enameloplasty of the affected proximal surface (usually described as "disking") to open the proximal contact and to remove most, if not all, of the cavitation, followed by topical treatments with fluoride varnish, will often suffice until the teeth exfoliate naturally. Extraction is usually indicated when mandibular primary incisors have extensive caries.

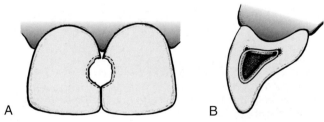

Figure 18-11 A, Schematic drawing of carious lesions on the mesial surfaces of maxillary primary central incisors that do not undermine the mesial angles of the teeth. The dotted line indicates the proposed labial outline of the class III cavity preparation. **B,** Proximal view illustrates that the class III preparation is limited to the cervical two thirds of the primary incisor. (From Roche JR. Restorative dentistry. In Goldman HM et al, eds. Current Therapy in Dentistry, vol 4. St Louis, Mosby, 1970.)

MODIFIED CLASS III CAVITY PREPARATION

The distal surface of the primary canine is a frequent site of caries attack in patients at high risk for caries if the canine is in proximal contact with the first molar. The position of the tooth in the arch, the characteristically broad contact between the distal surface of the canine and the mesial surface of the primary molar, and the height of the gingival tissue sometimes make it difficult to prepare a typical class III cavity and restore it adequately. The modified class III preparation uses a dovetail on the lingual or occasionally on the labial surfaces of the tooth. A lingual lock is normally considered for the maxillary canine, whereas a labial lock may be more conveniently prepared on the mandibular teeth for which the esthetic requirement is not so important (Figs. 18-12 and 18-13). The preparation allows for additional retention and access necessary to insert the restorative material properly.

Trairatvorakul and Piwat have compared 31 paired slot preparations to dovetail class III preparations in primary anterior teeth in a well controlled clinical study in children 2 years 6 months to 5 years 3 months of age.[19] All teeth were restored with composite and evaluated for marginal adaptation, anatomic form, secondary caries, and marginal discoloration at 6 months, 12 months, and 24 months. Twenty-two pairs of restorations were available at the end of the study. Only one restoration in the slot group was unacceptable and three in the dovetail group were unacceptable.

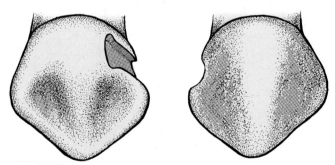

Figure 18-12 Lingual and labial views of a modified class III preparation for a maxillary primary canine. The dovetail improves retention form of the preparation and allows access for placing the restorative material to ensure adequate contact with the adjacent tooth.

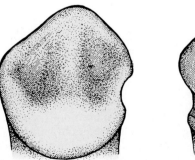
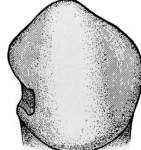

Figure 18-13 Lingual and labial views of a modified class III preparation for a mandibular primary canine.

There was no statistical significance between the two groups. These results suggest that the simpler and more conservative slot preparation may often be preferred.

RESTORATION OF PROXIMAL INCISAL CARIES IN PRIMARY ANTERIOR TEETH

ESTHETIC RESIN RESTORATION

One type of preparation used for the esthetic restoration of primary incisors in which dental caries approximates or involves the incisal edge of the teeth is illustrated in Fig. 18-14. As with other operative procedures for the pediatric patient, the use of the rubber dam aids in maintenance of a dry field, provides better vision, and facilitates control of the lips and tongue.

The preparation includes a proximal reduction through the incisal angle and the carious lesion, and ends at the established cervical seat. Labial and lingual locks are then prepared in the cervical third of the tooth. The remaining caries is removed, the tooth is etched, and a bonding agent is applied.

A properly placed matrix tightly wedged at the cervical seat aids the operator in placing, shaping, and holding the composite resin during the curing process. A good matrix also simplifies the finishing procedures.

McEvoy has described a similar preparation and restoration for primary incisors, except that the retentive locking component is placed on the labial surface only in the gingival one third of the tooth.[20] The lock extends minimally across two thirds of the labial surface and may extend even farther to include decalcified enamel in the cervical area. We would also recommend slightly beveling the enamel margins before etching to further improve the marginal bonding of the restoration.

Initial shaping of the restoration may be accomplished with a flame-shaped finishing bur. The excess resin is removed, and the contour of the restoration is established. The gingival margins may be finished with a sharp scalpel blade. Final polishing may be accomplished with the rubber cup and a fine, moist abrasive material or one of the composite polishing systems (Fig. 18-15).

STAINLESS STEEL CROWNS

Primary incisors or canines that have extensive proximal lesions involving the incisal portion of the tooth may be restored with stainless steel crowns.

A steel crown of appropriate size is selected, contoured at the cervical margin, polished, and cemented into place. The crown technique is discussed in detail later in this chapter. Although the crown will be well retained even on teeth that require removal of extensive portions of carious

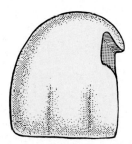
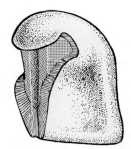
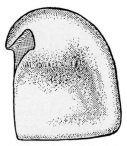

Figure 18-14 Labial, proximolingual, and lingual views of a preparation for an esthetic resin restoration in a primary incisor. The preparation includes a proximal reduction and the establishment of a definitive cervical seat that extends to labial and lingual locks in the cervical third of the tooth.

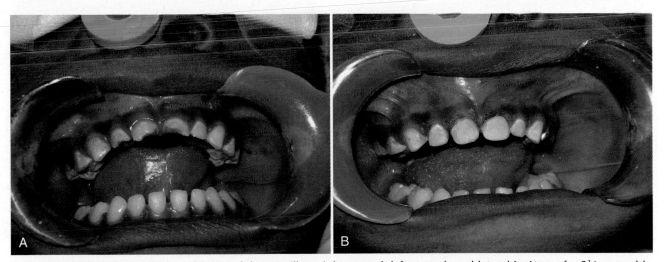

Figure 18-15 A, Extensive carious lesions of the maxillary right central, left central, and lateral incisors of a 3½-year-old patient. **B,** Postoperative view of the restored teeth. The restorations are retained with labial and lingual locks incorporated in the preparations. The maxillary lateral preparation was designed as illustrated in Fig. 18-14.

tooth structure, the esthetic requirements of some children may not be met by this type of restoration.

Most of the labial metal may be cut away, leaving a labial "window" that is then restored with composite resin (Fig. 18-16). This restoration is called an open-face stainless steel crown.

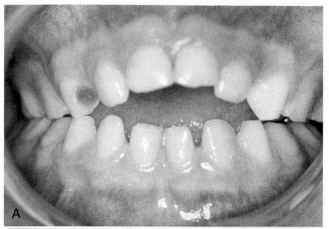

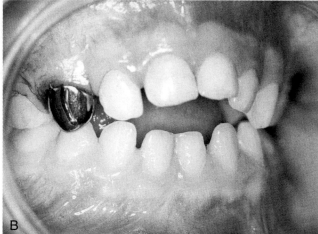

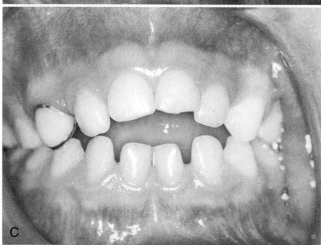

Figure 18-16 A, An extensive carious lesion is evident in the maxillary right primary canine. **B,** After the removal of caries and preparation of the tooth, a stainless steel crown was fitted to the tooth. **C,** The labial portion of the steel crown was removed and restored with resin. (Courtesy of Dr. Lionel Traubman.)

Several brands of stainless steel crowns with esthetic facings pre-veneered to the labial surfaces are also available to restore primary anterior teeth (Fig. 18-17). Such crowns are available for direct adaptation to the prepared teeth and have had a significant amount of success. One retrospective study of 226 crowns has shown an overall 91% of crowns retained good to excellent clinical appearance.[21] Alternatively, the restorations may be completed in two appointments, with the labial veneers added in the laboratory after the bare steel crowns are adapted to the teeth but before final cementation.

Croll recommends that an anterior alginate impression be made before the restorative appointment.[22] The crown preparations can then be simulated on a stone model, and most of the crown adaptation can be achieved in advance. This procedure enables the clinician to cement the crowns at the same appointment at which the preparations are made (rather than waiting for laboratory veneering of the adapted bare crowns). Croll's technique also gives the clinician a better opportunity to focus on fitting the crowns so that optimal tooth alignment will result, which further enhances the esthetic outcome.

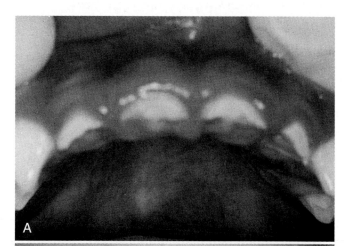

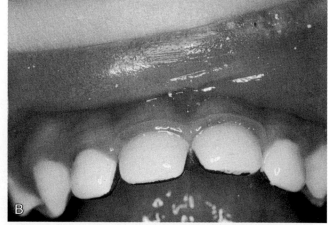

Figure 18-17 A, Extensive caries and coronal destruction of the maxillary incisors in a child 21 months of age. **B,** After pulp therapy, the teeth were restored with veneered stainless steel crowns. (Courtesy of Dr. Gary J. Hinz.)

DIRECT RESIN CROWNS

Webber and associates[23] described the resin crown technique wherein the tooth is restored with composite resin using a celluloid crown form as a matrix. They point out that very little finishing of the restoration is required when the celluloid crown has been properly fitted.

The jacket crown technique illustrated in Fig. 18-18 incorporates the use of a celluloid crown form and composite resin as advocated by Webber and associates[23] and today is commonly called a "strip crown." In a retrospective study by Kupietzky and others, strip crowns were shown to perform well for restoring primary incisors with large or multisurface caries for periods of more than 3 years. There was an 80% overall retention rate for the 145 restorations.[24]

Celluloid crown forms are also available for primary posterior teeth. These crown forms are useful matrices for some posterior bonded restorations. A good example of an indication for using such a crown form is to provide a bonded crown buildup to temporarily reestablish arch integrity and occlusion of an ankylosed (submerged) primary molar.

PREPARATION OF CAVITIES IN YOUNG PERMANENT TEETH

Many of the caries management procedures presented in this textbook also often apply to young permanent teeth. Entire textbooks are devoted to operative dentistry procedures, and the primary focus of these books is restoration of permanent teeth. Repeating all that information (or portions thereof) in this chapter is impractical and realistically impossible. For detailed information about the various cavity preparation designs for permanent teeth and the matrix systems to facilitate the placement and contour of restorations, please consult a standard textbook of operative dentistry listed in the references, such as the text by Roberson and colleagues.[25]

INTERIM RESTORATION FOR HYPOPLASTIC PERMANENT MOLARS

The dentist who routinely treats children occasionally faces a difficult restorative problem when severely hypoplastic first permanent molars erupt. Often the teeth are so defective that they require restoration at a very early stage of eruption. Many of these teeth have been saved by early restoration with stainless steel crowns as an interim procedure. However, this procedure may require sacrificing sound tooth surfaces to provide adequate space for the crown. Such full-coverage restorations are sometimes difficult to fit.

The composite materials have proved to be a more satisfactory interim restoration for many of these teeth. Such a bonded composite buildup restoration allows preservation of all sound tooth structure and depends on the presence of some enamel surfaces to provide bonded retention for the restorative material. Any soft defective areas are excavated, but little or no additional tooth preparation is done. Usually even undermined enamel surfaces are preserved for additional retention and support of the restorative material. In some cases gingivoplasty around the erupting tooth may first be necessary to allow adequate access to and isolation of the defective areas. Even if the restoration requires occasional repair, it still often provides a more satisfactory interim result than the stainless steel crown. Some of the newer restorative materials on the glass ionomer–composite resin continuum may provide an even better interim restoration for hypoplastic teeth because of their ability to release fluoride and to bond to hypoplastic enamel.

In situations in which a stainless steel crown is required to restore a young permanent molar, Radcliffe and Cullen have noted the importance of conservative tooth preparation to preserve better options for future restoration of the same tooth.[26] They advocate a preparation similar to that described in the following section.

STAINLESS STEEL CROWNS FOR POSTERIOR TEETH

Chrome steel crowns, as introduced by Humphrey in 1950, have proved to be serviceable restorations for children and adolescents and are now commonly called stainless steel crowns.[27] There are a number of indications for the use of stainless steel crowns in pediatric dentistry, including the following:

1. Restorations for primary or young permanent teeth with extensive and/or multiple carious lesions (Fig. 18-19)
2. Restorations for hypoplastic primary or permanent teeth that cannot be adequately restored with bonded restorations
3. Restorations for teeth with hereditary anomalies, such as dentinogenesis imperfecta or amelogenesis imperfecta
4. Restorations for pulpotomized or pulpectomized primary or young permanent teeth when there is increased danger of fracture of the remaining coronal tooth structure
5. Restorations for fractured teeth
6. Restorations for primary teeth to be used as abutments for appliances
7. Attachments for habit-breaking and orthodontic appliances

Randall published an extensive review of the literature that reports on the use of preformed metal crowns for primary and permanent molars.[28] She found five clinical studies that have compared the performance of crown restorations with that of multisurface amalgam restorations. The five studies included a total of 1210 crowns and 2201 amalgams that were followed from a minimum of 2 years to a maximum of 10 years. The findings in all five studies were in agreement that the crown restorations were superior to the amalgam restorations in the treatment of multisurface cavities in primary molars. Randall's review was followed by a position paper prepared by Seale that included additional scientific evidence favoring the use of stainless steel crown restorations, especially in children at high risk for caries.[29] Seale's published abstract states in part:

> The stainless steel crown (SSC) is an extremely durable restoration...Children with extensive decay, large lesions or multiple surface lesions in primary molars should be treated with stainless steel crowns. Because of the protection from future decay provided by their feature of full coverage and their increased durability and longevity, strong consideration should be given to the use of SSCs in children who require general anesthesia. Finally, a strong argument for the use of the SSC restoration is its cost effectiveness based on its durability and longevity.

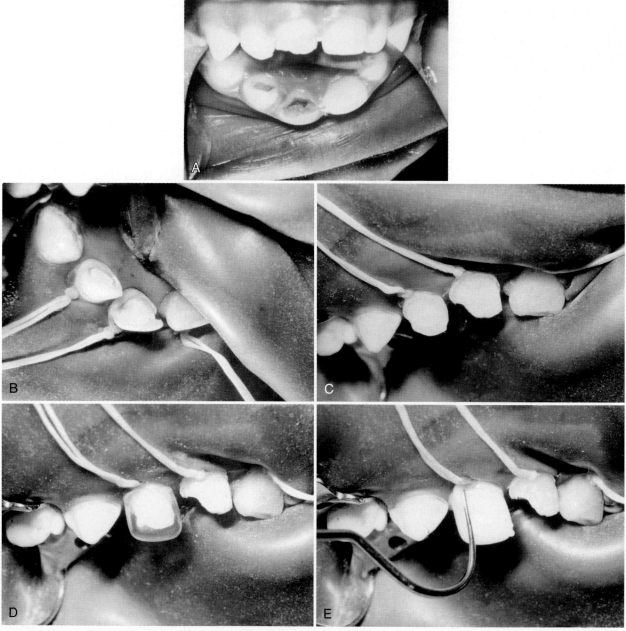

Figure 18-18 A, Extensive caries on the lingual surfaces of the maxillary right primary central and lateral incisors in a 2½-year-old patient. The caries has also severely undermined the proximal and incisal surfaces of the teeth. The maxillary left central incisor had been previously restored. **B,** The carious lesions have been excavated, and the exposed dentin has been covered with calcium hydroxide. **C,** Completed jacket preparations with cervical shoulders, slightly undercut walls at the cervical areas, and preservation of as much enamel and incisal tooth structure as possible. The enamel has been etched. **D,** Fitted celluloid crown form on the lateral incisor. The crown form should be trimmed to fit snugly and to just cover all cervical margins of the preparation. A snug fit at the cervical margin is desirable, even if the incisal is too long, to minimize cervical finishing of the restoration. **E,** The crown form filled with composite resin has been seated, and the excess material is being carefully removed at the cervical margins with an explorer. Note the excess material exuding from the vent hole placed on the mesial incisal of the crown form.

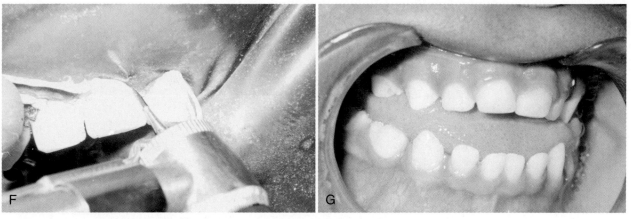

Figure 18-18 cont'd F, The central incisor was restored in a similar fashion. The incisal edges of the restorations have been trimmed back to the natural tooth structure with a No. 7901 finishing bur, which is also being used to trim the cervical margins and embrasure areas before polishing. **G,** The resin jacket crown restorations 2 months postoperatively. (Courtesy of Dr. Robert Rust.)

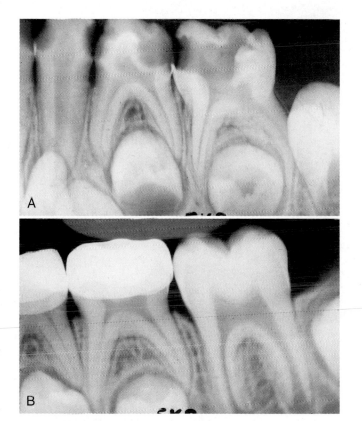

Figure 18-19 A, Primary molars with extensive carious lesions. **B,** Adequately contoured steel crowns have maintained function and the relationship of the primary teeth in the arch.

PREPARATION OF THE TOOTH

A local anesthetic should be administered and a rubber dam placed as for other restorative procedures. The proximal surfaces are reduced using a No. 69L bur at high speed (Fig. 18-20). Care must be taken not to damage adjacent tooth surfaces during the proximal reductions. A wooden wedge may be placed tightly between

the surface being reduced and the adjacent surface to provide a slight separation between the teeth for better access. Near-vertical reductions are made on the proximal surfaces and carried gingivally until the contact with the adjacent tooth is broken and an explorer can be passed freely between the prepared tooth and the adjacent tooth. The gingival margin of the preparation on the proximal surface should be a smooth feathered edge with no ledge or shoulder present. The cusps and the occlusal portion of the tooth may then be reduced with a No. 69L bur revolving at high speed. The general contour of the occlusal surface is followed, and approximately 1 mm of clearance with the opposing teeth is required.

The No. 69L bur at high speed may also be used to remove all sharp line and point angles. It is usually not necessary to reduce the buccal or lingual surfaces; in fact, it is desirable to have an undercut on these surfaces to aid in the retention of the contoured crown. In some cases, however, it may be necessary to reduce the distinct buccal bulge, particularly on the first primary molar.

If any carious dentin remains after these steps in crown preparation are completed, it is excavated next. In the event that a vital pulp exposure is encountered, a pulpotomy procedure is usually carried out.

SELECTION OF CROWN SIZE

The smallest crown that completely covers the preparation should be chosen. Spedding has advocated adhering to two important principles that will help consistently to produce well-adapted stainless steel crowns.[30] First, the operator must establish the correct occlusogingival crown length; and second, the crown margins should be shaped circumferentially to follow the natural contours of the tooth's marginal gingivae. The crown should be reduced in height, if necessary, until it clears the occlusion and is approximately 0.5 to 1 mm beneath the free margin of the gingival tissue. The patient can force the crown over the preparation by biting an orangewood stick or a tongue depressor. After making a

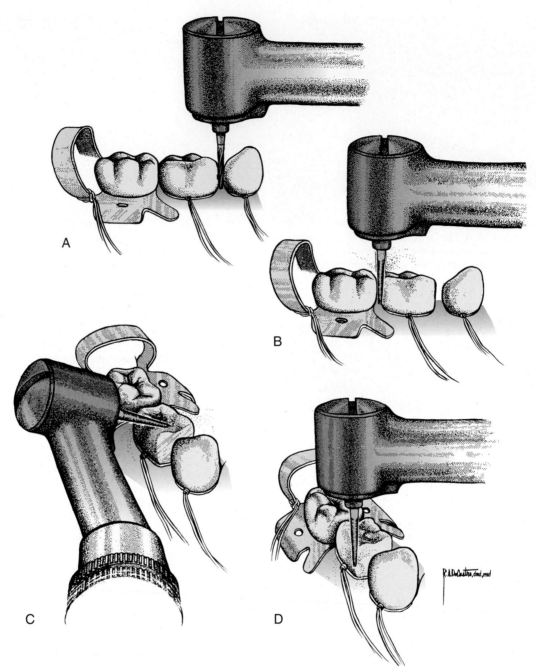

Figure 18-20 Steps in the preparation of a primary molar for a steel crown restoration using a No. 69L bur in the high-speed handpiece. **A,** Mesial reduction. **B,** Distal reduction. **C,** Occlusal reduction. **D,** Rounding of the line angles.

scratch mark on the crown at the level of the free margin of the gingival tissue, the dentist can remove the crown and determine where additional metal must be cut away with a No. 11B curved shears or a rotating stone (Fig. 18-21).

With a curved-beak pliers, the cut edges of the crown are redirected cervically and the crown is replaced on the preparation. The child is again directed to bite on an orangewood stick to forcibly seat the crown so that the gingival margins may be checked for proper extension.

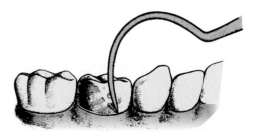

Figure 18-21 A scratch is made at the level of the free margin of the gingival tissue as an aid in determining where additional metal must be removed.

The precontoured and festooned crowns currently available often require very little, if any, modification before cementation.

CONTOURING OF THE CROWN (WHEN NECESSARY)

A crown-contouring pliers with a ball-and-socket design is used at the cervical third (if loosely fitting, start at the middle third) of the buccal and lingual surfaces to help adapt the margins of the crown to the cervical portion of the tooth. The handles of the pliers are tipped toward the center of the crown, so that the metal is stretched and curled inward as the crown is moved toward the pliers from the opposite side. A curved-beak pliers is used to further improve the contour on the buccal and lingual surfaces (Fig. 18-22). The curved-beak pliers may also be used to contour the proximal areas of the crown and develop desirable contact with adjacent teeth. Many clinicians prefer to complete the crown contouring procedures with a crown-crimping pliers (Fig. 18-23). If necessary, solder may be added to the proximal surfaces of the crown to improve the proximal contacts and contour. Trimming and contouring are continued until the crown fits the preparation snugly and extends under the free margin of the gingival tissue.

The crown should be replaced on the preparation after the contouring procedure to see that it snaps securely into place. The occlusion should be checked at this stage to make sure that the crown is not opening the bite or causing a shifting of the mandible into an undesirable relationship with the opposing teeth (Fig. 18-24).

The final step before cementation is to produce a beveled gingival margin that may be polished and that will be well tolerated by the gingival tissue. A rubber abrasive wheel can be used to produce the smooth margin.

On occasion, the best-fitting crown may need to be modified to produce a more desirable adaptation to the prepared cervical margin. Mink and Hill have referred to methods of modifying steel crowns for primary and permanent teeth.[31] The oversized crown may be cut as illustrated in Fig. 18-25 and the cut edges overlapped. The crown is replaced on the tooth to ensure that it now fits snugly at the cervical region, and a scratch is made at the overlapped margin. The crown is removed from the tooth and the overlapped material repositioned and welded. A small amount of solder is flowed over the outside margin. The crown is finished in the previously recommended manner and cemented to the prepared tooth.

If the dentist encounters a tooth that is too large for the largest crown, a similar technique may be helpful. The crown may be cut on the buccal or lingual surface. After the crown has been adapted to the prepared tooth, an additional piece of 0.004-inch stainless steel band material may be welded into place. A small amount of solder should be added to the outer surface of the margins. The crown may then be contoured in the usual manner, polished, and cemented into place.

Finally, just as with crowns for anterior teeth, preveneered stainless steel crowns for posterior primary teeth have been developed. These crowns require considerably

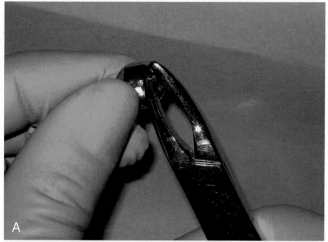

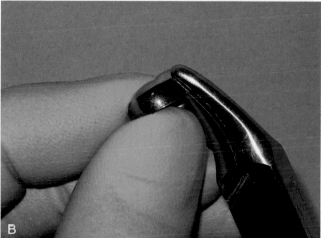

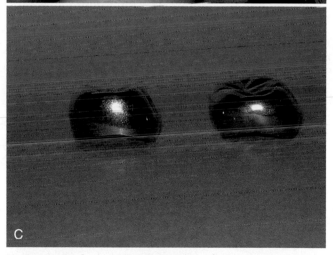

Figure 18-22 A, A crown-contouring pliers is used to contour the buccal and lingual surfaces of the crown. The crown is held firmly with the pliers, and pressure is exerted with the finger from the opposite side of the crown to bend the surface inward. **B,** The curved-beak pliers is "walked" completely around the cervical margins of the crown to direct all margins inward with smooth, flowing contour. **C,** The crown on the right was the same size and shape as the crown on the left before it was contoured. This illustrates the effectiveness of the contouring procedures with the pliers as described.

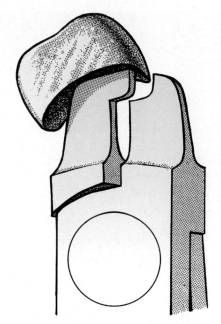

Figure 18-23 A crown-crimping pliers may also be used for crown contouring.

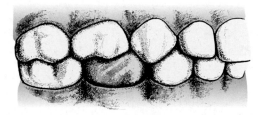

Figure 18-24 Final adaptation of the crown should result in good occlusion before cementation.

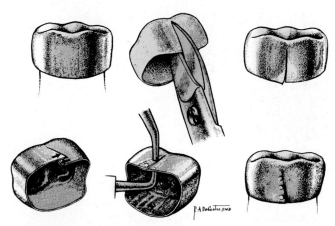

Figure 18-25 Technique for adapting an oversized crown to a prepared tooth.

more crown preparation than conventional stainless steel crowns, but Yilmaz and Kocogullari have reported success rates as high as 80%.[32]

ALTERNATIVE RESTORATIVE TREATMENT

Alternative or atraumatic restorative treatment, or *ART,* has become a popular descriptive term to describe a conservative method of managing both small and large carious lesions when treating the disease by more traditional restorative procedures is impossible or impractical for many reasons, including lack of access to traditional dental settings. This method may prevent pain and preserve teeth in individuals who do not have access to regular and conventional oral health care. ART may be performed with only hand instruments when no other dental equipment is available, but it may be useful sometimes in the conventional dental setting as well. ART does not require the complete excavation of dentinal caries before placement of the restorative material. This is not a totally new concept in dentistry, but it has enjoyed renewed recognition as a viable restorative approach because of the development of the more durable fluoride-releasing glass ionomer and resin-modified glass ionomer restorative materials. The principles validating this technique are discussed in the section Treatment of the Deep Carious Lesion in Chapter 19.

This technique is promoted and endorsed by the World Health Organization with the goals of preserving tooth structure, reducing infection, and avoiding discomfort. The International Association for Dental Research held a symposium on ART in June 1995 recognizing the technique as a means of restoring and preventing dental caries. The procedure does not require a traditional dental setting. Preventive measures to control the bacterial infection and the causative agents of the disease should also be used for optimal results following treatment.

In 2008, the American Academy of Pediatric Dentistry added the term *interim therapeutic technique (IRT).* Their reference manual differentiates the alternative restorative treatment from the interim therapeutic restorations as follows[33]:

> Because circumstances do not allow for follow-up care, ART mistakenly has been interpreted as a definitive restoration. ITR utilizes similar techniques, but has different therapeutic goals. ITR more accurately describes the procedure used in contemporary dental practice.

COSMETIC RESTORATIVE PROCEDURES FOR YOUNG PERMANENT ANTERIOR TEETH

A common problem confronting dentists who treat children is the esthetic management of anterior teeth that are discolored, developmentally undersized or malformed, malposed, or fractured. Dentists recognize that esthetic impairments of the teeth often adversely affect the social and psychologic development of the growing child. Esthetic restorative systems and bonding techniques are usually employed when restorations are indicated in these situations. Although bonding procedures are also applicable to primary tooth restorations (as described earlier in this chapter), the following discussion applies primarily to permanent anterior teeth simply because few indications are encountered in the primary dentition. However, Aron has reported the successful use of bonded porcelain veneers for primary incisors in a young patient.[34]

The following discussion assumes that one understands dental bonding principles and has a working knowledge of the process. These principles and procedures are similar for sealants, restorative resins, and resin luting agents (see Chapter 17). Some tooth preparation confined to enamel (as much as possible) is often indicated, although not always required, before cosmetic bonding procedures are performed.

BONDED COMPOSITE VENEER RESTORATIONS (COMPOSITE RESIN BONDING)

Composite restorative resins (and bonding agents) are frequently applied directly to etched enamel. The restorative resin simply becomes a veneer to improve tooth color or contour. Restorative resin-bonding techniques are particularly useful for restoring anterior crown fractures (see Chapter 21) and for cosmetically increasing the mesial-distal widths of young permanent anterior teeth (Fig. 18-26). Bonded composite veneers are also useful for restoring small hypoplastic or discolored areas on visible tooth surfaces. Many dentists also use this type of restoration to mask intrinsic discolorations by veneering the entire labial surfaces of the discolored anterior teeth. This approach may provide satisfactory cosmetic restorations for teeth with mild to moderate discolorations that will not respond to the bleaching or microabrasion procedures discussed in Chapter 7.

BONDED LAMINATE VENEER RESTORATIONS (DENTAL LAMINATES OR LAMINATE VENEERS)

The use of thin, prefitted porcelain facings (laminate veneers) that are bonded to enamel surfaces has become commonplace in cosmetic dentistry. Interest in laminate veneer restorations has grown steadily since their introduction by Faunce and Faunce.[35] Such restorations for

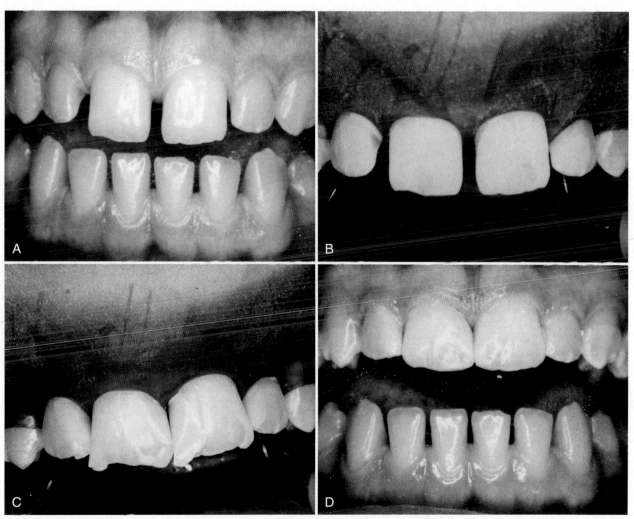

Figure 18-26 Composite resin bonding. **A,** Preoperative appearance of a 15-year-old girl who said, "I hate the spaces between my teeth." **B,** Maxillary anterior teeth isolated and etched. **C,** Composite restorative material bonded to teeth 7, 8, 9, and 10 before finishing. **D,** Postoperative appearance of finished restorations. (Courtesy of Dr. Wayne A. Moldenhauer.)

maxillary anterior teeth are recognized as conservative, esthetically satisfactory restorations, especially in children and young adults. Laminate veneer restorations have also been used successfully on mandibular anterior teeth.

The laminate veneer technique offers esthetic improvement because the restored teeth simulate the natural hue and appearance of normal, healthy tooth structure. When properly finished, the laminate restorations are well tolerated by the gingival tissues even though their contour may be slightly excessive. Immaculate oral hygiene is essential, but experience has shown that the maintenance of gingival health around the restorations is certainly possible in cooperative patients (Fig. 18-27).

The luting materials are tooth-colored resin systems designed for use in bonding techniques. If the teeth being treated are severely discolored, tinting or opaquing agents also may be required (Fig. 18-28). The laminate veneer procedure is not complicated, but it requires meticulous attention to detail for success.

The bonding procedure for a laminate veneer restoration requires proper preparation of the inside laminate surface and proper etching of the outer enamel surface. The inside of the porcelain laminate surface is etched with a hydrofluoric acid etchant and then coated with silane, which results in a bond with the resin luting agent similar to that achieved on etched enamel but also enhanced chemically by the silane. Excellent bond strengths to the porcelain surface have been reported by Lee and colleagues.[36]

The intraenamel preparation includes removal of 0.5 to 1 mm of facial enamel, tapering to about 0.25 to 0.5 mm at the cervical margin. This margin is finished in

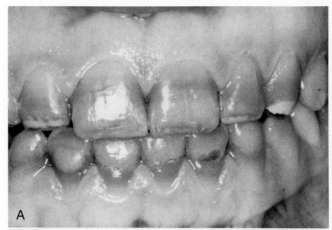

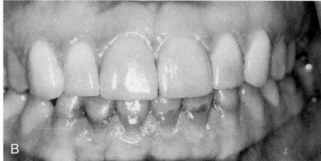

Figure 18-28 A, Severe intrinsic tooth discoloration in a teenager. **B,** Porcelain-bonded laminate veneer restorations have been placed onto the maxillary anterior teeth for a more natural appearance. The laminates were intentionally lengthened incisally to provide more coverage of the discolored lower incisors and to improve the patient's smile line.

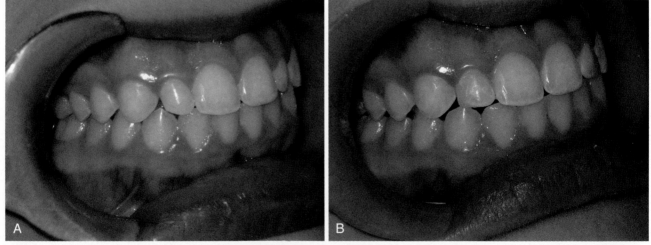

Figure 18-27 A, Undersized maxillary right lateral incisor in a young patient. **B,** Improved appearance of tooth after restoration with a bonded laminate veneer restoration.

a well-defined chamfer level with the crest of the gingival margin or not more than 0.5 mm subgingivally. The incisal margin may end just short of the incisal edge, or it may include the entire incisal edge ending on the lingual surface (Fig. 18-29). It is better not to place incisal margins where direct incising forces occur. Bonded porcelain techniques have significant value in cosmetic dental procedures (Fig. 18-30).

Refer to the text by Nixon[37] for additional information on the many varieties of materials and techniques available for dental cosmetic procedures.

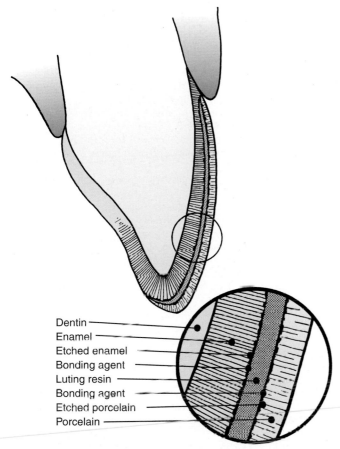

Dentin
Enamel
Etched enamel
Bonding agent
Luting resin
Bonding agent
Etched porcelain
Porcelain

Figure 18-29 Cross-sectional sketch of the intraenamel preparation and the precision-fitted porcelain laminate veneer that had been fabricated in the laboratory to restore the natural tooth contours when bonded in place.

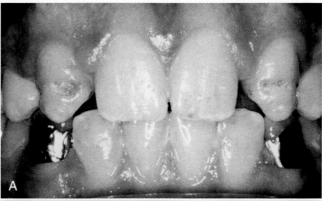
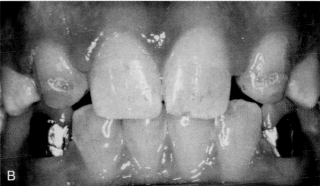
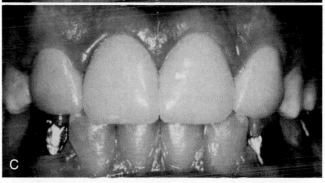

Figure 18-30 A, Anterior teeth of a teenaged patient immediately after the removal of bonded orthodontic appliances. Maxillary canines have been orthodontically positioned forward because of the congenital absence of the lateral incisors. Notice the interdental spaces distal to the central incisors and also the enlarged gingival tissues secondary (at least in part) to many months of orthodontic appliance therapy. The hypoplastic defects are obvious on the canines, and the central incisors are mildly affected as well. **B,** Photograph of same patient after completion of the intraenamel preparation of the canines. The central incisors received only minimal preparation so that the final restorations would provide slightly more support to the upper lip. No anesthesia was required during the tooth preparations, and no temporary restorations were necessary during the time the porcelain laminates were being fabricated in the laboratory. **C,** Bonded porcelain laminate restorations were placed several days later. The restored canines now resemble lateral incisors, and the interdental spaces are closed. Although the gingival tissues are somewhat irritated because of manipulation during the bonding procedures, some spontaneous reduction of the gingival enlargements are noticeable since better brushing and flossing were instituted.

REFERENCES

1. American Academy of Pediatric Dentistry. Reference Manual 31:06. Chicago: Author; 2009-2010, pp 172-179.
2. Berg JH. The continuum of restorative materials in pediatric dentistry: a review for the clinician, *Pediatr Dent* 20:93-100, 1998.
3. Bonilla E, White SN. Fatigue of resin-bonded amalgam restorations, *Oper Dent* 21:122-126, 1996.
4. Mahler DB, et al. One-year clinical evaluation of bonded amalgam restorations, *J Am Dent Assoc* 127:345-349, 1996.
5. Heise AL. Time required in rubber dam placement, *J Dent Child* 38:116-117, 1971.
6. Croll TP. Restorative dentistry for preschool children, *Dent Clin North Am* 39:737-770, 1995.
7. Suwatviroj P, et al. The effects of cavity preparation and lamination on bond strength and fracture of tooth-colored restorations in primary molars, *Pediatr Dent* 25(6):534-540, 2003.
8. Croll TP. Lateral-access class II restoration using resin-modified glass-ionomer or silver-cermet cement, *Quintessence Int* 26:121-126, 1995.
9. Vaikuntam J. Resin-modified glass ionomer cements (RM GICs): implications for use in pediatric dentistry, *J Dent Child* 64:131-134, 1997.
10. Marks LA, et al. Dyract versus Tytin class II restorations in primary molars: 36 months evaluation, *Caries Res* 33:387-392, 1999.
11. Welbury RR, et al. Clinical evaluation of paired compomer and glass ionomer restorations in primary molars: final results after 42 months, *Br Dent J* 189:93-97, 2000.
12. Hubel S, Mejare I. Conventional versus resin-modified glass-ionomer cement for class II restorations in primary molars. A 3-year clinical study, *Int J Paediatr Dent* 13:2-8, 2003.
13. Paquette DE, et al. Modified cavity preparations for composite resins in primary molars, *Pediatr Dent* 5:246-251, 1983.
14. Oldenburg TR, Vann WF Jr, Dilley DC. Composite restorations for primary molars: two-year results, *Pediatr Dent* 7:96-103, 1985.
15. Tonn EM, Ryge G. Two-year clinical evaluation of light-cured composite resin restorations in primary molars, *J Am Dent Assoc* 111:44-48, 1985.
16. Dilley DC, et al. Time required for placement of composite versus amalgam restorations, *J Dent Child* 57:177-183, 1990.
17. Donly KJ, et al. Clinical performance and caries inhibition of resin-modified glass ionomer cement and amalgam restorations, *J Am Dent Assoc* 130:1459-1466, 1999.
18. dos Santos MPA, et al. A randomized trial of resin-based restorations in class I and class II beveled preparations in primary molars, *J Am Dent Assoc* 140(2):156-166, 2009.
19. Trairatvorakul C, Piwat S. Comparative clinical evaluation of slot versus dovetail class III composite restorations in primary anterior teeth, *J Clin Pediatr Dent* 28(2):125-130, 2004.
20. McEvoy SA. A modified class III cavity preparation and composite resin filling technique for primary incisors, *Dent Clin North Am* 28:145-155, 1984.
21. MacLean JK, et al. Clinical outcomes for primary anterior teeth treated with preveneered stainless steel crowns, *Pediatr Dent* 29(5):377-381, 2007.
22. Croll TP. Primary incisor restoration using resin-veneered stainless steel crowns, *J Dent Child* 65:89-95, 1998.
23. Webber DL, et al. A method of restoring primary anterior teeth with the aid of a celluloid crown form and composite resins, *Pediatr Dent* 1:244-246, 1979.
24. Kupietzky A, et al. Long-term photographic and radiographic assessment of bonded resin composite strip crowns for primary incisors: results after 3 years, *Pediatr Dent* 27(3):221-225, 2005.
25. Roberson TM, et al. Sturdevant's Art & Science of Operative Dentistry, 5th ed. St. Louis, 2006, Mosby.
26. Radcliffe RM, Cullen CL. Preservation of future options: restorative procedures on first permanent molars in children, *J Dent Child* 58:104-108, 1991.
27. Humphrey WP. Uses of chrome steel in children's dentistry, *Dent Surv* 26:945-949, 1950.
28. Randall RC. Preformed metal crowns for primary and permanent molar teeth: review of the literature, *Pediatr Dent* 24:489-500, 2002.
29. Seale NS. The use of stainless steel crowns, *Pediatr Dent* 24:501-505, 2002.
30. Spedding RH. Two principles for improving the adaptation of stainless steel crowns to primary molars, *Dent Clin North Am* 28:157-175, 1984.
31. Mink JR, Hill CJ. Modification of the stainless steel crown for primary teeth, *J Dent Child* 38:61-69, 1971.
32. Yilmaz Y, Kocogullari ME. Clinical evaluation of two different methods of stainless steel esthetic crowns, *J Dent Child (Chic)* 71(3):212-214, 2004.
33. American Academy of Pediatric Dentistry: Reference Manual. Chicago: Author; 2008-2009;30:38-39.
34. Aron VO. Porcelain veneers for primary incisors: a case report, *Quintessence Int* 26:455-457, 1995.
35. Faunce FR, Faunce AR. The use of laminate veneers for restoration of fractured or discolored teeth, *Tex Dent J* 93(8):6-7, 1975.
36. Lee JG, et al. Bonding strengths of etched porcelain discs and three different bonding agents, *J Dent Child* 53:409-414, 1986.
37. Nixon RL. Masking severely tetracycline-stained teeth with ceramic laminate veneers, *Pract Periodontics Aesthet Dent* 8:227-235, 1996.

CHAPTER 19

Treatment of Deep Caries, Vital Pulp Exposure, and Pulpless Teeth

▲ Ralph E. McDonald, David R. Avery, and Jeffrey A. Dean

CHAPTER OUTLINE

*T*he treatment of the dental pulp exposed by the caries process, by accident during cavity preparation, or even as a result of injury and fracture of the tooth has long presented a challenge in treatment. As early as 1756, Pfaff reported placing a small piece of gold over a vital exposure in an attempt to promote healing.

Although it has been established that the pulp is capable of healing, there is still much to learn regarding the control of infection and inflammation in the vital pulp. Current methods of diagnosing the extent of pulpal injury are inadequate. More effective methods of pulp therapy are still needed, and more research is necessary.

DIAGNOSTIC AIDS IN THE SELECTION OF TEETH FOR VITAL PULP THERAPY

HISTORY OF PAIN

The history of either presence or absence of pain may not be as reliable in the differential diagnosis of the condition of the exposed primary pulp as it is in permanent teeth. Degeneration of primary pulp even to the point of abscess formation without the child's recalling pain or discomfort is not uncommon. Nevertheless, the history of a

toothache should be the first consideration in the selection of teeth for vital pulp therapy. A toothache coincident with or immediately after a meal may not indicate extensive pulpal inflammation. The pain may be caused by an accumulation of food within a carious lesion, by pressure, or by a chemical irritation to vital pulp protected by only a thin layer of intact dentin.

A severe toothache at night usually signals extensive degeneration of the pulp and calls for more than a conservative type of pulp therapy. A spontaneous toothache of more than momentary duration occurring at any time usually means that pulpal disease has progressed too far for treatment with even a pulpotomy.

CLINICAL SIGNS AND SYMPTOMS

A gingival abscess or a draining fistula associated with a tooth with a deep carious lesion is an obvious clinical sign of an irreversibly diseased pulp. Such infections can be resolved only by successful endodontic therapy or extraction of the tooth.

Abnormal tooth mobility is another clinical sign that may indicate a severely diseased pulp. When such a tooth is evaluated for mobility, the manipulation may elicit localized pain in the area, but this is not always the case. If pain is absent or minimal during manipulation of the diseased mobile tooth, the pulp is probably in a more advanced and chronic degenerative condition. Pathologic mobility must be distinguished from normal mobility in primary teeth near exfoliation.

Sensitivity to percussion or pressure is a clinical symptom suggestive of at least some degree of pulpal disease, but the degenerative stage of the pulp is probably of the acute inflammatory type. Tooth mobility or sensitivity to percussion or pressure may be a clinical signal of other dental problems as well, such as a high restoration or advanced periodontal disease. However, when this clinical information is identified in a child and is associated with a tooth having a deep carious lesion, the problem is most likely to be caused by pulpal disease and possibly by inflammatory involvement of the periodontal ligament.

RADIOGRAPHIC INTERPRETATION

A recent x-ray film must be available to examine for evidence of periradicular or periapical changes, such as thickening of the periodontal ligament or rarefaction of the supporting bone. These conditions almost always rule out treatment other than an endodontic procedure or extraction of the tooth. Radiographic interpretation is more difficult in children than in adults. The permanent teeth may have incompletely formed root ends, giving an impression of periapical radiolucency, and the roots of the primary teeth undergoing even normal physiologic resorption often present a misleading picture or one suggestive of pathologic change.

The proximity of carious lesions to the pulp cannot always be determined accurately in the x-ray film. What often appears to be an intact barrier of secondary dentin protecting the pulp may actually be a perforated mass of irregularly calcified and carious material. The pulp beneath this material may have extensive inflammation (Fig. 19-1). Radiographic evidence of calcified masses within the pulp chamber is diagnostically important. If the irritation to the pulp is relatively mild and chronic, the pulp will respond with inflammation and will attempt to eliminate the irritation by blocking with irregular dentin the tubules through which the irritating factors are transmitted. If the irritation is intense and acute and if the carious lesion is developing rapidly, the defense mechanism may not have a chance to lay down the reparative dentin barrier, and the disease process may reach the pulp. In this instance the pulp may attempt to form a barrier at some distance from the exposure site. These calcified masses are sometimes evident in the pulp horn or even in the region of the pulp canal entrance. A histologic examination of these teeth shows irregular, amorphous masses of calcified material that are not like pulp stones (Fig. 19-2). The masses bear no resemblance to dentin or to a dentinal barrier. In every instance they are associated with advanced degenerative changes of the coronal pulp and inflammation of the tissue in the canal.

PULP TESTING

The value of the electric pulp test in determining the condition of the pulp of primary teeth is questionable, although it will give an indication of whether the pulp is

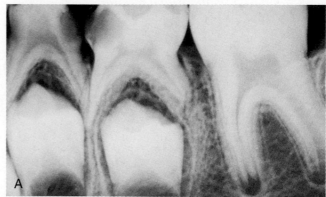

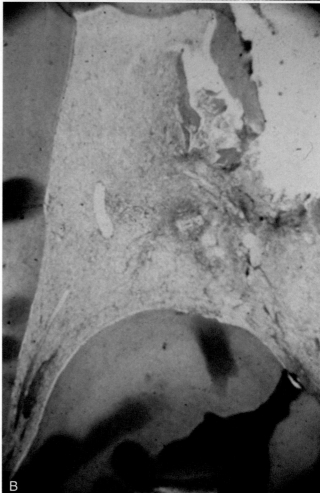

Figure 19-1 A, First primary molar appears to have an intact dentinal barrier beneath the carious lesion. **B,** Histologic section shows a perforation of the barrier with necrotic material at the exposure site. There is advanced inflammation of the pulp tissue, which is likely to evoke a spontaneous pain response.

vital. The test does not provide reliable evidence of the degree of inflammation of the pulp. A complicating factor is the occasional positive response to the test in a tooth with a necrotic pulp if the content of the canals is liquid. The reliability of the pulp test for the young child can also be questioned sometimes because of the child's

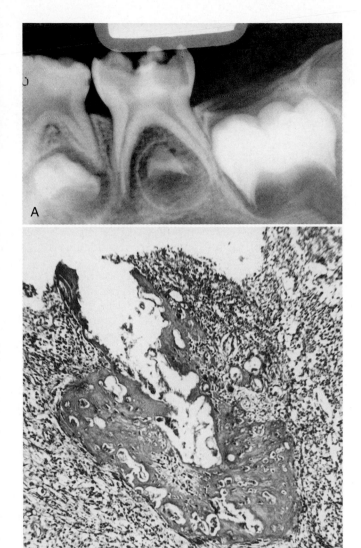

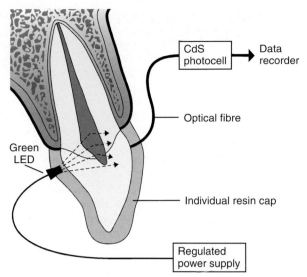

Figure 19-3 Schematic drawing of transmitted-light photo-plethysmography. LED, light-emitting diode. (Adapted from Miwa Z, et al. Pulpal blood flow in vital and nonvital young permanent teeth measured by transmitted-light photople-thysmography: A pilot study. Pediatr Dent 2002;24[6]: 594-598.)

Figure 19-2 A, Calcified mass in the pulp chamber beneath the exposure site is associated with extensive inflammation of the pulp in the coronal area and in the pulp canals. **B,** The amorphous mass is surrounded by pulp tissue with advanced inflammation.

apprehension associated with the test itself. Thermal tests have reliability problems in the primary dentition, too. The lack of reliability is possibly related to the young child's inability to understand the tests.

Several methods have been developed and advocated as noninvasive techniques for recording the blood flow in human dental pulp. Two of these methods include the use of a laser Doppler flowmeter and transmitted-light photoplethysmography. As shown in the schematic in Fig. 19-3, these methods essentially work by transmitting a laser or light beam through the crown of the tooth; the signal is picked up on the other side of the tooth by an optical fiber and photocell. A distinct advantage of this technique is its noninvasive nature, particularly in comparison to electric pulp testing. Not only is there inaccuracy in the response of the pulp to electric stimuli, but the electric pulp tester may elicit pain. Because the testing may be uncomfortable for young patients, further dental treatment may be affected. A study by Miwa and colleagues suggests that the transmitted-light technique can detect pulpal blood flow in young permanent teeth and is thus applicable to the assessment of pulp vitality.[1]

PHYSICAL CONDITION OF THE PATIENT

Although the local observations are of extreme importance in the selection of cases for vital pulp therapy, the dentist must also consider the physical condition of the patient. In seriously ill children, extraction of the involved tooth after proper premedication with antibiotics, rather than pulp therapy, should be the treatment of choice. Children with conditions that render them susceptible to subacute bacterial endocarditis or those with nephritis, leukemia, solid tumors, idiopathic cyclic neutropenia, or any condition that causes cyclic or chronic depression of granulocyte and polymorphonuclear leukocyte counts should not be subjected to the possibility of an acute infection resulting from failed pulp therapy. Occasionally, pulp therapy for a tooth of a chronically ill child may be justified, but only after careful consideration is given to the prognosis of the child's general condition, the prognosis of the endodontic therapy, and the relative importance of retaining the involved tooth.

EVALUATION OF TREATMENT PROGNOSIS BEFORE PULP THERAPY

The diagnostic process of selecting teeth that are good candidates for vital pulp therapy has at least two dimensions. First, the dentist must decide that the tooth has a good chance of responding favorably to the pulp therapy procedure indicated. Second, the advisability of performing the pulp therapy and restoring the tooth must be weighed against extraction and space management. For example, nothing is gained by successful pulp therapy if the crown of the involved tooth is nonrestorable or the periodontal structures are irreversibly diseased. By the same rationale, a dentist is likely to invest more time and effort to save a pulpally involved second primary molar in a 4-year-old child with unerupted first permanent molars than to save a pulpally involved first primary molar in an 8-year-old child.

Other factors to consider include the following:

1. The level of patient and parent cooperation and motivation in receiving the treatment
2. The level of patient and parent desire and motivation in maintaining oral health and hygiene
3. The caries activity of the patient and the overall prognosis of oral rehabilitation
4. The stage of dental development of the patient
5. The degree of difficulty anticipated in adequately performing the pulp therapy (instrumentation) in the particular case
6. Space management issues resulting from previous extractions, preexisting malocclusion, ankylosis, congenitally missing teeth, and space loss caused by the extensive carious destruction of teeth and subsequent drifting
7. Excessive extrusion of the pulpally involved tooth resulting from the absence of opposing teeth

These examples, in any combination, illustrate the almost infinite number of treatment considerations that could be important in an individual patient with pulpal pathosis.

TREATMENT OF THE DEEP CARIOUS LESION

Children and young adults who have not received early and adequate dental care and optimal systemic fluoride and do not have adequate oral hygiene often develop deep carious lesions in the primary and permanent teeth. Many of the lesions appear radiographically to be dangerously close to the pulp or to actually involve the dental pulp. Approximately 75% of the teeth with deep caries have been found from clinical observations to have pulpal exposures. Work by Dimaggio and Hawes supports this observation.[2,3] They also showed that well over 90% of the asymptomatic teeth with deep carious lesions could be successfully treated without pulp exposure using indirect pulp therapy techniques. This procedure is described herein.

If a carious exposure discovered at the time of the initial caries excavation could be routinely treated with consistently good results, a major problem in dentistry would be solved. Unfortunately, the treatment of vital exposures, especially in primary teeth, has not been entirely successful. For this reason, clinicians prefer to avoid pulp exposure during the removal of deep caries whenever possible.

INDIRECT PULP TREATMENT (GROSS CARIES REMOVAL OR INDIRECT PULP THERAPY)

The procedure in which only the gross caries is removed from the lesion and the cavity is sealed for a time with a biocompatible material is referred to as indirect pulp treatment (Fig. 19-4). Indirect pulp treatment is not a new procedure but has attracted renewed interest. Laboratory studies and favorable clinical evidence justify its routine use. Teeth with deep caries that are free of symptoms of painful pulpitis are candidates for this procedure.

The clinical procedure involves removing the gross caries but allowing sufficient caries to remain over the pulp horn to avoid exposure of the pulp. The walls of the cavity are extended to sound tooth structure because the presence of carious enamel and dentin at the margins of the cavity will prevent the establishment of an adequate seal (extremely important) during the period of repair. The remaining thin layer of caries in the base of the cavity is covered with a radiopaque biocompatible base material and sealed with a durable interim restoration (Fig. 19-5). Some interim restorative materials may also serve as the base material. It is sometimes helpful to adapt and cement a preformed stainless steel band to the tooth to support the interim restoration during the observation period (Fig. 19-6).

Other operative procedures can be performed at subsequent visits. However, the treated teeth should not be reentered to complete the removal of caries for at least 6 to 8 weeks. During this time the caries process in the deeper layer is arrested.

At the conclusion of the minimum 6- to 8-week waiting period, the tooth is reentered. Careful removal of the remaining carious material, now somewhat sclerotic, may reveal a sound base of dentin without an exposure of the pulp. If a sound layer of dentin covers the pulp, the tooth

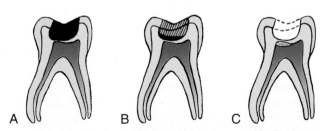

Figure 19-4 Indirect pulp therapy. **A,** A primary or permanent tooth with deep caries. **B,** The gross caries has been removed and the cavity sealed with durable biocompatible cement or restorative material. **C,** Six to 8 weeks later the cavity is reopened and the remaining caries excavated. A sound dentin barrier protects the pulp, and the tooth is ready for final restoration. (Courtesy of Dr. Paul E. Starkey.)

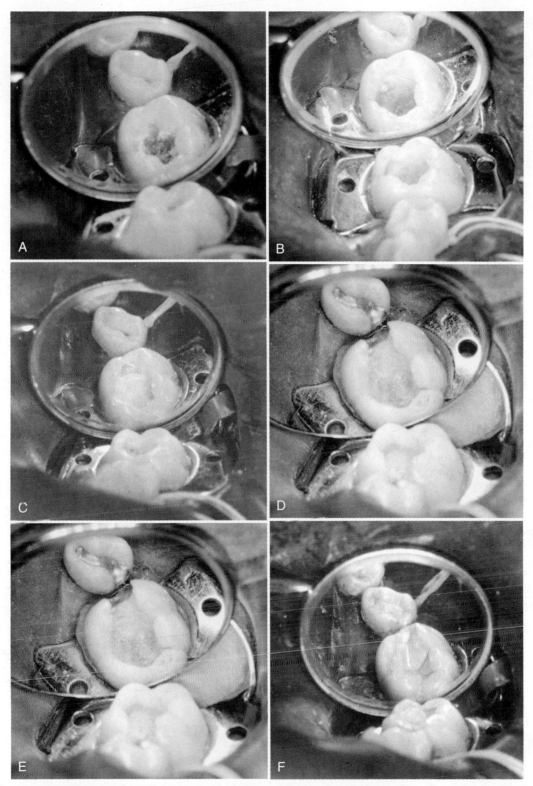

Figure 19-5 A, Second primary molar with deep occlusal caries. Because the tooth was free of symptoms of painful pulpitis, indirect pulp therapy was completed. **B,** The gross caries has been removed. A small amount of soft carious dentin remains at the base of the cavity. **C,** Calcium hydroxide has been placed over the remaining caries. The cavity may be sealed with a durable intermediate restorative material. **D,** After 6 to 8 weeks, the intermediate restorative material is removed. The caries in the base of the cavity appears arrested and dry. **E,** The remaining caries has been removed. **F,** After placement of a biocompatible base, the primary second molar has been restored with amalgam.

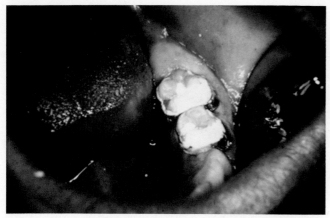

Figure 19-6 Preformed steel band has been cemented to the tooth to support the indirect pulp treatment material.

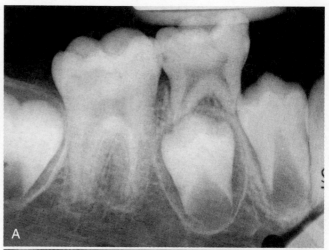

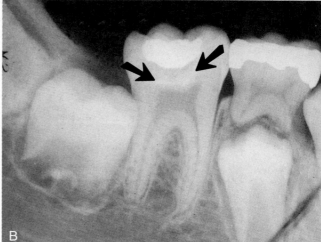

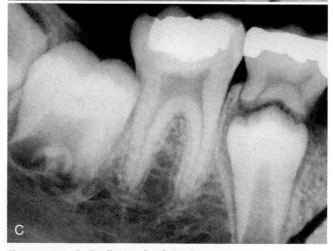

is restored in the conventional manner (Fig. 19-7). Al-Zayer and associates reported that the use of a base over the calcium hydroxide liner, in addition to a stainless steel crown, dramatically increases the success rate.[4] If a small pulp exposure is encountered, a different type of treatment, based on the clinical signs and symptoms and local conditions, must be used.

Studies by Traubman, who used television linear and density measurement instrumentation, indicated that the rate of regular dentin formation during the indirect pulp treatment was highest during the first month, but dentin formation continued during the year of experimental observation.[5] At the end of the 1-year observation period, some teeth had formed as much as 390 μm of new dentin on the pulpal floor. This observation provides justification for leaving the sealed interim restoration in place for longer than the minimal 6 weeks.

Nirschl and Avery performed indirect pulp therapy on 38 carefully selected primary and young permanent teeth.[6] Gross caries removal under rubber dam isolation was accomplished, calcium hydroxide was used in each tooth as a sedative base, and the teeth were restored with amalgam.

Successful treatment occurred in 32 (94.1%) of the 34 teeth that were available for the 6-month evaluation procedure. In all cases of successful treatment the base material and the residual carious dentin were observed to be dry on reentry and clinical examination. Of the successfully treated teeth, only four had residual carious dentin that felt somewhat soft when probed with an explorer; in the remainder the dentin felt hard. Pinto and colleagues showed similar dentin consistency results, as well as significantly decreased bacterial counts at the end of treatment.[7]

Indirect pulp therapy has been proved to be a valuable therapeutic procedure in treating asymptomatic teeth with deep carious lesions. The procedure reduces the risk of direct pulp exposure and preserves pulp vitality. One may question the need to reenter the tooth if it has been properly selected and monitored, if a durable restoration is placed initially, and if no adverse signs or symptoms develop. Most clinicians are successfully practicing

Figure 19-7 A, Radiograph of the first permanent molar revealed a deep carious lesion. Gross caries was removed, and calcium hydroxide was placed over the remaining caries. The tooth was restored with amalgam and was not reentered for complete caries removal for 3 months. **B,** Sclerotic dentin can be seen beneath the remaining caries and the covering of calcium hydroxide *(arrows)*. **C,** The tooth was reentered, and the remaining caries was removed. A sound dentin barrier was observed at the base of the cavity. A new amalgam restoration was placed after complete caries removal.

indirect pulp treatment without reentry after the initial caries excavation. The inexperienced dentist, however, may want to consider performing the treatment in two appointments until confidence in proper case selection has been achieved.

VITAL PULP EXPOSURE

Although the routine practice of indirect pulp therapy in properly selected teeth will significantly reduce the number of direct pulp exposures encountered, all dentists who treat severe caries in children will be faced with treatment decisions related to the management of vital pulp exposures.

The appropriate procedure should be selected only after a careful evaluation of the patient's symptoms, results of diagnostic tests, and conditions at the exposure site. The health of the exposed dental pulp is sometimes difficult to determine, especially in children, and there is often lack of conformity between clinical symptoms and histopathologic condition.

SIZE OF THE EXPOSURE AND PULPAL HEMORRHAGE

The size of the exposure, the appearance of the pulp, and the amount of bleeding are valuable observations in diagnosing the condition of the primary pulp. For this reason the use of a rubber dam to isolate the tooth is extremely important; in addition, with the rubber dam the area can be kept clean and the work can be done more efficiently.

The most favorable condition for vital pulp therapy is the small pinpoint exposure surrounded by sound dentin. However, a true carious exposure, even of pinpoint size, will be accompanied by inflammation of the pulp, the degree of which is usually directly related to the size of the exposure (Fig. 19-8).

A large exposure—the type that is encountered when a mass of leathery dentin is removed—is often associated with a watery exudate or pus at the exposure site. These conditions are indicative of advanced pulp degeneration and often of internal resorption in the pulp canal. In addition, excessive hemorrhage at the point of carious exposure or during pulp amputation is invariably associated with hyperemia and generalized inflammation of the pulp. When a generalized inflammation of the pulp is observed, endodontic therapy or extraction of the tooth is the treatment of choice.

DENTAL HEMOGRAM

Guthrie's findings have substantiated the previously mentioned observations.[8] His study was designed to investigate the value of a white blood cell differential count (hemogram) of the dental pulp as a diagnostic aid in determining pathologic or degenerative changes in the pulp. The first drop of blood from an exposed pulp was used for making the hemogram. The teeth were subsequently extracted. Based on a histologic examination it was decided whether they would have been good candidates for a pulpotomy procedure. Those teeth in which the inflammatory process was localized to the coronal pulp area were classified as good candidates for a pulpotomy. If the inflammation extended into the pulp canal beyond the area of convenient amputation, the tooth was considered a poor candidate. Although there was no consistent blood picture throughout the group, the teeth considered to be poor risks all had an elevated neutrophil count and gave evidence of profuse bleeding and pain other than at mealtime. In the histologic examination, numerous teeth in the poor risk group showed evidence of internal resorption in the pulp canal.

The use of the dental hemogram is not a practical diagnostic method in the routine clinical management of vital pulp exposures. However, experimental use of the dental hemogram has confirmed that a history of spontaneous pain and clinical evidence of profuse pulpal hemorrhage tend to correlate well with significant inflammation of pulpal tissue.

VITAL PULP THERAPY TECHNIQUES

For many centuries, and probably from almost the beginning of time for human beings, there has been a search for the best (safe and effective) methods of managing pulpal disease and traumatic pulpal exposure. During the twentieth century a significant share of the total dental research effort was devoted to finding better treatments and prevention methods for pulpal problems. These efforts have generated considerable controversy and debate as proponents of specific materials and methods attempt to justify their chosen techniques. These controversies are unsettled even now in the twenty-first century, despite many impressive scientific advancements. Identifying the best formulation of ingredients and techniques to predictably produce pulpal healing remains elusive. To further complicate this issue, the predominant belief is that pulp therapies appropriate for permanent teeth may not always be equally effective in treating similar pulpal conditions in primary teeth.

It is generally agreed that the prognosis after any type of pulp therapy improves in the absence of contamination by pathogenic microorganisms. Thus biocompatible neutralization of any existing pulpal contamination and

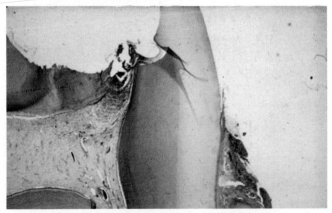

Figure 19-8 Pulp exposed by caries will show inflammation at the exposure site. Fragments of necrotic dentin will be introduced into the pulp during the excavation of the caries.

prevention of future contamination (e.g., microleakage) are worthy goals in vital pulp therapy. If the treatment material in direct contact with the pulp also has some inherent quality that promotes, stimulates, or accelerates a true tissue-healing response, so much the better; however, it is recognized that vital pulp tissue can recover from a variety of insults spontaneously in a favorable environment.

The techniques and procedures discussed in the following pages represent the standards as we perceive them at this writing. Some go back to the time when treatment decisions were made empirically. Their effectiveness has been proved over time, if not by science, and they represent the benchmarks with which newer techniques are compared. We look forward to having more effective, biologically compatible, and scientifically sound methods in the future.

DIRECT PULP CAPPING

The pulp-capping procedure has been widely practiced for years and is still the favorite method of many dentists for treating vital pulp exposures. Although pulp capping has been condemned by some, others report that, if the teeth are carefully selected, excellent results are obtained.

It is generally agreed that pulp-capping procedures should be limited to small exposures that have been produced accidentally by trauma or during cavity preparation or to true pinpoint carious exposures that are surrounded by sound dentin (Fig. 19-9). Pulp capping should be considered only for teeth in which there is an absence of pain, with the possible exception of discomfort caused by the intake of food. In addition, there should be either no bleeding at the exposure site, as is often the case in a mechanical exposure, or bleeding in an amount that would be considered normal in the absence of a hyperemic or inflamed pulp.

All pulp treatment procedures should be carried out under clean conditions using sterile instruments. Use of the rubber dam will help keep the pulp free of external contamination. All peripheral carious tissue should be excavated before excavation is begun on the portion of the carious dentin most likely to result in pulp exposure. Thus most of the bacterially infected tissue will have been removed before actual pulp exposure occurs. The work of Kakehashi and colleagues[9] and of Walshe,[10] which is described later in this chapter, supports the desirability of using a surgically clean technique to minimize bacterial contamination of the pulpal tissue.

Calcium hydroxide remains the standard material for pulp capping normal vital pulp tissue. The possibility of its stimulating the repair reaction is good. A hard-setting calcium hydroxide capping material should be used. If the tooth is small (such as a first primary molar), the hard-setting calcium hydroxide may also be used as the base for the restoration. Some studies have shown successful results with direct capping of exposed pulps with adhesive bonding agents, whereas others have reported pulp inflammation and unacceptable results using this technique.[11] In addition, the use of mineral trioxide aggregate has shown promise, but further research would be helpful.[12] Therefore the traditional practice of using calcium hydroxide can be maintained.

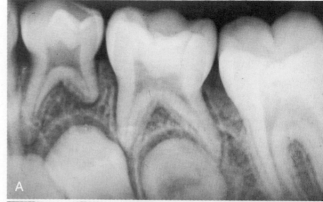

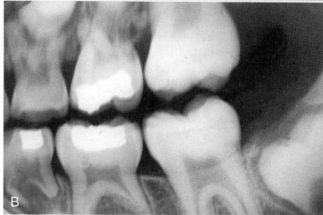

Figure 19-9 A, Mesial pulp horn of the mandibular second primary molar accidentally exposed during cavity preparation was covered with calcium hydroxide. **B,** Dentinal bridge across the mesial pulp horn is evidence of pulp healing.

PULPOTOMY

The removal of the coronal portion of the pulp is an accepted procedure for treating both primary and permanent teeth with carious pulp exposures. The justification for this procedure is that the coronal pulp tissue, which is adjacent to the carious exposure, usually contains microorganisms and shows evidence of inflammation and degenerative change. The abnormal tissue can be removed, and the healing can be allowed to take place at the entrance of the pulp canal in an area of essentially normal pulp. Even the pulpotomy procedure, however, is likely to result in a high percentage of failures unless the teeth are carefully selected.

In the pulpotomy procedure the tooth should first be anesthetized and isolated with the rubber dam. A surgically clean technique should be used throughout the procedure. All remaining dental caries should be removed, as well as the overhanging enamel, to provide good access to coronal pulp. Pain during caries removal and instrumentation may be an indication of faulty anesthetic technique. More often, however, it indicates pulpal hyperemia and inflammation, which makes the tooth a poor risk for vital pulpotomy. If the pulp at the exposure site bleeds excessively after complete removal of caries, the tooth is also a poor risk for vital pulpotomy.

The entire roof of the pulp chamber should be removed. No overhanging dentin from the roof of the pulp chamber or pulp horns should remain. No attempt is made to control the hemorrhage until the coronal pulp has been amputated. A funnel-shaped access to the entrance of the root canals should be produced. A sharp discoid spoon excavator, large enough to extend across the entrance of the individual root canals, may be used to amputate the coronal pulp at its entrance into the canals. The pulp stumps should be cleanly excised with no tags of tissue extending across the floor of the pulp chamber. The pulp chamber should then be irrigated with a light flow of water from the water syringe and evacuated. Cotton pellets moistened with water should be placed in the pulp chamber and allowed to remain over the pulp stumps until a clot forms (Fig. 19-10).

Laboratory and clinical observations indicate that a different technique and capping material are necessary in the treatment of primary teeth than in treatment of permanent teeth. As a result of these observations, two specific pulpotomy techniques have evolved and are in general use.

Pulpotomy Technique for Permanent Teeth

The calcium hydroxide pulpotomy technique is recommended in the treatment of permanent teeth with carious pulp exposures when there is a pathologic change in the pulp at the exposure site, although the use of mineral trioxide aggregate deserves further study. This procedure is particularly indicated for permanent teeth with immature root development but with healthy pulp tissue in the root canals. It is also indicated for a permanent tooth with a pulp exposure resulting from crown fracture when the trauma has also produced a root fracture of the same tooth. The procedure is completed during a single appointment. Only teeth free of symptoms of painful pulpitis are considered for treatment. The procedure involves the amputation of the coronal portion of the pulp as

described, the control of hemorrhage, and the placement of a calcium hydroxide capping material over the pulp tissue remaining in the canals (Fig. 19-11). A protective layer of hard-setting cement is placed over the calcium hydroxide to provide an adequate seal. The tooth is subsequently prepared for full-coverage restoration. However, if the tissue in the pulp canals appears hyperemic

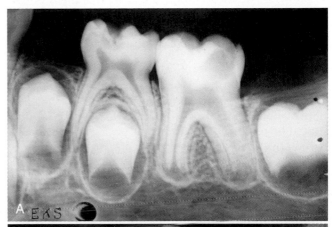
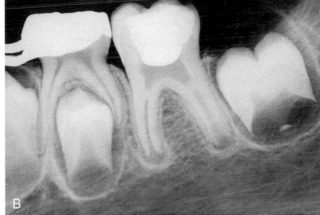
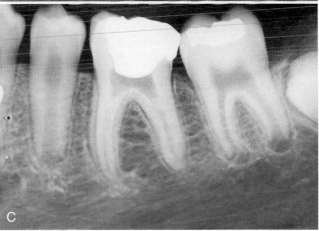

Figure 19-11 A, Pulp of the first permanent molar was exposed by caries. The tooth was considered a candidate for the calcium hydroxide pulpotomy technique. **B,** Calcified bridge has formed over the vital pulp in the canals. **C,** Continued root development and pulpal recession are indicative of continuing pulpal vitality. The crown should be supported with a full-coverage restoration.

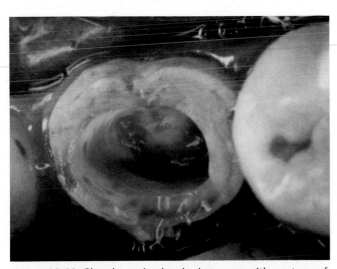

Figure 19-10 Cleanly excised pulpal stumps with no tags of tissue across the floor or along the walls of the chamber. The hemorrhage has been controlled. Notice also that the roof of the pulp chamber has been completely removed to provide total access to the pulp canals.

after the amputation of the coronal tissue, a pulpotomy should no longer be considered. Endodontic treatment is indicated if the tooth is to be saved.

After 1 year, a tooth that has been treated successfully with a pulpotomy should have a normal periodontal ligament and lamina dura, radiographic evidence of a calcified bridge if calcium hydroxide was used as the capping material, and no radiographic evidence of internal resorption or pathologic resorption. The treatment of permanent teeth by the calcium hydroxide method has resulted in a higher rate of success when the teeth are selected carefully based on existing knowledge of diagnostic techniques.

Pulpotomy Technique for Primary Teeth

The same diagnostic criteria recommended for the selection of permanent teeth for the pulpotomy procedure should be used in the selection of primary teeth for the pulpotomy procedure. The treatment is also completed during a single appointment. A surgically clean technique should be used. The coronal portion of the pulp should be amputated as described previously, the debris should be removed from the chamber, and the hemorrhage should be controlled. If there is evidence of hyperemia after the removal of the coronal pulp, which indicates that inflammation is present in the tissue beyond the coronal portion of the pulp, the technique should be abandoned in favor of the partial pulpectomy or the removal of the tooth. If the hemorrhage is controlled readily and the pulp stumps appear normal, it may be assumed that the pulp tissue in the canals is normal, and it is possible to proceed with the pulpotomy.

Although the formocresol pulpotomy technique has been recommended for many years as the principal method for treating primary teeth with carious exposures, a substantial shift away from use of this medicament has occurred because of concerns about its toxic effects. Many alternatives have been investigated to replace formocresol as the medicament of choice for a pulpotomy technique. Despite this, formocresol continues to be a very commonly used pulpotomy medicament. Indeed, Milnes' reevaluation of earlier and more recent research about formaldehyde metabolism, pharmacokinetics, and carcinogenicity led him to suggest that there is an inconsequential risk associated with formocresol's use in pediatric pulp therapy.[13] The pulp chamber is dried with sterile cotton pellets. Next, a pellet of cotton moistened with a 1:5 concentration of Buckley's formocresol and blotted on sterile gauze to remove the excess is placed in contact with the pulp stumps and is allowed to remain for 5 minutes. Because formocresol is caustic, care must be taken to avoid contact with the gingival tissues. The pellets are then removed, and the pulp chamber is dried with new pellets. A thick paste of hard-setting zinc oxide–eugenol is prepared and placed over the pulp stumps. The tooth is then restored with a stainless steel crown (Fig. 19-12).

Although the recommendation is that the blotted cotton pellet moistened with a 1:5 concentration of formocresol be applied to the pulp stumps for 5 minutes, the 5-minute application time has been determined somewhat arbitrarily. Few data are available to verify the optimal application time. García-Godoy and colleagues

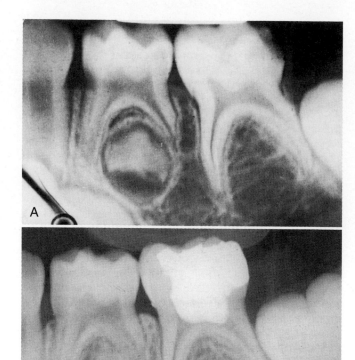

Figure 19-12 A, Formocresol pulpotomy technique was completed. **B,** Normal appearance of the supporting tissues is indicative of a successful treatment. The tooth should now be restored with a stainless steel crown.

have suggested that a 1-minute application time may be adequate and perhaps superior to the recommended 5 minutes based on their limited work with pulpotomies in dogs.[14] These authors agree, however, that further studies are needed for verification.

A series of research studies by Loos, Straffon, and Han,[15-17] have led to the conclusion that a dilute (1:5 concentration) of Buckley's formocresol applied to tissue achieves the desired cellular response as effectively as the full-strength formocresol agent, yet allows a faster recovery of the affected cells. The researchers suggested that the 1:5 concentration is a safer medicament that would produce equally good results with fewer postoperative problems in pulpotomy procedures. The original Buckley's formula for formocresol calls for equal parts of formaldehyde and cresol (Sultan Chemists, Inc., Englewood, NJ). The 1:5 concentration of this formula is prepared by first thoroughly mixing three parts of glycerin with one part of distilled water, then adding four parts of this diluent to one part of Buckley's formocresol, and thoroughly mixing again.

Some dentists prefer to make the pulp-capping material by mixing the zinc oxide powder with equal parts of eugenol and formocresol. There are no proved contraindications to adding formocresol to the mixture; however, neither are there any proven benefits. In view of the caustic nature of formocresol and the concern of some regarding the toxic and mutagenic potential from the excessive use of formocresol, its use in zinc oxide–eugenol paste is discouraged.

PARTIAL PULPECTOMY

A partial pulpectomy may be performed on primary teeth when coronal pulp tissue and the tissue entering the pulp canals are vital but show clinical evidence of hyperemia (Fig. 19-13). The tooth may or may not have a history of painful pulpitis, but the contents of the root canals should not show evidence of necrosis (suppuration). In addition, there should be no radiographic evidence of a thickened periodontal ligament or of radicular disease. If any of these conditions is present, a complete pulpectomy (described later) or an extraction should be performed.

The partial pulpectomy technique, which may be completed in one appointment, involves the removal of the coronal pulp as described for the pulpotomy technique. The pulp filaments from the root canals are removed with a fine barbed broach; considerable hemorrhage will occur at this point. A Hedström file will be helpful in the removal of remnants of the pulp tissue. The file removes tissue only as it is withdrawn and penetrates readily with a minimum of resistance. Care should be taken to avoid penetrating the apex of the tooth.

Many dentists prefer to use root canal instruments placed in a special handpiece for root canal débridement. Root canal instrumentation may be facilitated with the judicious use of this mechanical technique, especially in canals that are difficult to negotiate with hand instruments. Cautious manipulation is important, however, to prevent breaking the file or overinstrumenting the canal and apical tissues.

After the pulp tissue has been removed from the canals, a syringe is used to irrigate them with 3% hydrogen peroxide followed by sodium hypochlorite. The canals should then be dried with sterile paper points. When hemorrhaging is controlled and the canals remain dry, a thin mix of unreinforced zinc oxide–eugenol paste may be prepared (without setting accelerators), and paper points covered with the material are used to coat the root

canal walls. Small Kerr files may be used to file the paste into the walls. The excess thin paste may be removed with paper points and Hedström files. A thick mix of the treatment paste should then be prepared, rolled into a point, and carried into the canal. Root canal pluggers may be used to condense the filling material into the canals. An x-ray film may be necessary to allow evaluation of the success in filling the canals (Fig. 19-14). Further

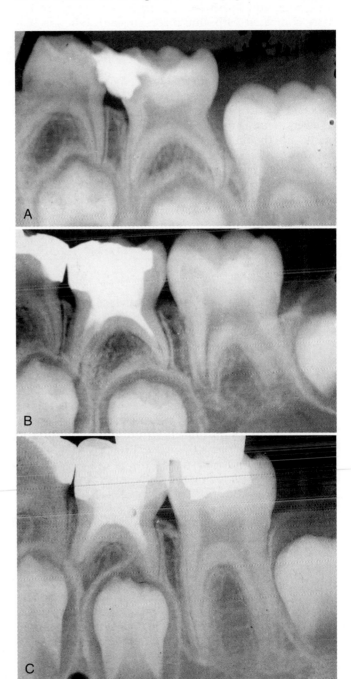

Figure 19-14 A, Pulp in the second primary molar showed evidence of inflammation. The tooth was treated with the partial pulpectomy technique. **B,** Thirteen months after treatment, the second primary molar was asymptomatic and the supporting tissues appeared normal. **C,** Three years after the initial treatment, the radiograph of the second primary molar appears normal. The first permanent molar has erupted into a good position.

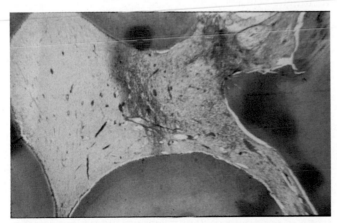

Figure 19-13 Histologic section of a second primary molar with a carious pulp exposure. There was clinical evidence of hyperemia and inflammation of the pulp. Inflammation is evident in half the coronal pulp and into the pulp canal. This condition may be treated using the partial pulpectomy technique.

condensation may be carried out if required. The tooth should be restored with full coverage.

Although zinc oxide–eugenol paste is viewed as the traditional root canal filling material for primary teeth, multiple studies[18-23] suggest that KRI paste (Pharmachemie AG, Drusberstr. 125, CH-8053 Zurich, Switzerland) may be preferable. Excellent results have been observed in many cases. The primary components of KRI paste are zinc oxide and iodoform. The main advantages of KRI paste compared with zinc oxide–eugenol paste are that KRI paste resorbs in synchrony with primary roots and is less irritating to surrounding tissues if a root is inadvertently overfilled.

Another popular root canal filling material for primary teeth is Vitapex (Dia Dent Group International, Inc., Vancouver, British Columbia, Canada), a product that has received many favorable anecdotal reports about its successful use in infected primary teeth. The primary components of Vitapex are calcium hydroxide and iodoform. Considerable laboratory and animal research has been reported. Vitapex may be at least as effective as KRI paste, and Nurko and García-Godoy[21,24] have published some human reports.

NONVITAL PULP THERAPY TECHNIQUE

COMPLETE PULPECTOMY

It is unwise to maintain untreated infected primary teeth in the mouth. They may be opened for drainage and often remain asymptomatic for an indefinite period. However, they are a source of infection and should be treated or removed. The morphology of the root canals in primary teeth makes endodontic treatment difficult and often impractical. Mature first primary molar canals are often so small that they are inaccessible even to the smallest barbed broach. If the canal cannot be properly cleansed of necrotic material, sterilized, and adequately filled, endodontic therapy is more likely to fail.

Hibbard and Ireland studied the primary root canal morphology by removing the pulp from extracted teeth, forcing acrylic resin into the pulp canals, and dissolving the covering of tooth structure in 10% nitric acid.[25] It was apparent that initially only one root canal was present in each of the mandibular and maxillary molar roots. The subsequent deposition of secondary dentin throughout the life of the teeth caused a change in the morphologic pattern of the root canal, producing variations and eventual alterations in the number and size of the canals. The variations included lateral branching, connecting fibrils, apical ramifications, and partial fusion of the canals. These findings explain the complications often encountered in root canal therapy.

Endodontic procedures for the treatment of primary teeth with necrotic pulps are indicated if the canals are accessible and if there is evidence of essentially normal supporting bone. Aminabadi and colleagues have demonstrated that while primary second molars are more accessible than first molars, all of them are negotiable.[26] In addition, other studies have looked at ultrasonic instrumentation[27] and root apex locators[28] in the root canal

treatment of primary teeth. If the supporting bone is also compromised, the likelihood of successful endodontic therapy is lower. If the second primary molar is lost before the eruption of the first permanent molar, the dentist is confronted with the difficult problem of preventing the first permanent molar from drifting mesially during its eruption. Special effort should be made to treat and retain the second primary molar even if it has a necrotic pulp. Similarly, longer than normal retention of a second primary molar may be desired when the succedaneous second premolar is congenitally missing (Fig. 19-15).

Starkey developed the following complete pulpectomy technique for primary molars.[29] The rubber dam should be applied, and the roof of the pulp chamber should be removed to gain access to the root canals as described previously in the pulpotomy technique. The contents of the pulp chamber and all debris from the occlusal third of the canals should be removed, with care taken to avoid forcing any of the infected contents through the apical foramen. A pellet moistened with camphorated monochlorophenol (CMCP) or a 1:5 concentration of Buckley's formocresol, with excess moisture blotted, should be placed in the pulp chamber. The chamber may be sealed with zinc oxide–eugenol. At the second appointment, several days later, the tooth should be isolated with a rubber dam and the treatment pellet removed. If the tooth has remained asymptomatic during the interval, the remaining contents of the canals should be removed using the technique described for the partial pulpectomy. The apex of each root should be penetrated slightly with the smallest file. (The dentist should experiment with dissociated primary molars to develop a feel for the instrument as it just penetrates the apex.) A treatment pellet should again be placed in the pulp chamber and the seal completed with zinc oxide–eugenol. After another few days the treatment pellet should be removed. If the tooth has remained asymptomatic, the canals may be prepared and filled as described for the partial pulpectomy. However, if the tooth has been painful and there is evidence of moisture in the canals when the treatment pellet is removed, the canals should again be mechanically cleansed and the treatment repeated.

Currently, pulpectomies in primary teeth are commonly completed in a single appointment (Fig. 19-16). If the tooth has painful necrosis with purulence in the canals, however, completing the pulpectomy procedure over two or three visits should improve the likelihood of success.

SUMMARY OF PULP THERAPY

The preceding discussion of various pulp therapies conforms, in principle, to the Guidelines for Pulp Therapy for Primary and Young Permanent Teeth as reaffirmed by the American Academy of Pediatric Dentistry in 2004.[30]

When one encounters clinical problems that will likely require pulp therapy to return the patient to satisfactory oral health, treatment decisions are not always clear-cut. Proper diagnosis of the pulpal problem is important to allow the dentist to select the most conservative treatment procedure that offers the best chance of

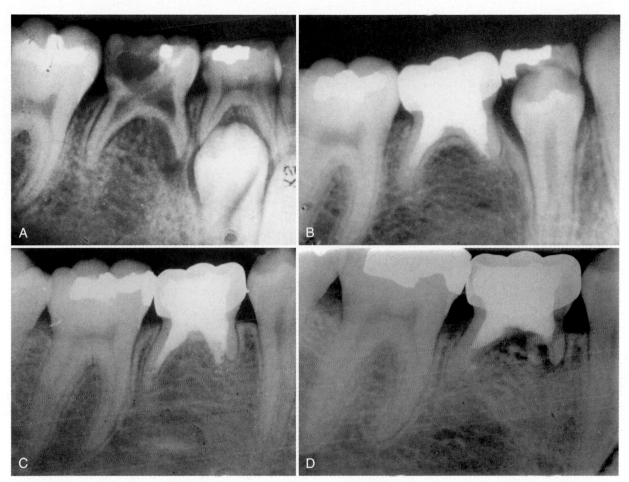

Figure 19-15 A, Necrotic tooth resulting from a carious exposure of the pulp of the second primary molar. Because the succedaneous second premolar was congenitally missing, a decision was made to attempt to save the tooth as a functional space maintainer through the growing years, if possible. Note the evidence of internal resorption at the floor of the pulp chamber. **B,** Radiograph made 1 year and 7 months after the pulp canals were treated and filled. The mesial canal was treated with complete pulpectomy; the distal canal was treated with partial pulpectomy. **C,** Six years and 7 months after treatment, the tooth is asymptomatic; the supporting tissues appear normal but some root resorption has occurred. **D,** Fourteen years and 6 months postoperatively, the tooth was extracted because of the development of symptoms and loss of bone support. At this time, the patient was a young adult and a fixed bridge was made.

long-term success with the least chance of subsequent complications. The dentist should think of the possible treatment options in a progressive manner that takes into account both treatment conservatism (e.g., a pulpotomy is more conservative than a partial pulpectomy) and post-treatment problems (Fig. 19-17). The most conservative treatment possible may not always be the indicated procedure after the dentist also weighs the risks of posttreatment failure in a particular case.

RESTORATION OF THE PULPALLY INVOLVED TOOTH

It has been a common practice for some dentists to delay for weeks or months the permanent restoration of a tooth that has undergone vital pulp therapy. The purpose has been to allow time to determine whether the treatment procedure will be successful. However, failures in pulp therapy are usually not evident for many months. Rarely

does a failure in pulp therapy or an endodontic procedure on a primary tooth cause the child to experience acute symptoms. Failures are usually evidenced by pathologic root resorption or rarefied areas in the bone and are discovered during regular recall appointments.

Primary and permanent molars that have been treated by the pulpotomy or pulpectomy technique have a weak, unsupported crown that is liable to fracture. Often a failure of the buccal or lingual plate occurs below the gingival attachment or even below the crest of the alveolar bone. This type of fracture makes subsequent restoration of the tooth impractical. Also, a delay in restoring the tooth with a material that will adequately seal the tooth and prevent an ingress of oral fluids is one cause for failure of pulp therapy. Application of a layer of hard-setting cement over the capping material followed by a substantial restoration will adequately protect the pulp against contaminating oral fluids during the healing process.

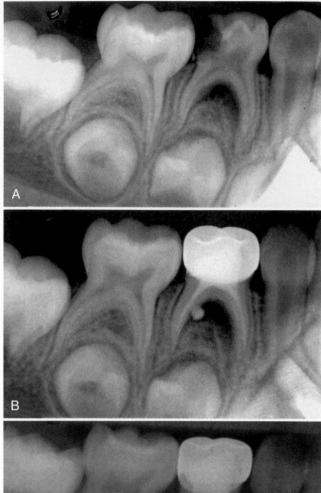

Figure 19-16 Successful single-appointment complete pulpectomy. Note extrusion of zinc oxide–eugenol into furcal area from distal root accessory canal, but adequate subsequent healing. **A,** Pretreatment. **B,** Immediately after treatment. **C,** 10 months after treatment.

An amalgam restoration, a composite resin restoration, or a glass ionomer restoration may serve as the immediate restoration and often the final restoration for teeth with pulp caps and well-supported crowns. As soon as it is practical, however, other pulpally treated posterior teeth should be prepared for stainless steel or cast crowns. Pulp treatment of a primary molar is often followed by placement of a stainless steel crown restoration during the same appointment.

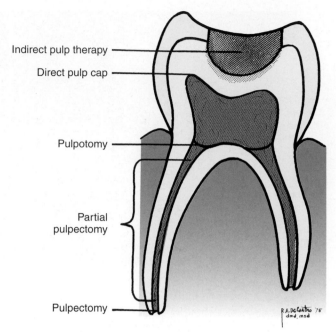

Figure 19-17 Pulp therapy progression.

REACTION OF THE PULP TO VARIOUS CAPPING MATERIALS

ZINC OXIDE–EUGENOL

Before calcium hydroxide came into common use, zinc oxide–eugenol was used more often than any other pulp-capping material. Many dentists have apparently had good clinical results with the use of zinc oxide–eugenol, but it is no longer recommended as a direct pulp-capping material.

CALCIUM HYDROXIDE

Herman first introduced calcium hydroxide as a biologic dressing.[31] Because of its alkalinity (pH of 12), it is so caustic that when it is placed in contact with vital pulp tissue the reaction produces a superficial necrosis of the pulp. The irritant qualities seem to be related to its ability to stimulate development of a calcified barrier. The superficial necrotic area in the pulp that develops beneath the calcium hydroxide is demarcated from the healthy pulp tissue below by a new, deeply staining zone comprising basophilic elements of the calcium hydroxide dressing. The original proteinate zone is still present. However, against this zone is a new area of coarse fibrous tissue likened to a primitive type of bone. On the periphery of the new fibrous tissue, cells resembling odontoblasts appear to be lining up. One month after the capping procedure, a calcified bridge is evident radiographically. This bridge continues to increase in thickness during the next 12 months (Fig. 19-18). The pulp tissue beneath the calcified bridge remains vital and is essentially free of inflammatory cells.

Many research studies can be cited regarding the use of calcium hydroxide as a pulp-capping material, and a few are included in the references for this chapter. Investigators who evaluate experimental pulp-capping

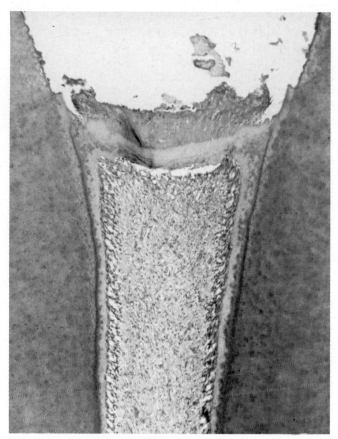

Figure 19-18 Calcified bridge covering an amputated pulp that was capped with calcium hydroxide.

agents commonly compare their results with the agent being tested to the results they can obtain with calcium hydroxide under similar conditions. Thus calcium hydroxide currently serves as the standard or control material for experimentation related to pulp-capping agents.

PREPARATIONS CONTAINING FORMALIN

The belief that exposing the pulp to formocresol or capping it with materials that contain formocresol will promote pulp healing or even maintain the pulp in a healthy state has not been adequately substantiated. Some studies have indicated that the formocresol pulpotomy technique may be applied to permanent teeth, but its use in permanent teeth remains an interim procedure to be followed by conventional endodontic therapy. The clinical success experienced in the treatment of primary pulps with these materials is possibly related to the drug's germicidal action and fixation qualities rather than to its ability to promote healing.

Doyle and associates compared the success of the full-strength formocresol pulpotomy technique with the success of the calcium hydroxide pulpotomy technique.[32] Experimental pulpotomies were performed on 65 normal human primary teeth, many of which could later be extracted for histologic examination. The formocresol technique was used on 33 teeth, and the calcium hydroxide technique was used in the treatment of the other 32. Under the conditions of this study the formocresol

pulpotomy technique yielded outcomes superior to those of the calcium hydroxide technique for at least the first 18 months after treatment. The results of the combined methods of evaluation indicated that the calcium hydroxide pulpotomy technique for primary teeth was successful in 61% of cases. The formocresol pulpotomy resulted in success in 95% of cases at the end of 1 year.

Formocresol did not stimulate the healing response of the remaining pulp tissue but rather tended to fix essentially all the remaining tissue (Figs. 19-19 and 19-20). Use of calcium hydroxide was associated with the formation of a dentin bridge and the complete healing of the amputated primary pulp in 50% of the cases that were available for histologic study.

GLUTARALDEHYDE

Glutaraldehyde has received attention as a potential pulp-capping agent for pulpotomy techniques in primary teeth. It is an excellent bactericidal agent and seems to offer some advantages compared with formocresol.

Berson and Good have reported that glutaraldehyde appears to be superior to formaldehyde preparations for pulp therapy in the following ways[33]:

1. Formaldehyde reactions are reversible, but glutaraldehyde reactions are not.

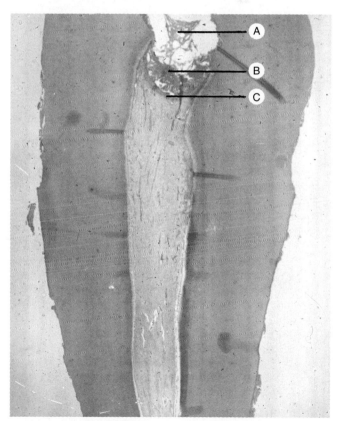

Figure 19-19 Histologic section of a primary pulp exposed to formocresol for 4 days. The medicament contacted the pulp at *A*, the debris and blood clot are evident at *B*, and a noticeably eosinophilic, compressed line is evident at *C*. The underlying pulp was a pale, homogeneously stained tissue with a loss of basophilic nuclei. (Courtesy of Dr. Walter A. Doyle.)

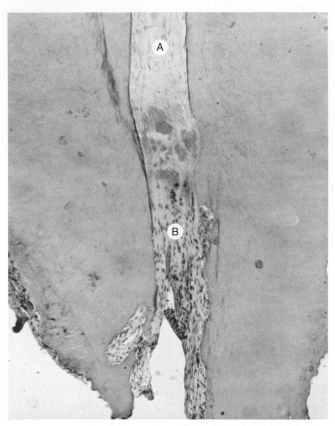

Figure 19-20 Histologic section of a primary pulp exposed to formocresol for 41 days. The pulp, *A*, appeared pale and pink, and there was a loss of cellular definition. Vital tissue can be seen in the apical portion, *B*. (Courtesy of Dr. Walter A. Doyle.)

2. Formaldehyde is a small molecule that penetrates the apical foramen, whereas glutaraldehyde is a larger molecule that does not.
3. Formaldehyde requires a long reaction time and an excess of solution to fix tissue, whereas glutaraldehyde fixes tissue instantly and an excess of solution is unnecessary.

Although glutaraldehyde seems to compare favorably with formocresol as a pulp-capping agent, it has not consistently demonstrated significant superior results in clinical trials. One clinical study by Fuks and associates found an 18% failure rate after 25 months in pulpotomized primary molars.[34] They concluded that their results did not justify substituting glutaraldehyde for formocresol treatment in primary tooth pulpotomies. Feigal and Messer have questioned the rationale for using glutaraldehyde as an alternative to formocresol after conducting a review of the available data for both agents.[35]

FERRIC SULFATE

Considerable interest and research have been devoted to investigating the effectiveness of ferric sulfate to treat the surface of the remaining pulp tissue after pulpotomy of primary teeth. Ferric sulfate agglutinates blood proteins and controls hemorrhage in the process without clot formation. Landau and Johnsen,[36] Davis and Furtado,[37] and

Fei and colleagues[38] called attention to the potential use of ferric sulfate for pulp capping after pulpotomies in animal and short-term clinical studies.

Fuks and two groups of coworkers have also contributed favorable data in an animal study and a longer-term clinical human study (mean observation period, 20.5 months).[39,40] Their success rates for ferric sulfate pulpotomies were very similar to those for dilute formocresol pulpotomies (control condition). More long-term clinical studies are needed, but currently it appears that ferric sulfate could be a better choice for treating primary teeth needing pulpotomy (equal results to dilute formocresol but with less toxicity). Ferric sulfate is available in a 15.5% solution under the trade name of Astringedent (Ultradent Products, Inc., South Jordan, Utah).

A study by Casas and colleagues compared the outcome of ferric sulfate pulpotomy with that of primary tooth root canal therapy (pulpectomy) on cariously exposed vital pulps of primary molars.[41] Although their study showed that root canal therapy had produced more acceptable treatment outcomes than ferric sulfate pulpotomy in vital pulp treatment of primary molars at a 2-year follow-up visit, the survival rates for the two techniques were not statistically different. There was no clinical evidence of pathosis in 96% of the ferric sulfate pulpotomies and 98% of the molars undergoing root canal therapy. They suggest that, for clinicians who wish to avoid aldehydes in vital molar pulp therapy for children, either one of these two alternatives is feasible. Of course, the main advantage of the ferric sulfate pulpotomy over a pulpectomy when working with children is the considerably faster speed with which a pulpotomy can be performed.

OTHER CAPPING MATERIALS (MINERAL TRIOXIDE AGGREGATE, BONE MORPHOGENETIC PROTEIN, AND OTHERS)

Pulp-capping experiments in animals have tested a variety of antibiotics and corticosteroids, alone or in combination with calcium hydroxide. Some of the earlier experiments were reported by Kutscher and Yigdall,[42] Seltzer and Bender,[43] Fiore-Donno and Baume,[44] and Baker.[45] These experiments were followed later by a study by Gardner and colleagues that tested vancomycin in combination with calcium hydroxide as a pulp-capping agent in monkeys.[46] The results of their tests, in a relatively small sample, suggested that the combination of these agents was somewhat more successful in stimulating the formation of regular reparative dentin bridges than calcium hydroxide alone. However, this work has not been expanded or repeated by others.

In the 1970s, interest in pulp-capping research shifted to other experimental materials. Tricalcium phosphate was evaluated by several investigators, including Boone and El-Kafrawy[47] and Heys and colleagues.[48] Dickey and associates[49] tested a crystalline form of pure calcium hydroxyapatite, and Ibarra[50] evaluated an experimental synthetic hydroxyapatite used in combination with chlorhexidine gluconate solution and distilled water as vehicles. None of these were as satisfactory as calcium hydroxide as a pulp-capping material. In addition, they were somewhat difficult to manipulate.

In other investigations in search of improved pulp-capping materials, agents that showed at least promising preliminary results include freeze-dried bone, chlorhexidine, feracrylum, calcium phosphate ceramics, tetracalcium phosphate cement, dentin-bonding agents in combination with bonded resin or glass ionomer materials, mineral trioxide aggregate, and bone morphogenetic proteins.[51-62]

Pulp-capping with dentin-bonding agents combined with bonding restorative materials has created considerable debate and controversy among dental investigators. Perhaps the most exciting and promising areas of pulp-capping research are the investigations underway with mineral trioxide aggregate and bone morphogenetic proteins. Both pulp treatment approaches seem to stimulate natural dentin repair at pulpal exposure sites. In research by Agamy and associates, gray mineral trioxide aggregate, white mineral trioxide aggregate, and formocresol were compared as pulp dressings in pulpotomized primary teeth.[63] Sixty pulpotomized teeth in 20 patients were studied. In both the clinical and histologic portions of the study, the gray mineral trioxide aggregate appeared to be superior to the white mineral trioxide aggregate and to formocresol as a pulp dressing for pulpotomized primary teeth.

In an excellent review on pulpotomies in primary teeth, Ranly suggested that pulpotomy modalities in primary teeth can be classified by treatment objective into three categories: devitalization, preservation, and regeneration.[64] He noted that the treatment objective of an ideal pulpotomy agent is to leave the radicular pulp vital and healthy and completely enclosed within an odontoblast-lined dentin chamber. The regeneration modality most closely resembles this ideal. Through the use of a family of bone morphogenetic proteins, it may be possible to induce reparative dentin formation with recombinant dentinogenic proteins similar to the native proteins of the body. Fuks suggests that, because the specificity of growth factors such as transforming growth factor b and bone morphogenetic protein in inducing reparative processes is not clear, further studies are required to fully understand the kinetics of growth factor release and the sequence of growth factor–induced reparative dentinogenesis.[11] Commercially available recombinant human bone morphogenetic proteins for pulp therapy are now available for experimentation and clinical trials. In addition, Sabbarini and others have demonstrated the effective use, both histologically and clinically, of an enamel matrix derivative as a pulpotomy agent in primary teeth.[65,66]

OTHER EXPERIMENTAL CAPPING METHODS

The pulp response to formocresol has been compared with electrosurgical coagulation after pulpotomies in the teeth of monkeys by Ruemping and associates.[67] The sample size was not large, and the observation periods were relatively short (maximum was 2 months after the operation), but the results of their histologic study showed the electrosurgical technique to be as favorable as the full-strength formocresol technique. Shaw and associates have also demonstrated favorable results lasting up to 6 months with electrosurgical pulpotomies in monkeys.[68]

Mack and Dean reported the results of a retrospective human study of electrosurgical pulpotomies performed on primary molars.[69] The mean postoperative observation time for the 164 teeth studied was 2 years, 3 months. They reported a 99.4% success rate (one failure) for this pulpotomy technique. In addition, Dean et al demonstrated no statistically significant difference between the electrosurgical and formocresol pulpotomy techniques in a prospective clinical study involving 50 children requiring at least one pulpotomy.[70] The children were randomly divided into two groups, with 25 undergoing the electrosurgical technique and 25 undergoing the formocresol technique. The mean age at treatment was 63.6 months and the mean postoperative observation time was 10.9 months. The clinically and radiographically determined success rates were 96% and 84%, respectively, for the electrosurgical group, and 100% and 92%, respectively, for the formocresol group. There was no statistically significant difference between results for the two techniques, although the electrosurgical group did have four failures whereas two failures occurred in the formocresol group. These researchers concluded that the results of their study support the use of electrosurgical pulpotomy as a viable alternative to formocresol pulpotomy. Rivera and colleagues[71] obtained results similar to those of Dean and associates; however, Fishman and colleagues[72] found considerably lower success rates with the use of electrosurgical pulpotomy.

Shoji and colleagues reported the results of some preliminary studies on the treatment of amputated pulps (pulpotomies) in dogs by CO_2 laser radiation.[73] Wilkerson and colleagues reported favorable pulpal responses of healing and repair in swine following pulpotomies using an argon laser.[74] Moritz and associates applied 200 direct pulp caps in adult patients after mechanical pulp exposures.[75] Half of the teeth (control group) received a conventional calcium hydroxide pulp cap. The other half (experimental group) received a calcium hydroxide cap after first undergoing CO_2 laser radiation until the "exposed pulps were completely sealed." The teeth were monitored monthly. One year after treatment, the success rate for teeth in the experimental group was 89%, whereas the success rate in the control group was 68%. Both the electrosurgical and the laser techniques seem to be favorable areas for further research in pulp therapy.

SUMMARY OF PULP-CAPPING MATERIALS

Clarity does seem to be developing regarding some research results that should allow the use of successful alternatives to formocresol.[76] However, the following survey conclusions by Dunston and Coll[77] show that we continue to lack uniformity in agreement:

Conclusions from 2005 versus 1997 survey of U.S. dental schools and diplomates of the American Board of Pediatric Dentistry:

1. For indirect pulp therapy, there has been significantly more use of glass ionomer and less zinc oxide–eugenol or calcium hydroxide liners; and most do not reenter a tooth following indirect pulp therapy.
2. Formocresol is still the preferred pulpotomy medicament but ferric sulfate use has increased. Zinc

oxide–eugenol remains the base of choice after a pulpotomy.

3. Slightly less pulpectomy therapy was advocated for abscessed teeth. When done, more were advocating iodoform and calcium hydroxide combined paste fillers. Few advocate a two-appointment pulpectomy procedure.

4. Disagreements continue and the AAPD pulp therapy guidelines and pulpal research were not always applied.

5. Diplomates tended to practice pulpal therapy similar to the way program directors teach.

FAILURES AFTER VITAL PULP THERAPY

Failure in the formation of a calcified bridge across the vital pulp has often been related to the age of the patient, degree of surgical trauma, sealing pressure, improper choice of capping material, low threshold of host resistance, and presence of microorganisms with subsequent infection. Kakehashi and colleagues studied the effect of surgical exposures of dental pulps in germ-free and conventional laboratory rats.[9] The injured pulpal tissue contaminated with microorganisms failed to show evidence of repair; especially lacking were matrix formation and attempted dentinal bridging. In the germ-free animals, bridging began in 14 days and was complete in 28 days regardless of the severity of the exposure. The major determinant in the healing of exposed rodent pulps appeared to be the presence or absence of microorganisms. These findings were later corroborated by Watts and Paterson.[78]

Walshe provided further evidence that the success of vital pulp therapy depends on adherence to a surgically aseptic technique. In his experiment the teeth of monkeys were capped with bovine dentin mixed with methylcellulose, and histologic observations were made 42 days postoperatively.[10] Approximately half the teeth capped with the experimental material were successfully repaired with atubular dentin (Fig. 19-21). The remaining teeth showed varying degrees of inflammation and repair. The Brown and Bren staining technique demonstrated the presence of microorganisms in the pulp of the teeth that failed to repair (Figs. 19-22 and 19-23). The stain also revealed microorganisms between the dentin walls and the filling material. The microorganisms were apparently introduced at the time of the pulp-capping procedure, or leakage of the restoration allowed them to gain entrance to the pulp chamber. This study likewise supports the need for a good surgical technique and the placement of a restoration that will provide the best possible seal.

INTERNAL RESORPTION

Radiographic evidence of internal resorption occurring within the pulp canal several months after the pulpotomy procedure is the most frequently seen evidence of an abnormal response in primary teeth (Fig. 19-24). Internal resorption is a destructive process generally believed to be caused by odontoclastic activity, and it may progress slowly or rapidly. Occasionally, secondary repair of the resorbed dentinal area occurs.

No satisfactory explanation for the postpulpotomy type of internal resorption has been given. It has been demonstrated, however, that with a true carious exposure of the pulp, an inflammatory process of some degree will be present. The inflammation may be limited to the exposure site, or it may be diffuse throughout the coronal portion of the pulp. Amputation of all the pulp that shows the inflammatory change may be difficult or impossible, and abnormal pulp tissue may be allowed to remain. If the inflammation extended to the entrance of the pulp canal, odontoclasts may have been attracted to the area; if it were possible to examine the tooth histologically, small bays of resorption would be evident. This condition may exist at the time of pulp therapy, although there is no way to detect it. The only indication would be the clinical evidence of a hyperemic pulp.

Inflammatory cells drawn to the area as a result of the placement of an irritating capping material might well attract the odontoclastic cells and initiate the internal resorption. This may explain the occurrence of internal resorption even though the pulp is normal at the time of treatment.

Because the roots of primary teeth are undergoing normal physiologic resorption, vascularity of the apical region is increased. Odontoclastic activity is present in the area. This may predispose the tooth to internal resorption when an irritant in the form of a pulp-capping material is placed on the pulp.

ALVEOLAR ABSCESS

An alveolar abscess occasionally develops some months after pulp therapy has been completed. The tooth usually remains asymptomatic, and the child is unaware of the infection, which may be present in the bone surrounding the root apices or in the area of the root bifurcation. A fistulous opening may be present, which indicates the chronic condition of the infection. Primary teeth that show evidence of an alveolar abscess should be removed. Permanent teeth that have previously been treated by pulp capping or by pulpotomy and later show evidence of pulpal necrosis and apical infection may be considered for endodontic treatment.

EARLY EXFOLIATION OR OVERRETENTION OF PRIMARY TEETH WITH PULP TREATMENTS

Occasionally a pulpally treated tooth previously believed to be successfully managed will loosen and exfoliate (or require extraction) prematurely for no apparent reason. It is believed that such a condition results from low-grade, chronic, asymptomatic, localized infection. Usually, abnormal and incomplete root resorption patterns of the affected teeth are also observed. When this occurs, space management must be considered.

Another sequela requiring close observation is the tendency for primary teeth undergoing successful pulpotomies or pulpectomies to be overretained. This situation may have the untoward result of interfering with the normal eruption of permanent teeth and

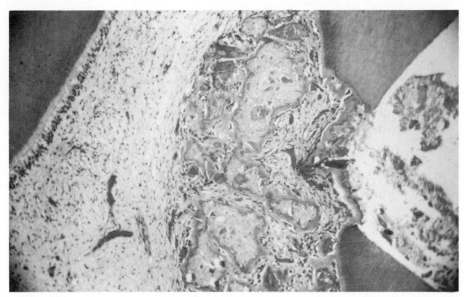

Figure 19-21 Surgical exposure of the pulp of a monkey was capped with powdered bovine dentin. Atubular dentin bridging the exposure site was evident 42 days postoperatively.

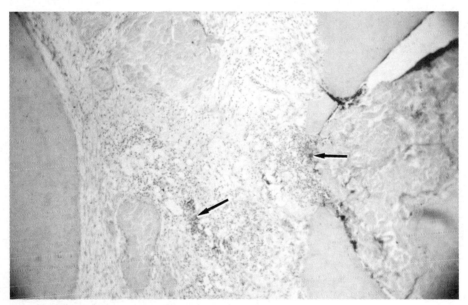

Figure 19-22. Pulps capped with bovine dentin failed to undergo calcific repair and demonstrated microorganisms *(arrows)* in the pulp. (Courtesy of Dr. Martin Walshe.)

adversely affecting the developing occlusion. Close periodic observation of pulpally treated teeth is necessary to intercept such a developing problem. Extraction of the primary tooth is usually sufficient. Starkey believes that this phenomenon occurs when normal physiologic exfoliation is delayed by the bulky amount of cement contained in the pulp chamber.[29] Even though the material is resorbable, its resorption is slowed significantly when large quantities are present (Fig. 19-25).

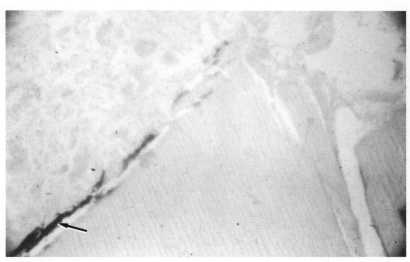

Figure 19-23 Microorganisms *(arrow)* may be seen between the dentin walls and the filling material. (Courtesy of Dr. Martin Walshe.)

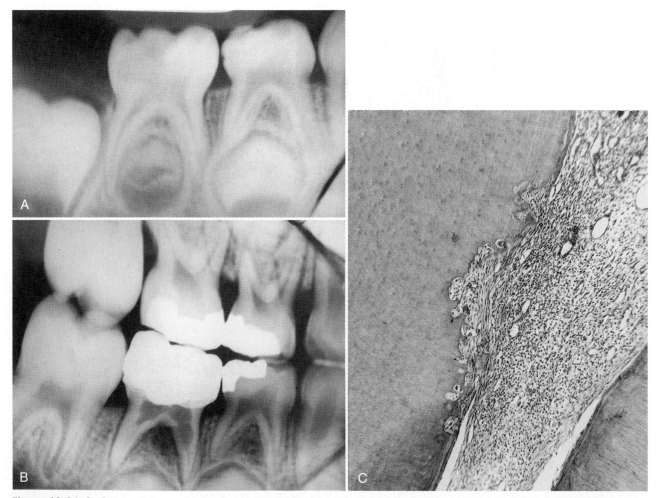

Figure 19-24 A, Preoperative radiograph of a second primary molar treated with the calcium hydroxide pulpotomy technique. **B,** Two years after treatment, internal resorption and bone rarefaction are evident. **C,** There may have been inflammation of the pulp apical to the amputation site and beginning internal resorption at the time of the initial treatment.

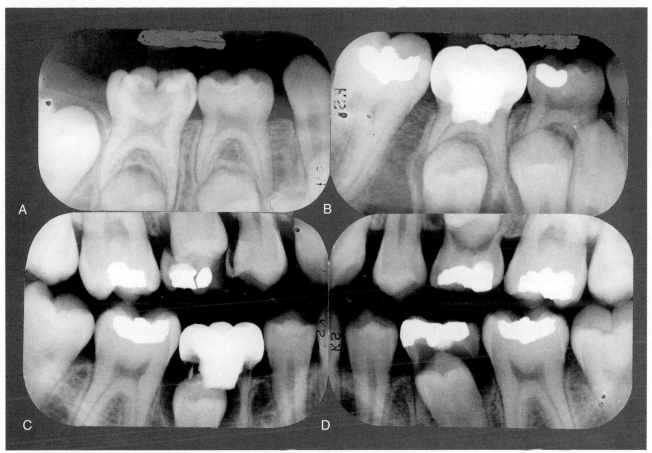

Figure 19-25 A, A pulpally involved second primary molar was successfully treated with a formocresol pulpotomy and restored with a steel crown. **B,** This 4-year posttreatment radiograph reveals long-term successful management. **C** and **D,** Bilateral bite-wing radiographs for the same patient 7 years after the pulpotomy reveal that the resorption of the pulpotomized molar is falling behind compared with its antimere. The eruption of the permanent second premolar is also being delayed. The pulpally treated tooth should be extracted at this time. (Courtesy of Dr. Wayne A. Moldenhauer.)

REFERENCES

1. Miwa Z, et al. Pulpal blood flow in vital and nonvital young permanent teeth measured by transmitted-light photoplethysmography: a pilot study, *Pediatr Dent* 24(6):594-598, 2002.
2. Dimaggio JJ, Hawes RR. Evaluation of direct and indirect pulp capping. *IADR* abstr no 40, 1962:24.
3. Dimaggio JJ, Hawes RR. Continued evaluation of direct and indirect pulp capping, *IADR* abstract no 41, 1963:380.
4. Al-Zayer MA, et al. Indirect pulp treatment of primary posterior teeth: a retrospective study, *Pediatr Dent* 25(1):29-36, 2003.
5. Traubman L 2nd. A critical clinical and television radiographic evaluation of indirect pulp capping. Master's thesis. Indianapolis, University School of Dentistry, 1967.
6. Nirschl RF, Avery DR. Evaluation of a new pulp capping agent in indirect pulp therapy, *J Dent Child* 50:25-30, 1983.
7. Pinto AS, et al. Clinical and microbiological effect of calcium hydroxide protection in indirect pulp capping in primary teeth, *Am J Dent* 19(6):382-386, 2006.
8. Guthrie TJ. An investigation of the dental pulp hemogram as a diagnostic aid for vital pulp therapy. Master's thesis. Indianapolis, Indiana University School of Dentistry, 1959.
9. Kakehashi S, et al. The effects of surgical exposure of dental pulps in germ-free and conventional laboratory rats, *Oral Surg* 20:340-349, 1965.
10. Walshe MJ. Pulp reaction to anorganic bovine dentin. Master's thesis. Indianapolis, Indiana University School of Dentistry, 1967.
11. Fuks AB. Current concepts in vital primary pulp therapy, *Eur J Paediatr Dent* 3(3):115-120, 2002.
12. Caicedo R, et al. Clinical, radiographic and histological analysis of the effects of mineral trioxide aggregate used in direct pulp capping and pulpotomies of primary teeth, *Aust Dent J* 51(4):297-305, 2006.
13. Milnes AR. Is formocresol obsolete? A fresh look at the evidence concerning safety issues, *Pediatr Dent* 30(3):237-246, 2008.
14. García-Godoy F, et al. Pulpal response to different application times of formocresol, *J Pedod* 6:176-193, 1982.
15. Loos PJ, Han SS. An enzyme histochemical study of the effect of various concentrations of formocresol on connective tissues, *Oral Surg* 31:571-585, 1971.
16. Loos PJ, et al. Biological effects of formocresol, *J Dent Child* 40:193-197, 1973.
17. Straffon LH, Han SS. Effects of varying concentrations of formocresol on RNA synthesis of connective tissues in sponge implants, *Oral Surg* 29:915-925, 1970.

18. Holan G, Fuks AB. A comparison of pulpectomies using ZOE and KRI paste in primary molars: a retrospective study, *Pediatr Dent* 15:403-407, 1993.

19. Ranly DM, García-Godoy F. Current and potential pulp therapies for primary and young permanent teeth, *J Dent* 28:153-161, 2000.

20. Ranly DM, García-Godoy F. Reviewing pulp treatment for primary teeth, *J Am Dent Assoc* 122(10):83-85, 1991.

21. García-Godoy F. Evaluation of an iodoform paste in root canal therapy for infected primary teeth, *J Dent Child* 54:30-34, 1987.

22. Rifkin A. A simple, effective, safe technique for the root canal treatment of abscessed primary teeth, *J Dent Child* 47:435-441, 1980.

23. Rifkin A. The root canal treatment of abscessed primary teeth—a three to four year follow-up, *J Dent Child* 49: 428-431, 1982.

24. Nurko C, García-Godoy F. Evaluation of the calcium hydroxide/iodoform paste (Vitapex) in root canal therapy for primary teeth, *J Clin Pediatr Dent* 23:289-294, 1999.

25. Hibbard ED, Ireland RL. Morphology of the root canals of the primary molar teeth, *J Dent Child* 24:250-257, 1957.

26. Aminabadi NA, et al. Study of root canal accessibility in human primary molars, *J Oral Sci* 50(1):69-74, 2008.

27. da Costa CC, et al. Endodontics in primary molars using ultrasonic instrumentation, *J Dent Child* 75(1):20-23, 2008.

28. Bodur H, et al. Accuracy of two different apex locators in primary teeth with and without root resorption, *Clin Oral Invest* 12(2):137-141, 2008.

29. Starkey PE. Treatment of pulpally involved primary molars. In McDonald RE, et al, eds. *Current therapy in dentistry*, vol 7. St Louis, 1980, Mosby.

30. American Academy of Pediatric Dentistry. Special issue: reference manual 2008-2009, *Pediatr Dent* 30(7 suppl): 170-174, 2004.

31. Herman B. Biologische Wurzelbehandlung. Frankfurt, Germany, 1936, W Kramer.

32. Doyle WA, et al. Formocresol versus calcium hydroxide in pulpotomy, *J Dent Child* 29:86-97, 1962.

33. Berson RB, Good DL. Pulpotomy and pulpectomy for primary teeth. In Stewart RE, et al, eds. *Pediatric dentistry: scientific foundations and clinical practice*. St Louis, 1981, Mosby.

34. Fuks AB, et al. Assessment of a 2% buffered glutaraldehyde solution in pulpotomized primary teeth of schoolchildren, *J Dent Child* 57:371-375, 1990.

35. Feigal RJ, Messer HH. A critical look at glutaraldehyde, *Pediatr Dent* 12:69-71, 1990.

36. Landau MJ, Johnsen DC. Pulpal response to ferric sulfate in monkeys, *J Dent Res* 67:215 (abstract 822), 1988.

37. Davis JM, Furtado LB. Ferric sulfate: a possible new medicament for pulpotomies in the primary dentition: the first year results from a four year study in Fortaleza, Brazil. Proceedings of the Thirteenth Congress of the International Association of Dentistry for Children, Kyoto, Japan, 1991.

38. Fei AL, et al. A clinical study of ferric sulfate as a pulpotomy agent in primary teeth, *Pediatr Dent* 13:327-332, 1991.

39. Fuks AB, et al. Pulp response to ferric sulfate, diluted formocresol and IRM in pulpotomized primary baboon teeth, *J Dent Child* 64:254-259, 1997.

40. Fuks AB, et al. Ferric sulfate versus dilute formocresol in pulpotomized primary molars: long-term follow-up, *Pediatr Dent* 19:327-330, 1997.

41. Casas MJ, et al. Two-year outcomes of primary molar ferric sulfate pulpotomy and root canal therapy, *Pediatr Dent* 25(2):97-102, 2003.

42. Kutscher AH, Yigdall I. Bacteriologic evaluation of the compatibility of antibiotics and other therapeutic agents, *Oral Surg* 5:1096-1098, 1952.

43. Seltzer S, Bender IB. Some influences affecting repair of the exposed pulps of dogs' teeth, *J Dent Res* 37:678-687, 1958.

44. Fiore-Donno G, Baume LJ. Effects of capping compounds containing corticosteroids on the human dental pulp, *Helv Odontol Acta* 6:23-32, 1962.

45. Baker GR. Topical antibiotic treatment of infected dental pulps of monkeys. Master's thesis. Indianapolis, Indiana University School of Dentistry, 1966.

46. Gardner DE, et al. Treatment of pulps of monkeys with vancomycin and calcium hydroxide, *J Dent Res* 50: 1273-1277, 1971.

47. Boone ME II, El-Kafrawy AH. Pulp reaction to a tricalcium phosphate ceramic capping agent, *Oral Surg* 47:369-371, 1979.

48. Heys DR, et al. Histologic considerations of direct pulp capping agents, *J Dent Res* 60:1371-1379, 1981.

49. Dickey DM, et al. Pulp reactions to a calcium hydroxyapatite in monkeys, *J Dent Res* 59(special issue A):360 (abstract 371), 1980.

50. Ibarra AJ. Pulp reactions to a synthetic hydroxyapatite and chlorhexidine in monkeys. Master's thesis. Indianapolis, Indiana University School of Dentistry, 1980.

51. Fadavi S, et al. Freeze-dried bone in pulpotomy procedures in monkeys, *J Pedod* 13:108-122, 1989.

52. Thomas GP, et al. Histologic study of pulp capping using chlorhexidine in dogs, *NDA J* 46:17-20, 1995.

53. Prabhu NT, Munshi AK. Clinical, radiographic and histologic observations of the radicular pulp following "feracrylum" pulpotomy, *J Clin Pediatr Dent* 21:151-156, 1997.

54. Higashi T, Okamoto H. Influence of particle size of calcium phosphate ceramics as a capping agent on the formation of a hard tissue barrier in amputated dental pulp, *J Endod* 22:281-283, 1996.

55. Yoshimine Y, Maeda K. Histologic evaluation of tetracalcium phosphate–based cement as a direct pulp-capping agent, *Oral Surg Oral Med Oral Pathol Oral Radiol Endod* 79:351-358, 1995.

56. Cox CF, et al. Biocompatibility of primer, adhesive and resin composite systems on non-exposed and exposed pulps of non-human primate teeth, *Am J Dent* 11(special issue):S55-S63, 1988.

57. Cox CF, Suzuki S. Re-evaluating pulp protection: calcium hydroxide liners vs. cohesive hybridization, *J Am Dent Assoc* 125:823-831, 1994.

58. Pameijer CH, Stanley HR. The disastrous effects of the "total etch" technique in vital pulp capping in primates, *Am J Dent* 11(special issue):S45-S54, 1988.

59. Ford TR, et al. Using mineral trioxide aggregate as a pulp capping material, *J Am Dent Assoc* 127:1491-1494, 1996.

60. Rutherford B, Fitzgerald M. A new biological approach to vital pulp therapy, *Crit Rev Oral Biol Med* 6:218-229, 1995.

61. Jepsen S, et al. Recombinant human osteogenic protein-1 induces dentin formation: an experimental study in miniature swine, *J Endod* 23:378-382, 1997.

62. Calland JW, et al. Human pulp cells respond to calcitonin gene–related peptide in vitro, *J Endod* 23:485-489, 1997.

63. Agamy HA, et al. Comparison of mineral trioxide aggregate and formocresol as pulp-capping agents in pulpotomized primary teeth, *Pediatr Dent* 26(4):302-309, 2004.

64. Ranly DM. Pulpotomy therapy in primary teeth: New modalities for old rationales, *Pediatr Dent* 16:403-409, 1994.

65. Sabbarini J, et al. Histological evaluation of enamel matrix derivative as a pulpotomy agent in primary teeth, *Pediatr Dent* 29(6):475-479, 2007.

66. Sabbarini J, et al. Comparison of enamel matrix derivative versus formocresol as pulpotomy agents in the primary dentition, *J Endod* 34(3):284-287, 2008.
67. Ruemping DR, et al. Electrosurgical pulpotomy in primates—a comparison with formocresol pulpotomy, *Pediatr Dent* 5:14-18, 1983.
68. Shaw DW, et al. Electrosurgical pulpotomy: a 6-month study in primates, *J Endod* 13:500-505, 1987.
69. Mack RB, Dean JA. Electrosurgical pulpotomy: a retrospective human study, *J Dent Child* 60:107-114, 1993.
70. Dean J, et al. Comparison of electrosurgical and formocresol pulpotomy procedures in children, *Int J Paediatr Dent* 12:177-182, 2002.
71. Rivera N, et al. Pulpal therapy for primary teeth: formocresol vs electrosurgery: a clinical study, *J Dent Child* 70(1):71-73, 2003.
72. Fishman SA, et al. Success of electrofulguration pulpotomies covered by zinc oxide and eugenol or calcium hydroxide: a clinical study, *Pediatr Dent* 18:385-390, 1996.
73. Shoji S, et al. Histopathological changes in dental pulps irradiated by CO_2 laser: a preliminary report on laser pulpotomy, *J Endod* 11:379-384, 1985.
74. Wilkerson MK, et al. Effects of the argon laser on primary tooth pulpotomies in swine, *J Clin Laser Med Surg* 14:37-42, 1996.
75. Moritz A, et al. The CO_2 laser as an aid in direct pulp capping, *J Endod* 24:248-251, 1998.
76. Fuks AB. Vital pulp therapy with new materials for primary teeth: new directions and treatment perspectives, *Pediatr Dent* 30(3):211-219, 2008.
77. Dunston B, Coll JA. A survey of primary tooth pulp therapy as taught in US dental schools and practiced by diplomates of the American Board of Pediatric Dentistry, *Pediatr Dent* 30(1):42-48, 2008.
78. Watts A, Paterson RC. Bacterial contamination as a factor influencing the toxicity of materials to the exposed dental pulp, *Oral Surg* 64:466-474, 1987.

SUGGESTED READINGS

Buckley J. Practical therapeutics: a rational treatment for putrescent pulps, *Dent Rev* 18:1193-1197, 1904.

Fadavi S, Anderson AW. A comparison of the pulpal response to freeze-dried bone, calcium hydroxide, and zinc oxide–eugenol in primary teeth in two cynomolgus monkeys, *Pediatr Dent* 18:52-56, 1996.

Farooq NS et al. Success rates of formocresol pulpotomy and indirect pulp therapy in the treatment of deep dentinal caries in primary teeth, *Pediatr Dent* 22:278-286, 2000.

Fuks AB. Pulp therapy for the primary and young permanent dentitions, *Pediatr Dent* 44:571-596, 2000.

Fuks AB, Bimstein E. Clinical evaluation of diluted formocresol pulpotomies in primary teeth of schoolchildren, *Pediatr Dent* 3:321-324, 1981.

Lazzari EP, et al. Biochemical effects of formocresol on bovine pulp tissue, *Oral Surg* 45:796-802, 1978.

Morawa AP et al. Clinical evaluation of pulpotomies using dilute formocresol, *J Dent Child* 42:360-363, 1975.

Myers DR et al. Distribution of 14C formaldehyde after pulpotomy with formocresol, *J Am Dent Assoc* 96:805-813, 1978.

Myers DR et al. The acute toxicity of high doses of systemically administered formocresol in dogs, *Pediatr Dent* 3:37-41, 1981.

Myers DR et al. Tissue changes induced by the absorption of formocresol from pulpotomy in dogs, *Pediatr Dent* 5:6-8, 1983.

Ranly DM, et al. The loss of 3H-formaldehyde from zinc oxide–eugenol cement: an in vitro study, *J Dent Child* 42:128-132, 1975.

CHAPTER 20

Gingivitis and Periodontal Disease

▲ Ralph E. McDonald, David R. Avery, James A. Weddell, and Vanchit John

CHAPTER OUTLINE

The gingiva is the part of the oral mucous membrane that covers the alveolar processes and the cervical portions of the teeth. It has been divided traditionally into the free and the attached gingiva.[1] The free gingiva is the tissue coronal to the bottom of the gingival sulcus. The attached gingiva extends apically from the free gingival groove to the mucogingival junction.

The gingival tissues are normally light pink, although the color may be related to the complexion of the person, the thickness of the tissue, and the degree of keratinization. The gingival color of the young child may be more reddish due to increased vascularity and thinner epithelium. The surface of the gingiva of a child appears less stippled or smoother than that of an adult. In the healthy adult, the marginal gingiva has a sharp, knifelike edge.[2] During the period of tooth eruption in the child, however, the gingivae are thicker and have rounded margins due to the migration and cervical constriction of the primary teeth.

Delaney reports probing depths around primary teeth to be approximately 2 mm, with the facial and lingual probe sites shallower than the proximal sites.[3] Children have a wider periodontal ligament than the adult. The width of the attached gingiva is narrower in the mandible than in the maxilla, and both widths increase with the transition from the primary to permanent dentition in the child. The alveolar bone surrounding the primary dentition demonstrates fewer trabeculae, less calcification, and larger marrow spaces.

Recent recognition that periodontal disease may have its origins in childhood has led dentists to be more aggressive in treatment. Studies confirm a high prevalence of gingival inflammation in children. Periodontal conditions that progress rapidly and result in the loss of primary and permanent teeth have been noted with increased frequency. Therefore, the American Academy of Pediatric Dentistry's recommendations for children and adolescents includes placing greater emphasis on the prevention, early diagnosis, and treatment of gingival and periodontal disease in children.[4] By establishing excellent oral hygiene habits in children, which will carry over to adulthood, the risk of periodontal disease is lowered.

Gingivitis is an inflammation involving only the gingival tissues next to the tooth. Microscopically, it is characterized by the presence of an inflammatory exudate and edema, some destruction of collagenous gingival fibers, and ulceration and proliferation of the epithelium facing the tooth and attaching the gingiva to it. Numerous studies indicate that marginal gingivitis is the most common form of periodontal disease and starts in early childhood.

Severe gingivitis is relatively uncommon in children, although numerous surveys have shown that a large portion of the pediatric population has a mild, reversible type of gingivitis. The major etiologic factors associated with gingivitis and more significant periodontal disease are uncalcified and calcified bacterial plaque. However, gingivitis rarely progresses to periodontitis in the preschool and grade school child.

Bacterial plaque, which is composed of soft bacterial deposits that adhere firmly to the teeth, is considered to be a complex, metabolically interconnected, highly organized bacterial system consisting of dense masses of microorganisms embedded in an intermicrobial matrix (biofilm). In sufficient concentration it can disturb the host-parasite relationship and cause dental caries and periodontal disease.

Eastcott and Stallard have observed that plaque begins to form within 2 hours after the teeth are brushed.[5] Coccal forms of bacteria form first on a thin fenestrated pellicle (organic bacteria-free film deposited on the tooth surface). The surface is completely covered with a smooth material 3 hours after brushing. Within 5 hours, plaque microcolonies develop, apparently by cell division. Between 6 and 12 hours, the covering material becomes thinner and is reduced to discontinuous small scattered areas. About 30% of the coccus bacteria are in various stages of division by 24 hours. Rod-shaped bacteria appear for the first time in 24-hour-old plaque. Within 48 hours the surface of the plaque is covered with a mass of rods and filaments.

Dental calculus, which is considered to be calcified dental plaque, is discussed later in the chapter. It is classified as supragingival or subgingival, depending on its location on the tooth. Supragingival calculus occurs as hard, firmly adherent masses on the enamel of teeth. Subgingival calculus is found as a concretion on the tooth in the confines of the periodontal pocket. The surface of dental calculus is always covered by uncalcified plaque. Calculus is an important factor in the development of gingival and periodontal disease.

Suomi and colleagues, in a study of approximately 1700 children 9 to 14 years of age, found that a relatively high percentage of children of all racial-ethnic groups had calculus (both supragingival and subgingival).[6] From 56% to 85% of the children in the various age, sex, and racial-ethnic groups had supragingival calculus. The findings of this study indicate that most children 9 to 14 years of age who are of low socioeconomic status would benefit from inclusion in a preventive periodontal disease program based on improvement of oral hygiene.

ERUPTION GINGIVITIS

A transitory type of gingivitis is often observed in young children when the primary teeth are erupting. This gingivitis, often localized and associated with difficult eruption, subsides after the teeth emerge into the oral cavity.

Weddell and Klein conducted a study to determine the prevalence of gingivitis in a group of children between 6 and 36 months of age.[7] The children, patients of pediatricians in the Indianapolis area, had been born in the area, which has a fluoridated water supply. Among 299 white children, gingivitis was present in 13% of those 6 to 17 months of age, 34% of those in the 18- to 23-month age group, and 39% of those in the 24- to 36-month age group. Black children were not included in the study because of the inconsistency of their gingival colors. The gingivitis observed by Weddell and Klein was for the most part eruption gingivitis. Nevertheless, their findings support the view that an oral hygiene program should be initiated by parents when the child is very young.

The greatest increase in the incidence of gingivitis in children is often seen in the 6- to 7-year age group when the permanent teeth begin to erupt. This increase in gingivitis apparently occurs because the gingival margin receives no protection from the coronal contour of the tooth during the early stage of active eruption, and the continual impingement of food on the gingivae causes the inflammatory process.

Food debris, materia alba, and bacterial plaque often collect around and beneath the free tissue, partially cover the crown of the erupting tooth, and cause the development of an inflammatory process (Fig. 20-1). This inflammation is most commonly associated with the eruption of the first and second permanent molars, and the condition can be painful and can develop into a pericoronitis or a pericoronal abscess. Mild eruption gingivitis requires no treatment other than improved oral hygiene. Painful pericoronitis may be helped when the area is irrigated with a counterirritant, such as Peroxyl (Colgate-Palmolive Co., New York, NY). Pericoronitis accompanied by swelling and lymph node involvement should be treated with antibiotic therapy.

DENTAL PLAQUE INDUCED GINGIVITIS

The degree of dental cleanliness and the condition of the gingival tissues in children are related. Horowitz and associates observed significant improvements in the gingivitis

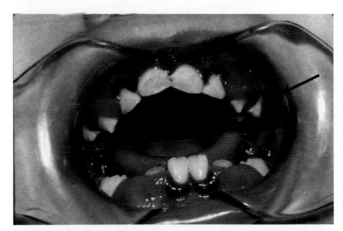

Figure 20-1 Mild inflammation *(arrow)* is evident in the tissue partially covering the crown of the erupting first permanent molar.

scores of schoolchildren after the initiation of a supervised daily plaque removal program.[8] Children in grades 5 to 8 participated in the program, and successful results were maintained during three school years. The mean gingivitis scores were reduced 40% among girls and 17% among boys during the program period, whereas the children in the control group maintained essentially the same gingivitis scores for the period of the study. Adequate mouth hygiene and cleanliness of the teeth are related to frequency of brushing and the thoroughness with which bacterial plaque is removed from the teeth. Favorable occlusion and the chewing of coarse, detergent-type foods, such as raw carrots, celery, and apples, have a beneficial effect on oral cleanliness.

In a study of 2876 children residing in a naturally fluoridated area, Murray confirmed the high prevalence of gingivitis in the young population.[9] He observed that inflammation of one or more papillae or margins associated with the incisor and canine teeth occurred in 90% of children 8 to 18 years of age. He, too, pointed to the importance of a good standard of oral cleanliness in reducing gingivitis and, ideally, preventing the progression of the disease in later life.

Gingivitis associated with poor oral hygiene is usually classified as early (slight), moderate, or advanced. Early gingivitis is quickly reversible and can be treated with a good oral prophylactic treatment and instruction in good toothbrushing and flossing techniques to keep the teeth free of bacterial plaque (Figs. 20-2 and 20-3). Gingivitis is generally less severe in children than in adults with similar plaque levels.

ALLERGY AND GINGIVAL INFLAMMATION

Matsson and Moller studied the degree of seasonal variation of gingival inflammation in children with allergies to birch pollen.[10] Thirty-four allergic children were examined during two successive spring seasons and the one intervening fall. Age- and sex-matched controls were also examined in the fall. Gingival inflammation

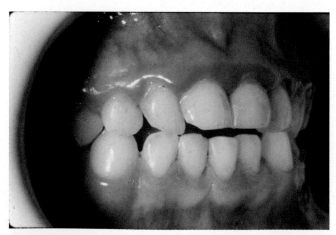

Figure 20-2 Gingivitis resulting from poor oral hygiene and reduced function in the area. A painful second primary molar has interfered with normal function on this side of the mouth.

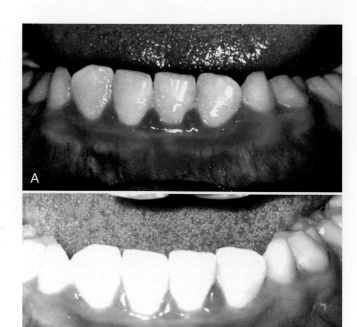

Figure 20-3 A, Localized gingival inflammation and recession associated with minimal plaque accumulation on mandibular right central incisor. **B,** Gingival health was greatly improved after a thorough plaque removal regimen was initiated at home.

and the presence or absence of plaque were recorded, and a bleeding/plaque ratio was calculated for each subject. The results indicated an enhanced gingival inflammatory reaction in the allergic children during the pollen seasons. Although the authors acknowledge that the significance of gingival reaction during short allergic seasons is difficult to assess, they speculate that patients with complex allergies who have symptoms for longer periods may be at higher risk for more significant adverse periodontal changes.

ACUTE GINGIVAL DISEASE

HERPES SIMPLEX VIRUS INFECTION

Herpes virus causes one of the most widespread viral infections. The primary infection usually occurs in a child younger than 6 years of age who has had no contact with the type 1 herpes simplex virus (HSV-1) and who therefore has no neutralizing antibodies. It is believed that 99% of all primary infections are of the subclinical type. The infection may also occur in susceptible adults who have not had a primary infection (Fig. 20-4).

In some preschool children the primary infection may be characterized by only one or two mild sores on the oral mucous membranes, which may be of little concern to the child or may go unnoticed by the parents. In other

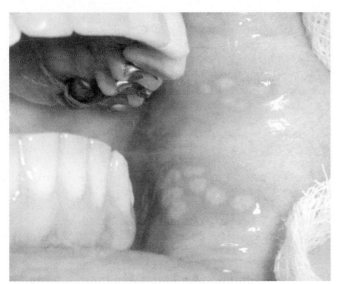

Figure 20-4 Ulcerated stage of primary herpes in a young adult. Notice the circumscribed confluent areas of inflammation.

children, the primary infection may be manifested by acute symptoms (acute herpetic gingivostomatitis). The active symptoms of the acute disease can occur in children with clean mouths and healthy oral tissues. In fact, these children seem to be as susceptible as those with poor oral hygiene. The symptoms of the disease develop suddenly and include, in addition to the fiery red gingival tissues, malaise, irritability, headache, and pain associated with the intake of food and liquids of acid content. A characteristic oral finding in the acute primary disease is the presence of yellow or white liquid-filled vesicles. In a few days the vesicles rupture and form painful ulcers, 1 to 3 mm in diameter, which are covered with a whitish gray membrane and have a circumscribed area of inflammation (Figs. 20-5 and 20-6). The ulcers may be observed on any area of the mucous membrane, including buccal mucosa, tongue, lips, hard and soft palate, and the tonsillar areas. Large ulcerated lesions may occasionally be observed on the palate or gingival tissues or in the region of the mucobuccal fold. This distribution makes the differential diagnosis more difficult. An additional diagnostic criterion is a fourfold rise of serum antibodies to HSV-1. The lesion culture also shows positive results for HSV-1.

Treatment of acute herpetic gingivostomatitis in children, which runs a course of 10 to 14 days, should include specific antiviral medication as well as provision for the relief of the acute symptoms so that fluid and nutritional intake can be maintained. The application of a mild topical anesthetic, such as dyclonine hydrochloride (0.5%) (Dyclone) before mealtime temporarily relieves the pain and allows the child to take in soft food. Another topical anesthetic, lidocaine (Xylocaine Viscous), can be prescribed for the child who can hold 1 teaspoon of the anesthetic in the mouth for 2 to 3 minutes and then expectorate the solution. Schaaf recommends as an alternative to the anesthetic a mixture of equal parts of diphenhydramine (Benadryl) elixir and Kaopectate.[11] This material can be compounded

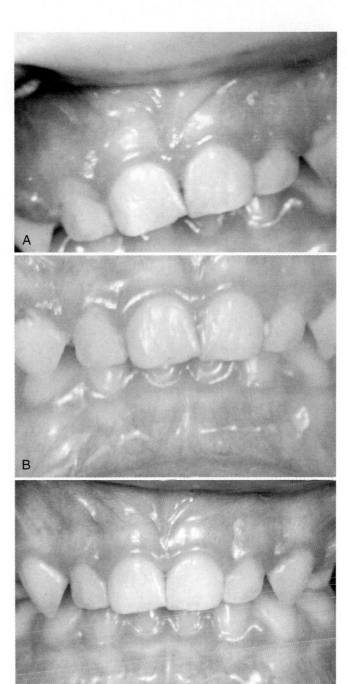

Figure 20-5 A, Acute herpetic gingivostomatitis in an 18-month-old child. The fiery red gingival tissues and the presence of ulcers on the mucous membrane are characteristic findings. **B,** Considerable improvement is evident within a week after the occurrence of the acute symptoms. **C,** Symptoms of the disease have subsided in 2 weeks. Mild inflammation of isolated gingival papillae is still evident.

by the pharmacist or mixed by the parent. The diphenhydramine has mild analgesic and antiinflammatory properties, whereas the kaolin-pectin compound coats the lesions. Because fruit juices are usually irritating to the ulcerated area, ingestion of a vitamin supplement during the course of the disease is indicated.

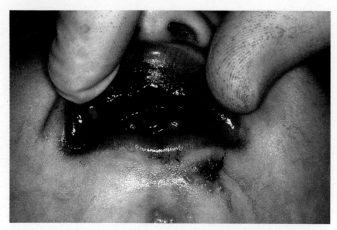

Figure 20-6 Several large, painful ulcers are evident on the tongue of a preschool child with acute herpetic gingivostomatitis.

Although the treatments described may be useful, they are only palliative. The mainstay of definitive therapy is regular doses of specific systemic antiviral medication combined with systemic analgesics (acetaminophen or ibuprofen) during the course of the disease.[12] The antiviral medications currently available are acyclovir, famciclovir, and valacyclovir. These medications inhibit viral replication in cells infected with the virus. Acyclovir (Zovirax; GlaxoSmithKline, Inc., Research Triangle Park, NC) should be administered in five daily doses to equal 1000 mg per day for 10 days. Acyclovir is available in capsules or suspension. Acyclovir therapy has been successfully used in infants and children.[13] Famciclovir (Famvir; Novartis Pharmaceuticals Corporation, East Hanover, NJ) and valacyclovir (Valtrex; GlaxoSmithKline, Inc., Research Triangle Park, NC) are newer and possibly more effective antiviral agents, but their use in pediatric populations has not yet been studied. Food and Drug Administration (FDA) approved treatment for recurrent herpes simplex labialis (cold sore, fever blister) in children 12 years and older is valacyclovir 2 g, initially and 2 g 12 hours later. Famciclovir 1500 g one dose with prodrome (earliest sign of the lesions) is a FDA-approved treatment for herpes simplex labialis in adults, but it has not been studied in children. Bed rest and isolation from other children in the family are also recommended. Hale and colleagues reported an outbreak of herpes simplex infection in a group of 13 children occupying one floor in an orphanage.[14] The children ranged in age from 11 to 35 months. In three of the children, a mild fever of brief duration and small oral lesions were the only signs of infection; these might easily have been unobserved in a situation different from that of an institutional study. The remaining children had symptoms of acute infection.

After the initial primary attack during early childhood, the herpes simplex virus becomes inactive and resides in sensory nerve ganglia. The virus often reappears later as the familiar cold sore or fever blister, usually on the outside of the lips (Fig. 20-7). Thus the disease has been commonly referred to as *recurrent herpes labialis* (RHL). However, approximately 5% of recurrences are intraoral.

With the recurring attacks, the sores develop in essentially the same area. Kleinman and colleagues published the results of a national survey of 39,206 schoolchildren aged 5 to 17 years.[15] A history of RHL was reported by 33% of the children.

The recurrence of the disease has often been related to conditions of emotional stress and lowered tissue resistance resulting from various types of trauma. Excessive exposure to sunlight may be responsible for the appearance of the recurrent herpetic lesions on the lip. Use of sunscreen can prevent sun-induced recurrences. Lesions on the lip may also appear after dental treatment and may be related to irritation from rubber dam material or even routine daily procedures.

The most effective treatment for these recurrences is the use of the specific systemic antiviral medications already discussed in connection with the treatment of the primary herpetic infection (acyclovir, famciclovir, and valacyclovir).[12] The medication should be taken immediately after the prodromal symptom of recurrence. The daily dosages are the same as those for the primary infection, but the course of treatment is usually 5 days instead of 10. One-day therapy for recurrent herpes labialis is a total of 4 g valacyclovir given in a divided dose; 2 g initially with the prodrome, followed 12 hours later with another 2 g. This regimen has been approved for children 12 years of age and older. Another topical antiviral agent, penciclovir cream (Denavir; Novartis Consumer Health, Inc., Parsippany, NJ), may be applied to perioral lesions but should not be applied to intraoral lesions. The penciclovir cream and systemic antivirals should not be prescribed for concurrent use. The penciclovir cream can be applied every 2 hours while awake for 4 days, and it is approved for use in children 12 years of age and older. Topical 5% acyclovir cream may be prescribed for use five times daily for 4 days in children 12 years of age and older.

Other remedies for herpes simplex infection also include the amino acid lysine. The oral therapy is based on lysine's antagonistic effect on another amino acid, arginine. Griffith and associates conducted an initial study in which 250 patients were given daily lysine doses of 1000 mg and were told to avoid eating arginine-rich foods, such as chocolate and nuts.[16] The lysine therapy was continued until the patients had been lesion free for 6 months. L-Lysine monohydrochloride is available commercially in capsule form or tablets containing 100 or 312 mg of L-Lysine (General Nutrition Corp., Pittsburgh, Pa.). The patients reported that pain disappeared overnight in virtually every instance. New vesicles failed to appear, and a majority considered the resolution of the lesions to be more rapid than in the past. There was also a reduction in frequency of occurrences. Griffith and colleagues concluded that improper food selection may make adequate lysine intake precarious for some persons.[16] Ingestion of cereals, seeds, nuts, and chocolate would produce a high arginine/lysine ratio and favor the development of herpetic lesions. Similar results are obtained when arginine is added to the medium in the laboratory to induce herpes proliferation. The avoidance of these foods, coupled with the selection of foods with adequate lysine, such as dairy products and yeast, should discourage herpes infection.

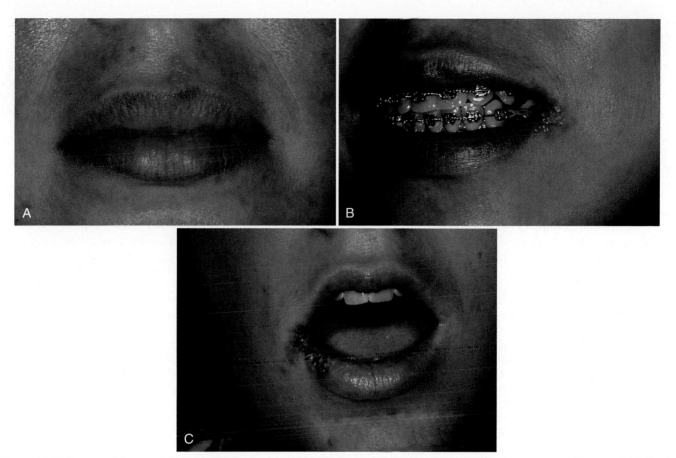

Figure 20-7 Recurrent herpes labialis. **A,** Early vesicular lesions. **B,** Mature vesicular lesion. **C,** Appearance of herpes labialis after rupture of vesicles and crusting of the lesion. (**A, B,** and **C** Courtesy of Dr. Susan L. Zunt.)

These authors postulate that this may explain the low incidence of herpes in infants before they are weaned from a predominantly milk diet. Prophylactic lysine is apparently useful in managing selected cases of RHL if serum lysine is maintained at adequate concentrations.

Brooks and associates have reported that dentists are frequently exposed to HSV-1.[17] They evaluated the risk of infection with the virus by assessing disease experience, comparing the individual's history with the results of a complement fixation or antibody titration test, or both. Their study group consisted of 525 dental students, 94 dental faculty members, and 23 staff members. Although almost all of those with a history of herpetic infection showed antibodies to HSV-1, only 57% of those lacking such a history had neutralizing antibody titers of 1:10 or higher. This finding suggests that a significant portion of practicing dentists risk primary herpetic infection. Consequently, dentists and dental auxiliaries without a history of herpetic lesions might benefit from serologic testing. Considering the occupational disability that often accompanies HSV-1 infection of the finger or eye, effective barrier protection for health professionals is important.

Primary herpetic infection has been observed on the dorsal surface of the thumb of a pediatric patient (Fig. 20-8). The child was a thumb sucker, and the acute primary infection was present in the mouth. The dorsal surface of the thumb, which rested on the lower incisor

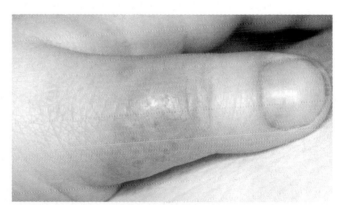

Figure 20-8 Primary herpetic infection involving the dorsal surface of the thumb of a 3-year-old child. An acute primary infection was present in the mouth.

teeth, apparently became irritated, and an inoculation of the virus took place. The oral condition and the lesions on the thumb subsided in 2 weeks.

RECURRENT APHTHOUS ULCER (CANKER SORE)

The recurrent aphthous ulcer (RAU)—also referred to as recurrent aphthous stomatitis (RAS)—is a painful ulceration on the unattached mucous membrane that occurs in school-aged children and adults. The peak age for RAU is between 10 and 19 years of age. It has been reported to be the most common mucosal disorder in people of all ages and races in the world. This disorder, according to definitions adopted in the epidemiologic literature, is characterized by recurrent ulcerations on the moist mucous membranes of the mouth, in which both discrete and confluent lesions form rapidly in certain sites and feature a round to oval crateriform base, raised reddened margins, and pain. They may appear as attacks of minor or single, major or multiple, or herpetiform lesions. They may or may not be associated with ulcerative lesions elsewhere.[18] In the national survey reported by Kleinman and colleagues, a history of RAU was reported by 37% of the schoolchildren and occurred approximately three times more often in white than in black schoolchildren.[15] Ship and colleagues reported the prevalence estimates of RAU to range between 2% and 50% with most estimates between 5% and 25% (among medical and dental students, estimated prevalence is between 50% and 60%).[19] Lesions persist for 4 to 12 days and heal uneventfully, leaving scars only rarely and only in cases of unusually large lesions. The description of RAU frequently includes the term *canker sores* (Fig. 20-9). The major form (RAS) is less common and has been referred to as *periadenitis mucosa necrotica recurrens* and *Sutton disease*. RAS has been associated with other systemic diseases: PFAPA (periodic fever, aphthous stomatitis, pharyngitis, adenitis), Behçet disease, Crohn disease, ulcerative colitis, celiac disease, neutropenia, immunodeficiency syndromes, Reiter syndrome, systemic lupus erythematosus, and MAGIC (mouth and genital ulcers with inflamed cartilage) syndrome.

The cause of RAU is unknown. Local and systemic conditions along with a genetic predisposition, as well as immunologic and infectious microbial factors, have been identified as potential causes. The condition may be caused by a delayed hypersensitivity to the L form of *Streptococcus sanguis,* which is a common constituent of the normal oral microbiota of humans. It is also possible that the lesions are caused by an autoimmune reaction of the oral epithelium. Epidemiologic studies by Ship and colleagues provide evidence for this hypothesis.[19] These data indicate that both RHL and RAU may be produced by the same mechanism, despite the known infectious agent of RHL and the absence of any known virus for RAU. Scully and Porter reported strong associations with interleuken genotypes.[18]

Local factors include trauma, allergy to toothpaste constituents (sodium lauryl sulfate), and salivary gland dysfunction. In a review of the clinical problem, Antoon and Miller suggested that minor trauma is a common precipitating factor accounting for as many as 75% of the episodes.[20] Injuries caused by cheek biting and minor facial irritations are probably the most common precipitating factors. Nutritional deficiencies are found in 20% of persons with aphthous ulcers. The clinically detectable deficiencies include deficiencies of iron, vitamin B_{12}, and folic acid. While screening patients with aphthous ulcers, Wray and associates observed a history of unusually high incidence of gastrointestinal disorders.[21] Stress may prove to be an important precipitating factor, particularly in stress-prone groups, such as students in professional schools and military personnel.

According to Greenspan and colleagues, either nonspecific factors (trauma, food allergy) or specific factors (bacterial or viral infection) may trigger a temporary imbalance in various cell subpopulations.[22] This imbalance could then upset immune regulation and result in local destruction of the oral epithelium and thus ulceration. Ship and colleagues also suggested herpes simplex virus, human herpesvirus type 6, cytomegalovirus, Epstein-Barr virus, and varicella-zoster virus as possible causes of RAS.[19]

Current treatment is focused on promoting ulcer healing, reducing ulcer duration and patient pain, maintaining the patient's nutritional intake, and preventing or reducing the frequency of recurrence of the disease.

A variety of treatments have been recommended for RAU, but a completely successful therapy has not been

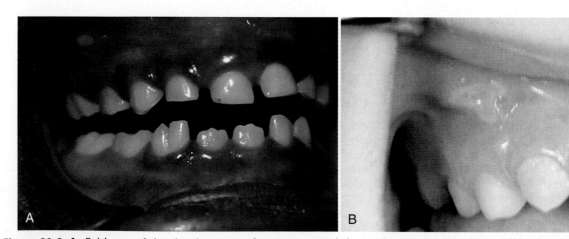

Figure 20-9 A, Evidence of the development of a recurrent aphthous ulcer in the mucobuccal fold above the primary canine. An area of inflammation and vesicle formation is apparent *(arrow).* **B,** Five days later the lesion is a well-developed ulcer with a circumscribed area of inflammation.

found. Topical antiinflammatory and analgesic medicines and/or systemic immunomodulating and immunosuppression agents have been used for RAU. The primary line of treatment uses topical gels, creams, and ointments as antiinflammatory agents. Currently, a topical corticosteroid (e.g., 0.5% fluocinonide, 0.025% triamcinolone, 0.5% clobetasol) is applied to the area with a mucosal adherent (e.g., isobutyl cyanoacrylate, Orabase). For example, the application of triamcinolone acetonide (Kenalog in Orabase) to the surface of the lesions before meals and before sleeping may also be helpful. Binnie and colleagues reported that an antiinflammatory and antiallergic medication in the form of a topical paste is effective in reducing pain and accelerating healing of RAU ulcers.[23] The active ingredient in the paste is 5% amlexanox and it is available under the trade name Aphthasol (Access Pharmaceuticals, Dallas, Texas). The paste is applied to the ulcer four times daily, after meals and at bedtime, until the ulcer heals. Zilactin (Zila Pharmaceuticals, Phoenix, Ariz), a topical paste with hydroxypropyl cellulose film, has also been used to adhere to the mucosa and cover the ulcer while providing pain relief for an extended period of time. Occlusive topical 2-otylcyanoacrylate adheres for 6 hours. Aloe vera freeze-dried gel extract adheres and forms an occlusive protective patch. In severe cases, oral prednisone has been prescribed.

Topical rinses have also been helpful for relief of RAU. Sucralfate has proved useful by coating the area. The topical application of tetracycline to the ulcers is often helpful in reducing the pain and in shortening the course of the disease. A mouthwash containing suspension of one of the tetracyclines has been helpful to some, but the mouthwash should not be swallowed. Chlorhexidine mouthwash has also been known to alleviate the symptoms of RAU. Swished dexamethasone elixir is useful to treat ulcerations in areas of the mouth that are difficult to access. Other findings that may be of significance include those of the two following studies: Meiller and associates have reported that the duration and severity of RAU lesions can be significantly reduced by vigorous twice-daily rinsing with an antimicrobial mouthwash (Listerine Antiseptic, Pfizer Warner Lambert Division, Morris Plains, NJ).[24] Pedersen reported that some of her recent work suggests that varicella-zoster virus may be of etiologic importance in RAU.[25] Furthermore, she found that six of eight patients with chronic severe RAU who were treated with acyclovir responded favorably within 2 days.

ACUTE NECROTIZING ULCERATIVE GINGIVITIS (VINCENT INFECTION)

The infectious disease commonly referred to as acute necrotizing ulcerative gingivitis (ANUG) is rare among preschool children in the United States, occurs occasionally in children 6 to 12 years old, and is common in young adults. Reade reported one instance of the typical picture of ulcerative gingivitis in a 15-month-old infant.[26] *Treponema vincentii* and gram-negative fusiform bacilli were demonstrated in a smear. Recovery occurred within 36 hours after initiation of penicillin therapy and the application of hydrogen peroxide.

ANUG can be easily diagnosed because of the involvement of the interproximal papillae and the presence of a pseudomembranous necrotic covering of the marginal tissue (Fig. 20-10). Two microorganisms, *Borrelia vincentii* and fusiform bacilli, referred to as spirochetal organisms, are generally believed to be responsible for the disease. The clinical manifestations of the disease include inflamed, painful, bleeding gingival tissue, poor appetite, temperature as high as 40°C (104°F), general malaise, and a fetid odor.

The disease responds dramatically within 24 to 48 hours to subgingival curettage, débridement, and the use of mild oxidizing solutions. If the gingival tissues are acutely and extensively inflamed when the patient is first seen, antibiotic therapy is indicated. Improved oral hygiene, the use of mild oxidizing mouth rinses after each meal, and twice-daily rinsing with chlorhexidine will aid in overcoming the infection.

There should be no difficulty in distinguishing ANUG from acute herpetic gingivostomatitis, although the two are sometimes confused. Round ulcers with red areolae on the lips and cheeks are characteristic of herpetic gingivostomatitis. Therapeutic prophylaxis and débridement bring about a favorable response in cases of ANUG but not in acute herpetic gingivostomatitis. A therapeutic trial of antibiotics reduces the acute symptoms in

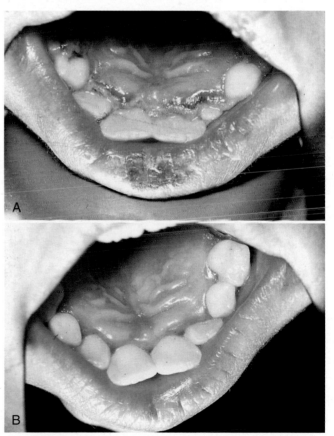

Figure 20-10 A, A rare example of necrotizing ulcerative gingivitis in an 8-year-old boy. **B,** Local treatment and improved oral hygiene produced a dramatic recovery from the infection.

ANUG but not in the viral infection. Acute herpetic gingivostomatitis is most frequently seen in preschool children, and its onset is rapid. As stated earlier, ANUG rarely occurs in the preschool-aged group and develops over a longer period, usually in a mouth in which irritants and poor oral hygiene are present. On the other hand, acute oral infections initially diagnosed as ANUG have frequently been found later to be an oral manifestation of one of the xanthomatoses. The early stages of conditions such as Hand-Schüller-Christian disease and Letterer-Siwe disease are associated with many of the symptoms of ANUG.

ACUTE CANDIDIASIS (THRUSH, CANDIDOSIS, MONILIASIS)

Candida (Monilia) albicans is a common inhabitant of the oral cavity but may multiply rapidly and cause a pathogenic state when host resistance is lowered. Young children sometimes develop thrush after local antibiotic therapy, which allows the fungus to proliferate. The lesions of the oral disease appear as raised, furry, white patches, which can be removed easily to produce a bleeding underlying surface (Fig. 20-11). Neonatal candidiasis, contracted during passage through the vagina and erupting clinically during the first 2 weeks of life, is a common

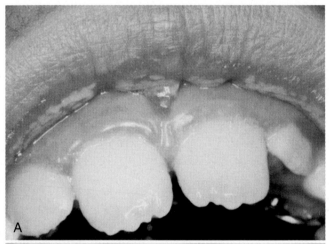

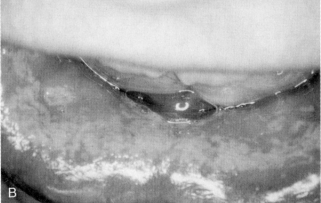

Figure 20-11 A, The characteristic appearance of acute candidiasis on the upper and lower lips of a young patient. The hard and soft palates were also severely affected. **B,** The infection was controlled with a 7-day regimen of nystatin.

occurrence. This infection is also common in immunosuppressed patients (see Chapter 24).

Antifungal antibiotics control thrush. For infants and very young children, a suspension of 1 mL (100,000 U) of nystatin (Mycostatin) may be dropped into the mouth for local action four times a day. The drug is nonirritating and nontoxic. Clotrimazole suspension (10 mg/mL), 1 to 2 mL applied to affected areas four times daily, is an effective antifungal medication. Systemic fluconazole suspension (10 mg/mL) is safe to use in infants at a total dosage of 6 mg/kg or less per day. For children old enough to manage solid medication allowed to dissolve in the mouth, clotrimazole troches or nystatin pastilles are recommended, because the therapeutic agent remains in the saliva longer than with the liquid medication. For children old enough to swallow, systemic fluconazole (100-mg tablets) in a 14-day course may be prescribed for patients whose infection has not responded to topical antifungal agents.

ACUTE BACTERIAL INFECTIONS

The prevalence of acute bacterial infection in the oral cavity is unknown. Blake and Trott reported acute streptococcal gingivitis with painful, vivid red gingivae that bled easily.[27] The papillae had enlarged, and gingival abscesses had developed. Cultures showed a predominance of hemolytic streptococci. Acute infections of this type may be more common than was previously realized. Littner and associates reported five cases, all in adults between 20 and 27 years of age.[28] The diagnosis is difficult to make, however, without extensive laboratory tests. Broad-spectrum antibiotics are recommended if the infection is believed to be bacterial in origin. Improved oral hygiene is important in treating the infection. As with any acute microbial oral infection, chlorhexidine mouth rinses are also appropriate. The placement of dental restorations to restore adequate function and contour after the reduction of acute symptoms is equally important.

CHRONIC NONSPECIFIC GINGIVITIS

A type of gingivitis commonly seen during the preteen-age and teenage years is often referred to as *chronic nonspecific gingivitis*. The chronic gingival inflammation may be localized to the anterior region, or it may be more generalized. Although the condition is rarely painful, it may persist for long periods without much improvement (Fig. 20-12).

Glauser and colleagues observed an unusual gingivitis in Navajo Indians between 12 and 18 years of age, similar to that seen in Fig. 20-13, in which the fiery red gingival lesion is not accompanied by enlarged interdental labial papillae or closely associated with local irritants.[29] The gingivitis showed little improvement after a prophylactic treatment. The age of the patients involved and the prevalence of the disease in girls suggested a hormonal imbalance as a possible factor. Histologic examination of tissue sections and the use of special stains ruled out a bacterial infection. Inadequate oral hygiene, which allows food impaction and the accumulation of materia

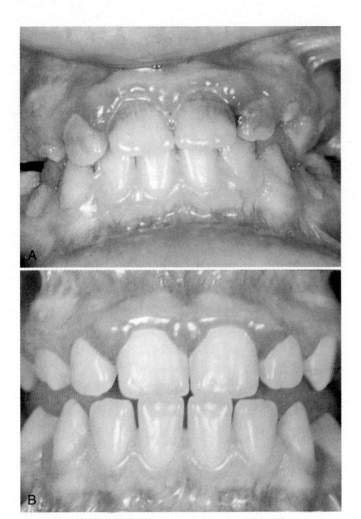

Figure 20-12 A, Chronic nonspecific gingivitis. The cause of this type of gingivitis is complex, and it often persists for prolonged periods without significant improvement. **B,** After 9 months of treatment, hyperplastic gingival tissue is still evident in the anterior maxillary region.

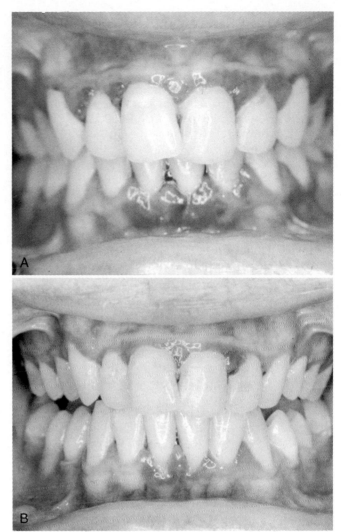

Figure 20-13 A, Fiery red gingival lesions essentially limited to the anterior labial tissues. Only minimum local deposits were evident. The gingivitis was classified as the chronic nonspecific type. **B,** Limited improvement was evident after 6 months of local treatment. A hormonal imbalance and vitamin deficiency were suspected as contributing etiologic factors.

alba and bacterial plaque, is undoubtedly the major cause of this chronic type of gingivitis.

Kaslick and colleagues studied 238 young adults and looked for a correlation between their periodontal status and their ABO blood type.[30] They discovered that the chronic gingivitis group had a larger percentage of AB blood types and a smaller percentage of O blood type than the control group.

The cause of gingivitis is complex and is considered to be based on a multitude of local and systemic factors. Because dietary inadequacies are often found in the preteenage and teenage groups, the 7-day diet survey described in Chapter 10 is an important diagnostic aid. Insufficient quantities of fruits and vegetables in the diet, leading to a subclinical vitamin deficiency, may be an important predisposing factor. An improved dietary intake of vitamins and the use of multiple-vitamin supplements will improve the gingival condition in many children.

Malocclusion, which prevents adequate function, and crowded teeth, which make oral hygiene and plaque removal more difficult, are also important predisposing factors in gingivitis. Carious lesions with irritating sharp margins, as well as faulty restorations with overhanging margins (both of which cause food accumulation), also favor the development of the chronic type of gingivitis.

A wide variety of local irritants can produce a hyperplastic type of gingivitis in children and young adults. The irritation to the gingival tissue produced by mouth breathing is often responsible for the development of the chronic hyperplastic form of gingivitis, particularly in the maxillary arch. All these factors should be considered contributory to chronic nonspecific gingivitis and should be corrected in the treatment of the condition. The importance of thorough daily oral hygiene must be emphasized repeatedly to the patients.

CHLORHEXIDINE AS A THERAPEUTIC PLAQUE CONTROL AGENT

Chlorhexidine (CH) is a chlorophenyl biguanide with broad antimicrobial activity. It has been used commonly as an antiseptic skin and wound cleanser for presurgical preparation of the patient and as a handwash and surgical scrub for health care personnel. It has also been added as a preservative to ophthalmic products and has been used internally in very dilute concentrations in the peritoneal cavity and urinary bladder.

In dentistry, CH has been studied for control of smooth surface caries, for use as a denture disinfectant, and as a plaque control agent. Its use in controlling dental plaque accumulations has received the most attention in dental research. Mouth rinses containing CH have been popular as therapeutic agents in several countries for some time, and in 1986 CH was approved for use in the United States. Two products under the trade names Peridex (Colgate-Palmolive Co., New York, NY) and PerioGard (Zila Pharmaceuticals, Phoenix, Ariz) have received FDA approval as prescription agents. This mouth rinse contains 0.12% CH gluconate as the active ingredient.

Widespread use of CH mouth rinses over many years, especially in Europe, has had an excellent safety record. Few adverse side effects have been reported with CH mouth rinses, but their use has been linked to mouth dryness and burning sensations in some persons due to the alcohol base. An alcohol-free product is available. Generalized staining over long-term use and taste alterations have been reported. Poorly defined desquamative lesions have been observed in others after the mouth rinse was used. Allergic reactions to CH are rare. If the rinse is inadvertently swallowed, it has essentially little systemic effect due to poor absorption in the gastrointestinal system.

Löe and Schiött reported highly significant inhibition of plaque formation and the prevention of gingivitis with use of an aqueous solution of 0.2% CH digluconate as a mouth rinse twice daily with swishing for 1 minute.[31] Yankell and associates have shown that dental stain from CH mouth rinse can be significantly reduced with regular use of a tartar-control dentifrice.[32]

It is important to recognize that the beneficial use of CH as a therapeutic mouth rinse should be considered adjunctive to the practice of sound conventional plaque control measures as presented in Chapter 11 and elsewhere in this text. A study by Brecx and colleagues regarding the efficacy of Listerine, Meridol, and chlorhexidine (CH) mouth rinses found CH to be the most effective to supplement habitual mechanical oral hygiene.[33] They also found a combination of habitual self-performed and nonsupervised oral hygiene with Listerine or Meridol is more beneficial for plaque control than the use of mechanical oral hygiene alone. Its adjunctive use would also seem most appropriate for therapy in cases in which attaining adequate plaque control is more difficult, such as during illness or convalescence after serious injuries.

The rationale to include use of daily antimicrobial mouth rinse to the child and adolescent's oral hygiene regimens when inadequate plaque control exists to control and prevent periodontal disease and deliver antimicrobial agents to mucosal sites harboring bacteria throughout the mouth thereby complementing plaque control is widely accepted.[34,35]

GINGIVAL DISEASES MODIFIED BY SYSTEMIC FACTORS

GINGIVAL DISEASES ASSOCIATED WITH THE ENDOCRINE SYSTEM

Puberty gingivitis is a distinctive type of gingivitis that occasionally develops in children in the prepubertal and pubertal period. Cohen, in a study of 270 boys and girls in the 11- to 14-year age group, observed that gingival enlargement in the anterior segment occurred with regularity in the prepubertal and premenarcheal period, as well as in pubescence.[36] The gingival enlargement was marginal in distribution and, in the presence of local irritants, was characterized by prominent bulbous interproximal papillae far greater than gingival enlargements associated with local factors. Nakagawa and colleagues found a statistically significant increase in gingival inflammation, sex hormones, and the occurrence of *Prevotella intermedia* in adolescents during puberty.[37]

Sutcliffe's survey of a group of children between 11 and 17 years of age revealed an initial high prevalence of gingivitis that tended to decline with age.[38] In both sexes the prevalence of gingivitis tended to decrease with age. Initially, 89% of 11-year-olds and 92% of 12-year-olds were affected.

The enlargement of the gingival tissues in puberty gingivitis is confined to the anterior segment and may be present in only one arch. The lingual gingival tissue generally remains unaffected (Fig. 20-14). Treatment of puberty gingivitis should be directed toward improved oral hygiene, removal of all local irritants, restoration of carious teeth, and dietary changes necessary to ensure an adequate nutritional status. Cohen observed a sharp improvement in gingival inflammation and enlargement after the oral administration of 500 mg of ascorbic acid.[36] However, the improvement did not occur until the vitamin had been taken for approximately 4 weeks.

Severe cases of hyperplastic gingivitis that do not respond to local or systemic therapy should be treated by gingivoplasty. Surgical removal of the thickened fibrotic marginal and interproximal tissue has been found effective. Recurrence of any hyperplastic tissue will be minimal if adequate oral hygiene is maintained.

GINGIVAL LESIONS OF GENETIC ORIGIN

Hereditary gingival fibromatosis (HGF) is characterized by a slow, progressive, benign enlargement of the gingivae. Genetic and pharmacologically induced forms of gingival enlargement are known. The most common genetic form, HGF, usually has an autosomal dominant mode of inheritance. Hart and colleagues identified the first polymorphic marker for HGF phenotype on chromosome band 2p21.[39] This rare type of gingivitis has been referred to as *elephantiasis gingivae* or *hereditary hyperplasia*

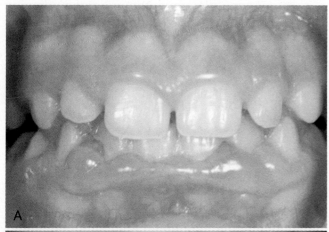

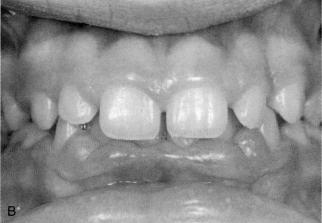

Figure 20-14 A, Puberty gingivitis. The enlargement of the gingival tissues was limited to the mandibular anterior region. **B,** Local treatment resulted in only a slight improvement of the condition. A persistence of the hyperplastic enlargement would indicate the need for gingivoplasty.

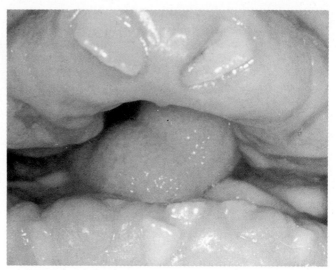

Figure 20-15 Fibromatosis in a 14-year-old girl. The gingival tissues have enlarged to the extent that they almost cover the crowns of the teeth.

of the gums. The gingival tissues appear normal at birth but begin to enlarge with the eruption of the primary teeth. Although mild cases are observed, the gingival tissues usually continue to enlarge with eruption of the permanent teeth until the tissues essentially cover the clinical crowns of the teeth (Fig. 20-15). The dense fibrous tissue often causes displacement of the teeth and malocclusion. The condition is not painful until the tissue enlarges to the extent that it partially covers the occlusal surface of the molars and becomes traumatized during mastication.

Zackin and Weisberger described fibromatosis histologically as a moderate hyperplasia of the epithelium, with hyperkeratosis and elongation of the rete pegs.[40] The increase in tissue mass is primarily the result of an increase and thickening of the collagenous bundles in the connective tissue stroma. The tissue shows a high degree of differentiation, and a few young fibroblasts are present.

Surgical removal of the hyperplastic tissue achieves a more favorable oral and facial appearance. However, hyperplasia can recur within a few months after the surgical procedure and can return to the original condition within a few years. Although the tissue usually appears pale and firm, the surgical procedure is accompanied by excessive hemorrhage. Therefore quadrant surgery is usually recommended. Brown and colleagues have reported a case in which apically positioned flap surgery and CO_2 laser evaporation were used to reduce the gingival tissue.[41] The importance of excellent plaque control should be stressed to the patient because this delays the recurrence of the gingival overgrowth.

PHENYTOIN-INDUCED GINGIVAL OVERGROWTH

Phenytoin (Dilantin, or diphenylhydantoin), a major anticonvulsant agent used in the treatment of epilepsy, was first introduced in the late 1930s with common side effects of varying degrees of gingival hyperplasia first described by Kimball in 1939.[42] He reported that 57% of 119 patients taking phenytoin for the control of seizure activity experienced some degree of gingival overgrowth.

Today an estimated 2 million persons use this medication because of its comparative safety and broad therapeutic range. The incidence of phenytoin-induced gingival overgrowth (PIGO) in patients undergoing long-term phenytoin therapy has been reported as ranging between 0% and 95%, with numerous investigators reporting figures at the 40% to 50% level.

Early research showed an increase in the number of fibroblasts in patients receiving Dilantin; thus the condition was termed Dilantin hyperplasia. Now the term *phenytoin-induced gingival overgrowth* is preferred because Hassell and colleagues found true hyperplasia not to exist.[43] There was no excessive collagen accumulation per unit of tissue, nor did the fibroblasts appear abnormal in number or size.

The influence of serum and salivary levels of phenytoin on the development of PIGO has also been investigated.

Some authors report a positive relationship between the level of phenytoin in serum and saliva and the severity of PIGO in some cases.[44-46] Other investigators have reported that no such correlation exists.[47,48] It is generally agreed that a relationship exists between dosage and PIGO when the level of phenytoin per unit body weight or actual serum level is considered. Sasaki and Maita reported a significant correlation between the degree of gingival overgrowth and a high level of basic fibroblast growth factor in serum.[49] No such correlations were observed for patient age, daily or total phenytoin dose, duration of therapy, or serum phenytoin level.

Most investigators agree on the existence of a close relationship between oral hygiene and PIGO. PIGO can be decreased or prevented by scrupulous oral hygiene and dental prophylaxis. The relationship between plaque, local irritants, and PIGO is also supported by the observation that patients without teeth almost never develop PIGO.

PIGO, when it does develop, begins to appear as early as 2 to 3 weeks after initiation of phenytoin therapy and peaks at 18 to 24 months. The initial clinical appearance is painless enlargement of the interproximal gingiva. The buccal and anterior segments are more often affected than the lingual and posterior segments (Figs. 20-16 and 20-17). The affected areas are isolated at first but can become more generalized later. Unless secondary infection or inflammation is present, the gingiva appears pink and firm and does not bleed easily on probing. As the interdental lobulations grow, clefting becomes apparent at the midline of the tooth (see Fig. 20-17). With time the lobulations coalesce at the midline, forming pseudopockets and covering more of the crown of the tooth. The epithelial attachment level usually remains constant. In some cases, the entire occlusal surface of the teeth becomes covered. These lesions may remain purely fibrotic in nature or may be combined with a noticeable inflammatory component.

PIGO may impose problems of esthetics, difficulty in mastication, speech impairment, delayed tooth eruption, tissue trauma, and secondary inflammation leading to periodontal disease.[50] No cure exists and treatment is often symptomatic in nature. Antihistamines, topical corticosteroids, ascorbic acid (vitamin C) supplements, topical antibiotics, and alkaline mouthwashes have been used with limited success and are considered to be ineffective.

Steinberg and Steinberg describe current recommended dental treatment based on clinical oral signs and symptoms.[51] Patients with mild PIGO (i.e., less than one third of the clinical crown is covered) require daily meticulous oral hygiene and more frequent dental care. For patients with moderate PIGO (i.e., one third to two thirds of the clinical crown is covered) meticulous oral home care and the judicious use of an irrigating device may be needed. Use of an antiplaque mouth rinse (0.12% chlorhexidine gluconate) in the device further helps control bacterial growth. Initially, a series of four consecutive weekly office visits for prophylaxis and topical stannous fluoride application is recommended. The fifth week is used to

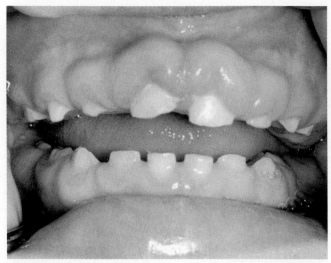

Figure 20-16 Phenytoin gingivitis in a preschool child. The enlarged gingival tissue covers two thirds of the maxillary primary lateral incisors and canines.

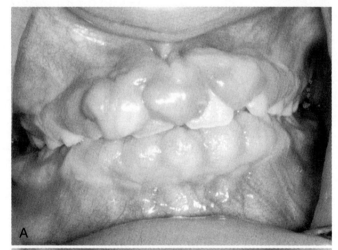

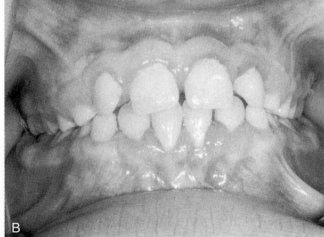

Figure 20-17 **A,** Phenytoin gingivitis of the severe generalized type. **B,** Surgical removal of the overgrowth of hyperplastic gingival tissue results in temporary improvement of the condition. Excellent oral hygiene is essential in controlling the gingival enlargement.

evaluate the gingivae and note any change in size. Phenytoin levels should be checked (normal therapeutic range is 10 to 15 mg/mL). If there has been no change, consultation with the patient's physician concerning the possibility of using a different anticonvulsant drug may be helpful. If no improvement occurs, surgical removal of the overgrowth may be recommended. For patients with severe PIGO (i.e., more than two thirds of the tooth is covered) who do not respond to the previously mentioned therapeutic regimens, surgical removal is necessary. As in any periodontal surgery, scaling and root planing before surgery and meticulous oral hygiene after surgery are essential to minimize the overgrowth, which can occur as early as 3 to 4 weeks after surgery. Donnenfeld and colleagues found no PIGO recurrence for as long as 9 months postoperatively.[52] If surgery is required a second time and the patient has a history of rapid recurrence, a pressure appliance should be considered as an adjunct to home oral care. If the patient has multiple gingivectomies, clinical management becomes one of postponing repeat surgery for as long as possible.

Specific surgical approaches for PIGO include gingivectomy with periodontal knives, laser, or electrosurgery, and internal bevel flap surgery. The use of periodontal knives allows the tissue to heal more quickly, but more operative and postoperative bleeding occurs, and the procedure requires more time and patient cooperation. Electrosurgery is less time consuming, decreases blood loss, improves visibility, allows superior control for areas of limited access, is self-sterilizing, and does not always require the use of periodontal packs. Disadvantages include its contraindication in patients with cardiac pacemakers, unpleasant odor, delayed healing, and the potential for error in application that results in undesired bone or tissue loss. Advantages of the surgical laser include lack of hemorrhage, which yields a dry field; noncontact during surgery; sterilization of the surgical area; prompt healing; minimal postoperative discomfort; and minimal time spent in performing the procedures. Disadvantages include cost and size of equipment, necessity for hospitalization, potential for delayed healing of some tissues, greater degree of expertise required, loss of tactile feedback, requirement for eye protection, ability of the laser to ignite a plastic or rubber endotracheal tube, and a need to cover the nonsurgical field with moist sponge shields to prevent penetration of the laser beam. Internal bevel flap surgery can also be used for PIGO patients and has some advantages over the previously mentioned treatment modalities. The internal bevel flap promotes faster healing (stimulates primary healing), controls postoperative bleeding, minimizes postoperative pain, and allows the optional use of a periodontal pack. The choice of surgical approach must be left to the operator and is based on patient cooperation and compliance, the degree of gingival overgrowth, and operator expertise. Healing is usually rapid with all these modalities.

The surgical removal of severely overgrown tissue in PIGO and good oral hygiene after surgery are generally considered to be the most effective treatment. However, even these procedures have often been followed by a gradual recurrence of the fibrous tissue.

A preliminary study of use of a pressure appliance for PIGO hyperplasia has been reported by Davis and colleagues.[53] Immediately after the surgical removal of hyperplastic tissue, an impression was taken and a positive-pressure splint was constructed. Periodontal dressings were removed at the end of 1 week, and the positive-pressure appliance was inserted. Seven of the nine members of the experimental group had no recurrence of gingival hyperplasia, one had a slight recurrence, and one had a moderate recurrence. The natural rubber, mouth-protector type of appliance and the type with a cast chromium-cobalt framework lined with soft plastic were equally effective. The appliance is generally used only at night but may be worn night and day if such a schedule is required. Sheridan and Reeve[54] has also reported success in controlling the gingival overgrowth with positive-pressure appliances.

Steinberg suggested that use of a series of pressure appliances may help reduce the size of the gingival overgrowth without surgery.[55] He reported one case in which existing systemic conditions contraindicated surgical removal of the gingival tissue. After oral hygiene was improved, pressure appliances were made on stone casts of the patient's upper and lower arches after trimming away 2 mm of the stone in the gingival overgrowth areas. The patient wore the appliance about 12 hours each day for 4 weeks; then a new pressure device was made. Steinberg observed a pronounced decrease in the size of the gingival lesions after 8 weeks of therapy. He suggested that a series of such appliances could succeed in gradually reducing gingival overgrowth to clinically tolerable limits. He also pointed out that this therapeutic approach is not practical for the average patient but that it may prove valuable for patients with contraindications to oral surgery.

Drew and colleagues[56] and Bäckman and associates[57] have reported that patients with PIGO or patients at risk for developing it may benefit from receiving folate therapy. Their work demonstrated a reduction in the severity of PIGO in patients who received systemic folic acid supplementation. The work of Drew and colleagues further demonstrated that twice-daily oral rinsing with a topical folic acid solution resulted in significantly better tissue responses than systemic folic acid therapy.[56] Their studies suggest that folic acid therapy may inhibit PIGO and that additional related studies are indicated.

Other drugs that have been reported to induce gingival overgrowth in some patients include cyclosporin, calcium channel blockers, valproic acid, and phenobarbital. As with all disorders affecting periodontal tissues, maintaining excellent oral hygiene is the primary key to successful therapy.

ASCORBIC ACID DEFICIENCY GINGIVITIS (SCORBUTIC GINGIVITIS)

Scorbutic gingivitis is associated with vitamin C deficiency and differs from the type of gingivitis related to poor oral hygiene. The involvement is usually limited to the marginal tissues and papillae. The child with scorbutic gingivitis may complain of severe pain, and spontaneous hemorrhage is evident. Fain and colleagues believe that bleeding and gingivitis occur in some adult cancer patients because of scurvy rather than because of their malignant disease or chemotherapy.[58]

Severe clinical scorbutic gingivitis is rare in children. However, it may occur in children allergic to fruit juices when provision of an adequate dietary supplement of vitamin C is neglected (Fig. 20-18). When blood studies indicate a vitamin C deficiency and exclude other possible systemic conditions, the gingivitis responds dramatically to the daily administration of 250 to 500 mg of ascorbic acid. Older children and adults may require 1 g of vitamin C for 2 weeks to speed recovery.

A less severe type of gingivitis resulting from vitamin C deficiency is probably much more common than most dentists realize. Inflammation and enlargement of the marginal gingival tissue and papillae in the absence of local predisposing factors are possible evidence of scorbutic gingivitis (Figs. 20-19 and 20-20).

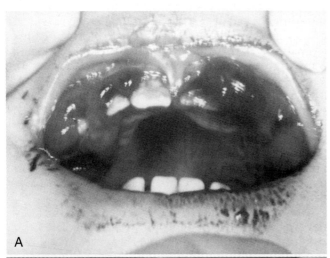

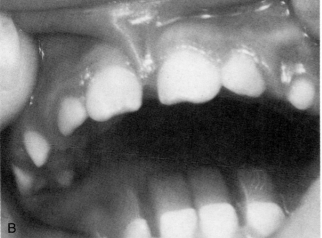

Figure 20-18 A, Severe scorbutic gingivitis in a 16-month-old child. Large hematomas were evident in the maxillary arch. The condition was initially incorrectly diagnosed as Vincent infection. **B,** Daily administration of 400 mg of ascorbic acid resulted in a dramatic recovery.

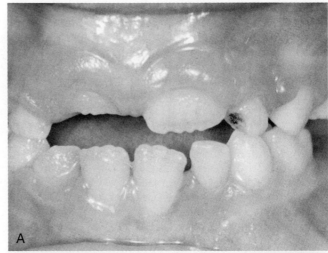

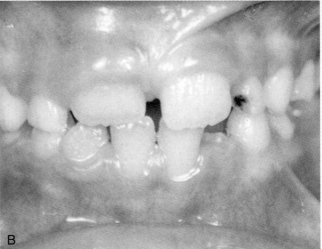

Figure 20-19 A, Mild gingivitis caused by a vitamin C deficiency. The marginal tissue and papillae were painfully enlarged. A dietary history revealed that the child's diet was grossly deficient in fruits and vegetables. **B,** Improvement in diet and greater emphasis on oral hygiene resulted in a great improvement in the oral health.

Questioning the child and parents regarding eating habits and using the 7-day diet survey frequently reveals that the child is receiving inadequate amounts of foods containing vitamin C. Complete dental care, improved oral hygiene, and supplementation with vitamin C and other water-soluble vitamins will greatly improve the gingival condition.

PERIODONTAL DISEASES IN CHILDREN

Periodontitis, an inflammatory disease of the gingiva and deeper tissues of the periodontium, is characterized by pocket formation and destruction of the supporting alveolar bone. Bone loss in children can be detected in bite-wing radiographs by comparing the height of the alveolar bone to the cementoenamel junction. Distances between 2 and 3 mm can be defined as questionable bone loss and distances greater than 3 mm indicate definite bone loss.

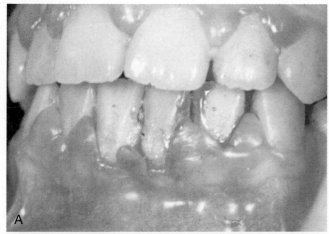

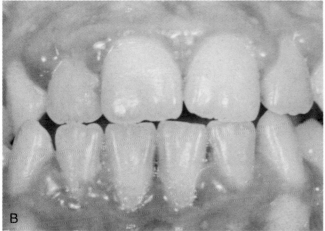

Figure 20-20 A, Scorbutic gingivitis in a 13-year-old girl. The diet was almost entirely lacking in foods containing vitamin C. **B,** An improved diet, supplemental amounts of fresh fruit juices, and toothbrushing instruction resulted in an improved gingival condition in 2 weeks.

According to Delaney, in preschool children with periodontitis, recession, gingival erythema, and edema are not usually found unless the child is neutropenic.[3] Periodontal probing for attachment loss and bite-wing radiography are often used to clinically confirm the diagnosis. Bone loss is usually between the primary first and second molars. Binstein and colleagues demonstrated abnormal alveolar bone resorption in 7.6% of 4-year-old children and in 5.9% of 5-year-old children of primarily Hispanic origin with high caries.[59]

In its classification of periodontitis, the American Academy of Periodontology categorized the early-onset form under Aggressive Periodontitis.[60,61]

EARLY-ONSET PERIODONTITIS (AGGRESSIVE PERIODONTITIS)

Albandar and associates proposed the term *early-onset periodontitis* (EOP).[62] This term has been replaced by *aggressive periodontitis* following the classification proposed by the American Academy of Periodontology in 1999. *Aggressive periodontitis* is used as a generic term to describe a heterogeneous group of periodontal disease occurring in younger individuals who are otherwise healthy. Aggressive periodontitis can be viewed as two categories of periodontitis that may have overlapping etiologies and clinical presentations: (1) a localized form (localized aggressive periodontitis [LAP]), (2) a generalized form (generalized aggressive periodontitis [GAP]). Albandar and colleagues, using data from a 1986-87 survey, estimated the prevalence of aggressive periodontitis in adolescent schoolchildren in the United States to be 10% in blacks, 5% in Hispanics, and 1.3% in whites.[63]

Löe and Brown have reported observations from a periodontal assessment of 1107 adolescents aged 14 to 17 years.[64] Approximately 0.53% were estimated to have LAP, 0.13% to have GAP, and 1.61% to have incidental loss of attachment. Boys were more likely to have GAP than girls (ratio, 4.3:1).

Page and colleagues believe that there are four different forms of periodontitis: prepubertal, juvenile, rapidly progressing, and adult.[65] However, as mentioned earlier, the classification of periodontal disease recommends that EOP be recategorized as aggressive periodontitis and that its subclassifications be discarded.

Aggressive periodontitis of the primary dentition can occur in a localized form but usually is seen in the generalized form. Localized aggressive periodontitis (LAP) is localized attachment loss and alveolar bone loss only in the primary dentition in an otherwise healthy child. The exact time of onset is unknown, but it appears to arise around or before 4 years of age, when the bone loss is usually seen on radiographs around the primary molars and/or incisors. Abnormal probing depths with minor gingival inflammation, rapid bone loss, and minimal to varying amounts of plaque have been demonstrated at the affected sites of the child's dentition. Abnormalities in host defenses (e.g., leukocyte chemotaxis), extensive proximal caries facilitating plaque retention and bone loss, and a family history of periodontitis have been associated with LAP in children.[66,67] As the disease progresses, the child's periodontium shows signs of gingival inflammation with gingival clefts and localized ulceration of the gingival margin.

The onset of GAP is during or soon after the eruption of the primary teeth. It results in severe gingival inflammation and generalized attachment loss, tooth mobility, and rapid alveolar bone loss with premature exfoliation of the teeth (Fig. 20-21). The gingival tissue may initially demonstrate only minor inflammation with a minimum of plaque material. Chronic cases display the presence of clefting and pronounced recession with associated acute inflammation. Testing may reveal a high prevalence of leukocyte adherence abnormalities and an impaired host response against bacterial infections. Alveolar bone destruction proceeds rapidly, and the primary teeth may be lost by 3 years of age. Microorganisms predominating in the gingival pockets include *Aggregatibacter actinomycetemcomitans* (Aa), *Porphyromonas (Bacteroides) gingivalis*, *Bacteroides melaninogenicus*, *Prevotella intermedia*, *Capnocytophaga sputigena*, and *Fusobacterium nucleatum*. Recent findings of Asikainen and associates suggest that the major periodontal pathogens are transmitted among family members.[68,69] Often the past medical history of the child reveals a history of recurrent infections. (e.g., otitis media, skin infections, upper respiratory tract infections).

Consultation with a pediatrician is needed to rule out systemic diseases. Treatment of LAP or GAP depends on early diagnosis, dental curettage, root planing, prophylaxis, oral hygiene instruction, restoration of decayed teeth, removal of the primary teeth that have lost bony support, and more frequent recalls. Use of antimicrobial rinses (chlorhexidine) and therapy with broad-spectrum antibiotics are effective in eliminating the periodontal pathogens. Amoxicillin has been used in children (250-mg liquid three times a day for 10 days). Treatment of GAP is less successful overall and sometimes requires extraction of all primary teeth. Delaney reported that children affected with LAP or GAP may experience severe periodontitis of the permanent teeth.[3]

See the later section Premature Bone Loss in the Primary Dentition.

LOCALIZED AGGRESSIVE PERIODONTITIS

The previously described condition of localized juvenile periodontitis has also been replaced by the term *localized aggressive periodontitis* (LAP). This condition presents a classic pattern and occurs in otherwise healthy children and adolescents without clinical evidence of systemic disease. It is characterized by the rapid and severe loss of alveolar bone around more than one permanent tooth, usually the first molars and incisors (Fig. 20-22). It appears self-limiting, and retrospective data obtained from LAP patients suggest that bone loss around the primary teeth can be an early finding in this disease. Reported estimates of the prevalence of LAP range from 0.1% to 1.5% with a bilaterally symmetric pattern of bone loss in a geographically diverse adolescent population. The prevalence in the black population is greater—2.5%. Clinically, LAP patients have less tissue inflammation and very little supragingival dental plaque or calculus. However, they do present with evidence of subgingival plaque accumulation, both tissue-associated and tooth-associated plaque. Progression of bone loss is three to four times faster than in chronic periodontitis.

LAP is not thought to be a single disease entity. The probable causative microbial species are Aa or Aa in combination with *Porphyromonas*-like species. A variety of neutrophil defects have been reported in patients with LAP. According to Page and colleagues, most patients with LAP manifest abnormalities in peripheral blood neutrophil (polymorphonuclear leukocyte) chemotaxis and in some cases in monocyte chemotaxis.[70] Also, anomalies of phagocytosis, bacterial activity, leukotriene B$_4$ generation, and other defects have been reported. Page and colleagues suspect a hereditary basis for LAP; some believe the mode of transmission is autosomal recessive, but others have provided evidence that the pattern is typical of an X-linked dominant mode.

GENERALIZED AGGRESSIVE PERIODONTITIS

The generalized form of aggressive periodontitis occurs at or around puberty in older juveniles and young adults. It often affects the entire periodontium of the dentition.

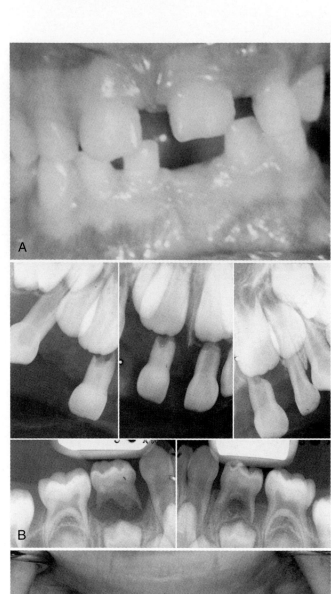

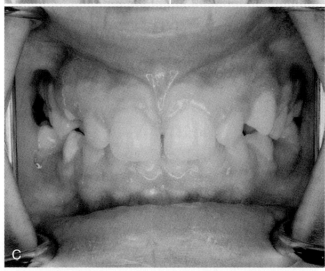

Figure 20-21 A, Prepubertal periodontitis in a 4½-year-old girl. Loosening, migration, and spontaneous loss of the primary teeth occurred. **B,** A generalized loss of alveolar bone can be seen in the radiographs. **C,** Eight years after the initial observation of an involvement of the supporting tissues, there is evidence of normal gingival tissues. It is believed that dietary counseling and excellent oral hygiene contributed to the success of the treatment.

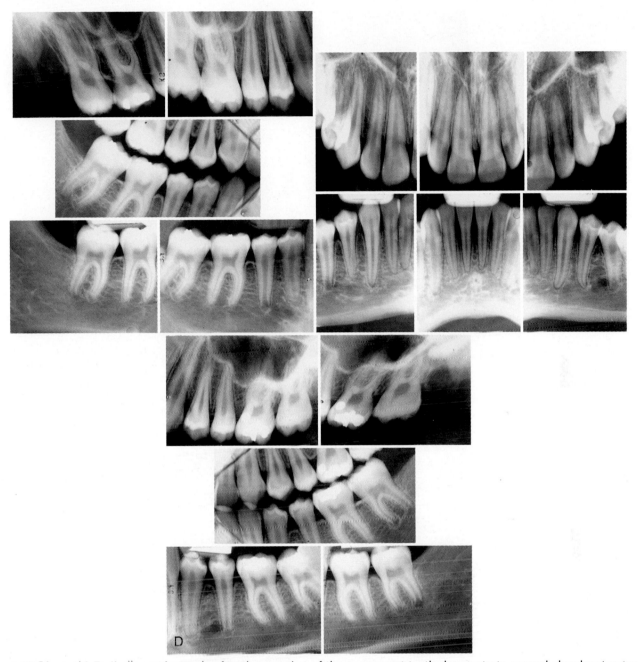

Figure 20-21 cont'd **D,** Radiographs made after the eruption of the permanent teeth demonstrate normal alveolar structures.

Because of its wide distribution and rapid rate of alveolar bone destruction, the generalized form of aggressive periodontitis has also been referred to by the terms such as *generalized juvenile periodontitis* (GJP), *severe periodontitis,* and *rapidly progressive periodontitis.* Affected teeth harbor more nonmotile, facultative, anaerobic, gram-negative rods (especially *Porphyromonas gingivalis*) in GAP than in LAP. The localized and generalized forms of aggressive periodontitis are distinctly different radiographically and clinically. Neutrophils in GAP patients have suppressed chemotaxis. Individuals with GAP exhibit marked periodontal inflammation and have heavy accumulations of plaque and calculus. Löe and Brown reported a 0.13% prevalence of GAP among adolescents in the United States.[64]

TREATMENT OF AGGRESSIVE PERIODONTITIS

Successful treatment of aggressive periodontitis depends on early diagnosis, use of antibiotics against the infecting microorganisms, and provision of an infection-free environment for healing. Treatment of aggressive periodontitis, both the localized and generalized types (LAP and GAP), includes surgery (Fig. 20-23) and the use of tetracyclines (sometimes in combination with metronidazole). In patients with LAP, Aa organisms penetrate into the crevicular epithelium. Treatment with antibiotics alone, such as a 2-week course of doxycycline (a synthetic tetracycline), has been shown to reduce the Aa population. Surgical removal of infected crevicular

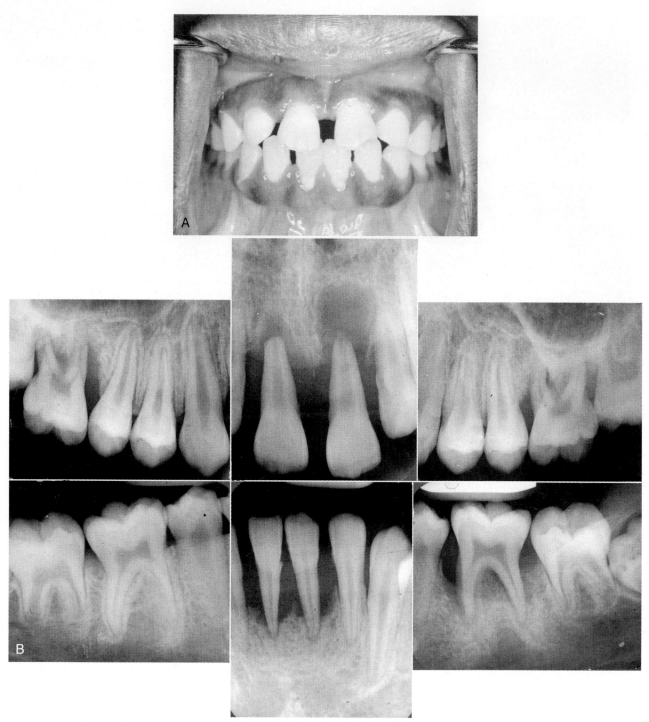

Figure 20-22 A, Evidence of mild gingivitis in a 12-year-old boy with the localized form of early-onset periodontitis. Clinical examination revealed extensive mobility of the anterior teeth. **B,** Radiographs revealed loss of support in the incisor and first permanent molar areas. The maxillary central incisors, mandibular incisors, and first permanent molars were removed. Partial dentures were constructed.

epithelium and débridement of root surfaces during surgery while the patient is on a 14-day course of doxycycline hyclate (100 mg per day) is considered the best effective treatment modality. In a study of deep periodontal lesions, Christersson and colleagues demonstrated that scaling and root planing alone were ineffective for the elimination of Aa.[71]

Microdentex manufactures the DMDx (Microdentex, Fort Myers, Fla) test, a DNA test kit for periodontal pathogens. The test aids in establishing the risk of aggressive periodontitis and confirms that the child has responded favorably to the use of adjunctive antibiotics. Retesting in 4 to 6 weeks after the completion of antibiotic therapy determines the patient's response to the treatment.

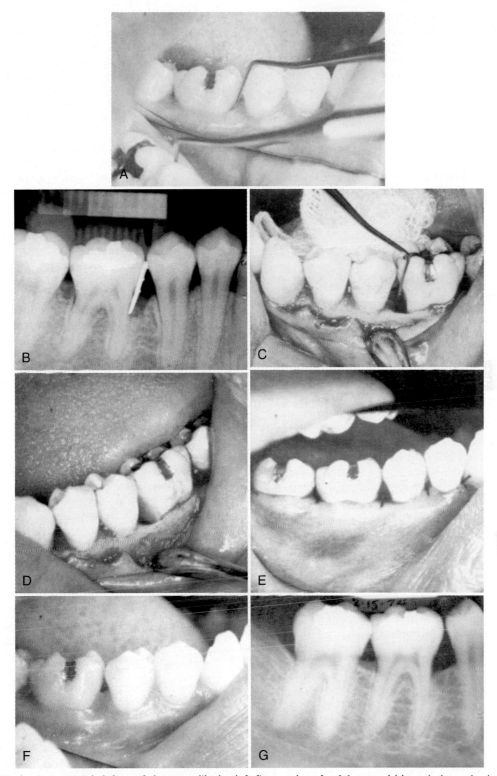

Figure 20-23 A, Probe in a mesial defect of the mandibular left first molar of a 16-year-old boy *(mirror view).* **B,** Radiograph showing depth of osseous defect. **C,** Periodontal probe showing depth of osseous defect. **D,** Defect completely débrided. **E,** Area sutured *(mirror view).* **F,** Area 6 months after surgery *(mirror view).* **G,** Radiograph 15 months after surgery. (Courtesy of Dr. Timothy J. O'Leary.)

The test involves collecting a plaque specimen by inserting a paper point provided in the kit into a periodontal pocket for 10 seconds. The paper point is placed into a test vial and returned for the microbial test. Although the Pedo Probe test provides a detailed analysis only for Aa, the laboratory will also perform a more detailed microbial analysis.

Rams and colleagues described the Keyes technique as effective in treating LAP.[72] The treatment involves meticulous scaling and root planing of all teeth, with concomitant irrigation to probing depth of saturated inorganic salt solutions and 1% chloramine T. In addition, they recommended administration of systemic tetracycline (1 g per day) for 14 days. We agree this dose is appropriate for patients 12 years of age and older. Patient home care treatment included daily application of a paste of sodium bicarbonate and 3% hydrogen peroxide and inorganic salt irrigations.

Treatment of GAP is often less predictable. Alternative antibiotics directed at the specific pathogenic flora may be required when there is no response to traditional therapies. The multidisciplinary approach combines clinical laboratory evaluation with conventional periodontal therapeutic methods for diagnosis and treatment of severe GAP cases.

PERIODONTITIS AS A MANIFESTATION OF SYSTEMIC DISEASE

The American Academy of Periodontology introduced a new classification in 1999, classifying periodontitis as a manifestation of systemic disease as a separate category. Several of these conditions are identified in the pediatric population:

A. Associated with hematological disorders
   1. Acquired neutropenia
   2. Leukemias
   3. Other
B. Associated with genetic disorders
   1. Familial and cyclic neutropenia
   2. Down syndrome
   3. Leukocyte adhesion deficiency syndromes
   4. Papillon-Lefèvre syndrome
   5. Chédiak-Higashi syndrome
   6. Histiocytosis syndromes
   7. Glycogen storage disease
   8. Infantile genetic agranulocytosis
   9. Cohen syndrome
   10. Ehlers-Danlos syndrome (types IV and VIII)
   11. Hypophosphatasia
   12. Other
C. Not otherwise specified (NOS)

PREMATURE BONE LOSS IN THE PRIMARY DENTITION

Advanced alveolar bone loss associated with systemic disease occurs in children and adolescents as well as adults. In the primary dentition, this is rare. Although most premature tooth loss from nonsystemic disease results from trauma or caries, the cause of advanced alveolar bone loss is often not readily apparent. Local factors (periodontitis, trauma, and infection secondary to caries) account for the majority of cases of premature bone loss. Goepferd reports that bony destruction in the primary dentition in the absence of local factors is highly suggestive of systemic disease.[73] Many possibilities exist; some of them are hypophosphatasia, Papillon-Lefèvre syndrome, histiocytosis X, agranulocytosis, leukocyte adherence deficiency, neutropenias, leukemias, diabetes mellitus, scleroderma, fibrous dysplasia, acrodynia, Down syndrome, and Chédiak-Higashi syndrome. The defect in immune and neutrophil cell function associated with these diseases is thought to increase patient susceptibility to infectious periodontitis causing alveolar bone loss and to other infections.

PAPILLON-LEFÈVRE SYNDROME

Coccia and colleagues observed Papillon-Lefèvre syndrome (precocious periodontosis) in a 2½-year-old child.[74] The syndrome is rare and the cause unknown. However, in the families of affected children (1 to 4 per 1,000,000) in which a familial predisposition to the disorder is noted, an autosomal recessive mode of inheritance has been identified.[75] Hart and colleagues recently narrowed the search for the causative gene for the syndrome by linking it to chromosome band 11q14-q21.[76] There is no racial or gender predominance.

The observations made in the young child in Fig. 20-24 are typical of those reported by Gorlin and associates.[77] The primary teeth erupted at the normal time. However, as early as 2 years of age, the child rubbed the gingival tissues and acted as if they were painful. There was a tendency toward gingival bleeding when the teeth were brushed. Hyperkeratosis of the palms and soles was present (Fig. 20-25); the first evidence was erythema and scaliness noted initially at 8 months of age. Delaney noted that hyperkeratotic lesions of the elbows and knees may be observed.[3] Repeated laboratory tests, including

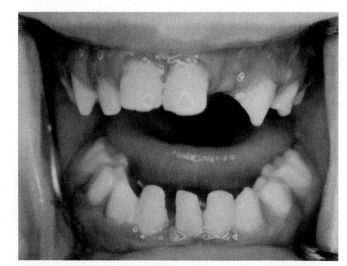

Figure 20-24 Intraoral condition of a 2½-year-old child who had Papillon-Lefèvre syndrome. Inflammatory gingival engorgement and accumulated accretions were present, especially in the mandibular incisor area.

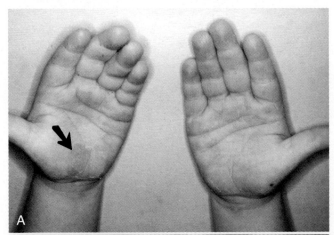

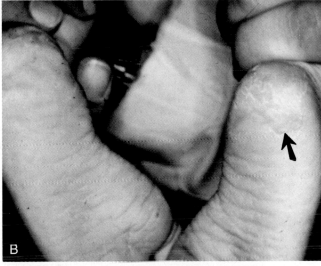

Figure 20-25 A, Hyperkeratosis of the palmar surfaces of the hands *(arrow)*. Erythema and scaliness were noted initially at 8 months of age. **B,** Hyperkeratosis of the plantar surfaces of the feet *(arrow)*.

complete blood count, urinalysis, and microserum calcium and phosphorus determinations, yielded essentially normal results.

At 2½ years of age, all the primary teeth showed looseness, and full-mouth radiographs revealed severe horizontal bone resorption (Fig. 20-26). Because of gingival inflammation, patient discomfort, and the presence of infected periodontal pockets, all the primary teeth were removed by 3 years of age. Histologic sections of the teeth displayed a premature resorption pattern with essentially normal pulp tissue. Cementum was apparently normal and covered the root structure. An accumulation of adherent basophilic plaque, made up of a mass of filamentous microorganisms, was noted on almost the entire length of the root surface. Periodontal pathogens (*Aggregatibacter actinomycetemcomitans, Fusobacterium nucleatum, Capnocytophaga* species, and *Eikenella corrodens*) have been isolated in the dental plaque of patients with Papillon-Lefèvre syndrome, according to Tinamoff and colleagues.[78,79]

Complete dentures were constructed 3 months after the removal of the primary teeth. The child tolerated the dentures well, both functionally and psychologically (Figs. 20-27 and 20-28). The first permanent molars and mandibular central incisors erupted at the expected time, and the denture base was adjusted to allow for the emergence of the teeth.

Although previous reports have indicated that the permanent dentition will also be affected, the child whose history is reported here has been followed into young adulthood, and the dentition, including the supporting tissues, appears normal (Fig. 20-29). The patient has successfully undergone orthodontic treatment.

Reports of the effectiveness of tetracycline therapy as an adjunct to meticulous subgingival débridement in the management of periodontal disease prompted McDonald to reinvestigate the history in the reported case of Papillon-Lefèvre syndrome. The father, a physician, reported that tetracyclines were given to the child repeatedly for ear infections between 3 and 6 years of age. This regimen may have been responsible for eliminating pathogens and preventing the destructive process from being carried into the permanent dentition. However, attempts at conventional therapy have been unsuccessful in preventing tooth loss. Delaney reports that periodontal treatment for these young children includes identification of specific pathogens, specific antibiotic therapy against these organisms, and full-mouth extractions early enough to provide an edentulous period before permanent tooth eruption.[3]

GINGIVAL RECESSION

Gingival recession is often observed in children.[80] Several factors predispose patients to gingival recession. These factors include presence of a narrow band of attached or keratinized gingiva, alveolar bony dehiscence, toothbrush trauma, tooth prominence, impinging frenum attachment, soft tissue impingement by opposing occlusion, orthodontic tooth movement, use of impression techniques including subgingival tissue retraction, oral habits, periodontitis, and pseudorecession (extrusion of teeth). Recession is dealt with conservatively by elimination of the stimulus if possible, while excellent oral hygiene is maintained in the affected areas. If the recession of the affected area remains unchanged (nonprogressive) or improves (less recession observed) over time, continued periodic monitoring is recommended. If the recession has progressed after a 4- to 8-week period of observation, other periodontal procedures may be required based on the identified predisposing factor.

SELF-MUTILATION

Although there has been infrequent reference to self-mutilation in the dental literature, occasionally children purposely traumatize their oral structures. Plesset reported observing a 9-year-old girl of apparently normal intelligence who worked her maxillary primary canine and mandibular permanent incisors loose from their supporting tissues and removed them.[81]

Self-mutilation probably occurs more frequently than is realized because relatively few children will admit to

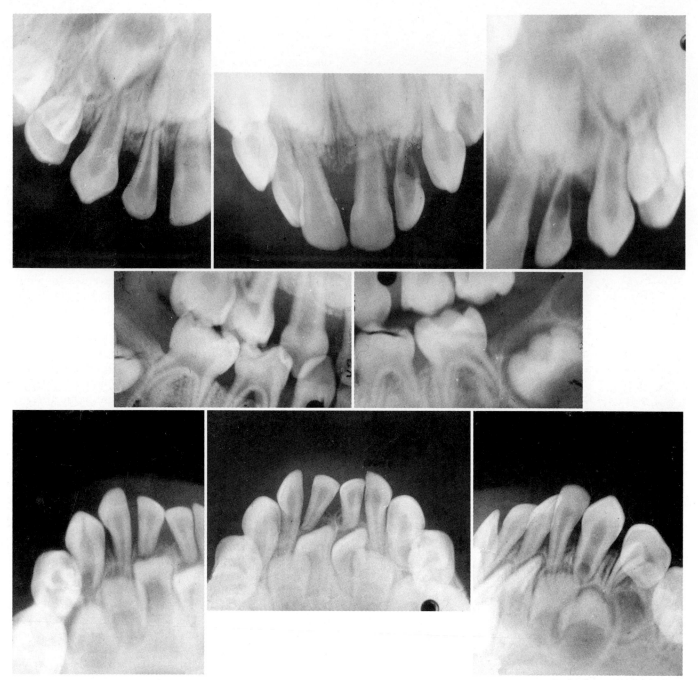

Figure 20-26 Full-mouth and bite-wing radiographs of the child with Papillon-Lefèvre syndrome. Severe horizontal bone resorption is readily detected in all four quadrants. The incisor areas display extreme alveolar bone loss to the extent that only the apical third of the root remains supported.

the act unless they are observed practicing it. Therefore the self-inflicted lesions may be incorrectly diagnosed. Dentists should be aware of the possibility of this condition and should approach the problem in the same manner as they do thumbsucking. An attempt should be made to determine the cause. If it is found to be the result of local dental factors, it can be corrected. However, in the majority of children an emotional problem is involved, and the family must be directed to competent counseling services.

Children as young as 4 years of age have been observed who have traumatized the free and attached gingival tissues with a fingernail, occasionally to the extent that the supporting alveolar bone has been destroyed (Fig. 20-30). A 14-year-old girl produced bilateral stripping of the buccal tissue in the maxillary premolar areas (Fig. 20-31) with her fingernail and a bobby pin. In addition, she bit the inner surface of her cheek and produced large necrotic areas. The parents were unaware of the habit and of the cause of the ulcerated areas in her

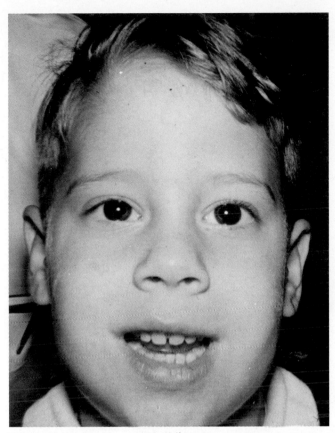

Figure 20-27 Three-year-old child with complete dentures.

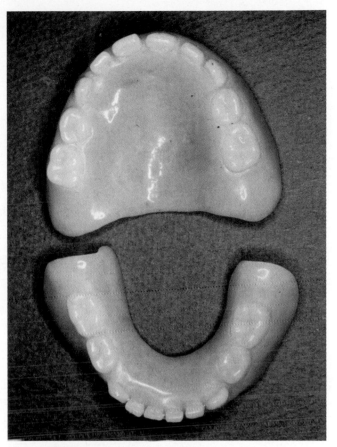

Figure 20-28 Constructed complete dentures, which were later modified to allow the eruption of the mandibular incisors and the first permanent molars.

mouth, because the daughter did not reveal that they were self-inflicted. The history revealed an unhappy child who was poorly adjusted to the home and school environments. Referral to a child guidance clinic was accepted by the child and the parents and resulted in a solution to the problem. The self-mutilation was apparently an escape from reality.

Traumatic gingival recession in infants resulting from a dummy (pacifier) sucking habit has been observed by Stewart and Kernohan.[82] In the unconventional sucking habit a segment of the plastic shield is embraced by the infant's lower lip so that the inner surface of the shield bears against the labial aspect of the incisors and the gingival tissues (Fig. 20-32). If the shield is held in this position, the edge of the shield moves with an abrasive action during sucking, which leads to gingival injury, recession, and loss of alveolar bone.

Self-mutilation by biting has been associated with severe emotional disturbances such as Lesch-Nyham syndrome (LNS), congenital insensitivity to pain, and autism. Friedlander and colleagues report autistic children with facial bruising, abrasions, and intraoral traumatic ulcerations are most often the result of self-injurious behaviors rather than abuse by parents or caretakers.[83] Management requires a choice between protective appliances initially versus surgical procedures. Littlewood and Mitchell report that mouthguards are helpful for children with congenital indifference to pain until they are

mature enough to appreciate and avoid self-mutilating behaviors, a learning process normally acquired by painful experiences.[84] Cusumano and colleagues report that the use of carbamazepine may be beneficial for children with LNS.[85]

ABNORMAL FRENUM ATTACHMENT

A frenum is a membranous fold that joins two parts and restricts the individual movement of each. Henry and colleagues describe a frenum as a mucous membrane fold containing epithelium and connective tissue fibers but no muscle.[86] A normal frenum attaches apically to the free gingival margin so as not to exert a pull on the zone of the attached gingiva, usually terminating at the mucogingival junction. Although a wide variety of aberrant positions occur, commonly observed locations of frenums in the child are on the facial gingival surface of the anterior midline of the maxilla, on the facial and lingual gingival surfaces of the anterior midline of the mandible, and on the mandibular and maxillary premolar facial area. Some frenums have bifid and trifid attachments to the alveolar process.

An abnormal or high frenum is present when there is inadequate attached gingiva in the terminal insertion area. A frenum attached too closely to the gingival margin may interfere with proper toothbrush placement, may

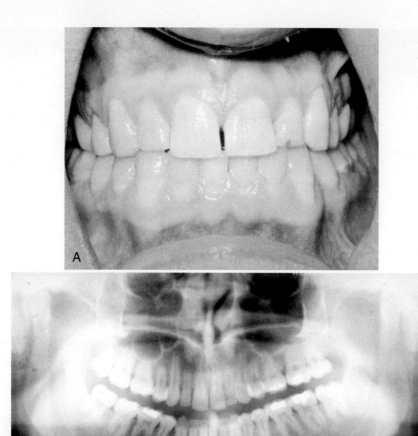

Figure 20-29 Photographs 15 years after initial diagnosis of Papillon-Lefèvre syndrome at 2½ years of age. **A,** Functional occlusion is noted after 18 months of orthodontic treatment. The clinical examination revealed good oral hygiene and normal gingival tissues. **B,** Panoramic radiographic survey revealed normal alveolar bone. Some apical root resorption related to orthodontic treatment can be seen in the mandibular incisors.

cause opening of the gingival crevice during function, or may interfere with speech. High frenum attachments may also be associated with isolated gingival recessions and diastemas, although a cause-and-effect relationship may or may not exist.

An abnormally short lingual frenum and the inability to extend the tongue is a congenital condition known as ankyloglossia (tongue-tie). Normal function can occur with this mild form, and the frenum may lengthen with normal growth and maturation of the child.

A mandibular anterior frenum occasionally inserts into the free or marginal gingival tissue and causes subsequent recession and pocket formation. The abnormal frenum attachment is most often observed in the central incisor area (Fig. 20-33), although it may involve the labial tissue in the canine areas. The abnormal attachment is frequently associated with a vestibular trough throughout the anterior region that is more shallow than normal.

Movements of the lip cause the abnormal frenum to pull on the fibers inserting into the free marginal tissue. Food accumulates and causes inflammation and eventually the development of a pocket between the labial surface of the tooth and the vestibular mucosa. Early

treatment of the abnormal frenum attachment is indicated to prevent continued stripping of the labial tissue, subsequent loss of alveolar bone, and possible eventual loss of the tooth. Although traumatic occlusion and poor oral hygiene are occasionally associated with the gingival stripping condition, the abnormal frenum attachment is more often the offender.

The maxillary anterior frenum connects the upper lip to the suture line areas between the central incisors. The importance of a frenum that prevents esthetic contact of the central incisors has been the subject of debate. The literature indicates that a diastema may be considered normal as the upper central incisors erupt and can be expected to close as the other permanent front teeth erupt. Seldom has any correlation been found between a maxillary frenum problem and recession.

FRENOTOMY AND FRENECTOMY

A frenotomy involves incision of the periosteal fiber attachment and possibly suturing of the frenum to the periosteum at the base of the vestibule. It is associated with less postoperative discomfort than a frenectomy and will usually suffice.

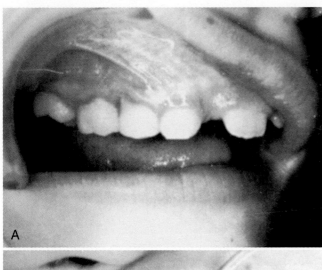

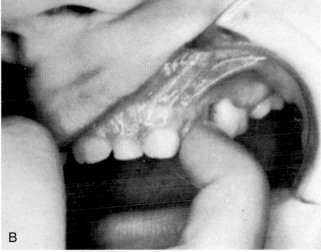

Figure 20-30 Traumatization of the gingiva between the maxillary primary molars with the index fingernail in a 6-year-old child.

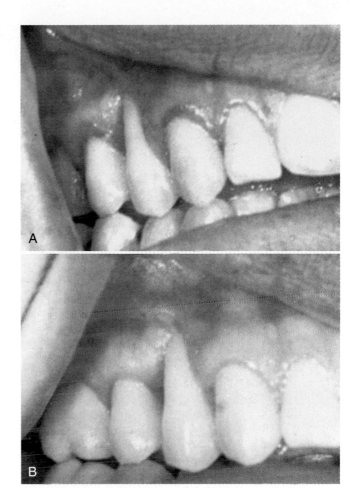

Figure 20-31 **A,** Stripping of the free and attached tissue from the buccal side of the premolar and exposure of the root surface were accomplished with a fingernail and a hairpin. The patient had a psychological problem and was referred to a child guidance clinic. **B,** After treatment of the emotional problem, the habit was discontinued. Although the soft tissue inflammation was reduced, there was no re-generation of tissue over the root surface.

A frenectomy involves complete excision of the frenum and its periosteal attachment. A frenectomy is indicated when large, fleshy frenums are involved. The need for a frenectomy or frenotomy should be based on the ability to maintain gingival health. The surgical management of the abnormal maxillary labial frenum is presented in Chapter 7 (see Figs. 7-50 to 7-52).

Indications for treating a high frenum include the following:

1. A high frenum attachment associated with an area of persistent gingival inflammation that has not responded to root planing and good oral hygiene.
2. A frenum associated with an area of recession that is progressive.
3. A high maxillary frenum and an associated midline diastema that persists after complete eruption of the permanent canines.
4. A mandibular lingual frenum that inhibits the tongue from touching the maxillary central incisors. This would interfere with the child's ability to make /t/, /d/, and /l/ sounds. As long as the child has enough range of motion to raise the tongue to the roof of the mouth,

no surgery would be indicated. Most children cannot normally make these sounds until after 6 or 7 years of age. Speech therapy may be indicated (see Fig. 7-45).

If a high frenum is associated with an area of no or minimal keratinized gingiva and a frenotomy or frenectomy is indicated, a gingival graft or vestibular extension should be used to augment the procedure. Under these circumstances, a frenotomy or frenectomy often does not create stable long-term results. Bohannan indicated that, if there is an adequate band of attached gingiva, high frenums and vestibular depth do not pose a problem.[87-89] Use of the latter procedures to accomplish elimination of the frenum pull is considered a more standard approach.

TECHNIQUES FOR MANDIBULAR FRENECTOMY AND VESTIBULAR DEPTH INCREASE

Bohannan has published a series of reports of his studies in the alteration of vestibular depth and frenectomy.[87-89] Three different surgical procedures, which he refers to as

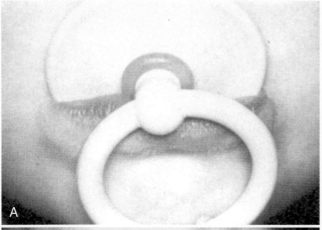

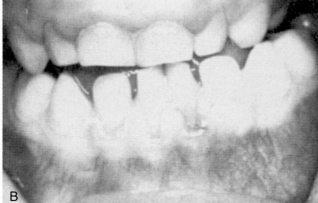

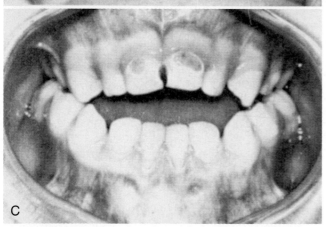

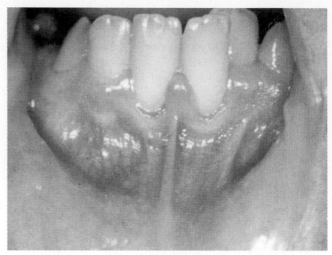

Figure 20-33 Abnormal attachment of the frenum. The fibers can be seen extending to the papilla between the central incisors with branching auxiliary fibers inserting into the marginal tissue.

Figure 20-32 A, An unconventional manner of pacifier sucking may lead to gingival trauma and recession. **B** and **C,** Gingival recession in the lower incisor region in two children. Note anterior open bite in **C.** (From Stewart DJ, Kernohan DC. Traumatic gingival recession in infants: The result of a dummy sucking habit, *Br Dent J* 135: 157-158, 1973.)

complete denudation, periosteum retention, and vestibular incision, were studied as methods to produce increased vestibular depth and frenum alteration.

Complete Denudation

The complete denudation procedure is preceded by a routine gingivectomy extending laterally to the first premolars. By blunt dissection, the periosteum and adherent fibrous tissue are detached apically, and the labial plate is exposed to a depth of approximately 12 mm. The resulting soft tissue flap is removed by excision. A rapid-setting dressing is placed directly over the osseous tissue and is changed at 7-day intervals for 4 weeks.

Periosteum Retention

The periosteum retention procedure, as carried out by Bohannan, does not always result in maintenance of the desirable amount of vestibular depth.[89] The procedure is essentially the same as that described previously, except that the periosteum is allowed to remain.

Vestibular Incision

The vestibular incision method (mandibular frenectomy) is a surgical procedure that we have used with success. The elimination of the abnormal frenum should remain the objective of the procedure, although it is often desirable also to alter the vestibular depth. However, the frenum is the primary etiologic factor in the stripping of the gingival tissue and labial pocket formation.

A preliminary prophylactic procedure should be performed to remove hard deposits, debris, and plaque material from the teeth. The surgical procedure should be more extensive than a conservative incision of the frenum. Such a procedure would allow the muscle fibers to reattach, with resultant scar tissue formation, and would perhaps make the condition more severe (Fig. 20-34).

A local anesthetic is given before the surgical procedure. A right and left inferior alveolar injection is the method of choice. Some dentists prefer to inject the local anesthetic solution throughout the operative field. However, caution should be exercised because the anesthetic may distend the tissue, which makes it more difficult to find landmarks during the surgical procedure.

The lower lip should be stretched outward and downward, and an incision approximately 1 cm in depth

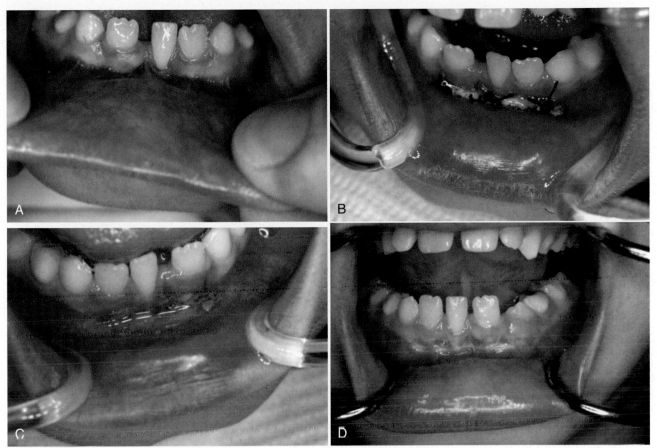

Figure 20-34 A, Tissue has been stripped and a pocket formed on the labial surface of the right central incisor. Frenectomy and procedure to increase the depth of the vestibular trough are indicated. **B,** An incision has been made and a pack has been placed and secured with three sutures. **C,** Five days after the operation, the pack was removed. Granulation tissue has formed, and normal healing is taking place. **D,** Three months after the operation, improvement in the health of the gingival tissue in the mandibular anterior region is evident.

beyond the level of the vestibular trough should be made at a right angle to the underlying bone. The incision is made at the junction of the mucobuccal fold and attached gingiva, and should extend at least two teeth on either side of the attachment. If the abnormal attachment is on the incisor area, an incision is often made from an area opposite one canine to the canine on the other side of the mouth. The connective tissue and muscle attachments are then freed by blunt dissection with a periosteal elevator. No attempt is made to strip the underlying periosteum.

A periodontal pack or some type of splint must be used to prevent reattachment of the tissue and to allow granulation to occur at a greater depth. A piece of rubber tubing 2 to 3 mm in diameter and the exact length of the incision can be coated with surgical paste and sutured in the trough. The patient is seen 24 hours postoperatively, and any granulation tissue that has developed over the ends of the tubing is removed. The pack is normally removed after 4 to 5 days, and the wound is irrigated as necessary until healing occurs.

As an alternative method of encouraging healing at a new depth, the entire surgical wound is filled with a stiff periodontal dressing of the zinc oxide–eugenol type. The pack, which extends over the labial surface of the anterior teeth, may be covered with dry foil and allowed to remain for 3 to 4 weeks with only weekly changes (Fig. 20-35). Some dentists ligate an acrylic splint to the teeth after surgery to aid in the reestablishment of the new depth of the sulcus.

FREE GINGIVAL AUTOGRAFT PROCEDURE

The free gingival autograft procedure (FGG) may be considered for children and young adults when there is a prominent tooth position that is complicated by absence of attached gingiva, a shallow vestibular fornix, and a high midline frenum attachment (Fig. 20-36). FGG is also indicated when there are areas of root exposure that are an esthetic concern to the patient, when the labial gingivae of some teeth require subgingival crown margins, when teeth are clasped by a removable partial denture having a narrow zone of gingiva, and when teeth that have no labial keratinized gingiva need orthodontic movement, which makes them more prominent in the arch. When these indications are kept in mind, it will be apparent that FGG is not always the best procedure. There may be an esthetic concern with the surrounding gingiva because the autograft will remain the same color

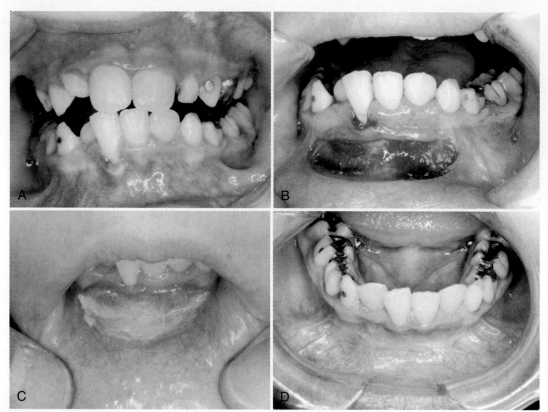

Figure 20-35 A, Stripping of the tissue and loss of alveolar bone from the labial aspect of the lower right central incisor are related to an abnormal frenum attachment and shallow vestibule. **B,** An incision has been made and the connective tissue and muscle attachments have been freed by blunt dissection. **C,** One week after the operation there is evidence of granulation tissue. **D,** An improvement is evident in the gingival contour of the tissue surrounding the right central incisor.

and texture as the palatal donor site (Fig. 20-37). FGG will not cover the area of recession but rather will prevent its progression. If root coverage is a goal, the laterally positioned pedicle graft and coronally positioned flap procedures are more predictable. When the amount of attached gingiva is adequate, FGG is not indicated. If pocket elimination is a concern, an apically repositioned flap should be a choice.

In the FGG procedure, the receptor site is first prepared. When a high frenum attachment has contributed to the mucogingival problem, tension is placed on the lower lip to activate the frenum and trace its insertion into the marginal tissue. A horizontal incision is made at the mucogingival junction, including the attachment of the frenum into the gingiva. The mucosa is displaced apically by blunt dissection, and a nonmovable receptor site is left consisting of periosteum and a thin covering of firm connective tissue. Any gingival epithelium coronal to the primary incision is trimmed away, which leaves a receptor bed of connective tissue with an adequate blood supply.

The next step is to fenestrate the periosteum to help prevent mobility of the graft after healing. To do this, two horizontal incisions, 1 mm apart, are made through the periosteum at the apical boundary of the displaced mucosa. The isolated periosteum between the two horizontal incisions is peeled away, so that the facial cortical plate of bone is exposed. A template of adhesive foil slightly larger than the mandibular receptor site is made, and the

palatal donor site is anesthetized. The template is placed on the anesthetized tissue and is outlined with a shallow incision. The graft is freed from the underlying submucosa by sharp dissection. The operator should strive to secure an intermediate-thickness graft (approximately 1 mm thick).

After the graft is removed from the palate, the connective tissue side is inspected to ensure that no fatty tissue remains on it (adherent fatty tissue would prevent revascularization of the graft from the connective tissue of the receptor site). If present, the fatty tissue is cut away. The graft is carried to the receptor site, and any final trimming is done to secure an approximation of the donor tissue to the receptor site. The graft is sutured into position with a 5-0 Dacron suture and an atraumatic (taper) needle. Normally a suture at the coronal aspect of each end of the graft is enough to secure it. The graft is covered with adhesive foil, which in turn is covered with a hard-setting periodontal dressing. When the patient returns 7 to 10 days after surgery, the dressing is removed, the area is débrided and irrigated, and the sutures are removed. A second dressing is usually placed for another 5 to 7 days.

When the second dressing is removed, the area is again débrided, and the teeth are polished. At this time the graft should be firmly fixed to the underlying receptor site, and the epithelial covering should be continuous with that of the contiguous gingiva and oral mucosa. The

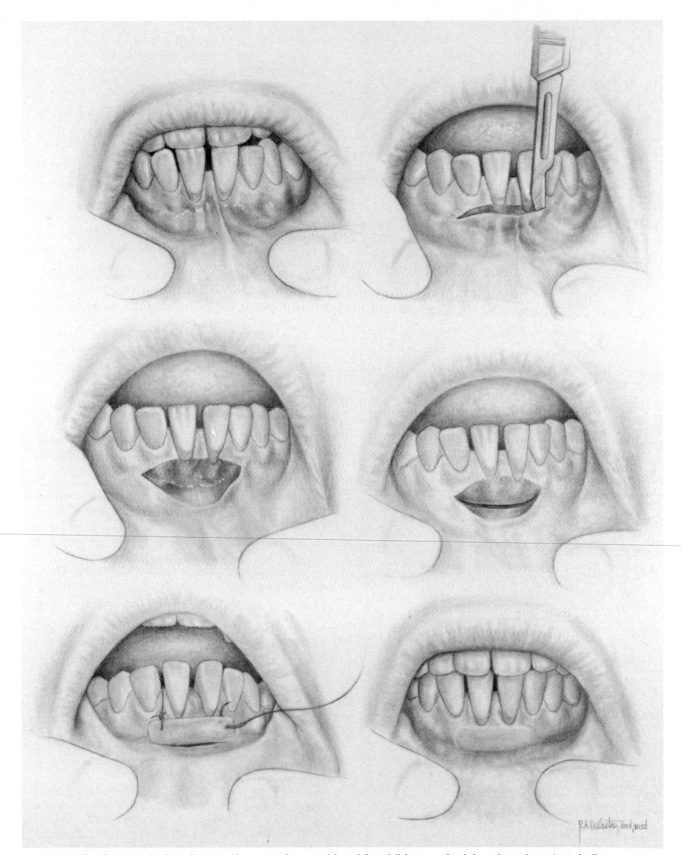

Figure 20-36 The free gingival graft procedure may be considered for children and adults when there is a shallow vestibular fornix and a high midline frenum attachment.

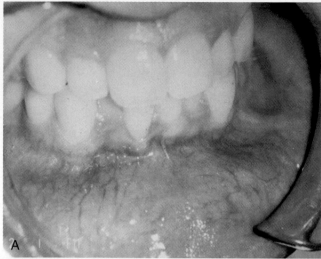

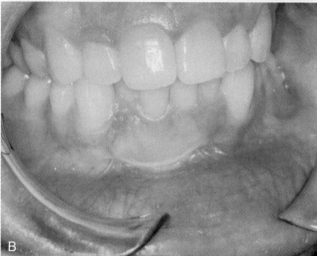

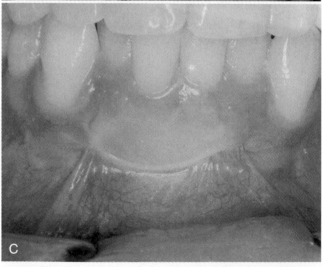

Figure 20-37 A, Initial presentation of patient to receive a mandibular free gingival graft. **B,** Postoperative appearance 3½ years later. **C,** Higher-magnification photograph of graft 5 years postoperatively.

patient is instructed to gently clean away any debris from the area with a cotton ball soaked in warm water and to continue the interdental flossing routine. Normal brushing can usually be reintroduced between 21 and 25 days after the graft is placed.

CLINICAL ASSESSMENT OF ORAL CLEANLINESS AND PERIODONTAL DISEASE

PLAQUE CONTROL RECORD

O'Leary and colleagues developed the plaque control record to give the dentist, hygienist, and dental educator a simple method of recording the presence of plaque on individual tooth surfaces (mesial, distal, facial, and lingual).[90]

At the initial appointment, a suitable disclosing solution, such as Bismarck brown, is painted on all exposed tooth surfaces. After the patient has rinsed, the operator, using an explorer, examines each stained surface for soft accumulations at the dentogingival junction. When found, these accumulations are recorded by making a dash in the appropriate spaces on the record form. Fig. 20-38A, shows a form completed at the patient's first appointment for learning plaque control. No attempt is made to differentiate between varying amounts of plaque on tooth surfaces.

After all teeth are examined and scored, an index can be derived when the number of plaque-containing surfaces is divided by the total number of available surfaces. The same procedure is carried out at subsequent appointments to determine the patient's progress in learning and carrying out the prescribed oral hygiene procedures. Fig. 20-38B, shows a patient's progress from the initial assessment to the point (fifth session) at which plaque control is deemed satisfactory.

A detailed approach to teaching toothbrushing, flossing, and plaque control is described in Chapter 11.

PERIODONTAL SCREENING AND RECORDING

As we noted in Chapter 1, we endorse the use of the periodontal screening and recording (PSR) method to facilitate the early detection of periodontal diseases in children. Clerehugh and Tugnait recommend using the PSR for pediatric dental patients following the eruption of the permanent incisors and first molars.[91] They suggest routine screening for new pediatric patients and at regular recare appointments so that periodontal problems are detected early and treated appropriately. Immunodeficient children are especially vulnerable to early loss of bone support.

Although the PSR was originally designed for use in adults, it has been found to be an effective method of detecting early signs of periodontal disease among certain children who may be at higher risk. Piazzini provided a favorable report on the application of PSR in children and adolescents.[92] The PSR is not a substitute for a comprehensive periodontal examination, but it should help the clinician efficiently identify the few child or adolescent patients who need a comprehensive

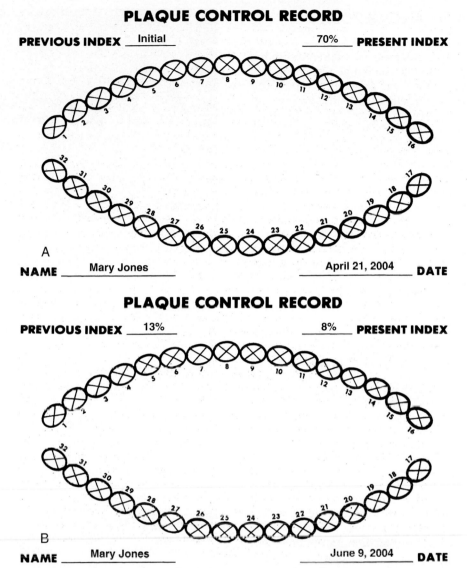

Figure 20-38 A, Plaque accumulations recorded at the initial control appointment. **B,** Plaque accumulations recorded at the fifth session.

periodontal evaluation. In addition, the possibility of false readings caused by gingival pseudopocketing must be considered, because pseudopocketing is more frequent in young patients.

For purposes of recording the results of the PSR, the dentition is divided into six areas (sextants): two anterior sextants (maxillary and mandibular) and four posterior sextants (right and left maxillary and mandibular). The gingival sulcus depth of each tooth or implant is measured in at least six areas (three facial and three lingual areas) by gentle probing with a periodontal probe in the standard manner. Each sextant is scored for periodontal health based on a code number from 0 to 4 as follows:

Code 0 indicates that all sulcus depths in the sextant are 3.5 mm or less, and no calculus is present and no gingival bleeding occurred from the gentle probing.

Code 1 indicates that all sulcus depths are 3.5 mm or less, and no calculus is present but some bleeding occurred from the gentle probing.

Code 2 indicates that all sulcus depths are 3.5 mm or less and some calculus is present.

Code 3 indicates that one or more sulcus depths are between 3.5 and 5.5 mm.

Code 4 indicates that one or more sulcus depths are more than 5.5 mm.

In addition to the code number, an asterisk (*) may accompany the code score to indicate furcation involvement, abnormal tooth mobility, mucogingival problems, or significant gingival recession.

Appropriate preventive care, oral hygiene instruction, and therapy (plaque and calculus removal) are indicated, as required, for patients who receive PSR code scores of 2, 1, or 0. Patients receiving code scores of 3 or 4 require more comprehensive periodontal evaluation and treatment.

EXTRINSIC STAINS AND DEPOSITS ON TEETH

Previous work regarding the staining of children's teeth has been related primarily to studies of orange and green stain of the extrinsic type. It has been generally accepted this stain has a microbial origin, although some reports have indicated that oral iron preparations or other medications may be responsible for an additional type of extrinsic staining. Woodall and colleagues report the accumulation of dental deposits and stains are effected by salivary composition and flow rates, poor oral hygiene, enamel defects and aging with exposed extrinsic factors (medications, coffee, tea, tobacco, and intrinsic physiological changes).[93] Extrinsic stains are identified by color, distribution, and tenaciousness along with age, sex, and home care.[94]

Staining is generally believed to be caused by extrinsic agents, which can be readily removed from the surface of the teeth with an abrasive material. The agents that are responsible for staining are deposited in enamel defects or become attached to the enamel without bringing about a change in its surface.

Pigmentation, in contrast to extrinsic staining, is associated with an active chemical change in the tooth structure, and the resultant pigment cannot be removed without alteration of the tooth structure.

GREEN STAIN

The cause of green stain, which is most often seen on the teeth of children, is unknown, although it is believed to be the result of the action of chromogenic bacteria on the enamel cuticle. Boys are more frequently affected than girls. The color of the stain varies from dark green to light yellowish green. This tenacious deposit is seen most often in the gingival third of the labial surface of the maxillary anterior teeth. The stain collects more readily on the labial surface of the maxillary anterior teeth in mouth breathers. It tends to recur even after careful and complete removal. The enamel beneath the stain may be roughened or may have undergone initial demineralization. The roughening of the surface is believed to be related to the frequency of recurrence of the stain (Fig. 20-39). Fungi (*Penicillium* and *Aspergillus*) and fluorescent bacteria have been associated with the discoloration.[94]

ORANGE STAIN

The cause of orange stain is likewise unknown. Orange stain occurs less frequently and is more easily removed than green or brown stain. Chromogenic bacteria (*Serratia marcescens* and *Flavobacterium lutescens*) have been reported to be implicated as a probable cause.[95] The stain is most often seen in the gingival third of the tooth and is associated with poor oral hygiene (Fig. 20-40).

BLACK STAIN

A black stain occasionally develops on the primary or permanent teeth of children, but it is much less common than the orange or green type (Fig. 20-41). A thin black line of dots or band of stain may be seen following the gingival contour or it may be apparent in a more generalized pattern on the clinical crown, particularly if there are roughened or pitted areas. The black type of stain is difficult to

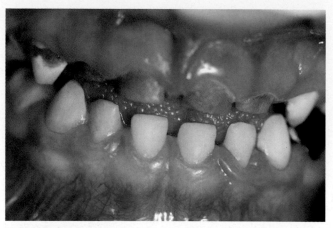

Figure 20-39 Dark green stain is evident on maxillary anterior teeth. Papillary and marginal gingivitis is also present. The patient had poor oral hygiene and was a mouth breather.

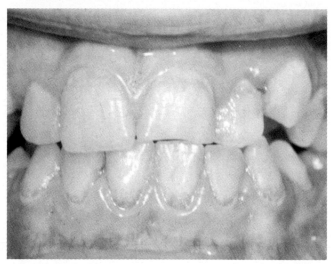

Figure 20-40 Orange stain is evident in the gingival third of the mandibular anterior teeth.

remove, especially if it collects in pitted areas. It has been reported more frequently in females. Many children who have black stain are relatively free of dental caries and have excellent oral hygiene. The chromogenic bacteria primarily associated with this stain is *Actinomyces*.[96]

REMOVAL OF EXTRINSIC STAINS

Extrinsic stains can be removed by polishing with a rubber cup and flour pumice. If the stain is resistant and difficult to remove, the excess water should be blotted from the pumice and the teeth should be dried before the polishing procedure is performed. Because stains are most often seen in a mouth in which there is poor oral hygiene, improving the oral hygiene minimizes the recurrence of the stain.

PIGMENTATION CAUSED BY STANNOUS FLUORIDE APPLICATION

During the first clinical trials involving the topical application of an 8% stannous fluoride solution, certain areas of the tooth became discolored. A characteristic pigmentation of both carious and precarious lesions has been found to be associated with exposure to stannous fluoride (Fig. 20-42).

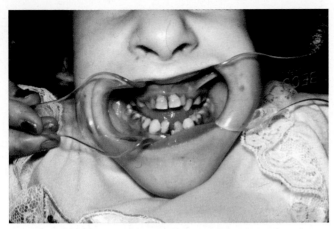

Figure 20-41 Black stain is evident on the primary teeth. The stain is difficult to remove, particularly when it collects in roughened areas of the tooth.

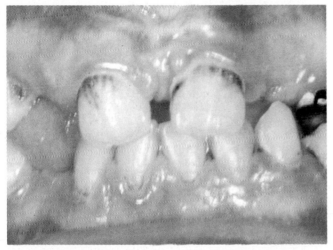

Figure 20-42 Pigmentation of carious and precarious enamel. The color ranges from light brown to black, the darker pigmentation being evident in the area of greatest caries involvement. The pigmentation is evidence of caries arrest following stannous fluoride application.

CALCULUS

Calculus is not often seen in preschool children, and even in children of grade school age it occurs with much lower frequency than in adult patients. A low caries incidence is related to high calculus incidence.

Bhat reported findings in 14- to 17-year-old children who participated in the 1986-1987 National Survey of Oral Health.[97] Supragingival calculus was observed in nearly 34% of the children and subgingival calculus in approximately 23%. Both types show a predilection for molars in the maxilla and incisors and canines in the mandible.

Children with mental retardation often have accumulations of calculus on their teeth. This accumulation may be related to abnormal muscular function, a soft diet, poor oral hygiene, and stagnation of saliva.

The observations of Turesky and colleagues regarding early calculus formation in children and adults substantiate those of others and indicate that calculus begins as a soft, adherent, bacteria-laden plaque that undergoes progressive calcification.[98] They observed calculus formation on cellulose acetate strips that were fixed in children's mouths. Plaque material that accumulated on the strips underwent progressive hardening. A soft plaque material consisted for the most part of bacteria appearing as a dense meshwork of diffusely distributed gram-negative cocci with occasional rod forms. Filamentous or thread-shaped organisms were scarce. Leukocytes and epithelial cells were also scattered within the amorphous matrix.

Gross accumulations of calculus are occasionally seen in teenaged and preteenaged children (Figs. 20-43 and 20-44). Traiger reported on a 14-year-old girl who had excessive deposits of supragingival and subgingival calculus.[99] The calculus covered the labial surfaces of the anterior teeth, extended into the mucobuccal fold, and covered the attached gingiva.

Supragingival deposits of calculus occur most frequently and in greater quantity on the buccal surfaces of the maxillary molars and the lingual surfaces of the mandibular anterior teeth. These areas are near the openings of the major salivary glands. Local factors are unquestionably important in the initiation of calculus formation.

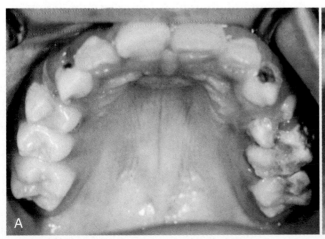

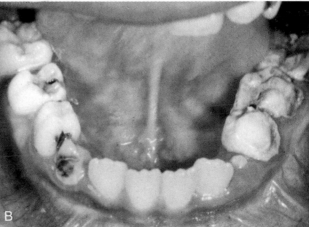

Figure 20-43 Gross accumulations of calculus are seen on the clinical crowns of the posterior teeth on the left side of the mouth. The fact that the child chewed mostly on his right side accounts partially for the greater cleanliness on that side.

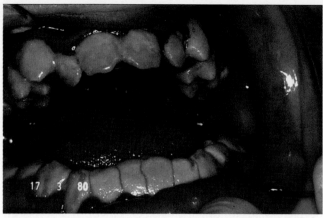

Figure 20-44 Young adult with calculus covering the labial and lingual surfaces of the mandibular anterior teeth. After the calculus was removed, amelogenesis imperfecta was apparent. The rough surface of the crown favorably influenced the deposition of calculus.

REFERENCES

1. Löe H, et al. The gingiva: structure and function. In Genco RJ, et al, eds. *Contemporary periodontics*. St Louis, 1990, Mosby.
2. Delaney JE, Keels MA. Pediatric oral pathology. Soft tissue and periodontal conditions, *Pediatr Clin North Am* 47(5):1125-1147, 2000.
3. Delaney JE. Periodontal and soft-tissue abnormalities, *Dent Clin North Am* 39:837-850, 1995.
4. American Academy of Pediatric Dentistry: Special issue: Reference manual 2008-2009, *Pediatr Dent* 30(7 Suppl): 7, 236-253, 2008.
5. Eastcott AD, Stallard RE. Sequential changes in developing human dental plaque as visualized by scanning electron microscope, *J Periodontol* 44:218-224, 1973.
6. Suomi JD, et al. Oral calculus in children, *J Periodontol* 42:341-345, 1971.
7. Weddell JA, Klein AI. Socioeconomic correlation of oral disease in 6- to 36-month children, *Pediatr Dent* 3:306-310, 1981.
8. Horowitz AM, et al. Effects of supervised daily dental plaque removal by children after 3 years, *Community Dent Oral Epidemiol* 8:171-176, 1980.
9. Murray JJ. The prevalence of gingivitis in children continuously resident in a high fluoride area, *J Dent Child* 41: 133-139, 1974.
10. Matsson L, Moller C. Gingival inflammatory reactions in children with rhinoconjunctivitis due to birch pollinosis, *Scand J Dent Res* 98:504-509, 1990.
11. Schaaf JE. Non-dental pharmacotherapeutics, *Alumni Bull Sch Dent Indiana Univ, Spring* 48-53, 1984.
12. Zunt SL. Personal communication, 2003.
13. Faden H. Management of primary herpetic gingivostomatitis in young children, *Pediatr Emerg Care* 22(4):268, 2006.
14. Hale BD, et al. Epidemic herpetic stomatitis in orphanage children, *Dent Abst* 8:556, 1963.
15. Kleinman DV, et al. Epidemiology of oral mucosal lesions in United States schoolchildren: 1986-87, *Community Dent Oral Epidemiol* 22:243-253, 1994.
16. Griffith RS, Norins AL, Kagan C. A multicentered study of lysine therapy in herpes simplex infection, *Dermatologica* 156:257-267, 1978.
17. Brooks SL, et al. Prevalence of herpes simplex virus disease in a professional population, *J Am Dent Assoc* 102:31-34, 1981.
18. Scully C, Porter S. Oral mucosal disease: recurrent aphthous stomatitis, *Br J Oral Maxill Surg* 46:198-206, 2008.
19. Ship JA, et al. Recurrent aphthous stomatitis, *Quintessence Int* 31:95-112, 2000.
20. Antoon JW, Miller RL. Aphthous ulcers: a review of the literature on etiology, pathogenesis, diagnosis, and treatment, *J Am Dent Assoc* 101:803-808, 1980.
21. Wray D, et al. Recurrent aphthae: Treatment with vitamin B12, folic acid and iron, *Br Med J* 2:490-493, 1975.
22. Greenspan JA, et al. Lymphocyte function in recurrent aphthous ulceration, *J Oral Pathol* 14:592-602, 1985.
23. Binnie WH, et al. Amlexanox oral paste: a novel treatment that accelerates the healing of aphthous ulcers, *Compendium Contin Educ Dent* 18:1116-1118, 1120-1122, 1124-1126, 1997.
24. Meiller TF, et al. Effect of an antimicrobial mouth rinse on recurrent aphthous ulcerations, *Oral Surg Oral Med Oral Pathol* 72:425-429, 1991.
25. Pedersen A. Acyclovir in the prevention of severe aphthous ulcers, *Arch Dermatol* 128:119, 1992.
26. Reade PC. Infantile acute ulcerative gingivitis: a case report, *J Periodontol* 34:387-390, 1963.
27. Blake GC, Trott JR. Acute streptococcal gingivitis, *Dent Pract* 10:43-45, 1959.
28. Littner MM, et al. Acute streptococcal gingivostomatitis, *Oral Surg Oral Med Oral Pathol* 53:144-147, 1982.
29. Glauser RO, et al. An unusual gingivitis among Navajo Indians, *Periodontics* 1:255-259, 1963.
30. Kaslick RS, et al. Association between ABO blood groups, HL-A antigens and periodontal diseases in young adults: a follow-up study, *J Periodontol* 51:339-342, 1980.
31. Löe H, Schiött CR. The effect of mouthrinses and topical application of chlorhexidine on the development of dental plaque and gingivitis in man, *J Periodontal Res* 5:79-83, 1970.
32. Yankell SL, et al. Laboratory and clinical stain removal evaluations of two tartar control dentifrices, *J Clin Dent* 6:207-210, 1995.
33. Brecx M, et al. Efficacy of Listerine, Meridol and chlorhexidine mouthrinses as supplements to regular tooth-cleaning measures, *J Clin Periodontal* 19:202-207, 1992.
34. Barnett ML. The rationale for the daily use of an antimicrobial mouthrinse, *JADA* 137(7 Suppl):16S-21S, 2006.
35. Silverman S, Wilder R. Antimicrobial mouthrinse as part of a comprehensive oral care regimen, *JADA* 137 (11 Suppl):22S-26S, 2006.
36. Cohen MM. The effect of large doses of ascorbic acid on gingival tissue at puberty, *J Dent Res* 34:750-751 (abstract), 1955.
37. Nakagawa S, et al. A longitudinal study from prepuberty to puberty of gingivitis, *J Clin Periodontol* 21:658-665, 1994.
38. Sutcliffe P. A longitudinal study of gingivitis and puberty, *J Periodontal Res* 7:52-58, 1972.
39. Hart TC, et al. Genetic linkage of hereditary gingival fibromatosis to chromosome 2p21, *Am J Hum Genet* 62:876-883, 1998.
40. Zackin SJ, Weisberger D. Hereditary gingival fibromatosis: report of a family, *Oral Surg Oral Med Oral Pathol* 14:825-835, 1961.
41. Brown RS, et al. Treatment of a patient with hereditary gingival fibromatosis: a case report, *Spec Care Dentist* 15:149-153, 1995.
42. Kimball OP. Treatment of epilepsy with sodium diphenyl-hydantoinate, *JAMA* 112:1244-1245, 1939.

43. Hassell T, et al. Diphenylhydantoin (Dilantin) gingival hyperplasia: drug-induced abnormality of connective tissue, *Proc Natl Acad Sci U S A* 73:2909-2912, 1976.
44. Addy V, et al. Risk factors in phenytoin-induced gingival hyperplasia, *J Periodontol* 54:373-377, 1983.
45. Kapur RN, et al. Diphenylhydantoin-induced gingival hyperplasia: its relationship to dose and serum level, *Dev Med Child Neurol* 15:483-487, 1973.
46. Little RM, et al. Diphenylhydantoin-induced gingival hyperplasia: its response to changes in drug dosage, *Dev Med Child Neurol* 17:421-424, 1975.
47. Livingston S, et al. The medical treatment of epilepsy: managing side effects of antiepileptic drugs, *Pediatr Ann* 8:261-266, 1979.
48. Ciancio SG, et al. Gingival hyperplasia and diphenylhydantoin, *J Periodontol* 43:411-414, 1972.
49. Sasaki T, Maita E. Increased BfGF level in the serum of patients with phenytoin-induced gingival overgrowth, *J Clin Periodontol* 25:42-47, 1998.
50. Jones JE, et al. Incidence and indications for surgical management of phenytoin-induced gingival overgrowth in a cerebral palsy population, *J Oral Maxillofac Surg* 46:385-390, 1988.
51. Steinberg SC, Steinberg AD. Phenytoin-induced gingival overgrowth control in severely retarded children, *J Periodontol* 53:429-433, 1982.
52. Donnenfeld OW, et al. A nine-month clinical and histological study of patients on diphenyl hydantoin following gingivectomy, *J Periodontol* 45:547-557, 1974.
53. Davis RK, et al. A preliminary report on a new therapy for Dilantin gingival hyperplasia, *J Periodontol* 34:17-22, 1963.
54. Sheridan PJ, Reeve CM. Effective treatment of Dilantin gingival hyperplasia, *Oral Surg Oral Med Oral Pathol* 35:42-46, 1973.
55. Steinberg AD. Clinical management of phenytoin-induced gingival overgrowth in handicapped children, *Pediatr Dent* 3(special issue):130-136, 1981.
56. Drew HJ, et al. Effect of folate on phenytoin hyperplasia, *J Clin Periodontol* 14:350-356, 1987.
57. Bäckman N, et al. Folate treatment of diphenylhydantoin-induced gingival hyperplasia, *Scand J Dent Res* 97:222-232, 1989.
58. Fain O, et al. Lesson of the week: scurvy in patients with cancer, *Br Med J* 316:1661-1662, 1998.
59. Bimstein E, et al. Radiographic assessment of the alveolar bone in children and adolescents, *Pediatr Dent* 10:199, 1988.
60. American Academy of Periodontology. Parameter on aggressive periodontitis, *J Periodontol* 71(suppl):867, 2000.
61. Armitage GC. Development of a classification system for periodontal diseases and conditions, *Ann Periodontal* 4:1-6, 1999.
62. Albandar JM, et al. Clinical classification of periodontitis in adolescents and young adults, *J Periodontol* 68:545-555, 1997.
63. Albandar JM, et al. Clinical features of early-onset periodontitis, *J Am Dent Assoc* 128:1393-1399, 1997.
64. Löe H, Brown LJ. Early onset of periodontitis in the United States of America, *J Periodontol* 62:608-616, 1991.
65. Page RC, et al. Rapidly progressive periodontitis: a distinct clinical condition, *J Periodontol* 54:197-209, 1983.
66. Buchmann R, et al. Aggressive periodontitis: 5 year follow-up of treatment, *J Periodontol* 73:675, 2002.
67. Deas DE, et al. Systemic disease and periodontitis: manifestations of neutrophil dysfunction, *Periodontology* 2000:32, 82, 2003.
68. Asikainen S, et al. Can one acquire periodontal bacteria and periodontitis from a family member? *J Am Dent Assoc* 128:1263-1270, 1997.
69. Yang ET, et al. Periodontal pathogen detection in gingival/tooth and tongue flora samples from 18-48 month old children and periodontal status of their mothers, *Oral Microbiol Immunol* 17:55, 2002.
70. Page RC, et al. Clinical and laboratory studies of a family with a high prevalence of juvenile periodontitis, *J Periodontol* 56:602-610, 1985.
71. Christersson LA, et al. Microbiological and clinical effects of surgical treatment of localized juvenile periodontitis, *J Clin Periodontol* 12:465-476, 1985.
72. Rams TE, et al. Treatment of juvenile periodontitis with microbiologically modulated periodontal therapy (Keyes technique), *Pediatr Dent* 7:259-270, 1985.
73. Goepferd SJ. Advanced alveolar bone loss in the primary dentition: a case report, *J Periodontol* 52:753-757, 1981.
74. Coccia CT, et al. Papillon-Lefèvre syndrome: precocious periodontosis with palmar-plantar hyperkeratosis, *J Periodontol* 37:408-414, 1966.
75. Canger EM, et al. Intraoral findings of Papillon-Lefevre syndrome, *J Dent Child* 75:99-103, 2008.
76. Hart TC, et al. Sublocalization of the Papillon-Lefèvre syndrome locus on 11q14-q21, *Am J Med Genet* 79:134-139, 1998.
77. Gorlin RJ, et al. The syndrome of palmar-plantar hyperkeratosis and premature periodontal destruction of the teeth, *J Pediatr* 65:895-908, 1964.
78. Tinanoff N, et al. Treatment of the periodontal component of Papillon-Lefèvre syndrome, *J Clin Periodontal* 13:6, 1986.
79. Tinanoff N, et al. Dental treatment of Papillon-Lefèvre syndrome: 15-year follow-up, *J Clin Periodontol* 22:609-612, 1995.
80. Bimstein E, et al. Prevalence of gingival stippling in children, *J Clin Pediatr Dent* 27:163, 2003.
81. Plesset DN. Auto-extraction, *Oral Surg Oral Med Oral Pathol* 12:302-303, 1959.
82. Stewart DJ, Kernohan DC. Traumatic gingival recession in infants: The result of a dummy sucking habit, *Br Dent J* 135:157-158, 1973.
83. Friedlander AH, et al. the neuropathology, medical management and dental implications of autism, *JADA* 137:1517-1527, 2006.
84. Littlewood SJ, Mitchell L. The dental problems and management of a patient suffering from congenital insensitivity to pain, *Int J Paediatr Dent* 8:47-50, 1998.
85. Cusumano FJ, et al. Prevention of self-mutilation in patients with Lesch-Nyham syndrome: review of literature, *J Dent Child* 68:175-178, 2001.
86. Henry SW, et al. Histologic features of the superior labial frenum, *J Periodontol* 47:25-28, 1976.
87. Bohannan HM. Studies in the alteration of vestibular depth. I, Complete denudation, *J Periodontol* 33:120-128, 1962.
88. Bohannan HM. Studies in the alteration of vestibular depth. II, Periosteum retention, *J Periodontol* 33:354-359, 1962.
89. Bohannan HM III. Vestibular incision, *J Periodontol* 34:209-215, 1963.
90. O'Leary TJ, et al. The plaque control record, *J Periodontol* 43:38, 1972.
91. Clerehugh V, Tugnait A. Periodontal diseases in children and adolescents: I. Aetiology and diagnosis, *Dent Update* 28:222-230, 232, 2001.

92. Piazzini LF. Periodontal screening and recording (PSR) application in children and adolescents, *J Clin Pediatr Dent* 18:165-171, 1994.

93. Woodall IR, et al. *Polishing the teeth in comprehensive dental hygiene care*, 3rd ed. St Louis, 1989, CV Mosby, pp 507-520.

94. Hattabfn Qudeimat MA, Al-Rimawi HS. Dental discoloration: an overview, *J Esthet Dent* 11:291-310, 1999.

95. Carranza FA, Newman MG. Dental calculus. In Carranza FA Jr, ed. *Clinical periodontology*, 8th ed. Philadelphia, 1996, WB Saunders, pp 158-159.

96. Slots J. The microflora of black stain on primary teeth, *Scand J Dent Res* 82:484-490, 1974.

97. Bhat M. Periodontal health of 14- to 17-year-old US schoolchildren, *J Public Health Dent* 51:5-11, 1991.

98. Turesky S, et al. Histologic and histochemical observations regarding early calculus formation in children and adults, *J Periodontol* 32:7-14, 1961.

99. Traiger J. Unusual deposition of calculus: report of a case, *Oral Surg Oral Med Oral Pathol* 14:623-624, 1961.

SUGGESTED READINGS

Anderson HH, et al. Gingival overgrowth with valproic acid: a case report, *J Dent Child* 64:294-297, 1997.

Christersson LA, Zambon JJ. Suppression of *Actinobacillus actinomycetemcomitans* in localized juvenile periodontitis with systemic tetracycline, *J Clin Periodontol* 20:395-401, 1993.

Delaney JE, Kornman KS. Microbiology of subgingival plaque form children with localized prepubertal periodontitis, *Oral Microbiol Immunol* 2:71-76, 1987.

Flaitz CM. Oral pathologic conditions and soft tissue anomalies. In Pinkham JR, et al, ed. *Pediatric dentistry: infancy through adolescence*, 4th ed. Philadelphia, 2005, WB Saunders.

Greenberg MS. Herpesvirus infections, *Dent Clin North Am* 40:359-368, 1996.

Haffajee AD, et al. Clinical and microbiological changes associated with the use of combined antimicrobial therapies to treat 'refractory periodontitis', *J Clin Periodontol* 31:869, 2004.

Herman W et al. Over-the-counter preparations for recurrent aphthous stomatitis, *J Pract Hyg* 12(4):17-20, 2003.

Kamma JJ, Behni PC. Five-year maintenance follow-up of early-onset periodontitis patients, *J Clin Periodontol* 30:562, 2003.

Maynard JG, Ochsenbein C. Mucogingival problems, prevalence, and therapy in children, *J Periodontol* 46:543-552, 1975.

Modeer T, Wondimu B. Periodontal diseases in children and adolescents, *Dent Clin North Am* 44:633, 2000.

Neely AL. Prevalence of juvenile periodontitis in a circumpubertal population, *J Clin Periodontol* 19:367-372, 1992.

Oh TJ, et al. Periodontal diseases in the child and adolescent, *J Clin Periodontol* 29:400, 2002.

Sanders BJ, Weddell JA, Dodge NN. Managing patients who have seizure disorders: dental and medical issues, *J Am Dent Assoc* 126:1641-1647, 1995.

Seymour RA, et al. Risk factors for drug-induced gingival overgrowth, *J Clin Periodontal* 27:217-223, 2000.

Spruance SL et al. Acyclovir cream for treatment of herpes simplex labialis: results of two randomized, double-blind, vehicle-controlled, multicenter clinical trials, *Antimicrob Agents Chemother* 46(7):2238-2243, 2002.

Van Dyke TE, et al. The role of host response in periodontal disease progression: Implications for future treatment strategies, *J Periodontol* 64:792-806, 1993.

Vandana KL, et al. Clinical and radiographic evaluation of Emdogain as a regenerative material in the treatment of interproximal vertical defects in chronic and aggressive periodontitis patients, *Int J Periodont Restor Dent* 24:185, 2004.

Worch KP, et al. A multidisciplinary approach to the diagnosis and treatment of early-onset periodontitis: a case report, *J Periodontol* 72(1):96-106, 2001.

CHAPTER 21

Management of Trauma to the Teeth and Supporting Tissues

▲ Ralph E. McDonald, David R. Avery, Jeffrey A. Dean and James E. Jones

CHAPTER OUTLINE

A trauma with accompanying fracture of a permanent incisor is a tragic experience for the young patient and is a problem whose management requires experience, judgment, and skill perhaps unequaled by any other portion of the dentist's practice. The dentist whose counsel and treatment are sought after a trauma is obligated either to treat the patient with all possible means or to immediately refer the patient to a specialist. The oral and emotional health of the young patient is involved, and the child's appearance, marred by an unsightly oral injury, must be restored to normal as soon as possible to relieve the consciousness of being different from other children. Slack and Jones observed that the progress of children in school and their behavior elsewhere, as well as their psychological well-being, can be adversely influenced by an injury to the teeth that causes an unsightly fracture.[1] In addition, the short- and long-term costs associated with managing trauma to the oral and perioral structures can be large. Borum and Andreasen estimate that the yearly cost from traumatic dental injuries in Denmark ranges from US $2 million to US $5 million per 1 million inhabitants per year.[2]

Injuries to the teeth of children or adults present unique problems in diagnosis and treatment. The diagnosis of the extent of the injury after a blow to a tooth, regardless of loss of tooth structure, is difficult and often inconclusive. Trauma to a tooth is invariably followed by pulpal hyperemia, the extent of which cannot always be determined by available diagnostic methods. Congestion and alteration in the blood flow in the pulp may be sufficient to initiate irreversible degenerative changes, which over time can cause pulpal necrosis. In addition, the apical vessels may have been severed or damaged enough to interfere with the normal reparative process. Treatment of injuries causing pulp exposure or tooth displacement are particularly challenging, because the prognosis of the involved tooth is often uncertain.

The treatment of fractured teeth, particularly in young patients, is further complicated by the often difficult but extremely important restorative procedure. Although the dentist may prefer to delay the restoration because of a questionable prognosis for the pulp, often a malocclusion can develop within a matter of days as a result of a break in the normal proximal contact with adjacent teeth. Adjacent teeth may tip into the area created by the loss of tooth structure. This loss of space will create a problem when the final restoration is contemplated. There must often be a compromise of an ideal esthetic appearance, at least in the initial restoration, because the prognosis is questionable or because the tooth is young and has a large pulp or is still in the stage of active eruption.

Often the likelihood of success depends on the rapidity with which the tooth is treated after the injury, regardless of whether the procedure involves protecting a large area of exposed dentin or treating a vital pulp exposure. Several factors can be considered common to all types of injury to the anterior teeth. These important considerations should become a checklist invariably used by the dentist in the diagnosis of and treatment planning for traumatic injuries.

The International Association of Dental Traumatology reports that one out of every two children sustains a dental injury, most often between the ages of 8 and 12. They suggest that in most cases of dental trauma a rapid and appropriate treatment can lessen its impact from both an oral and an esthetic standpoint. To that end, the association has developed guidelines for the evaluation and management of traumatic dental injuries, which is available at the following website: http://www.iadt-dentaltrauma.org.

HISTORY AND EXAMINATION

The routine use of a clinical evaluation sheet for injured anterior teeth is helpful during the initial examination and subsequent examinations of an injured tooth (Fig. 21-1). The form, which becomes a part of the patient's record, serves as a checklist of important questions that must be asked and observations that must be made by the dentist and the auxiliary personnel during the examination of the child.

HISTORY OF THE INJURY

The time of the injury should first be established. Unfortunately, many patients do not seek professional advice and treatment immediately after an injury. Occasionally the accident is so severe that dental treatment cannot be started immediately because other injuries have higher priority. Davis and Vogel emphasized that a force strong enough to fracture, intrude, or avulse a tooth is also strong enough to result in cervical spine or intracranial injury. The dentist must be particularly alert to such potential problems, be prepared ahead of time to make a neurologic assessment, and make appropriate medical referral when indicated without delay.[3] The patient should be assessed for nausea, vomiting, drowsiness, or possible cerebral spinal fluid leakage from the nose and ears, which would be indicative of a skull fracture. In addition, the patient should be evaluated for lacerations and facial bone fractures. Obtaining a baseline temperature, pulse, blood pressure, and respiratory rate should be considered as information to be gathered before addressing the dental

needs of the patient. Finally, Davis[4] recommends a quick cranial nerve evaluation involving the following four areas:

1. Extraocular muscles are intact and functioning appropriately; that is, the patient can track a finger moving vertically and horizontally through the visual field with the eyes remaining in tandem.
2. Pupils are equal, round, and reactive to light with accommodation.
3. Sensory function is normal as measured through light contact to various areas of the face.
4. Symmetry of motor function is present, as assessed by having the patient frown, smile, move the tongue, and perform several voluntary muscular movements.

The prognosis of an injured tooth depends logically, often to a great extent, on the time that has elapsed between the occurrence of the accident and the initiation of emergency treatment. This is particularly true in cases of pulp exposure, for which pulp capping or pulpotomy would be the procedure of choice. Rusmah treated 123 traumatized permanent incisors and monitored them over a 24-month period. His findings suggest that the interval between trauma and emergency treatment is directly related to the severity of the injury and the dental awareness of the patients.[5] Furthermore, the prognosis of the injured teeth maintaining pulpal vitality diminished when treatment was delayed. The loss of vitality of some injured teeth occurred as early as 3 months and as late as 24 months after the injury, which justifies a long follow-up period after injury.

For practical and especially economic reasons, Andreasen and colleagues have attempted to classify pulpal and periodontal healing of traumatic dental injuries based on the effect of treatment delay.[6] They developed three major categories of treatment timing: acute treatment (i.e., within a few hours), subacute treatment (i.e., within the first 24 hours), and delayed treatment (i.e., after the first 24 hours). Unfortunately, there is limited knowledge of the effect of treatment delay on wound healing available in the literature.

Taking a complete dental history can help the dentist learn of previous injuries to the teeth in the area. Repeated injuries to the teeth are not uncommon in children with protruding anterior teeth and in those who are active in athletics. In these patients the prognosis may be less favorable. The dentist must rule out the possibility of a degenerative pulp or adverse reaction of the supporting tissues as a result of previous trauma.

The patient's complaints and experiences after the injury are often valuable in determining the extent of the injury and in estimating the ability of the injured pulp and supporting tissues to overcome the effects of the injury. Pain caused by thermal change is indicative of significant pulpal inflammation. Pain occurring when the teeth are brought into normal occlusion may indicate that the tooth has been displaced. Such pain could likewise indicate an injury to the periodontal and supporting tissues. The likelihood of eventual pulpal necrosis increases if the tooth is mobile at the time of the first examination; the greater the mobility, the greater the chance of pulp death.

Trauma to the supporting tissues may cause sufficient inflammation to initiate external root resorption. In instances of severe injury, teeth can be lost as a result of pathologic root resorption and pulpal degeneration.

CLINICAL EXAMINATION

The clinical examination should be conducted after the teeth in the area of injury have been carefully cleaned of debris. When the injury has resulted in a fracture of the crown, the dentist should observe the amount of tooth structure that has been lost and should look for evidence of a pulp exposure. With the aid of a good light, the clinical crown should be examined carefully for cracks and craze lines, the presence of which could influence the type of permanent restoration used for the tooth. With light transmitted through the teeth in the area, the color of the injured tooth should be carefully compared with that of adjacent uninjured teeth. Severely traumatized teeth often appear darker and reddish, although not actually discolored, which indicates pulpal hyperemia (Fig. 21-2). This appearance suggests that at some later time the pulp may undergo degenerative change terminating in pulpal necrosis.

Historically, the Ellis and Davey classification of crown fractures is useful in recording the extent of damage to the crown.[7] The following is a modification of their classification (Fig. 21-3):

Class I— Simple fracture of the crown involving little or no dentin

Class II—Extensive fracture of the crown involving considerable dentin but not the dental pulp

Class III—Extensive fracture of the crown with an exposure of the dental pulp

Class IV—Loss of the entire crown

A vitality test of the injured tooth should be performed, and the teeth in the immediate area, as well as those in the opposing arch, should be tested. The best prediction of continued vitality of the pulp of a damaged or traumatized tooth is the vital response to electric pulp testing at the time of the initial examination. A negative response, however, is not reliable evidence of pulp death because some teeth that give such a response soon after the injury may recover vitality after a time. When the electric pulp tester is used, the dentist should first determine the normal reading by testing an uninjured tooth on the opposite side of the mouth and recording the lowest number at which the tooth responds. If the injured tooth requires more current than does a normal tooth, the pulp may be undergoing degenerative change. If less current is needed to elicit a response from a traumatized tooth, pulpal inflammation is usually indicated.

Many practitioners question the need for the electric vitality test immediately after the injury. Because the electrical stimulus has been shown to produce negligible additional pulpal irritation, its use is not contraindicated on this basis. However, the patient's measured responses to the test may be almost meaningless. The reliability of the electric pulp test depends on eliciting valid responses from the patient. The mere presence of this new, unknown instrument may create anxiety in children that hampers their ability to respond accurately to the test.

Because an unscheduled emergency appointment for treatment of an injury is a new experience, it seems reasonable to introduce the child to the instrument during the first emergency visit when the child does not know what to expect. This gives the dentist an opportunity to allay the child's anxiety about the instrument during a time when the responses are not as important as they will be on subsequent visits. Furthermore, the electric pulp test is frequently unreliable even on normal teeth when apices are incompletely formed.

The thermal test is also somewhat helpful in determining the degree of pulpal damage after trauma. Although there are difficulties with the thermal test, it is probably more reliable in testing primary incisors in young children than the electric pulp test. Failure of a tooth to respond to heat is indicative of pulpal necrosis. The response of a tooth to a lower degree of heat than is necessary to elicit a response in adjacent teeth is an indication of inflammation. Pain occurring when ice is applied to a normal tooth will subside when the ice is removed. A more painful and often lingering reaction to cold indicates a pathologic change within the pulp, the nature of which can be determined when the reaction is correlated with other clinical observations.

Failure of a recently traumatized tooth to respond to the pulp test is not uncommon and may indicate a previous injury with a resulting necrotic pulp. However, the traumatized tooth may be in a state of shock and as a result may fail to respond to the accepted methods of determining pulp vitality. The failure of a pulp to respond immediately after an accident is not an indication for endodontic therapy. Instead, emergency treatment should be completed, and the tooth should be retested at the next follow-up visit.

Laser Doppler flowmetry has been reported to be a significant aid in determining vascular vitality of traumatized teeth by Olgart and associates[8] and more recently by Mesaros and Trope.[9] Although this technology is not yet affordably priced for dental offices, it may be in the future.

RADIOGRAPHIC EXAMINATION

The examination of traumatized teeth cannot be considered complete without a radiograph of the injured tooth, the adjacent teeth, and sometimes the teeth in the opposing arch. It may even be necessary to obtain a radiograph of the soft tissue surrounding the injury site in search of a fractured tooth fragment (Fig. 21-4). The relative size of the pulp chamber and canal should be carefully examined. Irregularities or an inconsistency in the size of the chamber or canal compared with that of adjacent teeth may be evidence of a previous injury. This observation is important in determining the immediate course of treatment. In young patients, the stage of apical development often indicates the type of treatment, just as the size of the coronal pulp and its proximity to the area of fracture influence the type of restoration that can be used. A root fracture as a result of the injury or one previously sustained can be detected by a careful examination of the radiograph. However, the presence of a root fracture may not influence the course of treatment, particularly if the

ASSESSMENT OF ACUTE TRAUMATIC INJURIES	PATIENT NAME:_____ DATE OF BIRTH:_____
DATE: TIME:	REFERRED BY:

MEDICAL HISTORY:	
ALLERGIES:	**DATE OF LAST TETANUS INNOCULATON:**
DATE AND TIME OF INJURY:	**TIME LAPSED SINCE INJURY:**
WHERE INJURY OCCURRED:	
HOW INJURY OCCURRED:	

HISTORY

Check if present and describe	**MANAGEMENT PRIOR TO EXAM** By whom: Describe:
Nondental injuries	
Loss of consciousness	
Altered orientation/mental status	
Hemorrhage from nose/ears	
Headache/nausea/vomiting	
Neck pain	
Spontaneous dental pain	
Pain on mastication	
Reaction to thermal changes	
Previous dental trauma	
Other complaints	

EXTRAORAL EXAM

Check if present and describe	**OTHER FINDINGS/COMMENTS:**
Facial fractures	
Lacerations	
Contusions	
Swelling	
Abrasions	
Hemorrhage/drainage	
Foreign bodies	
TMJ deviation/asymmetry	

INTRAORAL EXAMINATION

Check if injured and describe	**DIAGRAM OF INJURIES**
Lips	
Frenae	
Buccal mucosa	
Gingivae	
Palate	
Tongue	
Floor of mouth	
Occlusion	
Molar classification R___ L___	
Canine classification R___ L___	
Overbite (%)_____	
Overjet (mm)_____	
Crossbite Y N	
Midline deviation Y N	
Interferences Y N	

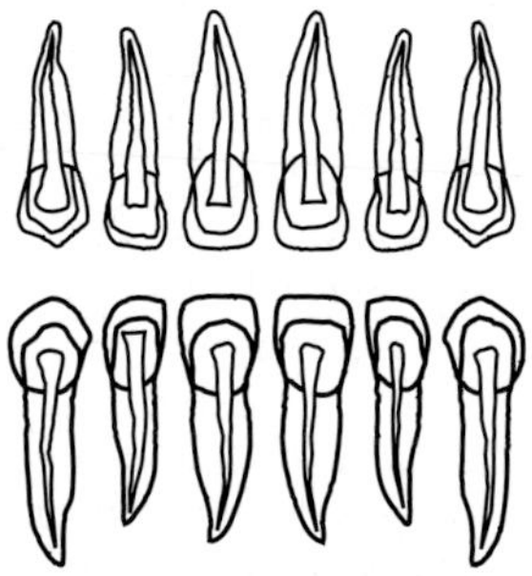

Figure 21-1 Clinical evaluation sheet for injured anterior teeth. (Adapted from American Academy of Pediatric Dentistry. *Pediatr Dent* 24(7 suppl):95-96, 2002.)

	TOOTH NUMBER					
DENTAL INJURIES	AVULSION — Extraoral time					
	Storage medium					
	INFRACTION					
	CROWN FRACTURE					
	PULP EXPOSURE — Size					
	Appearance					
	COLOR					
	MOBILITY (mm)					
	PERCUSSION					
	LUXATION — Direction					
	Extent					
	PULP TESTING — Electric					
	Thermal					
	CARIES/PREVIOUS RESTORATIONS					
RADIOGRAPHS	PULP SIZE					
	ROOT DEVELOPMENT					
	ROOT FRACTURE					
	PERIODONTAL LIGAMENT SPACE					
	PERIAPICAL PATHOLOGY					
	ALVEOLAR FRACTURE					
	FOREIGN BODY					
	DEVELOPMENTAL ANOMALY					
	OTHER					

TREATMENT

Check if performed and describe
- Soft tissue management
- Medication
- Pulp therapy
- Repositioning
- Stabilization
- Restoration
- Extraction
- Prescription
- Referral
- Other

SUMMARY

INSTRUCTIONS AND DISPOSITION

Check if discussed
- Diet
- Hygiene
- Pain
- Swelling
- Infection
- Prescription
- Complications:
  - Damage to developing teeth
  - Abnormal position/ankylosis
  - Tooth loss
  - Pulp damage to injured teeth
- Other:
- Follow-up:
- Other

Subsequent visit No. 1   Date _____

1. Pulpal response   7 8   9 10 ☐ ☐ | ☐ ☐
2. Radiographic exam   ☐ ☐ | ☐ ☐ 26 25 24 23
3. Treatment and comments: _____
_____

                             Date _____
Subsequent visit No. 2

1. Pulpal response   7 8   9 10 ☐ ☐ | ☐ ☐
2. Radiographic exam   ☐ ☐ | ☐ ☐ 26 25 24 23
3. Treatment and comments: _____
_____

Subsequent visit No. 3   Date _____

1. Pulpal response   7 8   9 10 ☐ ☐ | ☐ ☐
2. Radiographic exam   ☐ ☐ | ☐ ☐ 26 25 24 23
3. Treatment and comments: _____
_____

                             Date _____
Subsequent visit No. 4

1. Pulpal response   7 8   9 10 ☐ ☐ | ☐ ☐
2. Radiographic exam   ☐ ☐ | ☐ ☐ 26 25 24 23
3. Treatment and comments: _____
_____

Figure 21-1 cont'd

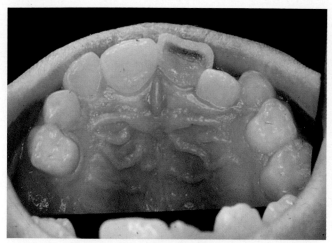

Figure 21-2 The reddish appearance of the exposed dentin is evidence of severe hyperemia within the pulp tissue. The prognosis for retaining vitality of the pulp is poor.

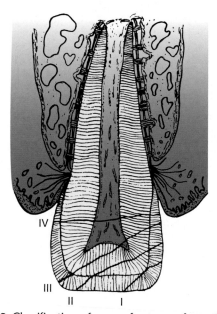

Figure 21-3 Classification of crown fractures of anterior teeth.

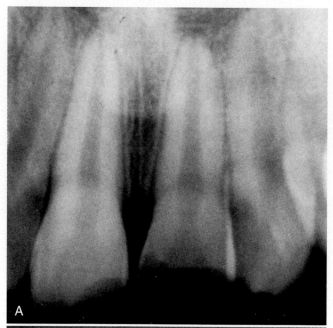

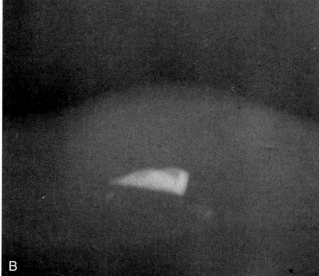

Figure 21-4 A radiograph with a reduced exposure time (25% of the usual time) was useful in detecting where this fractured tooth fragment was located within the patient's lip.

fracture line is in the region of the apical third. Teeth with root fractures in this area rarely need stabilization, and a fibrous or calcified union usually results. If teeth have been discernibly dislocated, with or without root fracture, two or three radiographs of the area at different angles may be needed to clearly define the defect and aid the dentist in deciding on a course of treatment.

Another value of the radiograph is that it provides a record of the tooth immediately after the injury. Frequent, periodic radiographs reveal evidence of continued pulp vitality or adverse changes that take place within the pulp or the supporting tissues. In young teeth in which the pulp recovers from the initial trauma, the pulp chamber and canal decrease in size coincident with the normal formation of secondary dentin. After a period of time, an inconsistency in the true size or contour of the pulp chamber or canal compared with that

of adjacent teeth may indicate a developing pathologic condition.

When more complex facial injuries have occurred or jaw fractures are suspected, extraoral films may also be necessary to identify the extent and location of all injury sequelae. Oblique lateral jaw radiographs and panoramic films are often useful adjuncts to this diagnostic process.

EMERGENCY TREATMENT OF SOFT TISSUE INJURY

Injury to the teeth of children is often accompanied by open wounds of the oral tissues, abrasion of the facial tissues, or even puncture wounds. The dentist must recognize the possibility of the development of tetanus after the injury and must carry out adequate first aid measures.

Children with up-to-date active immunization are protected by the level of antibodies in their circulation produced by a series of injections of tetanus toxoid. Primary immunization is usually a part of medical care during the first 2 years of life. However, primary immunization cannot be assumed but must be confirmed by examining the child's medical record.

When the child who has had the primary immunization receives an injury from an object that is likely to have been contaminated, the antibody-forming mechanism may be activated with a booster injection of toxoid. An unimmunized child can be protected through passive immunization or serotherapy with tetanus antitoxin (tetanus immune globulin, or TIG).

The dentist examining the child after an injury should determine the child's immunization status, carry out adequate débridement of the wound, and, when indicated, refer the child to the family physician. Tetanus is often fatal, and preventive measures must be taken if there is a possibility that an injured child is not adequately immunized.

Débridement, suturing, and/or hemorrhage control of open soft tissue wounds should be carried out as indicated. Working with an oral and maxillofacial surgeon or a plastic surgeon may also be indicated.

EMERGENCY TREATMENT AND TEMPORARY RESTORATION OF FRACTURED TEETH WITHOUT PULP EXPOSURE

A trauma to a tooth that causes a loss of only a small portion of enamel should be treated as carefully as one in which greater tooth structure is lost. The emergency treatment of minor injuries in which only the enamel is fractured may consist of no more than smoothing the rough, jagged tooth structure. However, without exception, a thorough examination should be conducted as previously described. The patient should be reexamined at 2 weeks and again at 1 month after the injury. If the tooth appears to have recovered at that time, continued observation at the patient's regular recall appointments should be the rule.

Sudden injuries with a resultant extensive loss of tooth structure and exposed dentin require an immediate temporary restoration or protective covering, in addition to the complete diagnostic procedure. In this type of injury, initial pulpal hyperemia and the possibility of further trauma to the pulp by pressure or by thermal or chemical irritants must be reduced. In addition, if normal contact with adjacent or opposing teeth has been lost, the temporary restoration or protective covering can be designed to maintain the integrity of the arch. Because providing an adequate permanent restoration may depend on maintaining the normal alignment and position of teeth in the area, this part of the treatment is as important as maintaining the vitality of the teeth. Several restorations that will satisfy these requirements can easily be fabricated.

FRAGMENT RESTORATION (REATTACHMENT OF TOOTH FRAGMENT)

Occasionally the dentist may have the opportunity to reattach the fragment of a fractured tooth using resin and bonding techniques. Tennery reported the successful reattachment of tooth fragments for eight teeth in five patients.[10] One reattached fragment was subsequently lost as the result of a second traumatic episode. Starkey reported successful reattachment of one tooth fragment on a lower central incisor 2 days after the injury.[11]

This procedure is atraumatic and seems to be the ideal method of restoring the fractured crown. Sealing the injured tooth and esthetically restoring its natural contour and color are accomplished simply and constitute an excellent service to the patient. The procedure provides an essentially perfect temporary restoration that may be retained a long time in some cases.

It is not often that the fractured tooth fragment remains intact and is recovered after an injury, but when this happens, the dentist may consider the reattachment procedure. The tooth requires no mechanical preparation because retention is provided by enamel etching and bonding techniques. If little or no dentin is exposed, the fragment and the fractured tooth enamel are etched and reattached with bonding agents and materials. Farik and colleagues have tested the use of the new single-bottle dentin adhesives with and without unfilled resins in the fragment-bonding technique.[12] Their hypothesis was that the amount of resin in single-bottle dentin adhesives might not be sufficient to secure an adequate fragment bond. The results of their study showed that all but one of the seven dentin adhesive systems tested should be used with an additional unfilled resin when fractured teeth are restored by reattachment.

For cases in which considerable dentin is exposed or a direct pulp cap is indicated, some controversy exists about the best treatment to enhance the likelihood of maintaining pulpal vitality. Some believe that the meticulous use of bonding agents and materials to directly cap the exposed dentin and the pulp (if exposed) is best, whereas others believe that calcium hydroxide should be applied to the exposed dentin and pulp before completing the bonding procedure. The former method has been called the *total-etch technique*.

Fig. 21-5 illustrates the successful management of a class II fracture of the maxillary left central incisor in a 6-year-old boy who was treated approximately 1 hour after the injury. After the fragment was trial-seated to confirm a precise fit, the exposed dentin of the fractured tooth was covered with a thin layer of hard-setting calcium hydroxide that was allowed to remain as a sedative dressing between the tooth and the restored fragment. A portion of the dentin in the fragment was removed to provide space for the calcium hydroxide. The fragment was then soaked in etchant, and the fractured area of the tooth was also etched well beyond the fracture site. After thorough rinsing and drying of all etched enamel, the fragment and the etched portion of the tooth were painted with a light-curing sealant material. Although no bonding agent was used here, its use is currently recommended. The selected shade of

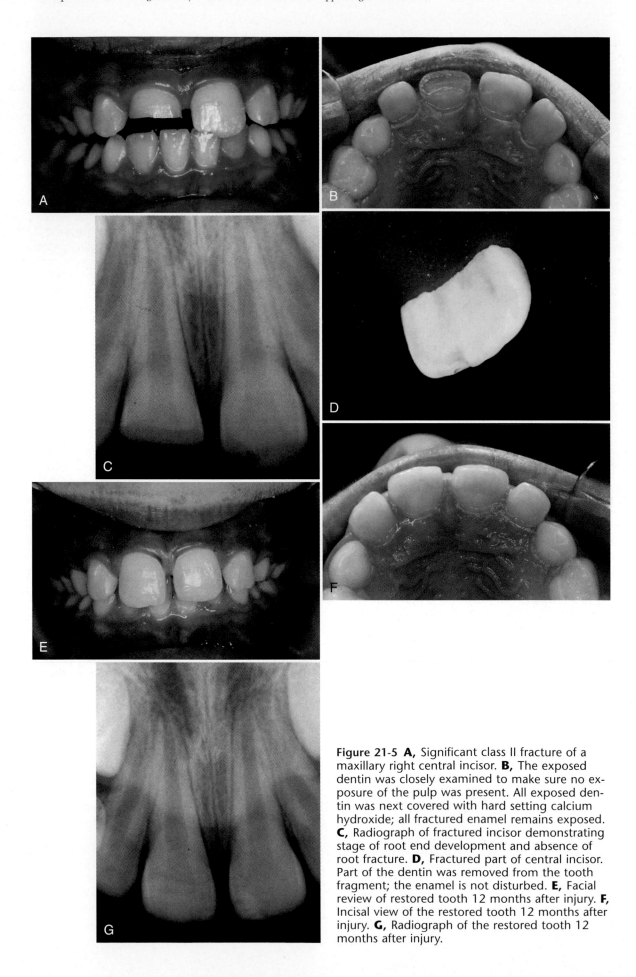

Figure 21-5 A, Significant class II fracture of a maxillary right central incisor. **B,** The exposed dentin was closely examined to make sure no exposure of the pulp was present. All exposed dentin was next covered with hard setting calcium hydroxide; all fractured enamel remains exposed. **C,** Radiograph of fractured incisor demonstrating stage of root end development and absence of root fracture. **D,** Fractured part of central incisor. Part of the dentin was removed from the tooth fragment; the enamel is not disturbed. **E,** Facial review of restored tooth 12 months after injury. **F,** Incisal view of the restored tooth 12 months after injury. **G,** Radiograph of the restored tooth 12 months after injury.

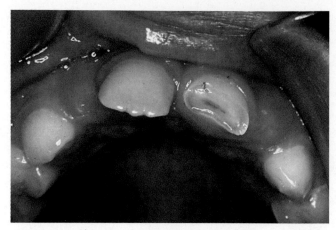

Figure 21-7 Class III injury to a permanent central incisor. A small pulp exposure is evident that should be capped and protected with a bonded restoration.

inflammation is not widespread and if a deeper access opening is not needed to help retain the coronal restoration.[16] Pulpotomy is also indicated for immature permanent teeth if necrotic pulp tissue is evident at the exposure site with inflammation of the underlying coronal tissue, but a conventional or cervical pulpotomy would be required. Yet another indication is trauma to a more mature permanent (closed apex) tooth that has caused both a pulp exposure and a root fracture. In addition, a shallow pulpotomy may be the treatment of choice for a class III fracture of a tooth with a closed apex when definitive treatment can be provided soon after the injury (Fig. 21-10).

The exposure site should be conservatively enlarged, and 1 to 2 mm of coronal pulp tissue should be removed for the shallow pulpotomy or all pulp tissue in the pulp chamber removed for the conventional pulpotomy. When

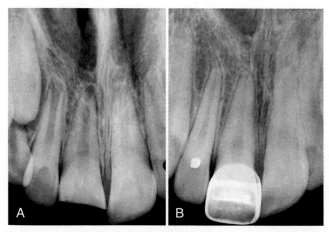

Figure 21-8 A, The pulp of a permanent central incisor has been exposed as a result of trauma. The pulp was capped with calcium hydroxide. **B,** A successful pulp capping has been accomplished. Continued root end development indicates pulp vitality. The tooth was restored with an esthetic resin-faced steel crown, but a bonded resin restoration is currently recommended.

pulp amputation has been completed to the desired level, the pulp chamber should be thoroughly cleaned with copious irrigation. No visible dentin chips or pulp tissue tags should remain. If the remaining pulp is healthy, hemorrhage will be easy to control with a pledget of moist cotton lightly compressed against the tissue. The pulp should also have a bright reddish pink color and a concave contour (meniscus). A deeper amputation may be necessary if the health of the pulp is questionable. A dressing of calcium hydroxide is gently applied to the vital pulp tissue so that it is in passive contact with the pulp. The remaining access opening is filled with a hard-setting, biocompatible material with excellent marginal sealing capability. Then the crown may be restored with a separate bonding procedure.

Some experts on pulp therapy recommend conventional pulpectomy and root canal fillings for all teeth treated with calcium hydroxide pulpotomies soon after the root apices close. They view the calcium hydroxide pulpotomy as an interim procedure performed solely to achieve normal root development and apical closure. They justify the pulpectomy and root canal filling after apical closure as necessary to prevent an exaggerated calcific response that may result in total obliteration of the root canal (calcific metamorphosis or calcific degeneration).

We have observed this calcific degenerative response and agree that it should be intercepted with root canal therapy if possible after apical closure (Fig. 21-11). However, long-term successes after calcium hydroxide pulpotomy in which no calcific metamorphosis has been observed can be documented. We have followed such successful cases for more than 10 years without seeing any adverse results. McCormick has reported one case of a tooth successfully treated with a calcium hydroxide pulpotomy that was observed for more than 19 years and never required further pulp therapy.[17]

If healthy pulp tissue remains in the root canal, if the coronal pulp tissue is cleanly excised without excessive tissue laceration and tearing, if the calcium hydroxide is placed gently on the pulp tissue at the amputation site without undue pressure, and if the tooth is adequately sealed, there is a high probability that long-term success can be achieved without follow-up root canal therapy.

PULPECTOMY WITH ENDODONTIC TREATMENT

One of the most challenging endodontic procedures is the treatment and subsequent filling of the root canal of a tooth with an open apex. The lumen of the root canal of such an immature tooth is largest at the apex and smallest in the cervical area and is often referred to as a *blunderbuss canal*. Hermetic sealing of the apex with conventional endodontic techniques is usually impossible without apical surgery. This surgical procedure is traumatic for the young child and should be avoided if possible.

In instances of class III or class IV fractures of young permanent teeth with incomplete root growth and a vital pulp, the pulpotomy technique (as just described) is the procedure of choice. The successful pulpotomy allows the pulp in the root canal to maintain its vitality and also

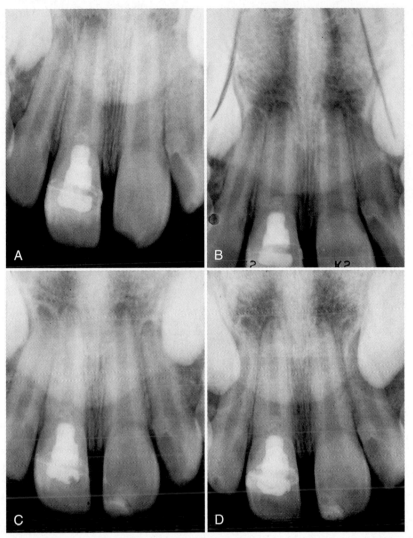

Figure 21-9 A, Radiographic appearance of the restored maxillary right central incisor 10 days after the class IV crown fracture occurred and the calcium hydroxide pulpotomy was performed. A fragment restoration was also used to restore the class II fracture of the maxillary left central incisor at this same appointment, but after this radiograph was obtained. **B,** This radiograph made 7½ weeks after the pulpotomy shows evidence of a calcified bridge developing at the level of the pulpal amputation. **C,** Eight months after initial treatment, it appears that root development is progressing normally for both maxillary central incisors. **D,** Root completion has been achieved on both maxillary central incisors 20 months after the original injury. The root canals exhibit normal anatomic configuration.

allows the apical portion to continue to develop (apexogenesis). For class IV fractures, the eventual restoration may require a post in the root canal. Before this type of restoration is completed, the dentinal bridge that has formed after the pulpotomy can be perforated and routine endodontic procedures can be undertaken in a now completely developed root canal.

Occasionally a patient has an acute periapical abscess associated with a traumatized tooth. The trauma may have caused a very small pulp exposure that was overlooked, or the pulp may have been devitalized as a result of injury or actual severing of the apical vessels. A loss of pulp vitality may have caused interrupted growth of the root canal, and the dentist is faced with the task of treating a canal with an open apex.

If an abscess is present, it must be treated first. If there is acute pain and evidence of swelling of the soft tissues,

drainage through the pulp canal will give the child almost immediate relief. A conventional endodontic access opening should be made into the pulp chamber. If pain is caused by the pressure required to make the opening into the pulp, the tooth should be supported by the dentist's fingers. Antibiotic therapy is also generally indicated.

THERAPY TO STIMULATE ROOT GROWTH AND APICAL REPAIR SUBSEQUENT TO PULPAL NECROSIS IN ANTERIOR PERMANENT TEETH (APEXIFICATION)

The conventional treatment of pulpless anterior teeth usually requires apical surgery if the teeth have open apices. Many young teeth have been saved in this manner. However, a less traumatic endodontic therapy called *apexification* has been found to be effective in the management of immature, necrotic permanent teeth. The

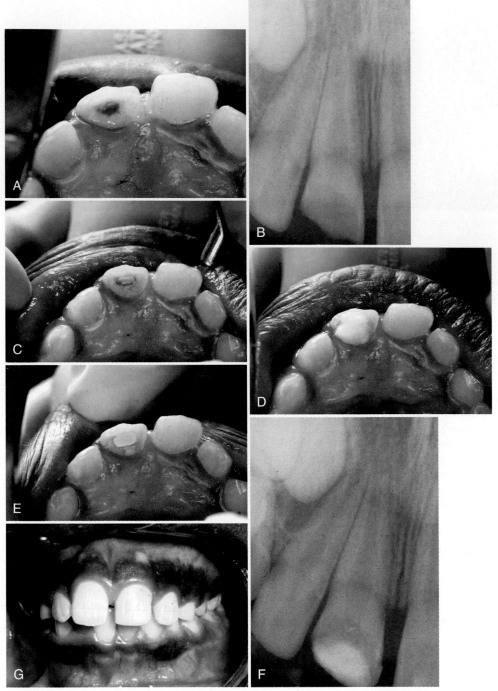

Figure 21-10 A, Severe class III fracture of the maxillary right central incisor. The trauma happened approximately 60 minutes earlier. **B,** Maxillary periapical radiograph of traumatized incisor. Note the apical closure of the root tip. **C,** After appropriate infiltration local anesthesia (no local anesthesia injected into the pulp tissue at the fracture site), approximately 2 mm in depth of pulpal tissue at the fracture was removed using a number 4 round diamond with gentle water irrigation. This creates an undercut in tooth structure facilitating retention of calcium hydroxide to be placed later during the procedure. Note the excellent hemostasis of the amputated pulp tissue. **D,** A cotton pellet, moistened with sterile saline, is placed over the pulpaltissue for 5 minutes. **E,** After verification of excellent hemostasis following use of the moistened cotton pellet, calcium hydroxide was used to fill the area created during pulp removal. **F,** Maxillary radiograph after placement of the calcium hydroxide. **G,** Clinical picture of incisor 3 months after the traumatic event. Normal pulp testing response to both electric and cold pulp testing was obtained at 1-, 2-, and 3-month observation intervals. A permanent restoration is planned.

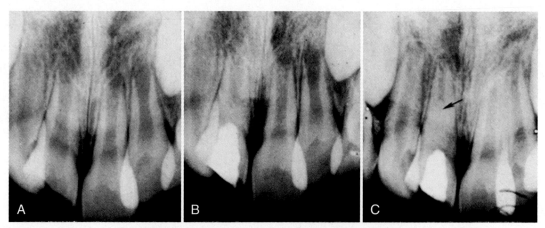

Figure 21-11 A, Pulp exposure was treated by the pulpotomy technique. **B,** A wider-than-normal dentin bridge has formed, an indication of possible calcific metamorphosis. **C,** Evidence of continued apical development. Two thirds of the pulp canal is filled with calcified material *(arrow).* This barrier would be difficult to penetrate if root canal therapy were attempted.

apexification procedure should precede conventional root canal therapy in the management of teeth with irreversibly diseased pulps and open apices.

Frank has described a technique based on the normal physiologic pattern of root development that brings about the resumption of apical development so that the root canal can be obliterated by conventional canal-filling techniques.[18] The procedure described by Frank and demonstrated to be successful in repeated clinical trials stimulates the process of root end development, which was interrupted by pulpal necrosis, so that it continues to the point of apical closure (Fig. 21-12).[18] Often a calcific bridge develops just coronal to the apex. When the closure occurs, or when the calcific "plug" is observed in the apical portion, routine endodontic procedures may be completed; the possibility of recurrent periapical pathosis is thus prevented.

The following steps are included in the technique:

1. The affected tooth is carefully isolated with a rubber dam, and an access opening is made into the pulp chamber.
2. A file is placed in the root canal, and a radiograph is made to establish the root length accurately. It is important to avoid placing the instrument through the apex, which might injure the epithelial diaphragm.
3. After the remnants of the pulp are removed using barbed broaches and files, the canal is flooded with hydrogen peroxide to aid in the removal of debris. The canal is then irrigated with sodium hypochlorite and saline.
4. The canal is dried with large paper points and loose cotton.
5. A thick paste of calcium hydroxide and camphorated mono-parachlorophenol (CMCP) or calcium hydroxide in a methylcellulose paste (Pulpdent Corp., Watertown, Mass) is transferred to the canal with the aid of an amalgam carrier. An endodontic plugger may be used to push the material to the apical end, but an excess of material should not be forced beyond the apex of the tooth.
6. A cotton pledget is placed over the calcium hydroxide, and the seal is completed with a layer of reinforced zinc oxide–eugenol cement.

Weine recommends that the apexification procedure be completed in two appointments.[19] After instrumentation, irrigation, and drying of the canal during the first appointment, he advises sealing a sterile, dry cotton pellet in the pulp chamber for 1 to 2 weeks. Placing a calcium hydroxide dressing in the canal is optional at the first appointment. During the second appointment, the débridement procedures are repeated before filling the canal with a thick paste of calcium hydroxide and CMCP or calcium hydroxide in a methylcellulose paste.

Whether the tooth is filled in one or two appointments (or more) should be determined to a large extent by the clinical signs and symptoms present and to a lesser extent by operator convenience. The signs and symptoms of active infection should be eliminated before the canal is filled with the treatment paste. Absence of tenderness to percussion is an especially good sign before filling the canal. Because of the wide-open communication to periapical tissues, it is not always possible to maintain complete dryness in the root canal. If the canal continues to weep but other signs of infection seem to be controlled after two or three appointments, the dentist may elect to proceed with the calcium hydroxide paste treatment.

As a general rule, the treatment paste is allowed to remain for 6 months. The root canal is then reopened to determine whether the tooth is ready for a conventional gutta-percha filling as determined by the presence of a "positive stop" when the apical area is probed with a file. Often there is also radiographic evidence of apical closure. Frank has described four successful results of apexification treatment[18]: (1) continued closure of the canal and apex to a normal appearance, (2) a dome-shaped apical closure with the canal retaining a blunderbuss appearance, (3) no apparent radiographic change but a positive stop in the apical area, and (4) a positive stop and radiographic evidence of a barrier coronal to the anatomic apex of the tooth.

If apical closure has not occurred in 6 months, the root canal is retreated with the calcium hydroxide paste. If weeping in the canal was not controlled before filling, retreatment is recommended 2 or 3 months after the first treatment.

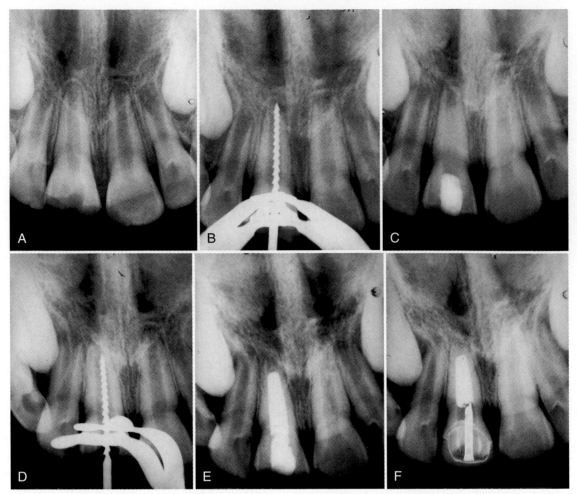

Figure 21-12 Series of radiographs demonstrating treatment to stimulate root end development of a pulpless young anterior permanent central incisor. **A,** An injury several months before had resulted in a pulp exposure. An acute abscess was present at the beginning of treatment. An opening to the pulp chamber was made to allow drainage. **B,** Four days after the initial treatment, the canal length was established. Files were used to clean the canal. After cleansing and irrigation of the canal, calcium hydroxide and camphorated mono-parachlorophenol were used to fill the canal. **C,** One month after initial treatment. **D,** Six months after initial treatment a definite calcified stop is encountered when the file is introduced. The canal was cleansed thoroughly, and gutta-percha was used to fill the canal. **E,** Five months after the placement of the gutta-percha canal filling. **F,** A 6-month postoperative radiograph. A tube and resin core was placed and the tooth was restored with a jacket crown. Currently, an esthetic bonded composite resin restoration (or a fragment restoration if possible) would probably be the preferred interim restoration until the patient has attained adulthood. (Courtesy Drs. Paul E. Starkey and Joe Camp.)

Although apical closure often occurs in a 6-month period, one of the authors (Avery) has monitored retreatment for more than 2½ years before favorable results were achieved. Retreatment of the canal at 3- to 6-month intervals for an extended period seems justified as long as the patient remains free of adverse signs and symptoms, because apical closure is likely to occur eventually.

Ideally the postoperative radiographs should demonstrate continued apical growth and closure as in a normal tooth. However, any of the other three previously described results are considered successful. When closure has been achieved, the canal is filled in the conventional manner with gutta-percha.

Currently there seems to be a trend away from incorporating antibacterial agents, such as CMCP, in the calcium hydroxide treatment paste. It is generally agreed that calcium hydroxide is the major ingredient responsible for

stimulating the desired calcific closure of the apical area. Calcium hydroxide is also an antibacterial agent. It may be that CMCP does not enhance the repair; on the other hand, its use as described here has not been shown to be detrimental. Certainly more than one treatment paste has been employed with success. Giuliani and associates have demonstrated the use of mineral trioxide aggregate (MTA) to form an apical plug for apexification in three clinical cases[20] (Fig. 21-13). The root canals of central incisors that had suffered premature interruption of root development as a consequence of trauma were rinsed with 5% sodium hypochloride. Calcium hydroxide was then placed in the canals for 1 week. Following this, the apical portion of the canal (4 mm) was filled with MTA and the remaining portion of the root canals were closed with thermoplastic gutta-percha. At 6-month and 1-year follow-up periods, the clinical and radiographic appearance of the teeth

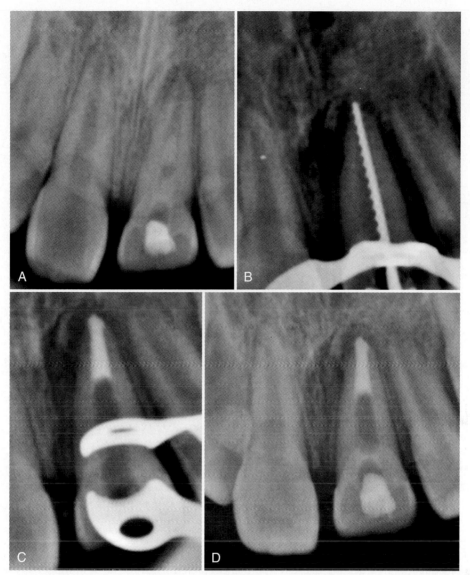

Figure 21-13 A, Maxillary right central incisor with periapical pathology secondary to trauma. The canal has been opened, rinsed with 5% sodium hypochlorite, dried, and filled with calcium hydroxide. **B,** Approximately 7 days after initial treatment with calcium hydroxide, the incisor is instrumented to remove all remaining tissue before further treatment. **C,** The apical 4 to 5 mm of the incisor root has been filled with mineral trioxide aggregate (MTA). **D,** The incisor has completed initial treatment with MTA. A temporary restoration has been placed to seal the canal opening. It was thought that several months of observation would be desired before the final gutta-percha placement on top of the MTA apical seal. (Courtesy Dr. Joseph Legan)

showed resolution of the periapical lesions. These researchers suggest that MTA is a valid option for apexification. They also suggest that long-term outcome studies are needed to test whether this treatment modality will be successful in a large group of teeth.

Trairatvorakul reported on a most interesting and unusual case in which a maxillary primary central incisor successfully responded to apexification therapy.[21] A 14-month-old child experienced early childhood caries to the extent that one maxillary central incisor was necrotic and the root of the tooth was not fully formed. The tooth was treated in a manner similar to that just described. The tooth was retreated with calcium hydroxide 3 months

later and restored with composite resin. An additional 3 months later (6 months after initial treatment), an apical stop was present when the area was probed from the root canal access opening. The root canal was then filled with zinc oxide–eugenol paste. The tooth remained functional and radiographically and clinically successful until its normal exfoliation 6 years after initial treatment.

Teeth treated by the apexification method are susceptible to fracture because of the brittleness that results from nonvitality and from the relatively thin dentinal walls of the roots. In addition, another important problem with the calcium hydroxide apexification technique is the duration of therapy, which often lasts many months.

REACTION OF THE TOOTH TO TRAUMA

PULPAL HYPEREMIA

The dentist must be cognizant of the inadequacies of present methods of determining the initial pulpal reaction to an injury and of the difficulty in predicting the long-range reaction of the pulp and supporting tissues to the insult. A trauma of even a so-called minor nature is immediately followed by a condition of pulpal hyperemia.

Congestion of blood within the pulp chamber a short time after the injury can often be detected in the clinical examination. If a strong light is directed to the labial surface of the injured tooth and the lingual surface is viewed in a mirror, the coronal portion of the tooth will often appear reddish compared with the adjacent teeth. The color change may be evident for several weeks after the accident and is often indicative of a poor prognosis.

INTERNAL HEMORRHAGE

The dentist will occasionally observe temporary discoloration of a tooth after injury. Hyperemia and increased pressure may cause the rupture of capillaries and the escape of red blood cells, with subsequent breakdown and pigment formation. The extravasated blood may be reabsorbed before gaining access to the dentinal tubules, in which case little if any color change will be noticeable and what appears will be temporary (Fig. 21-14). In more severe cases there is pigment formation in the dentinal tubules. The change in color is evident within 2 to 3 weeks after the injury, and although the reaction is reversible to a degree, the crown of the injured tooth retains some of the discoloration for an indefinite period. In cases of this type, there is some chance that the pulp will retain its vitality, although the likelihood of vitality is apparently low in primary teeth with dark gray discoloration. Croll and colleagues found that 33 of 51 traumatized teeth (65%) with gray-black discoloration were necrotic.[22] Holan and Fuks conducted a retrospective study of 88 pulpectomized primary incisors, of which 48 met their nine clinical and radiographic criteria for further investigation.[23] Briefly, their criteria included dark-gray coronal discoloration as the primary diagnostic sign before pulpectomy. The remaining criteria were indicative of normal conditions or conditions only somewhat suggestive of a pulpal problem. They found that 47 (98%) of the teeth included in the study were either necrotic (37, or 77%) or partially necrotic (10, or 21%). Because all of these teeth were previously determined to need pulpectomy, the 98% confirmation is not so surprising. However, the fact remains that all the teeth exhibited dark-gray discoloration and few, if any, other minor signs or symptoms of a problem. Discoloration that becomes evident for the first time months or years after an accident, however, is evidence of a necrotic pulp.

CALCIFIC METAMORPHOSIS OF THE DENTAL PULP (PROGRESSIVE CANAL CALCIFICATION OR DYSTROPHIC CALCIFICATION)

A frequently observed reaction to trauma is the partial or complete obliteration of the pulp chamber and canal (Fig. 21-15). Although the radiograph may give the illusion

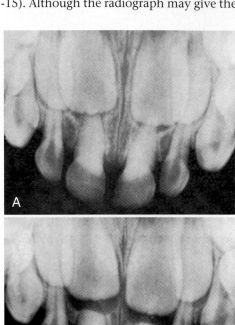
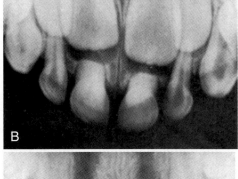
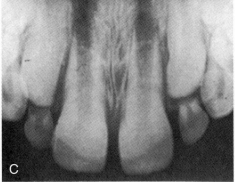

Figure 21-15 A, Radiograph demonstrates almost complete obliteration of the pulp chambers and canals. **B,** Normal root resorption of the primary incisors has occurred. **C,** The permanent incisors have erupted.

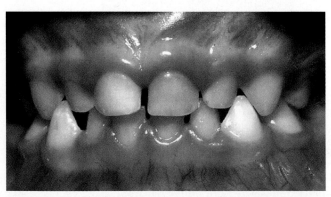

Figure 21-14 Maxillary left primary central incisor became discolored within 2 weeks after trauma. A pulp test indicated that the pulp was vital.

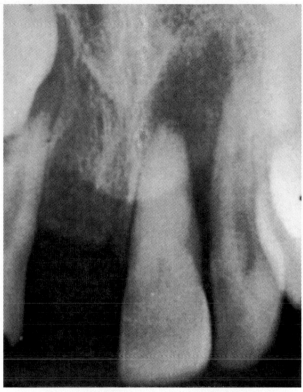

Figure 21-16 Trauma occurred 10 years before acute symptoms developed in the left central incisor. An apical lesion area may be seen. The right central incisor was lost at the time of the injury.

of complete obliteration, an extremely fine root canal and remnants of the pulp will persist.

The crowns of teeth that have undergone this reaction may have a yellowish, opaque color. Primary teeth demonstrating calcific metamorphosis will usually undergo normal root resorption, although Peterson and colleagues have reported observing one patient who exhibited calcific metamorphosis of a maxillary primary central incisor that subsequently showed evidence of significant internal resorption in the root.[24] They emphasize the need for careful monitoring of traumatized teeth that have undergone calcific metamorphosis.

Permanent teeth will often be retained indefinitely. However, a permanent tooth showing signs of calcific changes as a result of trauma should be regarded as a potential focus of infection. A small percentage demonstrate pathologic change many years after the injury (Fig. 21-16).

INTERNAL RESORPTION

Internal resorption is a destructive process generally believed to be caused by odontoclastic action. It may be observed radiographically in the pulp chamber or canal within a few weeks or months after an injury. The destructive process may progress slowly or rapidly. If progression is rapid, it may cause a perforation of the crown or root within a few weeks (Fig. 21-17). Mummery described this condition as "pink spot" because when the crown is affected, the vascular tissue of the pulp shines through the remaining thin shell of the tooth.[25] He referred to the

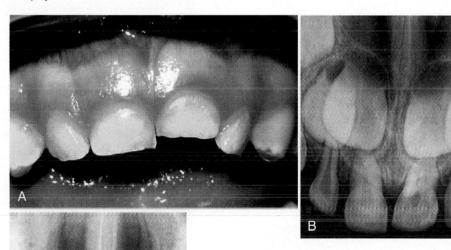

Figure 21-17 Internal resorption in a traumatized left primary incisor. **A,** The tooth 6 months after injury. The tooth has a slight color change as compared with the nontraumatized maxillary right primary incisor. **B,** A later radiograph shows internal resorption in the pulp chamber and canal and some evidence of attempted repair. **C,** This radiograph shows the subsequent degree of resorption. The tooth was extracted.

occurrence of a perforation as "perforating hyperplasia of the pulp." If evidence of internal resorption is detected early, before it becomes extensive with resulting perforation, the tooth may possibly be retained when endodontic procedures are instituted.

PERIPHERAL (EXTERNAL) ROOT RESORPTION

Trauma with damage to the periodontal structures may cause peripheral root resorption (Fig. 21-18). This reaction starts from without, and the pulp may not become involved. Usually the resorption continues unabated until gross areas of the root have been destroyed. In exceptional cases the resorption may become arrested, and the tooth may be retained. Peripheral root resorption is most often observed in cases of severe trauma in which there has been some degree of displacement of the tooth.

PULPAL NECROSIS

Little relationship exists between the type of injury to the tooth and the reaction of the pulp and supporting tissues. A severe blow to a tooth causing displacement often results in pulpal necrosis. The blow may cause a severance of the apical vessels, in which case the pulp undergoes autolysis and necrosis. In a less severe type of injury, the hyperemia and slowing of blood flow through the pulpal

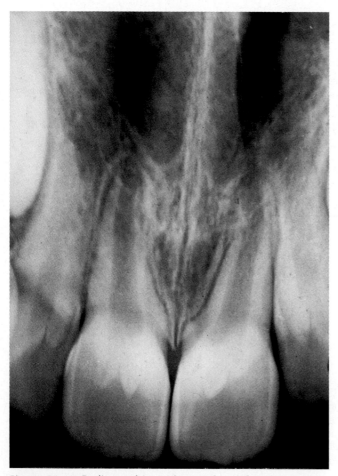

Figure 21-18 Radiographic evidence of peripheral resorption. In these teeth the pulpal vitality was retained and root resorption did not continue.

tissue may cause eventual necrosis of the pulp. In some cases the necrosis may not occur until several months after the injury.

A tooth receiving an injury that causes coronal fracture may have a better pulpal prognosis than a tooth that sustains a severe blow without fracturing the crown. Part of the energy of the blow dissipates as the crown fractures, rather than all of the energy's being absorbed by the tooth's supporting tissues. Thus the periodontium and the pulp of the injured tooth sustain fewer traumas when the crown fractures. The prognosis for long-term retention of the tooth and for maintenance of pulp vitality may then improve. However, because some teeth do not recover from traumatic blows that seem relatively minor, all injured teeth should be closely monitored.

Injured teeth with subsequent pulpal necrosis are commonly asymptomatic, and the radiograph is essentially normal. It should be realized, however, that these teeth are probably infected and that acute symptoms and clinical evidence of infection will inevitably develop at a later date. The tooth with a necrotic pulp should therefore be extracted or treated with endodontic procedures, whichever is indicated.

A necrotic pulp in an anterior primary tooth may be successfully treated if no extensive root resorption or bone loss has occurred (Fig. 21-19). The treatment technique is essentially the same as that for permanent teeth. However, trauma to the periapical tissues during canal instrumentation must be carefully avoided. After the canal has been properly prepared via a facial access in this example, it is filled with slow-setting zinc oxide–eugenol. The canal walls are first lined with a thin mix of the canal-filling material. A thicker mix should then be placed in the pulp chamber. Over this is placed a pledget of cotton, and the material is forced into the canal with a small amalgam plugger.

ANKYLOSIS

Another reaction observed after trauma to anterior primary or permanent teeth is ankylosis. The condition is caused by injury to the periodontal ligament and subsequent inflammation, which is associated with invasion by osteoclastic cells. The result is irregularly resorbed areas on the peripheral root surface. In histologic sections, repair can be seen that may cause a mechanical lock or fusion between alveolar bone and root surface. Clinical evidence of ankylosis is a difference in the incisal plane of the ankylosed tooth and adjacent teeth. The adjacent teeth continue to erupt, whereas the ankylosed tooth remains fixed in relation to surrounding structures. The radiograph shows an interruption in the periodontal membrane of the ankylosed tooth, and often the dentin may appear to be continuous with alveolar bone.

The ankylosed anterior primary tooth should be removed if there is evidence of its causing delayed or ectopic eruption of the permanent successor. If ankylosis of a permanent tooth occurs during active eruption, eventually a discrepancy between the position of this tooth and its adjacent ones will be obvious. The uninjured teeth will continue to erupt and may drift mesially with a loss of arch length. Therefore the removal of a permanent tooth

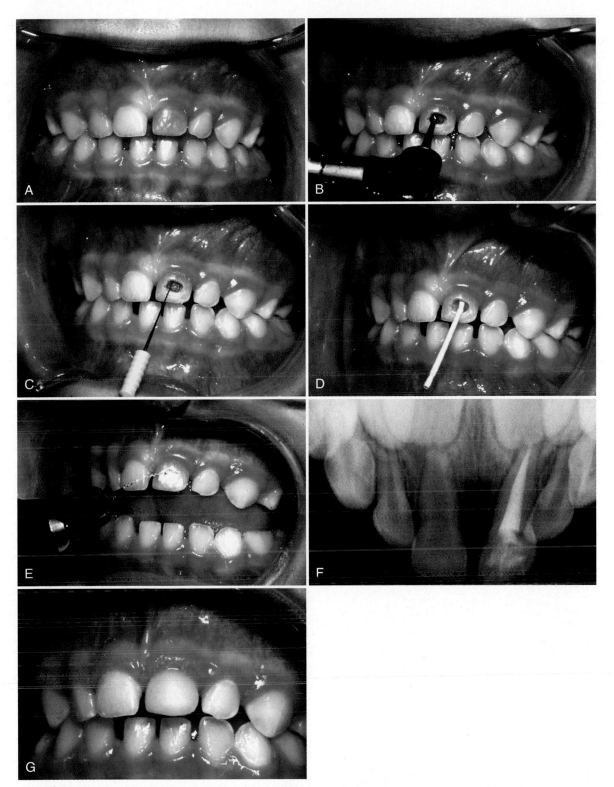

Figure 21-19 A, Evidence of dark crown for the maxillary left central incisor demonstrating possible pulpal necrosis. A pulp test indicated that the pulp was nonvital. **B,** A conservative facial access was used to enter the pulp chamber. This access helps maintain tooth structure for the final restoration. **C,** The canal is instrumented to remove all necrotic tissue. Special care is taken not to traumatize the periapical tissue during instrumentation. **D,** A paper point is used to thoroughly dry the canal before placement of the filling material. **E,** A slow-setting zinc oxide–eugenol mix is gently spun into the canal using rotary instrumentation. **F,** Postoperative radiograph showing excellent filling of the canal to the apex of the tooth. **G,** Final restoration after addressing the necrotic pulp. A facial composite restoration was used as a conservative restoration in this clinical presentation. (Courtesy Dr. James Weddell)

that becomes ankylosed is often necessary, especially if the ankylosis occurs during the preteenage or early teenage years.

RESTORATION OF FRACTURED TEETH

The restoration of a fractured tooth is as important as the emergency treatment designed to aid in the recovery of the pulp after the trauma. Several restorations have been advocated, and although the dentist has a wide choice of techniques and types of restorations, the circumstances surrounding the case often dictate the type of restoration for a given patient. The prognosis of pulp healing, the amount of tooth structure remaining, the stage of eruption of the tooth and adjacent teeth, the size of the dental pulp and degree of root closure, the normalcy of the occlusion, and the wishes of the patient must all be considered in the selection of a temporary restoration, an intermediate restoration, or the permanent restoration. In the young patient, although it is often desirable to wait for continued eruption of the tooth or to determine the outcome of a vital pulp procedure, a delay of even a few weeks is often sufficient to allow the tipping of adjacent teeth, overeruption of opposing teeth, or other undesirable changes in the occlusion.

ESTHETIC BONDED COMPOSITE RESIN RESTORATION

The feathered-edge restorative technique without mechanical tooth preparation is appropriate in some situations, but it requires excessive contour in the restoration. It offers the advantage of creating less irritation to the pulp, because little or no enamel modification is required. In some cases, the excess contour is relatively insignificant, but it may be more significant if the restoration is large (50% or more of the crown) or the fracture extends near or below gingival tissue. Excessive contour on the lingual surface of a maxillary anterior tooth may interfere with normal occlusion.

A beveled preparation affords the dentist the opportunity to reduce the amount of overcontouring of larger restorations, and it reduces contour in areas where the occlusion prohibits overcontouring. The dentist may elect the feathered-edge technique (no preparation) on the labial tooth surface and the beveled preparation on the proximal or lingual surfaces, or both. Both techniques are described in the following discussion.

When a beveled preparation is desired, the bevel is made in the enamel around the entire circumference or the selected part of the fracture (Figs. 21-20 and 21-21). The bevel should be about 1 to 2 mm incisocervically and about halfway (or more) through the thickness of the enamel at the fracture margins. The labial enamel margin should be irregular to provide a better esthetic blending of the resin with the tooth structure. This sequence may be altered if the practitioner uses some of the latest-generation bonding adhesive systems.

The exposed dentin from a recent injury may be covered with a calcium hydroxide liner. Dilute phosphoric acid (etchant or tooth conditioner) is applied to the enamel surface of the preparation for about 20 seconds

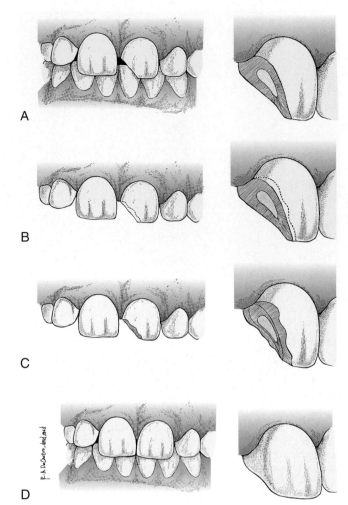

Figure 21-20 A, Typical class II fracture of a permanent incisor. **B,** Dotted line represents the approximate location of the irregular enamel margin to be placed on the labial surface in the bevel preparation. **C,** Bevel preparation complete and ready for etching. **D,** Bonded composite material restores natural contour and color.

(longer for primary teeth). The tooth is then thoroughly flushed with water, and excess moisture is removed with air. The etched area should appear frosty and opaque. Alternatively, the total-etch technique may be employed. In either case a bonding agent is applied to all etched tooth structure. Again, this sequence may be altered with the use of some of the latest bonding adhesive systems.

A celluloid matrix strip may be placed interproximally and wedged for close adaptation at the gingival margin. In large restorations a custom-cut celluloid crown form matrix may be used to help contour the restoration.

Often, little or no mechanical preparation of the fractured incisor is necessary with the feathered-edge technique. Instead, the resin margins are allowed to overlap the fractured edges to become feathered-edge margins on the etched sound enamel cervical to the fracture (Fig. 21-22). This procedure requires a slightly overcontoured restoration and therefore has limitations. (Fig. 21-23) The dentist should be alert to potential undesirable changes in gingival

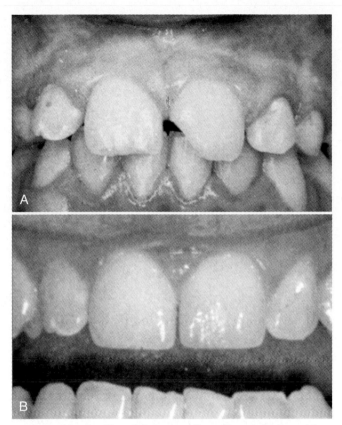

Figure 21-21 A, Class II fracture of maxillary left central incisor. **B,** This 7½-year postoperative photograph shows an acceptable esthetic and functional restoration, although close examination reveals loss of material along the incisal edge as a result of functional wear.

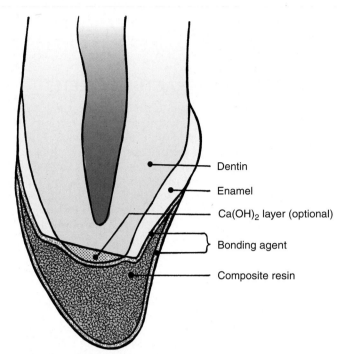

Figure 21-22 This sagittal drawing illustrates the application of a feathered-edge restoration on a fractured incisor. Little or no tooth preparation is required before calcium hydroxide (optional) is placed on the exposed dentin and the tooth is etched. Slight beveling of the fractured enamel margins is suggested. The drawing also illustrates the need to overcontour the labial and lingual surfaces with the feathered-edge restoration.

Figure labels:
- Dentin
- Enamel
- Ca(OH)₂ layer (optional)
- Bonding agent
- Composite resin

health or the creation of traumatic occlusion. Slight beveling of the fractured enamel margins is usually recommended with the feathered-edge technique to remove loose enamel rods and ensure a fresh surface for etching. The exposed dentin may be protected with a layer of hard-setting calcium hydroxide, and etching should extend 2 or 3 mm beyond the fracture to allow an adequate surface for feather-edging the resin restorative materials. Most manufacturers supply a kit, which usually includes an etchant, a bonding agent, the restorative materials, and a shade guide. The bonding agent is applied to the etched surfaces.

The light-polymerized materials offer the advantage of allowing the clinician to build or sculpt the restoration in small increments and minimize finishing time. Clinical studies have confirmed that excellent and durable restorations may be obtained. Finishing disks and large, round finishing burs or diamonds may be used to contour the labial and lingual surfaces.

REACTION OF PERMANENT TOOTH BUDS TO INJURY

The dentist who provides emergency care for a child after an injury to the anterior primary teeth must be aware of the possibility of damage to the underlying developing permanent teeth.

Andreasen and colleagues have reported on the effect of injuries to primary teeth on their permanent successors.[26] In a clinical and radiographic study of 213 teeth, these investigators reported that more than 40% of their young patients had changes in the permanent teeth that could be traced to injury to the primary dentition. The close anatomic relationship between the apices of primary teeth and their developing permanent successors explains why injuries to primary teeth may involve the permanent dentition (Fig. 21-24).

The dentist and the physician should also be aware of the possibility of trauma to permanent tooth buds from other unusual injuries so that parents may be informed of the possibility of defective permanent tooth development. Some injuries to the face and jaws may not appear to have caused any dental injuries initially, but the problem may be noticed several months or years later (Fig. 21-25).

HYPOCALCIFICATION AND HYPOPLASIA

Cutright's experiments with miniature pigs have shown many lesions similar to those seen in permanent human teeth as a result of trauma, infection, or both.[27] He observed small areas that showed destruction of the ameloblasts and a pitted area where a thin enamel layer had been laid down before the injury. In other teeth there was evidence of destruction of the ameloblasts before any enamel had been laid down, resulting in hypoplasia that clinically appeared as deep pitting.

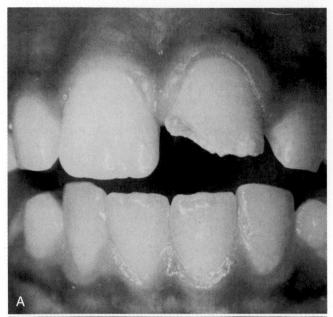

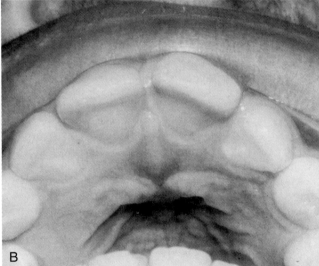

Figure 21-23 A, Incisal view of a class II crown fracture involving the entire incisal edge of the maxillary left central incisor. This view illustrates rotation and labial position of the tooth which makes it more susceptible to trauma. **B,** Six-month postoperative incisal view of the restored tooth. Note the illusion of better tooth alignment was achieved when the mesial half of the labial surface was deliberately undercontoured during finishing.

Erupted permanent teeth in the human may show a variety of these defects, including gross malformations of the crown (Figs. 21-26 and 21-27). The presence of a small, pigmented hypoplastic area has been referred to as *Turner tooth*. Small hypoplastic defects may be restored by the resin-bonding technique.

REPARATIVE DENTIN PRODUCTION

In cases in which the injury to the developing permanent tooth is severe enough to remove the thin covering of developing enamel or cause destruction of the ameloblasts, the subjacent odontoblasts have been observed to

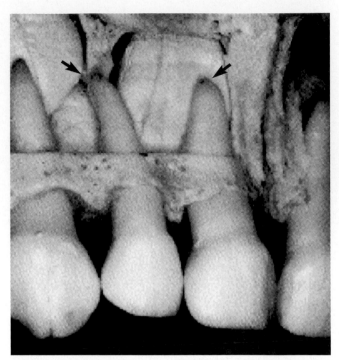

Figure 21-24 Skull of a 5-year-old child demonstrating the relationship between the position of the roots of the primary central and lateral incisors and the crowns of their permanent successors (see *arrows*).

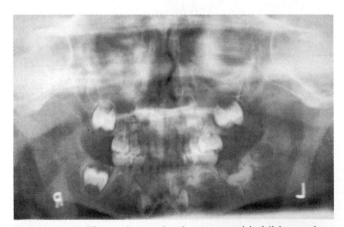

Figure 21-25 This radiograph of a 4-year-old child reveals improper formation of the mandibular left first permanent molar. At 18 months, the child had been viciously attacked by a dog. There had been a severe puncture wound of the lower left jaw from the dog's canines, although it was not known then that the injury involved the permanent molar tooth bud. The calcified lesion was removed and microscopically diagnosed as a developing tooth with displaced enamel matrix into follicular tissue. Early removal enhances the potential of the normally developing second permanent molar to eventually acquire an acceptable first permanent molar position.

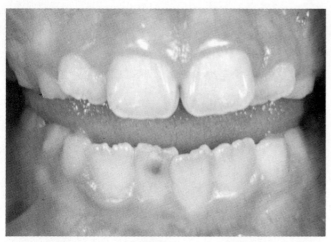

Figure 21-26 Isolated hypoplastic area on the labial surface of a maxillary right permanent central incisor. There was a history of a trauma to the primary tooth when the child was younger than 2 years old.

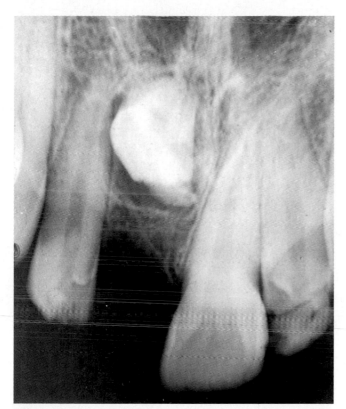

Figure 21-27 Radiograph of malformed central incisor. This condition can be traced to a severe trauma to the primary teeth.

produce a reparative type of dentin. The irregular dentin bridges the gap where there is no enamel covering to aid in protecting the pulp from further injury.

DILACERATION

The condition referred to as dilaceration occasionally occurs after the intrusion or displacement of an anterior primary tooth. The developed portion of the tooth is twisted or bent on itself, and in this new position growth

of the tooth progresses. Cases have been observed in which the crown of a permanent tooth or a portion of it develops at an acute angle to the remainder to the tooth (Fig. 21-28). Kilpatrick and colleagues reported a dilacerated root of a primary central incisor in a 6-year-old boy.[28] The tooth was necrotic, the root had not resorbed, and the apex of the root was exposed in the labial sulcus and was associated with a draining sinus. No specific history of trauma could be confirmed, but the child was prone to accidents. The authors speculate that this unusual dilaceration may have been due to injury soon after initial eruption of the tooth.

Rushton reported that an injury during development may cause the subsequent appearance of an additional cusp, crown, or denticle.[29] Partial duplication of the affected teeth may occur, with the appearance of gemination in the part of the tooth formed after the injury.

DISPLACEMENT OF PRIMARY AND PERMANENT ANTERIOR TEETH (LUXATION)

INTRUSION AND EXTRUSION OF TEETH

The displacement of anterior primary and permanent teeth presents a challenge in diagnosis and treatment for the dentist. Relatively few studies have been reported that can be used as a guide in treating injuries of this type.

Primary Teeth

The intrusion by forceful impaction of maxillary anterior primary teeth is a common occurrence in children during the first 3 years of life. Frequent falls and striking of the teeth on hard objects may force the teeth into the alveolar process to the extent that the entire clinical crown becomes buried in bone and soft tissue. Although there is a difference of opinion regarding treatment of injuries of this type, it is generally agreed that immediate attention

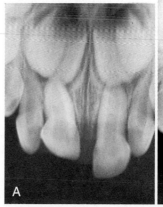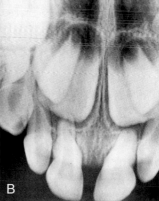

Figure 21-28 A, The degree of intrusion of the primary tooth. Damage to the permanent teeth often results from an injury of this type. **B,** Radiograph obtained 8 months after the injury shows that the injured tooth has re-erupted. The pulp has retained its vitality, although there is evidence of partial obliteration of the pulp canal. External root resorption has occurred on the adjacent central incisor.

should be given to soft tissue damage. Intruded primary teeth should be observed; with few exceptions, no attempt should be made to reposition them after the accident. Most injuries of this type occur at an age when it would be difficult to construct a splint or a retaining appliance to stabilize the repositioned teeth.

Normally the developing permanent incisor tooth buds lie lingual to the roots of the primary central incisors. Therefore, when an intrusive displacement occurs, the primary tooth usually remains labial to the developing permanent tooth (Fig. 21-29). If the intruded primary tooth is found to be in a lingual or encroaching relationship to the developing permanent tooth, it should be removed. Such a relationship may be confirmed from a lateral radiograph of the anterior segment.

The examination should be carried out as previously described, and radiographs should be made to detect evidence of root fracture, fracture of the alveolar bone, and damage to permanent teeth. However, predicting whether the permanent successors will show evidence of interrupted growth and development is impossible unless actual encroachment of their space can be seen radiographically.

Primary anterior teeth intruded as a result of a blow may often re-erupt within 3 to 4 weeks after the injury. In a study of the results of 248 traumatic episodes to primary incisors, Ravn reported 88 cases of intrusion.[30] Of these teeth, four were extracted within 2 weeks because of infection and four did not re-erupt and were extracted several months later, but the remaining 80 teeth fully re-erupted within 6 months. Incipient re-eruption was observed 14 days after the injury in a few instances. These teeth may even retain their vitality and later undergo normal resorption and be replaced on schedule by their permanent successors. During the first 6 months after the injury, however, the dentist often observes one or more of the reactions of the pulp and supporting tissues that have been mentioned previously in this chapter, the most common of which is pulpal necrosis. Even after re-eruption a necrotic pulp can be treated if the tooth is sound in the alveolus and no pathologic root resorption is evident.

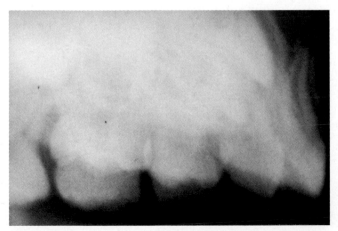

Figure 21-29 Radiograph of intruded primary central incisor with its root apex lying labial to the permanent central incisor.

Primary teeth that are displaced but not intruded should be repositioned by the dentist or parent as soon as possible after the accident to prevent interference with occlusion. The prognosis for severely loosened primary teeth is poor. Frequently the teeth remain mobile and undergo rapid root resorption.

Skieller observed 60 children treated for looseness of one or more young teeth.[31] Loosened teeth were divided into three groups: simple looseness, dislocation with impaction, and dislocation with extrusion. He concluded that the immediate and future prognosis for the pulp was more favorable if root formation was still incomplete at the time of the accident. Root resorption, which was observed in all three groups of loosened teeth, was most common in impaction cases. Teeth with complete root formation seemed to undergo resorption more frequently than those with incomplete root formation. However, when resorption did occur, it was more extensive and progressed more rapidly in teeth with incomplete root development.

Permanent Teeth

Intruded permanent teeth apparently have a poorer prognosis than similarly injured primary teeth. The tendency for the injury to be followed by rapid root resorption, pulpal necrosis, or ankylosis is greater. The treatment for a permanent tooth with a closed root end consists in gradually repositioning the tooth orthodontically over a 2- or 3-week period and then continuing to stabilize the tooth for 2 to 4 weeks. The pulp should be extirpated 2 weeks after the injury, and calcium hydroxide should be placed in the root canal as an interim dressing. This treatment approach is recommended by Malmgren and associates[32] and by Trope and colleagues.[33]

These same authors recommend that intruded immature permanent teeth be left to re-erupt spontaneously, unless the intrusion is severe. If the immature tooth does not show early evidence of spontaneous re-eruption (after 1 to 2 weeks) or if the intrusion is severe, orthodontic repositioning should be initiated. The clinician may elect to reposition the tooth orthodontically but delay endodontic therapy in the absence of unfavorable signs or symptoms. Endodontic therapy is often required, however, and the tooth should be monitored closely while a decision on endodontic therapy is pending.

Tronstad and associates have reported on the management of severely intruded mature maxillary central incisors in an 11-year-old patient in whom spontaneous re-eruption occurred.[34] Rather than repositioning the teeth to gain endodontic access, they performed a palatal gingivectomy and endodontic treatment 10 days after the injury while the teeth remained in their intruded position. Eight weeks after the injury the teeth had re-erupted naturally and were judged to be near their original position. Similar management of severely intruded immature central incisors has been reported by Shapira and colleagues.[35] In these cases, the palatal gingivectomies and endodontic treatment were performed 8 to 10 weeks after injury when periapical rarefactions and root resorption were noted radiographically. They noted accelerated spontaneous re-eruption of all treated teeth soon after the gingivectomies and calcium hydroxide endodontic treatments were performed. Complete re-eruption of the teeth and apparent periapical and periodontal healing had occurred 2 to 3 months after the surgical intervention.

It seems that both treatment approaches to treatment of severely intruded permanent teeth (early repositioning or waiting for spontaneous re-eruption) have demonstrated reasonably successful results. However, the affected teeth seem to benefit by early calcium hydroxide endodontic therapy with either treatment approach. The decision to reposition mechanically or hope for spontaneous re-eruption of intruded permanent teeth remains a matter of clinical judgment that may be based on several conditions associated with the particular case.

The extrusive luxation of a permanent tooth usually results in pulpal necrosis. The immediate treatment involves the careful repositioning of the tooth and stabilization following the technique described later in this chapter. If mature repositioned teeth do not respond to pulp vitality tests within 2 to 3 weeks after repositioning, endodontic treatment should be undertaken before there is evidence of root resorption, which often occurs after severe injuries of this type. The need for endodontic intervention is virtually certain in cases of significant extrusion (more than 2 mm) of mature teeth. With extruded immature teeth, the clinician should monitor the situation frequently and be prepared to intervene with endodontic therapy, as described later, if conditions warrant.

AVULSION AND REPLANTATION

Replantation is the technique in which a tooth, usually one in the anterior region, is reinserted into the alveolus after its loss or displacement by accidental means. There are few reports in the literature of this technique's proving successful for indefinite periods of time. For example, Barry reports on functioning teeth that were replanted 42 years earlier.[36] However, slow or even rapid root resorption often occurs with even the most precise and careful technique. Replantation of permanent teeth continues to be practiced and recommended, however, because prolonged retention is also achieved in many cases, especially when replantation occurs soon after the accident. The replanted tooth serves as a space maintainer and often guides adjacent teeth into their proper position in the arch, a function that is important during the transitional dentition period. The replantation procedure also has psychological value. It gives the unfortunate child and parents hope for success; even though they are told of the possibility of eventual loss of the tooth, the early result often appears favorable and softens the emotional blow of the accident (Figs. 21-30 and 21-31).

The success of the replantation procedure is undoubtedly related to the length of time that elapses between the loss of the tooth and its replacement in the socket. The condition of the tooth, and particularly the condition of the periodontal ligament tissue remaining on the root surface, are also important factors that influence the success of replantation. There have been reports that immediate replacement of a permanent tooth occasionally results in maintenance of vitality and indefinite retention. However, replantation should generally be viewed as a temporary measure. Under favorable conditions, many replanted teeth are retained for 5 or 10 years and a few for a lifetime. Others, however, fail soon after replantation.

Camp reports that the tooth most commonly avulsed in both the primary and the permanent dentition is a maxillary central incisor.[37] Most often an avulsion injury involves only a single tooth. Avulsion injuries are three times more frequent in boys than in girls and occur most commonly in children 7 to 9 years of age when permanent incisors are erupting. Andreasen suggests that the loosely structured periodontal ligament surrounding the erupting teeth favors complete avulsion.[38]

The sooner a tooth can be replanted in its socket after avulsion, the better the prognosis will be for retention without root resorption. Andreasen and Hjørting-Hansen

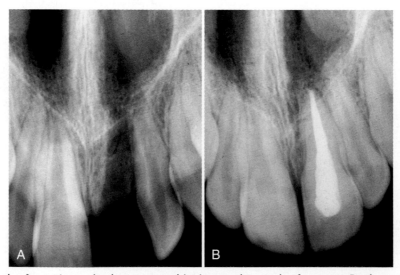

Figure 21-30 A, Radiograph of a patient who lost a central incisor as the result of trauma. Replantation was performed. **B,** After the replantation procedure, peripheral root resorption is evident along the mesial surface.

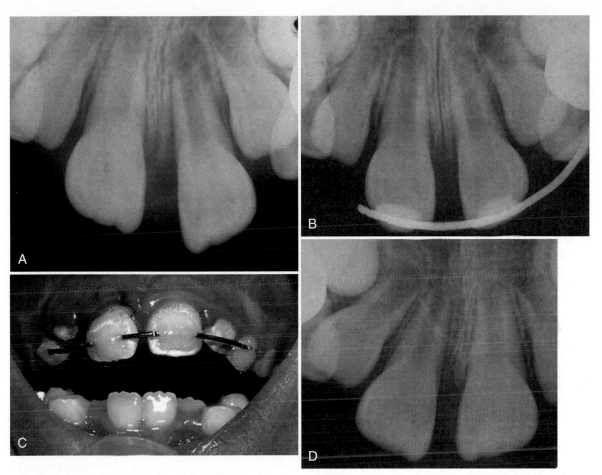

Figure 21-31 A, Radiograph of an avulsed maxillary right central incisor, with incomplete root development, that was positioned into canal immediately upon arrival at the office. The patient was seen within 20 minutes after tooth avulsion. Note the degree that the tooth must be repositioned to approximate the original position of the tooth. Gentle pressure is exerted to place the apex of the root to the ideal position. **B,** Radiograph of the avulsed central incisor showing it is now at the desired position and has been stabilized with a section of 0.028 stainless steel wire. Note that at least one nontraumatized tooth, on either side of the avulsed incisor, has been used to anchor the splint. The splint will remain in place for at least 7 to 10 days. **C,** Splint in place at the end of the initial appointment. **D,** Radiograph at the conclusion of 10 days of splint therapy. The incisor tested vital to both electric and cold pulp testing. The incisor, to this date, has received periodic evaluation and has not required follow-up pulp therapy.

reported a follow-up study of 110 replanted teeth. Of those replanted within 30 minutes, 90% showed no discernible evidence of resorption 2 or more years later.[39] However, 95% of the teeth replanted more than 2 hours after the injury showed root resorption. If the tooth has been out of the mouth for less than 30 minutes, the prognosis is therefore more favorable. Also, if the apical end of the tooth is incompletely developed at the time of the injury, there is a greater chance of regaining pulp vitality after replantation. If the apex is closed, the dentist should proceed with a pulpectomy a few days after the replantation, even if the extraoral time for the tooth was brief.

If a parent calls to report that a tooth has been avulsed and it can be determined that the injury is without other oral, neurologic, or higher-priority physical complications, the dentist may instruct the parent to replace it in the socket immediately and to hold it in place with light

finger pressure while the patient is brought to the dental office. If the avulsion occurred in a clean environment, nothing should be done to the tooth before the parent replants it. If the tooth is dirty, an attempt should be made to clean the root surface, but it is very important to preserve any remnants of the periodontal ligament that are still attached to the root. Therefore the parent would then be instructed to keep the tooth immersed in a suitable storage medium and bring the child and the tooth for immediate care.

Milk has been shown to be a suitable storage medium that is also often readily available (skim or low-fat milk, if available, is preferred). Isotonic saline is another excellent solution to use for this purpose if it is available. A commercial product designed specifically for storing avulsed teeth is the Emergency Medical Treatment Toothsaver (EMT Toothsaver; SmartPractice, Phoenix,

Ariz). The system includes an appropriate container for storage and transport of the tooth while immersed in a pH-balanced cell culture fluid (similar to Hanks balanced salt solution). This product has a 2-year shelf-life without refrigeration.

The tooth must be kept moist during the trip to the dental office if the parent cannot or will not replant it. Allowing the avulsed tooth to dehydrate before replantation is damaging to a favorable prognosis. Many studies, including that by Blomlöf and colleagues, have compared various storage solutions for avulsed teeth.[40] A compilation of this information indicates that Hanks buffered saline, isotonic saline, and pasteurized bovine milk may be the most favorable known storage media. If none of these solutions is readily available, human saliva is an acceptable short-term substitute storage liquid. Presumably, the patient's saliva (and perhaps blood) would be readily available to collect in a small container (or a cupped hand) in which to keep the tooth moist while transporting it to the dental office. Although tap water has been a commonly recommended storage solution (and its use would be preferable to allowing dehydration of the tooth), saliva is a better storage medium. Neither water nor saliva is as good as milk or saline, if the tooth must be stored for a long period (more than 30 minutes before replantation). Because water is hypotonic, its use leads to rapid cell lysis and increased inflammation on replantation.

The patient should receive immediate attention after arriving at the dental office. If the tooth has not already been replanted, the dentist should make every effort to minimize the additional time that the tooth is out of the socket. The patient's general status should be quickly assessed to confirm that there are no higher-priority injuries.

If an evaluation of the socket area shows no evidence of alveolar fracture or severe soft tissue injury, the tooth is intact, and only a few minutes have elapsed since the injury, the dentist should replant the tooth immediately. Under the conditions just described, every effort should be directed toward preserving a viable periodontal ligament. Trope correctly asserts that treatment is directed at avoiding or minimizing the resultant inflammation, which occurs as a direct result of the two main consequences of tooth avulsion: attachment damage and pulpal infection.[41] If the tooth was cleanly avulsed, it can probably be replanted without local anesthetic, and obtaining the initial radiograph can also be delayed until the tooth is replaced in the socket and held with finger pressure. The minutes saved may contribute to a more successful replantation. If a clot is present in the socket, it will be displaced as the tooth is repositioned; the socket walls should not be scraped with an instrument. If the tooth does not slip back into position with relative ease when finger pressure is used, local anesthesia and a radiographic evaluation are indicated. Local anesthetic should also be administered when fractured and displaced alveolar bone must be repositioned before the tooth is replanted. Soft tissue suturing may be delayed until the tooth has been replaced in the socket; however, the suturing should be performed to control hemorrhage before the tooth is

stabilized with a bonded splint. Splinting techniques are discussed in the next section of this chapter.

Sherman studied the mechanism by which the replanted tooth becomes secured in the alveolus.[42] Intentional replantation was performed on 25 incisors in dogs and monkeys. The root canals were hermetically sealed with guttapercha, and the teeth were splinted for 1 month. Subsequent microscopic examination under fluorescent and incandescent light revealed deposition of secondary cementum and new alveolar bone, which entrapped the periodontal fibers (Fig. 21-32).

The preservation of an intact and viable periodontal ligament is the most important factor in achieving healing without root resorption. Delicate handling of the tooth, storage in an appropriate moist environment, quick replantation, and appropriate stabilization are all important in preserving the periodontal ligament. Undesirable periodontal ligament reactions may result in replacement resorption (ankylosis) or inflammatory resorption of the root. Either reaction may cause eventual loss of the tooth unless the resorption can be controlled. Use of an enamel matrix derivative (Emdogain; Biora, Chicago, Ill, and Malmö, Sweden) has been shown to increase the incidence of healed periodontal ligament when this gel is applied to the root surface of the avulsed tooth and/or

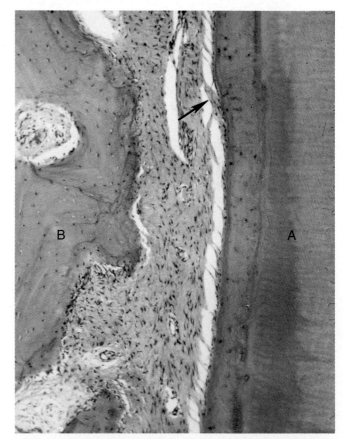

Figure 21-32 Microscopic section of a tooth replanted with the periodontal ligament intact. The reattachment of the periodontal fibers is illustrated by their crossing the tear in the periodontal ligament. **A,** Tooth. **B,** Alveolar bone. (Courtesy Dr. Philip Sherman Jr.)

inserted directly into the alveolar socket before implantation. It appears to aid in preventing or retarding resorption and ankylosis.

In the past, few attempts were made to replant avulsed primary teeth; however, there have been a few reports of success with this procedure. Andreasen and Andreasen have stated that replantation of primary teeth is contraindicated because of the poor prognosis for success and the additional risk of further injury to the succedaneous tooth.[43] We agree that, even under the most ideal conditions, replanting a primary tooth has higher risk and poorer prognosis despite the remote chance for a favorable outcome.

Stabilization of Replanted Teeth

After replantation of a tooth that has been avulsed, a splint is required to stabilize it during at least the first week of healing. Camp[37] has stated that an acceptable splint should meet the following criteria:
1. It should be easy to fabricate directly in the mouth without lengthy laboratory procedures.
2. It should be able to be placed passively without causing forces on the teeth.
3. It should not touch the gingival tissues, causing gingival irritation.
4. It should not interfere with normal occlusion.
5. It should be easily cleaned and allow for proper oral hygiene.
6. It should not traumatize the teeth or gingiva during application.
7. It should allow an approach for endodontic therapy.
8. It should be easily removed.

The splint should also allow mobility of the replanted tooth that is comparable with the normal mobility of a tooth. Rigid stabilization seems to stimulate replacement resorption of the root. Hurst has demonstrated that rigid stabilization of a replanted tooth is detrimental to proper healing of the periodontal ligament.[44]

The bonded resin and wire splint satisfies all the criteria just described. It can be used in most situations requiring the stabilization of one or more teeth if sufficient sound teeth remain for anchorage. Rectangular or round orthodontic wire is bent to approximate the arch configuration along the midportion of the labial surfaces of the teeth to be incorporated in the splint. At least one sound tooth on each side of the tooth to be stabilized is included. The size of the wire is not too critical, but rectangular wire should be at least 0.016 × 0.022 inch and round wire at least 0.018 inch. If three or four teeth must be stabilized, a stiffer wire (e.g., 0.028-inch round wire) is required. If round wire is used, a right-angle bend should be made near each end of the wire to prevent rotation of the wire in the resin. A 20- to 30-pound-test monofilament nylon line is an acceptable substitute for wire in the splint.

If the labial enamel surfaces to be etched are not plaque free, they should be cleaned with a pumice slurry, rinsed, thoroughly dried, and isolated with cotton rolls. The enamel surfaces are etched with a phosphoric acid etchant; the gel form is convenient. The enamel surfaces are thoroughly washed and dried again. The wire is then attached to the abutment teeth by placing increments of the resin material over the wire and onto the etched enamel. The resin should completely surround a segment of the wire, but it should not encroach on the proximal contacts or embrasures. The replanted tooth is then held in position while resin is used to bond it to the wire. The resin may be lightly finished if necessary after polymerization. The splint is easily removed (usually 7 to 10 days later) by cutting through the resin with a bur to uncover the wire. The remaining resin may then be removed with conventional finishing instruments. If the splint is used to stabilize lower teeth, it may be necessary to affix the wire to the lingual surfaces if placing it on the labial surfaces will interfere with natural occlusion. Because lingual surfaces are more likely to be contaminated with saliva during the procedure, however, labial placement is preferred whenever possible.

Direct-bonded orthodontic brackets may also be placed on the teeth, and a light labial archwire bent to accurately conform to the natural curvature of the arch is then ligated to the brackets. The brackets are properly aligned on the archwire and bonded to the abutment teeth first. Then the avulsed tooth is ideally positioned and additional bonding material is placed, if necessary, to fill any remaining small space between the tooth and the bracket before bonding it to the splint. If performed properly, this technique results in an excellent splint (Fig. 21-33). However, it requires much more accurate and precise wire bending than the bonded resin and wire technique (without brackets) to achieve a passive appliance.

If the patient is mentally disabled or has immature behavior and does not tolerate foreign objects in the mouth well, or if there are insufficient abutment teeth available for the bonded resin and wire splint, the suture and bonded resin splint advocated by Camp[37] may be an acceptable alternative (Fig. 21-34). Examples of other types of splint are shown in Fig. 21-35. The titanium trauma splint has been developed by von Arx and colleagues to ease the application and removal of the splint and to increase comfort for the patient.[45]

In general, stabilization for replanted teeth without other complications is required for 7 to 14 days. The periodontal ligament fibers should have healed sufficiently after the first week to remove the splint. However, the patient should be advised not to bite directly on the replanted tooth for 3 to 4 weeks after the injury and then

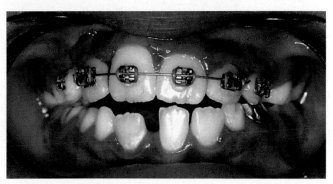

Figure 21-33 Bonded brackets and archwire splint.

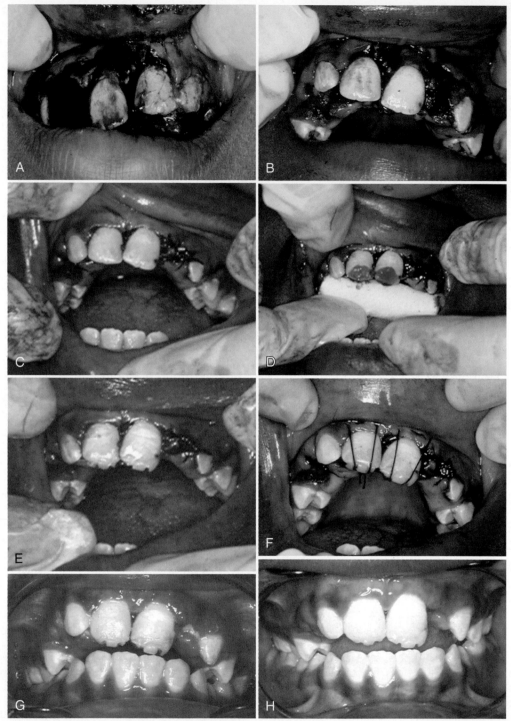

Figure 21-34 Suture and bonded resin splint. **A,** The maxillary central incisors as seen at the initial presentation at the office. The maxillary left central incisor was avulsed and placed in its socket by the parent (approximately 30 minutes after being avulsed) after instructed to do so by the front desk staff on the way to the office. **B** and **C,** The area has been initially cleansed and suturing has been accomplished to reapproximate the lacerated gingival tissue. There are not sufficient teeth to provide adequate anchorage adjacent to the replanted maxillary central incisors. **D,** The incisal edges of the maxillary central incisors are etched, per manufacturer's instruction, before resin placement. **E,** Retention grooves have been created in the resin on the incisal edges of the maxillary central incisors. **F,** A suture is placed over each tooth. Starting at the labial tissue, each suture crosses the incisal edge, enters and exits the lingual tissue, recrosses the incisal edge, and reenters the labial tissue. The ends are then tied. Care is taken to assure that no contact with the opposing occlusion is present. **G** and **H,** Clinical presentation at 7 (sutures removed) and 21 days after initial replantation. Both teeth are stable in their respective sockets, with minimal mobility, and gingival tissue health is improved. Pulp testing demonstrates necrosis in both maxillary central incisors, and root canal • therapy is scheduled.

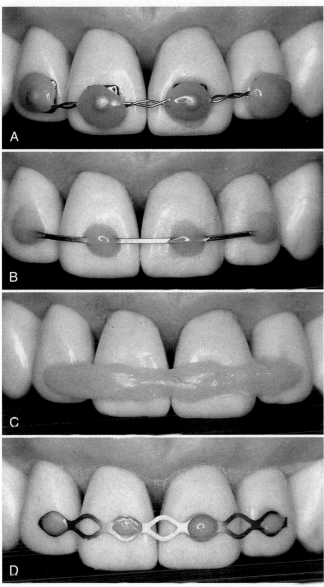

Figure 21-35 Examples of bonded splints. **A,** Button with stainless steel ligature and acrylic caps. **B,** Orthodontic archwire. **C,** Fiber-filled acrylic. **D,** Titanium trauma splint. (Courtesy Dr. Adreas Filippi.)

gradually to begin to return to normal use of the tooth. During this time, food may be cut into bite-size pieces and chewed carefully with unaffected teeth. The patient should maintain good oral hygiene by brushing and flossing normally and using chlorhexidine mouthrinses.

We recommend that systemic antibiotic therapy begin immediately and continue for at least a week following replantation. If the apex is closed, extending the antibiotic therapy until the pulp is extirpated seems to be a good way to determine the duration of antibiotic coverage. Research by Sae-Lim and associates has shown that antibiotic therapy is effective in preventing the development of external inflammatory root resorption of replanted teeth in which the pulps were not extirpated.[46] This finding suggests that antibiotic therapy may also be

helpful in those cases in which the pulps of immature replanted teeth are allowed to remain while hoping for revitalization. Additional studies in this area are indicated. In fact, research in this area is ongoing to find better storage and soaking media. Various antibiotics, fluoride liquids and gels, glucocorticoids, and a liver transport medium are being investigated. Krasner and Rankow have published detailed recommendations for replanting a tooth based on its status as judged by the clinician's determination of the physiologic condition of the root periodontal ligament cells, the development of the root apex, and the length of extraoral time.[47] Their recommendations recognize 10 different categories of avulsed teeth and detail a specific treatment regimen for each category. A modified version of Guidelines for the Management of Avulsed Permanent Teeth from the International Association of Dental Traumatology is shown in Box 21-1.[48] Of course, the dentist should confirm at the time of replantation that the patient is adequately immunized against tetanus.

Endodontic Management of Replanted Teeth
All replanted permanent teeth with complete apical root development should undergo a pulpectomy soon after replantation regardless of the length of time the tooth was out of the mouth. Even though a few reports of revitalization exist, the chances for revitalization are remote at best. Moreover, adverse reactions are virtually certain if degenerating pulp tissue is allowed to remain in the canals for more than a few days. The risk-benefit ratio for the patient favors pulpal extirpation.

Because replantation should be done as soon as possible after the injury, the dentist should not take time to extirpate the pulp before replantation. The pulp should be extirpated before the splint is removed, however, and preferably within 1 week after the injury. A sterile, dry cotton pellet or one dampened with CMCP and blotted on sterile gauze may be sealed in the pulp chamber after débridement and irrigation. The canal should be filled approximately 2 weeks after the injury. When the canal is filled, calcium hydroxide paste is the material of choice. However, Trope suggests that the pulp contents be removed at the emergency visit and a tetracycline-corticosteroid combination (Ledermix; Sigma Pharmaceuticals Pty Lid., Croydon, Victoria, Australia) be placed in the root canal.[41] He feels that this combination decreases the inflammatory response after replantation to allow for more favorable healing than in those teeth that do not receive the medicament.

Research by Andreasen indicates that early extirpation of the pulp may help to control the early onset of inflammatory root resorption.[38] Filling the root canal with calcium hydroxide also controls and may even arrest external inflammatory root resorption. If the calcium hydroxide is placed in the canal too soon (before adequate healing of the periodontal ligament), however, it may stimulate replacement root resorption. Andreasen suggested that 2 weeks after the replantation is the ideal time to fill the canal with calcium hydroxide. The use of calcium hydroxide as a root canal–filling material was described previously in the discussion of apexification.

Box 21-1

Categories for Treatment of Avulsed Teeth

Mature Apex

Less than 15 minutes out of mouth:
Rinse the tooth with physiologic solution to remove debris from the root surface.
Flush the socket with sterile water or saline.
Reimplant the tooth in the socket.

15 minutes to 6 hours in physiologic solution:
Place the tooth in Hank's balanced salt solution for 30 minutes.
Flush the socket with sterile water or saline.
Reimplant the tooth in the socket.
Splint the tooth in a functional position.

15 minutes to 1 hour in nonphysiologic solution:
Place the tooth in Hank's Balanced salt solution for 30 minutes.
Flush the socket with sterile water or saline.
Reimplant the tooth in the socket.
Splint the tooth in a functional position.

Greater than 1 hour dry storage:
Remove remnants of the periodontal ligament by soaking in sodium hypochlorite for 10 to 15 minutes.
Instrument the root canal with the tooth out of the mouth.
Soak the tooth in 2% stannous fluoride solution for 5 minutes.
Obturate the root canal with gutta-percha.
Coat the tooth root with Emdogain, and place Emdogain (Biora, Chicago, Ill, and Malmö, Sweden) in the socket.
Reimplant the tooth in the socket.
Splint the tooth in a functional position.

Immature Apex

Less than 15 minutes out of mouth:
Soak the tooth in doxycycline solution for 5 minutes.
Reimplant the tooth in the socket.
Splint the tooth in a functional position.
Check the tooth for vitality and apex closure every month.

15 minutes to 6 hours in physiologic solution:
Soak the tooth in doxycycline solution for 5 minutes.
Flush the socket with sterile water or saline.
Reimplant the tooth in the socket.
Splint the tooth in a functional position.

15 minutes to 1 hour in nonphysiologic solution:
Place the tooth in Hank's Balanced Salt Solution for 30 minutes.
Soak the tooth in doxycycline solution for 5 minutes.
Flush the socket with sterile water or saline.
Reimplant the tooth in the socket.
Splint the tooth in a functional position.

Greater than 1 hour dry storage:
Remove remnants of the periodontal ligament by soaking in sodium hypochlorite for 10 to 15 minutes.
Instrument the root canal with the tooth out of the mouth.
Soak the tooth in 2% stannous fluoride solution for 5 minutes.
Obturate the root canal with gutta-percha.
Coat the tooth root with Emdogain, and place Emdogain in the socket.
Reimplant the tooth in the socket.
Splint the tooth in a functional position.

Adapted from Krasner P: Advances in the treatment of avulsed teeth, *Dent Today* 22:84-87, 2003.

If the avulsed permanent tooth has immature root formation with an open apex, the chances of pulpal revitalization after replantation improve considerably, especially if replantation occurs less than 30 minutes after avulsion. If the avulsed tooth has been cared for properly, there is a small chance for revitalization even if the tooth is replanted 2 hours after the injury. However, many do not revitalize. Those that do respond favorably may still require root canal treatment several months later. During the time beyond 1 week that the pulp tissue is allowed to remain, evaluation of the tooth is recommended at weekly intervals until favorable signs of healing without pulp pathosis are conclusive (vitality tests are unreliable) or until a decision is made to extirpate the pulp. The pulp should be extirpated when the first signs of degeneration appear.

Rubber dam isolation is always desirable when performing pulp therapy. It can usually be employed even during the pulp extirpation procedure while several teeth are splinted together. Instead of separate holes in the rubber dam for each tooth, a slit is made so that the rubber can be placed over all teeth in the splinted segment. This does not afford ideal isolation, but it is generally better than the use of cotton rolls. In addition, the rubber dam helps prevent the swallowing or aspiration of foreign objects during treatment. If small endodontic instruments are used without rubber dam protection, they should be secured with a length of dental floss to facilitate retrieval in the unlikely event that they are dropped in the patient's mouth.

The calcium hydroxide material used to fill the root canal should be replaced every 3 to 6 months until a decision is made to fill the canal with gutta-percha. The optimum duration of the calcium hydroxide treatment is unknown, but generally calcium hydroxide should be kept in the canal for at least 6 months or until root end closure (apical plug) occurs beyond 1 year. In cases in which an adjacent tooth is still unerupted, Fountain and Camp recommend continuing the calcium hydroxide treatment until after the eruption of the adjacent tooth.[49] It is believed that eruption may stimulate or accelerate the resorptive process in a nearby replanted root.

MANAGEMENT OF ROOT FRACTURES

Root fracture of primary teeth is relatively uncommon because the more pliable alveolar bone allows displacement of the tooth. When root fracture does occur, it should be treated in the same manner as was recommended for permanent teeth; however, the prognosis is less favorable. The pulp in a permanent tooth with a fractured root has a better chance to recover.

Root fractures that occur in the apical half of the tooth are more likely to undergo repair (Fig. 21-36). Fractures in the apical third are often repaired without treatment. In fact, many apparently are undetected until evidence of a calcified repair is seen radiographically sometime after the injury.

Andreasen[43] has described four tissue reactions after root fracture: (1) healing with calcified tissue, which is characterized by a uniting callus of hard tissue that may consist of dentin, osteodentin, or cementum; (2) healing with interposition of connective tissue, in which the fractured root surfaces are covered by cementum with connective tissue fibers joining the two fragments; (3) healing with interposition of bone and connective tissue, in which a bony bridge and connective tissue are positioned between the fragments; and (4) interposition of granulation tissue.

The last is the least favorable form of attempted repair, and the fracture will not heal spontaneously. The teeth usually present unfavorable symptoms that may be accompanied by fistulas resulting from necrosis of the coronal portion and also sometimes the apical portion of the pulp. These teeth require follow-up endodontic treatment or extraction.

Gross separation of the root fragments invariably causes inflammation in the area and subsequent resorption of the approximating fractured surfaces. For repair to take place, the fragments must be maintained in apposition. Therefore splinting is usually necessary, particularly if the coronal fragment is mobile.

Although a relatively long stabilization period (3 months) has been previously recommended for teeth with fractured roots, Cvek and colleagues have cast doubts on the efficacy of long-term splinting and the types of splints used for root fracture healing.[50,51] Previously a longer stabilization period seemed necessary to encourage a more favorable type of healing of calcified tissue; however, their study showed no significant difference in the frequency of healing when short periods (less than 60 days) and long periods (60 to 90 days) of splinting were compared. They found that hard tissue healing also took place in teeth that were not even splinted. A comparison between nonsplinted and splinted teeth showed no difference in frequency of healing. They suggest that optimal positioning of dislocated fragments significantly increases the frequency of healing, particularly in mature teeth. Their study showed that, in immature teeth, healing took place even after suboptimal repositioning of dislocated coronal fragments and persistent diastases between the fragments after splinting. They conclude by suggesting that teeth with no or slight loosening of the fragment may not require splinting.

In addition, there is general agreement that splints for root fractures should be more rigid than the splints used for stabilization after other types of displacement injuries. Application of a more rigid splint is also believed to enhance the opportunity for a calcified tissue repair.

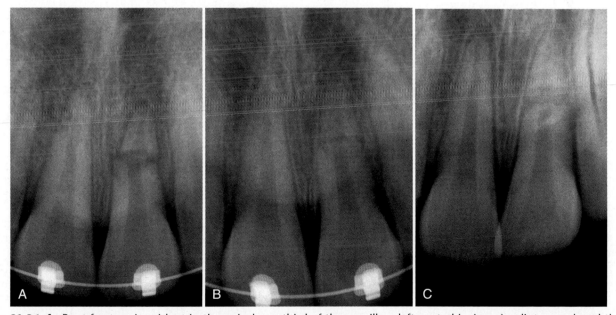

Figure 21-36 A, Root fracture is evident in the apical one third of the maxillary left central incisor. A splint was placed the day of the fracture. The patient reported that both teeth received trauma (via a baseball to the area) although only the root of the maxillary left central incisor was fractured. **B,** One month after initial splint placement. Both central incisors responded favorably to pulp testing and the splint was removed. Periodic evaluation and pulp testing was maintained. **C,** More than 2 years had elapsed when this radiograph revealed a normal periapical appearance to the maxillary left central incisor with the fractured root. Pulp testing for the incisor was normal. The patient complained of pain associated with the maxillary right central incisor (see developing periapical lesion) and was referred for endodontic evaluation.

Therefore use of heavier wires is recommended (0.032 to 0.036 inch) when one is stabilizing teeth with fractured roots.

The occlusion should be adjusted so that the injured tooth is not further traumatized during normal masticatory function. Follow-up radiographs should be obtained and pulp tests performed at frequent intervals during the first 6 months after the injury.

OTHER DISPLACEMENT INJURIES OF TEETH REQUIRING STABILIZATION

Teeth subjected to less severe luxation injuries may also benefit from stabilization with a bonded resin and wire splint during the recovery period. The severity of the injury will help determine the length of time the splint should remain in place. Splinting times may vary from 1 to 2 weeks for teeth that have been discernibly loosened (subluxation) to 4 to 6 weeks for teeth that have been laterally displaced, fracturing the alveolar process. As with all tooth injuries, frequent periodic evaluation is required for at least the first 6 months to afford the dentist the opportunity for early intervention if adverse sequelae develop; after this, evaluation at regular recall appointments should continue.

Nearly all significantly displaced teeth with closed apices and many with open apices will require follow-up endodontic therapy. As with many of the other injuries already discussed, calcium hydroxide paste is the currently recommended canal-filling material initially, and the canal should be recleaned and refilled with calcium hydroxide periodically if signs or symptoms warrant retreatment. This current recommendation of using calcium hydroxide may change in the relatively near future. Placement of a permanent gutta-percha filling should be delayed for at least 1 year (arbitrarily determined), and the calcium hydroxide should be replaced at least once (again arbitrarily determined) during this time. If the injured tooth had an open apex when endodontic therapy was initiated, the calcium hydroxide filling material should be used until the apexification process is complete or at least 1 year has elapsed, whichever is longer.

MANAGEMENT OF ORAL BURNS

As a result of secondary wound healing and scar contracture, burns involving the perioral and intraoral tissues can cause varying degrees of microstomia. A common cause of oral burns is electrical trauma. The most frequently encountered electrical injury to children is a burn about the mouth. These burns occur most often in children between 6 months and 3 years of age and are equally common among boys and girls.

Oral electrical burns occur when (1) the child places the female end of a "live" extension cord into the mouth, (2) the child places the female end of a "live" appliance cord (e.g., that for a hot plate, shaver, or portable radio) into the mouth, or (3) the child sucks or chews on exposed or poorly insulated electrical wires.

How does the burn occur? One plausible theory is that an electric arc is produced between a source of the current, such as the female end of an extension cord, and oral tissues. The electrolyte-rich saliva provides a short circuit between the cord terminals and the mouth, which results in the arc phenomenon. This type of burn characteristically involves intense heat that causes coagulation tissue necrosis.

NATURE OF THE INJURY

The clinical appearance of electrical burns is variable and depends on several factors: (1) the degree and duration of contact, (2) the source and magnitude of electric current, (3) the state of grounding, and (4) the relative degree of resistance at the point of contact. The wound may be superficial, involving only the vermilion border of one or both lips, or it may be a very destructive, full-thickness, third-degree burn. The more serious burns generally involve portions of the upper and lower lips and the commissure. Damage with more serious burns may extend intraorally to the tongue, the labial vestibule, the floor of the mouth, or the buccal mucosa. There have also been reports of damage to hard tissue, such as the mandible and the primary and permanent teeth.

With third-degree burns, subcutaneous tissues may be damaged. The tissue destruction may be much more extensive than is initially evident. Because nerves are frequently damaged, the patient will probably have paresthesia or anesthesia. Therefore pain is generally not a significant problem. Hemorrhage is usually inconsequential because blood vessels are cauterized when the injury is sustained. However, spontaneous arterial bleeding may occur anytime during the first 3 weeks of healing. The hemorrhage may be caused by the rupture of blood vessel walls weakened by the passage of current. Bleeding can also occur with sloughing of necrotic tissue that overlies regenerating granulation tissue.

The clinical appearance of an electrical burn involving the lips and commissures is characteristic of a wound caused by intense, localized heat, perhaps as high as 3000° C. Necrosis, in which there has been heat-induced coagulation of protein, liquefaction of fats, and vaporization of tissue fluids, is evident.

During the first few days after the accident, the center of the lesion is generally composed of grayish or yellowish tissue that may be depressed relative to a slightly elevated, narrow, erythematous margin of tissue that surrounds it (Fig. 21-37).

Within a few hours after the injury there may be a great increase in edema. The margins of the wound may become ill defined and the lips protuberant. The patient may drool uncontrollably because of the loss of sensation. In 7 to 10 days the edema begins to subside. The delineation between the central nonviable tissue and the surrounding viable tissue becomes more apparent. The necrotic tissue, known as eschar, becomes charred or crusty in appearance and begins to separate from the surrounding viable tissue (Fig. 21-38). The eschar sloughs off 1 to 3 weeks after the burn incident. Healing occurs by secondary intention as granulation tissue proliferates and matures. Two or 3 months after the accident the wound becomes indurated as a result of fibrous tissue formation. For an additional 6 months, the immature scar tissue may bind the lips, alveolar ridges, and other involved structures. If it is not treated, contraction of the fibrotic scar tissue results in unesthetic and functionally debilitating

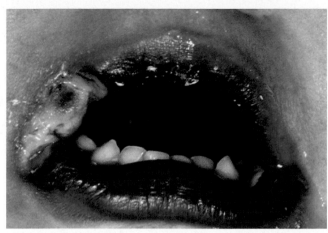

Figure 21-37 Appearance of injury to the upper lip and commissure 5 days after electrical burn. (Courtesy Dr. Theodore R. Lynch.)

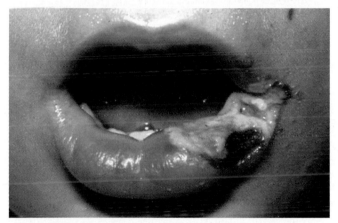

Figure 21-38 Appearance of injury to the lower lip and commissure 10 days after electrical burn. The dark lesion on the lower lip is an eschar. (Courtesy Dr. Theodore R. Lynch.)

microstomia. The scar tissue softens as it matures, and by 9 months to 1 year after the injury the potential for tissue contraction is greatly decreased. The duration of the healing process and the selected course of treatment depend on the extent and severity of tissue destruction. Because of the variable nature of burn injuries, surgery or appliance therapy may be used or no treatment may be needed.

TREATMENT

Assessing the general physical status of a patient who has sustained an electrical burn to the mouth is the first priority. Subsequently, the extent of the burn is carefully evaluated and local measures are initiated, such as control of minor hemorrhage or conservative débridement of nonviable tissue.

The immunization status of the patient must be ascertained, and tetanus toxoid or depot triple antigen (diphtheria-pertussis-tetanus vaccine) administered when appropriate. Many physicians prescribe a broad-spectrum antibiotic as prophylaxis. However, it may not be necessary or prudent to prescribe antibiotics in the absence of infection.

The parents should be informed of the possibility of spontaneous arterial hemorrhage during the first 3 weeks. They should be instructed to place firm pressure, with gauze, to the bleeding area for 10 minutes. If bleeding persists, they should take the child to the emergency department. Usually, hemorrhage is not a significant problem and does not warrant prophylactic hospitalization except for the most severe and extensive injuries.

The surgical management of burn injuries to the mouth, especially with regard to the time when such surgery should be performed, is controversial. Initially, no surgical intervention is generally warranted. Instead, the treatment of choice is the use of a prosthetic appliance. The primary functions of such an appliance are to prevent contracture of healing tissue and to serve as a framework on which a more normal-appearing commissure may be created and preserved after completion of the healing process. Many patients at James Whitcomb Riley Hospital for Children have been successfully treated with these appliances. Moreover, surgical procedures have not been needed in cases with good patient compliance in appliance use.

The major components of the burn appliance are illustrated in Fig. 21-39. The appliance is removed when the patient eats, when the teeth and appliance are cleaned, or when modifications of the wings are necessary. The appliance is a static base with wings extending

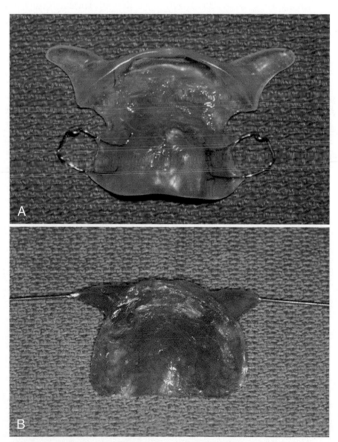

Figure 21-39 A, Example of a burn appliance designed for intraoral retention. **B,** Example of a burn appliance designed for intraoral and extraoral retention in combination with headgear.

laterally to provide contact with both commissures. If symmetry relative to the midline is to be maintained during the healing process, the wings must contact the commissures equidistant from the midline and must exert essentially equal pressure at these points.

The shape and location of the wings are important, not only in preventing contracture or cohesion of the lips during healing but also in shaping the affected commissure to duplicate the unaffected side. The wing is contoured so that it is thickest in its occlusocervical dimension on the labial aspect. It is tapered as thinly as possible at the point of contact with the commissure (Fig. 21-40). The wings should be large enough just to maintain the correct shape of the commissure. Wings of the proper size will look more pleasing during wear and will enhance acceptance and compliance by the child and parent.

If compliance is a problem with an acrylic appliance, a modified fixed appliance can be constructed and ligated in the mouth. Bands are adapted on the upper second primary molars, and an impression is made. Headgear tubes are welded on the bands, and a Nance appliance is constructed from 0.036- or 0.040-inch wire. If the Nance button is not used, the wire is contoured along the gingival portion of the teeth.

After the stabilizing framework is made, the outer portion of the appliance is formed. Using 0.045-inch wire, the anterior arch form is established. Horizontal loops are placed in the area approximating the location of the commissures, as determined by clinical measurements. The wire is continued posteriorly, and omega loops are placed mesial to the headgear tubes. Adjustments are made in the acrylic in one or both of the omega loops to achieve the correct fit. With the omega loops used as tiebacks, the appliance is ligated in the mouth. The patient should be evaluated as often as needed during the first month to make any necessary adjustments. Then the patient should be seen at least once a month.

Ideally the patient with an electrical burn to the mouth should be seen by the dentist between the fifth and tenth days after the accident. The initial appointment is probably the most crucial to the success or failure of treatment with the burn appliance. Parental apprehension and feelings of guilt are often high, and the trust and confidence of both the parents and the child must be acquired as soon as possible. They should be told in detail what they can expect from the dental services offered and

what is expected of them. The parents and the child should be shown pictures from previous cases. This not only demonstrates the appearance and purpose of the appliance but also emphasizes that they are not the only ones who have experienced the physical and psychological trauma associated with such an accident. Pictures of patients who did not have an appliance or who did not wear their appliance as instructed are also shown. The impact of such illustrative materials is dramatic.

After the consultation session, the initial data are recorded, photographs are taken, and alginate impressions are obtained for fabrication of the appliance. The appliance is generally delivered between the 10th and 14th days after the injury. At the delivery appointment and at each subsequent appointment, the information and instructions given in the initial consultation session are reinforced. Constant encouragement and positive reinforcement are important psychological aids in enhancing compliance.

After delivery of the appliance the patient is seen as often as needed during the first week, but at least once during that time. The patient is checked again 4 and 8 weeks after appliance delivery. During this period, most of the major modifications to the wings and other components of the appliance are made, and the patient's compliance is closely monitored. Once the appliance is properly modified and the patient is wearing the appliance as instructed, the appointments can be spaced out over 4- to 6-week intervals. The appliance should be worn 24 hours a day for 9 to 12 months except for eating and cleaning (Fig. 21-41).

The burn appliance may not eliminate the need for minor surgical revisions of the lips or surrounding cutaneous tissues. Its purpose is to obviate the necessity for more difficult surgical procedures, because good results are hard to achieve and maintain when one is surgically restoring the shape and location of the oral commissure. The appliance can prevent asymmetry of the commissures resulting from tissue cohesion and scar contracture. It can provide a more normal-appearing commissure after healing. The successful use of this appliance ultimately depends on patient compliance (Fig. 21-42).

Infants or toddlers who do not have primary molars that can be used for intraoral anchorage will not be able to retain the burn appliance without extraoral stabilization. Fig. 21-43 illustrates a headgear type of extraoral anchorage apparatus. It is made of durable cloth, such as denim lined with gingham, and provides a static base from which elastic material extends to the wings of the burn appliance. A well-fitted bonnet may also be used.

Patients with burns to the mouth who did not have access to appliance therapy or were noncompliant in wearing the burn appliance may have tissue cohesion, contraction, and deformation as a result of healing. Such patients may require a commissurotomy to reestablish the original dimensions and symmetry of the mouth. Unfortunately, with healing of the commissurotomy there is again a tendency for wound contraction and distortion. Therefore it may be necessary for the patient to undergo more than one such surgical procedure unless surgery is followed by appliance therapy.

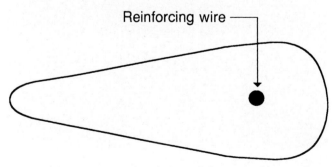

Reinforcing wire

Figure 21-40 Cross-sectional view of the commissure wing of the burn appliance.

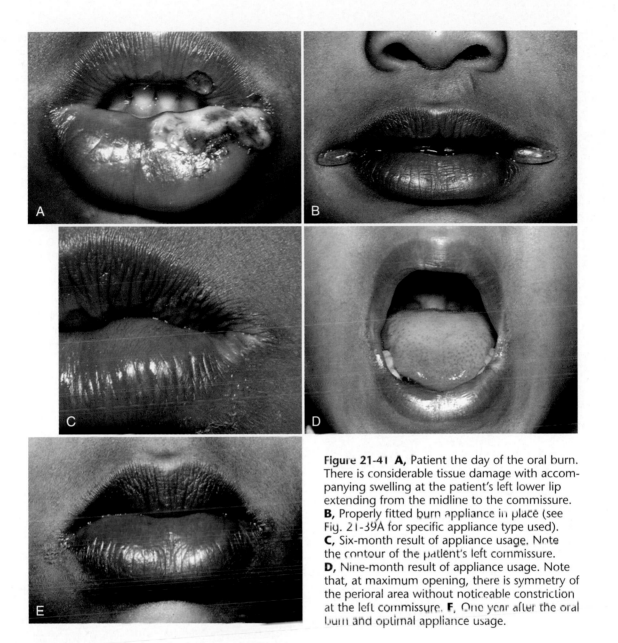

Figure 21-41 **A,** Patient the day of the oral burn. There is considerable tissue damage with accompanying swelling at the patient's left lower lip extending from the midline to the commissure. **B,** Properly fitted burn appliance in place (see Fig. 21-39A for specific appliance type used). **C,** Six-month result of appliance usage. Note the contour of the patient's left commissure. **D,** Nine-month result of appliance usage. Note that, at maximum opening, there is symmetry of the perioral area without noticeable constriction at the left commissure. **F,** One year after the oral burn and optimal appliance usage.

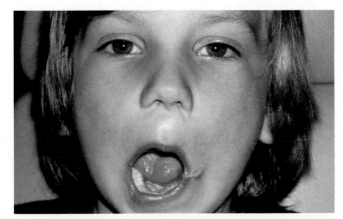

Figure 21-42 Burn patient who did not wear the appliance as recommended, shown 10 months after the injury. Surgical correction will be considerably more difficult in this patient.

Clinical management of the burn appliance after a commissurotomy differs from management of the appliance after a burn injury. First, the appliance must be delivered by the time the sutures are removed. By the second week after surgery there may already be a decrease in the lateral extension of the primary incision as a result of wound healing. Second, the total time the patient needs to wear the appliance may be less than 1 year, depending on the clinical course of the healing process. The patient still wears the appliance 24 hours a day except for eating and cleaning.

TRAUMA PREVENTION

Dental practitioners should be proud that we are a prevention-oriented profession. Prevention is especially predominant in dentistry for children. We strive to

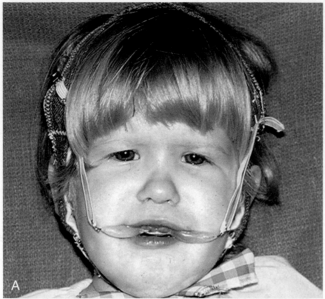

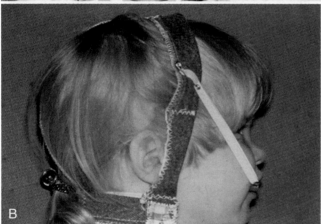

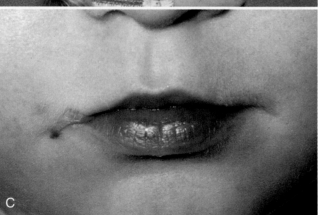

Figure 21-43 A and **B,** Properly fitted burn appliance with headgear to enhance stability and retention of the appliance. **C,** Nine-month result with appliance therapy.

prevent dental caries, periodontal disease, malocclusion, and anxiety about dental care. If disease is present, our treatment becomes part of an overall prevention plan designed to halt the progress of disease and prevent its recurrence. The success of the prevention plan, provided that there is parent and patient cooperation, is reasonably predictable.

Unfortunately, our ability to prevent injuries to oral structures is limited. Living and growing carry a high risk of trauma. A child will not learn to walk without falling, and few children reach 4 years of age without having received a blow to the mouth. We cannot totally prevent trauma. Moreover, the results of treatment of trauma are often less predictable than those of other types of dental treatment.

On the brighter side, there are preventive measures that have been proved to reduce the prevalence of traumatic episodes in certain environmental situations. For example, because the prevalence of fractured incisors is higher among those with protrusive anterior teeth, many dentists are recommending early reduction of excessive protrusion to reduce the susceptibility of such teeth to injury. The use of car safety seats and restraining belts has prevented many injuries to infants and young children. The protective mouthguard described in Chapter 22 has prevented or reduced the severity of countless injuries to the teeth of youngsters participating in organized athletic activities; active youngsters should be encouraged to wear their mouthguards during high-risk unsupervised athletic activities as well.

Parents should be reminded that accessible "live" electric cords are potentially dangerous, especially to small children who still use their mouths to evaluate their environment. In addition, anticipatory guidance and education are necessary to advise our patients regarding the negative health effects of intraoral and perioral body piercing. Possible problems that can occur include scar tissue formation, fracture of the dentition, allergic reactions, and bacterial endocarditis in susceptible patients. When we have the opportunity to save a child from pain and suffering, an ounce of prevention is worth a pound of cure.

REFERENCES

1. Slack GL, Jones JM. Psychological effect of fractured incisors, *Br Dent J* 99:386-388, 1955.
2. Borum MK, Andreasen JO. Therapeutic and economic implications of traumatic dental injuries in Denmark: an estimate based on 7549 patients treated at a major trauma center, *Int J Paediatr Dent* 11(4):249-258, 2001.
3. Davis MJ, Vogel L. Neurological assessment of the child with head trauma, *J Dent Child* 62:93-96, 1995.
4. Davis MJ. Orofacial trauma management. Patient assessment and documentation, *N Y State Dent J* 61(7):42-46, 1995.
5. Rusmah M. Traumatized anterior teeth in children: a 24-month follow-up study, *Aust Dent J* 35:430-433, 1990.
6. Andreasen JO, et al. Effect of treatment delay upon pulp and periodontal healing of traumatic dental injuries—a review article, *Dent Traumatol* 18(3):116-128, 2002.
7. Ellis RG, Davey KW. *The classification and treatment of injuries to the teeth of children*, ed 5, Chicago, 1970, Mosby.
8. Olgart L, et al. Laser Doppler flowmetry in assessing vitality in luxated permanent teeth, *Int Endod J* 21:300-306, 1988.
9. Mesaros SV, Trope M. Revascularization of traumatized teeth assessed by laser Doppler flowmetry: case report, *Endod Dent Traumatol* 13:24-30, 1997.
10. Tennery TN. The fractured tooth reunited using the acid-etch bonding technique, *Tex Dent J* 96:16-17, 1978.

11. Starkey PE. Reattachment of a fractured fragment to a tooth, *J Indiana Dent Assoc* 58(5):37-38, 1979.

12. Farik B, et al. Fractured teeth bonded with dentin adhesives with and without unfilled resin, *Dent Traumatol* 18:66-69, 2002.

13. Croll TP. Rapid reattachment of fractured crown segment: an update, *J Esthet Dent* 2:1-5, 1990.

14. Kanca J. Replacement of a fractured incisor fragment over pulpal exposure: a long-term case report, *Quintessence Int* 27:829-832, 1996.

15. Ludlow JB, LaTurno SA. Traumatic fracture—one-visit endodontic treatment and dentinal bonding reattachment of coronal fragment: report of a case, *J Am Dent Assoc* 110:341-343, 1985.

16. Cvek M. A clinical report on partial pulpotomy and capping with calcium hydroxide in permanent incisors with complicated crown fractures, *J Endod* 4:232-237, 1978.

17. McCormick FE. Calcium-hydroxide pulpotomy: report of a case observed for nineteen years, *J Dent Child* 48:222-225, 1981.

18. Frank AL. Therapy for the divergent pulpless tooth by continued apical formation, *J Am Dent Assoc* 72:87-93, 1966.

19. Weine FS. *Endodontic therapy*, ed 6, St Louis, 2004, Mosby.

20. Giuliani V, et al. The use of MTA in teeth with necrotic pulps and open apices, *Dent Traumatol* 18:217-221, 2002.

21. Trairatvorakul C. Apexification of a primary central incisor: 6-year follow up, *Pediatr Dent* 20:425-427, 1998.

22. Croll TP, et al. Traumatically injured primary incisors: a clinical and histological study, *J Dent Child* 54:401-422, 1987.

23. Holan G, Fuks AB. The diagnostic value of coronal dark-gray discoloration in primary teeth following traumatic injuries, *Pediatr Dent* 18:224-227, 1996.

24. Peterson DS, et al. Calcific metamorphosis with internal resorption, *Oral Surg* 60:231-233, 1985.

25. Mummery JH. Some further cases of chronic perforating hyperplasia of the pulp, the so-called "pink spot," *Br Dent J* 47:801-811, 1926.

26. Andreasen JO, et al. The effect of traumatic injuries to the primary teeth on their permanent successors, *Scand J Dent Res* 79:219-283, 1971.

27. Cutright DE. The reaction of permanent tooth buds to injury, *Oral Surg* 32:832-839, 1971.

28. Kilpatrick NM, et al. Dilaceration of a primary tooth, *Int J Paediatr Dent* 1:151-153, 1991.

29. Rushton MA. Partial duplication following injury to developing incisors, *Br Dent J* 104:12, 1958.

30. Ravn JJ. Sequelae of acute mechanical traumata in the primary dentition, *J Dent Child* 35:281-289, 1968.

31. Skieller V. The prognosis for young teeth loosened after mechanical injuries, *Acta Odontol Scand* 18:171-181, 1960.

32. Malmgren O, Malmgren B. Orthodontic management of the traumatized dentition. In Andreasen JO, Andreasen FM, eds. *Textbook and color atlas of traumatic injuries to the teeth*, ed 4, St Louis, 2007, Mosby.

33. Trope M, et al. Traumatic injuries. In Cohen S, Hargreaves KM, eds. *Pathways of the pulp*, 9th ed, St Louis, 2005, Mosby.

34. Tronstad L, et al. Surgical access for endodontic treatment of intruded teeth, *Endod Dent Traumatol* 2:75-78, 1986.

35. Shapira J, et al. Reeruption of completely intruded immature permanent incisors, *Endod Dent Traumatol* 2:113-116, 1986.

36. Barry GN. Replanted teeth still functioning after 42 years: report of a case, *J Am Dent Assoc* 92:412-413, 1976.

37. Camp JH. Replantation of teeth following trauma. In McDonald RE, et al, eds. *Current therapy in dentistry*, vol 7. St Louis, 1980, Mosby.

38. Andreasen JO. Effect of extra-alveolar period and storage media upon periodontal and pulpal healing after replantation of mature permanent incisors in monkeys, *Int J Oral Surg* 1:43-53, 1981.

39. Andreasen JO, Hjørting-Hansen E. Replantation of teeth. I. Radiographic and clinical study of 110 human teeth replanted after accidental loss, *Acta Odontol Scand* 24:263-286, 1966.

40. Blomlöf L, et al. Effect of storage in media with different ion strengths and osmolalities on human periodontal ligament cells, *Scand J Dent Res* 89:180-187, 1981.

41. Trope M. Clinical management of the avulsed tooth: present strategies and future directions, *Int Endod J* 18:1-11, 2002.

42. Sherman P Jr. A histologic study of intentional replantation of teeth in dogs and monkeys. Master's thesis. Indianapolis, Indiana University School of Dentistry, 1967.

43. Andreasen JO, Andreasen FM, eds. *Textbook and color atlas of traumatic injuries to the teeth*, ed 4, St Louis, 2007, Mosby.

44. Hurst RV. Regeneration of periodontal and transseptal fibers after autografts in rhesus monkeys: a qualitative approach, *J Dent Res* 51:1183-1192, 1972.

45. von Arx T, et al. Splinting of traumatized teeth with a new device: TTS (titanium trauma splint), *Dent Traumatol* 17:180-184, 2001.

46. Sae-Lim V, et al. Effect of systemic tetracycline and amoxicillin on inflammatory root resorption of replanted dogs' teeth, *Endod Dent Traumatol* 14:216-220, 1998.

47. Krasner P, Rankow HJ. New philosophy for the treatment of avulsed teeth, *Oral Surg Oral Med Oral Pathol Oral Radiol Endod* 9:616-623, 1995.

48. Flores MT, et al. Guidelines for the management of traumatic dental injuries. II, Avulsion of permanent teeth, *Dent Traumatol* 23:130-136, 2007

49. Fountain SB, Camp JH. Traumatic injuries. In Cohen S, Hargreaves KM, eds. *Pathways of the pulp*, 9th ed, St Louis, 2005, Mosby.

50. Cvek M, Andreasen JO, Borum MK. Healing of 208 intraalveolar root fractures in patients age 7-17 years, *Dent Traumatol* 17:53-62, 2001.

51. Cvek M, Mejare I, Andreasen JO. Healing and prognosis of teeth with intraalveolar fractures involving the cervical part of the root, *Dent Traumatol* 18:27-65, 2002.

SUGGESTED READINGS

Aeinehchi M, et al. Mineral trioxide aggregate (MTA) and calcium hydroxide as pulp-capping agents in human teeth: a preliminary report, *Int Endod J* 36(3):225-231, 2003.

American Academy of Pediatric Dentistry. Special Issue: Reference Manual 2002-2003, *Pediatr Dent* 24(7 suppl):91-96, 2002.

Flores MT. Traumatic injuries in the primary dentition, *Dent Traumatol* 18:287-298, 2002.

Clark JC, Jones JE. Tooth fragments embedded in soft tissue: A diagnostic consideration, *Quintessence Int* 18;653-665, 1987.

Garcia-Godoy F, Pulver F. Treatment of trauma to the primary and young permanent dentitions, *Pediatr Dent* 44(3):597-631, 2000.

Hammarström L et al. Replantation of teeth and antibiotic treatment, *Endod Dent Traumatol* 2:51-57, 1986.

Iqbal MK, Bamaas NS. Effect of enamel matrix derivative (EMDOGAIN®) upon periodontal healing after replantation of permanent incisors in Beagle dogs, *Dent Traumatol* 17:36-45, 2001.

Jones JE, Cooper MD. Tooth avulsion: a protocol for improved success, *Contemp Oral Hygiene* 2(4):40-43, 2002.

Kenny DJ, Barrett EJ. Recent developments in dental traumatology, *Pediatr Dent* 23(6):464-468, 2001.

Lee JY, et al. Management of avulsed permanent incisors: a decision analysis based on changing concepts, *Pediatr Dent* 23(4):357-360, 2001.

Linsuwanont P. MTA apexification combined with conventional root canal retreatment, *Aust Endod J* 29(1):45-49, 2003.

Palin WE, et al. Perioral electrical injury in a pediatric population, *J Oral Med* 42:17-21, 1987.

Rock WP, et al. The relationship between trauma and pulp death in incisor teeth, *Br Dent J* 136:236-239, 1974.

Sadove AM, et al. Appliance therapy for perioral electrical burns: a conservative approach, *J Burn Care Rehabil* 9: 391-395, 1988.

Taylor LB, Walker J. A review of selected microstomia prevention appliances, *Pediatr Dent* 19(6):413-418, 1997.

CHAPTER 22

Prosthodontic Treatment of the Adolescent Patient

▲ Robert J. Cronin Jr., David T. Brown, and Charles J. Goodacre

CHAPTER OUTLINE

RESTORATION OF SINGLE MAL-
FORMED, DISCOLORED, OR
FRACTURED TEETH
  All-Ceramic and Metal-Ceramic
  Crowns
  Teeth with Pulpal Involvement

FIXED PARTIAL DENTURES
  Resin-Bonded Retainers
  Complete Crown Retainers
  Fixed Partial Denture Pontics
REMOVABLE PARTIAL DENTURES
OVERDENTURES

IMPLANT PROSTHESES
  Implant Usage Before Growth
  Completion
  Implants for Orthodontic Anchorage
RECARE PROGRAM
PROTECTIVE MOUTHGUARDS

Scientific advancements in the areas of preventive dentistry, access to and use of dental services, water fluoridation, topical application of fluorides, and new commercial preventive dentistry products have led to substantial reductions in dental disease in developed countries. However, Caplan and Weintraub determined that adolescents are still affected by caries, particularly those who are minorities, rural inhabitants, have minimal fluoride exposure, and are from less educated and less affluent families.[1] Results of a more recent health and nutrition survey reported by Vargas and colleagues also supports a higher caries prevalence among lower-income children and minorities.[2] Assessments of periodontal health by Barmes and Leous[3] and by Bader and associates[4] show a decrease in severity but indicate that some adolescents are still affected.

Dental trauma continues to be a significant problem among adolescents as supported by Gift and Bhat's assessment of orofacial injury[5]; Bader and colleagues' estimates of the incidence and consequences of tooth fracture[6]; and Haug and associates' epidemiologic study of facial fractures and concomitant injuries.[7] Pilo and colleagues indicate that congenital anomalies continue to result in missing or malformed teeth.[8] In addition, bulimia, anorexia, and dietary habits have led to an increase in the erosion of tooth structure among teenagers, particularly in girls.

Some of the esthetic treatment needs resulting from these conditions can be managed with resin-bonding procedures and porcelain laminate veneers, and whenever possible these should be considered as the treatments of first choice. When these procedures have not provided a satisfactory result or when teeth are missing, then prosthodontics such as single crowns, fixed partial dentures, implant prostheses, or removable prostheses are indicated.

Because adolescents are often affected psychologically by the unacceptable appearance of diseased, damaged, or missing teeth, one should not allow chronologic age to preclude performance of whatever treatment is necessary to provide proper function and esthetics. If the teeth involved are fully erupted, have achieved complete root formation, and may be prepared without causing irreversible damage to the pulp, successful prosthodontic treatment can often be provided for patients as young as 12 to 14 years of age. Patient cooperation, however, is mandatory during and after treatment. Adolescent patients must be able to tolerate long appointments and remain still for extended periods while teeth are being prepared and impression materials are setting. Also, they must be able to achieve and maintain good oral hygiene around both the provisional and definitive restorations, as well as in the rest of the mouth. All these conditions make it highly desirable to perform the necessary treatment as expeditiously as possible. Finally, it must be understood that an adolescent is more likely to sustain trauma to the oral structures than is an adult and thus there is greater risk of damage to restorations and prostheses than in an adult patient.

Prosthodontic treatment of the adolescent patient often requires highly intricate procedures that go beyond the scope of this chapter. The goal of this chapter is to offer the reader an opportunity to develop a better appreciation of the achievable and available solutions for the young patient with a prosthodontic need. The interested reader should consult the prosthodontic literature and current textbooks on fixed, removable, and implant prosthodontics for more detailed information in this area of dentistry.

RESTORATION OF SINGLE MALFORMED, DISCOLORED, OR FRACTURED TEETH

ALL-CERAMIC AND METAL-CERAMIC CROWNS

Crowns are only indicated when more conservative treatments cannot be performed or have proven to be unsuccessful. All-ceramic crowns are the most esthetic complete-coverage restorations currently available in dentistry. The achievement of optimal longevity with all-ceramic crowns requires normal tooth preparation form because the prepared tooth must provide support for the restoration. Therefore, if a large portion of tooth structure is missing because of trauma or caries, or if previous restorations become dislodged during tooth reduction, then a separate restoration that is well retained in remaining tooth structure should be placed to establish an ideal preparation form (Fig. 22-1). Also, the fracture resistance of all-ceramic crowns is enhanced when other characteristics are present. Occlusal forces should be average or below-average. The centric occlusal contacts should ideally be located over the concave lingual portion of the prepared tooth and not cervical to the cingulum where fracture of the crown is more likely to occur. The prepared tooth should possess average or greater incisocervical length and should not be short, round, or overtapered in form.

The tooth preparation for an all-ceramic crown (Fig. 22-2) should possess a well-defined, smooth finish line that is 0.8 mm deep around the entire tooth, with the axial surfaces reduced to a depth of 0.8 mm. The lingual reduction for occlusal clearance should be 1 mm. An incisal edge reduction of 1.5 to 2 mm is required and is biologically acceptable even in the presence of large pulps. The use of resin cement and associated dentin bonding is recommended because crown strength is significantly improved. Both chamfer and shoulder finish lines can be used in conjunction with resin cement without compromising restoration strength. If zinc phosphate or glass ionomer cement is used, however, then a shoulder finish line should be used to optimize crown strength.

When the ideal tooth preparation form is seriously compromised or the magnitude of occlusal forces contraindicates restoration with an all-ceramic crown, use of the stronger metal-ceramic crown is indicated. The tooth preparation design and reduction depths for a metal-ceramic crown are shown in Fig. 22-3. When cervical esthetics must be optimized in a metal-ceramic restoration, one can use a collarless design that eliminates facial cervical metal and uses a porcelain facial margin (Figs. 22-4 and 22-5).

Whenever possible, cervical margins should not be extended into the gingival sulcus of an adolescent patient. If oral hygiene is inadequate, subgingival margins may produce accelerated gingival recession or interfere with the normal cervical relocation of the gingival tissues as the patient matures. Both occurrences produce an esthetic liability (Figs. 22-6 and 22-7).

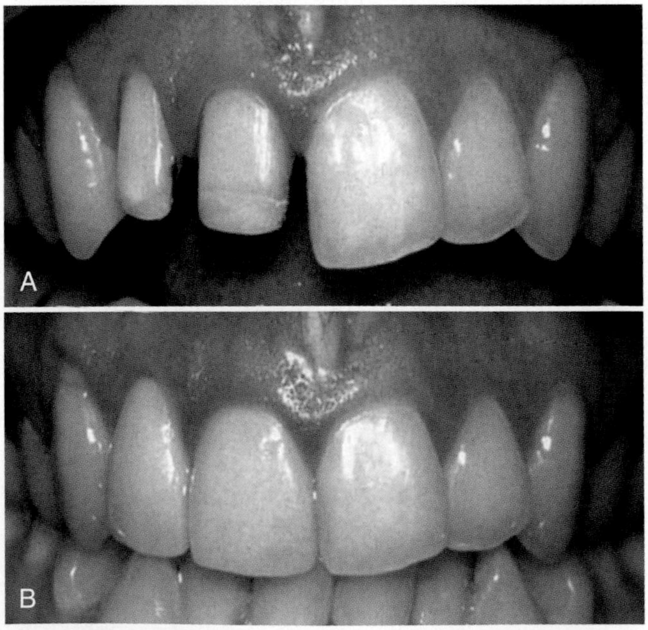

Figure 22-1 A, Traumatically injured central and lateral incisors that have been restored with bonded resins and then prepared to receive all-ceramic crowns. **B,** All-ceramic crowns have been cemented.

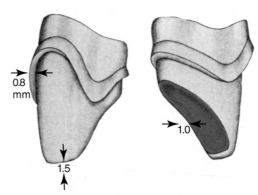

Figure 22-2 Two views of all-ceramic (porcelain jacket crown) preparation showing recommended reduction depths and shoulder finish line.

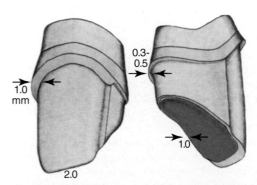

Figure 22-3 Two views of metal-ceramic crown preparation showing minimal facial reduction and shoulder finish line, minimal incisal reduction, lingual axial reduction depth and chamfer finish line, and lingual reduction for occlusal clearance.

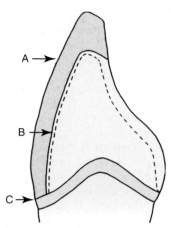

Figure 22-4 Collarless metal-ceramic framework design that eliminates visible cervical metal. *A* indicates porcelain; *B* indicates underlying metal framework that does not cover shoulder finish line; *C* is margin where porcelain contacts only prepared tooth.

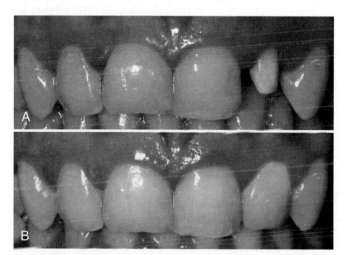

Figure 22-5 A, The maxillary lateral incisor was traumatically injured, resulting in loss of the incisal one-third and much of the lingual surface. The tooth has been prepared for a metal ceramic crown with a porcelain margin (collarless metal ceramic crown). **B,** The lateral incisor crown has been cemented.

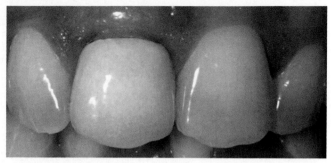

Figure 22-6 Gingival contour in 25-year-old patient resulting from placement of subgingival crown on maxillary right central incisor at 8 years of age. The gingival crest is not positioned as far apically on the restored central incisor, and its form is rounded and thick rather than the normal form of the gingival margin, which is thinner and sharper.

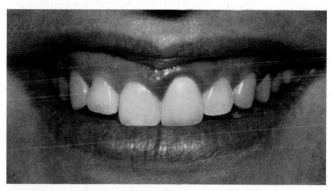

Figure 22-7 Accelerated gingival recession around maxillary left central incisor resulting from metal-ceramic crown with subgingival margins placed at a young age. The gingiva is edematous and red, and the gingival margin is rounded and thick.

TEETH WITH PULPAL INVOLVEMENT

When tooth fracture or caries involves the pulp and root development is complete, a routine pulpectomy and gutta-percha root canal filling should be completed. Because posts and cores do not strengthen endodontically treated teeth, their use is indicated only when remaining coronal tooth structure does not provide adequate retention for the definitive restoration.[9] Restorations that do not use a post should be used whenever possible to replace missing tooth structure and serve as a retentive foundation. It is particularly important that teeth in the mouths of accident-prone adolescents or those in whom athletic trauma has previously occurred be restored

without using a post, if possible. This practice helps avoid irreparable damage in the form of root fracture in case the restored tooth is once again subjected to trauma. Even though trauma may result in restoration dislodgment or perhaps even fracture of the tooth, the tooth will have survived at least one more traumatic experience.

In the case of pulpal involvement when the root is incompletely formed, a pulpotomy followed by placement of an appropriate restoration is indicated. Subsequently, when root formation is completed, a pulpectomy is performed, followed by placement of the definitive restoration or crown, if needed.

FIXED PARTIAL DENTURES

When a tooth is lost, space maintenance should be provided immediately after extraction to prevent tipping, tilting, or rotation of the abutment teeth or eruption of the opposing teeth. Space maintenance should be continued until the fixed prosthesis is completed. If the abutment teeth are malaligned and pulp size does not permit the amount of tooth reduction necessary to align the preparations, orthodontic repositioning of the abutment teeth should be initiated.

The use of conventional fixed partial dentures, requiring complete coverage tooth preparations, is decreasing in adult patients due to the use of dental implants and they are only sparsely used in adolescents. Contemporary treatment planning more frequently indicates that an interim fixed or removable prosthesis be used until such time as growth is completed and dental implants can be placed. When an interim fixed prosthesis is needed, resin-bonded fixed partial dentures are a good choice. When implants will not be used or have not been successful, fixed partial dentures become an appropriate definitive treatment. These fixed partial dentures can use conventional complete coverage retainers or they can use resin-bonded retainers designed for long-term service.

RESIN-BONDED RETAINERS

For reasons of pulpal and periodontal health and conservation of tooth structure, resin-bonded retainers are frequently used to replace missing teeth when dental implants are not being used (Fig. 22-8). Retention and resistance form is achieved through tooth preparations,

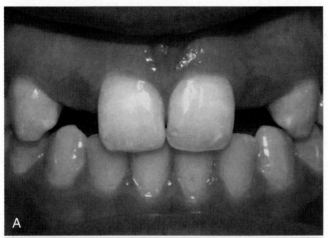

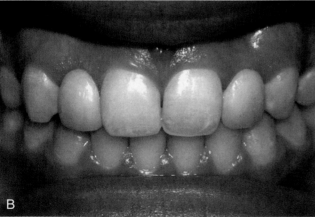

Figure 22-8 A, Congenitally missing maxillary lateral incisors. **B,** Resin-bonded prostheses were used instead of conventionally cemented prostheses to preserve as much tooth structure as possible on the central incisor and canine abutments.

terminating in enamel, coupled with acid etching of the enamel and fixation with resin cement. The conservative approach of using resin-bonded retainers does, however, require that the abutment teeth be intact or minimally restored, with substantial enamel present for bonding procedures. To produce an adequate area for resin bonding, the existing crown should be of average or greater length. A maximal amount of the nonvisible portions of the lingual and proximal surfaces should be covered by the retainers, because Pegoraro and Barrack have determined that bond strength increases with the area of enamel covered.[10] The existing crown form, color, and axial alignment must be satisfactory, because this prosthesis design does not permit the incorporation of changes in the facial enamel of abutment teeth. When abutment crown contours or color require esthetic changes, then complete-coverage retainers may produce a superior result.

These prostheses can be successful for many years, but suitable attention must be paid to four factors: (1) appropriate diagnosis and treatment planning, (2) correct tooth preparation, (3) good-fitting castings, and (4) meticulous adherence to the required resin-bonding procedures.

Several factors important to diagnosis and treatment planning have been identified in clinical studies. Because Dunne and Millar determined that prostheses with only one pontic have much higher success rates, the use of long-span prostheses should be avoided.[11] The use of multiple splinted retainers was associated with higher failure rates according to Marinello and colleagues.[12] As with any prosthesis, the presence of heavy occlusal forces reduces longevity.[13] The use of resin-bonded cantilevered prostheses (using only one retainer) has been reported, and data of Hussey and associates[14] and Leempoel and colleagues[15] indicate that this type of design can be used successfully in certain situations such as a missing maxillary lateral incisor (Fig. 22-9).

Preparation of abutment teeth for resin-bonded prostheses is not recommended for prostheses that will only be used on an interim basis. However, when long-term service is needed, tooth preparation has been found to substantially reduce debonding of retainers.

Barrack and Bretz determined that the successful use of resin-bonded prostheses requires establishment of retention and resistance form through tooth preparation (see Fig. 22-9B and Fig. 22-10).[16] Because the tooth preparation is limited principally to enamel, these retainers can be used without pulpal damage and the teeth can often be prepared without anesthesia. Besimo states that the proximal surfaces adjacent to the edentulous area should be reduced to remove interproximal undercuts and to provide parallel surfaces that aid retention.[17] One or two proximal grooves must be placed to enhance the resistance and retention form (see Fig. 22-10A). Proximal grooves have been identified as a key factor in the resistance to debonding in several studies.[16-20] The tooth preparation should include a small peripheral chamfer finish line (see Fig. 22-10B) formed with the tip of a rounded-end diamond instrument. The lingual surfaces of anterior teeth are reduced to create occlusal clearance with the opposing teeth. The minimal occlusal clearance space for short-span

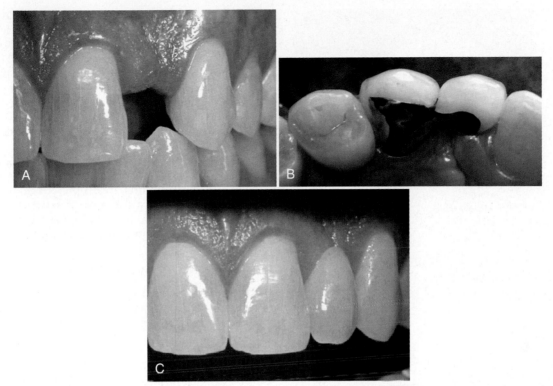

Figure 22-9 A, Congenitally missing maxillary lateral incisor. **B,** Incisal view of the bonded two-unit prosthesis where the lateral incisor pontic has been cantilevered from the maxillary canine. **C,** Facial view of the completed prosthesis.

(three-unit) prostheses with normal occlusal forces is 0.5 mm. It may not be necessary to reduce the abutment teeth lingually when there is existing occlusal clearance, whereas reduction of opposing teeth may be necessary when occlusal contact occurs over broad areas of the lingual surfaces. Multiple ledges, prepared across the reduced lingual surface (see Fig. 22-10C), increase the casting rigidity and, along with the proximal grooves, aid in retention and resistance form and in orientation of the casting during cementation.

The preparation of posterior abutment teeth should include reduction of the proximal surfaces to eliminate undercuts and to produce minimal occlusal convergence for retention and resistance form. The reduction should also include lingual surfaces and at least 180 degrees of circumferential reduction as determined by Creugers and colleagues[21] and by Crispin.[22] One or two proximal grooves are placed, one or two occlusal rest seats are prepared,[16] and a small chamfer finish line is formed. The use of an inlay-like occlusal rest has been advocated to increase resistance and retention form. The occlusal aspect of the lingual cusp can also be slightly reduced and covered with metal to increase the bonding area and prosthesis retention (Fig. 22-11).

A metal-ceramic alloy is used for the prosthesis framework, which allows porcelain to be bonded over the visible facial surface of pontics to meet esthetic requirements. Several design variations are used for the retainer castings, differing in the manner in which the resin mechanically

interlocks with the surface of the casting that contacts the prepared teeth.

The first prosthesis design, introduced by Rochette, employed retainer castings that were perforated lingually, which allowed resin to encompass the casting.[23] Subsequently, Livaditis and Thompson introduced a technique that uses a base metal alloy and thereby takes advantage of the ability of the alloy to be acid-etched to provide microscopic areas of retention (Fig. 22-12).[24] This technique is not suitable for use with gold-containing alloys because they cannot be etched in this manner.

An alternative method of treating the metal surface to provide retention for the resin is to subject the bonding surface to airborne-particle abrasion using 50-m aluminum oxide. This method has been shown to provide retention comparable to that of chemically etched metal and can be used with any casting alloy.[11,12,25,26]

The completed prosthesis is first trial-seated so that any required adjustments of form, color, occlusion, and glaze can be completed. The prosthesis then should be cleaned ultrasonically to remove debris that may be present in the retentive areas and dried thoroughly with clean, dry, compressed air.

Cementation of the prosthesis with the acid-etching and resin procedure requires optimal moisture control, which is best obtained with use of a rubber dam. Composite resins specially designed for cementation of this

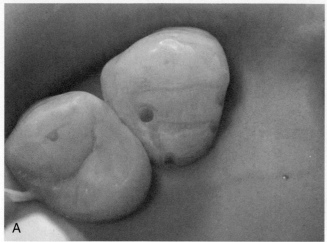

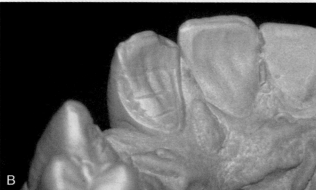

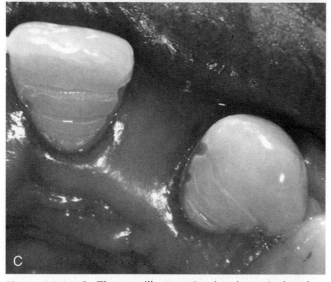

Figure 22-10 A, The maxillary canine has been isolated for prosthesis cementation using a rubber dam, which affords a good view of the well-defined proximal grooves. **B,** Cast of prepared maxillary central incisor and canine. Note the small peripheral chamfer, the lingual ledges, and the small proximal grooves. **C,** Another patient in whom the maxillary central incisors and canine have been prepared using multiple lingual ledges and multiple proximal grooves.

type of prosthesis are employed. After isolation of the prepared teeth (Fig. 22-13), the enamel is acid-etched in the usual manner, rinsed, and dried. The resin is applied to the casting and the prosthesis seated (see Fig. 22-13B). Excess cement is quickly removed, and the prosthesis is held motionless until polymerization is complete. Resin cement left in interproximal undercut areas until hard can be very difficult to remove.

Opaque resins can be used to help mask the metal when abutment teeth are very translucent. This procedure helps reduce the darkening effect of lingual metal showing through the incisal aspect of a tooth. Also, when adequate bonding area is present lingually, it may be possible to reduce the area of retainer coverage by cutting away lingual metal before cementation so that none is located behind thin translucent areas of the tooth.

COMPLETE CROWN RETAINERS

When a resin-bonded retainer cannot be used because of the tooth condition, crown form, crown length, axial alignment, occlusal forces, or conditions requiring maximal retention and resistance form, use of complete-coverage retainers is indicated.

Cast metal retainers should be used posteriorly wherever esthetically possible, since they require less tooth reduction than a metal-ceramic retainer. When short clinical crowns are encountered, it may be necessary to use auxiliary grooves or boxes in the axial surfaces to achieve the required degree of retention and resistance form. It may also be necessary to perform a gingivoplasty so that more tooth structure is exposed.

When esthetic requirements demand and pulp size permits, metal-ceramic restorations are indicated. When complete-coverage retainers are indicated but pulp size allows only minimal reduction, an all-resin fixed prosthesis may be the best choice. The all-resin restoration offers good esthetics initially and requires only minimal axial tooth reduction (0.5 mm), but because it has less wear resistance, strength, and color stability than porcelain, it must be replaced periodically. All-resin prostheses rarely last more than a few years without significant wear, color change, or fracture. If the casts and records are retained, however, additional replacement prostheses can be made and several additional years of service obtained. Subsequent treatment may permit the use of metal-ceramic retainers because enough pulpal recession may have occurred so that additional tooth reduction can be safely accomplished. The development of new resins and fiber reinforcement may extend the longevity of such prostheses.

Complete crown retainers can also be used in conjunction with cantilevered prostheses, so that tooth preparation is limited to one tooth. Schwartz and associates[27] and Foster[28] have shown use of the cantilever design to be a viable treatment alternative. The absence of a maxillary lateral incisor, which is encountered in adolescents because of congenital abnormality, is a situation well suited to this design. A two-unit fixed prosthesis can be fabricated with a lateral incisor pontic cantilevered from the canine retainer (Fig. 22-14). The positional stability of the canine is important to the success

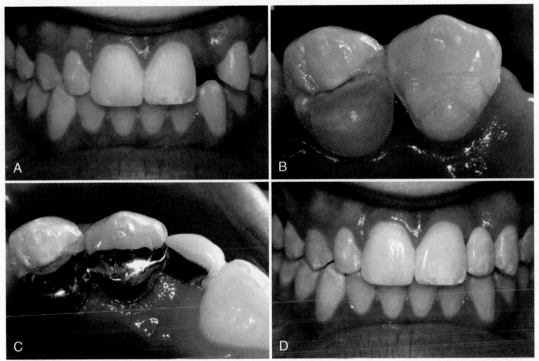

Figure 22-11 A, Congenitally missing maxillary lateral incisor. **B,** Mirror view of the canine and first premolar, which have been prepared for a resin-bonded prosthesis. The lingual cusp of the premolar has been reduced so the retainer can be bonded over the cusp. **C,** Mirror view of bonded prosthesis showing coverage of the premolar lingual cusp. **D,** Facial view of completed prosthesis.

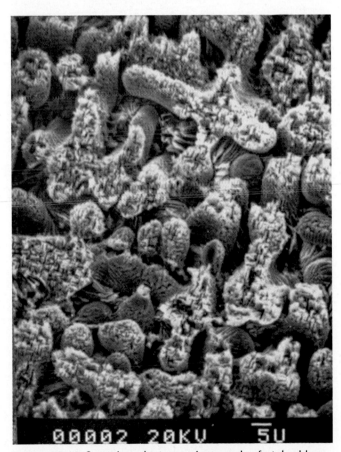

Figure 22-12 Scanning electron micrograph of etched base metal (×1000). (Courtesy of B. K. Moore.)

of this design. The canine should not be mobile, and the arch form should be stable (i.e., teeth have not and are not shifting position). The canine should not have recently undergone orthodontic repositioning that involved significant rotation.

FIXED PARTIAL DENTURE PONTICS

Pontics are usually of an all-metal or metal-ceramic design, depending on esthetic requirements. The metal-ceramic pontic is a highly versatile replacement, combining the esthetic benefits of porcelain with the strength of metal, and is widely adaptable to edentulous spaces of varying sizes.

Pontic design must include meticulous attention to the amount of ridge coverage; the area of contact must be minimized and the embrasures must be as large as possible while meeting esthetic demands. These procedures are mandatory to provide soft tissue access for oral hygiene aids.

REMOVABLE PARTIAL DENTURES

When the number of missing teeth prevents use of a fixed partial denture, a removable partial denture becomes a restoration of necessity. Indications for a removable partial denture include excessive span length, the inability to achieve adequate retention for a fixed prosthesis, congenital malformations that result in only a few widely spaced permanent teeth, and injuries that have caused multiple teeth and often alveolar bone to be lost (Figs. 22-15 and 22-16).

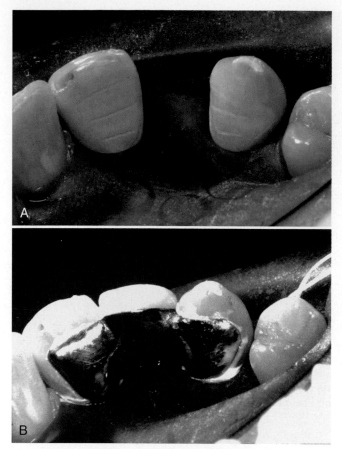

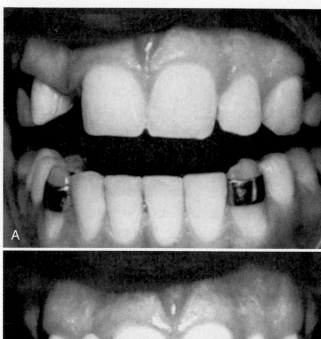

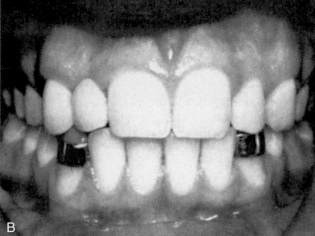

Figure 22-13 A, Teeth isolated with rubber dam in preparation for resin bonding procedures. **B,** Prosthesis bonded with resin.

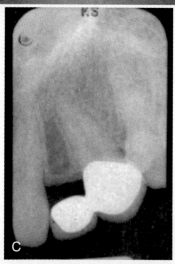

Figure 22-14 A, Maxillary canine has been prepared for metal-ceramic cantilevered prosthesis. Notice discrepancy in path of insertion with central incisor, which necessitated cantilever design. **B,** Facial view of cemented prosthesis. **C,** Postinsertion periapical radiograph showing malalignment of canine and central incisor roots.

When treatment is planned for an adolescent patient who needs a removable partial denture, there are three major objectives: (1) the restoration of the functions of mastication and speech, (2) the restoration of dental and facial esthetics, and (3) the preservation of the remaining teeth and their supportive tissues.

The function of mastication can be restored when correct, harmonious, and nondestructive occlusal relationships are provided between the supplied teeth and the opposing remaining natural dentition. The development of proper speech can be ensured if the parts of the partial denture are given correct form, dimension, and position in their relationships to the tongue, cheek, and lips.

The restoration of esthetics is often the most important personal consideration for adolescent patients. Artificial teeth of compatible color, size, and form, naturally arranged and positioned, enhance dental esthetics. In addition, the form and size of the base of a partial denture must be correct to ensure the restoration of normal facial contours.

The preservation of the remaining teeth and their supportive tissues is the most important objective of all but will not be achieved without adequate mouth preparation, correct partial denture design, accurate fabrication

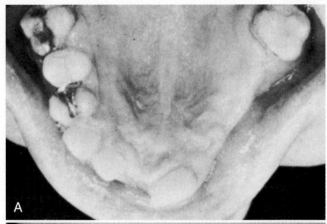

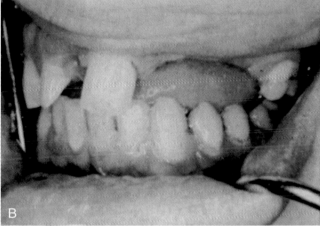

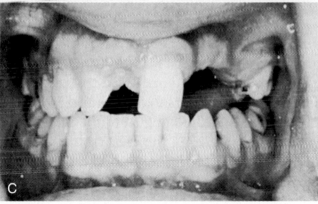

Figure 22-15 A, Mirror view of maxillary arch. Multiple teeth have been lost in this young adult as a result of a gunshot accident. **B,** Left lateral view in centric occlusion. **C,** Anterior view in centric occlusion.

of that design, periodic professional follow-up care, and continued proper home care by the patient.

Additional dental procedures may be required to create an oral environment that will furnish proper support and retention for the removable partial denture and that will prevent the development of forces or processes that are harmful to the remaining teeth and their supportive tissues. These preparatory procedures may involve all phases or branches of dentistry. Adolescents may require periodontal procedures, particularly to increase crown length for crown or fixed partial denture retention or to

improve tissue contours so that more ideal results can be achieved.

Orthodontic procedures can be used to reposition severely malpositioned teeth that would otherwise require extraction. Orthodontic procedures are particularly indicated for malpositioned teeth that are vital to an adequate plan of treatment (Fig. 22-17).

OVERDENTURES

Occasionally, congenital abnormalities or trauma result in the loss of multiple teeth and the resulting interarch relationship does not allow a conventional removable partial denture to reestablish proper occlusion with opposing teeth. This situation may necessitate fabrication of a prosthesis that overlays all or part of the remaining teeth so that proper function and facial esthetics are established (Fig. 22-18).[29]

IMPLANT PROSTHESES

An understanding of dental development and craniofacial growth is certainly a prerequisite for anyone anticipating the use of dental implants in growing patients.[30] Growth and development in the maxilla and mandible are essentially quite different, as are growth and development in the specific areas of each arch.[31-34] In the maxilla, growth is intimately associated with the growth of the cranial base in early childhood, whereas later growth primarily occurs by enlargement of the maxilla. This growth is extremely variable and can be observed as vertical growth, transverse growth, and anteroposterior growth. Transverse growth occurs primarily at the midpalatal suture of the maxilla. The sutural growth site is extremely important and poses a risk to the placement of an implant-supported prosthesis that crosses this suture and could limit its growth potential. The maxilla also grows vertically by passive displacement as well as by alveolar appositional growth. It is the vertical component of maxillary growth that causes the most concern in the long-term positional stability of the individual implant and its effect on restorative function and esthetics.

Mandibular growth differs greatly from the complex growth in the maxilla. Not closely associated with major cranial passive growth, mandibular growth is primarily downward and forward, mediated by appositional condylar growth. This growth is not purely linear but can be rotational secondary to the precise direction of condylar growth patterns. The appositional growth is also refined by certain areas of resorption, primarily seen on the anterior aspect of the ramus. As the mandible increases in length, it also increases in width, secondary to the flaring of posterior growth direction. This allows the mandible to accommodate to the increased maxillary width caused by the growth in the palatal suture area. Anterior stabilization is accomplished by the early closure of the mandibular synthesis. Although less dynamic than maxillary growth, mandibular growth can create many complexities that could place dental implants at positional risk, especially in the posterior mandible, secondary to vertical changes and resorptive processes.

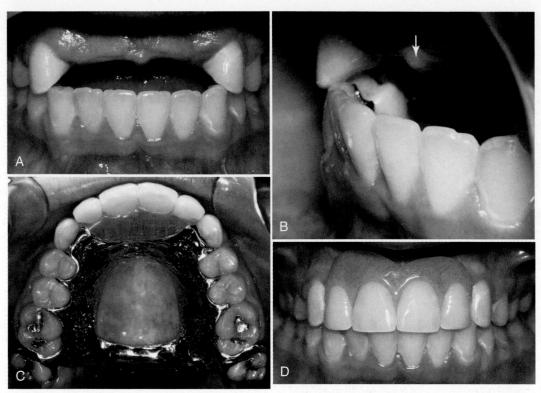

Figure 22-16 A, The four maxillary incisors have been lost as a result of traumatic injury. Note the long span, short clinical crowns, and facial flare to the canines, which make retention and resistance form difficult to achieve for a conventional fixed partial denture. **B,** Lateral view showing the relationship of the mandibular incisors to the residual alveolar ridge. The trauma caused substantial bone loss, and the ridge is located lingual to the mandibular incisors (*arrow* indicates the position of the incisive papilla on the crest of the residual alveolar ridge), which necessitates use of a removable partial denture base for lip support and proper esthetics. **C,** Occlusal view of maxillary removable partial denture. **D,** Facial view of completed prosthesis.

In addition to understanding growth and development, the clinician must also comprehend the dynamics of the positional relationship between the dental implant and its biologic environment in the growing patient. A wealth of dental literature using in vivo evidence-based studies attests to the long-term success of dental implants

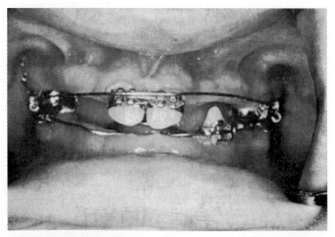

Figure 22-17 Orthodontic treatment is in progress to erupt the molars, depress the mandibular left canine, and close the maxillary central incisor diastema.

and their associated prostheses in adults. Such a wealth of knowledge does not exist, however, for the growing patient. The behavior of an osseointegrated dental implant essentially resembles that of an ankylosed tooth and the latter therefore provides an accurate model of the behavior of an implant in a growing patient. Two facets of the relationship of ankylotic teeth to their actively growing environment must be understood. First, the ankylotic tooth, lacking the adaptive mechanisms of a healthy tooth, does not erupt normally and becomes buried. Second, failing to participate in vertical growth, it often creates severe malocclusions secondary to tipping and associated growth changes in normal teeth adjacent to the affected ankylotic tooth It seems logical that an osseointegrated implant placed prematurely could elicit the same negative growth effects.

The routine successful use of osseointegrated dental implants in total or partial support of prostheses in adults has heightened interest in their use in younger patients. Adolescents are frequently seen who have congenital anomalies, have undergone ablative surgical procedures or radiation therapy, or have experienced traumatic tooth loss, and the use of dental implants would greatly assist prosthesis support (Figs. 22-19 and 22-20). Replacement of congenitally missing teeth with implants can often be accomplished in an esthetic

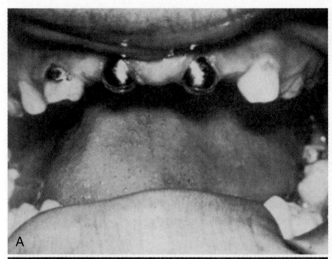

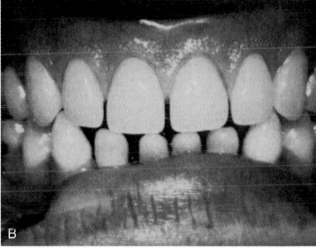

Figure 22-18 A, Facial view of maxillary arch where remaining primary and permanent teeth were improperly spaced and lacked adequate bone support for a fixed prosthesis. Lip support, facial esthetics, and proper occlusal interdigitation with the opposing mandibular teeth could be achieved only by use of an overdenture. Central incisors required endodontic treatment and have been restored with cast posts and cores. **B,** Facial view of overdenture.

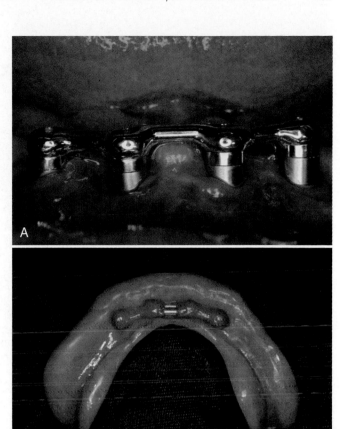

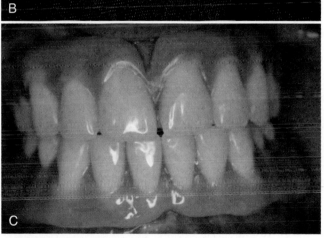

Figure 22-19 A, A congenital condition resulted in extensive and aggressive bone changes and loss of the teeth. Four implants were placed at age 12. This treatment greatly enhances prosthesis stability and will help preserve the remaining mandibular anterior bone. Because the mandibular symphysis fuses at birth or shortly thereafter, early implant placement in this area is less affected by future growth. **B,** Mandibular overdenture prosthesis that will be supported by the four implants and bar. **C,** Facial view of the completed prostheses.

manner that preserves the integrity of adjacent teeth. However, dental and skeletal growth is a major confounding variable related to the use of dental implants in adolescent patients.[35]

There are two primary concerns related to the placement of implants before growth is completed: (1) the effect of growth on the long-term relative position of the dental implant, and (2) the effect of the implant-supported prosthesis on future dental and skeletal growth.

An understanding of growth and development and its variability in the male and female adolescent population raises serious concern about the premature placement of implants. Refer to Chapter 25 for a more in-depth discussion of this topic.

IMPLANT USAGE BEFORE GROWTH COMPLETION

Although it is best to wait until maxillary and mandibular growth is completed before placing osseointegrated implants, dentists are constantly faced with apparent

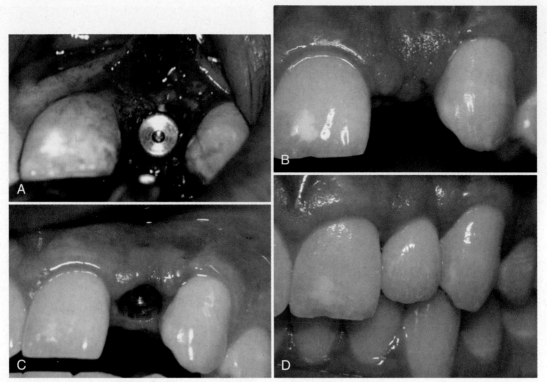

Figure 22-20 A, A 16-year-old boy traumatically fractured the maxillary left lateral incisor, rendering it nonrestorable. An implant is being placed in the socket immediately after extraction. **B,** Edentulous ridge following implant placement. **C,** Incisal view of the implant after appropriate bone and soft tissue healing has occurred. **D,** Completed metal-ceramic restoration.

indications for implant treatment. The clinician must understand the disadvantages of early placement and weigh those factors against the functional and esthetic advantages afforded by implants. If a determination is made that implants are needed before growth completion, it is more predictable to restore larger edentulous areas with implants than to place a single implant-supported crown in a growing patient (Figs. 22-21 and 22-22). The successful use of implant-assisted prostheses in patients with multiple missing teeth has been reported.[36-38] Implants have been placed in the anterior mandible in patients as young as 5 years of age (Fig. 22-23). Often, the placement of implants in this area will diminish the residual alveolar resorption anticipated from many years of removable prosthesis wear. Unfortunately, one of the most frequently encountered implant indications is treatment of the traumatic loss or congenital absence of a single anterior maxillary tooth. The placement of dental implants in this area should not be attempted until the accelerated phase of peripubertal growth is close to complete.

IMPLANTS FOR ORTHODONTIC ANCHORAGE

Osseointegrated implants have been used as valuable adjuncts to orthodontic treatment when there is a need for anchorage but no conventional tooth anchorage is available.[39,40-43] Because the implants act as ankylosed teeth and are incapable of being moved by orthodontic or orthopedic forces, they serve as ideal anchorage units.[44]

Their use has produced tooth movements that otherwise would not be possible, particularly when a large number of teeth are missing as a result of trauma or congenital anomalies. Implants are especially valuable when their postorthodontic positioning permits them to be used to support a future prosthesis.

RECARE PROGRAM

The prosthodontic treatment of an adolescent does not end with the placement of the prosthesis. Periodic recare appointments for inspection, maintenance, repair, or replacement are a necessity. For patients who have removable partial dentures, relining or rebasing should be performed when indicated. When all-ceramic crowns or metal-ceramic restorations are used in an adolescent patient, replacement may be needed periodically as the gingival tissue assumes its adult position. Patients with fixed partial dentures should be examined periodically for soft tissue health, evidence of occlusal wear, and response of the supportive tissues to the added stress loads. Patients with implant-assisted restorations should be evaluated frequently to ensure the health of the osseointegrated implant and its surrounding tissue, as well as to assess the effect of the implant-supported prosthesis on the overall growth and development of the patient. The use of dental implants to assist in the support of a prosthesis necessitates an extremely vigilant recare program.

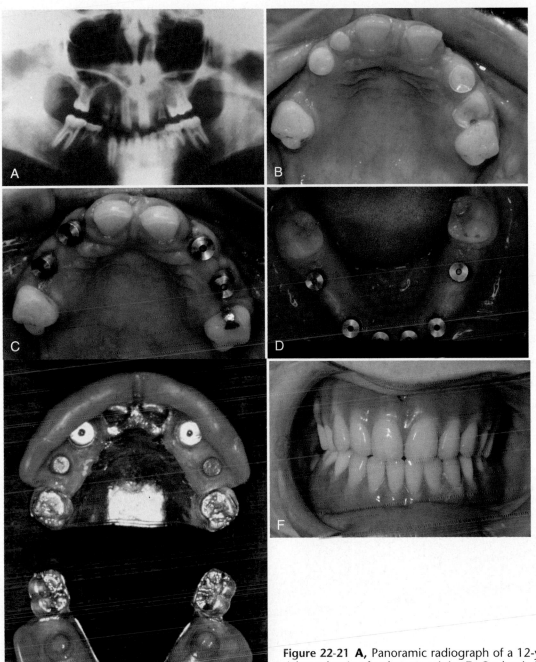

Figure 22-21 A, Panoramic radiograph of a 12-year-old with partial anodontia of unknown origin. **B,** Occlusal view of maxillary arch showing primary teeth that will be extracted. **C,** Four maxillary implants have been placed. **D,** Six mandibular implants have been placed to provide prosthesis stability and preserve bone. **E,** Maxillary and mandibular overdentures using magnets to augment stability and retention. **F,** Facial view of completed overdentures.

Every adolescent patient must be taught proper oral hygiene and home care for his or her prosthodontic restorations and must be motivated until adequate performance is routinely achieved. Each patient with fixed or implant-supported prostheses should be taught the use of aids such as the floss threader and inter proximal brush to enhance oral hygiene efforts. Only with regular recare programs can maximum longevity of service can be realized.

PROTECTIVE MOUTHGUARDS

Although this chapter is concerned with the prosthodontic treatment of adolescents, emphasis should always be placed on the prevention of oral disease and injury. The number and severity of injuries to the teeth and jaws can be significantly reduced through the faithful use of protective mouthguards by athletes who are engaged in contact sports.[45,46]

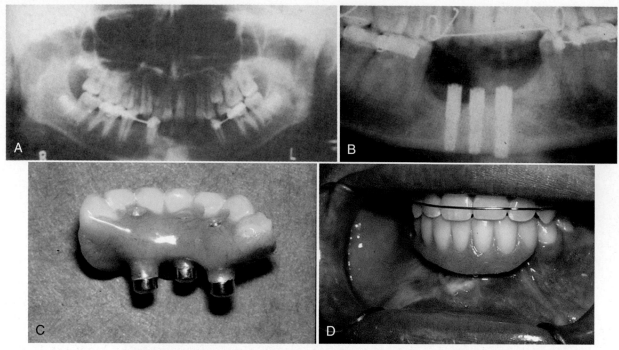

Figure 22-22 A, Panoramic radiograph of a 13-year-old patient after removal of a giant cell granuloma from the anterior mandible. **B,** Radiograph showing ridge defect and the location of the three implants. **C,** Fixed prosthesis that will be attached to the three implants. **D,** Prosthesis in place.

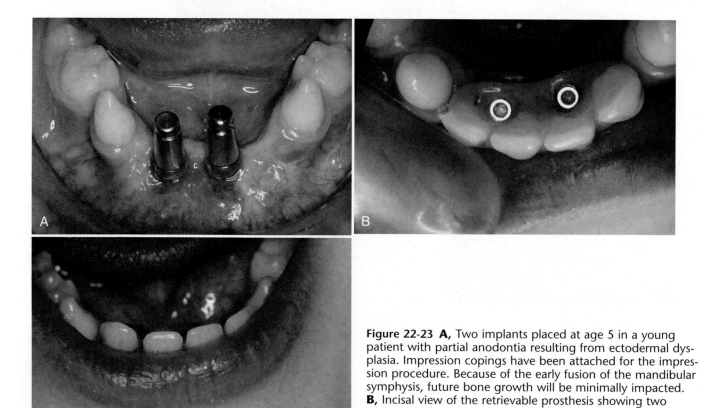

Figure 22-23 A, Two implants placed at age 5 in a young patient with partial anodontia resulting from ectodermal dysplasia. Impression copings have been attached for the impression procedure. Because of the early fusion of the mandibular symphysis, future bone growth will be minimally impacted. **B,** Incisal view of the retrievable prosthesis showing two lingually located screws. A retrievable design permits the prosthetic teeth to be replaced to accommodate future growth. **C,** Facial view of completed prosthesis.

Effective and relatively inexpensive prefabricated mouth-guards are available at sporting goods stores. A custom-made mouthguard may be fabricated, however, by vacuum-molding a sheet of thick, clear material over a stone cast of the maxillary arch. Seals and Dorrough have reviewed the advantages of custom-made mouth protectors.[47]

Studies comparing custom-made (laboratory) mouth-guards with standard (manufactured) or intraorally formed mouthguards have shown that the custom-made mouth-guards provide better fit and comfort, are less likely to adversely affect the player's speech, and are less likely to come loose.[48] In a study reported by Bass and Williams, the majority of athletes thought that they were more likely to wear their mouthguards if they fit better and were comfortable.[49]

Several materials have been suggested for use in mouthguards, including poly (vinyl acetate-ethylene) copolymer thermoplastic, polyurethane, and laminated thermoplastic.[50] Chaconas and colleagues demonstrated that the laminated thermoplastic underwent significantly less dimensional change than other materials.[51]

Because a custom-made mouthguard accurately fits individual tooth and arch form, it affords maximal resistance to dislodgment. The technique of fabrication involves placing the mouthguard material (Fig. 22-24A) in a molding machine, which softens the material by heat (see Fig. 22-24B) and closely adapts it to a dry stone cast by vacuum (see Fig. 22-24C). After the adapted material has cooled, the guard is removed from the cast and the excess peripheral material is trimmed off with scissors (see Fig. 22-24D). The borders are rounded by trimming the material with a resin-trimming bur and flaming with a torch or polishing with wet pumice on a rag wheel (see Fig. 22-24E).

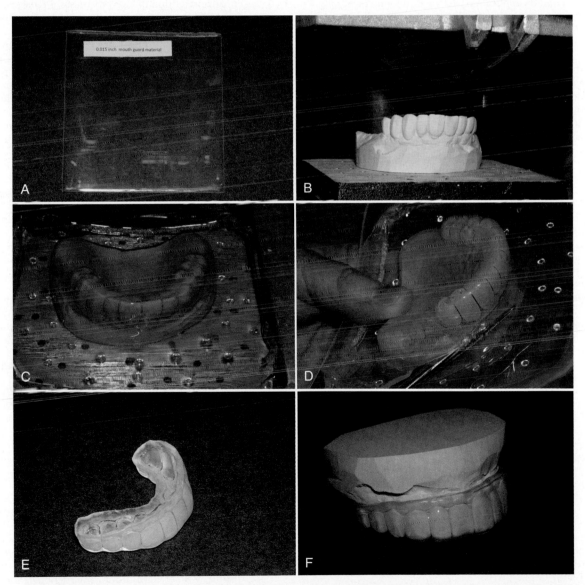

Figure 22-24 A, Clear material (0.150 inch) used to fabricate a mouthguard. **B,** Material clamped in machine and heated until it softens and droops. **C,** Material vacuum-adapted to dry stone cast. **D,** Guard being trimmed with scissors. **E,** Appearance of borders after being trimmed with acrylic bur and polished with pumice. **F,** Completed mouthguard on cast.

Maximum retention is obtained when the entire hard palate is covered. If the guard interferes with speech, however, a portion of the palatal area of the guard can be removed.

The successful use of mouthguards by many young athletes has proven that they can be worn with comfort and serve as effective safeguards against injuries to the teeth.

REFERENCES

1. Caplan DJ, Weintraub JA. The oral health burden in the United States: a summary of recent epidemiologic studies, *J Dent Educ* 57(12):853-862, 1993.
2. Vargas CM, et al. Sociodemographic distribution of pediatric dental caries: NHANES III, 1988-1994, *J Am Dent Assoc* 129:1229-1238, 1998.
3. Barmes DE, Leous PA. Assessment of periodontal status by CPITN and its applicability to the development of long-term goals on periodontal health of the population, *Int Dent J* 36:177-181, 1986.
4. Bader JD, et al. Periodontal status and treatment needs among regular dental patients, *Int Dent J* 38:255-260, 1988.
5. Gift HC, Bhat M. Dental visits for orofacial injury: defining the dentist's role, *J Am Dent Assoc* 124:92-98, 1993.
6. Bader JD, et al. Preliminary estimates of the incidence and consequences of tooth fracture, *J Am Dent Assoc* 126:1650-1654, 1995.
7. Haug RH, et al. An epidemiologic survey of facial fractures and concomitant injuries, *J Oral Maxillofac Surg* 48:926-932, 1990.
8. Pilo R, et al. Diagnosis of developmental dental anomalies using panoramic radiographs, *J Dent Child* 54:267-272, 1987.
9. Sorensen JA, Martinoff JT. Endodontically treated teeth as abutments, *J Prosthet Dent* 53:631-636, 1985.
10. Pegoraro LF, Barrack G. A comparison of bond strengths of adhesive cast restorations using different designs, bonding agents, and luting resins, *J Prosthet Dent* 57:133-138, 1987.
11. Dunne SM, Millar BJ. A longitudinal study of the clinical performance of resin bonded bridges and splints, *Br Dent J* 174:405-411, 1993.
12. Marinello CP, et al. First experiences with resin-bonded bridges and splints: a cross-sectional retrospective study, part II, *J Oral Rehabil* 15:223-235, 1988.
13. Williams V, et al. Acid-etch retained cast metal prostheses: a seven-year retrospective study, *J Am Dent Assoc* 108:629-631, 1984.
14. Hussey DL, et al. Performance of 400 adhesive bridges fitted in a restorative dentistry department, *J Dent* 19:221-225, 1991.
15. Leempoel PJ, et al. The survival rate of bridges: a study of 1674 bridges in 40 Dutch general practices, *J Oral Rehabil* 22:327-330, 1995.
16. Barrack G, Bretz WA. A long-term prospective study of the etched-cast restoration, *Int J Prosthodont* 6:428-434, 1993.
17. Besimo C. Resin-bonded fixed partial denture technique: results of a medium-term clinical follow-up investigation, *J Prosthet Dent* 69:144-148, 1993.
18. Simon JF, et al. Improved retention of acid-etched fixed partial denture: a longitudinal study, *J Prosthet Dent* 68:611-615, 1992.
19. Rammelsberg P, et al. Clinical factors affecting adhesive fixed partial dentures: a 6-year study, *J Prosthet Dent* 70:300-307, 1993.
20. Hansson O, Bergström B. A longitudinal study of resin-bonded prostheses, *J Prosthet Dent* 76:132-139, 1996.
21. Creugers NHJ, et al. Clinical performance of resin-bonded bridges: a 5 year prospective study. Part II: influence of patient dependent variables, *J Oral Rehabil* 16:521-527, 1989.
22. Crispin BJ. A longitudinal clinical study of bonded fixed partial dentures: the first 5 years, *J Prosthet Dent* 66:336-342, 1991.
23. Rochette AL. Attachment of a splint to enamel of lower anterior teeth, *J Prosthet Dent* 30:418-423, 1973.
24. Livaditis GJ, Thompson VP. Etched castings: an improved retentive mechanism for resin-bonded retainers, *J Prosthet Dent* 47:52-58, 1982.
25. Atta MO, Smith BGN. The bond strength of a new adhesive bridge cement to sand-blasted nickel-chromium alloy compared with composite to acid-etched alloy, *J Dent Res* 65(special issue, IADR Program and Abstracts):496 (abst no 74), 1986.
26. Covington JS, et al. Electrical vs. physical etching to enhance retention of cast prostheses, *J Dent Res* 66(special issue, IADR Program and Abstracts):199 (abst no 744), 1987.
27. Schwartz NL, et al. Unserviceable crowns and fixed partial dentures: life-span and causes for loss of serviceability, *J Am Dent Assoc* 81:1395-1401, 1970.
28. Foster LV. Failed conventional bridge work from general dental practice: clinical aspects and treatment needs of 142 cases, *Br Dent J* 168:199-201, 1990.
29. Esposito S, Vergo TJ. Removable overdentures in the oral rehabilitation of patients with dentinogenesis imperfecta, *J Pedod* 2:304-315, 1978.
30. Behrents RG. A treatise on the continuum of growth in the aging craniofacial skeleton. Ann Arbor, University of Michigan, Center for Human Growth and Development, 1985.
31. Björk A, Skieller V. Growth of the maxilla in three dimensions as revealed radiographically by the implant method, *Br J Orthod* 4:53-64, 1977.
32. Cronin RJ, Oesterle LJ. Implant use in growing patients: treatment planning concerns, *Dent Clin North Am* 42(1):1-34, 1998.
33. Cronin RJ, et al. Mandibular implants and the growing patient, *Int J Oral Maxillofac Implants* 9:55-62, 1994.
34. Oesterle LJ, et al. Maxillary implants and the growing patient, *Int J Oral Maxillofac Implants* 8:377-387, 1993.
35. Bergendal B, et al. Implant failure in young children with ectodermal dysplasia: a retrospective evaluation of use and outcome of dental implant treatment in children in Sweden, *Int J Oral Maxillofac Implants* 23(3):520-524, 2008.
36. Guckes AD, et al. Using endosseous dental implants for patients with ectodermal dysplasia, *J Am Dent Assoc* 122:59-62, 1991.
37. Ledermann PD, et al. Osseointegrated dental implants as alternative therapy to bridge construction or orthodontics in young patients: seven years of clinical experience, *Pediatr Dent* 15:327-333, 1993.
38. Westwood RM, Duncan JM. Implants in adolescents: a literature review and case reports, *Int J Oral Maxillofac Implants* 11:750-755, 1996.
39. Kokich VG. Managing complex orthodontic problems: the use of implants for anchorage, *Semin Orthod* 2:153-160, 1996.
40. Upadhyay M, et al. Mini-implant anchorage for en-masse retraction of maxillary anterior teeth: a clinical cephalometric study, *Am J Orthod Dentofacial Orthop* 134(6):803-810, 2008.

41. Iseri H, et al. Ten-year follow-up of a patient with hemifacial microsomia treated with distraction osteogenesis and orthodontics: an implant analysis, *Am J Orthod Dentofacial Orthop* 134(2):296-304, 2008.

42. Upadhyay M, et al. Mini-implants for en masse intrusion of maxillary anterior teeth in a severe Class II division 2 malocclusion, *J Orthod* 35(2):79-89, 2008.

43. Garfinkle JS, et al. Evaluation of orthodontic mini-implant anchorage in premolar extraction therapy in adolescents, *Am J Orthod Dentofacial Orthop* 133(5):642-653, 2008.

44. Roberts WE, et al. Rigid implant anchorage to close a mandibular first molar extraction site, *J Clin Orthod* 28: 693-704, 1994.

45. Garon MW, et al. Mouth protectors and oral trauma: a study of adolescent football players, *J Am Dent Assoc* 112:663-665, 1986.

46. Matalon V, et al. Compliance of children and youngsters in the use of mouthguards, *Dent Traumatol* 24(4):462-467, 2008.

47. Seals RR, Dorrough BC. Custom mouth protectors: a review of their applications, *J Prosthet Dent* 51:238-242, 1984.

48. Stokes ANS, et al. Comparison of laboratory and intraorally formed mouth protectors, *Endod Dent Traumatol* 3:255-258, 1987.

49. Bass EH, Williams FA. A comparison of custom vs. standard mouthguards: a preliminary study, *N Y State Dent J* 55: 74-76, 1989.

50. Geary JL, Kinirons MJ. Post thermoforming dimensional changes of ethylene vinyl acetate used in custom-made mouthguards for trauma prevention—a pilot study, *Dent Traumatol* 24(3):350-355, 2008.

51. Chaconas SJ, et al. A comparison of athletic mouthguard materials, *Am J Sports Med* 13:193-197, 1985.

CHAPTER 23

Dental Problems of Children with Special Health Care Needs

▲ **James A. Weddell, Brian J. Sanders,** and **James E. Jones**

CHAPTER OUTLINE

pproximately 52 million children and adults in the United States have a disabling condition.[1] The American Academy of Pediatric Dentistry defines individuals with special health care needs (SHCN) as those with "any physical, developmental, mental, sensory, behavioral, cognitive, or emotional impairment or limiting condition that requires medical management, health care intervention, and/or use of specialized services or programs."[2] Patients with SHCN are at increased risk for oral disease.[3]

Many children with SHCN are best managed initially by a multidisciplinary team in which a dentist is available to evaluate extraoral and intraoral findings of the child. A diagnosis is then established, and an impression is gained of the child's strengths and weaknesses and the team's recommendations for future care. The child may then be "mainstreamed" to a dental practitioner whom the family chooses, if a preference is indicated. The team is available to help the family practitioner or pediatric dentist treat the child and prepare the family for the child's future treatment needs because oral health is a vital part of the child's well being and general health.[3]

Children with SHCN may present challenges that require special preparation before the dentist and office staff can provide acceptable care. In addition, parental anxiety concerning the problems associated with a child's SHCN frequently delays dental care until significant oral disease has developed. Also, some dentists feel uncomfortable providing treatment for children with SHCN, which results in a loss of greatly needed services. Kane

and colleagues reported failure to obtain routine medical care as well as income below 400% of federal poverty guidelines as a barrier to receipt of dental care for children with SHCN.[4] Financing and reimbursement issues are other barriers for families with SHCN children and for dental practitioners.[5] Nonfinancial barriers such as language and psychosocial, structural, and cultural considerations also interfere with access to oral care.[5]

This chapter discusses disabling pediatric conditions that dentists sometimes encounter in practice. If a dentist becomes familiar with the special health care needs of a child and with the parents' concerns, the dental management of the child can be gratifying.

DENTAL ACCESS

Improving access to oral health care for those deprived of needed services should be of great concern to the dental profession. Large segments of the population do not have access to dental care. Children with SHCN, such as those who are chronically ill, homebound, developmentally disabled, and emotionally impaired, fall into this group. In addition, these groups have been identified as a significant portion of the 20% of the U.S. population who exhibit 80% of all caries.

The rapid expansion of the elderly population, the presence of children with SHCN, and the emergence of legislative guidelines for people of all ages with SHCN are three important factors that should prompt dentists to address cost-efficient ways to make their office facilities and operatory areas accessible for persons with SHCN. In August 1984, another federal-level cornerstone was laid for barrier-free facility access with the passage of the Uniform Federal Accessibility Standards.[6] Enacted in 1990, the Americans with Disabilities Act defines the dental office as a place of public accommodation.[7] Dental consumer populations are becoming more sensitive to the service needs and desires of people with SHCN by improving family conditions and public education. Failure to accommodate SHCN patients could be considered discrimination and a violation of state or federal law. Table 23-1 lists common minimum requirements needed to gain access.

In the dental operatory, doorways should be 4 inches (10 cm) wider than normal. In the dental suite where floor circulation space is at a premium, aisle passage in the operatory area should be planned with the dimensions shown in Fig. 23-1. The required wheelchair turning space and top space under furniture and fixtures may be more readily accommodated if one operatory is specifically designed with a movable dental chair, instrument control unit, and suction system. Movable equipment should enhance the opportunity to back the patient's wheelchair into the operatory and thus reduce the need for more wheelchair turning space. If possible, a wider radius for turning space is desirable to accommodate wheelchair

Table 23-1

Accessibility Guidelines

External/Internal Building Features	Gradient	Length	Width	Surface, Other Specifics
Parking space	1:50 max slope	Standard	Auto: 96 inches Van: 144 inches	Nonskid, paved, sign-posted, adjacent to walkway
Walkway	1:12 max slope	Not applicable	36 inches	Nonskid, no obstructions, overhangs, smooth
Passenger loading zone	Flat	20 feet	60 inches	Same as above
Curb ramps	1:12 max slope		36 inches	Nonskid, side flair <1:10 slope
Door	5-foot entrance and exit platform area	Standard	32-inch minimum; preferably 36 inches	Away from prevailing winds, lever with 10-lb pull, auto-assisted door available, kick plate
Interior ramp	1:20 max slope	72-inch minimum length if rise > 6 inches	36 inches	Nonskid, handrails
Wheelchair lift	Bilevel	8-foot max drop	36×48 inches	Nonskid, dependent on specific chair
Corridor		Standard	48 inches/64 inches	New facility, no obstacles
Flooring	Flat, firm carpet	Not applicable	½-inch maximum thickness	No doormats, level thresholds
Signs	Braille, raised letters	Above 5 feet	Readable	Near latch of office door
Waiting room	Flat	Standard	36-inch aisle One cleared area: 36×52 inches	No carpet pad, well insulated, minimum low-frequency background noise
Restrooms	Flat		32-inch stall min, preferably 36 inches	Nonskid, magnetic catch door
Public telephone	No higher than 4 feet	3 feet above floor	26-inch clearance	Phone directory near phone, adjustable volume control
Elevator	Flat		54×68 inches	Nonskid, call and control box 48 inches high, include Braille or incised letters
Operatory	Flat 8×10 feet	Standard	32- to 36-inch door	Nonskid, rotating or movable chair, drill, and suction

Adapted from Bill DJ, Weddell JA. Dental office access for patients with disabling conditions, *Spec Care Dentist* 6:246-252, 1986.

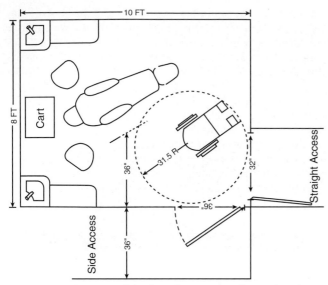

Figure 23-1 An accessible dental operatory floor plan designed for either a straight or side access doorway. (From Bill DJ, Weddell JA. Dental office access for patients with disabling conditions, *Spec Care Dentist* 6:246-252, 1986.)

extensions and adaptations that are required for some persons. Dental chairs should be adjustable for height to match different wheelchair designs.

FIRST DENTAL VISIT

Many people avoid dental treatment for themselves or their children because of their fear that dental visits are routinely painful. Dental professionals should use every opportunity to help patients or parents overcome this barrier into the mainstream of effective dental care and establish a "dental home" with them (see Chapter 1).

Upon scheduling an appointment, the dental receptionist should determine the presence and nature of any SHCN, should determine who the family's medical provider is, and should alert the dentist so adequate time can be allowed. The initial dental examination for a child with SHCN is like the initial examination described in Chapter 1. Special attention should be given to obtaining a thorough medical and dental history. The names and addresses of medical or dental personnel who have previously treated the patient are necessary for consultation purposes. Consultation with these specialists is common and helps provide insight in case management, planning, and avoiding unwanted outcomes. Health Insurance Portability and Accountability Act compliance is mandatory throughout this process.

The first dental appointment is very important and can set the stage for subsequent appointments. As previously noted, parental anxiety about a child's dental treatment may be a significant factor. In many situations, parents or guardians do not realize the importance of this visit and desire treatment immediately. By scheduling the patient at a designated time (early in the day) and allowing sufficient time to talk with the parents (or the guardian) and the patient before initiating any dental care, a practitioner can establish an excellent relationship with

them. Sending a letter before the appointment explaining the first visit to the family and sending another letter afterward letting them know how helpful they were is beneficial. This initial demonstration of sincere interest in the child often proves advantageous and saves time throughout the entire treatment process. Obtaining an informed consent is imperative. Many times dental treatment must be delayed until an informed consent is obtained through a guardian or court petition when no parents are legally accountable.

RADIOGRAPHIC EXAMINATION

Adequate radiographic records are often necessary in planning dental treatment for the child with SHCN. Through appropriate behavior management of the child, a dentist can usually perform a complete radiographic examination of the teeth when indicated. Occasionally, assistance from the parent and dental auxiliaries and the use of immobilization devices may be necessary to obtain the films. Better cooperation may be elicited from some children by delaying radiographs until the second visit, when they are familiar with the dental office and have found it a friendly place.

For patients with limited ability to control film position, intraoral films with bite-wing tabs are used for all bite-wing and periapical radiographs. An 18-inch (46-cm) length of floss is attached through a hole made in the tab, as shown in Fig. 23-2, to facilitate retrieval of the film if it falls toward the pharynx. Digital sensors can be cumbersome. Regardless of the types of radiographs to be made, the patient should wear a lead apron with a thyroid shield, and anyone who helps hold the patient and the film or sensor steady should wear a lead-lined apron and gloves (Fig. 23-3).

PREVENTIVE DENTISTRY

Preventing oral disease before it starts is the most desirable way of ensuring good dental health for any dental patient. An effective preventive dentistry program is important for a child with SHCN because of the predisposing factors that make restorative dental care harder to obtain when it is necessary. Dental diagnosis and treatment planning will

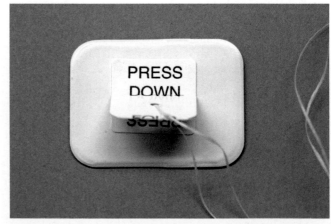

Figure 23-2 Bite-wing radiographic film secured with floss.

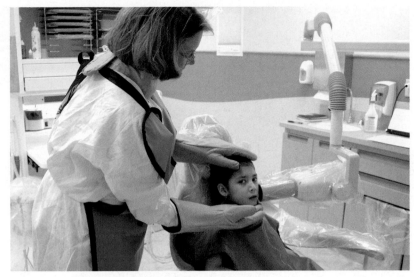

Figure 23-3 Extra assistance in holding the patient's head steady to prevent movement while a radiograph is being made.

necessitate an accurate, up-to-date medical history at each visit. After the diagnosis, the dentist should determine the patient's needs, assume the responsibility for formulating an individual program for the child, and adequately communicate to the parents and patient how such a program can be effected. Use of a Caries-Risk Assessment Tool (CAT) to integrate these dental risk factors may result in a more aggressive approach to the individual's dental treatment plan. A clear perception of the situation by everyone involved is essential for a successful preventive program; adequate communication is vital.

HOME DENTAL CARE

Dental education of parents/guardians/caregivers is important to ensure children with SHCN do not jeopardize their overall health by neglecting their oral health. The parents (or the guardian) are initially responsible for establishing good oral hygiene in the home. Reinforcement of good home dental care is provided through mass media (e.g., newspapers, radio, television, and internet), communication with other people, and school activities (e.g., health classes, parent-teacher association meetings, and observation of National Dental Health Month). This supplementary support relieves the dentist having sole responsibility for explaining the need for home dental care and reinforces the receptivity of the parent and child to such a program. The dentist or the hygienist is responsible for consulting with the caregiver of the child with SHCN (i.e., parent, guardian, or nursing home attendant) when continued oral hygiene problems occur. Regular follow-up supervision at home and in office is essential for effective implementation of the preventive dental treatment plan.

Home dental care should begin in infancy; the dentist should teach the parents to gently cleanse the incisors daily with a soft cloth or an infant toothbrush. For older children who are unwilling or physically unable to cooperate, the dentist should teach the parent or guardian to clean teeth twice a day using correct toothbrushing techniques, safely immobilizing the child when necessary. Figure 23-4 shows several positions for toothbrushing

that permit firm control and support of the child, adequate visibility, and convenient positioning of the adult, with reasonable comfort for both adult and child (also see Fig. 11-14). Positions most commonly used for children requiring oral care assistance are as follows:

- The standing or sitting child is placed in front of the adult so that the adult can cradle the child's head with one hand while using the other hand to brush the teeth.
- The child reclines on a sofa or bed with the head angled backward on the parent's lap. Again, the child's head is stabilized with one hand while the teeth are brushed with the other hand.
- The parents face each other with their knees touching. The child's buttocks are placed on one parent's lap, with the child facing that parent, while the child's head and shoulders lie on the other parent's knees; this allows the first parent to brush the teeth.
- The extremely difficult patient is isolated in an open area and reclined in the brusher's lap. The patient is then immobilized by an extra attendant while the brusher institutes proper oral care. If a child cannot be adequately immobilized by one person, then both parents and perhaps siblings may be needed to complete the home dental care procedures.
- The standing and resistive child is placed in front of the caregiver so that the adult can wrap his or her legs around the child to support the torso while using the hands to support the head and brush the teeth.

If a child with SHCN is institutionalized, the staff should be instructed in the proper dental care regimen for the child. Wrapped tongue blades may be of benefit in helping to keep a child's mouth open while plaque is being removed. Stabilization of the child's head prevents unnecessary trauma from sudden movements. Follow-up observation is carried out by the dentist or the hygienist, and it is appropriate to offer in-service training sessions and to check with the staff periodically to identify and solve the problems associated with an oral hygiene program in the institution.

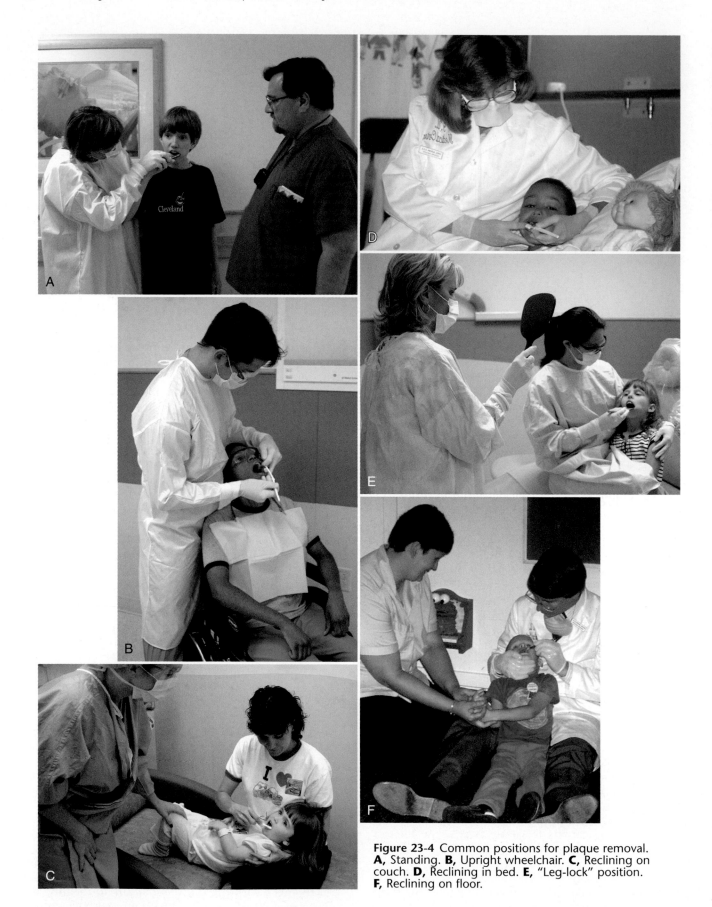

Figure 23-4 Common positions for plaque removal. **A,** Standing. **B,** Upright wheelchair. **C,** Reclining on couch. **D,** Reclining in bed. **E,** "Leg-lock" position. **F,** Reclining on floor.

Some parents and health centers have encouraged children with SHCN to assume the responsibility for their own oral hygiene, but the results are usually poor. Although independent brushing is not contraindicated, parents and staff should be aware that, without their follow-up, unsupervised oral hygiene procedures in children with SHCN can have serious dental consequences. The amount of supervision and assistance provided by the parents or staff should depend on the child's willingness to cooperate and ability to maintain good oral hygiene twice a day.

A plaque control program is essential in monitoring oral hygiene in the child with SHCN and determining the level of success achieved by each patient. The brushing technique for patients with SHCN who have fine or gross motor deficiencies limiting their ability to brush should be effective and yet simple for the person performing the brushing. One technique often recommended is the horizontal scrub method because it is easy to perform and can yield good results. This technique consists of performing gentle horizontal strokes on cheek, tongue, and biting surfaces of all teeth and gums. Other patients with SHCN without such motor problems can use age-appropriate techniques previously discussed in Chapter 11. A soft, multitufted nylon brush should be used.

Figure 23-5 illustrates some modifications that may be made to a toothbrush to help persons with poor fine motor skills improve their brushing techniques. Although many types of grips are available, using the patient's hand to custom-design a handle has often had good results (Fig. 23-6). Electric toothbrushes have also been used effectively by children with SHCN. The vibration and noise tend to desensitize the patient for future dental appointments if followed by positive reinforcement while the design and color is motivational for the child. Daily flossing, with supervision or the use of floss holders, is essential to maintain optimal gingival health.

DIET AND NUTRITION

Diet and nutrition influence dental caries by affecting the type and virulence of the microorganisms in dental plaque, the resistance of teeth and supporting structures, and the

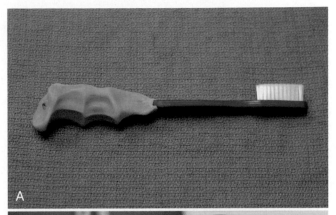

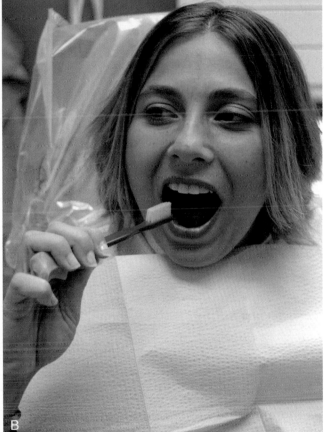

Figure 23-6 A, Custom-designed acrylic handle. **B,** Patient using the custom-handle toothbrush.

properties of saliva in the oral cavity. A proper noncariogenic diet, as outlined in Chapter 12, is essential to a good preventive program for a child with SHCN. As discussed in Chapter 10, one should assess the diet by reviewing answers on a diet survey with the parent, realizing that allowances must be made for certain conditions for which dietary modifications are required. For example, conditions associated with difficulty in swallowing, such as severe cerebral palsy, may require that the patient be on a pureed diet. Patients with certain metabolic disturbances or syndromes, such as phenylketonuria, diabetes, or Prader-Willi syndrome, have diets that restrict specific foods or total caloric consumption. Whatever the special circumstances,

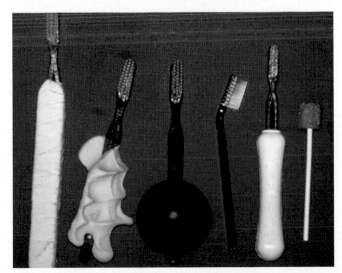

Figure 23-5 Various toothbrush handle modifications.

any dietary recommendations should be made individually after proper consultation with the patient's primary physician or dietitian. The oral side effects of their medications should be reviewed with the parents or guardians at each visit to identify specific concerns, for example, of increased caries or gingival overgrowth, to prevent or minimize these problems. Particular emphasis should be placed on discontinuation of the nursing bottle by 12 months of age and cessation of at-will breast-feeding after teeth begin to erupt to decrease the likelihood of early childhood caries.

FLUORIDE EXPOSURE

The judicious use of systemic fluoride is important in the comprehensive management of any dental patient. Special emphasis should be placed on ensuring adequate systemic fluoride for patients with disabilities. The dentist should first determine the concentration of fluoride in the patient's daily water supply. If the level of fluoride is between 0.7 and 1 ppm, no supplementation is normally required. If the dentist is not sure of the fluoride level of the patient's drinking water or other sources, an analysis to determine the level is indicated. Once the level has been documented, a determination of the need for fluoride supplementation can be made. The amount of systemic fluoride supplementation necessary, along with the various forms available (i.e., drops, tablets, and rinses), is outlined in Chapter 10.

Whether the patient lives in an area with a fluoridated or nonfluoridated water supply, a topical fluoride should be applied after a regularly scheduled professional prophylaxis. Also, 5% neutral sodium fluoride varnishes have been shown to be beneficial.[8] An American Dental Association–accepted dentifrice containing a therapeutic fluoride compound should also be used daily. Some clinicians treating patients with SHCN who have chronically poor oral hygiene and high decay rates suggest a daily regimen of rinsing with 0.05% sodium fluoride solution. Nightly application of a 0.4% stannous fluoride or 1.1% sodium fluoride brush-on gel has also been successfully used to decrease caries in children.

PREVENTIVE RESTORATIONS

Pit and fissure sealants have been shown to reduce occlusal caries effectively. Sealants are appropriate in patients with SHCN. For a patient who requires dental work under general anesthesia, deep occlusal pits and fissures should be restored with amalgam or long-wearing composites to prevent further breakdown and decay. Patients with severe bruxism and interproximal decay may need their teeth restored with stainless steel crowns to increase the longevity of the restorations.

REGULAR PROFESSIONAL SUPERVISION

Close observation of caries-susceptible patients and regular dental examinations are important in the treatment of patients with SHCN. Although most patients are seen semiannually for professional prophylaxis, examination, and topical fluoride application, certain patients can benefit from recall examinations every 2, 3, or 4 months. This is particularly true of patients who are confined to institutions in which dental health programs are inadequate. Transferring the " dental home" of an adult patient with SHCN to a

knowledgeable general dentist is recommended when dental care needs go beyond the scope of a pediatric dentist. If necessary, the pediatric dentist may refer the patient for "specialized care" (e.g., oral surgeon, orthodontist, periodontist).

MANAGEMENT OF A CHILD WITH SPECIAL HEALTH CARE NEEDS DURING DENTAL TREATMENT

The principles of behavior management discussed in Chapter 3 are even more important in treating a child with SHCN. Because hospital visits or previous appointments with a physician frequently result in the development of apprehension in the patient, additional time must be spent with the parent and the child to establish rapport and dispel the child's anxiety. If patient cooperation cannot be obtained, the dentist must consider alternatives such as protective stabilization, conscious sedation, or general anesthesia to allow performance of the necessary dental procedures.

PROTECTIVE STABILIZATION

Partial or complete protective stabilization of the patient is sometimes a necessary and effective way to diagnose and deliver dental care to patients who need help controlling their extremities, such as infants or patients with certain neuromuscular disorders. Protective stabilization is also useful for managing combative, resistant patients, so that the patient, practitioner, and/or dental staff may be protected from injury while care is being provided. This can be performed by the dentist, staff, or parent, with or without the aid of a stabilization device.

The parents, guardian, or patient (if an adult) must be informed and must give consent, and the consent must be documented, before protective stabilization is used. These individuals should have a clear understanding of the type of stabilization to be used, the rationale, and the duration of use. In many cases this information should be included in the explanation of the overall management approach for the child during the initial examination and conference with the parents.

In October 1990, the Omnibus Budget Reconciliation Act of 1987 became effective. It provided recommended guidelines to reduce the risk of injury and death from the use of patient restraints.

The American Academy of Pediatric Dentistry's *Behavior Guidance for the Pediatric Dental Patient Reference Manual 2008-09* indicates that the need to diagnose and treat, as well as to protect the safety of the patient, parent, staff and practitioner, must justify the use of stabilization.[9] This decision should take into consideration a careful review of the patient's emotional development, physical and medical conditions (e.g., asthma-compromised respiratory function), dental needs, other alternative behavioral modalities, and quality of dental care. Although the benefits and importance of protective stabilization have been documented, the use of behavioral management or sedation, as discussed in Chapter 14, can reduce the amount of stabilization required. This is only one means of behavior control to achieve an adequate level of dental treatment.

The use of protective stabilization is indicated in the following situations:

- A patient requires immediate diagnosis and/or limited treatment and cannot cooperate because of lack of maturity, mental or physical disability.
- A patient requires diagnosis or treatment and does not cooperate after other behavior management techniques have failed.
- The safety of the patient, staff, parent or practitioner would be at risk without the use of protective stabilization.

The use of stabilization is contraindicated in the following situations:

- A cooperative non-sedated patient.
- Patients who cannot be safely stabilized due to medical or physical conditions.
- Patients who have experienced previous physical or psychological trauma from protective stabilization (unless no other alternatives are available).
- Nonsedated patients with nonemergent treatment requiring lengthy appointments.

Protective stabilization should not be used as punishment and should not be used solely for the convenience of the staff. The patient's record should display an informed consent, the indications for use, the type of stabilization used, and the duration of application. The tightness and duration of stabilization must be monitored and reassessed at regular intervals. Stabilization around the extremities or chest must not actively restrict circulation or respiration. Stabilization should be terminated as soon as possible in a patient who is experiencing severe stress or hysterics to prevent possible physical or psychological trauma.

Common mechanical aids for maintaining the mouth in an open position are shown in Fig. 23-7. Padded and wrapped tongue blades are easy to use, disposable, and inexpensive. Frequently, parents of a child with disabilities are given wrapped tongue blades or Open Wide (Specialized Care Co., Hampton, NH) disposable mouth props to aid with home dental care. The Open Wide mouth prop has a durable foam core on the end of a tongue depressor. It is also easy to use, disposable, and available in two sizes, but it is slightly more expensive than wrapped tongue blades. The Molt Mouth Prop (Hu-Friedy, Chicago, Ill) can be very helpful in the management of a difficult patient for a prolonged period. It is made in both adult and child sizes, allows accessibility to the opposite side of the mouth, and operates on a reverse scissors action. Its disadvantages include the possibility of lip and palatal lacerations and luxation of teeth if it is not used correctly. Caution must be exercised to prevent injury to the patient, and the prop should not be allowed to rest on anterior teeth. The

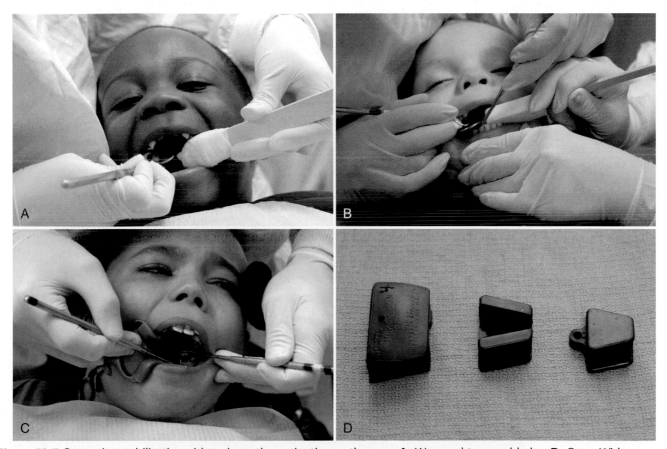

Figure 23-7 Protective stabilization aids to keep the patient's mouth open. **A,** Wrapped tongue blades. **B,** Open Wide (Specialized Care Co., Hampton, NH) disposable mouth prop in proper position. **C,** Molt Mouth Prop (Hu-Friedy, Chicago, Ill) in proper position. **D,** McKesson bite blocks.

patient's mouth should not be forced beyond its natural limits because patient discomfort and panic will result, which will cause further resistance and perhaps airway compromise.

Rubber bite blocks can be purchased in various sizes to fit on the occlusal surfaces of the teeth and stabilize the mouth in an open position. The bite blocks should have floss attached for easy retrieval if they become dislodged in the mouth.

Body control is gained through a variety of methods and techniques. For children who have a severe intellectual disability or very young, parents and dental assistants can assist in the control of movements during dental procedures, as shown in Fig. 23-8. Usually, however, for a child who has severe intellectual disability, better working conditions and a more predictable patient response are obtained through the combined use of psychological management techniques, parental assistance, pharmacologic aids, and stabilization.

The following are commonly used for protective stabilization:

Body
Papoose Board (Olympic Medical Corp., Seattle, Wash)
Triangular sheet
Pedi-Wrap (The Medi•Kid Co., Hemet, Calif)
Beanbag dental chair insert
Safety belt
Extra assistant

Extremities
Posey straps (Posey Co., Arcadia, Calif)
Velcro straps
Towel and tape
Extra assistant

Head
Forearm-body support
Head positioner
Plastic bowl
Extra assistant

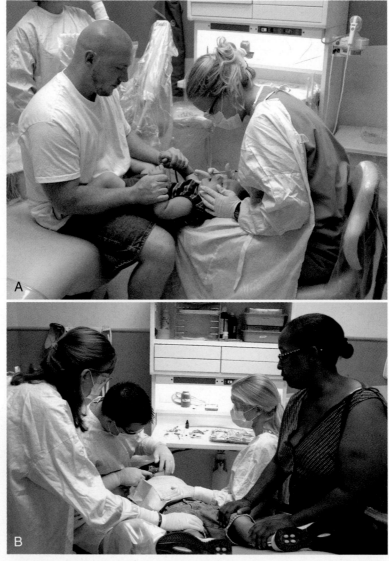

Figure 23-8 Assistance for protective stabilization. **A,** Parental aid during an examination. **B,** Additional assistance during the dental procedure.

The Papoose Board (Fig. 23-9) has several advantages. Simple to store and use, it is available in sizes to hold both large and small children. It has attached head stabilizers and is reusable. It does not always fit the contours of a dental chair, however, and sometimes a supporting pillow is needed. Because it covers the patient's diaphragm, a pretracheal stethoscope is necessary to monitor respiration if it is used in combination with sedation. An extremely resistant patient may develop hyperthermia if immobilized too long, and, of course, any restrained patient requires constant attendance and supervision.

Mink[10] describes the bedsheet (triangular sheet) technique and its use in controlling an extremely resistant child (Fig. 23-10A). This economical method allows the patient to sit upright during radiographic examinations. Its disadvantages include the frequent need for straps to maintain the patient's position in the chair, the difficulty of its use with small patients, and the possibility of airway impingement if the patient slips downward unnoticed. Hyperthermia may be another problem during long periods of stabilization. Again, the need for constant supervision is emphasized so that these problems may be avoided.

The Rainbow Stabilizing System or "Pedi-Wrap" (Specialized Care Co., Hampton, NH ; see Fig. 23-10B), which is available with or without the backboard, also comes in various sizes and allows some movement while still confining the patient. Its mesh fabric permits better ventilation, lessening the chances of the patient developing hyperthermia. It, too, requires straps to maintain body position in the dental chair and constant supervision to prevent the patient from rolling out of the chair.

The beanbag dental chair insert was developed to help comfortably accommodate hypotonic and severely spastic persons who need more support and less stabilization in a dental environment (see Fig. 23-10C). It is reusable and washable, and one size fits most people. Many patients with SHCN relax more in this setting.

The child's arms and legs can be stabilized with help from the parent or the dental assistant, with Posey straps, or with a towel and adhesive tape (Fig. 23-11). If movement of the extremities is the only problem, having a dental assistant stabilize the child is very helpful. Posey straps fasten to the arms of the dental chair and allow limited movement of the patient's forearm and hand. This limited movement frequently prevents overaction by resistant or combative patients. Wrapping a towel wrapped around the patient's forearms and fastening it with adhesive tape (without impeding circulation) is often helpful for an athetoid-spastic cerebral palsy patient who tries desperately, but without success, to control body movements. Protective stabilization actually encourages relaxation and prevents undesired reflexes by keeping the patient's arms in the midline of the body.

A patient's head position can usually be successfully maintained through the use of forearm-body pressure by the dentist. Other options include presence of an additional assistant to stabilize the child's head or use of a Papoose Board head positioner or a plastic bowl (doggie bowl) to provide position guidance (Fig. 23-12).

An explanation of the benefits of protective stabilization should be presented by the dentist before used if communication with the patient is possible. The mouth prop can be identified as a "tooth chair," the Pedi-Wrap as a "safety robe," and a stabilization strap as a "safety belt," which allows the patient to feel secure rather than threatened. The parents should be given a careful explanation about how protective stabilization allows the needed dental work to be done while minimizing the possibility of accidental injury to the patient, parent, staff, or dentist. If a child requires extensive dental treatment and cooperation cannot be achieved by routine psychological, physical, or pharmacologic measures, the use of general anesthesia in a controlled atmosphere, as discussed in Chapter 15, is recommended.

INTELLECTUAL DISABILITY

Intellectual disability is a general term used when an individual's intellectual development is significantly lower than average and his or her ability to adapt to the environment is consequently limited.[11] The condition varies in severity and cause. A classification of intellectual disability is presented in Table 23-2. Intellectual disability has been identified in approximately 3% of the U.S. population. For many years the potential abilities of people with intellectual disabilities were poorly understood, and such individuals were often treated as inferior. They were described using the terms *idiot* (IQ [intelligence quotient] below 25), *imbecile* (IQ of 25 to 50), and *moron* (IQ of 50 to 70). With the formation of the President's Committee on Mental Retardation in 1968, emphasis was placed on education of individuals with intellectual disabilities to increase their social and civic responsibilities, motor skills, and independence within society.

Although a child who scores 2 standard deviations below the mean on the Stanford-Binet Intelligence Scale or the Wechsler Intelligence Scale for Children may have some degree of retardation, a diagnosis of intellectual disability is not made based on IQ alone. Both inadequate adaptive functioning and intellectual deficiency are required to fulfill a diagnosis of intellectual disability.

A child with mild intellectual disability is one who, because of low intelligence, requires special supports in the school environment. In the academic environment these children may be eligible for special education services for students with mild intellectual disability. Educational programs for such children are generally simplified versions of regular school programs and usually lead to literacy and attainment of skills necessary for employment. Most children in this group, which accounts for approximately 80% of all persons with intellectual disability, will function acceptably as adults.

Children who are capable of some education and partial independence but who are not expected to experience full independence as adults may be eligible for special education services for students with moderate intellectual disability. Classroom activities may focus on attainment of daily living skills. Classrooms are often designed and furnished like a home, and the curriculum includes dressing, grooming, cooking, table setting, feeding, and cleaning. Individuals with moderate intellectual

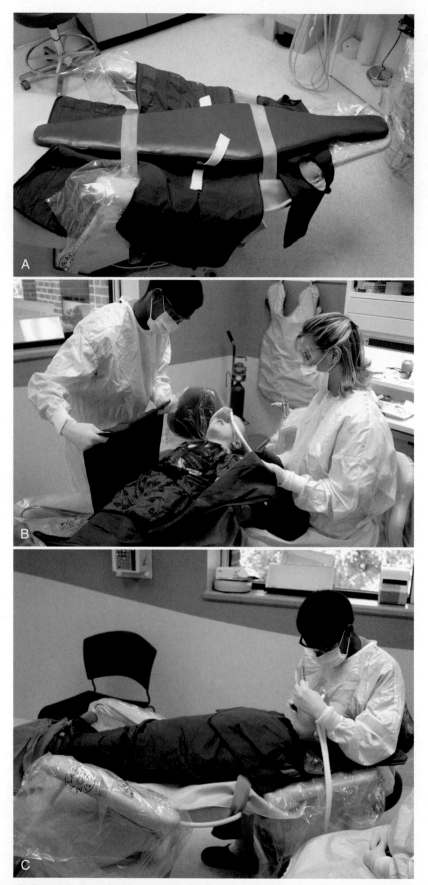

Figure 23-9 A, The Olympic Papoose Board (Olympic Medical Corp., Seattle, Wash) secured to a dental chair. **B,** Patient being placed in Papoose Board. **C,** Papoose Board in use.

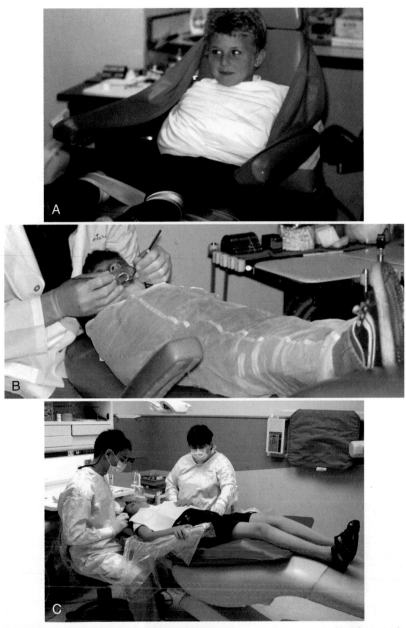

Figure 23-10 Protective stabilization for control of body and extremities. **A,** Patient confined in a triangular sheet with leg straps. **B,** Patient in a Pedi-Wrap. **C,** Patient lying in a beanbag dental chair insert. (**C** Courtesy Dr. Priscilla John Bond.)

Figure 23-12 |
B, Use of the

Table 23-2

Classificat

Degree of Men
Disability

Mild

Moderate

Severe or prof

SB-IV, Stanford-B

disability can be expected to master many vocational, leisure, and self-help skills within a supportive environment with trained personnel who help them with problems with which they may not be able to cope on their own.

A child with severe or profound intellectual disability may present a significant challenge and may be grouped in special education programs. A student with severe to profound intellectual disability can achieve success with self-help, leisure, and some vocational skills given sufficient training and support. Group home placement can allow individuals with severe to profound intellectual disability a measure of independence while providing sufficient support for safety and continuing reinforcement.

DENTAL TREATMENT OF A PERSON WITH INTELLECTUAL DISABILITY

Children with intellectual disability may have a higher incidence of poor oral hygiene, gingivitis, malocclusion, and untreated caries. As the severity of intellectual disability increases, typical oral signs of clenching, bruxing, drooling, pica, trauma, missing teeth, and self-injurious behaviors increase. Providing dental treatment for a person with intellectual disability requires adjusting to social, intellectual, and emotional delays. A short attention span, restlessness, hyperactivity, and erratic emotional behavior may characterize patients with intellectual disability undergoing dental care. The dentist should assess the degree of intellectual disability by consulting the board or electronic device, be sure it is available to assist with dental explanations and instructions.

3. Give only one instruction at a time. Reward the patient with compliments after the successful completion of each procedure.
4. Actively listen to the patient. People with intellectual disability often have trouble with communication, and the dentist should be particularly sensitive to gestures and verbal requests.
5. Invite the parent/guardian into the operatory for assistance and to aid in communication with the patient when helpful.
6. Keep appointments short. Gradually progress to more difficult procedures (e.g., anesthesia and restorative dentistry) after the patient has become accustomed to the dental environment.
7. Schedule the patient's visit early in the day, on a lightly scheduled day, when the dentist, the staff, and the patient will be less fatigued.

With adequate preparation the dentist and the staff can provide a valuable service. By thoroughly understanding the patient's degree of intellectual disability and abilities, and by exercising patience and understanding, the dentist should have no significant problems in delivering dental care. When cooperation does not exist, sedation or general anesthesia may be an option.

DOWN SYNDROME (TRISOMY 21 SYNDROME)

Down syndrome is the best-known chromosomal disorder and is caused by the presence of an extra copy of chromosome 21(trisomy 21). Medical conditions that occur more frequently in infants and children with Down syndrome and increase the mortality of these individuals include cardiac defects, leukemia, and upper respiratory infections. The incidence of congenital cardiac defects is about 40%, and because of these patients' high susceptibility to periodontal disease, knowledge of a heart condition is essential for dental treatment. Children with Down syndrome have a 10- to 20-fold greater incidence of leukemia during infancy compared with the general population. This increased incidence of leukemia is not maintained later in life.

Skeletal findings are an underdeveloped midface, creating a prognathic occlusal relationship. Oral findings include mouth breathing, open bite, appearance of macroglossia, fissured lips and tongue, angular cheilitis, delayed eruption times, missing and malformed teeth, oligodontia, small roots, microdontia, crowding, and low level of caries. Children with Down syndrome experience a high incidence of rapid, destructive periodontal disease, which may be related to local factors such as tooth morphology, bruxism, malocclusion, and poor oral hygiene. Certain systemic factors are also believed to contribute to periodontal disease, including poor circulation, decreased humoral response, general physical deterioration at an early age, and genetic influences. Bell, and colleagues reported that severity of tooth wear (both attrition and erosion) was significantly greater in children with Down syndrome than in children without the syndrome.[12]

Many children with Down syndrome are affectionate and cooperative, and dental procedures can be provided without compromise if the dentist works at a slightly slower pace. Emphasis should be placed on preventive dental care with frequent follow-up visits to monitor oral hygiene. A recent study by Cheng and colleagues documented periodontal healing responses in adult patients with Down syndrome using nonsurgical periodontal therapy in conjunction with the use of chlorhexidine rinse twice a day and chlorhexidine gel and monthly recalls.[13] Comprehensive dental care is an overall goal with alteration based on the individual's level of functioning. Light sedation and immobilization may be indicated in those children who are moderately apprehensive. Severely resistive patients may require general anesthesia.

Delayed tooth eruption frequently occurs in children with Down syndrome. For this reason, additional discussion of this disorder is presented in Chapter 9.

LEARNING DISABILITIES

For years, students who consistently had difficulty achieving a level of academic performance concomitant with their intellectual capacity were unfortunately labeled as *retarded*. Today the term *learning disabled* is applied to children who exhibit a disorder in one or more of the basic psychological processes involved in understanding or using spoken or written language. Learning disabilities affect between 3% and 15% of the population. They occur four times more frequently among boys than among girls.

In 1968 the National Advisory Committee on Handicapped Children of the U.S. Department of Health, Education, and Welfare stated that learning disabilities "may be manifested in disorders of listening, thinking, talking, reading, writing, spelling, or arithmetic. They include conditions that have been referred to as perceptual handicaps, brain injury, minimal brain dysfunction, dyslexia, and developmental aphasia."[14] It should be emphasized that learning disabilities do not include learning problems caused mainly by hearing, visual, or motor handicaps, mental disability, emotional disturbance, or environmental conditions.

The cause of learning disabilities remains unclear. Physiologic factors, such as minimal brain injury or damage to the central nervous system, have been implicated. Because learning disabilities appear more frequently in some families than in others, a genetic factor has also been suggested. The possibility exists that severe emotional disturbances can develop as a result of learning disabilities. This potential has prompted early diagnosis and treatment of affected persons.

Most children with learning disabilities accept dental care and cause no unusual management problems for the dentist. If a child is resistant, behavioral management and conscious sedation techniques can be used with success.

FRAGILE X SYNDROME

Fragile X is an X-linked developmental disorder. It accounts for 30% to 50% of cases of X-linked mental disability. The defect is an abnormal gene on the terminal

Figure 23
on foreai

patient's
coordina
The f
establish
ducing t
1. Give
tempt
(parer

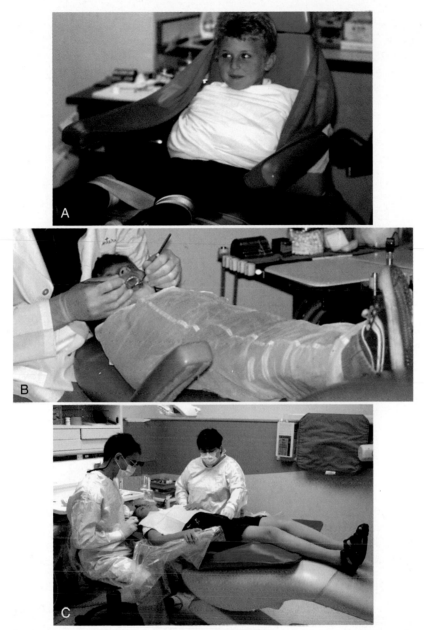

Figure 23-10 Protective stabilization for control of body and extremities. **A,** Patient confined in a triangular sheet with leg straps. **B,** Patient in a Pedi-Wrap. **C,** Patient lying in a beanbag dental chair insert. (**C** Courtesy Dr. Priscilla John Bond.)

disability can be expected to master many vocational, leisure, and self-help skills within a supportive environment with trained personnel who help them with problems with which they may not be able to cope on their own.

A child with severe or profound intellectual disability may present a significant challenge and may be grouped in special education programs. A student with severe to profound intellectual disability can achieve success with self-help, leisure, and some vocational skills given sufficient training and support. Group home placement can allow individuals with severe to profound intellectual disability a measure of independence while providing sufficient support for safety and continuing reinforcement.

DENTAL TREATMENT OF A PERSON WITH INTELLECTUAL DISABILITY

Children with intellectual disability may have a higher incidence of poor oral hygiene, gingivitis, malocclusion, and untreated caries. As the severity of intellectual disability increases, typical oral signs of clenching, bruxing, drooling, pica, trauma, missing teeth, and self-injurious behaviors increase. Providing dental treatment for a person with intellectual disability requires adjusting to social, intellectual, and emotional delays. A short attention span, restlessness, hyperactivity, and erratic emotional behavior may characterize patients with intellectual disability undergoing dental care. The dentist should assess the degree of intellectual disability by consulting the

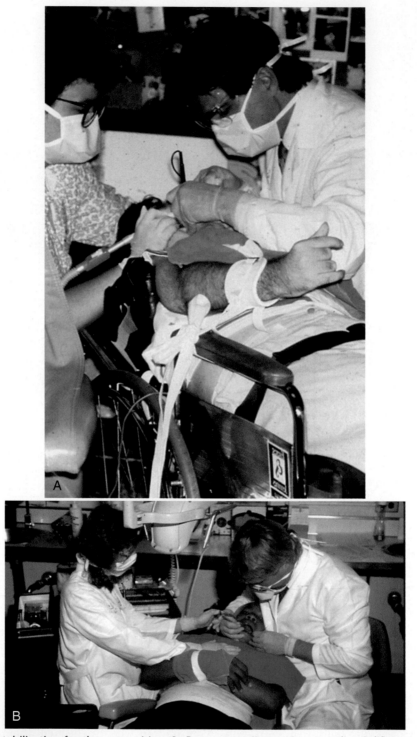

Figure 23-11 Protective stabilization for the extremities. **A,** Posey strap (Posey Co., Arcadia, Calif) on wrist. **B,** Towel and tape on forearm.

patient's physician for frequent medical assessment and coordinate care when appropriate.

The following procedures have proved beneficial in establishing dentist-patient-parent-staff rapport and reducing the patient's anxiety about dental care:

1. Give the family a brief tour of the office before attempting treatment. Introduce the patient and family (parent/caretaker/guardian) to the office staff. This will familiarize the patient with the personnel and facility and reduce the patient's fear of the unknown. Allow the patient to bring a favorite item (stuffed animal, blanket, or toy) to hold for the visit.

2. Be repetitive; speak slowly and in simple terms. Make sure explanations are understood by asking the patient if there are any questions. If the individual has an alternative communication system, such as a picture

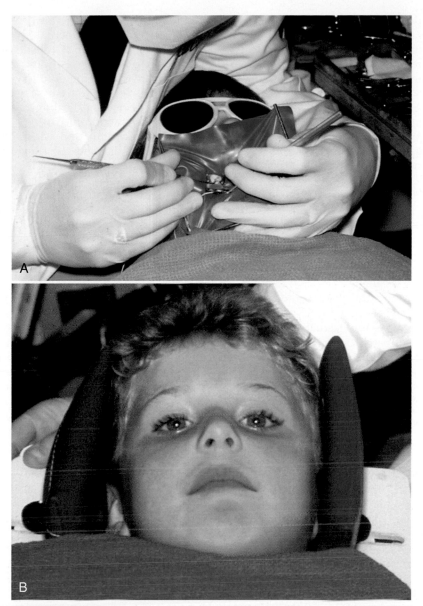

Figure 23-12 Protective stabilization aids for the head. **A,** Proper positioning of the dentist's hands, forearm, and body. **B,** Use of the Olympic Papoose Board head positioner.

Table 23-2

Classification of Intellectual Disability

Degree of Mental Disability	SB-IV	WISC-III	Communication	Special Requirements for Dental Care
Mild	67-52	69-55	Should be able to speak well enough for most communication needs	Treat as normal child; mild sedation or nitrous oxide–oxygen analgesia may be beneficial
Moderate	51-36	54-40	Has vocabulary and language skills such that the child can communicate at a basic level with others	Mild to moderate sedation may be beneficial; use restraints and positive reinforcement; general anesthesia may be indicated in cases of severe, generalized, dental decay
Severe or profound	35 and below	39 and below	Mute or communicates in grunts; little or no communication skills	Same as for moderately intellectually disabled

SB-IV, Stanford-Binet Intelligence Scale, 4th ed; WISC-III, Wechsler Intelligence Scale for Children, 3rd ed.

board or electronic device, be sure it is available to assist with dental explanations and instructions.

3. Give only one instruction at a time. Reward the patient with compliments after the successful completion of each procedure.
4. Actively listen to the patient. People with intellectual disability often have trouble with communication, and the dentist should be particularly sensitive to gestures and verbal requests.
5. Invite the parent/guardian into the operatory for assistance and to aid in communication with the patient when helpful.
6. Keep appointments short. Gradually progress to more difficult procedures (e.g., anesthesia and restorative dentistry) after the patient has become accustomed to the dental environment.
7. Schedule the patient's visit early in the day, on a lightly scheduled day, when the dentist, the staff, and the patient will be less fatigued.

With adequate preparation the dentist and the staff can provide a valuable service. By thoroughly understanding the patient's degree of intellectual disability and abilities, and by exercising patience and understanding, the dentist should have no significant problems in delivering dental care. When cooperation does not exist, sedation or general anesthesia may be an option.

DOWN SYNDROME (TRISOMY 21 SYNDROME)

Down syndrome is the best-known chromosomal disorder and is caused by the presence of an extra copy of chromosome 21(trisomy 21). Medical conditions that occur more frequently in infants and children with Down syndrome and increase the mortality of these individuals include cardiac defects, leukemia, and upper respiratory infections. The incidence of congenital cardiac defects is about 40%, and because of these patients' high susceptibility to periodontal disease, knowledge of a heart condition is essential for dental treatment. Children with Down syndrome have a 10- to 20-fold greater incidence of leukemia during infancy compared with the general population. This increased incidence of leukemia is not maintained later in life.

Skeletal findings are an underdeveloped midface, creating a prognathic occlusal relationship. Oral findings include mouth breathing, open bite, appearance of macroglossia, fissured lips and tongue, angular cheilitis, delayed eruption times, missing and malformed teeth, oligodontia, small roots, microdontia, crowding, and low level of caries. Children with Down syndrome experience a high incidence of rapid, destructive periodontal disease, which may be related to local factors such as tooth morphology, bruxism, malocclusion, and poor oral hygiene. Certain systemic factors are also believed to contribute to periodontal disease, including poor circulation, decreased humoral response, general physical deterioration at an early age, and genetic influences. Bell, and colleagues reported that severity of tooth wear (both attrition and erosion) was significantly greater in children with Down syndrome than in children without the syndrome.[12]

Many children with Down syndrome are affectionate and cooperative, and dental procedures can be provided without compromise if the dentist works at a slightly slower pace. Emphasis should be placed on preventive dental care with frequent follow-up visits to monitor oral hygiene. A recent study by Cheng and colleagues documented periodontal healing responses in adult patients with Down syndrome using nonsurgical periodontal therapy in conjunction with the use of chlorhexidine rinse twice a day and chlorhexidine gel and monthly recalls.[13] Comprehensive dental care is an overall goal with alteration based on the individual's level of functioning. Light sedation and immobilization may be indicated in those children who are moderately apprehensive. Severely resistive patients may require general anesthesia.

Delayed tooth eruption frequently occurs in children with Down syndrome. For this reason, additional discussion of this disorder is presented in Chapter 9.

LEARNING DISABILITIES

For years, students who consistently had difficulty achieving a level of academic performance concomitant with their intellectual capacity were unfortunately labeled as *retarded*. Today the term *learning disabled* is applied to children who exhibit a disorder in one or more of the basic psychological processes involved in understanding or using spoken or written language. Learning disabilities affect between 3% and 15% of the population. They occur four times more frequently among boys than among girls.

In 1968 the National Advisory Committee on Handicapped Children of the U.S. Department of Health, Education, and Welfare stated that learning disabilities "may be manifested in disorders of listening, thinking, talking, reading, writing, spelling, or arithmetic. They include conditions that have been referred to as perceptual handicaps, brain injury, minimal brain dysfunction, dyslexia, and developmental aphasia."[14] It should be emphasized that learning disabilities do not include learning problems caused mainly by hearing, visual, or motor handicaps, mental disability, emotional disturbance, or environmental conditions.

The cause of learning disabilities remains unclear. Physiologic factors, such as minimal brain injury or damage to the central nervous system, have been implicated. Because learning disabilities appear more frequently in some families than in others, a genetic factor has also been suggested. The possibility exists that severe emotional disturbances can develop as a result of learning disabilities. This potential has prompted early diagnosis and treatment of affected persons.

Most children with learning disabilities accept dental care and cause no unusual management problems for the dentist. If a child is resistant, behavioral management and conscious sedation techniques can be used with success.

FRAGILE X SYNDROME

Fragile X is an X-linked developmental disorder. It accounts for 30% to 50% of cases of X-linked mental disability. The defect is an abnormal gene on the terminal portion of the long arm of an X chromosome. Males are more vulnerable because they have only one X chromosome and are more significantly affected than females. Numerous studies have investigated fragile X syndrome in males, but fragile X syndrome in females has not been investigated as extensively because the physical and cognitive deficits in females are usually less severe. It is one of the most common genetic causes of learning disability, but because it is less phenotypically recognizable, reports of orofacial findings are limited.

A history of developmental delay and hyperactivity, and physical features such as prominent ears, long face, prominent jaw, flattened nasal bridge, hyperextensible joints, flat feet, mitral valve prolapse (MPV), simian creases of the palms, and postadolescent macroorchidism in males should be considered potential indicators for fragile X syndrome. A higher incidence of malocclusions including an open bite and crossbites have been reported

Behavioral features such as hand slapping, hand biting, and poor eye contact are frequently seen. Fragile X syndrome may be diagnosed in individuals with another diagnosis such as Down syndrome or cerebral palsy.

Treatment of children with fragile X syndrome is multidisciplinary, and speech, language, and occupational therapy are required to address the cognitive, language, and sensory integration problems. Medical intervention can be useful in decreasing the hyperactivity and improving the attention span. Females with fragile X syndrome have a more favorable outcome with appropriate intervention than males with fragile X syndrome.

Mode of dental treatment depends on the level of developmental delay, cognitive ability, and degree of hyperactivity. Those with mild cases may be treated by scheduling short appointments and using immobilization and/or conscious sedation. Severely affected individuals must be treated in the operating room under general anesthesia.

FETAL ALCOHOL SPECTRUM DISORDER

Fetal alcohol spectrum disorder (FASD) is an umbrella term that describes the range of effects that may occur with maternal consumption of alcohol during pregnancy. Its occurrence is about 40,000 babies per year and it is likely that the alcohol affects the normal development of the neural crest cells. The Centers for Disease Control and Prevention requires three facial findings, growth deficits, and central nervous system abnormalities to make the diagnosis but that even in the absence of the characteristic findings, FASD should be suspected in children with growth deficits, central nervous system abnormalities, and a history of prenatal alcohol exposure. Physical findings may include moderate to severe growth retardation with persistent microcephaly. There are often eye abnormalities, short palpebral fissures, a smooth philtrum, and a thin vermillion border. Cardiac malformations include ventricular septal defects, pulmonary artery hypoplasia, and interruption of the aortic arch. Hearing and vestibular problems are also seen and because the development of speech is dependent upon an intact hearing apparatus, children with FASD may have slurred speech, and poor

receptive and language skills. The vestibular damage may result in postural disturbances. Other associated abnormalities such as skeletal, urinary, and immune system impairment have also been reported.

Craniofacial features include midface underdevelopment, small teeth, absent teeth, high arched palate, delayed dental development, enamel anomalies, cleft lip or palate, crowded incisors, excessive maxillary overjet, and open bite.

AUTISM SPECTRUM DISORDER

Autism spectrum disorder (ASD) is an incapacitating disturbance of mental and emotional development that causes problems in learning, communicating, and relating to others. This lifelong developmental disability manifests itself during the first 3 years of life, is difficult to diagnose, and has no cure. In the past, autism was believed to be an emotional disability. The Diagnostic and Statistical Manual of Mental Disorders, published by the American Psychiatric Association, has listed ASD as a neurologic disorder. It is now believed to be caused by a physical disorder of the brain.

The prevalence of ASD is about 6 per 1000 people, with approximately four times more common in boys as girls. The number of people known to have ASD has increased dramatically since the 1980s, partly due to changes in diagnostic practice; the question of whether actual prevalence has increased is not clear.[15] Children with ASD look like unaffected children and have normal life spans. However, they have a limited capacity to communicate, socialize, and learn. Approximately 60% of persons diagnosed with ASD have IQ scores below 50, 20% have scores between 50 and 70, and only 20% have scores greater than 70. Special educational programs that use behavior modification techniques designed for the specific individual have proved helpful in training children with ASD. Counseling the family on effective management techniques in the home is essential in the overall training of persons with ASD.

Children with ASD have multiple medical and behavioral problems that make dental treatment difficult. These children often have poor muscle tone, poor coordination, drooling, a hyperactive knee jerk, and strabismus; 30% eventually develop epilepsy. Children with ASD may have strict routines and prefer soft foods and sweetened foods. Because of poor tongue coordination, children with ASD tend to pouch food instead of swallowing. This habit, combined with the desire for sweetened foods, leads to increased susceptibility to caries.

Because of their tendency to adhere to routines, children with ASD may require several dental visits to acclimate to the dental environment. The use of a Papoose Board or Pedi-Wrap and preappointment conscious sedation may be necessary and in some instances has a calming effect on the child.

CEREBRAL PALSY

Cerebral palsy is one of the primary handicapping conditions of childhood. The incidence of cerebral palsy in the United States, for all ages, is 1.5 to 3 cases per 1000 individuals. One newborn in approximately 200 live births will be affected with this condition. Cerebral palsy is not a specific disease entity but rather a collection of disabling disorders caused by insult and permanent damage to the brain in the prenatal and perinatal periods, during which time the central nervous system is still maturing. This disability might involve muscle weakness, stiffness, or paralysis; poor balance or irregular gait; and uncoordinated or involuntary movements.

Although many recognized conditions result in damage to the motor centers of the brain, in at least one third of the cases of cerebral palsy no discernible cause is found. It has been well established that any factor contributing to decreased oxygenation of the developing brain can be responsible for brain damage. In addition, causal relationships have been established between cerebral palsy and complications of labor or delivery; infections of the brain, such as meningitis and encephalitis; toxemias of pregnancy; congenital defects of the brain; kernicterus; poisoning with certain drugs and heavy metals; and accidents resulting in trauma to the head. There is a high correlation between premature birth and cerebral palsy. (Approximately one third of all infants born prematurely have a demonstrable nervous system abnormality.)

There are various types of cerebral palsy, which are distinguished according to the neuromuscular dysfunctions observed and the extent of anatomic involvement. Some persons may have almost imperceptible symptoms. Others are severely disabled, with no appreciable use of the muscles of their limbs and other voluntary muscles. It is imperative to keep in mind that two patients with the same type of cerebral palsy may show very disparate symptoms. The following terms are commonly used to designate involved areas of the body:

1. Monoplegia—involvement of one limb only
2. Hemiplegia—involvement of one side of the body
3. Paraplegia—involvement of both legs only
4. Diplegia—involvement of both legs with minimum involvement of both arms
5. Quadriplegia—involvement of all four limbs

The following outline provides a classification of cerebral palsy according to the type of neuromuscular dysfunction and lists a few of the basic characteristics of each type:

I. *Spastic* (approximately 70% of cases)
   A. Hyperirritability of involved muscles, resulting in exaggerated contraction when stimulated
   B. Tense, contracted muscles (e.g., Spastic hemiplegia affects one third of all children with cerebral palsy. The hand and arm are flexed and held in against the trunk. The foot and leg may be flexed and rotated internally, which results in a limping gait with circumduction of the affected leg.)
   C. Limited control of neck muscles, which results in head roll
   D. Lack of control of the muscles supporting the trunk, which results in difficulty in maintaining upright posture
   E. Lack of coordination of intraoral, perioral, and masticatory musculature; possibility of impaired chewing and swallowing, excessive drooling,

persistent spastic tongue thrust, and speech impairments

II. *Dyskinetic* (athetosis and choreoathetosis) (approximately 15% of cases)
   A. Constant and uncontrolled motion of involved muscles
   B. Succession of slow, twisting, or writhing involuntary movements (athetosis) or quick, jerky movements (choreoathetosis)
   C. Frequent involvement of neck musculature, which results in excessive movement of the head (Hypertonicity of these muscles may cause the head to be held back, with the mouth constantly open and the tongue positioned anteriorly or protruded.)
   D. Possibility of frequent, uncontrolled jaw movements, causing abrupt closure of the jaws or severe bruxism
   E. Frequent hypotonicity of perioral musculature with mouth breathing, tongue protrusion, and excessive drooling
   F. Facial grimacing
   G. Chewing and swallowing difficulties
   H. Speech problems

III. *Ataxic* (approximately 5% of cases)
   A. Inability of involved muscles to contract completely, so that voluntary movements can be only partially performed
   B. Poor sense of balance and uncoordinated voluntary movements (e.g., stumbling or staggering gait or difficulty in grasping objects)
   C. Possibility of tremors and an uncontrollable trembling or quivering on attempting voluntary tasks

IV. *Mixed* (approximately 10% of cases)
   A. Combination of characteristics of more than one type of cerebral palsy (e.g., mixed spastic-athetoid quadriplegia)

Two additional forms of cerebral palsy have been described but occur infrequently. In hypotonia, the muscles are flaccid (i.e., there is an inability to elicit muscle activity on volitional stimulation). In rigidity the muscles are in a constant state of contraction. The condition is characterized by prolonged periods in which the muscles of the extremities or trunk remain rigid, resisting any effort to move them.

In many patients with cerebral palsy, certain neonatal reflexes may persist long after the age at which they normally disappear. These primitive reflexes are usually modified or are progressively replaced as the subcortical dominance of the infant's behavior is suppressed by higher centers of the maturing central nervous system. Three of the most common reactions, which a dentist should recognize, are the following:

1. *Asymmetric tonic neck reflex.* If the patient's head is suddenly turned to one side, the arm and leg on the side to which the face is turned extends and stiffens. The limbs on the opposite side flex.
2. *Tonic labyrinthine reflex.* If the patient's head suddenly falls backward while the patient is supine, the back may assume the position known as *postural extension*; the legs and arms straighten out, and the neck and back arch.

3. *Startle reflex.* This reflex, which is frequently observed in persons with cerebral palsy, consists of sudden, involuntary, often forceful bodily movements. This reaction is produced when the patient is surprised by stimuli, such as sudden noises or unexpected movements by other people.

Because the motor involvement in cerebral palsy results from irreversible damage to the developing brain, other symptoms of organic brain damage may also be present. The fact that these other symptoms are frequently seen underscores the premise that cerebral palsy does not denote one specific disease entity. Rather, it is a complex of disabling conditions, the clinical manifestations of which depend on the extent and location of damage to the brain. The following are some common manifestations:

1. *Intellectual disability.* Approximately 60% of persons with cerebral palsy demonstrate some degree of intellectual disability.
2. *Seizure disorders.* Seizures are an accompanying condition in 30% to 50% of cases; they occur primarily during infancy and early childhood. Most seizures can be controlled with anticonvulsant medications.
3. *Sensory deficits or dysfunctions.* Impairment of hearing is more common than in the normal population, and eye disorders affect approximately 35% of persons with cerebral palsy. The most common visual defect is strabismus.
4. *Speech disorders.* More than half of patients with cerebral palsy have some speech problem—usually dysarthria, an inability to articulate well because of lack of control of the speech muscles.
5. *Joint contractures.* Persons with spasticity and rigidity demonstrate abnormal limb postures and contractures during growth and at maturity, primarily because of disuse of muscle groups.

No intraoral anomalies are unique to persons with cerebral palsy. However, several conditions are more common or more severe than in the general population. These conditions are as follows:

1. *Periodontal disease.* Periodontal disease and poor oral hygiene occurs with great frequency in persons with cerebral palsy. Often the patient will not be physically able to brush or floss adequately. When oral hygiene measures must be provided for the person by another individual, they may be performed infrequently and inadequately. Diet may also be significant; children who have difficulty chewing and swallowing tend to eat soft foods, which are easily swallowed and are high in carbohydrates. Patients with cerebral palsy who take phenytoin to control seizure activity will generally have a degree of gingival hyperplasia.
2. *Dental caries.* The data are conflicting regarding the incidence of dental caries in patients with cerebral palsy compared with the incidence in the general population. Except among institutionalized patients, the incidence of caries does not seem to be significantly greater among persons with cerebral palsy.
3. *Malocclusions.* The prevalence of malocclusions in patients with cerebral palsy is approximately twice that in the general population. Commonly observed conditions include noticeable protrusion of the maxillary anterior teeth, excessive overbite and overjet, open bites, and unilateral crossbites. A primary cause may be a disharmonious relationship between intraoral and perioral muscles. Uncoordinated and uncontrolled movements of jaws, lips, and tongue are observed with greater frequency in patients with cerebral palsy. This may result in impaired chewing and swallowing, excessive drooling, tongue thrust and speech impairment.
4. *Bruxism.* Bruxism is commonly observed in patients with athetoid cerebral palsy. Severe occlusal attrition of the primary and permanent dentition may be noted, with the resulting loss of vertical interarch dimension. Temporomandibular joint disorders may be sequelae of this condition in adult patients.
5. *Trauma.* Persons with cerebral palsy are more susceptible to trauma, particularly to the maxillary anterior teeth. This situation is related to the increased tendency to fall, along with a diminished extensor reflex to cushion such falls, and the frequent increased flaring of the maxillary anterior teeth. Susceptibilities also include aspiration and ingestion of a foreign body.

To an uninformed dentist, a person with cerebral palsy who has involuntary movements of the limbs and head might be perceived as an uncooperative and unmanageable patient. In addition, patients who have unintelligible speech, uncontrollable jaw movements, and spastic tongue are often erroneously assumed to be intellectually delayed. A clinician who is not knowledgeable about cerebral palsy and other physically and intellectually disabling conditions may feel uncomfortable about treating such patients and may refuse to do so.

In providing treatment for children with cerebral palsy, it is imperative that a dentist evaluate each patient thoroughly in terms of personal characteristics, symptoms, and behavior and then proceed as conditions and needs dictate.

The dentist should never make assumptions about the degree of a child's physical or intellectual impairments without first acquiring the facts. Taking a thorough medical and dental history is very important, and the parent or guardian should be interviewed before the initiation of any treatment. It may also be beneficial to consult the patient's physician regarding the patient's medical status.

A patient with cerebral palsy who has involuntary head movements may be cognizant of the need to minimize these movements while receiving dental care. Paradoxically, the patient's own endeavors to control these movements may only exacerbate the problem. Therefore it is imperative that all dental personnel be empathic about the fears and frustrations that such a person experiences. The importance of maintaining a calm, friendly, and professional atmosphere cannot be overemphasized.

The following suggestions are offered to the clinician as being of practical significance in treating a patient with cerebral palsy:

1. Consider treating a patient who uses a wheelchair in the wheelchair. Many patients express such a preference, and it is frequently more practical for the

dentist. For a young patient, the wheelchair may be tipped back into the dentist's lap.

2. If a patient is to be transferred to the dental chair, ask about a preference for the mode of transfer. If the patient has no preference, the two-person lift is recommended.

3. Make an effort to stabilize the patient's head throughout all phases of dental treatment.

4. Try to place and maintain the patient in the midline of the dental chair, with arms and legs as close to the body as feasible.

5. Keep the patient's back slightly elevated to minimize difficulties in swallowing. (It is advisable not to have the patient in a completely supine position.)

6. On placing the patient in the dental chair, determine the patient's degree of comfort and assess the position of the extremities. Do not force the limbs into unnatural positions. Consider the use of pillows, towels, and other measures for trunk and limb support.

7. Use stabilization judiciously to control flailing movements of the extremities.

8. For control of involuntary jaw movements, choose from a variety of mouth props. Patient preference should weigh heavily, since a patient with cerebral palsy may be very apprehensive about the ability to control swallowing. Such appliances may also trigger the strong gag reflex that many of these patients possess. Allow frequent time-outs for patient to regroup, relax and breath normally.

9. To minimize startle reflex reactions, avoid presenting stimuli such as abrupt movements, noises, and lights without forewarning the patient.

10. Introduce intraoral stimuli slowly to avoid eliciting a gag reflex or to make it less severe.

11. Consider the use of the rubber dam, a highly recommended technique, for restorative procedures.

12. Work efficiently, quickly and minimize patient time in the chair to decrease fatigue of the involved muscles.

13. Sedation or general anesthesia may be an option for more complex patients.

SPINA BIFIDA AND LATEX ALLERGY

Although the etiology of spina bifida is unknown, it is thought to be the result of a genetic predisposition whose manifestation is triggered by the environment. There are two common forms of this neural tube defect, spina bifida occulta and myelomeningocele. Spina bifida occulta (i.e., closed) presents with skin covering an area where tissue protrudes through a bony cleft in the vertebral column. These children may develop foot weakness or bowel and bladder sphincter disturbances. Myelomeningocele (spina bifida aperta, i.e., open) is the most severe because the spinal cord, spinal fluid, and membranes protrude in a sac through the defect. These children can suffer from hydrocephalus, paralysis, orthopedic deformities, and genitourinary abnormalities. Taking folic acid during the first 6 weeks of pregnancy can prevent over 50% of neural tube defects.

Children with neural tube defects are at higher risk for caries secondary to poor hygiene, poor nutritional intake, and long-term drug therapy. They are also at higher risk for latex allergy because they are frequently exposed to latex as a result of undergoing procedures in which latex products are used. Therefore, Nettis and colleagues[16] recommend that all patients be screened for conditions such as spina bifida and exposure to recurrent surgical procedures, and for a history of atopy, cross-reactive food allergies (i.e., allergies to banana, avocado, kiwi, and chestnuts, which may sensitize allergic patients to latex exposure), and previous reactions to natural rubber latex.

For all patients with a latex allergy or latex allergy risk factors, all equipment that comes in intimate contact with the patient should be made of nonlatex substitutes. Nettis and colleagues[16] suggest avoiding handling of nonlatex products while wearing latex gloves or with unwashed hands to prevent the transfer of latex allergens to nonlatex products. They suggest that the ideal time to schedule dental appointments for such individuals is at the beginning of a working session, such as in the morning or after a vacation when the office has been closed. This will allow for settling of airborne latex particles. Another good scheduling time is after the office has been professionally vacuumed and cleaned to remove latex-tainted cornstarch. Mild irritant reactions to latex can be managed with immediate removal of the rubber object and administration of an antihistamine. However, acute systemic reactions (anaphylaxis) require immediate treatment with epinephrine injection 1:1000 USP and may necessitate emergency resuscitation (call 911).

RESPIRATORY DISEASES

ASTHMA (REACTIVE AIRWAY DISEASE)

Asthma is a common childhood disease, affecting 1 in 10 children. Although often thought of as acute respiratory distress brought on by environmental factors, asthma is a chronic airway disease characterized by inflammation and bronchial constriction.

Asthma is a diffuse obstructive disease of the airway caused by edema of the mucous membranes, increased mucous secretions, and spasm of smooth muscle. It is twice as common in prepubertal boys but affects both sexes equally during adolescence and adulthood. The etiology includes biochemical, immunologic, infectious, endocrine, and psychological factors. The typical symptoms of asthma are coughing, wheezing, chest tightness, and dyspnea. The clinical onset of an episode may occur over minutes (acute) or hours and days. An acute attack is associated with exposure to irritants such as cold air, fumes, or dust, and it may develop in minutes. An attack developing over days is usually precipitated by a viral respiratory infection. Severe bronchial obstruction results in labored breathing, wheezing, tachypnea, profuse perspiration, cyanosis, hyperventilation, tachycardia, and sometimes chest pain. A dental procedure constitutes an acute irritant to the airways of the asthmatic child and may precipitate an attack.

Fortunately, three fourths of childhood asthma is mild, with minimal daily symptoms and short-lived exacerbations. Before initiating dental treatment, the dentist should know what are the frequency and severity of the attacks, what are the triggering agents, when the patient was hospitalized and/or in the emergency department, when the last attack occurred, what medications the patient takes, and what limitations on activity the patient may have. Patients taking systemic corticosteroids and those who were hospitalized or in the emergency department in the past year should be treated with caution because they are at higher risk of morbidity and mortality. Sometimes, deferring the dental visit until the patient's asthma is controlled is the best approach.

Patients who use bronchodilators should take a dose before their appointment, and they should bring their inhalers or nebulizers into the dental office in case trouble arises. Acute symptoms may be prevented by the use of the child's bronchodilator (inhaled β2 receptor agonist such as albuterol or terbutaline sulfate). Behavioral methods are employed to reduce anxiety, and the use of nitrous oxide–oxygen analgesia may be helpful. Hydroxyzine hydrochloride (Vistaril) and diazepam (Valium) have been successful in alleviating anxiety. Barbiturates and narcotics are not indicated because of their potential for histamine release leading to a bronchospasm. Aspirin compounds and non steroidal antiinflammatory agents are contraindicated because about 4% of patients experience wheezing after taking these drugs. Acetaminophen is recommended. Positioning a child with mild asthmatic symptoms in an upright or semiupright position for the dental procedure may be beneficial.

Oral findings of children with moderate to severe asthma include higher caries rate, decreased salivary rate, increased prevalence of oral mucosal change characteristic of chronic mouth breathers, and increased levels of gingivitis. Increased incidence of orofacial abnormalities such as high palatal vault, more posterior crossbites, greater overjets, and increased facial height is also seen.

Dental goals are similar to those for other patients, with care taken to avoid the potential for dental materials and products to exacerbate the asthma. The patient's pulmonary function, propensity for developing an attack, immune status, and adrenal status should be evaluated prior to dental treatment. Emergency treatment for a person with asthma who is in respiratory distress requires discontinuing the dental procedure, reassuring the patient, and opening the airway. Administer 100% oxygen while placing the patient in an upright or comfortable position. Keeping the airway open, administer the patient's β2 agonist with an inhaler or nebulizer. If there is no improvement, administer subcutaneous epinephrine (0.01 mg/kg of 1:1000 solution) and obtain medical assistance immediately.

BRONCHOPULMONARY DYSPLASIA

Bronchopulmonary dysplasia is a chronic lung disease usually resulting from the occurrence during infancy of respiratory distress syndrome that requires prolonged ventilation with a high concentration of inspired oxygen. Chronic lung changes are more likely to occur in the premature infant. The incidence is 80% to 90% in infants weighing less than 1000 g at birth. With the increased survival of low-birth-weight infants, the prevalence of bronchopulmonary dysplasia has increased. The lung pathology of children with bronchopulmonary dysplasia shows evidence of bronchial ulceration, necrosis with plugging of bronchiolar lumina, and inflammatory cells. This bronchiolar injury compromises further lung development. Inflammatory changes and bronchiolar fibrosis lead to increased airway resistance and contribute to the hypoxemia seen in infants with bronchopulmonary dysplasia. Some children with bronchopulmonary dysplasia develop right ventricular hypertrophy (cor pulmonale). Other significant pulmonary complications include tracheal stenosis, upper airway obstruction secondary to subglottic cysts, and hoarseness because of partial or complete vocal cord paralysis. About 20% of infants with bronchopulmonary dysplasia die within the first year of life. The major causes of death are cor pulmonale, respiratory infections, and sudden death.

An increased oxygen supply must be provided to prevent hypoxic pulmonary vasoconstriction and to decrease the work of breathing. The nasal cannula provides continuous oxygen delivery, which results in fewer fluctuations in oxygen tension. Weaning off oxygen is possible with improved lung function and lung size. Children who develop cor pulmonale may require diuretic therapy to prevent congestive heart failure.

Dental care for children with bronchopulmonary dysplasia requires more chair time than usual. These children often spend a significant part of their early lives in the hospital and exhibit significant oral defensiveness.

After the initial dental evaluation, consultation with a pulmonologist is beneficial to plan safe dental treatment for the patient. If the dental patient is taking oxygen continuously via a nasal cannula, short appointments with frequent breaks are necessary to prevent the development of pulmonary vasoconstriction. Parents of children with bronchopulmonary dysplasia may need to provide additional oral hygiene for their children when these children are required to eat frequent small meals to maintain the proper caloric intake. Any nonemergent dental care should be avoided when the patient is not doing well medically.

CYSTIC FIBROSIS

Cystic fibrosis is an autosomal recessive disorder occurring in 1 of every 2000 births. It is the most common lethal genetic disorder affecting whites. The genetically altered protein affects exocrine gland function. The defective exocrine gland function leads to micro obstruction of the pancreas, which results in cystic degeneration of the pancreas and ultimately a digestive enzyme deficiency producing malabsorption of nutrients.

The defective gene products cause abnormal water and electrolyte transport across epithelial cells, which results in a chronic disease of the respiratory and gastrointestinal system, elevated levels of electrolytes in sweat, and impaired reproductive function.

In the lungs, retention of mucus occurs, which causes obstructive lung disease and increased frequency of infections. As the progressive lung disease develops, there is an increase in chest diameter, clubbing of the fingers and toes, decreased exercise tolerance, and a chronic productive cough. Before advances in antibiotic therapy, physical therapy, and nutritional supplementation, these individuals rarely survived childhood. The median life expectancy has been increased to 31 years. Death is most frequently the result of pneumonia and anoxia after a long period of respiratory insufficiency. Cystic fibrosis–related diabetes is becoming more common as patients live longer.

Children with cystic fibrosis have a high incidence of tooth discoloration when systemic tetracyclines are taken during tooth formation. With the advent of alternative antibiotics the incidence of tooth discoloration is decreasing. The incidence of dental caries in children with cystic fibrosis is low secondary to long-term antibiotic therapy, buffering capacity of excess calcium in the saliva, and pancreatic enzyme replacement therapy. There is a high incidence of mouth breathing and open-bite malocclusion associated with chronic nasal and sinus obstruction. Patients with cystic fibrosis may prefer to be treated in a more upright position to allow them to clear secretions more easily. The use of sedative agents that interfere with pulmonary function should be avoided, and the patient's physician should be contacted before using nitrous oxide–oxygen sedation in a patient exhibiting evidence of severe emphysema.

HEARING LOSS

Hearing loss (deafness) is a disability that is often overlooked because it is not obvious. Total hearing loss affects 1.8 million people, and there are 14 million hearing-impaired individuals in the United States. About 1 in 600 neonates has a congenital hearing loss. During the neonatal period, many more acquire hearing loss from other associated conditions. Almost inevitably, speech is affected. If an impairment is severe enough that dentist and child cannot communicate verbally, the dentist must use sight, taste, and touch to communicate and to allow the child to learn about dental experiences. Table 23-3 shows how speech and psychological problems relate to various degrees of hearing loss. Many times, mild hearing losses are not diagnosed, which leads to management problems because of the child's misunderstanding of instructions; children with more severe hearing losses already have psychological and social disturbances that make dental behavior management more complex. Parents may suspect profound hearing loss if their infant does not respond to ordinary sounds or voices. Early identification and correction of hearing loss is essential for normal development of communication skills. No abnormal dental findings are associated with hearing loss.

The following are known causes of hearing loss:
• Prenatal factors
• Viral infections, such as rubella and influenza
• Ototoxic drugs, such as aspirin, streptomycin, neomycin, kanamycin
• Congenital syphilis
• Heredity disorders (e.g., Alport, Arnold-Chiari, Crouzon, Hunter, Klippel-Feil, Stickler, Treacher Collins, and Waardenburg syndromes)
• Perinatal factors

Table 23-3

Implications of Auditory Disability Relative to International Standards Organization (ISO) Reference Levels*

Iso (DB)	Disability	Speech Comprehension	Psychological Problems in Children
0	Insignificant	Little or no difficulty	None
25	Slight	Difficulty with faint speech; language and speech development within normal limits	Child may show a slight verbal deficit
40	Mild-moderate	Frequent difficulty with normal speech at 3 feet (91.4 cm); language skills are mildly affected	Psychological problems can be recognized.
55	Marked	Frequent difficulty with loud speech at 3 feet (91.4 cm); difficulty understanding with hearing aid in school situation	Child is likely to be educationally retarded, with more pronounced emotional and social problems than in children with normal hearing.
70	Severe	May understand only shouts or amplified speech at 1 foot (30.5 cm) from ear	The prelingually deaf show pronounced educational retardation and evident emotional and social problems.
90	Extreme	Usually no understanding of speech even when amplified; child does not rely on hearing for communication	The prelingually deaf usually show severe intellectual disability emotional underdevelopment.

*Reference levels are in decibels relative to threshold in young patients with normal hearing.
Adapted from Goetzinger CP. The psychology of hearing impairment. In Katz J, ed. *Handbook of Clinical Audiology*, 2nd ed. Baltimore, 1978, Williams & Wilkins.

- Toxemia late in pregnancy
- Prematurity
- Birth injury
- Anoxia
- Erythroblastosis fetalis
- Postnatal factors
- Viral infections, such as mumps, measles, chickenpox, influenza, poliomyelitis, meningitis
- Injuries

The following should be considered when treating a hearing-impaired patient:

1. Prepare the patient and parent before the first visit with a welcome letter that states what is to be done and include a medical history form.
2. Let the patient and parent determine during the initial appointment how the patient desires to communicate (i.e., interpreter, lip-reading, sign language, note writing, or a combination of these). Look for ways to improve communication. It is useful to learn some basic sign language. Face the patient and speak slowly at a natural pace and directly to the patient without shouting. Exaggeration of facial expressions and the use of slang make lip-reading difficult. Even the best lip-readers comprehend only 30% to 40% of what is said.
3. Assess speech, language ability, and degree of hearing impairment when taking the patient's complete medical history. Identify the age of onset, type, degree, and cause of hearing loss, and determine whether any other family members are affected.
4. Enhance visibility for communication. Watch the patient's expression. Make sure the patient understands what the dental equipment is, what is going to happen, and how it will feel. Have the patient use hand gestures if a problem arises. Write out and display information.
5. Reassure the patient with physical contact; hold the patient's hand initially, or place a hand reassuringly on the patient's shoulder while the patient maintains visual contact. Without visual contact the child may be startled. Explain to the patient if you must leave the room.
6. Employ the tell-show-feel-do approach. Use visual aids and allow the patient to see the instruments, and demonstrate how they work. Hearing-impaired children may be very sensitive to vibration.
7. Display confidence; use smiles and reassuring gestures to build up confidence and reduce anxiety. Allow extra time for all appointments.
8. Avoid blocking the patient's visual field, especially with a rubber dam.
9. Adjust the hearing aid (if the patient has one) before the handpiece is in operation, because a hearing aid amplifies all sounds. Many times the patient will prefer to have it turned off.
10. Make sure the parent or patient understands explanations of diagnosis, treatment, and payment. Deaf persons have different levels of skill with English. Use of an interpreter is extremely helpful.

VISUAL IMPAIRMENT

Total visual impairment (blindness) affects more than 30 million people. The list that follows gives some of the known causes of visual impairment; however, in more than 35% of those affected the cause is either unknown or unreported. Blindness is not an all-or-nothing phenomenon; a person is considered to be affected by blindness if the visual acuity does not exceed 20/200 in the better eye with corrective lenses or if the acuity is greater than 20/200 but is accompanied by a visual field of no greater than 20 degrees.

The following are known causes of visual impairment:

- Prenatal causes
- Optic atrophy
- Microphthalmos
- Cataracts
- Colobomas
- Dermoid and other tumors
- Toxoplasmosis
- Cytomegalic inclusion disease
- Syphilis
- Rubella
- Tuberculous meningitis
- Developmental abnormalities of the orbit
- Postnatal causes
- Trauma
- Retrolental fibroplasia
- Hypertension
- Premature birth
- Polycythemia vera
- Hemorrhagic disorders
- Leukemia
- Diabetes mellitus
- Glaucoma

Visual impairment may be only one aspect of a child's disability. For example, a patient with congenital rubella may have deafness, mental retardation, congenital heart disease, and dental defects, as well as blindness resulting from congenital cataracts. Total visual impairment is one disorder that may result in frequent hospitalizations, separation from family, and slow social development. Because the capabilities of a child with blindness are difficult to assess, the child may be considered developmentally delayed.

Consideration must be given to every developmental aspect of a child with blindness. Early in development the parents may experience guilt and either overprotect or reject the child; this can result in a lack of development of self-help skills and delayed development in general, which is often misinterpreted as intellectually disabled. Assessment of parental attitudes is of primary importance in behavioral management. In addition, children with blindness may exhibit self-stimulating activities, such as eye pressing, finger flicking, rocking, and head banging. Therefore assessment of the child's socialization is useful in the management of dental behavior.

A distinction should be made between children who at one time had sight and those who have not and thus do not form visual concepts. More explanation is needed for children in the latter category to help them perceive the dental environment. Dentists should realize that congenitally visually impaired children need a greater display of affection and love early in life and that they differ intellectually from children who are not congenitally visually impaired. Although explanation is accomplished through touching and hearing, reinforcement takes place through smelling and tasting. The modalities of listening, touching, tasting, and smelling are extremely important for these children in helping to learn coping behavior. Reports indicate that, once speech is developed, the other senses assume heightened importance and other development can occur that is comparable to that in children with sight.

Reports also reveal that motor activity affects the development of language and perception. Visually impaired children tend to have more accidents than other children during the early years while they are acquiring motor skills.

Hypoplastic teeth and trauma to the anterior teeth have been reported to occur with greater than average frequency in visually impaired children. Such children are also more likely to have gingival inflammation because of their inability to see and remove plaque. Other dental abnormalities occur with the same frequency as in the general population.

Before initiating dental treatment for a visually impaired child, the dentist should keep the following points in mind:

1. Determine the degree of visual impairment. (Can the patient tell light from dark?)
2. If the patient is accompanied by a companion, find out if the companion is an interpreter. If he or she is not, address the patient.
3. Establish rapport; afterward offer verbal and physical reassurance. Avoid expressions of pity or references to visual impairment as an affliction.
4. In guiding the patient to the operatory, ask if the patient desires assistance. Do not grab, move, or stop the patient without verbal warning. Encourage the parent to accompany the child.
5. Paint a picture in the mind of the visually impaired child by describing the office setting and treatment. Always give the patient adequate descriptions before performing treatment procedures. It is important to use the same office setting for each dental visit to allay the patient's anxiety.
6. Introduce other office personnel very informally.
7. When making physical contact, do so reassuringly. Holding the patient's hand often promotes relaxation.
8. Allow the patient to ask questions about the course of treatment and answer them, keeping in mind that the patient is highly individual, sensitive, and responsive.
9. Allow a patient who wears eyeglasses to keep them on for protection and security.
10. Rather than using the tell-show-feel-do approach, invite the patient to touch, taste, or smell, recognizing that these senses are acute. Avoid sight references.
11. Describe in detail instruments and objects to be placed in the patient's mouth. Demonstrate a rubber cup on the patient's fingernail.
12. Because strong tastes may be rejected, use smaller quantities of dental materials with such characteristics.
13. Some patients may be photophobic. Ask parents about light sensitivity and allow these patients to wear sunglasses.
14. Explain the procedures of oral hygiene and then place the patient's hand over yours as you slowly but deliberately guide the toothbrush.
15. Use audiocassette tapes and braille dental pamphlets explaining specific dental procedures to supplement information and decrease chair time.
16. Announce exits from and entrances to the dental operatory cheerfully. Keep distractions to a minimum, and avoid unexpected loud noises.
17. Limit providers of the patient's dental care to one dentist whenever possible.
18. Maintain a relaxed atmosphere. Remember that your patient cannot see your smile.

The provision of dental care to a visually impaired child is facilitated by an in-depth understanding of the patient's background. A team approach by all health professionals involved in the care of the child is ideal. Disease prevention and continuity of care are of utmost importance.

HEART DISEASE

Heart disease can be divided into two general types: congenital and acquired. Because individuals with heart disease may require special precautions during dental treatment, such as antibiotic coverage for prevention of infective endocarditis (IE), a dentist should closely evaluate the medical histories of all patients to ascertain their cardiovascular status. In April 2007, the American Heart Association presented recommendations to conserve the use of antibiotics for the prevention of IE to minimize the risk of developing resistance to current regimens.[17]

CONGENITAL HEART DISEASE

The incidence of congenital heart disease is approximately 9 in 1000 births. The following is the relative incidence of congenital heart defects (Toronto Heart Registry):

Defect	Percent
Ventricular septal defect	22
Patent ductus arteriosus	17
Tetralogy of Fallot	11
Transposition of the great vessels	8
Atrial septal defect	7
Pulmonary stenosis	7
Coarctation of the aorta	6
Aortic stenosis	5
Tricuspid atresia	3
All others	14

The cause of a congenital heart defect is obscure. Generally it is a result of aberrant embryonic development of a normal structure or the failure of a structure to progress beyond an early stage of embryonic development. Only rarely can a causal factor be identified in congenital heart disease. Maternal rubella and chronic maternal alcohol abuse are known to interfere with normal cardiogenesis. If a parent or a sibling has a congenital heart defect, the chances that a child will be born with a heart defect are about 5 to 10 times greater than average. Congenital heart disease can be classified into two groups: acyanotic and cyanotic.

Acyanotic Congenital Heart Disease.

Acyanotic congenital heart disease is characterized by minimal or no cyanosis and is commonly divided into two major groups. The first group consists of defects that cause left-to-right shunting of blood within the heart. This group includes ventricular septal defect and atrial septal defect. Clinical manifestations of these defects can include congestive heart failure, pulmonary congestion, heart murmur, labored breathing, and cardiomegaly.

The second major group consists of defects that cause obstruction (e.g., aortic stenosis and coarctation of the aorta). The clinical manifestations can include labored breathing and congestive heart failure.

Cyanotic Congenital Heart Disease

Cyanotic congenital heart disease is characterized by right-to-left shunting of blood within the heart. Cyanosis is often observed even during minor exertion. Examples of such defects are tetralogy of Fallot, transposition of the great vessels, pulmonary stenosis, and tricuspid atresia. Clinical manifestations can include cyanosis, hypoxic spells, poor physical development, heart murmurs, and clubbing of the terminal phalanges of the fingers (Fig. 23-13).

ACQUIRED HEART DISEASE

Rheumatic Fever

Rheumatic fever is a serious inflammatory disease that occurs as a delayed sequela to pharyngeal infection with group A streptococci. Rheumatic fever is a commonly diagnosed cause of acquired heart disease in patients under 40 years of age. The mechanism by which the group A Streptococcus strains initiate the disease is unknown.

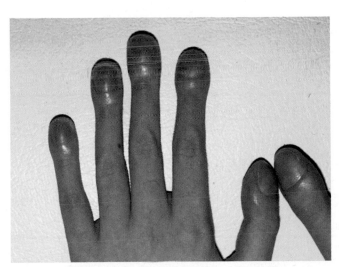

Figure 23-13 Hand of a 9-year-old boy with tetralogy of Fallot. Clubbing of the terminal phalanges is apparent.

The infection can involve the heart, joints, skin, central nervous system, and subcutaneous tissue. In general the incidence of rheumatic fever is decreasing. However, the incidence after exudative pharyngitis in epidemics is approximately 3%. (The incidence is much lower when the streptococcal pharyngitis is less severe.)

Although rheumatic fever can occur at any age, it is rare in infancy. It appears most commonly between the ages of 6 and 15 years. Rheumatic fever is most prevalent in temperate zones and at high altitudes and is more common and severe in children who live in substandard conditions. The clinical symptoms of rheumatic fever vary.

Cardiac involvement is the most significant pathologic sequela of rheumatic fever; carditis develops in approximately 50% of patients. Cardiac involvement can be fatal during the acute phase or can lead to chronic rheumatic heart disease as a result of scarring and deformity of heart valves.

Infective Endocarditis

Infective endocarditis (IE) is one of the most serious infections of humans. It is characterized by microbial infection of the heart valves or endocardium in proximity to congenital or acquired cardiac defects. IE has been classically divided into acute and subacute forms. The acute form is a fulminating disease that usually occurs when microorganisms of high pathogenicity attack a normal heart, causing erosive destruction of the valves. Microorganisms associated with the acute form include *Staphylococcus*, group A *Streptococcus*, and *Pneumonococcus*. In contrast, subacute IE usually develops in persons with preexisting congenital cardiac disease or rheumatic valvular lesions. Surgical placement of prosthetic heart valves can also predispose a patient to IE; heart valve infections occur in 1% to 2% of such patients. The subacute form is commonly caused by viridans streptococci, microorganisms common to the flora of the oral cavity.

Embolization is a characteristic feature of infective endocarditis. Microorganisms introduced into the bloodstream may colonize the endocardium at or near congenital valvular defects, valves damaged by rheumatic fever, or prosthetic heart valves. These vegetations, composed of microorganisms and fibrous exudate, may separate and, depending on whether the endocarditis involves the left or right side of the heart, be propelled into the systemic or pulmonary circulation.

The clinical symptoms of IE include low, irregular fever (afternoon or evening peaks) with sweating, malaise, anorexia, weight loss, and arthralgia. Inflammation of the endocardium increases cardiac destruction, and murmurs subsequently develop. Painful fingers and toes and skin lesions are also important symptoms. Laboratory findings can include leukocytosis and neutrophilia and normocytic, normochromic anemia. The erythrocyte sedimentation rate is rapid.

Infective Endocarditis Prophylaxis

Transient bacteremia is an important initiating factor in IE. Procedures known to precipitate transient bacteremias in dentistry and for which IE prophylaxis is or is not recommended are included in Box 23-1.

Dental Procedures for Which Endocarditis Prophylaxis Is Reasonable for Highest Risk Patients

All dental procedures that involve manipulation of gingival tissue or the periapical region of teeth or perforation of the oral mucosa*

*PRN prophylaxis: routine anesthetic injections through non-infected tissue, taking dental radiographs, placement of removable prosthodontic or orthodontic appliances, adjustment of orthodontic appliances, placement of orthodontic brackets, shedding of deciduous teeth, and bleeding from trauma to the lips or oral mucosa. From Wilson W, et al. Prevention of infective endocarditis: Guidelines from American Heart Association. Circulation 2007;116:1736-1754. Reprinted with permission ©2007, American Heart Association, Inc.

Certain heart conditions are associated with the highest risk of adverse outcomes from IE (Box 23-2). Any dental patient who has a history of congenital heart disease or rheumatic heart disease or who has a prosthetic heart valve should be considered susceptible. The American Heart Association's antibiotic recommendations for prevention of bacterial endocarditis are presented in Box 23-3.

The recent AHA revision concluded only a small number of cases of IE might be prevented by antibiotic prophylaxis for dental procedures even if such prophylactic therapy were 100% effective. IE prophylaxis for invasive dental procedures involving the manipulation of gingival tissue or the periapical region of teeth or perforation of the oral mucosa is only for patients with the highest risk of adverse outcome (see Box 23-2). Prophylaxis is not recommended.[16,17]

DENTAL MANAGEMENT

Parents of patients with cardiac risks typically lack knowledge about IE even after being informed during routine cardiology visits. Hayes and Fasules[18] report a deficiency of knowledge among dentists regarding the indications for prophylaxis and the antibiotic regimen required to prevent IE. Before initiating care, the dentist should obtain a thorough medical and dental history, perform a physical examination, formulate a complete treatment plan, and discuss the treatment with the child's physician or cardiologist. Behavior management techniques are useful, and conscious sedation and nitrous oxide–oxygen analgesia also have been proven beneficial in reducing anxiety in such patients. Conscious sedation monitoring and cardiopulmonary resuscitation equipment should be readily available during the appointment. If general anesthesia is indicated, the dental procedures should be completed in a hospital setting, where adequate supportive care is available if needed.

Other considerations are especially important in treating patients who are susceptible to IE:
- Pulp therapy is not recommended for primary teeth with a poor prognosis because of the high incidence of associated chronic infection. Extraction of such teeth with appropriate fixed-space maintenance is preferred.
- Endodontic therapy in the permanent dentition can usually be accomplished successfully if the teeth to be treated are carefully selected and the endodontic therapy is adequately performed.
- A dentist who feels uncomfortable in treating patients who are susceptible to IE has a responsibility to refer them to someone who will adequately care for them.

CARDIAC SURGERY PATIENTS

Patients who are to undergo cardiac surgery should first have a careful dental evaluation so that any needed dental treatment can be completed beforehand. This practice, along with an implemented preventive dental program, will decrease the incidence of postoperative IE from oral sources.

After dental radiographs are obtained and an evaluation is performed, a consultation with the patient's cardiologist is in order to plan required dental treatment

Cardiac Conditions Associated with the Highest Risk of Adverse Outcome from Endocarditis for Which Prophylaxis with Dental Procedures Is Reasonable

Prosthetic cardiac valve or prosthetic material used for cardiac valve repair
Previous infective endocarditis
Congenital heart disease (CHD)*
Unrepaired cyanotic CHD, including palliative shunts and conduits
Completely repaired congenital heart defect with prosthetic material or device, whether placed by surgery or by catheter intervention, during the first 6 months after the procedure†
Repaired CHD with residual defects at the site or adjacent to the site of prosthetic patch or prosthetic device (which inhibit endothelialization)
Cardiac transplantation recipients who develop cardiac valvulopathy

*Except for the conditions listed above, antibiotic prophylaxis is no longer recommended for any other form of CHD.
†Prophylaxis is reasonable because endothelialization of prosthetic material occurs within 6 months after the procedure.
From Wilson W, et al. Prevention of infective endocarditis: Guidelines from American Heart Association. Circulation 2007;116:1736-1754. Reprinted with permission ©2007, American Heart Association, Inc.

Box 23-3

Regimens for a Dental Procedure

Situation	Agent	Regimen: Single Dose 30 to 60 Minutes before Procedure	
		Adults	**Children**
Oral	Amoxicillin	2 g	50 mg/kg
Unable to take oral medication	Ampicillin OR	2 g IM or IV	50 mg/kg IM or IV
	Cefazolin or ceftriaxone	1 g IM or IV	50 mg/kg IM or IV
Allergic to penicillins or ampicillin— oral	Cephalexin *† OR	2 g	50 mg/kg
	Clindamycin OR	600 mg	20 mg/kg
	Azithromycin or clarithromycin	500 mg	15 mg/kg
Allergic to penicillin or ampicillin and unable to take oral medication	Cefazolin or ceftriaxone† OR	1g IM or IV	50 mg/kg IM or IV
	Clindamycin	600 mg IM or IV	20 mg/kg IM or IV

IM, intramuscular; IV, intravenous.
*Or other first-or second-generation oral cephalosporin in equivalent adult or pediatric dosage.
†Cephalosporins should not be used in an individual with a history of anaphylaxis, angioedema, or urticaria with penicillins or ampicillin.

before surgery. The cardiologist will indicate the specific desired antibiotic prophylaxis needed before the dental treatment. The dental examination and preventive dental program should be implemented before 6 months of age when possible. Ideally, dental treatment should be completed within 3 or 4 weeks of the planned surgery to allow for healing and the return of normal flora.

REFERENCES

1. University of Florida College of Dentistry. Oral health care for persons with disabilities. Available at: http://www.dental.ufl.edu/Faculty/PBurtner/Disabilities/English/titlepag.htm. Accessed Feb. 17, 2009.
2. American Academy of Pediatric Dentistry. Guideline on Management of Dental Patients with Special Health Care Needs. Pediatr Dent (Supp Issue: Ref. Manual, 2008-09) 2009;30:15.
3. US Dept of Health and Human Services. Oral health in America: a report of the Surgeon General, Rockville, MD: US Dept of Health and Human Services, National Institute of Dental and Craniofacial Research, National Institutes of Health, 2000.
4. Kane D, et al. Factors associated with access to dental care for children with special health care needs, *J Am Dent Assoc* 139:326-333, 2008.
5. Chen AY, Newacheck PW. Insurance coverage and financial burden for families of children with special health care needs, *Ambul Pediatr* 6(4):204-209, 2006.
6. Uniform Federal Accessibility Standards, part II, *Fed Reg* 153(49):31528-31613, 1984.
7. US Dept of Health and Human Services Health Insurance Portability and Accountability Act (HIPAA). Available at: http://aspe.hhs.gov/admnsimp/pl104191.htm. Accessed Feb. 17, 2009.
8. Beltran-Aguilar E, Goldstein J. Fluoride varnishes: a review of their clinical use, cariostatic mechanisms, efficacy, and safety, *J Am Dent Assoc* 131:589-596, 2000.
9. American Academy of Pediatric Dentistry. Behavior guidance for the pediatric dental patient (supplemental issue: Reference manual 2008-09), *Pediatr Dent* 30:125-133, 2009.
10. Mink JR. Dental care for the handicapped child. In Goldman HM et al, eds. *Current therapy in dentistry*, vol 2. St Louis, 1966, Mosby.
11. Schalock RL, et al. The renaming of mental retardation: understanding the change to the term intellectual disability, *Intellect Dev Disabil* 45(2):116-124, 2007.
12. Bell EJ, et al. Tooth wear in children with Down syndrome, *Aust Dent J* 47:30-35, 2002.
13. Cheng RH, et al. Non-surgical periodontal therapy chlorhexidine use in adults with Down syndrome, *J Periodontol* 79(2)379-385, 2008.
14. National Advisory Committee on Handicapped Children. Special Education for Handicapped Children, First Annual Report. Washington, DC, US Department of Health, Education and Welfare, 1968.
15. Newschaffer CJ, et al. The epidemiology of autism spectrum disorders, *Annu Rev Public Health* 28:235-258, 2007.
16. Nettis E, et al. Reported latex allergy in dental patients, *Oral Surg Oral Med Oral Pathol Oral Radiol Endod* 93(2):144-148 2002.
17. Wilson W, et al. Prevention of infective endocarditis: guidelines from American Heart Association, *Circulation* 116:1736-1754, 2007.
18. Hayes PA, Fasules J. Dental screening of pediatric cardiac surgical patients, *J Dent Child* 68:255-258, 2001.

SUGGESTED READINGS

Abman SH, Mourani PM, Sontag M. Bronchopulmonary dysplasia: a genetic disease, *Pediatrics* 122(3):658-659, 2008.
American Academy of Pediatric Dentistry. Reference manual 2008-09. Chicago, The Academy, 2009.
Aps JK, Van Maele GO, Martens LC. Oral hygiene habits and oral health in cystic fibrosis, *Eur J Paediatr Dent* 3(4):181-187, 2002.

Barnett ML. Dental treatment program for patients with mental retardation, *Ment Retard* 26:310, 1988.

Barnett ML et al. The prevalence of periodontitis and dental caries in the Down syndrome population, *J Periodontol* 57:288-293, 1986.

Behrman RE, et al. Nelson textbook of pediatrics, 18th ed. Philadelphia, 2007, WB Saunders.

Bill D, Weddell JA. Dental office access for the disabled, *Spec Care Dentist* 7:246-252, 1987.

Brown ER. Bronchopulmonary dysplasia. In Taeusch HW, Yogman MW, eds. *Follow-up management of the high-risk infant.* Boston, 1987, Little, Brown.

Clark CA et al. *Dental treatment for deaf patients, Spec Care Dentist* 6:102-106, 1986.

Danforth HA, et al. Dental management of the cerebral palsied patient. Project DECOD, Seattle, 1978, University of Washington.

Engar RC, Stiefel DJ. *Dental treatment of the sensory impaired patient.* Seattle, 1977, Disability Dental Instruction.

Fernald GW, et al. Cystic fibrosis: a current review, *Pediatr Dent* 12:72-77, 1990.

Hagerman RJ. Fragile X syndrome, *Curr Probl Pediatr* 17: 627-665, 1987.

Hagerman GW et al. Girls with fragile X syndrome: physical and neurocognitive status and outcome, *Pediatrics* 89: 395-400, 1992.

Hallett K et al. Medically compromised children. In Cameron AC, Widmer RP, eds. *Handbook of pediatric dentistry.* 2nd ed. London, 2003, Mosby.

Hennequin M, et al. Accuracy of estimation of dental treatment need in special care patients, *J Dent* 28:131-136, 2000.

Hobsen P. The treatment of medically handicapped children, *Int Dent J* 30:6-13, 1980.

Hudson M. Dental surgery in pediatric patients with spina bifida and latex allergy, *AORN J* 74(1):56-78, 2001.

Leslie ND, Sperling MA. Relation of metabolic control to complications in diabetes mellitus, *J Pediatr* 108:491-497, 1986.

McCrindle BW et al. An evaluation of parental concerns and misconceptions about heart murmurs, *Clin Pediatr* 34:25-31, 1995.

Morsey SL. Communicating with and treating the blind child, *Dent Hyg* 65:288-290, 1980.

Pope JEC, Curzon MEJ. The dental status of cerebral palsied children, *Pediatr Dent* 13(3):156-162, 1991.

Posnick WR, Feigal RJ. Cystic fibrosis and its dental implications, *J Dent Handicap* 5:21-23, 1980.

Rosenberg DJ et al. Estimating treatment and treatment times for special and nonspecial patients in hospital ambulatory dental clinics, *J Dent Educ* 50:665-672, 1986.

Sanders BJ, et al. Managing patients who have seizure disorders: Dental and medical issues, *J Am Dent Assoc* 126:1641-1647, 1995.

SantaAnna LB, Tosello DO. Fetal alcohol syndrome and developing craniofacial and dental structures: a review, *Orthod Craniofacial Res* 9:172-185, 2006.

Shelhart WC, et al. Oral findings in Fragile X syndrome, *Am J Med Genetics* 23:179-187, 1986.

Simko A et al. Fragile X: recognition in young children, *Pediatrics* 83:547-551, 1989.

Steinbacher DM, Glick M. The dental patient with asthma: an update and oral health consideration, *J Am Dent Assoc* 132:1229-1239, 2001.

Stensson M, et al. Oral health in preschool children with asthma, *Int J Paediatr Dent* 18(4):243-250, 2008.

Terzian EC, Schneider RE. Management of the patient with cystic fibrosis in oral and maxillofacial surgery, *J Oral Maxillofac Surg* 66(2):349-354, 2008.

Tesini DA, Fenton SJ. Oral health needs of persons with physical or mental disabilities, *Dent Clin North Am* 38:483-498, 1994.

Waldman BH, et al. Children with mental retardation and epilepsy: demographics and general concerns, *J Dent Child* 67:268-274, 2000.

Wandera A, Conry JP. Aspiration and ingestion of a foreign body during dental examination by a patient with spastic quadriparesis: case report, *Pediatr Dent* 15:362-363, 1993.

Zhu J et al. Dental management of children with asthma, *Pediatr Dent* 18:363-370, 1996.

CHAPTER 24

Management of the Medically Compromised Patient: Hematologic Disorders, Cancer, Hepatitis, and AIDS

▲ Brian J. Sanders, Amy D. Shapiro, Randy A. Hock, James A. Weddell, and Christopher Edward Belcher

CHAPTER OUTLINE

*T*o achieve optimal oral health for the medically compromised patient, the dentist and physician must establish a close working relationship. Because of the complexity of many of these medical conditions additional treatment time may be needed to provide services. To minimize the risk for potential complications that may affect the physical health of medically compromised patients, an aggressive prevention-oriented program is required. Each patient presents a unique set of challenges to the dentist, but achieving a successful outcome can be a rewarding experience. This chapter discusses major medical conditions and their dental management.

HEMOPHILIA

DISORDERS OF HEMOSTASIS

The hemophilias are disorders of hemostasis resulting from a deficiency of a procoagulant. Hemophilia is an inherited bleeding disorder affecting approximately 1 in 7500 males.[1] Hemophilia A, or classic hemophilia, is a deficiency of factor VIII, also known as *antihemophilic factor.* Factor VIII deficiency is the most common of the hemophilias and is inherited as an X-linked recessive trait. Therefore males are affected, females are carriers, and there is no male-to-male transmission. If a normal male has children with a carrier of hemophilia, there is a 50%

chance that hemophilia will occur in each male offspring and a 50% chance that each female offspring will be a carrier. If a male hemophilic has children with a normal female, all male offspring will be normal, and all female offspring will be carriers. Hemophilia B, or Christmas disease, is caused by a deficiency of factor IX (plasma thromboplastin component) and is also inherited as an X-linked recessive trait. Factor IX deficiency is one-fourth as prevalent as factor VIII deficiency.[2,3]

Factor XI (plasma thromboplastin antecedent) deficiency, also referred to as *hemophilia C* or *Rosenthal's' disease,* is inherited as an autosomal recessive trait, with male and female offspring equally affected. This disorder is most frequently observed in those of Ashkenazi Jewish descent. Other factor deficiencies, such as those of factors II, V, and XIII (one case per 1 million population) and factor VII (one case per 500,000 population) are rare and are inherited as autosomal recessive traits.[4,5]

Von Willebrand disease is a hereditary bleeding disorder resulting from an abnormality of the Von Willebrand factor (VWF) found in plasma, platelets, megakaryocytes, and endothelial cells. VWF circulates in conjunction with factor VIII and is important in platelet adhesion to the subendothelium via collagen and therefore in the formation of the primary platelet plug. In von Willebrand disease, the VWF may have a quantitative or qualitative abnormality. The VWF is composed of subunits called *multimers.* Von Willebrand disease is divided into subtypes based on the platelet and plasma multimeric VWF structure. Optimal treatment of this disorder is dependent upon the subtype.[6]

Impaired formation of the platelet plug may result in bleeding from the skin and mucosa, bruising, epistaxis, prolonged bleeding after surgical procedures, and menorrhagia (Fig. 24-1). This is in contrast to hemophilia involving deficiencies of factors VIII and IX, in which the hallmark bleeding events involve muscles and joints (Fig. 24-2).

PROCOAGULANT CLASSIFICATION

Hemophilia A (factor VIII deficiency) and hemophilia B (factor IX deficiency) are classified based on the level of the procoagulant present with normal levels ranging from 55% to 100%:

- Severe deficiency: levels less than 1%
- Moderate deficiency: levels between 1% and 5%
- Mild deficiency: levels greater than or equal to 5% to less than 50%

Patients with severe deficiency may experience frequent bleeding episodes, often occurring two to four times per month. Bleeding episodes may be spontaneous, without a specific history of injury or trauma. Common sites of bleeding include joints, muscles, and skin. Hemarthroses (joint hemorrhages) are common, and symptoms include pain, stiffness, and limited motion. Repeated episodes of hemarthroses or muscle hemorrhage result in chronic musculoskeletal disease and culminate in debilitating painful arthritis. Commonly

affected joints include knees, elbows, ankles, hips, and shoulders. Pseudotumors (hemorrhagic pseudocysts) may occur in several locations including the jaw, in which case curettage is indicated.[7,8]

Patients with moderate deficiency experience less frequent bleeding episodes (approximately four to six times per year). However, if a target joint (a joint with repeated episodes of bleeding) develops in a patient with moderate deficiency, spontaneous bleeding may occur. Patients with mild deficiency bleed infrequently and only in association with surgery or injury. The diagnosis of a mild deficiency may occur when an abnormality is found during presurgical evaluation or when bleeding occurs in association with surgery or trauma. The dental care provider may be the first health care provider to identify a patient with mild deficiency as interventions or injury in the oral cavity may unmask a previously undiagnosed individual.

Mouth lacerations are a common cause of bleeding in children with all severities of hemophilia. Sonis and Musselman evaluated 132 patients with factor VIII–deficient hemophilia and noted that "persistent oral bleeding resulted in the diagnosis of 13.6% of all cases of hemophilia."[9] About 29% of cases of mild hemophilia observed were discovered as a result of bleeding from the oral cavity. Of the cases diagnosed secondary to oral bleeding, 78% were the result of bleeding from the maxillary frenum, and 22% resulted from tongue bleeds. Thus initial diagnosis of hemophilia, especially in moderate or mild disease, may directly involve the dentist.

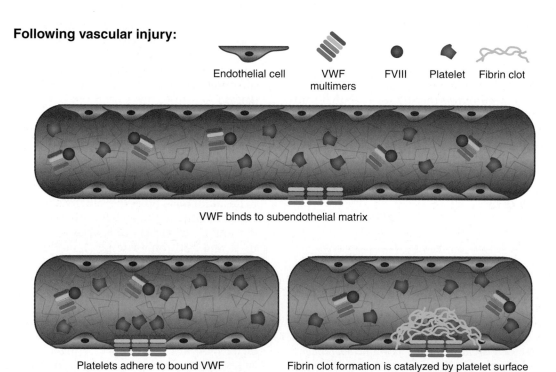

Following vascular injury:

Endothelial cell   VWF multimers   FVIII   Platelet   Fibrin clot

VWF binds to subendothelial matrix

Platelets adhere to bound VWF

Fibrin clot formation is catalyzed by platelet surface

Figure 24-1 Primary hemostatic response to vascular injury with evolution into secondary hemostasis. This figure shows the primary hemostatic response to vascular injury involving the endothelial cell and platelet; primary hemostasis leads to and is an integral part of secondary hemostasis involving coagulation factors, including Von Willebrand factor, factor VIII culminating in the generation of fibrin. (With permission from CSL Behring and Robert Montgomery.)

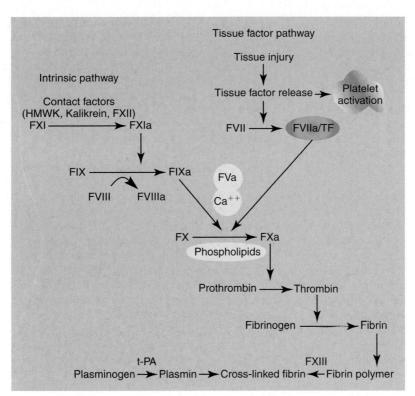

Figure 24-2 Coagulation cascade. This figure shows the complex interplay between the plasma coagulation factors and the fibrinolytic pathway (plasminogen and end enzyme plasmin) responsible for clot lysis after healing. The importance of the role of the tissue factor pathway and cellular systems (platelets) in initiating physiologic hemostasis is highlighted. The factors deficient in hemophilia A and B (factors VIII and IX, respectively) are shown in relationship to their role in the coagulation pathway. (Courtesy Anjali Sharathkumar.)

TREATMENT

The mainstay of therapy for hemophilia is replacement of the deficient coagulation factor, through the use of purified concentrates either manufactured through recombinant technology or from pooled plasma. In the past, whole blood, plasma, or cryoprecipitate was used for replacement therapy. Factor concentrates are advantageous as they are generally accessible, easily handled and stored, virally inactivated, and commonly result in consistent hemostatic results. The dosage, frequency of administration, and duration of therapy depend on the activity level required, the half life of the procoagulant, the intervention or procedure contemplated, or the location and severity of the bleeding episode. The half-life of factor VIII is approximately 12 hours, whereas for factor IX it is approximately 18 hours.[10]

Hemophilia A

Factor VIII concentrate is used for treatment of hemophilia A. Vials of factor concentrate are labeled with the number of international activity units contained, where 1 IU is the amount of activity of the procoagulant present in 1 mL of normal plasma. For routine hemorrhagic episodes, such as early joint, soft tissue, and oral bleeds, a one-time correction to approximately a level of 40% to 50% will achieve hemostasis and resolution of the bleeding episode. For mild factor VIII–deficient hemophilia, DDAVP (1-deamino-8-D-arginine vasopressin) (Sanofi-Aventis, Bridgewater, NJ)

may be used for minor hemorrhagic episodes to achieve hemostasis. DDAVP (desmopressin acetate) is a synthetic analogue of the natural pituitary hormone 8-arginine vasopressin (antidiuretic hormone) affecting renal water conservation. This drug, when given intravenously, subcutaneously, or intranasally (Stimate) causes a rise in factor VIII activity and VWF through release from stored sites in endothelial cells, often to the hemostatic range. An appropriate rise in factor VIII activity to hemostatic levels should be documented for any given patient before therapeutic use of this agent, because response may vary among individuals. Peak levels are obtained approximately 1 hour after administration via intravenous and subcutaneous routes and 90 minutes after administration intranasally. The intranasal form of this medication, which is used to treat patients with bleeding disorders, has a more concentrated form of DDAVP compared with the preparation used to treat diabetes insipidus or enuresis. Therefore this preparation should be written for brand name only or in conjunction with the stated concentration of 1.5 mg/mL of desmopressin acetate. Repeated administration of DDAVP may result in tachyphylaxis, a reduction in expected response with sequential dosing due to depletion of storage sites. Use of DDAVP to treat hemorrhagic disorders may also be associated with water retention, hyponatremia, and rarely seizures; therefore monitoring of electrolytes may be required in some circumstances, especially in surgical situations.[11-13]

Hemophilia B

Factor IX–deficient hemophilia is treated with purified coagulation factor IX concentrate (monoclonal and recombinant). In the past, less pure products in the class of prothrombin complex concentrate (PCC) were used. PCCs contained other vitamin K–dependent coagulation factors in addition to factor IX, including some activated forms of these procoagulants. Individuals who require high doses or repeated infusions of PCC are at risk for development of disseminated intravascular coagulation and thrombosis. The minimal desired level for hemostasis is the same for factor IX as for factor VIII (40%). However, the number of units required to achieve that level is different as the volume of distribution of plasma-derived factor IX (1.0) is greater than that for factor VIII (0.5). The volume of distribution of recombinant factor IX is greater than that of plasma-derived factor IX (estimated minimum volume of 1.2 compared with 1, respectively, whereas in infants and young children a minimum volume of distribution of 1.4 should be used for dose calculation). Because interindividual variability of volume of distribution is wide, measurement of activity levels may be required to document a hemostatic level.[14-17]

Clotting factor concentrates are administered in different regimens depending on the patient's level of severity, number of bleeding episodes, and the treating physician's recommendations. Treatment regimens may be divided into replacement therapy administered after a bleeding episode has occurred (on-demand therapy) or as administered on a regular scheduled basis to prevent or suppress bleeding episodes (prophylaxis). Prophylactic regimens are further subdivided into primary and secondary. Primary prophylaxis is a long-term treatment for prevention of joint disease instituted before or after minimal hemarthrosis has occurred; secondary prophylaxis may be long or short term, but is instituted after hemarthrosis has occurred or to interrupt a bleeding pattern to rest a joint. Primary prophylactic therapy has been shown in a prospective randomized study to be the most effective regimen to prevent joint disease in patients with severe hemophilia and is now considered the standard of care for these patients.[18] Therefore dental care providers should schedule dental evaluations and interventions on regularly planned infusion days, whereas patients treated with on-demand regimens require discussion regarding the need to administer replacement therapy specifically for dental interventions. Patients using regimens of prophylaxis may have a central venous catheter placed due to the need for frequent venous access. The use of antibiotic prophylaxis to protect the central venous access device may be considered although is not recommended by the Centers for Disease Control and Prevention (see Antibiotic Prophylaxis in the section on Dental Management).

WOMEN WITH BLEEDING DISORDERS

Von Willebrand Disease

Patients with von Willebrand disease should undergo subtyping to determine optimal therapy. DDAVP may be used to achieve hemostasis in most patients with type I von Willebrand disease, where type I VWD represents a quantitative VWF deficiency with intact multimers.

When DDAVP is used, a test dose should be administered to document an adequate hemostatic response. For patients with less common subtypes of VWD, patients who do not respond to DDAVP, or patients for whom DDAVP is inappropriate, or in bleeding events for which DDAVP should not be used, other therapeutic modalities may be required, including replacement with exogenous intact VWF through the use of a concentrate. Interventions and therapeutic approaches should be discussed with a hemophilia-comprehensive treatment center.[19,20]

Female carriers of hemophilia A and B may have decreased levels of factors VIII and IX, respectively, that place them in the mild range of deficiency. It is recommended that all carriers of hemophilia have an evaluation to determine their baseline activity level specific to the type of hemophilia carried to determine bleeding risk. Women who are carriers of hemophilia should be treated as potential mild-deficient patients and their hematologist contacted to determine the baseline factor activity level and need for treatment before or after specific dental interventions.[21,22]

COMPLICATIONS

Inhibitors are antibodies that neutralize the replaced coagulation factor and are one of the most severe complications for patients. Inhibitors may develop in approximately 28% of patients with severe factor VIII deficiency and in 3% to 5% of patients with severe factor IX deficiency. The key to successful treatment of patients with inhibitors is accurate knowledge of the classification and level of the inhibitor. Patients with inhibitors are divided into two general groups, high responders and low responders, based on the past peak anamnestic response of the inhibitor titer. Inhibitor levels are measured in Bethesda units (BU), a measurement that reflects the ability of the antibody to neutralize a specific amount of procoagulant.[23,24]

Patients in the low-responding group have peak levels at any time less than 5 BU, and may continue to be treated with factor concentrate, whereas those in the high-response group have peak titers greater than or equal to 5 BU and require use of bypassing products (either PCC, activated PCC, or recombinant factor VIIa). Hemophilic patients with inhibitors pose considerable treatment challenges and should be managed only in conjunction with a hemophilia-comprehensive treatment center, because hemostasis is often difficult to achieve or maintain.

Other complications of hemophilia include arthritis and degenerative joint disease secondary to recurrent bleeding.[25] Blood-borne viral infections represent an important complication of treatment of these disorders and may have been transmitted via required blood or blood products. Hepatitis, including both B and C and resultant liver disease have been a significant source of morbidity and mortality in this patient population.[26] The human immunodeficiency virus (HIV) has also been a major source of morbidity and mortality since approximately 1979. Before 1985, there was no antibody test for HIV and no consistent method of viral inactivation in the manufacture of factor concentrates. Therefore between 1979 and 1985, factor concentrates and blood products may have been contaminated with HIV. Approximately 90% of hemophilic patients with severe factor VIII deficiency and 30% of those with severe factor IX deficiency who received factor concentrate during the at-risk period may have become infected with HIV. HIV infection is a sensitive issue to these individuals, who may now bear the burden of two chronic conditions.[27] Currently available treatments of factor concentrates made through recombinant technology or pooled plasma have effectively eliminated transmission of HIV and hepatitis B and C. Nevertheless, universal precautions should be followed when treating all hemophilic patients with a history of receiving either factor concentrate.

RISKS TO DENTAL STAFF

The risk for acquiring hepatitis B virus infection following an accidental stick with a needle used by a hepatitis B virus carrier ranges from 6% to 30%, far higher than the risk for transmission of HIV infection (less than 1%) following a stick with a needle used by an HIV-infected patient. Moreover, although HIV antibodies have been isolated in saliva and other body fluids, there is no evidence to suggest that HIV is easily transmitted through saliva alone.

A study by Klein and colleagues demonstrated a less than 0.5% occupational risk for HIV infection among dental professionals despite their infrequent compliance with recommended infection control precautions, frequent occupational exposure to persons at increased risk for HIV infection, and frequent accidental parenteral inoculations with sharp instruments.[28] These data are reassuring but do not obviate the need for appropriate universal precautions with all patients.

DEVELOPMENT OF A TREATMENT PLAN

With recent advances in treatment, most hemophilic patients can receive outpatient dental care routinely. With a thorough understanding of the patient's hemostatic disorder, the dentist, in conjunction with the hematologist, is able to make safe and appropriate treatment decisions.

The dentist must be fully aware of the procedures that can be safely performed and those in which complications may arise. The dentist should confer with the patient's physician and hematologist to formulate an appropriate treatment plan. The dentist should know the specific type of bleeding disorder, the severity of the disorder, the frequency and treatment of bleeding episodes, and the patient's inhibitor status. Many individuals with hemophilia self-administer infusion products at home and are therefore able to treat themselves when required. The dentist should be prepared to discuss with the hematologist the type of anesthetic anticipated to be administered, the invasiveness of the dental procedure, the amount of bleeding anticipated, and the time involved in oral wound healing to help establish an appropriate treatment plan including the need for replacement and adjunctive therapies.[29]

USE OF ANTIFIBRINOLYTIC AGENTS

Antifibrinolytic agents are an adjunctive therapy for dental management of patients with bleeding disorders and are important for prevention or treatment of oral bleeding. These agents include ε-aminocaproic acid (Amicar, Xanodyne Pharmaceuticals, Florence, KY) and tranexamic acid (Cyklokapron, Pfizer, New York). Hemophilic patients form loose, friable clots that may be readily dislodged or quickly dissolved, especially in the oral cavity where local fibrinolysis is increased. Antifibrinolytics prevent clot lysis within the oral cavity. They are often used as an adjunct to factor concentrate replacement. For some dental procedures in which minimal bleeding is anticipated, they may be used alone.

Dosages

In children, ε-aminocaproic acid is given immediately before dental treatment in an initial loading dose of 100 to 200 mg/kg by mouth up to a maximum total dose of 10 g. Subsequently, 50 to 100 mg/kg per dose up to a total maximum dose of 5 g is administered orally every 6 hours for 5 to 7 days. Alternatively, for patients of approximately adult size or heavier than 30 kg, a regimen of 3 g by mouth four times daily without a loading dose may be used. The advantage of ε-aminocaproic acid for children is that it is available in both tablet and liquid form.

The adult and pediatric dosage of tranexamic acid is 25 mg/kg given immediately before dental treatment. The same dose is continued every 8 hours for 5 to 7 days. The oral preparation of tranexamic acid is not available in the United States but the intravenous formulation is. The intravenous formulation may be administered orally if required.[30]

Side Effects

The common side effects associated with the use of antifibrinolytics include headache, nausea, and dry mouth. These side effects are usually tolerable and, unless severe, do not require discontinuation of the medication. Other less common side effects have also been reported. To avoid thrombosis, antifibrinolytics should not be used when renal or urinary tract bleeding is present or when there is any evidence of disseminated intravascular coagulation. Repeated use of PCC or bypassing products (activated PCC) in patients with inhibitors should also be avoided during a course of antifibrinolytic therapy because they may predispose to thrombotic episodes.

PAIN CONTROL

Analgesia

If patient apprehension is significant, sedation or nitrous oxide–oxygen inhalation analgesia may be considered. Hypnosis has also proved beneficial for some individuals. Intramuscular injections of hypnotic, tranquilizing, or analgesic agents are contraindicated due to the risk of hematoma formation. Analgesics containing aspirin or anti-inflammatory agents (e.g., ibuprofen) may affect platelet function and should be avoided. Acute pain of moderate intensity can frequently be managed using acetaminophen (Tylenol, McNeil Pharmaceuticals, Washington, PA). Propoxyphene hydrochloride (Darvon, aaiPharmp, Wilmington, NC), another analgesic, is acceptable for use in patients with hemophilia whereas Darvon Compound-65 contains aspirin and should be avoided. For severe pain, narcotic analgesics may be required and are not contraindicated in the hemophilic patient.

Local Anesthesia

In the absence of factor replacement, periodontal ligament (PDL) injections may be used. The anesthetic is administered along the four axial surfaces of the tooth by placement of the needle into the gingival sulcus and the periodontal ligament space. Infiltration anesthesia can generally be administered without pretreatment with either ε-aminocaproic acid or replacement therapy. However, if the infiltration injection is into loose connective tissue or a highly vascularized area, then factor concentrate replacement to achieve a level of approximately 30% to 40% activity is recommended.

One must proceed with caution when considering block anesthesia. The loose, connective, nonfibrous, and highly vascularized tissue at the sites of inferior alveolar nerve injection and posterior superior alveolar injections are predisposed to development of a dissecting hematoma, which potentially may cause airway obstruction and create a life-threatening bleeding episode. Therefore a minimum of a 40% factor correction is mandatory with block anesthesia. The dentist must carefully aspirate to ensure that the needle has not entered a blood vessel. If there is bloody aspirate, further factor replacement may be required, and the attending hematologist should be notified immediately following the operative procedure. All patients should be observed for development of a hematoma and immediately referred for treatment in case hematoma forms after the administration of local anesthesia.

DENTAL MANAGEMENT

Most hemophilic patients can receive outpatient dental care routinely. Appointments should be arranged so that maximum treatment is accomplished per visit to minimize the need for unscheduled factor infusions and hence cost. Patients with inhibitors are best treated at a center with experience in dealing with this complication.[31-33]

The dental procedures used in treating a patient with hemophilia do not differ significantly from those used for unaffected individuals.

Prevention of Dental Disease

A program that includes toothbrushing, flossing, appropriate topical fluoride exposure, and adequate systemic fluoride administration, as well as consumption of a proper diet and professional examination at regular intervals are effective measures that prevent dental problems. Rubber cup prophylaxis and supragingival scaling may be safely performed without prior factor replacement therapy. Minor bleeding can be readily controlled with local measures, such as direct pressure with a moistened gauze square. If bleeding persists for several minutes, the topical application of bovine thrombin,* microfibrillar collagen (Avitene, Medchem Products, Inc., Woburn, MA), and local fibrin glue may be of value.

Periodontal Therapy

Patients who require deep scaling because of gross calculus should initially undergo supragingival scaling. The tissue should be allowed to heal for 7 to 14 days, during which time the gingiva recede as edema and hyperemia diminish. Subsequent treatments to remove calculus and irritants therefore incur decreased bleeding risk from the tissue. If subgingival scaling is planned, replacement therapy may be considered, depending on the amount of anticipated bleeding and the severity of the factor deficiency. It is imperative that periodontal patients be placed on a maintenance schedule for proper management.[34,35]

An abnormal frenum attachment may cause gingival recession and pocket formation. Early treatment is indicated to prevent continued gingival recession and alveolar bone loss. All appropriate frenectomy techniques are surgically acceptable for hemophilic patients; both factor concentrate replacement and antifibrinolytic therapy are required before frenum or other periodontal surgery. If a large amount of bleeding is anticipated, these procedures should be performed in a hospital environment, with the requisite preparation. The hematologist or attending physician must be contacted to determine the appropriate factor correction required and the possible need for subsequent hospital management.

Restorative Procedures

The patient with hemophilia should be allowed to consider the prospect of all restorative procedures. Most restorative procedures on primary teeth are successfully completed without factor concentrate replacement using PDL injections of local anesthesia or local infiltration. Small lesions may be restored using nitrous oxide–oxygen inhalation analgesia alone. The use of acetaminophen with codeine may also decrease discomfort in the child.

Most operative procedures for adults may also be completed using local infiltration of anesthetic, a procedure that usually does not require factor concentrate replacement. If a mandibular block or a posterior superior alveolar injection is anticipated, factor concentrate replacement to a level of 40% and antifibrinolytic therapy are required before injection. If factor concentrate replacement is required, all possible restorative treatment should be completed in one visit to minimize the number of infusions required to complete the restorative treatment plan.

A rubber dam should be used to isolate the operating field and to retract and protect the cheeks, lips, and tongue. These soft tissues are highly vascular, and accidental laceration may present a difficult management problem. A thin rubber dam is preferred because there is a decreased tendency to torque the rubber dam retainer and cause gingival tissue abrasion. The retainer should be placed carefully so that it is stable. If a retainer slips, it may lacerate the gingival papilla. Retainers with subgingival extensions should be avoided.

Wedges and matrices can be used conventionally. During proximal preparation, the wedge retracts the papilla, thus protecting it. A properly placed matrix should not cause bleeding.

High-speed vacuum and saliva ejectors must be used with caution so that sublingual hematomas do not occur. Care must also be used in the placement of intraoral

---

*Although not reported in the dental literature, bovine thrombin–induced factor V deficiency, a rare, acquired coagulopathy, has been reported.

radiographic films, particularly in highly vascular sublingual tissues.

The preparation of a tooth for a cast crown requires caution in gingival preparation, as does placement of retraction cord and impression material. Periphery wax is used on the impression tray to prevent possible intraoral laceration during tray placement. Undue trauma should be avoided in cementing or finishing a crown.

Pulpal Therapy.

At times, pulp exposures in primary and permanent teeth may be avoided if carious dentin is not entirely removed in one procedure (indirect pulp therapy). A pulpotomy or pulpectomy is preferable to extraction. The extraction of a tooth in an individual with hemophilia involves more complicated treatment and expense to the patient. Most vital pulpotomy and pulpectomy procedures can be successfully completed using local infiltration anesthesia. Nitrous oxide–oxygen inhalation analgesia may also help alleviate discomfort. If the pulp of a vital tooth is exposed, an intrapulpal injection may be used safely to control pain. Bleeding from the pulp chamber does not present a significant problem in that it is readily controlled with pressure from cotton pledgets. If pulp tissue is necrotic, local anesthetic is usually unnecessary.

Oral Surgery

Preoperative evaluation and postoperative management of the hemophilic patient undergoing extractions must be coordinated with the hematologist. The dentist should discuss with the hematologist the surgical procedure, including the anesthetic technique, the degree of anticipated surgical trauma, and the expected duration for healing. The hematologist can then determine the amount and duration of factor concentrate replacement and adjunctive therapies required for surgery and postoperative management. Today it is possible to perform oral surgery in the hemophilic patient on an outpatient basis.[36,37] Requirements include an experienced dentist and hematologist, a facility available for the patient to receive infusions if home infusion is not performed, and a coagulation laboratory capable of timely needed laboratory evaluations. Patients with inhibitors should only be treated in a hospital setting by those experienced in their management.

For simple extractions of erupted permanent teeth and multirooted primary teeth, a 30% to 40% factor correction is administered within 1 hour before dental treatment. Antifibrinolytic therapy should be started immediately before or after the procedure and should be continued for 5 to 10 days. The patient should be placed on a clear liquid diet for the first 72 hours. For the next week, a soft, pureed diet is recommended. During this time, the patient should not use straws, metal utensils, pacifiers, or bottles. After 10 days, the patient may begin to consume a more normal diet. Specific postoperative instructions should be provided to the patient and parent. Factor concentrate is extremely costly, therefore all extractions should be completed in one appointment if possible.

After extractions are completed, the direct topical application of hemostatic agents, such as thrombin or microfibrillar collagen hemostat (Avitene), may assist with local hemostasis. The socket should be packed with an absorbable gelatin sponge (e.g., Gelfoam, Pharmacia and Upjohn Co., Kalamazoo, MI). Microfibrillar collagen or topical thrombin or fibrin glue may then be placed in the wound. Direct pressure with gauze should then be applied to the area.

Stomahesive (J. Knipper and Company, Inc., Lakewood, NJ) may be placed over the wound for additional protection from the oral environment. In general, the use of sutures should be avoided unless suturing is expected to markedly enhance healing, in which case resorbent sutures are recommended. The patient must be given specific and thorough postoperative instructions.

For surgical extractions of impacted, partially erupted, or unerupted teeth, a higher factor activity level may be targeted before surgery. This should be discussed with the hematologist, due to the increased likelihood of surgical trauma and a longer healing period. The hematologist may also elect to administer factor replacement to the patient postoperatively. Antifibrinolytic therapy should be started immediately before or after the procedure and continued for 7 to 10 days.

For simple extractions of single-rooted primary teeth (i.e., incisors and canines), one must evaluate the amount of root development present to determine whether factor replacement therapy is required. If there is complete root development, factor replacement therapy may be required, whereas if there is only partial root formation, antifibrinolytic therapy along with local hemostatic agents may be all that is required.

The normal exfoliation of primary teeth does not usually result in bleeding or require factor replacement. Bleeding in these circumstances can generally be controlled with direct finger and gauze pressure maintained for several minutes. The direct topical application of an adjunctive agent may also help with local hemostasis. If there is continuous slow bleeding, antifibrinolytic therapy may be initiated. In rare circumstances, most commonly when the gingival tissue is repeatedly traumatized during exfoliation, use of factor replacement therapy may be required. In this circumstance, dental evaluation should be performed and consideration given to removal of the exfoliating tooth if repeated trauma cannot be avoided.

Surgical Complications

Despite all precautions, bleeding may occur 3 to 4 days postoperatively when the clot begins to break down. Both systemic and local treatment should be used for hemostatic control. Sufficient replacement factor should be administered to control recurrent bleeding.

It is not prudent to protect a loose clot. The typical clot in this situation is characterized as a "liver clot" and is dark red, usually protruding from the surgical site, and often covers the surfaces of several teeth. Following adequate replacement with factor concentrate, usually to a 30% to 40% activity level, the abnormal clot should be removed and the area cleansed to help isolate the source of bleeding. The socket should then be repacked and use of antifibrinolytic agents considered.

Antibiotic Prophylaxis

Total joint replacement, usually of the hip or knee, is often performed in adult patients with severe hemophilia to restore function and alleviate pain associated with degenerative arthritis due to multiple hemarthroses. Antibiotic prophylaxis is required for patients with artificial joints before invasive dental procedures. The American Heart Association recommendations for bacterial endocarditis prophylaxis, last updated in 2007, are commonly followed. Antibiotic prophylaxis is no longer recommended for patients with central venous access devices, although each particular patient's circumstance should be considered.[38] If the patient is immunocompromised because of HIV infection, intravenous antibiotic prophylaxis may be considered.

Orthodontic Treatment

Early recognition of an orthodontic problem is important, in that selective guidance can diminish or eliminate complex orthodontic problems. Both interceptive and full-banded orthodontics may be performed if required. Care must be taken in the adaptation and placement of bands and avoidance of protruding sharp edges and wires to prevent laceration of oral mucosa. Bleeding caused by an accidental scratch or minor laceration of the gingiva usually responds to applied pressure for 5 minutes. The use of preformed orthodontic bands and brackets, which can be bonded directly to the teeth, almost totally eliminates contact of orthodontic appliances with gingiva during placement. Longer-acting wires and springs require less frequent adjustment of orthodontic appliances. Oral hygiene is particularly important to avoid inflamed, edematous, and hemorrhagic gingival tissues. A water-irrigating device may be helpful for home dental care.

Dental Emergencies

Oral trauma is a common occurrence during childhood. Management of bleeding injuries, including hematomas, in the oral cavity of the patient with a bleeding disorder may require a combination of factor replacement and antifibrinolytic therapy, as well as treatment with local hemostatic agents. Blood loss from the oral cavity is easily underestimated or overestimated. The patient's hemoglobin may be checked to ensure that the patient is not anemic in these circumstances.

VIRAL HEPATITIS

Viral hepatitis is an infection that produces inflammation of liver cells, which may lead to necrosis or cirrhosis of the liver. Acute hepatitis classically presents with lethargy, loss of appetite, nausea, vomiting, abdominal pain, and ultimately jaundice.

Acute viral hepatitis may be caused by any of the following: hepatitis A virus (HAV), hepatitis B virus (HBV), hepatitis delta virus (HDV), and two forms of non-A, non-B hepatitis virus (NANB)—parenterally transmitted NANB or hepatitis C virus (HCV), and enterically transmitted NANB or hepatitis E virus.

Infection with hepatitis A virus results in an acute febrile illness with jaundice, anorexia, nausea, and malaise. Most HAV infections in infants and children cause mild, nonspecific symptoms without jaundice. HAV is spread by the fecal-oral route and is endemic in developing areas. Spread occurs readily in households and day-care centers, where symptomatic illness occurs primarily among adult contacts of children. No HAV carrier state exists, and the presence of immunoglobulin G–anti-HAV indicates past infection and lifelong immunity to HAV. The risk for transmission in a dental setting is low.

Hepatitis B transmission is of major concern to the dentist. Members of the dental profession assume a risk for acquiring HBV that is at least three times higher than that in the general population. An additional concern, beyond that of acquiring HBV, is the potential of becoming an asymptomatic yet infectious carrier of HBV and of having the capability of transmitting the disease to patients and dental staff members and family.

HBV is transmitted from person to person by parenteral, percutaneous, or mucous membrane inoculation. It can be transmitted by the percutaneous introduction of blood, administration of certain blood products, or direct contact with secretions contaminated with blood containing HBV. Infection may also result from inoculation of mucous membranes, including sexual transmission. Wound exudates contain HBV, and open-wound to open-wound contact can transmit infection. There can also be vertical transmission from an infected mother to her baby, and this frequently leads to chronic infection.

A medical history is unreliable in identifying patients who have HBV infection, because approximately 80% of all HBV infections are undiagnosed. However, the medical history is useful in identifying groups of patients who are at higher risk of being undiagnosed carriers. Among populations at high risk for HBV infection are patients undergoing hemodialysis, patients requiring frequent large-volume blood transfusions or administration of clotting factor concentrates, residents of institutions for the mentally disabled, and users of illicit injectable drugs.

In 2006, an estimated 46,000 people in the United States became infected with HBV, and an estimated 1.25 million chronically infected people live in the United States. Overall, chronic liver disease from hepatitis B claims 5000 lives a year in the United States.[39]

Chronic active hepatitis develops in more than 25% of carriers and often progresses to cirrhosis. Furthermore, HBV carriers have a risk of developing primary liver cancer that is between 12 and 300 times higher than that of uninfected individuals.

For detection of acute or chronic HBV infection, the serologic test for hepatitis B surface antigen (HepBsAg) is most commonly used. The antibody to surface antigen (HepBsAb or anti-HepBsAg) is protective and indicates a resolved natural infection or successful vaccination. Antibody to the core antigen (HepBcAb or anti-HepBc) indicates exposure to natural hepatitis B virus but can be present in either resolved or chronic infection. The hepatitis Be antigen (HepBeAg) is a useful marker for infectivity. Patients who test positive for HepBeAb and HepBsAg are most likely to transmit the disease. If the patient still shows a positive test result for HepBsAg 6 months after an acute HBV infection, the patient is considered to be chronically infected.

The availability of a safe, effective hepatitis B vaccine affords the dentist and staff additional protection against acquiring HBV infection. HBV vaccine is recommended for all health care personnel. The vaccine is derived using recombinant DNA and therefore does not have the potential to transmit the disease. When administered in a three-dose injection regimen (0, 1, 6 months), the recombinant DNA vaccine induced protective antibody (anti-HepBs) in 95% to 100% of adults.

A fulminant type of hepatitis occurs with infection by HDV but only with coexisting or simultaneous infection with HBV. HDV is defective in that it requires HBV for outer coat proteins (HepBsAg), as well as requiring HBV for replication. Transmission is similar to that of HBV, by parenteral, percutaneous, or mucous membrane inoculation.

According to Cottone,[40] HDV infection occurs in two primary modes:

The first is simultaneous infection with HBV and HDV. When simultaneous infection occurs, the acute clinical course of hepatitis often is limited with resolution of both hepatitis B and HDV infections. The second mode of transmission, acute delta super-infection, involves those with chronic Hepatitis B infection. In this situation, the patient already has a high titer of circulating HepBsAg; thus HDV can rapidly replicate. These patients are more likely to have a serious and possibly acute fulminant form of hepatitis that more often leads to chronic HDV.

Hepatitis C (formerly known as parenterally transmitted NANB hepatitis) is of great concern to the dentist, because it can be transmitted by needle stick (risk of about 1.8% with a range of 0% to 10%) and no immunization is available. Patients at risk for hepatitis C include those who received blood transfusions or organ transplants before 1992, those who received clotting factors before 1987, those on long-term dialysis, and most commonly those who have experimented with illicit intravenous drugs regardless of how many times or how long ago. Of those infected, chronic infection develops in 70% to 85%, and chronic liver disease develops in about 70%. Although only 3% of infected people die of liver failure, hepatitis C is the leading reason for liver transplantation in adults in the United States.

In 1989, parenterally transmitted NANB was identified as HCV. Subsequently, three genotypes have been identified. Diagnosis is made by detection of antibody to hepatitis C virus (anti-HCV) in the serum and can be confirmed by radioimmunoblot assay. Polymerase chain reaction (PCR) testing can be done in a qualitative fashion to confirm diagnosis or in a quantitative fashion to assess response to treatment. Treatment, when indicated, includes administration of interferon or pegylated interferon with or without ribavirin. Response rates vary from 50% for type 1 infection to 80% for types 2 and 3.

In 2006, the Centers for Disease Control and Prevention estimated that there were 19,000 new cases of infection with hepatitis C in the United States, down from 240,000 per year in the 1980s.[41] There are 4.1 million people infected with hepatitis C in the United States (1.6%). Of the 3.2 million who are chronically infected, 8000 to 10,000 patients die per year. Infection associated with injection drug use accounts for more than 50% of the new cases in the United States.

As noted earlier, of concern to dentists and staff is the lack of immunization against HCV. Antibodies formed in patients with HCV are not protective antibodies. However, the use of universal precautions provides adequate protection.

Enterically transmitted NANB has now been identified as the hepatitis E virus. Transmission is by the fecal-oral route. Large, well-documented outbreaks have been seen in India, the former Soviet Union, North America, Mexico, and Southeast Asia. There appears to be a 6- to 8-week incubation period and a low incidence of carrier state after infection. However, a high fatality rate (10% to 20%) is seen in women in their third trimester of pregnancy who contract this virus. There is no immunization available against this pathogen.

SICKLE CELL ANEMIA

Patients with sickle cell anemia have an autosomal recessive hemolytic disorder that occurs predominantly in persons of African descent but is also found among Italian, Arabian, Greek, and Indian people.

Patients with sickle cell anemia produce hemoglobin S instead of the normal hemoglobin A. Hemoglobin S has a decreased oxygen-carrying capacity. Decreased oxygen tension causes the sickling of cells. These patients are susceptible to recurrent acute infections, which result in an "aplastic crisis" caused by decreased red blood cell production and in subsequent joint and abdominal pain with fever. Over time there is a progressive deterioration of cardiac, pulmonary, and renal function.

Many factors can precipitate a sickle cell crisis, including acidosis, hypoxia, hypothermia, hypotension, stress, hypovolemia, dehydration, fever, and infection.

Radiographic changes are associated with sickle cell anemia. There is a generalized radiolucency and loss of trabeculae with prominent lamina dura, caused by increased erythropoietic demands that result in expansion of the marrow spaces. Bone growth may be decreased in the mandible, resulting in retrusion, and the teeth may be hypomineralized. Occasionally, patients with sickle cell anemia have infarcts in the jaw, which may be mistaken for a toothache or osteomyelitis. The patients experience dental pain with absence of pathology.

Dental appointments should be short to reduce potential stress on the patient. The importance of an aggressive preventive program cannot be understated, and such a program should have the goal of maintaining excellent oral health and decreasing the possibility of oral infection. Dental treatment should not be initiated during a sickle cell crisis. If emergency treatment is necessary during a crisis, only treatment that will make the patient more comfortable should be provided. Patients with sickle cell anemia may have skeletal changes that make orthodontic treatment beneficial. Special care must be taken to avoid tissue irritation, which may induce bacteremias, and the disease process may compromise the proposed treatment. Careful monitoring is a necessity when proposing elective orthodontic treatment in patients with sickle cell anemia.

Many patients with sickle cell anemia have defective spleen function or undergo a splenectomy, which leaves them more vulnerable to infection because immunoglobulin production is decreased and phagocytosis of foreign antigens is thus impaired. Most patients with sickle cell anemia are taking low-dose daily prophylactic antibiotics, and the need for additional antibiotics for dental procedures is debatable. Some authors have recommended the use of antibiotics for all dental procedures, whereas others recommend the administration of additional antibiotics when there is obvious dental or periodontal infection. The selection of an antibiotic is usually similar to that in cases of heart defect.

The use of local anesthetics with a vasoconstrictor is not contraindicated in patients with sickle cell anemia. Some textbooks do recommend against the use of vasoconstrictors, although there is no evidence to support this practice. Similarly, the use of nitrous oxide is not contraindicated in these patients. Care must be taken in treating patients with sickle cell anemia to avoid diffusion hypoxia at the completion of the dental procedure.

The restoration of teeth, including pulpotomies, is preferable to extraction. Pulpectomy in a nonvital tooth is reasonable if the practitioner is fairly confident that the tooth can remain noninfected. If the tooth is likely to persist as a focus of infection, then extraction is indicated.

The use of general anesthesia for dental procedures must be approached cautiously in consultation with the hematologist and anesthesiologist. Previously, the standard protocol was to perform a direct transfusion (immediate introduction of whole blood or blood components) or an exchange transfusion (repetitive withdrawal of small amounts of blood and replacement with donor blood until a large portion of the patient blood has been exchanged) before general anesthesia. The goal of the transfusion is to increase the patient's hemoglobin level to higher than 10 g/dL and to decrease the hemoglobin S level below 40%. Transfusions do not provide complete protection against venous complications, but they may temporarily improve the patient's condition and reduce the hazards of surgery.

The current thinking is to weigh the risks associated with transfusion prior to anesthesia induction. Suggested guidelines for performing a prophylactic transfusion before general anesthesia have been proposed. Patients with a hemoglobin level of less than 7 g/dL and a hematocrit of less than 20% may require a transfusion. Pediatric patients are usually less likely to have post-transfusion complications than are adults. A high frequency of hospitalizations is indicative of a more severe anemia, and such patients may require transfusion before surgery. Minor surgeries may not require a transfusion.

ACQUIRED IMMUNODEFICIENCY SYNDROME

Acquired immunodeficiency syndrome (AIDS) is a clinically defined condition caused by infection with HIV type 1 or, much less commonly, type 2. Estimates at the end of 2003 were that, in the United States, between 1,039,000 to 1,185,000 people are infected with HIV and one fourth of them do not know they are infected. Glynn and Rhodes estimated HIV prevalence in the United States at the end of 2003.[42] Worldwide in 2007, 33.2 million adults and 2.5 million children were infected with HIV.[43]

The incubation period from the time of infection to the appearance of symptoms of AIDS is approximately 11 years in adults. Therefore HIV-infected individuals can unknowingly spread the virus to sexual or needle-sharing partners or, in the case of infected mothers, to their children.

HIV infects cells of the immune system, specifically lymphocytes and macrophages. These white blood cells contain the greatest number of CD4 cell surface receptors (glycoproteins), which permit attachment with viral surface proteins (GP120) and enhance host-cell invasion and infection. Under the control of the HIV "pol" gene, the virus produces the enzyme reverse transcriptase, which is essential for incorporating viral RNA into host nuclear DNA. The viral genome is integrated into the host-cell genome and leads to progressive and eventually irreversible immunosuppression by producing more virus and further killing the CD4 (T4) helper-inducer lymphocytes that are important modulators of the immune system. The subsequent immunodeficiency results in a variety of opportunistic infections, malignancies (e.g., Kaposi sarcoma and lymphoma), and autoimmune diseases. Diagnosis is made by screening the serum for antibodies to HIV and is confirmed by a second methodology such as Western blot analysis or PCR. Ongoing management is guided by the patient's CD4$^+$ cell count and viral load as measured by PCR. The former is an indication of the patient's immune status, whereas a higher viral load is associated with a more accelerated disease. The current antiretroviral drugs target the virus at several steps: (1) the adhesion of the virus to the chemokine receptor CCR5, (2) the fusion of the virus to the host cell (fusion inhibitors), (3) the integration of viral genes into the target cell (integrase inhibitors), (4) the transcription of DNA from viral RNA by reverse transcriptase (nucleoside, nonnucleoside, and nucleotide reverse transcriptase inhibitors), and (5) the cleavage of viral proteins by the viral protease enzyme (protease inhibitors) . The most effective treatment strategies use a combination of several drugs to inhibit the virus at several steps.

In the United States, 67% of newly infected men diagnosed in 2006 acquired HIV through homosexual contact, infection from illicit drug use accounted for 12% of new cases, and 16% of infections were acquired through heterosexual contact.[44] Among infected women in the United States, 80% acquired HIV through heterosexual contact and 19% through intravenous drug use. Almost 30% of newborns of untreated HIV-infected mothers can acquire the HIV virus through vertical transmission. However, treatment of pregnant women with antiretroviral medications, including azidothymidine (AZT), has decreased the rate of transmission by 70%. The onset of symptoms is shortened in children who have acquired their infection prenatally and go untreated. Only 75% of untreated babies survive to age 5 years, and by that age 50% have severe symptoms.

Infants and children with AIDS have clinical findings similar to those in adults. Early manifestations of HIV infection include *Pneumocystis jirovecii* pneumonia, interstitial pneumonitis, weight loss and failure to thrive, hepatomegaly or splenomegaly, generalized lymphadenopathy, and chronic diarrhea. Unlike in adults, recurrent and severe bacterial infections are common in pediatric patients with HIV infection.

ORAL MANIFESTATIONS OF HIV INFECTION

The types of oral lesions seen in HIV infection may be caused by fungal, viral, or bacterial infections, as well as neoplastic and idiopathic processes.

Fungal Infection

Pindborg stated that the most common HIV-associated infection of the mouth is caused by the fungus *Candida albicans*.[45] Oral candidiasis is frequently present and may lead to esophageal or disseminated candidiasis. There are four major types of oral candidiasis: (1) pseudomembranous, (2) hyperplastic, (3) erythematous (atrophic), and (4) angular cheilotic.

The pseudomembranous lesion is characterized by the presence of creamy white or yellow plaques that can easily be removed from mucosa, leaving a red, bleeding surface. The most common locations for these lesions are the palate, buccal and labial mucosa, and dorsum of the tongue.

The hyperplastic lesion is characterized by white plaques that cannot easily be removed. The most common location is the buccal mucosa.

The erythematous (atrophic) lesion is characterized by a red appearance. Common locations are the palate and the dorsum of the tongue. The lesion may also appear as spotty areas on the buccal mucosa.

Angular cheilitis is characterized by fissures radiating from the commissures of the mouth, often associated with small, white plaques.

The treatment of *C. albicans* infection can be either systemic or topical. Topical therapy involves the use of nystatin (Mycostatin) rinses (100,000 U, three to five times daily) or clotrimazole (Mycelex) troches. Treatment for 1 to 2 weeks is usually effective. Systemic therapy calls for ketoconazole (Nizoral) 200 or 400 mg daily with food, or fluconazole (Diflucan), 100 mg daily. Amphotericin B and its lipid preparations, azoles such as fluconazole (administered intravenously), and echinocandins are used when candidal infection has become systemic.

Candidal infections frequently recur. Therefore patients may remain on antifungal medication indefinitely. As an adjunctive measure, mouth rinses with Peridex (0.12% chlorhexidine digluconate) (Zila Pharmaceuticals, Phoenix, AZ) may be used. Chronic oral candidiasis may be a poor prognostic sign indicating a phase of more rapid decline of immune function to the terminal phase of AIDS.

Viral Infection

In the same way that fungi can cause oral disease because of the immune dysfunction induced by HIV infection, several viruses can produce lesions in the mouth following colonization or reactivation. These include herpes group viruses and papillomaviruses according to Greenspan.[46]

Oral warts may be seen in the HIV-infected patient, with human papillomavirus as the etiologic agent. Some warts have a raised, cauliflower-like appearance, whereas others are well circumscribed, have a flat surface, and almost disappear when the mucosa is stretched.

Herpes simplex virus (HSV) can produce recurrent episodes of painful ulceration. Intraorally the lesions appear most commonly on the palate. Typically these lesions present as vesicles that break open to form ulcers. However, they may also have an atypical appearance as slitlike lesions on the tongue or may mimic other diseases. Diagnosis can be made from culture, PCR, or fluorescent antibody testing.

Herpetic lesions may be treated with oral acyclovir and its relatives valacyclovir and famciclovir. Acyclovir may also be administered intravenously (750 mg/m^2 in divided doses three times a day until lesions clear) in individuals with more severe oropharyngeal lesions or in those unable to swallow.

Herpes zoster (shingles) is caused by varicella-zoster virus (VZV), the chickenpox virus. Varicella-zoster virus can produce oral ulcerations, which are usually accompanied by skin lesions generally restricted to one side of the face. These lesions are also treated with acyclovir.

Oral hairy leukoplakia (HL) is a white lesion that does not rub off, located on the lateral margins of the tongue. The surface may be smooth, corrugated, or markedly folded. HL is seen only in patients who are HIV infected. HL is a virally induced lesion caused by the Epstein-Barr virus. Treatment may include the use of high-dose acyclovir. However, the lesions usually recur.

Bacterial Infection

Bacteria causing oral lesions may include *Mycobacterium avium-intracellulare* and *Klebsiella pneumoniae*. Many of the oral lesions seen in association with HIV infection are not new entities; rather, they are known diseases that either follow an atypical course or that show an unusual response to treatment. This is frequently the case with neoplasms as well.

Neoplasms

Kaposi sarcoma is the most common malignancy seen in AIDS and occurs in 15% to 20% of AIDS patients according to Silverman.[47] Intraoral lesions may occur alone or along with skin, visceral, and lymph node lesions. Often the first lesions of Kaposi sarcoma appear in the mouth. They may be red, blue, or purple, flat or raised, and solitary or multiple. The most common oral site is the hard palate, although lesions may be found on any part of the oral mucosa. Treatment for aggressive lesions involves radiation, laser surgery, or chemotherapy. Conventional surgery may be appropriate for small lesions.

The group of malignancies whose incidence is growing the fastest among patients with AIDS is the lymphomas, most commonly the non-Hodgkin's lymphomas. The first manifestation may be a firm, painless swelling in the mouth. Biopsies of these growths are indicated to establish a diagnosis. Treatment includes multidrug chemotherapy and radiation. Less than 20% of patients survive 2 years; the mean survival time is approximately 6 months from diagnosis.

Oral squamous cell carcinomas also occur more frequently in the HIV-infected population.

Idiopathic Lesions

According to Greenspan, oral ulcers of unknown etiology are being reported with increasing frequency in people with HIV infection.[46] The ulcers resemble aphthous lesions, appearing as well-circumscribed ulcers with an erythematous margin. Patients sometimes exhibit extremely large and painful necrotic ulcers that may persist for several weeks.

Salivary gland swelling has been seen in both adults and children with HIV infection. The cause of the swelling is unknown. It usually involves the parotid glands and is also accompanied by xerostomia.

HIV-infected patients may develop autoimmune disorders, including immune thrombocytopenic purpura. Oral lesions appear as small, blood-filled purpuric lesions or petechiae. Spontaneous gingival bleeding may also occur.

HIV-Associated Gingivitis and HIV-Associated Periodontitis

Progressive and premature periodontal disease is seen relatively frequently in HIV-infected individuals and may even be the first sign of HIV infection. Unlike conventional periodontal disease, these lesions do not respond effectively to standard periodontal therapy. There may be a rapid progression from mild gingivitis to advanced, painful, spontaneously bleeding periodontal disease in a few months. Treatment includes aggressive curettage, Peridex (0.12% chlorhexidine digluconate) rinses three times daily, and possibly antibiotic treatment.

LEUKEMIA

Malignancy is second only to accidents as the leading cause of death in children. Leukemias are hematopoietic malignancies in which there is a proliferation of abnormal leukocytes in the bone marrow and dissemination of these cells into the peripheral blood. The abnormal leukocytes (blast cells) replace normal cells in bone marrow and accumulate in other tissues and organs of the body.

Leukemia is classified according to the morphology of the predominant abnormal white blood cells in the bone marrow (Table 24-1). These types are further categorized as acute or chronic, depending on the clinical course and the degree of differentiation, or maturation, of the predominant abnormal cells.

In the United States, about 6550 new cases of cancer are diagnosed each year in children under the age of 15. Acute leukemia is the most common malignancy in children, with about 2500 new cases diagnosed annually in the United States.

Thus acute leukemia accounts for about one third of all childhood malignancies; of these, approximately 80% are lymphocytic (acute lymphocytic leukemia, or ALL).

Chronic leukemia in children is rare, accounting for less than 2% of all cases.

Leukemia affects about one of every 29,000 children each year in the United States. The peak incidence is between 2 and 5 years of age. Although the cause of leukemia is unknown, ionizing radiation, certain chemical agents, and genetic factors have been implicated. For example, children with chromosomal abnormalities (Down syndrome and Bloom syndrome), children with an identical twin who has leukemia, and children with immunologic disorders have an increased risk for leukemia. In the US leukemia rates for white children are nearly double that for black children.[48]

The clinical manifestations of acute leukemia are caused by the infiltration of leukemia cells into tissues and organs. Infiltration and proliferation of leukemia cells in the bone marrow lead to anemia, thrombocytopenia, and granulocytopenia. Because these cytopenias develop gradually, the onset of the disease is frequently insidious. The history at presentation may reveal increased irritability, lethargy, persistent fever, vague bone pain, and easy bruising. Some of the more common findings on initial physical examination are pallor, fever, tachycardia, adenopathy, hepatosplenomegaly, petechiae, cutaneous bruises, gingival bleeding, and evidence of infection.

In approximately 90% of the cases of acute leukemia a peripheral blood smear reveals anemia and thrombocytopenia. In about 65% of cases the white blood cell count is low or normal, but it may be greater than 50,000 cells/mm^3.

When a new case of leukemia is diagnosed, the patient is hospitalized and therapy is directed toward stabilizing the patient physiologically, controlling hemorrhage, identifying and eliminating infection, evaluating renal and hepatic functions, and preparing the patient for chemotherapy.

These interventions proceed while the definitive studies to determine the exact type of leukemia are undertaken. These include performing a bone marrow aspiration to obtain marrow for microscopic analysis, special cytochemical staining, immunophenotyping by flow cytometry, and cytogenetic analysis.

The goal of treatment is to induce and maintain a complete remission, which is defined as resolution of the physical findings of leukemia (e.g., adenopathy, hepatosplenomegaly, petechiae) and normalization of peripheral blood counts and bone marrow (less than 5% blasts).

A new term minimal residual disease (MRD) has been applied when using multiple parameter flow cytometry and less than 0.1% blasts are found. Remission with MRD is better prognostically than the old definition of remission.

The basic principle of treatment of ALL is substantially different from that of acute myelogenous or nonlymphocytic leukemia (ANLL). In general, the treatment of ANLL is very intense and results in profound bone marrow hypoplasia, but the treatment duration is usually short (less than 1 year). For ALL, the treatment is less intense but more prolonged (2½ to 3½ years).

Table **24-1**			

Childhood Leukemias

Type	Age and White Blood Cell Count (WBC) at Onset	Prognosis	Treatment
Acute lymphocytic (ALL)	Peak age 3-6 years	>94% remission induction, varies with age and presenting WBC count	Vincristine, L-asparaginase, prednisone, dexamethasone, 6-mercaptopurine, methotrexate, daunomycin, doxorubicin, cytosine arabinoside [araC], cyclophosphamide
Standard risk	1-9 years with WBC <50,000/mm^3	80%-90% EFS at 60 months	
Poor risk	>10 years or any age with WBC >50,000/mm^3	50%-60% EFS at 60 months	
Infants	<1 year, any WBC	20%-30% EFS at 60 months	
Acute myelogenous (AML)		80% remission induction; 40% EFS at 36 months; >95% EFS in children with Down syndrome younger than 2 years of age	Cytosine arabinoside, daunomycin, VP-16, 6-thioguanine, idarubicin, dexamethasone; hemopoietic stem cell transplantation*
Myelocytic (AML)	Older children and adolescents	Presence of (t8;21) cytogenetic abnormality yields better outcome ~70% survival while abnormalities of 11q23, monosomy 5 or 7 portend poor prognosis (20%)	
Monocytic or myelomonocytic (AmoL; AMML)	Infants and young children more common	Presence of cytogenetic abnormality (inv 16) yields better outcome ~70 % survival	
Promyelocytic (APL)	Uncommon; seen in older children	Presence of cytogenetic abnormality (t15,17) yields better outcome ~70 % survival	Responds to all trans-retinoic acid and arsenic trioxide
Erythroleukemia	Very rare	Generally very poor	
Megakaryocytic leukemia	Very rare	Generally very poor, in young Down syndrome patients—excellent prognosis	
Chronic myelocytic (CML)			
Juvenile, Philadelphia chromosome negative	Infants and toddlers very rare	Median survival <9 months	Hematopoietic stem cell transplantation†

continued

Table 24-1—cont'd
Childhood Leukemias

Type	Age and White Blood Cell Count (WBC) at Onset	Prognosis	Treatment
Adult, Philadelphia chromosome positive	Older children and adolescents	Chronic phase about 2-4 years, then death in blast crisis, usually of AML, which is resistant to therapy; great improvement with Imatinib	Imatinib (Gleevec), hydroxyurea; interferon alpha; hematopoietic stem cell transplantation[†]
Chronic lymphocytic	Not seen in children		

*Sibling HLA-matched hematopoietic stem cell transplantation (HSCT) is considered the treatment of choice for most subtypes of acute myelogenous leukemia. Each sibling has one chance in four of being a perfect match. The patient is put into remission using standard chemotherapy before bone marrow transplantation. Of AML patients undergoing transplantation in first remission, 60% show no evidence of disease after 2 years.

†Hematopoietic stem cell transplantation has been the treatment of choice for adult and juvenile chronic myelocytic leukemia. Response to standard chemotherapy is generally poor. Imatinib, a selective inhibitor of tyrosine kinase at the breakpoint cluster region on the ABL gene (causative abnormality in CML), is highly effective and well tolerated in all phases of CML when taken orally. Because long-term oral imatinib has been successful in children, the role and timing of HSCT is somewhat controversial in the treatment of childhood Philadelphia chromosome-positive CML. Transplantation for adult-type CML in first chronic phase using a matched sibling donor gives 60% disease-free survival at 2 years.

EFS, Event-free survival.

Courtesy Dr. Randy Hock and Dr. Alexandra Cheerua.

Overall, the treatment regimens vary considerably depending on prognostic factors and the parameters being evaluated by the strategists' cooperative group (e.g., Children's Oncology Group). The initial phase of treatment, induction, incorporates the use of a combination of antileukemic drugs at staggered intervals during a 4-week regimen (Table 24-2). This combination of drugs should rapidly destroy the leukemic cells, yet maintain the regenerative potential of the nonmalignant hematopoietic cells within the bone marrow. About 95% of patients with ALL will be in complete remission at day 28 of therapy.

The second phase of ALL treatment, consolidation, attempts to consolidate remission and intensify prophylactic central nervous system (CNS) treatment. Prevention of CNS relapse uses intrathecally administered chemotherapy (methotrexate with or without cytosine arabinoside and hydrocortisone) to destroy leukemic cells within the CNS. This chemotherapeutic agent is instilled directly into the lumbar spinal fluid because most antileukemic drugs do not readily cross the blood-brain barrier. Intensive intrathecal chemotherapy to prevent CNS relapse has replaced cranial irradiation for patients in the good and intermediate-risk groups of ALL patients. However, both cranial irradiation and intrathecal chemotherapy are still used to prevent CNS relapse in high-risk ALL patients.

The third phase of treatment, interim maintenance, uses a combination of agents that are relatively nontoxic and require only monthly visits to the outpatient clinic. In most cases, another phase, delayed intensification, follows interim maintenance. This serves to intensify antileukemic therapy again after a short period of less intensive therapy. The addition of a late phase of intensive therapy substantially improves survival in patients with ALL. Following delayed intensification, therapy continues for 2 years for girls and 3 years for boys (maintenance phase), with chemotherapeutic agents given as in interim maintenance.

The prognosis for a child with acute leukemia has improved dramatically over the past several decades. Thirty-five years ago, there would have been little need to discuss dental treatment for a child with leukemia because the disease was invariably fatal, in most cases within 6 months of diagnosis. Today, with the development of new and better antileukemia drugs, the use of intensive combination drug therapy, the incorporation of radiation therapy, and improvements in diagnostic techniques and general supportive care, the overall survival for all children with ALL is now about 80%.

Pretreatment prognostic factors identify patients who are likely to benefit from either standard or more intensive therapy. Factors that identify patients who are likely to benefit from the type of therapy just outlined, which causes relatively minimal toxicity, are patient age between 1 and 10 years, a white blood cell count of less than 50,000/mm^3, lymphoblast morphology that is not of the Burkitt type, and the absence of certain cytogenetic abnormalities [t(4;11); t(9;22)] (also known as the Philadelphia chromosome) or hypoploidy in the lymphoblast. The presence of either the TEL-AML1 fusion [t(12;21)(p13;q22)] or the simultaneous trisomies of chromosomes 4, 10, and 17 in the lymphoblasts correlates with an improved prognosis and may qualify these children for less strenuous therapy.

Children with ALL who are at particularly high risk are those who are younger than 1 year of age at diagnosis,

Table **24-2**

Major Chemotherapeutic Agents and Their Side Effects

Agent	Nausea*	Bone Marrow Suppression	Hair Loss	Stomatitis/Ulcers	Renal	Neurologic
Alkylating Agents						
Carboplatin	Yes	Yes	Yes	No	No	No
Cisplatin	Yes (severe)	Yes	Yes	No	No	Peripheral neuropathy
Cyclophosphamide	Yes	Yes	Yes	No	No	Seizures (rare)
Ifosfamide	Yes	Yes	Yes	No	No	Somnolence
Antibiotics						
Actinomycin D	Yes	Yes	Yes	Yes	No	No
Vincristine[†]	No	No	Yes	No; jaw pain	No	Peripheral neuropathy, seizures (rare)
Daunomycin[‡]	Yes	Yes	Yes	Yes	No	No
Doxorubicin[‡]	Yes	Yes	Yes	Yes	No	No
Idarubicin[‡]	Yes	Yes	Yes	Yes	No	No
Antimetabolites						
Cytosine arabinoside (araC)	Yes	Yes	Yes	Yes	No	Cerebellar dysfunction
Methotrexate	Yes	Yes	Yes	Yes	Yes	Leukoencephalopathy[§]
6-Mercaptopurine	Yes	Yes	Mild	Rare	No	No
Plant alkaloids						
Etoposide	Yes	Yes	Yes	No	No	No
Miscellaneous Dexamethasone	No	No	No	No	No	Pseudotumor; psychoses
Prednisone	No	No	No	No	No	Pseudotumor; psychoses
L-Asparaginase[¶]	No	No	No	No	No	Seizures (rare), thrombosis

*Nausea is substantially alleviated by judicious use of antiemetics.
†These agents cause severe skin burns if they extravasate from the vein.
‡High cumulative doses may result in cardiac toxicity.
§Leukoencephalopathy is usually seen with methotrexate in conjunction with whole-brain radiation.
¶L-Asparaginase may cause pancreatitis and diabetes.

have a high white blood cell count, or have the cytogenetic abnormalities mentioned above. More intrusive treatment regimens are used for these patients.

The early response to induction chemotherapy is also a strong predictor of outcome for patients with ALL.[49] Current clinical trials in leukemia are using flow cytometry and molecular techniques to detect blast cells not visible morphologically in bone marrow aspirates.

Quantification of this MRD is being used as an additional tool to direct therapy so that children can receive risk-based adjusted therapy.

The prognosis for children with acute myelogenous leukemia (AML) has improved significantly over the past several years, with event-free survivals of approximately 50% (at 3 years) for children receiving chemotherapy and somewhat higher percentages for patients undergoing allogeneic hematopoietic stem cell transplantation from a matched sibling after achieving remission with chemotherapy.[50] The treatment regimens are intrusive and result in profound bone marrow suppression. These patients have severe prolonged neutropenia, necessitating long hospitalizations. They often have serious infections and severe mucositis.

ORAL MANIFESTATIONS OF LEUKEMIA

Pathologic changes in the oral cavity as a result of leukemia occur frequently. Oral signs or symptoms suggestive of leukemia have been reported in as many as 75% of adults and 29% of children with leukemia. The lower incidence of oral manifestations in children can be attributed in part to the early age at diagnosis and the high percentage of ALL in the pediatric age group. The incidence of ALL peaks at 3 years of age, when preexisting inflammatory and degenerative changes are comparatively less frequent.

Abnormalities in or around the oral cavity occur in all types of leukemia, and in all age groups. However, oral pathoses are more commonly observed in acute leukemias than in chronic forms of the disease. Oral findings suggestive of leukemia are also more common in AML than in ALL.

The most frequently reported oral abnormalities attributed to the leukemic process include regional lymphadenopathy, mucous membrane petechiae and ecchymoses, gingival bleeding, gingival hypertrophy, pallor, and nonspecific ulcerations. Manifestations seen occasionally are cranial nerve palsies, chin and lip paresthesias, odontalgia, jaw pain, loose teeth, extruded teeth, and gangrenous stomatitis. Each of these findings has been reported in all types of leukemia. Regional lymphadenopathy is the most frequently reported finding. Gingival abnormalities, including hypertrophy and bleeding, are more common in patients with AML, whereas petechiae and ecchymoses are more common in those with ALL.

Like the systemic manifestations of leukemia, oral changes can be attributed to anemia, granulocytopenia, and thrombocytopenia, all of which result from the replacement of normal bone marrow elements by undifferentiated blast cells, or to direct invasion of tissue by these leukemic cells. Very high circulating white blood cell numbers in the peripheral blood can lead to stasis in small vascular channels. The subsequent tissue anoxia results in areas of necrosis and ulceration that can readily become infected by opportunistic oral microorganisms in patients with neutropenia. A person with severe thrombocytopenia, having lost the capacity to maintain vascular integrity, is likely to bleed spontaneously. Clinical manifestations are petechiae or ecchymoses of the oral mucosa or frank bleeding from the gingival sulcus (Figs. 24-3 and 24-4). The propensity for gingival bleeding is greatly increased in persons with deficient oral hygiene, because accumulated plaque and debris are significant local irritants.

Direct invasion of tissue by an infiltrate of leukemic cells can produce gingival hypertrophy. Such gingival changes can occur despite excellent oral hygiene. Infiltration of leukemic cells along vascular channels can result

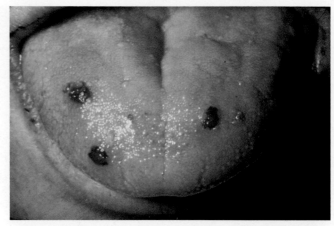

Figure 24-3 Several small ecchymoses on the dorsal surface of the tongue in a 10-year-old girl with acute lymphocytic leukemia. (Courtesy Dr. Bruce W. Vash)

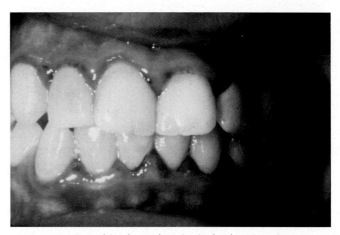

Figure 24-4 Petechia along the gingival sulcus in a 14-year-old female with acute lymphocytic leukemia. (Courtesy Dr. Bruce W. Vash)

in strangulation of pulpal tissue and spontaneous abscess formation as a result of infection or focal areas of liquefaction necrosis in the dental pulp of clinically and radiographically sound teeth. In a similar fashion, the teeth may rapidly loosen as a result of necrosis of the periodontal ligament.

Skeletal lesions caused by leukemic infiltration of bone are common in childhood leukemia. The most common finding is a generalized osteoporosis caused by enlargement of the Haversian canals and Volkmann canals. Osteolytic lesions resulting from focal areas of hemorrhage and necrosis and leading to loss of trabecular bone are also common.

Evidence of skeletal lesions is visible on dental radiographs in up to 63% of children with acute leukemia. Manifestations in the jaws include generalized loss of trabeculation, destruction of the crypts of developing teeth, loss of lamina dura, widening of the periodontal

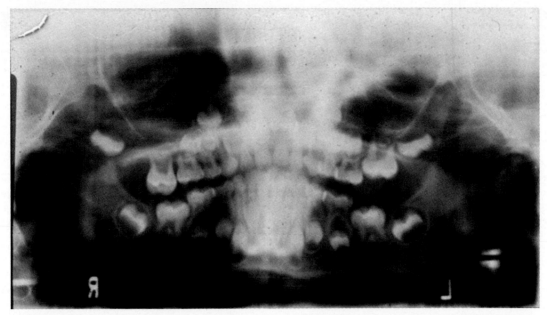

Figure 24-5 Panoramic radiograph of a patient with acute mylocytic leukemia resulting in the displacement of the maxillary right permanent molar. (Courtesy Dr. Bruce W. Vash)

ligament space, and displacement of teeth and tooth buds (Fig. 24-5). Because none of the oral changes is a pathognomonic sign of leukemia and all can be associated with numerous local or systemic disease processes, a diagnosis of leukemia cannot be based on oral findings alone. Such changes should, however, alert the clinician to the possibility of malignancy as the underlying cause.

DENTAL MANAGEMENT OF PATIENTS WITH LEUKEMIA

Before any dental treatment is administered to a child with leukemia, the child's hematologist/oncologist or primary care physician should be consulted. The following information should be ascertained:

1. Primary medical diagnosis
2. Anticipated clinical course and prognosis
3. Present and future therapeutic modalities
4. Present general state of health
5. Present hematologic status

It is also important to establish, by consultation with the patient's physician, when dental treatment may be most propitious, and to schedule the patient's treatment accordingly. The proposed procedures should be discussed to determine if they are appropriate.

For a child whose first remission has not yet been obtained, or one who is in relapse, all elective dental procedures should be deferred. However, it is essential that potential sources of systemic infection within the oral cavity be controlled or eradicated whenever they are recognized (e.g., immediate extraction of carious primary teeth with pulpal involvement).

Routine preventive, restorative, and surgical procedures can usually be provided for a patient who is in complete remission yet is undergoing chemotherapy. The time when

such procedures may be completed without complications will depend on the specific agents administered and the time of administration. Before the appointment—preferably the same day—a blood cell profile (complete blood count) and platelet count should be taken to confirm that the patient is not unexpectedly at undue risk for hemorrhage or infection. A patient who has been in complete remission for at least 2 years and no longer requires chemotherapy may be treated in an essentially normal manner. A preappointment blood workup is not necessary.

Pulp therapy on primary teeth is contraindicated in any patient with a history of leukemia. Endodontic treatment for permanent teeth is not recommended for any patient with leukemia who may have a chronic, intermittent suppression of granulocytes. Even with the most exacting technique, an area of chronic inflammatory tissue may remain in the periapical region of endodontically treated teeth. An area of low-grade, chronic inflammation in a healthy patient is generally well tolerated, but in an immunosuppressed, neutropenic patient the same area can act as an anachoretic focus with devastating sequelae. The decision to perform an endodontic procedure on a patient who has been in prolonged complete remission and who is not undergoing chemotherapy must be made by the dentist.

A platelet level of 100,000/mm³ is adequate for most dental procedures (Table 24-3). Routine preventive and restorative treatment, including nonblock injections, may be considered when the platelet count is at least 50,000/mm³. With inadequate oral hygiene, unhealthy periodontal tissues, and the presence of local irritants, hemorrhage from the gingival sulcus may be observed when platelet counts are between 20,000 and 50,000/mm³. Such hemorrhaging is usually noted only after

Table 24-3

Clinical Importance of Platelet Count*

Count (cells/mm³)	Significance
150,000-400,000	Normal
50,000-150,000	Bleeding time is prolonged, but patient would tolerate most routine procedures
20,000-50,000	At moderate risk for bleeding; defer elective surgical procedures
<20,000	At significant risk for bleeding; defer elective dental procedures

*An absolute indication for platelet transfusion is significant bleeding. If the count is <20,000 to 30,000 cells/mm³, the patient should probably be given prophylactic platelet transfusion before dental procedures. Prophylactic platelet transfusions are given for platelet levels below 10,000 cells/mm³. Indiscriminate use of platelet therapy may lead to the development of antiplatelet antibodies.
Courtesy Dr. Thomas D. Coates.

manipulation of the tissues, such as during toothbrushing. If the platelet count is lower than 20,000/mm³, all the intraoral mucosal tissues may show clinical evidence of spontaneous hemorrhaging (e.g., petechiae, ecchymoses, or frank hemorrhage). No dental treatment should be performed at such a time without a preceding prophylactic platelet transfusion. Good oral hygiene must be maintained while the platelet count is at this level, but it may be necessary to discontinue the use of a toothbrush and to substitute cleaning with moist gauze wipes, supplemented by frequent saline rinses.

The absolute neutrophil count (ANC) is an indicator of the host's ability to suppress or eliminate infection. It is calculated using the following formula:

$$\text{ANC} = (\% \text{ of neutrophils} + \% \text{ of bands}) \times \text{total white count} \div 100$$

The clinical significance of the ANC is presented in Table 24-4. If the ANC is less than 1000/mm³, elective dental treatment should be deferred. A leukemic patient with a low ANC may require prophylactic broad-spectrum antibiotic therapy before certain dental procedures. The patient's physician should be consulted regarding the appropriate drugs and dosages.

Infection and hemorrhage are the primary causes of death other than resistant disease or relapse in children with leukemia. Therefore the primary objective of dental treatment in a child with leukemia should be the prevention, control, and eradication of oral inflammation, hemorrhage, and infection.

Frequently, initial oral manifestations of bleeding or infection are observed in association with an unhealthy periodontium. In patients with leukemia who are neutropenic or who are being treated with corticosteroids, the true degree of periodontal inflammation or infection may be masked, because the cardinal signs of inflammation may not be apparent. There is a much greater propensity for gingival bleeding when the periodontium is unhealthy. When oral hygiene is neglected and local irritants are present, spontaneous hemorrhaging from the gingival sulcus may be observed if the patient is thrombocytopenic.

It is imperative that a patient who is diagnosed as having leukemia be enrolled in a good preventive dental care program in which special emphasis is placed on the initiation and maintenance of a comprehensive oral

Table 24-4

Clinical Importance of White Blood Cell Count

ANC*	Significance
>1500	Normal
500-1000	Patient at some risk for infection; defer elective procedures that could induce significant transient bacteremia
200-500	Patient must be admitted to hospital if febrile and given broad-spectrum antibiotics; at moderate risk for sepsis; defer all elective dental procedures
<200	At significant risk for sepsis

Courtesy Dr. Thomas D. Coates
*All values refer to absolute neutrophil count (ANC) and compute as follows:
ANC = (% of polymorphonuclear leukocytes + % of bands) × total white count ÷ 100

hygiene regimen. The use of a soft nylon toothbrush for the removal of plaque is recommended, even if the patient is thrombocytopenic. As long as the gingiva remains in a healthy state and its manipulation by brushing does not induce significant hemorrhage, it is not appropriate to discontinue the use of a toothbrush because of the platelet level alone. The practicality of flossing must be assessed on an individual basis.

It is important that significant local irritants, including orthodontic appliances, be removed. Scaling and subgingival curettage should not necessarily be perceived as elective dental treatment in all patients. This is especially true if the anticipated clinical course may place the patient at high risk for hemorrhage and infection. Patients with classic leukemic gingivitis experience varying degrees of discomfort. The use of warm saline rinses several times each day may assist in the relief of symptoms.

Erosive or ulcerative lesions are common in children with leukemia. These lesions are often associated with the use of certain chemotherapeutic agents (see Table 24-2), especially methotrexate and the anthracycline antibiotics daunomycin and doxorubicin. The lesions may be an early indicator of drug toxicity. After administration of the drug is discontinued and the ANC has recovered, these lesions usually disappear within a few days. Treatment is directed toward the relief of discomfort (Table 24-5).

In a patient who is granulocytopenic, trauma may result in the occurrence of ulcerative lesions, especially along the lateral border of the tongue and buccal mucosa. The clinical course of these ulcerations is generally benign, although the time necessary for healing may be prolonged. Use of topical obtundents for pain may be the only treatment indicated.

Infrequently, deep lesions will bleed spontaneously or as a result of trauma. Local measures, such as the topical application of either bovine thrombin or Avitene, and the placement of an oral adhesive for protection, may be beneficial.

In a patient who is physically debilitated or who is in relapse, septic, and severely granulocytopenic, ulcerative lesions require close observation. Such lesions may serve as a nidus for the proliferation of microorganisms, which can lead to potentially fatal viral, fungal, or bacterial infection. Therefore specimens from these ulcerative lesions should be cultured and subsequent sensitivity testing performed, and antibiotic therapy should be initiated or modified accordingly.

Candidiasis is common in children with leukemia. They are especially susceptible to this fungal infection because of (1) general physical debilitation, (2) immunosuppression, (3) prolonged antibiotic therapy, (4) chemotherapy, and (5) poor oral hygiene. The following topical use of nystatin can be particularly beneficial:
- Nystatin oral suspension, 100,000 U/mL
- Swish 5 mL for 5 minutes and then swallow
- Repeat every 6 hours; continue for 48 hours after lesions disappear

Table 24-5

Topical Obtundents for Oral Pain (Frequently Used at James Whitcomb Riley Hospital for Children and St. Vincent Children's Hospital)

Combination	Administration	Indications
Benacort-Tetrastat (Mary's Magic Potion)		
Hydrocortisone poser 60 mg	Swish 5-10 mL for 1 minute; then expectorate	Generalized stomatitis and mild discomfort
Tetracycline 1.5 g		
Nystatin suspension 100,000 U/mL 60 mL		
Benadryl elixir qs 240 L		
Philadelphia Mouthwash*		
Benadryl elixir 90 mL	Swish 5-10 mL for 1 minute; then expectorate	Generalized stomatitis and mild discomfort
Maalox suspension 90 mL		
Viscous lidocaine 2% 90 mL		
Distilled water 180 mL		
Cherry or vanilla flavoring to taste		
Orabase with Benzocaine, or Viscous lidocaine 2%, or Dyclonine HCL 0.5%	Apply locally to lesions with cotton swab	Discrete, painful lesions

*Use should be supervised to prevent lidocaine toxicity.

In more resistant cases of oral candidiasis, fluconazole may be useful, administered once daily either orally or intravenously (in young children 6 mg/kg on day 1, then 3 mg/kg to a maximum of 12 mg/kg per day; in older children and adults 200 mg on day 1, then 100 mg).

For patients who are thrombocytopenic or at risk for intermittent episodes of thrombocytopenia because of chemotherapy or active disease, the dentist should avoid prescribing drugs that may alter platelet function, such as salicylates (aspirin) and nonsteroidal anti-inflammatory drugs.

HEMATOPOIETIC STEM CELL TRANSPLANTATION

The transplantation of hemopoietic stem cells can be curative for a variety of disorders, including aplastic anemia, thalassemia, and severe combined immunodeficiency. Stem cell transplantation has also been shown to be effective as rescue therapy for patients undergoing extremely aggressive treatment for leukemia in which both lethal doses of chemotherapy and total-body irradiation are used to destroy all bone marrow elements, including normal marrow cells. Intensive chemotherapy, total-body irradiation, and stem cell rescue are being used in experimental treatment protocols for children with very aggressive malignancies (e.g., advanced neuroblastoma and Ewing sarcoma).

As with any organ transplantation, hemopoietic stem cell transplantation candidates must have a compatible donor. The ideal donor, in most cases, is a healthy identical twin, which would result in a syngeneic recipient and donor. Next best is an HLA-compatible sibling yielding an allogeneic transplant. In the absence of a related HLA-compatible donor, stem cells from matched unrelated donors or from placental cord blood can sometimes be used. In certain cases, autologous transplantation is performed in which the patient's own bone marrow or peripheral blood stem cells are harvested and stored and then returned to the patient after intensive treatment and after remission has been achieved.

In almost all organ transplantation procedures, host rejection of the transplanted organ and infection are prime reasons for treatment failure. An additional complication in allogeneic hemopoietic stem cell transplantation is graft-versus-host disease (GVHD) in which immunocompetent donor lymphocytes attack the recipient host cells.

During and after hemopoietic stem cell transplantation, the most common cause of serious morbidity and mortality is infection. The risk for infection from exogenous sources is reduced by good hand washing. Despite multiple-agent antibacterial, antifungal, and antiviral therapy, endogenous opportunistic organisms are usually the cause of life-threatening infection in hemopoietic stem cell transplantation patients, who, because of ablated bone marrow function, are unable to mount protective inflammatory and immune responses before engraftment of donor bone marrow.

ORAL COMPLICATIONS OF BONE MARROW TRANSPLANTATION

The oral complications of bone marrow transplantation differ from those seen during conventional therapy for malignant disease only in degree and duration. Oral ulceration, mucositis, and transient salivary gland dysfunction are frequent consequences of stomatotoxic chemotherapy and total-body irradiation. Minor trauma to atrophic mucous membranes often results in self-induced ulceration of the buccal mucosa, lips, and tongue. Thrombocytopenic gingival bleeding and bleeding from oral ulcerations are also frequently encountered.

Oral bleeding responds well to platelet transfusions and intravenous aminocaproic acid (Amicar). Topical application of Avitene (bovine corium collagen hydrochloride), powdered thrombin, and pressure are often effective for control of localized bleeding and often must be relied on in those cases in which the patient fails to respond to transfused platelets.

Oral ulceration and mucositis resolve with the return of bone marrow function and rising absolute neutrophil counts. Interim treatment is directed toward palliation and prevention of secondary infection. Any of the topically applied obtundent solutions or topical local anesthetics mentioned previously may be used. The efficacy of each will vary among patients, and in some cases only potent systemic analgesics will provide relief. In all cases, however, infection must be suspected, and specimens from all lesions should be cultured and growing organisms tested for antibiotic susceptibility.

GRAFT-VERSUS-HOST DISEASE

A major problem of allogeneic bone marrow transplantation is the development of GVHD. This disorder appears to result from an interaction between donor immunocompetent cells and recipient cells that display disparate antigens. The acute form of the disease involves the lymphoid system, skin, liver, and gastrointestinal tract. Cutaneous and oral mucosal involvement in chronic GVHD is common and is manifested as painful overt mucosal erythema, reticular or lichenoid eruptions, or desquamation and ulceration. Treatment with dexamethasone oral rinses may be helpful in cases of severe mucosal involvement in chronic GVHD. Mucosal involvement may be accompanied by salivary gland dysfunction with xerostomia, dysphagia, and dysgeusia.

Treatment of both acute and chronic GVHD is directed at correcting, masking, or preventing disordered immune regulation. Therapies with low- and high-dose steroids (prednisone, dexamethasone), antithymocyte globulin, cyclosporin, azathioprine, or methotrexate have been attempted with mixed results. Although severe acute GVHD can be rapidly fatal, chronic GVHD is usually transient and controllable with systemic therapy. The goals of therapy for mucosal and salivary gland manifestations, which relies on abundant rinses, are palliation and prevention of secondary infection.

Of note, the positive side of GVHD is an associated graft-versus-leukemia effect. In both acute and chronic GVHD, the immune response associated with GVHD appears to affect leukemia cells in that there is an inverse relationship between the severity of GVHD and the incidence of relapse.

PRETRANSPLANTATION PREPARATION

Bone marrow transplantation programs place a high priority on pretransplantation dental care and daily mouth care in the transplant unit. The primary goal of this oral health care protocol is to prevent, reduce in severity, or palliatively relieve oral problems involved in the oral care of patients receiving oncologic therapy. The integrity of the oral cavity is maintained by keeping the oral structures, both hard and soft tissues, clean, moist, and free of infection. The resultant decrease in septic episodes in the oral cavity should diminish the patient's morbidity and mortality because the mouth is the most common source of infection in these patients.

Four weeks before bone marrow transplantation, all candidates for this procedure should receive a thorough clinical and radiographic oral examination during the workup phase initiated from the oncology physician's consult. The resultant dental treatment plan, along with the primary goals of oral health care, are discussed with the patient's oncologist, the patient, and the parents. Each patient is also informed of all potential oral complications of bone marrow transplantation and GVHD.

Along with professional preventive dental care, each patient should receive instruction in daily mouth care, including brushing and flossing. The daily use of self-applied topical fluoride gel and Peridex rinse (every 12 hours) is recommended. Dental appointments are scheduled for any necessary periodontal, restorative, or oral surgery treatment, if indicated, to eliminate and control oral infections or conditions that may lead to episodic problems. Potential foci of infection or bleeding, such as pulpally involved teeth, periodontally involved teeth, partially erupted teeth, exfoliating primary teeth and carious teeth, or teeth with defective restorations, must be treated before admission to the transplant unit. Recommended treatment should ideally be completed at least 2 weeks before admission to allow for healing of violated tissues and the reestablishment of optimal oral hygiene.

Unfortunately, there are times when the patient's medical status necessitates admission for transplantation before all dental treatment can be completed. Therefore the minimum preadmission dental requirement is a mouth free of foci of acute infection and free of physical irritants. Each patient must receive thorough supragingival and subgingival scaling and prophylaxis; open carious lesions and carious lesions approaching the pulp must be restored, and abscessed teeth and teeth with severe periodontal involvement, as well as exfoliating primary teeth causing gingival irritation, must be removed.

ADMISSION AND NURSING INTERVENTIONS

Peridex has been shown to be effective in minimizing the septic episodes in the oral cavity when used with other chemotherapeutic agents. On admission, the patient should be instructed to brush his or her teeth three times a day with a Peridex-soaked ultrasoft toothbrush (e.g.,

Sensodyne Gentle). When the platelet count is less than 20,000/mm^3 and gum bleeding is apparent, a toothette should be used in place of a toothbrush. The patient may not eat or drink for 1 hour following the use of Peridex. Surgilube may be applied to the lips following each rinse session and every 4 hours for dryness.

Allogeneic and autologous transplant patients are started on antifungal prophylaxis with fluconazole (5 mg/kg per day by mouth, maximum dose 200 mg per day). The condition of the oral cavity should be monitored and charted on each shift. Doctors should be notified of any change in the oral cavity from the previous day or shift.

The treatment of mucositis is described in Box 24-1. Mild mucositis is defined as mild erythema, no mucosal ulcerations, and no pain; the patient is able to swallow, and no local analgesia is required. Moderate mucositis is defined as moderate erythema, multiple mucosal ulcerations with pain that may or may not require analgesics; the patient can swallow but it may be painful. Severe mucositis is defined as erythema, multiple ulcerations, severe pain requiring analgesia, and difficulty in or inability to swallow. Although the regimens shown are not always successful in cases of moderate or severe

---

Box 24-1

Treatment of Mucositis and Candidiasis (Guidelines for Nursing Staff)

Mild mucositis
- Continue same oral regimen and add 2% sodium bicarbonate.
- Chart condition of oral cavity each shift; notify doctor of any change from the previous day or shift.

Moderate or severe mucositis
- Obtain order for pain medication to be administered either before oral care or as a continuous drip (i.e., morphine sulphate); may require bolus administration in addition to continuous drip.
- Follow same regimen as with mild mucositis using both 2% sodium bicarbonate and Peridex with toothette.
- Use Peridex every 4 hours; if patient is having difficulty rinsing with full-strength Peridex, dilute Peridex 1:1 with sterile water.

Candida infection
- Contact dentist to examine and obtain a culture specimen. Hold one dose of Peridex and nystatin until culture is obtained.
- Patient must be started on additional antifungal therapy once culture results show evidence of yeast infection.
- If oral candidiasis is documented by culture, nystatin should be applied with a toothette, swished for 30 to 60 seconds, then swallowed.
- Chart condition of oral cavity; each shift should notify doctor of any change from the previous day shift.

mucositis, consistent follow-through minimizes many signs and symptoms.

The presence of white patches (i.e., candidal infection) may occur. Care must be taken in obtaining culture specimens and providing specific antifungal therapy.

REMISSION PHASE

During the remission phase of post–bone marrow transplantation therapy, consistent oral hygiene should be provided by the patient or parent. For the first 90 days, the dental staff should provide maintenance oral evaluations and preventive oral care reinforcement for the bone marrow transplantation patient when he or she returns for periodic hospital oncologic evaluations.

Afterward, the patient should be referred to his or her private dentist for continuity of oral health care. If the patient has no dentist, referral should be made to a dental diagnostic clinic at the patient's medical center for dental health status evaluation and dental care.

SOLID TUMORS

Solid tumors account for approximately half of the cases of childhood malignancy. The most common tumors include brain tumors, lymphoma, neuroblastoma, Wilms tumor, osteosarcoma, and rhabdomyosarcoma. Because many of the malignancies can involve bone marrow and their treatment with chemotherapy and radiation can suppress marrow function, many of the complications seen in acute leukemia are also seen with these patients. Bleeding diatheses and the propensity to infection are the most notable medical complications seen. In general, the dental management of patients with solid tumors is similar to that of patients with acute leukemia.

REFERENCES

1. Soucie JM, et al. Occurrence of hemophilia in the United States. The Hemophilia Surveillance System Project Investigators, *Am J Hematol* 59(4):288-294, 1998.
2. Miller R. Counseling about diagnosis and inheritance of genetic bleeding disorders: haemophilia A and B, *Haemophilia* 5(2):77-83, 1999.
3. Ljung R, Tegård U. Genetic counseling of hemophilia carriers, *Semin Thromb Hemost* 29(1):31-36, 2003.
4. Gomez K, Bolton-Maggs P. Factor XI deficiency, *Haemophilia* Feb 27 [Epub ahead of print.], 2008
5. Peyvandi F, et al. Rare bleeding disorders, *Haemophilia* 14(Suppl 3):202-210, 2008.
6. Nichols WL, et al. Von Willebrand disease (VWD): evidence-based diagnosis and management guidelines, the National Heart, Lung, and Blood Institute (NHLBI) Expert Panel report (USA), *Haemophilia* 14(2):171-232, 2008.
7. World Health Organization. Delivery of Treatment for Haemophilia. Report of a Joint WHO/WFH/ISTH Meeting; London, United Kingdom, 11-13 February 2002. World Health Organization. Available at: http://whqlibdoc.who.int/hq/2002/WHO_WFH_ISTH_WG_02.6.pdf.
8. de Sousa SO, et al. Hemophilia pseudotumor of the jaws: report of two cases, *Oral Surg Oral Med Oral Pathol Oral Radiol Endod* 79(2):216-219, 1995.
9. Sonis AL, Musselman RJ. Oral bleeding in classic hemophilia, *Oral Surg* 53:363-366, 1982.
10. Kessler CM. Advances in the treatment of hemophilia, *Clin Adv Hematol Oncol* 6(3):184-187, 2008.
11. Gill JC, et al. Evaluation of high concentration intranasal and intravenous desmopressin in pediatric patients with mild hemophilia A or mild-to-moderate type 1 von Willebrand disease, *J Pediatr* 140(5):595-599, 2002.
12. Castaman G. Desmopressin for the treatment of haemophilia, *Haemophilia* 14(Suppl 1):15-20, 2008.
13. Rodeghiero F, et al. How to estimate bleeding risk in mild bleeding disorders, *J Thromb Haemost* 5(Suppl 1): 157-166, 2007
14. Pipe SW. Recombinant clotting factors, *Thromb Haemost* 99(5):840-850, 2008.
15. Young G, Aledort L. Therapy for haemophilia: recent advances and goals for the future, *Expert Opin Emerg Drugs* 10(1):173-184, 2005.
16. Giangrande P. Haemophilia B: Christmas disease, *Expert Opin Pharmacother* 6(9):1517-1524, 2005.
17. Björkman S, et al. Pharmacokinetics of recombinant factor IX in relation to age of the patient: implications for dosing in prophylaxis, *Haemophilia* 7(2):133-139, 2001.
18. Manco-Johnson MJ, et al. Prophylaxis versus episodic treatment to prevent joint disease in boys with severe hemophilia, *N Engl J Med* 357(6):535-544, 2007.
19. Byams VR. Women with bleeding disorders, *J Womens Health* 16(9):1249-1251, 2007.
20. Federici AB, Mannucci PM. Management of inherited von Willebrand disease in 2007, *Ann Med* 39(5):346-358, 2007.
21. Plug I, et al. Bleeding in carriers of hemophilia, *Blood* 108(1):52-56, 2006.
22. Street AM, et al. Management of carriers and babies with haemophilia, *Haemophilia* 14(Suppl 3):181-187, 2008.
23. DiMichele DM. Inhibitor treatment in haemophilias A and B: Inhibitor diagnosis, *Haemophilia* 12(Suppl 6):37-41, 2006.
24. Astermark J. Overview of inhibitors, *Semin Hematol* 43(2 Suppl 4):3-7, 2006.
25. Luck JV Jr, et al. Hemophilic arthropathy, *J Am Acad Orthop Surg* 12(4):234-245, 2004.
26. Goedert JJ, et al. Human immunodeficiency and hepatitis virus infections and their associated conditions and treatments among people with haemophilia, *Haemophila.*, 10(Suppl 4):205-210, 2004.
27. Evatt BL. The tragic history of AIDS in the hemophilia population, 1982-84, *J Thromb Haemost* 4(11):2295-2301, 2006.
28. Klein RS, et al. Low occupational risk of human immuno deficiency virus infection among dental professionals, *N Engl J Med* 318:89-90, 1988.
29. Kumar JN, et al. Specialty dentistry for the hemophiliac: is there a protocol in place? *Indian J Dent Res* 18(2): 48-54, 2007.
30. Lee AP, et al. Effectiveness in controlling haemorrhage after dental scaling in people with haemophilia by using tranexamic acid mouthwash, *Br Dent J* 198(1):33-38; discussion 26, 2005.
31. Vinall C, Stassen LF. The dental patient with a congenital bleeding disorder, *J Ir Dent Assoc* 54(1):24-28, 2008.
32. Jover-Cerveró A, et al. Dental treatment of patients with coagulation factor alterations: an update, *Med Oral Pathol Oral Cir Bucal* 12(5):E380-E387, 2007.
33. Israels S, et al. Bleeding disorders: characterization, dental considerations and management, *J Can Dent Assoc* 72(9):827, 2006.
34. Azhar S, et al. Periodontal status and IOTN interventions among young hemophiliacs, *Haemophilia* 12(4): 4011-4, 2006. Erratum in *Haemophilia* 12(5):559, 2006.

35. Correa ME, et al. Clinical impact of oral health indexes in dental extraction of hemophilic patients, *J Oral Maxillofac Surg* 64(5):785-788, 2006.

36. Brewer AK. Advances in minor oral surgery in patients with congenital bleeding disorders, *Haemophilia* 14(Suppl 3): 119-121, 2008.

37. Piot B, et al. Management of dental extractions in patients with bleeding disorders, *Oral Surg Oral Med Oral Pathol Oral Radiol Endod* 93(3):247-250, 2002.

38. O'Grady NP, et al. Guidelines for the prevention of intravascular catheter-related infections. MMWR. August 9, 2002;51(RR10):1-26. Available at: http://www.cdc.gov/mmwr/preview/mmwrhtml/rr5110a1.htm.

39. CDC MMWR March 21, 2008/ 57(SS02);1-24 and http://www.cdc.gov/ncidod/disease/hepatitits/b/fact.htm accessed 6/14/2008.

40. Cottone JA. Recent developments in hepatitis: new virus, vaccine, and dosage recommendations, *J Am Dent Assoc* 20:501-508, 1990.

41. Centers for Disease Control and Prevention. Viral hepatitis. Available at: http://www.cdc.gov/ncidod/diseases/hepatitis/c/fact.htm. Accessed June 14, 2008.

42. Glynn M, Rhodes P. Estimated HIV prevalence in the United States at the end of 2003. National HIV Prevention Conference. Abstract 595. Atlanta, June 2005.

43. UNAIDS. AIDS epidemic update: December 2007. "UNAIDS/07.27E / JC1322E"

44. Centers for Disease Control and Prevention. HIV/AIDS Surveillance Report, 2006. Vol. 18. Atlanta: US Department of Health and Human Services, Centers for Disease Control and Prevention, 2008.

45. Pindborg JJ. Oral candidiasis in HIV infection. In Robertson PB, Greenspan JS, eds. *Perspectives on oral manifestations of AIDS. Diagnosis and management of HIV-associated infections.* Littleton, MA, 1988, PSG Publishing.

46. Greenspan D. Oral manifestations of HIV infection. In Robertson PB, Greenspan JS, eds. *Perspective on oral manifestations of AIDS. Diagnosis and management of HIV-associated infections.* Littleton, MA, 1988, PSG Publishing.

47. Silverman S. AIDS, HIV Infection and Dentistry. Part I: Epidemiology, Pathogenesis and Transmission. Part II: Oral Manifestations, Diagnosis and Management, Vol 7. Fairfax, VA, California and American Dental Institutes for Continuing Education, 1991.

48. National Cancer Institute, SEER Program, NIH Pub No. 99-4649. Bethesda, MD, NCI, 1999.

49. Donadieu J, Hill C. Early response to chemotherapy as a prognostic factor in childhood acute lymphoblastic leukaemia: a methodological review, *Br J Haemtol* 115:34-45, 2001.

50. Meschinchi S, Arceci RJ. Prognostic factors and risk-based therapy in acute myeloid leukemia, *Oncologist* 12:341-355, 2007.

SUGGESTED READINGS

Aach RD. Management update: the emerging clinical significance of hepatitis C. Hosp Pract 1992;27:19-22.

Alter H et al. Detection of antibody to hepatitis C virus in prospectively followed transfusion recipients with acute and chronic non-A, non-B hepatitis, *N Engl J Med* 321:1494-1500, 1989.

Alter M. Risk factors for acute non-A, non-B hepatitis in the United States and association with hepatitis C virus infection, *JAMA* 264:2231-2235, 1990.

American Academy of Pediatric Dentistry. Dental management of pediatric dental patients receiving chemotherapy, hematopoietic cell transplantation, and/or radiation, *Pediatr Dent* 30(7 suppl):219-225, 2008-2009; Reference manual.

Barnett HX et al. Natural history of human immune deficiency virus disease in perinatally infected children: an analysis from the pediatric spectrum of disease project, *Pediatrics* 97:710-715, 1996.

Choo Q-L et al. Isolation of a CDNA clone derived from a blood non-A, non-B viral hepatitis genome, *Science* 244: 359-362, 1989.

Conner EM et al. Reduction of maternal infant transmission of human immune deficiency virus type I with zidovudine treatment, *N Engl J Med* 331:1173-1180, 1994.

da Fonseca MA. Pediatric bone marrow transplantation: oral complications and recommendations for care, *Pediatr Dent* 20(7):386-397, 1988.

Duggal MS et al. The dental management of children with sickle cell disease and B thalassaemia: a review, *Int J Paediatr Dent* 6:227-237, 1996.

Feinstone S. Non-A, non-B hepatitis. In Mandell G, ed. *principle and practice of infectious diseases,* 3rd ed. New York, 1990 Churchill Livingstone.

Flemming PL et al. HIV prevalence in the United States. Presented at the Ninth Conference on Retrovirus and Opportunistic Infections, Seattle, WA, February, 2002.

Fox PC, Janson CC, eds. Consensus development conference on oral complications of cancer therapies: diagnosis, prevention, and treatment. NCI Monographs, No 9, Bethesda, MD; 1990, US Dept of Health and Human Services, Public Health Service, National Institutes of Health.

Hsla PC, Seett LB. Non-A, non-B hepatitis: impact of the emergence of the hepatitis C virus, *Adv Intern Med* 37:197-223, 1991.

Ketchmen L et al. Human immunodeficiency virus infection in children, *J Pediatr* 12:143-146, 1990.

Kuo G et al. An assay for circulating antibodies to a major etiologic virus of human non-A, non-B hepatitis, *Science* 244:362-364, 1989.

Piot P et al. The global impact of HIV/AIDS, *Nature* 410: 968-973, 2001.

Pizzo PA, Poplack DG, eds. Principles and Practice of Pediatric Oncology, London, 1989, JB Lippincott.

Sams DR, Thornton JB, Amamoo PA. Managing the dental patient with sickle cell anemia: a review of the literature, *Pediatr Dent* 12:316-319, 1990.

Taylor LB et al. Sickle cell anemia: a review of dental concerns and a retrospective study of dental and bony changes, *Spec Care Dentist* 15:38-42, 1995.

Thornton JB, Sams DR. Preanesthesia transfusion and sickle cell anemia patients: case report and controversies, *Spec Care Dentist* 13:254-257, 1993.

CHAPTER 25

Growth of the Face and Dental Arches

▲ Donald J. Ferguson

CHAPTER OUTLINE

*H*istorically, patient care in medicine and dentistry has been oriented toward the elimination of disease and the resolution of debilitating conditions. Competent care in dentistry today includes issues related not only to disease and functional disability but also to the patient's well-being. The appearance of the face and dentition is recognized with increasing frequency as a major factor in human psychosocial health.[1]

This chapter is about dental and facial malocclusion—the recognition and anticipation of malocclusion during the growing years. The dentofacial pattern can be easily and accurately assessed at chairside. In clinical terms, pertinent growth issues are discussed in relation to how growth changes the pattern of the face, occlusion, and dental arches. Knowledge of pattern appraisal and growth can be integrated into efficacious clinical decisions about a young patient. This chapter enhances the reader's diagnostic and treatment planning skills with reference to malocclusion in the pediatric patient.

The clinician treating malocclusion is primarily interested in the growth and development of craniofacial tissues as they result in facial and dentoalveolar pattern. Our understanding of how genes express their influence on dentofacial pattern and how environment influences gene expression has advanced at a remarkable pace. How molecular mechanisms are implicated at a clinically relevant level, however, has yet to be elucidated. Mao pointed out that what we understand about induced treatment effects at the macroscopic phenotype level has been described in moderate detail at the cellular level but is only beginning to be described at the level of protein and peptide production.[2] For this reason, this chapter discusses dentofacial growth and development at a macroscopic level, from the perspective of the practicing clinician.

THE NATURE OF GROWTH

Growth refers to an increase in anatomic size. Three parameters commonly used in growth literature to assess craniofacial size increase are magnitude, velocity, and direction. Magnitude refers to the linear dimension overall or the dimension of a part. Direction means the vector of size increase as might be described on a three-dimensional coordinate system. Velocity is defined as the amount of change per unit of time.

Size increase is typically illustrated in one of two ways. When growth is measured periodically and measurements are plotted as percentages of total growth, the result is a cumulative or distance curve (Fig. 25-1). A human postnatal cumulative curve is characterized by two plateaus and one period of accelerated growth. A second method of graphically demonstrating growth change is by use of an incremental or velocity growth curve (Fig. 25-2). A velocity curve plots growth increments (e.g., centimeters per year) as a function of time. Characteristic of an incremental human growth curve is rapid accelerating prenatal growth, rapid decelerating postnatal growth for the first 2 or 3 years, and a period of relatively slow incremental growth during childhood

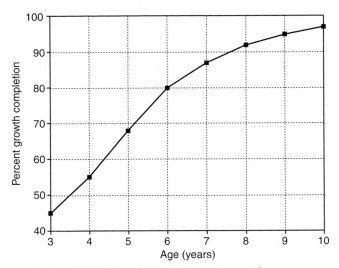

Figure 25-1 Cumulative (distance) growth curve.

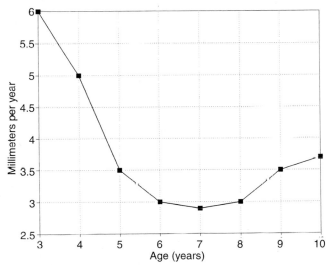

Figure 25-2 Incremental (velocity) growth curve.

followed by growth acceleration for 2 or 3 years during pubertal adolescence.

Three observations are central to a clinically relevant understanding of growth. First, growth implies change, a transition from one condition to another. This broader meaning of growth helps define growth as a concept. Conceptual growth refers to a passage from one anatomic form (i.e., size and shape) to another. Transitions in functional stage or activity refer to development. Development, in biologic literature, usually means increased specialization or a higher order of organization and also connotes an interaction of functioning parts. Development means increased organization or specialization of functioning (physiologic) parts.

Growth is more readily understood when a physical pattern is used to describe the effects of growth change. Growth, by nature, is a relational concept. Without reference to a structural model, growth has little clinical utility or meaning. This chapter discusses growth with

reference to "ideal" facial, occlusion, and dental arch paradigms.

Growth is a complex phenomenon. There is a large volume of information available on craniofacial growth. Moreover, there is little consensus in the literature as to which data or combination of data is most useful to the practitioner committed to making competent decisions about direct patient care. In light of these prevailing circumstances, the following concepts and principles about craniofacial growth are presented in a way that should be clinically useful and difficult to refute. These postulates are derived and adapted in part from widely held tenets about general human growth and development presented by Valadian and Porter.[3] The discussion of general craniofacial principles is followed by application of the principles to three areas of craniofacial growth: the face, occlusion, and dental arches. The goal of this chapter is to integrate growth principles in patient appraisal to enhance diagnostic and treatment planning efficacy.

BASIC CONCEPTS OF HUMAN GROWTH

1. Growth disposition is similar for all healthy individuals. Healthy individuals go through growth stages that are the same for everyone, according to Valadian and Porter.[3] The prenatal period, from conception to birth, averages 40 weeks in length. Infancy includes the first 2 years of life after birth, and childhood ranges from 2 to 10 years for girls and 2 to 12 years for boys. The length of adolescence is the same for both sexes but comprises different years, 10 to 18 years for females and 12 to 20 years for males (Fig. 25-3).

   Each growth stage is unique. Rate of size increase is most remarkable during the prenatal period and declines substantially during infancy. Generally, growth velocity plateaus during childhood and increases again during adolescence. All healthy individuals experience these growth cycles, although the various basic tissues and body parts are affected differently.
2. Different body parts increase in length at different rates. From birth to adulthood, the head increases about twice in length, the trunk about three times, the arms about four times, and the legs about five times. Different parts of the body grow at different times and at different rates. For example, the head increases in size very early in life, and its rate of increase is very rapid during the prenatal and early postnatal periods.
3. The overall potential for growth is determined primarily by intrinsic or genetic factors. Genetic endowment is the main determinant of growth potential. Intrinsic factors are also those conditions and events that occur from conception to birth. Maternal nutrition or disease can modify child development before birth. Some tissues tend to demonstrate high genetic predilection. Neural and primary cartilage tissue growth seems genetically predisposed in size and growth timing. Tooth size appears to be under strict genetic control.[4,5]
4. The extent to which an individual attains his or her potential for growth is determined predominately by extrinsic or environmental factors. Extrinsic factors include all postnatal environmental conditions, such as nutrition, illness, exercise, and climate. Environmental

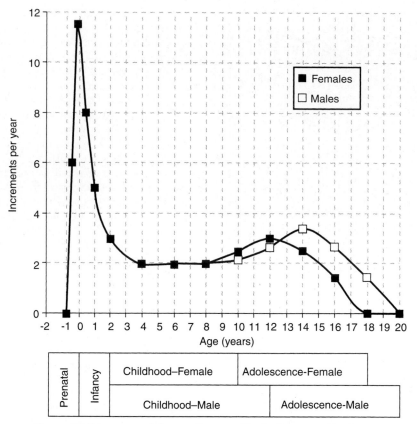

Figure 25-3 Incremental growth curve illustrating growth stages.

factors of particular interest to the dental clinician are oral habits, pathology, caries, premature loss of teeth, and metabolic disease. In the absence of detrimental extrinsic factors, the dentofacial complex will tend to attain its maximum potential in growth.

CRANIOFACIAL GROWTH PRINCIPLES

1. The basic tissue types and functioning spaces that comprise the head and face are subject to growth timing differences. The human head is composed of a variety of basic tissue types; the relative percentage of these types, at any given age, depends on timing of their growth. Neural tissue completes its growth at an early age. By contrast, general somatic tissues, such as muscle, bone, and connective tissue, mature at a slower rate. Neural tissue has attained about 60% to 70% of adult size by birth and its growth is about 95% completed by middle childhood. This is in sharp contrast to growth of other craniofacial soft tissues (Fig. 25-4). Muscle tissue is only 40% to 45% of its adult size by birth, and its growth is approximately 70% completed by 7 years of age. The size of craniofacial lymphoid tissue (tonsils and adenoids) is about 125% of adult size at 5 years of age and decreases gradually to adulthood. Linder-Aronson and Leighton have shown that functional pharyngeal space increases in relation to decreased tonsillar-adenoid mass.[6]

Growth timing of skeletal tissues also demonstrates variation. Craniofacial bone growth is about 45% completed by birth and 70% completed by 7 years of age. In

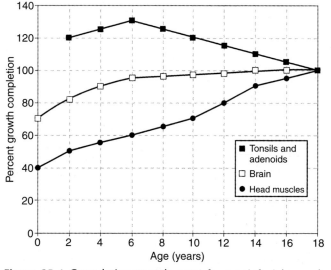

Figure 25-4 Cumulative growth curve for craniofacial neural, muscle, and lymphoid tissues. (From Linder-Aronson S, Leighton BC. A longitudinal study of the development of the posterior nasopharyngeal wall between 3 and 6 years of age, *Eur J Orthod* 5:47-58, 1983.)

contrast, primary cartilage of the head and face has achieved approximately 75% of adult size by birth and 95% by 7 years of age (Fig. 25-5). The small amount of primary cartilage remaining in the head and face after middle childhood, however, continues to grow through puberty.

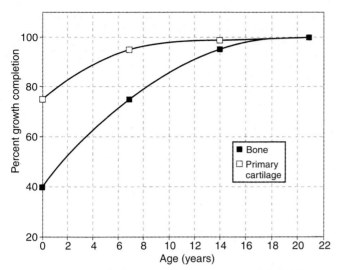

Figure 25-5 Cumulative growth curve for craniofacial bone and primary cartilage.

2. Growth of primary cartilage and functioning spaces has a directing influence on craniofacial pattern change. Primary cartilage is a tissue of particular interest to craniofacial growth theorists. According to Enlow and Hans, it is singular in form; has the capacity to grow from within (interstitial growth); is pressure tolerant, noncalcified, flexible, and nonvascular; and does not require a covering nutrient membrane for survival.[7] Primary cartilage found in the head and face is identical to the growth plate cartilage of long bones. Scott contends that primary cartilage is genetically predisposed, acts during growth as an autonomous tissue, and is able to directly influence the craniofacial pattern.[8]

Sperber documents that primary cartilage first appears in the head during the fifth week prenatally.[9] By the eighth prenatal week, a cartilaginous mass called the *chondrocranium* is present and is the precursor to the adult cranial base and nasal and otic structures. By middle childhood, most primary cartilage is replaced by bone in a process called *endochondral bone formation*.

The overall growth-directing influence of primary cartilage on craniofacial pattern change is most profound in early life. By birth, cartilage comprises a substantial portion of the nasal septum and cranial base. Interstitial expansion of primary cartilage probably has a direct influence on the position of the maxilla by way of the septopremaxillary suspensory ligament, as suggested by Latham[10] and later contended by Gange and Johnston.[11] The maxilla is most likely thrust downward and forward during infancy and early childhood. The contributions to midface growth of primary cartilage is greatly diminished after middle childhood.

The development of functioning spaces has also received considerable attention as a key concept among craniofacial growth theories.[12] The head carries out numerous functions. Some functions are more essential than others, but all require the development and maintenance of spaces. Neural integration is a critical function,

and space is required for the brain and central and peripheral nervous system expansion. Respiration and deglutition are also essential to life and require development of nasal, pharyngeal, and oral spaces. Sight, olfaction, hearing, and speech are important but less critical craniofacial functions that also require development of functioning spaces for operation.

According to Moss and Salentijn, a likely craniofacial growth scenario of functioning space development in head and facial patterns includes the following sequence of events.[13] Rapid size increase of the brain during prenatal and early postnatal life thrusts the calvarial bony plates outward and the midface forward. Birth invokes a set of functional processes previously not essential for life (i.e., breathing and swallowing). Repositioning of the mandible and tongue takes place to ensure patency of nasal-oral-pharyngeal spaces. The mandible is depressed and thrust forward for these functions to be supported and maintained.

3. Mandibular condylar cartilage, craniofacial sutures, and appositional-resorptive bone change facilitate pattern growth of the head and face. Koski identifies the mandibular condyles, once considered growth centers with directive capacity, as an adaptive growth mechanism.[14] Cartilage found at the head of the condyle is a secondary, fibrous cartilage and differs significantly from the primary, growth plate cartilage considered to be under high genetic control.[15] During craniofacial growth, the mandible is repositioned continuously to its best functional advantage. Reposturing alters the anatomic position of condyle to glenoid fossa. Compensatory growth of secondary condylar cartilage is one mechanism that facilitates maintenance of mandibular position.

Koski also points out that craniofacial sutures are important growth sites that serve to facilitate calvarial and midface growth.[14] Calvarial sutures close by 5 years of age, but some facial sutures remain patent through puberty. Craniofacial bones are thrust apart by primary cartilage and functioning space increases. Sutures enable osseous deposition at bone edges, which allows bones of the face and skull to adapt.

Enlow and Hans have shown that bone, unlike primary cartilage, is subject to environmental controls.[16] Bone may assume many forms during growth; it is pressure sensitive, calcified, vascular, and relatively inflexible, and requires a covering membrane for survival. The craniofacial skeleton increases in size by way of surface addition only and increases in shape through differential appositional-resorptive bone growth. This differential growth process accounts for a considerable amount of size increase after middle childhood.

Growth theorists Moss and Salentijn[12] believe that the general somatic tissues (i.e., bone, muscle, and connective tissue) demonstrate growth change as a consequence of supporting the functioning operations of the head. Indeed, the research evidence of Linder-Aronson[17] and of Harvold and associates[18] are convincing in that bone and muscle, as basic tissues, are adaptive and compensatory in nature. Understanding bone and muscle growth may come through understanding the temporal development of functioning spaces and the effects of interstitial cartilage expansion on surrounding tissues.

4. Growth of the head and face tends to demonstrate relative equivalency. Humans tend to grow with relative consistency. A percentile growth chart is a valuable instrument for assessing growth consistency over a time period (Fig. 25-6). Percentile charts are customarily divided into the following seven percentile levels: 97th, 90th, 75th, 50th, 25th, 10th, and 3rd. Healthy children tend to maintain a similar percentile level through successive stages of development. Deviations during growth of more than two percentile levels may indicate developmental problems, such as illness or disease.

Attributes (craniofacial parts) that are structurally related also maintain a consistent relationship throughout successive stages of growth after infancy. Enlow and Hans[16] identify the dental arches of the maxilla and mandible as an example of a structural part-counterpart relationship. An Angle class II skeletal pattern at 3 years of age is maintained into adulthood without corrective therapy. Both dental arches in healthy individuals tend to increase in size at about the same rate. Hence, balanced or equivalent growth tends to maintain architecturally related structures of any craniofacial pattern that is present after 2 years of age.

BASIC CONCEPTS OF CRANIOFACIAL GROWTH

1. Different parts of the craniofacial complex grow at different times. The head takes on appearance characteristics unique to each particular growth stage. Different parts of the face experience differences in growth timing as well. The infant has a disproportionately large calvaria and forehead compared with the adult because growth of the neural tissue takes place earlier in life than facial growth.

Size increase of the face and calvaria in the three spatial planes is a differential growth process. Scott,[19] Meredith,[20] and Ranly[21] have contributed to an understanding of this process. By birth, the cranial height dimension has attained about 70% of its adult status; cranial width, 65%; and cranial length or depth, 60% (Fig. 25-7). In contrast, only 40% of facial height and 45% of facial length (depth) has been achieved by birth. Face width (i.e., bizygomatic and bigonial), on the other hand, has attained about 60% of adult stature. Growth in face width actually falls between the classic neural and general somatic growth curves.

After birth, a pattern in facial growth timing emerges. The anterior cranial base completes most of its growth during infancy and early childhood, but frontal and nasal bones continue outward expansion through appositional-resorptive bone growth.[22] Growth magnitude and duration are greater for the anterior maxilla than for the forehead but less than for the anterior mandible. The posterior face demonstrates the greatest incremental growth during late puberty.

2. Differences in growth size, direction, velocity, and timing are observed among individuals. Bergersen has also noted large variations in growth patterns among individuals and has shown that any measured attribute will demonstrate a range of expression about a central tendency.[23] Incremental growth curves for healthy males and females will demonstrate the same general disposition but may show marked differences in maturation timing (Fig. 25-8). Generally, females mature 2 years earlier than males, but Valadian and

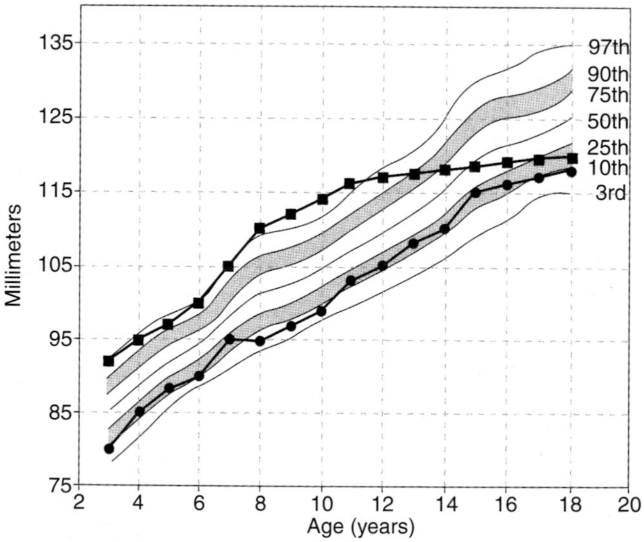

Figure 25-6 Cumulative growth chart for male face height (hard tissue nasion to menton), illustrating seven percentile levels. • Relatively normal growth; ▪ deviation of several percentile levels during growth, suggestive of abnormalcy. (From Broadbent BH, et al. *Bolton standards of dentofacial developmental growth.* St Louis, 1975, Mosby.)

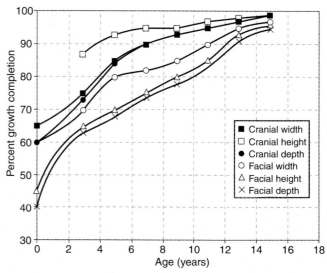

Figure 25-7 Cumulative growth curve for calvaria and face in width, height, and depth. (From Scott JH. The growth of the human face, *Proc R Soc Med* 47:5, 1954; Meredith HV. Changes in form of the head and face during childhood, *Growth* 24:215-264, 1960; Ranly DM. *A synopsis of craniofacial growth.* New York, 1980, Appleton & Lange.)

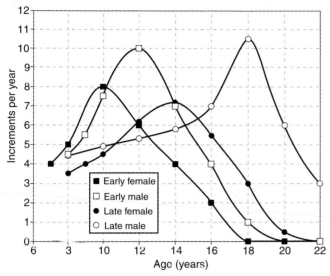

Figure 25-8 Incremental growth curves for early- and late-maturing males and females.

Porter have indicated that variations are so great that an early-maturing boy may mature earlier than a late-maturing girl.[3] Males tend to grow larger in size than females.

3. The heads and faces of no two humans are exactly the same. Brodie pointed out that no two humans are exactly the same.[24] This fact is no more clearly evident than when one compares, at any given age, a measured attribute shared by healthy individuals. Most attributes have a range of expression that can be graphically illustrated by a normal distribution curve (Fig. 25-9).

If the same attribute was measured in a population of individuals, the most frequently occurring value (mode), middle value in the series (median), or arithmetic average of all the measured values combined (mean) would represent the central tendency of the population. Central tendency is often referred to as *normalcy*. Another way to describe attribute distribution is by using percentile equivalents. The 50th percentile indicates the center of the distribution, the 25th percentile the lower one fourth, and so on.

A third statistical parameter often used in growth literature to indicate distribution is the standard deviation.

A standard deviation (SD) of ±1 includes about 68% of the entire population; ±2 SD and ±3 SD are equivalent to approximately 95% and 99% of the distribution, respectively. The mean values and SDs for a normative population are invaluable aids in describing a patient's condition. By comparing a patient's value to a population value for the same trait, the clinician can make statements about relative largeness or smallness. Generally, measurements beyond ±2 SD are considered clinically important because those values fall outside 95% of the population on which the normative value is based.

In the remainder of this chapter, references are made to craniofacial growth principles and concepts in discussing growth of the face, occlusion, and dental arches.

CRANIOFACIAL PATTERN

In clinical assessment and treatment planning for the young patient, information about growth is often not considered to the degree that it should be. Craniofacial growth issues can be made more central to patient care concerns when a physical model is used to help visualize growth effects. For this reason, a particularly strong effort is made here to define physical craniofacial pattern.

There are two methods commonly used in dentistry to gather information about craniofacial pattern. One method is to examine the patient physically at chairside. Information collected in this fashion is based on criteria contrived and established in the practitioner's mind. The second method is to analyze dental records. Historically, cephalometric analysis has been a particularly useful tool for collecting objective information about craniofacial patterns. Generally, the patient's radiographic values measured on the cephalogram are compared with normative values derived from a population database. In this way, degrees of normalcy can be estimated by the clinician. One database is unique in its composition in that only individuals presenting with optimal or ideal craniofacial pattern were included in the study.[25] This unique conceptual approach to defining craniofacial pattern enables the practitioner to make assessments about patient optimality. Patient-measured values are compared with values from cephalograms that have relatively ideal patterns. Cephalometric analysis is discussed in Chapter 26. Darwis and colleagues suggest that using a combination of methods, such as three-dimensional facial morphometry and Fourier analysis, can provide a more comprehensive knowledge of growth and development of craniofacial structures and thus may allow improved prediction of clinical outcomes.[26] Fourier analysis is a mathematical curve-fitting procedure that can represent boundaries so that the outlines of objects can be addressed.

IDEAL PARADIGMS FOR DENTOFACIAL PATTERN

Standards for chairside facial appraisal have been offered by Ackerman and Proffit,[27] Angle,[28] Bell and colleagues,[29] Cox and van der Linden,[30] Lucker and coworkers,[1] and Patterson and Powell.[31] Most of these physical appraisal models refer to the adult face. Horowitz and Hixon[32] describe idealized facial pattern as "the way things ought to

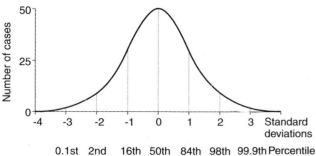

Figure 25-9 Normal distribution curve illustrating standard deviations and percentile equivalents.

be." Models available for examining the face espouse an assessment of proportion, balance, and harmony— concepts that help define overall facial attractiveness. The concept of an ideal face can be a useful clinical tool if it is used properly and its limitations are acknowledged. The first limitation is the fact that an ideal has little or no biologic basis. Biologic data can neither refute nor support the contention that the face should be ideal. Second, faces do not need to be ideal to work properly; ideal pattern, for the most part, has little connection with physiologic function. Third, an ideal model is simply a mental construct, a fiction. The words *ideal paradigm* mean "perfect example."

A perfect example can, on the other hand, be a powerful diagnostic and treatment-planning tool. The patient's facial pattern can be compared with criteria for idealness, the differences noted, and hence a problem list constructed. Criteria for an ideal face can help organize a vast array of information that is readily available to the clinician through physical observation. An ideal facial paradigm can serve as a treatment planning tool as well. Although the concept of an ideal face is fictitious and biologically unsupported, it can serve as a guide by providing an example toward which treatment may be directed. Ideal paradigms for dental occlusion and dental arch pattern are also represented in dental literature; good examples may be found in the works of Angle,[28] Andrews,[33] and Roth.[34] The purposes served by these paradigms are the same as for ideal facial models; they are powerful diagnostic and treatment-planning aids.

GROWTH AND FACIAL PATTERN

CONSISTENCY IN PATTERN MATURATION

Following birth, the face increases in size to a greater extent than does the calvaria. Bell and associates propose that, by adulthood, the ideal face should be equally proportioned in forehead, midface, and lower face heights.[29] Enlow demonstrated that the facial profile flattens as the face ages. Nose and chin become more prominent, and lips become less pronounced[35] (Fig. 25-10). Every healthy individual, regardless of the overall craniofacial pattern, experiences profile flattening and face height increases relative to cranium.

IDEAL FRONTAL FACIAL PATTERN

Criteria for facial idealness are age dependent. Because the face elongates and the profile becomes less convex with maturity, ideal criteria appropriate for the adult face would not necessarily apply to the younger face. The ideal frontal facial pattern for a 7-year-old child might include the following criteria (Fig. 25-11):
1. Right and left face halves are symmetrical.
2. Glabella (midpoint between eyebrows) to subnasale (point where columella merges with upper lip) equals subnasale to menton (inferior aspect of chin).
3. Subnasale to lower border of upper lip represents one-third the distance from subnasale to menton.
4. Upper central incisor edge is 2 mm inferior to lower border of upper lip.
5. Alar base width equals inner canthal width.

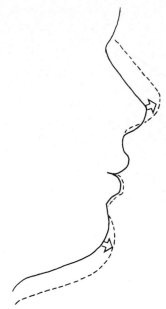

Figure 25-10 Graphic illustration of facial profile flattening from 6 years of age *(solid line)* to 18 years of age *(broken line).*

IDEAL FACIAL PROFILE PATTERN

Use of a reference plane is very helpful for evaluation of the facial profile at chairside. The Frankfort horizontal plane is an anthropometric reference line frequently used for analysis of the lateral face. It is defined by Farkas as the superior limit of the external auditory meatus and the palpated border of the infraorbital bony rim.[36] A second reference line constructed perpendicular to the Frankfort horizontal plane and through the glabella (FHP) has been used in lateral profile assessment by Legan and Burstone.[37]

The ideal profile pattern for a 7-year-old child might include the following criteria (Fig. 25-12):
1. Chin 5 mm behind FHP
2. Most anterior aspect of lower lip on FHP
3. Most anterior aspect of upper lip 5 mm ahead of FHP
4. Nasolabial angle of 100 degrees
5. No more than 2 mm lip separation when relaxed

MAINTENANCE OF OVERALL PATTERN

The overall pattern presented by the individual at an early age will be maintained into adulthood. Although every individual experiences profile flattening and facial elongation as the face matures, Enlow and colleagues demonstrated that the magnitude of these changes is not great enough to offset disharmonies in overall facial structure.[38] Discrepancies between the position of the maxilla and mandible persist throughout life unless clinical therapy is employed to rectify the disharmonies.

At chairside, disharmony between the maxilla and the mandible can be simply and readily identified. A list of differences can be formulated by comparing the patient's facial measurements with the criteria of an ideal face. The differences serve as a patient problem list. Adding average growth change (i.e., magnitude, direction, and velocity)

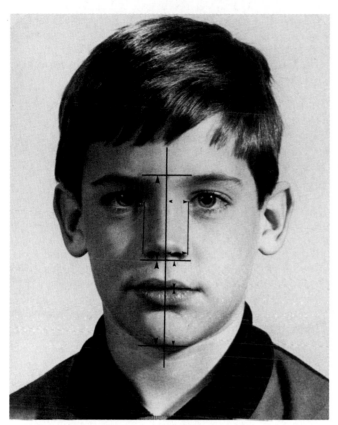

Figure 25-11 Ideal frontal facial pattern for a 7-year-old child.

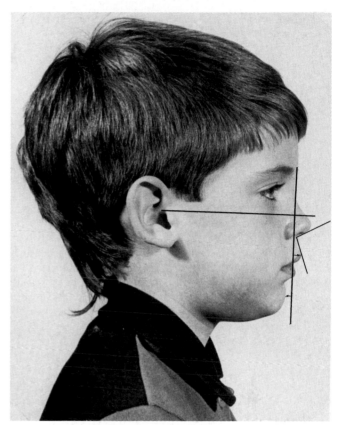

Figure 25-12 Ideal profile facial pattern for a 7-year-old child.

to the pattern presented by the individual will give an estimate of how facial patterns will look at a later age. This growth scheme is known as a *mean-change-expansion scheme*.[32] Balbach demonstrated it to be the most useful to predict the effects of growth on facial pattern.[39] The mean-change-expansion scheme is useful for evaluation of almost all patients routinely seen in the dental office. Balanced or average growth affecting all aspects of the head and face relatively equally, however, cannot be assumed for all patients. The heads and faces of individuals who have some craniofacial congenital anomalies, hypoplastic defects, or acquired deformities that alter primary or compensatory craniofacial growth mechanisms do not grow in a typical manner.

Because growth change in healthy children affects the face in a relatively consistent and predictable way, the key to facial diagnosis and treatment planning is the clinician's ability to identify and diagnostically describe facial pattern. Identification of balanced, proportional facial pattern, as well as recognition of facial imbalance, should be routine during patient assessment. The use of criteria related to ideal facial pattern can be helpful.

The goal in treating facial imbalance in children is to establish architectural balance in the facial pattern. If corrective measures include compensation for the effects from treatment rebound or relapse, the facial pattern established by therapy will be maintained. As the face continues to grow and increase in size, all structurally related parts of the treated face will undergo relative growth equality.

Correction of facial imbalance in the child is achieved through clinical manipulation of the means by which adaptive, compensatory facial growth occurs. Some sutures of the upper face remain patent into adolescence. Application of forces through orthopedic headgear, controlled in direction and amount, can result in an alteration of maxillary growth direction and ultimately of maxillary position. Also maxillary transverse size can be increased by judicious expansion of the palatal suture. The secondary cartilage of the mandibular condyle remains responsive to mechanical stimulation throughout life, but appositional response of this fibrocartilage decreases with age, as shown by McNamara and Carlson.[40] Facial bones respond to changes in microenvironmental stress and strain by changing form. Patterns of osseous deposition and resorption can be altered by using appliances that carefully load bone with physiologically compatible biomechanical forces.

Successful treatment of a child with facial imbalance secondary to mandibular retrognathia, for example, involves manipulation of several growth mechanisms. Mandibular anterior repositioning with a functional appliance probably affects many sites. Graber and Swain[41] believe that modification of the dentofacial complex occurs by the following means:

1. Condylar growth (secondary cartilage growth)
2. Glenoid fossa adaptation (apposition-resorption bone growth)
3. Elimination of functional retrusion
4. More favorable mandibular growth direction

5. Withholding of downward and forward maxillary arch movement (apposition-resorption bone growth)
6. Differential upward and forward eruption of lower buccal segment (apposition-resorption bone growth)
7. Orthopedic movement of maxilla and upper dentition (maxillary suture system growth)

FACIAL GROWTH EMULATES GENERAL SOMATIC GROWTH

The degree to which the facial pattern can be altered through biomechanical therapy depends on the amount of growth potential remaining. In general, the magnitude of facial pattern alteration possible is inversely proportional to age; the older the individual, the less the facial pattern can be therapeutically modified. The opportunity to alter compensatory, adaptive growth mechanisms is also greater in a rapidly growing individual. The adolescent growth spurt is characterized by increased growth velocity at about 10 to 12 years of age for girls and 12 to 14 years of age for boys. The maximum velocity or peak height velocity of growth is attained approximately 2 years after pubertal onset. Cumulative facial growth closely parallels general somatic growth (Fig. 25-13). Analysis of skeletal hand development can be helpful in estimating general skeletal maturation and, hence, facial skeletal maturation. It is relevant to evaluate a child's maturity in direct relation to the child's own pubertal growth spurt to assess whether maximum pubertal growth is imminent, has been reached, or has been passed.

GROWTH AND PATTERN OF OCCLUSION

CONSISTENCY IN PATTERN DEVELOPMENT

Usually, no teeth are clinically visible at birth. Leighton has shown that the upper anterior gum pad (intercuspid width) is typically wider than the lower anterior pad, and the upper anterior gum pad protrudes (overjet) about

5 mm relative to the lower anterior gum pad.[42] The upper anterior gum pad usually overlaps (overbite) the lower anterior pad by about 0.5 mm. In the first 6 months of postnatal life, there is marked palatal width increase, and the overjet decreases rapidly.

PRIMARY DENTITION TERMINUS

By 3 years of age, the occlusion of 20 primary teeth is usually established. The relationship of the distal terminal planes of opposing second primary molar teeth can be classified into one of three categories (Fig. 25-14). A flush terminal plane (flush terminus) means that the anterior-posterior positions of the distal surfaces of opposing primary second molars are in the same vertical plane. A mesial-step terminus is defined as a lower second primary molar terminal plane that is mesial to the maxillary primary terminus. Distal-step terminal plane is descriptive of the situation in which the mandibular second primary molar terminus is distal to the upper second primary molar terminus.

Statistical studies of primary terminal plane status report that 49% of the time, the terminal plane of the lower

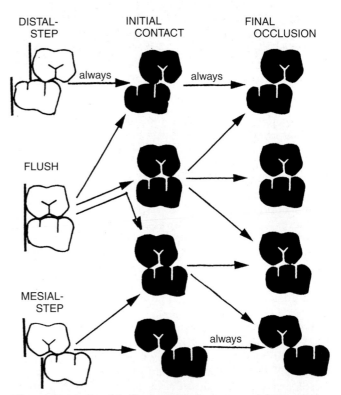

Figure 25-14 Graphic illustration of permanent first molar occlusion development. Outlined crown images represent three terminal plane relationships of primary second molars at about 5 years of age. Darkened images represent various permanent first molar relationships at initial occluding contact (about 6½ years of age) and at full occlusion contact (about 12 years of age). (From Arya BS, et al. Prediction of first molar occlusion, *Am J Orthod* 63:610-621, 1973; Carlsen DB, Meredith HV. Biologic variation in selected relationships of opposing posterior teeth, *Angle Orthod* 30:162-173, 1960; Moyers RA. *Handbook of orthodontics,* 3rd ed. Chicago, 1973, Mosby.)

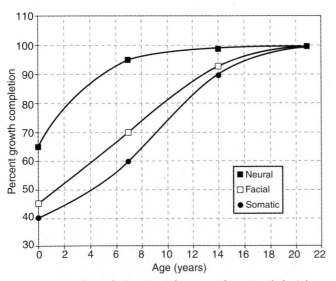

Figure 25-13 Cumulative growth curves for neural, facial, and general somatic tissues.

primary second molar is mesial to the upper terminus (mesial step); the lower terminus is flush with the upper terminus 37% of the time; and the distal-step primary terminus is seen in approximately 14% of cases. These data are derived from studies reported by Arya and associates[43] and by Carlsen and Meredith.[44]

OPPOSING FIRST MOLARS AT INITIAL CONTACT

The permanent first molars are clinically visible at about 6 years of age and are the first permanent teeth to emerge. The relationship of permanent first molars when initial occluding contact occurs during eruption may be represented by one of four categories (see Fig. 25-14). A class I relationship means that the mesial-buccal (m-b) cusp of the upper permanent molar contacts at or very near the buccal groove of the lower permanent first molar. This occurs approximately 55% of the time. An end-on relationship means that m-b cusps of both molars oppose one another. The incidence of this situation is about 25%. A class II relationship, occurring 19% of the time, is one in which an upper m-b cusp is anterior to the lower m-b cusp. Class III represents the situation in which an upper m-b cusp is distal to the lower buccal groove. This occurs in only 1% of the population.[44] Table 25-1 shows the incidence of medial-step, flush, and distal-step primary terminus and end-on, class I, class II, and class III permanent first molar occlusions during three stages of occlusion development.[43-45]

IDEAL STATIC OCCLUSION PATTERN

The concept of ideal occlusion development has been described by Friel[46] and by Lewis and Lehman.[47] Sanin and Savara have also shown that, to a considerable extent, ideal occlusion at a young age predisposes to an ideal adult occlusion.[48] The most desirable occlusion in the permanent dentition is a class I interdigitation, and certain features in the primary and mixed dentitions, if observed accurately, can provide clinical clues as to whether a class I relationship of the dentition will eventually develop.

The major difference between ideal adult and child occlusions is the teeth present. By 7 years of age, the primary central and lateral incisors have been or are in the process of being replaced by their permanent successors, and the permanent first molars have already erupted. The primary dentition remaining usually includes the canine and first and second molars of both arches. Criteria for ideal dental occlusion for a 7-year-old child might include the following:
1. Class I molar and canine interdigitation
2. 2-mm anterior and posterior overjet
3. 2-mm anterior overbite
4. Coincident dental midlines

MAINTENANCE OF OVERALL PATTERN

Gum pad relationships at birth cannot be used as reliable diagnostic criteria for predicting subsequent arch relationship. The primacy of life-supporting functions (i.e., respiration and swallowing) is so great at birth that major unpredictable adjustments in maxillary and mandibular positions take place in the first few years of life. By 3 years of age, however, the relationship of maxilla to mandible is well established, and overall maxillomandibular pattern does not change significantly thereafter.

One key diagnostic feature regarding future occlusion status is the relationships of the primary terminal planes. The likelihood of developing a class I relationship in the permanent dentition is greatest when a mild mesial-step terminus exists during the primary dentition stage (see Fig. 25-14). If an exaggerated mesial step exists, a class III permanent molar relationship will develop. The possibility that a class I relationship will develop from a distal-step primary terminus is virtually nonexistent. Hence, the presence of a distal step is highly predictive of a developing class II permanent molar relationship.

Another important diagnostic feature that is predictive of later occlusion status is the relationships of the first permanent molars during initial occluding contact. The first permanent molars erupt between 5 and 7 years of age. The chance that a class I interdigitation of the dentition

---

Table 25-1

Incidence of Terminal Molar Relationships at Three Stages of Occlusion Development

Primary Terminal Plane at Age 5 Years	Initial Permanent First Molar Occlusion at Age 6½ Years	Final Occlusion at About Age 12 Years
	1% Class III	3% Class III
49% Class I (ms)	27% Class I	59% Class I
37% Flush	49% End-on	
14% Class II (ds)	23% Class II	39% Class II

ms, Medial step; ds, distal step.
Arya BS, et al. Prediction of first molar occlusion, *Am J Orthod* 63:610-621, 1973; Carlsen DB, Meredith HV. Biologic variation in selected relationships of opposing posterior teeth, *Angle Orthod* 30:162-173, 1960; HEW reports on occlusion: Summary and discussion, *J Clin Orthod* 12:849-862, 1978.

will evolve is best when a class I relationship is represented at initial permanent first molar occluding contact. A class II first permanent molar occlusion at initial occluding contact will predictably remain a class II occlusion into the complete adult dentition. Also indicative of a developing malocclusion are some initially occluding end-to-end relationships. Three quarters of initial contacting end-on first molar occlusions will shift toward a class I during the transition dentition phase. However, 25% of these end-on relationships will shift into a class II relationship. A class III occlusion at initial contact will predictably lead to a future class III molar relationship. This discussion regarding diagnostic and predictive information is based on the work of Arya and associates,[43] Carlsen and Meredith,[44] and Moyers.[49]

The development of the transitional phase occlusion and malocclusion is graphically illustrated in Fig. 25-14. Note that distal-step terminus always leads to class II initial contact and final permanent first molar occlusions. The probability that a class III final first permanent molar relationship will develop from a class III initial contact occlusion is also very high. Development of the occlusion from flush terminus, end-on, and class I initial contact molar relationships is highly variable.

The occlusion relationship of upper to lower dentition remains nearly the same throughout the growing period.[50] Exceptions are cases in which environmental factors, such as premature loss of primary teeth, are superimposed on the developing occlusion, as shown by Northway and associates.[51] Carlsen and Meredith demonstrated that, 70% of the time, the lower permanent first molars move mesially relative to the upper permanent first molar during the transition occlusion phase.[44] The magnitude of this shift, however, typically does not compensate for a permanent first molar malocclusion. Overall occlusion pattern is maintained during growth.

GROWTH AND DENTAL ARCH PATTERN

SIMILAR STAGE SEQUENCING

The stage sequence of dental arch development is the same for everyone. According to Nery and Oka, the crowns of primary teeth begin calcification between 3 and 4 months prenatally.[52] The calcification of mandibular teeth usually precedes that of the maxillary dentition; the central incisors typically show first evidence of calcification and the second molars last. Boys typically begin calcification before girls.

The first primary tooth to erupt is the central incisor at about 7½ months, and the last to erupt is the second primary molar at about 2½ years. Closure of root apex occurs at 3 years for the second primary molar. The usual sequence of primary dentition eruption is the central incisor (in Palmer notation designated by the letter A), the lateral incisor (B), the first primary molar (C), and the canine (D), followed by the second primary molar (E). Hence, the typical eruption sequence is A-B-D-C-E.

Calcification of the permanent teeth does not begin until after birth.[52] The first permanent molar is the first to

show evidence of calcification, which takes place during the second postnatal month. The third molar is the last to begin calcification, which occurs at about 9 years.

The typical eruption sequence for the mandibular arch is as follows: first molar (in Palmer notation, designated by the number 6), central incisor (1), lateral incisor (2), canine (3), first premolar (4), second premolar (5), and second molar (7), followed by the third molar (8). For the maxillary arch, the usual sequence of eruption for the permanent teeth is as follows: 6-1-2-4-5-3-7-8. Eruption timing in girls generally precedes that in boys by an average of 5 months.

Eruption times for permanent teeth can vary considerably depending on the specific tooth. According to Garn, eruption time for the lower incisor varies the least; 90% of lower permanent incisors erupt within a span of 3 years. In contrast, eruption time varies the most for the lower second permanent premolar, which shows a 6½-year span.[4]

Dimensional changes for dental arch length, circumference, and intermolar and intercanine widths during childhood and adolescence have been compiled by Moorrees.[53,54] Average dimensional dental arch changes from age 6 to 18 years for maxillary and mandibular arches are as follows:

Lower Arch	
Arch width:	Bicanine: 3-mm increase
	Bimolar: 2-mm increase
Arch length:	1-mm decrease because of up-righting of incisors
Arch circumference:	Decrease of 4 mm
Upper Arch	
Arch width:	Bicanine: 5-mm increase
	Bimolar: 4-mm increase
Arch length:	Slight decrease because of up-righting of incisors
Arch circumference:	Increase of 1 mm

IDEAL DENTAL ARCH PATTERN

Development of dental arch malocclusion is predictable. Development of a clinically acceptable dental arch likewise can be predicted. The status of the dental arch at mid-adolescence is contingent on clinical features that can be easily recognized during the transition phase dentition. The simplest method of evaluating the dental arch for factors predisposing to malocclusion is to compare the patient's mixed dentition dental arch with an ideal dental arch pattern.

For the dental arch, the ideal pattern for a 7-year-old child might meet the following criteria:
1. Tight proximal contacts
2. No rotations
3. Specific buccal-lingual axial inclinations
4. Specific mesial-distal axial inclinations
5. Even marginal ridges vertically
6. Flat occlusal plane
7. Excess (positive) leeway space

Ethnic background can make a difference in the dentition and occlusal development. An interesting study by Anderson[55] showed that the primary dental arch dimensions of African-American children were significantly larger than those of European-American children in arch width, length, perimeter and interdental space.

TOOTH SIZE/ARCH SIZE RATIO AS PATTERN DETERMINANT

Tooth size and alveolar size are the primary factors that determine the status of the permanent dental arch. If tooth size and arch size are not balanced, the effect on the permanent dental arch is crowding or spacing. Crowding is the most common feature of dental arch malocclusion. Only when the combined size of the permanent teeth is balanced with the size of the alveolar apical area is an ideal dental arch possible.

Van der Linden referred to the alveolar bone surrounding the dental apex regions as the *apical area*.[56] Ten Cate reported evidence that the alveolus probably forms as a result of inductive action from cells of the dental follicle.[57] The size of alveolar bone is influenced by the many environmental factors that affect intra membranous bone growth. It is possible to clinically increase or decrease the size of the alveolar apical area during growth. Fränkel has demonstrated that alveolar arch size can be increased dramatically during childhood and that the increases are stable into adulthood.[58]

Tooth size, for the purpose of discussing dental arch development, refers to the mesial-distal dimensions of each tooth. According to Garn[4] and Potter and colleagues,[5] mesial-distal tooth size is determined primarily by genetic factors. Four chromosomal gene loci appear responsible for mesial-distal maxillary tooth size, and the mandibular dentition seems to be under the genetic control of six loci. Tooth size is polygenically determined and continuously variable (i.e., a wide range of individuality exists in terms of the width of any single tooth). Dental size is expressed through X-linked inheritance, and racial differences are known. The upper lateral incisor shows the most variability in tooth size.

Tooth size and alveolar apical area size are the most pertinent factors in the determination of the intra-arch component of malocclusion. Therefore, it is relevant to consider these factors at length. The alveolar apical area will respond to biomechanical stimulation from orthodontic appliances, because intramembranous bone is adaptive and compensatory in nature. Crown size, on the other hand, cannot be predictably influenced during growth by clinical therapy.

The clinical crowns of all permanent teeth, except for the third molar, are completely formed by middle childhood. Mesial-distal crown widths will not change after crown formation unless affected by factors such as caries. Hence, mesial-distal crown dimension is a stable factor in the tooth size/arch size ratio. In an attempt to exploit the clinical usefulness of crown dimension stability, tooth size relationships are examined.

Comparison of primary to permanent mesial-distal tooth sizes is one such consideration. Studies by Moorrees revealed that there is little about primary dentition size that predicts permanent dentition size.[53] Correlation coefficient (r) values ranging from r = 0.2 to r = 0.6 are indicative of the poor predictive relationship between primary mesial-distal tooth size and the size of

their permanent successors. Correlation coefficients of r = 0.8 or higher are required to make predictions for the individual patient at chairside.[32] The combined mesial-distal sizes of all primary teeth and the combined sizes for the permanent teeth show a correlation of r = 0.5. Hence, Moorrees concluded that the size of the primary teeth is of little predictive value in estimating the size of their permanent successors.[53]

The strength of the size relationships among the permanent teeth, however, is clinically important for some comparisons. Potter and Nance demonstrated that the size of an individual tooth is highly correlated with the size of the contralateral tooth in the same arch, as reflected in an r value of around 0.9.[59] The combined mesial-distal dimensions of contralateral quadrants of teeth show a slightly higher correlation of r = 0.95. Intra-arch comparisons of tooth groupings, such as mesial-distal size of the lower incisors versus mesial-distal sizes of the lower canine and premolars combined, show only moderate correlation (r = 0.6) and therefore are not useful clinically.[60]

COMPUTATION OF TOOTH SIZE/ARCH SIZE BALANCE

The primary reason for dental arch malocclusion is imbalance between tooth size and alveolar apical size. In the transition (mixed) dentition, it is possible to accurately determine if combined mesial-distal tooth size will be balanced with alveolar arch size in later life. This process of determination is called *mixed dentition space analysis*. Many methods of mixed dentition space analysis are available.[61,62] Common to all of these methods is the attempt to determine the combined mesial-distal size of the unerupted permanent canine and first and second premolars. According to Horowitz and Hixon, the lower dental arch is the focus for space analysis and the basis of orthodontic diagnosis and treatment planning.[32] The mandibular alveolar base can be modified less therapeutically than can the upper alveolus and therefore restricts treatment possibilities. The mandibular arch also undergoes less growth change than does the upper arch.

Efficacy studies by Gardner,[63] Kaplan and colleagues,[64] and Staley and colleagues[65-67] revealed one method to be the most accurate in predicting the combined size of the unerupted canine and premolars during the mixed dentition. This method, originally devised by Hixon and Oldfather,[60] has been refined by Bishara and Staley.[68] In summary, the analysis involves the following steps:

1. Measure the combined width of the lower lateral and central incisors on one side.
2. Measure directly from the radiograph the crown sizes of the unerupted 4-5 on the same side.
3. Add together the incisor and the premolar sizes.
4. Refer to the prediction chart to determine the sizes of the unerupted 3-4-5.

Techniques of mixed dentition space analysis allow estimation of the sizes of the unerupted canine and premolars on the lower arch. This size estimate must then be compared with a measurement of the arch space available between the mesial aspect of the lower molar and the distal aspect of the lateral incisor in the same quadrant. The difference between the combined width of the three unerupted permanent teeth and this arch space has been called *leeway space.*

The most favorable dental arch pattern is one in which leeway space is excessive (i.e., combined size of unerupted canine and premolars is smaller than arch space available). If leeway space is deficient, dental arch crowding predictably results. Average growth changes in the dental arch are not great enough to compensate for leeway deficiencies.

COMPENSATIONS IN DENTAL ARCH DEVELOPMENT

Tooth size/arch size imbalances result in dental arch conditions that are less than ideal. When combined mesial-distal tooth size exceeds alveolar arch size, compensatory adjustments occur, which results in dental arch crowding, excessive curve of Spee, or deviant axial tooth inclinations. Dental spacing results when alveolar arch size exceeds the combined mesial-distal size of the teeth.

Competent treatment planning during the mixed dentition must account not only for differences between the size of unerupted canine and premolars and the space available for them, but also for compensating dental factors. Ideal dental arch status provides a model for such planning. Each compensating factor (i.e., crowding, spacing, excess occlusal curve, or deviant axial tooth position) can be appraised relative to an ideal dental arch. Alteration of a crowded arch to an ideally aligned arch is not possible without creating extra space to resolve the crowding. Consequently, a competent dental arch treatment plan must specify the manner in which space will be clinically created. Several means are available for creating dental arch space. They include the following:
1. Move molars distally.
2. Decrease the mesial-distal dimension of the teeth present in the arch.
3. Increase the buccal-lingual axial inclination of the incisors.
4. Reduce the number of teeth in the arch by extraction.

Resolution of excessive occlusal curve also requires more space. Merrifield indicated that generally, for each millimeter of excessive occlusal curve, 1 mm of arch length space is required.[69] To upright labially inclined incisors, arch length space is also required. In contrast, more arch length is created when retroclined incisors are proclined through therapy; the length of the arch is increased by repositioning the incisal edges from a lingual to a more labial position.

MAINTENANCE OF OVERALL PATTERN

Space analysis combined with evaluation of the impact of compensating factors on dental arch status is the means by which overall space requirements for the lower arch can be determined during the mixed dentition phase. Overall space appraisal during the mixed dentition is highly indicative of future arch status. The condition presented during the mixed dentition will, to a high degree, be maintained in the permanent dental arch. For this reason, a nonideal adult arch status can be anticipated early, and many undesirable conditions can be resolved during the transition from the primary to the permanent dental arch.

Overall space appraisal is typically expressed as millimeters of arch length space excess or deficiency. Dental arch space excess (1 to 2 mm) is a relatively ideal situation. Clinically, little intervention is usually required because mesial drifting of the permanent teeth often results in little or no crowding or residual spacing. Space excess exceeding 3 to 4 mm, however, can lead to dental arch problems. For example, congenital absence of one or more teeth can leave so much arch space that mesial drifting cannot compensate. Decisions favoring retention of primary teeth as long as possible, extraction of primary teeth and retention of space for later restorative prosthesis, or extraction followed by space closure must be made as long-term planning decisions.

Space deficiencies less than −2 mm can usually be managed with a lower lingual holding arch. Arch space deficiencies of −3 to −6 mm should be scrutinized carefully. Typically, a space-regaining lower lingual arch or arch length expansion treatment measure is indicated. Arches with deficiencies in excess of −6 mm are candidates for aggressive space-regaining techniques, dental arch expansion treatment, or one of a number of serial extraction sequences. Clinical approach to various conditions of space excess and deficiency is based on overall space appraisal (space analysis plus compensating factors) as shown in Table 25-2.

EFFECT OF ENVIRONMENTAL FACTORS ON DENTAL ARCH PATTERN

The primary determinant of dental arch malocclusion is mesial-distal tooth size/arch size imbalance. Nevertheless, secondary factors can dramatically influence the disposition of the dental arch during childhood. Dental arch status is subject to the ravaging effects of environmental factors that include early loss of primary teeth, interproximal caries, pathology, ankylosis of primary teeth, oral habits, trauma, and early eruption of permanent second molars.

The environmental factors most commonly affecting dental arch status are probably caries and premature loss of primary teeth. Early primary tooth loss and caries can have a profound effect on dental arch status. Caries and early loss of the primary first molars (D), second molars (E), or both (D + E) result in a decrease in dental arch length. A study by Northway and colleagues[51] showed the following specific details:
1. E loss had the most deleterious effect on dental arch length.
2. Early posterior primary loss resulted in 2- to 4-mm space closure per quadrant in both arches.
3. Space loss was age related in the upper but not in the lower arch.
4. Upper D loss typically resulted in blocked-out canines; upper E loss usually led to an impacted second permanent premolar.
5. The greatest space loss was caused by mesial molar movement.
6. More space was lost in the first year after premature tooth loss than in successive years.
7. No recovery of space was demonstrated during growth in the upper arch, and little was found in the lower arch.

Table **25-2**		
Clinical Disposition Guidelines for Various Dental Arch Space Conditions Resulting from Overall Mixed Dentition Space Appraisal		
Overall Appraisal	**mm**	**Clinical Disposition**
Large space excess	Greater than +3	Long-term planning
Space excess	Less than +3 to 0	No action; observation
Equivalency	0	Careful observation
Deficiency	Less than −3 to 0	Lower lingual holding arch
Moderate deficiency	−3 to −6	Space regaining or arch expansion
Large deficiency	Greater than −6	Space regaining, arch expansion, or extraction

SUMMARY

This chapter integrates basic growth principles with patient appraisal to enhance diagnostic and treatment-planning efficacy. Merging growth principles with dentofacial pattern brings to light specific growth features pertinent to clinical patient-care decision making. This chapter focused on growth events germane to a better understanding of malocclusion as it affects the face, occlusion, and dental arches. Two themes were consistent throughout the chapter. First, overall pattern is maintained from early childhood until growth completion. Growth change affects architecturally equivalent structures in a balanced way. For this reason, craniofacial pattern can be predicted to a great extent. The best estimation of future status is obtained by taking the pattern present at an early age and adding the average growth change. Second, dentofacial pattern changes regionally as an individual matures, and these maturation changes are common in all healthy individuals. Regional variation introduced by the maturing process, however, is not great enough to alter overall dentofacial pattern.

REFERENCES

1. Lucker GW, et al, eds. Psychological aspects of facial form. Monograph No 11, *Craniofacial growth series*. Ann Arbor, 1980, University of Michigan.
2. Mao JJ. Mechanobiology of craniofacial sutures, *J Dent Res* 81:810-816, 2002.
3. Valadian I, Porter D. *Physical growth and development: from conception to maturity*. Boston, 1977, John Wright-PSG.
4. Garn SM. Genetics of dental development. In McNamara JA Jr, ed. *The biology of occlusal development*. Monograph No 7. *Craniofacial growth series*. Ann Arbor, 1977, University of Michigan.
5. Potter RH, et al. A twin study on dental dimension. II, Independent genetic determinants, *Am J Phys Anthropol* 44:397-412, 1976.
6. Linder-Aronson S, Leighton BC. A longitudinal study of the development of the posterior nasopharyngeal wall between 3 and 6 years of age, *Eur J Orthod* 5:47-58, 1983.
7. Enlow DH, Hans MG. *Essentials of facial growth*. Philadelphia, 1996, WB Saunders.
8. Scott JH. The nasal septum, *Br Dent J* 95:37, 1953.
9. Sperber GH. *Craniofacial embryology*, 3rd ed. Boston, 1981, John Wright-PSG.
10. Latham RA. Maxillary development and growth: the septopremaxillary ligament, *J Anat* 107:471, 1974.
11. Gange RJ, Johnston LE. The septopremaxillary attachment and midfacial growth, *Am J Orthod* 66:71-81, 1979.
12. Moss ML, Salentijn L. The primary role of functional matrices in facial growth, *Am J Orthod* 55:566-577, 1969.
13. Moss ML, Salentijn L. The capsular matrix, *Am J Orthod* 56:474-490, 1969.
14. Koski KL. Cranial growth centers: facts or fallacies? *Am J Orthod* 54:566-583, 1968.
15. Dixon AD, et al. *Fundamentals of craniofacial growth*. Boca Raton, FL, 1997, CRC Press. p. 121-124.
16. Enlow DH, Hans MG. *Handbook of facial growth*. Philadelphia, 1996, WB Saunders.
17. Linder-Aronson S. Effects of adenectomy on dentition and nasopharynx, *Am J Orthod* 65:1-15, 1974.
18. Harvold EP, et al. Primate experiments on oral respiration, *Am J Orthod* 79:359-372, 1981.
19. Scott JH. The growth of the human face, *Proc R Soc Med* 47:5, 1954.
20. Meredith HV. Changes in form of the head and face during childhood, *Growth* 24:215-264, 1960.
21. Ranly DM. *A synopsis of craniofacial growth*. New York, 1980, Appleton & Lange.
22. Stramud L. External and internal cranial base, *Acta Odontol Scand* 17:239, 1959.
23. Bergersen EO. The directions of facial growth from infancy to adulthood, *Angle Orthod* 36:18-43, 1960.
24. Brodie AG. Facial patterns: a theme on variation, *Angle Orthod* 16:75-87, 1946.
25. Broadbent BH Sr, et al. *Bolton standards of dentofacial developmental growth*. St Louis, 1975, Mosby.
26. Darwis WE, et al. Assessing growth and development of the facial profile, *Pediatr Dent* 25:103-108, 2003.

27. Ackerman JL, Proffit WR. The characteristics of malocclusion: a modern approach to classification and diagnosis, *Am J Orthod* 56:443-454, 1969.

28. Angle EH. *Treatment of malocclusion of the teeth,* 7th ed. Philadelphia, 1907, SS White Dental Mfg.

29. Bell WH, et al. *Surgical correction of dentofacial deformities,* Vol 1. Philadelphia, 1980, WB Saunders.

30. Cox NH, van der Linden F. Facial harmony, *Am J Orthod* 60:175-183, 1971.

31. Patterson CN, Powell DG. Facial analysis in patient evaluation for physiologic and cosmetic surgery, *Laryngoscope* 84:1004-1019, 1979.

32. Horowitz SL, Hixon EH. *The nature of orthodontic diagnosis.* St Louis, 1966, Mosby.

33. Andrews LF. Six keys to normal occlusion, *Am J Orthod* 62:296-309, 1972.

34. Roth RH. Functional occlusion for the orthodontist. Part III, *J Clin Orthod* 15:174, 1981.

35. Enlow DH. A morphogenetic analysis of facial growth, *Am J Orthod* 52:283-299, 1966.

36. Farkas LG. *Anthropology of the head and face in medicine.* New York, 1981, Elsevier.

37. Legan HL, Burstone CJ. Soft tissue cephalometric analysis for orthognathic surgery, *J Oral Surg* 38:744-752, 1980.

38. Enlow DH, et al. A procedure for the analysis of intrinsic facial form and growth, *Am J Orthod* 56:6-23, 1969.

39. Balbach DR. The cephalometric relationship between the morphology of the mandible and its future occlusal position, *Angle Orthod* 39:29-41, 1969.

40. McNamara JA, Carlson DS. Quantitative analysis of temporomandibular joint adaptations to protrusive function, *Am J Orthod* 76:593-611, 1979.

41. Graber TM, Swain BF. *Orthodontics: current principles and techniques.* St Louis, 1985, Mosby.

42. Leighton BC. Early recognition of normal occlusion. In McNamara JA, ed. *The biology of occlusion development,* Monograph No 7. *Craniofacial growth series.* Ann Arbor, 1977, University of Michigan.

43. Arya BS, et al. Prediction of first molar occlusion, *Am J Orthod* 63:610-621, 1973.

44. Carlsen DB, Meredith HV. Biologic variation in selected relationships of opposing posterior teeth, *Angle Orthod* 30:162-173, 1960.

45. HEW reports on occlusion: summary and discussion, *J Clin Orthod* 12:849-862, 1978.

46. Friel S. Occlusion: observations on its development from infancy to old age, *Int J Orthod* 13:322-341, 1927.

47. Lewis SJ, Lehman IA. Observations of the growth changes in the teeth and dental arches, *Dent Cosmos* 70:480, 1929.

48. Sanin C, Savara BS. The development of excellent occlusion, *Am J Orthod* 61:345-352, 1972.

49. Moyers RA. *Handbook of orthodontics,* 3rd ed. Chicago, 1973, Mosby.

50. da Silva LP, Gleiser R. Occlusal development between primary and mixed dentitions: a 5-year longitudinal study, *J Dent Child* 75(3):287-294, 2008.

51. Northway WM, et al. Effects of premature loss of deciduous molars, *Angle Orthod* 54:295-329, 1984.

52. Nery EB, Oka SW. Developmental stages of the human dentition. In Melmich M, et al, eds. *Clinical dysmorphology of oro-facial structures.* Boston, 1982, John Wright-PSG.

53. Moorrees CFA. *The dentition of the growing child.* Cambridge, MA, 1959, Harvard University Press.

54. Moorrees CFA. Growth studies of the dentition: a review, *Am J Orthod* 55:600-616, 1969.

55. Anderson AA. The dentition and occlusal development in children of African American descent, *Angle Orthod* 77(3):421-429, 2007.

56. Van der Linden FPGM. Transition of the human dentition, Monograph No 13. *Craniofacial growth series.* Ann Arbor, 1982, University of Michigan.

57. Ten Cate AR. Formation of supporting bone in association with periodontal ligament organization in the mouse, *Arch Oral Biol* 20:137-138, 1975.

58. Fränkel R. Decrowding during eruption under the screening influence of vestibular shields, *Am J Orthod* 65:372-406, 1974.

59. Potter RH, Nance WE. A twin study on dental dimension. I, Discordance, asymmetry and mirror imagery, *Am J Phys Anthropol* 44:391-395, 1976.

60. Hixon EH, Oldfather RE. Estimation of the sizes of unerupted cuspid and bicuspid teeth, *Angle Orthod* 28:236-240, 1958.

61. Melgaco CA, et al. Mandibular permanent first molar and incisor width as predictor of mandibular canine and premolar width, *Am J Orthod Dentofacial Orthop* 132(3): 340-345, 2007.

62. Durgekar SC, Naik V. Evaluation of Moyers mixed dentition analysis in school children, *Indian J Dent Res* 20(1):26-30, 2009.

63. Gardner RB. A comparison of four methods of predicting arch length, *Am J Orthod* 75:387-398, 1979.

64. Kaplan RG, et al. An analysis of three mixed dentition analyses, *J Dent Res* 56:1337-1343, 1977.

65. Staley RN, Kerber PE. A revision of the Hixon and Oldfather mixed dentition prediction method, *Am J Orthod* 78:296-302, 1980.

66. Staley RN. Prediction of the widths of unerupted canines and premolars, *J Am Dent Assoc* 108:185-190, 1984.

67. Staley RN, et al. Prediction of lower canine and premolar widths in the mixed dentition, *Am J Orthod* 76:300-309, 1979.

68. Bishara SE, Staley RN. Mixed-dentition mandibular arch length analysis: a step-by-step approach using the revised Hixon-Oldfather prediction method, *Am J Orthod* 86: 130-135, 1984.

69. Merrifield LL. Differential diagnosis with total space analysis, *J Charles Tweed Foundation* 6:10-15, 1978.

CHAPTER 26

Cephalometrics and Facial Esthetics: The Key to Complete Treatment Planning

▲ John T. Krull, George E. Krull, Thomas H. Lapp, and David A. Bussard

CHAPTER OUTLINE

In studying a case of malocclusion, give no thought to the methods of treatment or appliances until the case shall have been classified and all peculiarities and variations from the normal in type, occlusion, and facial lines have been thoroughly comprehended. Then the requirements and proper plan of treatment become apparent.

—**Edward H. Angle**

Cephalometrics, the assessment of craniofacial dimensions, particularly the ethnographic determination of cranial morphology, is an ancient skill practiced by anthropologists for centuries.

Beauty and harmony are the traditional guiding principles used to assess facial proportions, although the definition of beauty may change as civilizations change. Greek sculpture during the golden age of art (fourth century BC) shows facial proportions very similar to those found desirable today. Basic facial features of Greek male and female figures appear to be depicted identically, with most sculpture angles within 5 degrees of contemporary standards; the exceptions are a more acute mentolabial sulcus and nasofacial angle for the ancient Greek ideal.

In the early twentieth century, dentistry began to include the concepts of facial harmony and balance in the theory and practice of cephalometrics. In 1922, Simon introduced this modern era with the development of gnathostatics, a photographic technique that related the teeth and their respective bony bases to each other, as well as to specific craniofacial structures. Although Pacini and Carrera obtained the first x-ray films of the skull by the standard lateral view in 1926, it was not until the introduction of the cephalometer by Broadbent in 1931 that the science of cephalometrics became standardized. This sophisticated form of radiography enabled the practitioner to identify specific problem areas of craniofacial disproportion and devise detailed therapeutic interventions. Through the contributions of investigators such as Brodie, Downs, Reidel, Steiner, Tweed, and Ricketts, the clinical application of cephalometrics has developed the techniques that permit the observation of discrepancies observed in the mandible, maxilla, dental units, and soft tissue profile.

The primary aim of cephalometric analysis is to localize malocclusion within a tracing of facial bone and soft tissue structures. The analysis is performed by using standardized cephalometric landmarks to construct lines, angles, and imaginary planes, which permits linear and angular assessments of dental and facial relationships as seen on radiographic films of the head and face. These findings are compared with established normal values, and an individualized treatment protocol is developed for orthopedic, orthodontic, and orthognathic therapies.

The science of cephalometrics has often been referred to as a "numbers game" and has the reputation of being difficult to master. There appears to be a universal search for a reliable group of numbers that will ultimately lead one to an accurate diagnosis. Such a search is futile, because all cephalometric measurements may at times lead one to an erroneous conclusion. However, an accurate, in-depth analysis provides one with an assessment of dentofacial and craniofacial morphology. A cephalometric radiograph furnishes one with a static analysis, whereas subsequent films allow the clinician to follow the growth patterns of the adolescent patient on a longitudinal basis. In addition, comparison of serial cephalograms of the same patient may allow some developmental predictions to be made.

The use of cephalometrics serves to confirm the diagnosis and makes it possible to include the morphology of the cranium when alternative treatment modalities are considered. In patient care, cephalometrics can provide valuable data when treatment is first initiated and can serve a monitoring function during the course of orthodontic care. On completion of treatment, cephalometric radiology allows assessment of the relative degree of posttreatment stability and evaluation of treatment results produced by various mechanical and appliance selections.

Cephalometric numbers or central tendencies have been developed to serve as guidelines in evaluation of the patient. Dentists must keep in mind that they are treating individuals, not averages, and that the numbers merely help or guide in the formulation of an accurate diagnosis and treatment plan. Because of individual anatomic, biologic, and environmental variations, it is imperative that the clinician consider several factors to achieve a comprehensive case analysis. Any attempt to simplify the analysis is likely to lead to an erroneous conclusion.

The norm is commonly referred to as the *mean* or *average*. On the contrary, however, the norm, as it is applied in cephalometrics, is not a set of averages. The average patient in any given population will generally deviate from the norm, because the norm is derived from samples demonstrating ideal dental occlusions of the class I variety.

Most biologic variables are randomly distributed in the population and can be graphically illustrated by a bell-shaped curve (Fig. 26-1). Within this curve, approximately 70% of any given population lies within 1 standard deviation of the mean, whereas 95% of the group falls within 2 standard deviations. Throughout this chapter, the statistical concept of standard deviation is referred to as *clinical deviation* (CD).

As a general rule, the goal in treatment planning is to treat in the direction of cephalometric norms. The clinical advantages include the following:
1. A more favorable and predictable esthetic result
2. Greater posttreatment stability
3. Improved function and periodontal health

RADIOGRAPHIC TECHNIQUE

The technique employed in cephalometric radiology has been standardized to permit the comparison of initial and subsequent films for the same patient so that growth can be assessed and treatment progress monitored.

This standardization requires that the equipment include a headholder (cephalostat) and an x-ray tube positioned at a distance of 60 inches from the mid sagittal plane of the subject and that the distance from the midsagittal plane of the patient to the film be approximately 7.5 inches (Fig. 26-2). The cephalostat maintains a reproducible spatial relationship with respect to the position of the patient's head, the film, and the x-ray source. The most common device uses a counterbalanced beam with the radiographic tube on one end and the cephalostat on the other. This entire unit can be adjusted vertically to compensate for variations in patient height.

The patient is positioned in the cephalostat by means of laterally adjusted ear rods and a vertically adjusted nasal piece (Fig. 26-3). The nasal piece allows the clinician to orient the patient's head so that the Frankfort horizontal plane (a plane extending from the tragus of the ear to the inferior border of the orbital rim) is parallel to the floor. The ear posts should be centrally aligned to the source of radiation so that a transporionic axis is established.

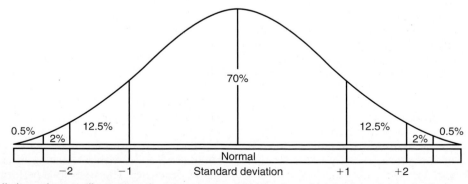

Figure 26-1 Bell-shaped curve illustrating the approximate distribution of biologic variables in the general population.

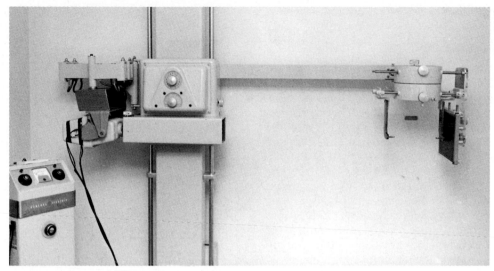

Figure 26-2 Wall-mounted, counterbalanced cephalometer. (Courtesy Dr. William W. Merow.)

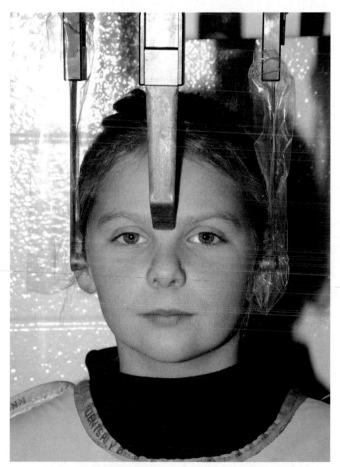

Figure 26-3 Patient positioned in the cephalostat.

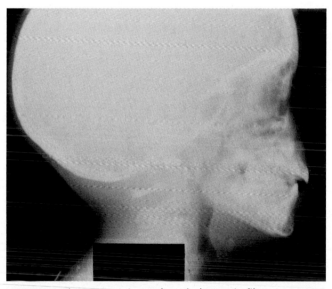

Figure 26-4 Lateral cephalometric film.

LATERAL HEAD FILM

For a lateral head radiograph, the patient is first positioned so that the left side of the face is tangent to an 8- by 10-inch film cassette, which permits less magnification and less distortion of the left-sided structures (Fig. 26-4).

The film cassette should be positioned as close as possible to the patient to minimize the effects of magnification, maximize resolution, and standardize the technique. The distance from the film cassette to the patient's midsagittal plane should be recorded to allow for comparison of serial films. Generally, the film is obtained with the mandible in its most retruded position and the lips in repose. Use of additional positions may be indicated. Once the patient has been positioned, the x-ray beam should enter through the ear rods perpendicular to the film.

Grids and intensifying screens are accessories used to improve the quality of the radiographic image. Rare-earth intensifying screens allow for a reduction of radiographic exposure while increasing the clarity of the radiographic image. Because the film range does not provide for sharp skeletal and soft tissue contrast, a movable aluminum screen attached to the cassette must be used over the soft tissue profile area to reduce the radiation and provide a better differential contrast between the two tissue types.

FRONTAL (POSTEROANTERIOR) FILM

Most diagnostic features related to vertical and anteroposterior (AP) problems are evident from the lateral film, though severe maxillary transverse deficiencies or facial asymmetries may be better diagnosed by the use of a posteroanterior (PA) film (Fig. 26-5). The patient is oriented facing the film cassette, with the ear rods and nasion piece positioning the patient so that the midsagittal and Frankfort planes are at right angles to the film cassette. After the patient's head is positioned so that the central x-ray beam passes through the head at the level of the transporionic axis and at its midpoint, the film cassette is moved into contact with the patient's nose. Because more radiation is required for this view, the milliamperage must be increased over that used in the lateral film technique.

CEPHALOMETRIC TRACING TECHNIQUE

Precise localization of the anatomic landmarks used in cephalometric analysis requires adequate knowledge of the radiographic and anatomic appearance of the facial bones and their relationships to adjacent structures. Various features are discernible: lines, shadows, the projections of bony structures, and contours of varying density. All of these make it difficult for the clinician to interpret and identify the anatomic relationships. A clear understanding of craniofacial structures and their relative spatial relationships is imperative before a lateral head film is traced.

Fig. 26-6 depicts a lateral cephalometric tracing. The lateral tracing should include the soft tissue outline, bony profile, outline of the mandible, posterior and anterior cranial base, odontoid process of the axis, anterior lip of the foramen magnum, clivus, planum orbitale, sella turcica, orbit, pterygomaxillary fissure, floor of the nose, roof of the palate, and body of the hyoid bone. In addition to the bony tissues, at least the first permanent molars as well as the most anterior maxillary and mandibular incisors are commonly included. In certain situations it may be desirable to trace other teeth or the complete dentition as shown in Fig. 26-6.

To make the tracing, the radiograph is placed on a view box with the facial profile to the right side. Acetate tracing paper (0.003 matte) is then placed over the radiograph with the matte side up. With a sharp No. 2 or 3H drawing pencil, all the necessary structures are traced. Because all x-rays become divergent once they emanate from the collimator, magnification of the subject will result, and a double-image effect will occur along the inferior border of the mandible and the area of the posterior teeth. All paired structures will produce double images on the head films. Because left-sided structures are magnified less by the radiographic beam and are considered more accurately rendered, the outline of these structures can be traced, although some prefer to make the tracing lines bisect bilateral images.

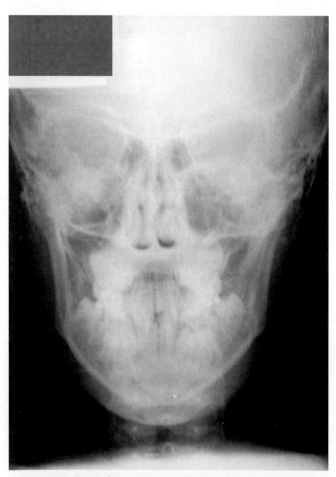

Figure 26-5 Frontal (posteroanterior) cephalometric film. (Courtesy Dr. William W. Merow.)

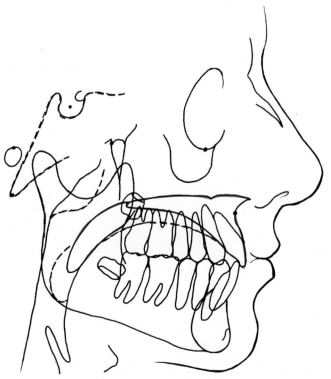

Figure 26-6 Lateral cephalometric tracing.

A PA cephalometric radiograph, as illustrated in Fig. 26-5, can be of significant diagnostic value in cases demonstrating mandibular displacement, facial asymmetry, severe posterior crossbite, or other types of bony dysplasia. Cephalometric analysis and a thorough and systematic clinical examination of these patients often reveal malocclusions accompanied by mandibular shifts when the patient is in maximum occlusion.

The PA radiograph is traced in the same manner as the lateral film. Fig. 26-7 illustrates the important skeletal and dental structures that must be traced for an accurate and complete analysis.

REFERENCE POINTS FOR LATERAL TRACING

The ultimate diagnostic value of the cephalometric analysis is dependent on the initial accurate identification and localization of anatomic and anthropologic points (Fig. 26-8). These landmarks are used to construct the lines, angles, and planes used to make a two-dimensional assessment of the patient's craniofacial and dental relationships. Although each analysis is completed in two dimensions, when the lateral analysis and the PA analysis for the same patient are considered together, a three-dimensional simulation emerges to contribute to the overall diagnosis and treatment plan. The following reference points are used in this chapter (see Fig. 26-8):

Sella turcica (S, or sella). The midpoint of the hypophyseal fossa. This is the ovoid area of the spheroid bone that contains the pituitary gland.

Nasion (N). The external junction of the nasofrontal suture in the median plane. If the suture is not visible,

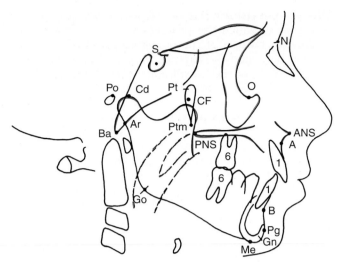

Figure 26-8 Lateral tracing with cephalometric reference points. (Adapted from Dr. William W. Merow.)

this point is located at the deepest concavity of the two bones.

Orbitale (O). The most inferior point on the external border of the orbit.

Condylion (Cd). The most superior point on the articular head of the condyle.

Anterior nasal spine (ANS). The most anterior projection of the anterior nasal spine of the maxilla in the median plane.

A point (subspinale, or A). The deepest point of the curvature of the anterior maxilla between the ANS and the alveolar crest. Although the A point may change with treatment, it represents the most forward point of the maxilla.

B point (supramentale, or B). The most posterior point on the outer curve of the mandibular alveolar process between the alveolar crest and the bony chin. The B point delineates the most anterior point of the mandible in the median plane.

Pogonion (Pg). The most anterior point on the midsagittal mandibular symphysis.

Menton (Me). The most inferior point of the mandibular symphysis.

Gnathion (Gn). A constructed point that is formed by the intersection of the facial and mandibular planes.

Gonion (Go). Another constructed point that is represented by the intersection of the lines tangent to the posterior margin of the ascending ramus and the mandibular plane.

Articulare (Ar). The point of intersection of the posterior margin of the ascending ramus and the outer margin of the cranial base.

Porion (Po). A point located at the most superior point of the external auditory meatus or the superior aspect of the metal ring that is a component of the left ear rod of the cephalostat.

Basion (Ba). The most inferior posterior point on the occipital bone that corresponds to the anterior margin of the foramen magnum.

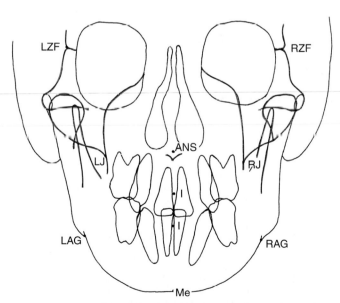

Figure 26-7 Frontal (posteroanterior) cephalometric tracing (see also Fig. 26-10). *ANS,* Anterior nasal spine; *I,* I (incisor) point; *LAG,* left antegonial notch; *LJ,* left jugal process of maxillary tuberosity; *LZF,* left zygomaticofrontal suture; *Me,* menton; *RAG,* right antegonial notch; *RJ,* right jugal process of maxillary tuberosity; *RZF,* right zygomaticofrontal suture.

Pterygomaxillary fissure (Ptm). A teardrop-shaped fissure of which the posterior wall is created by the anterior borders of the pterygoid plates of the sphenoid bone and the anterior wall represents the posterior border of the maxilla (maxillary tuberosity). The tip of this fissure denotes the posterior extent of the maxilla.

Posterior nasal spine (PNS). The tip of the posterior spine of the palatine bone. This landmark is usually not visible even on well-exposed lateral head films; therefore it is a constructed point that is represented by the intersection of a continuation of the anterior wall of the pterygopalatine fossa and the floor of the nose. It also denotes the posterior limit of the maxilla.

Pt point (Pt). The intersection of the inferior border of the foramen rotundum with the posterior wall of the Ptm.

CF point (center of face). The cephalometric landmark formed by the intersection of the Frankfort horizontal plane and a perpendicular line through Pt.

REFERENCE LINES, ANGLES, AND PLANES

Linear assessment is derived when two reference points are connected. Angular measurements are possible when three points are used. Planes (and some lines) are actually imaginary when the cephalometric tracing is viewed because the planes are at right angles to the tracing and can be seen only as a line on the two-dimensional tracing (Fig. 26-9). In cephalometric analysis, the dentist must become accustomed to thinking in three dimensions while viewing a two-dimensional representation. Therefore a point on the tracing may not only be a point but also may represent a line (or axis). A line on the tracing may actually be a line (or axis) or it may represent a plane.

Several lines or planes are used in the different cephalometric analyses, although one line or plane generally serves as the major reference on which the entire analysis is based. Two common references are the sella-nasion plane (anterior cranial base) and the Frankfort horizontal plane.

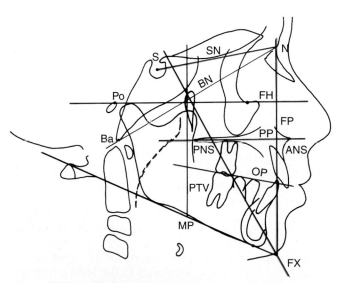

Figure 26-9 Cephalometric reference lines and planes. (Adapted from Dr. William W. Merow.)

The basic units of cephalometric analysis are angles and distances (lines). Measurements may be treated as absolute values, or they may be related to one another and expressed as relative proportions. These measurements and interrelationships provide the basic framework for describing craniofacial abnormalities. The following definitions help explain the planes of reference used in this chapter (see Fig. 26-9).

Frankfort horizontal plane (FH). This plane is constructed from porion (Po) to orbitale (O) and represents the basic horizontal plane of the head.

Sella-nasion plane (SN). This plane is represented by a line connecting the sella (S) and the nasion (N). It denotes the AP extent of the anterior cranial base. This reference plane is of questionable diagnostic value in true mandibular prognathism.

Occlusal plane (OP). This plane separates the maxillary and mandibular permanent molars (or in younger patients the primary second molars) and passes through the contact between the most anterior maxillary and mandibular incisors. If the incisors do not contact, the line passes midway between the incisal edges. Ideally, OP is nearly parallel to both the palatal plane (PP) and the FH.

Facial plane (FP). A line constructed through the nasion (N) perpendicular to the FH represents this plane.

Mandibular plane (MP). The mandibular plane is constructed as a tangent to the inferior border of the mandible.

Pterygoid vertical plane (PTV). This plane is represented by a line perpendicular to the FH through the Pt point. Studies have shown that the inter section of FH and PTV is extremely stable, because growth has little effect on this point. An overall view of patient growth may be gained by evaluation of serial cephalometric films on which FH and PTV are superimposed. PTV represents a basic vertical reference plane.

Basion-nasion plane (BN). This plane passes through the basion (Ba) and nasion (N). The plane represents cranial base and is the dividing plane between the cranium and the face.

Facial axis (FX). This line is constructed from the Pt point through the gnathion. FX ideally crosses BN at a right angle.

Palatal plane (PP). This plane extends through the anterior nasal spine (ANS) and posterior nasal spine (PNS). The relationship of this plane to FH is useful in evaluating treatment changes occurring in the maxilla.

INTERPRETATION OF MEASUREMENTS

The objectives of cephalometric interpretation are summarized as follows:
1. To define both the skeletal and facial types
2. To evaluate the relationship between the maxillary and mandibular basal bones
3. To assess the dental relationships (the spatial relationship between the teeth, maxilla, mandible, and cranial base)
4. To locate the malocclusion within the dentofacial complex and analyze its origin (skeletal or dentoalveolar)

5. To study the facial soft tissue contours with respect to the cause of the malocclusion
6. To consider the impact of the various options for correcting the malocclusion on the facial contours as well as on the skeletal and dental components
7. To facilitate selection of a treatment plan
8. To evaluate the results of various soft tissue surgical procedures

LATERAL CEPHALOMETRIC ASSESSMENT

MAXILLARY SKELETAL

SNA: The angle between SN and N–A point
Clinical norm: 82 degrees
Clinical deviation: 2 degrees
Interpretation: Establishes horizontal location of the maxilla. Deviation in cranial base (SN, angulation, or length) or vertical maxillary excess proves that this measurement is unreliable. Therefore reduced emphasis should be given in these instances.

Maxillary depth: The angle formed by the intersection of the FH and N–A point planes
Clinical norm: 90 degrees
Clinical deviation: 3 degrees
Interpretation: Indicates horizontal position of maxilla. Class II skeletal patterns caused by a prognathic maxilla show values exceeding 90 degrees. Chronic thumb suckers generally demonstrate large values.

Maxillary length: The measurement of the line extending from Cd to A point
Clinical norm: 85 mm female, 87 mm male
Clinical deviation: 6 mm
Interpretation: Increases 1 mm per year until adult size is attained (95 to 100 mm). This measurement determines if the class II or class III skeletal pattern is attributable to a long or short maxilla, respectively.

ANB: The difference between the SNA and SNB angles
Clinical norm: +2 degrees
Clinical deviation: 2 degrees
Interpretation: Indicates the horizontal relationship between maxilla and mandible. Positive values indicate that the maxilla is forward of the mandible, whereas negative values indicate a class III skeletal relationship.

MAXILLARY DENTAL

Maxillary incisor angulation: The angle formed by SN and the incisor long axis
Clinical norm: 102 degrees
Clinical deviation: 3 degrees
Interpretation: Relates the upper incisor angulation to the upper and middle face. Values well above 102 degrees indicate angular incisor protrusion, whereas values significantly less than that demonstrate angular retrusion.

Maxillary incisor AP position: The horizontal distance from the facial surface of the maxillary central incisors to the N–A point line

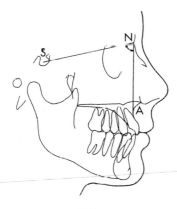

SNA

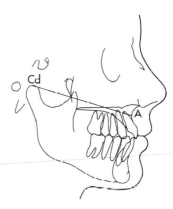

MAXILLARY LENGTH

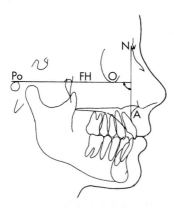

MAXILLARY DEPTH

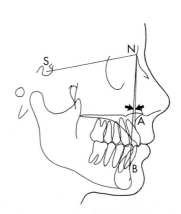

ANB

Clinical norm: 4 mm

Clinical deviation: 2 mm

Interpretation: Indicates horizontal position of the maxillary incisors. Values in excess of 6 mm indicate anterior dental protrusion, whereas values 1 mm or less show dental retrusion.

Upper molar position: The horizontal distance from PTV to the distal surface of the maxillary first molar

Clinical norm: Chronologic age of the patient + 3 mm (e.g., a 10-year-old has a clinical norm of 10 + 3 = 13 mm). The growth change is approximately 1 mm per year through the years of active growth.

Clinical deviation: 3 mm

Interpretation: Determines if the dental malocclusion is caused by the AP position of the maxillary molar. It is important in treatment planning considerations involving distal movement of the maxillary molars.

Maxillary incisor to upper lip: The vertical distance between the inferior border of the upper lip and the incisal edge of the maxillary incisor

Clinical norm: 3 mm

Clinical deviation: 1 mm

Interpretation: Gives an evaluation of the amount of upper incisor in repose. Values of 5 mm or more may be associated with vertical maxillary excess. This value must be compared with upper lip length. Patients with short upper lips will show more incisor at rest.

MANDIBULAR SKELETAL

SNB: The angle formed between the SN and N–B point planes

Clinical norm: 80 degrees

Clinical deviation: 2 degrees

Interpretation: Indicates horizontal location of the mandible. Abnormal cranial base angulation and vertical facial excess will adversely affect the reliability of this measurement.

Facial angle (depth): The angle formed between the N-Pg and FH planes

Clinical norm: 87 degrees at 9 years of age. Increases 0.33 degree per year.

Clinical deviation: 3 degrees

Interpretation: Locates the horizontal position of the chin. Determines if the skeletal class II or class III relation ship is attributable to a retrognathic or a prognathic mandible.

Mandibular length: The absolute distance between Cd and Gn

Clinical norm: 105 mm at 9 years of age with yearly growth increments of 2 to 2.5 mm, reaching a maximum of 120 to 130 mm. Generally 2 mm less in females than in males at 9 years of age.

Clinical deviation: 6 mm

Interpretation: Determines whether the skeletal class II or class III relationship is attributable to a small or large mandible.

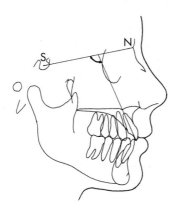

MAXILLARY INCISOR ANGULATION

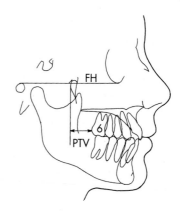

UPPER MOLAR POSITION

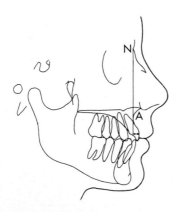

MAXILLARY INCISOR (A-P) POSITION

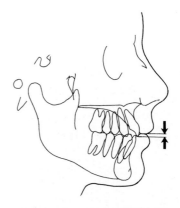

MAXILLARY INCISOR TO UPPER LIP

MANDIBULAR DENTAL

Mandibular incisor protrusion: The horizontal distance from the tip of the mandibular incisor to the A point–Pg line
Clinical norm: +2 mm
Clinical deviation: 2.3 mm
Interpretation: Defines the AP position of the mandibular dental unit and quantifies the reciprocal relationship of the maxillary and mandibular dental units. Not only is this a key esthetic relationship, but it also needs to be correlated with a functional arch length analysis.

Incisor mandibular plane angle (IMPA): The inner angle between the long axis of the mandibular incisor and MP
Clinical norm: 90 degrees
Clinical deviation: 4 degrees
Interpretation: Gives an evaluation of the angular position of the incisor to the mandibular basal bone.
Holdaway ratio: The ratio of the mandibular incisor and Pg to the N–B point line
Clinical norm: 1:1
Clinical deviation: 2 mm
Interpretation: The AP position of the mandibular incisor and Pg should project equally from the N–B point line for good facial balance.

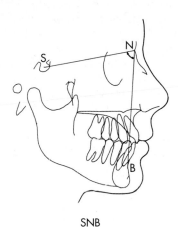

SNB

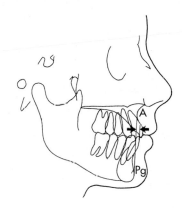

MANDIBULAR INCISOR PROTRUSION

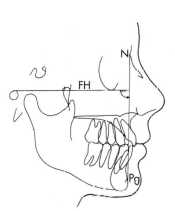

FACIAL ANGLE

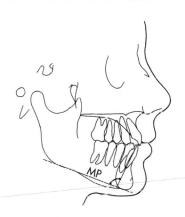

IMPA

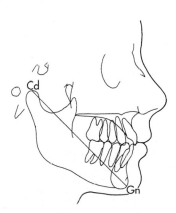

MANDIBULAR LENGTH

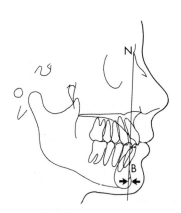

HOLDAWAY RATIO

VERTICAL

Posterior facial height: The linear distance between Go and the CF point

Clinical norm: 55 mm for the average-sized patient at 8.5 years of age. Increases 1 mm per year.

Clinical deviation: 3.3 mm

Interpretation: Measures vertical growth of the ramus and can therefore be of value in predicting clockwise or counterclockwise growth patterns. Values less than 51 mm represent a leaning toward dolichofacial patterns, whereas values in excess of 59 mm may indicate brachyfacial or counterclockwise growth trends.

Mandibular plane angle (FMA): The angle formed by the intersection of FH and MP

Clinical norm: 26 degrees. Decreases 1 degree every 4 years during normal growth.

Clinical deviation: 4 degrees

Interpretation: Values in excess of 31 degrees may indicate clockwise growth with dolichofacial growth trends, whereas values less than 21 degrees imply vertical deficiency as often seen in brachyfacial growth patterns.

Facial axis angle: The angle between FX and BN

Clinical norm: 90 degrees

Clinical deviation: 3.5 degrees. Changes 1 degree every 3 years in the average patient.

Interpretation: Expresses the ratio of facial height to depth and thus indicates the direction of growth of the chin. Values in excess of 94 degrees may indicate counterclockwise growth, whereas those less than 85 degrees may imply clockwise growth in brachyfacial and dolichofacial facial types, respectively.

Facial height: The vertical relationship between upper and lower facial height (N-ANS:ANS-M)

Clinical norm: Upper 53 mm; lower 65 mm

Interpretation: More important than the absolute value is the ratio between upper and lower facial height, which should be approximately 5:6 for a well-balanced face.

SOFT TISSUE

Nasolabial angle: The angle formed by the intersection of the lines tangent to the columella of the nose and the upper lip

Clinical norm: 90 to 110 degrees

Interpretation: Provides an assessment of the nose-to-upper-lip relationship. Values in excess of 114 degrees may indicate upper lip retrusion, whereas values of 96 degrees or less may be associated with dental protrusion.

Zero meridian: The horizontal distance from the chin to a line perpendicular to FH and tangent to the soft tissue nasion

Clinical norm: 0 mm

Clinical deviation: 2 mm

Interpretation: May be helpful in assessment of the projection of the chin relative to FH.

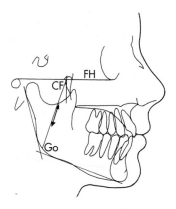

POSTERIOR FACIAL HEIGHT

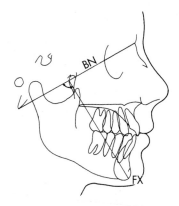

FACIAL AXIS ANGLE

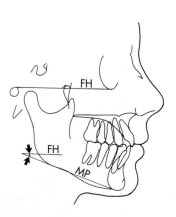

FMA

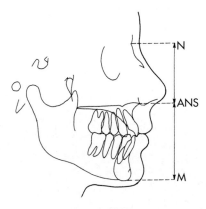

FACIAL HEIGHT

Interlabial distance: The vertical distance between the inferior aspect of the upper lip and the superior surface of the lower lip with the patient in repose

Clinical norm: 1.9 mm

Clinical deviation: 1.2 mm

Interpretation: High values indicate lip incompetence and are often associated with hyperactivity of the mentalis muscle. Low values may be associated with overclosure.

Lip protrusion: The horizontal distance between the lower lip and the esthetic plane (E plane). The esthetic plane is a line connecting the tip of the nose and the most anterior point on the soft tissue chin.

Clinical norm: –2 mm at 8.5 years of age; decreases 0.2 mm per year. The values tend to decrease with age until adult values of –5 mm are reached.

Clinical deviation: 2 mm

Interpretation: Indicates soft tissue balance between lips and profile (nose-chin).

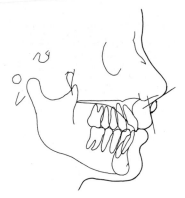

NASOLABIAL ANGLE

FRONTAL (POSTEROANTERIOR) CEPHALOMETRIC ASSESSMENT

Frontal cephalometric points and planes are used to evaluate the overall relationships of the cranium, maxilla, mandible, and denture from a frontal view. Fig. 26-10 is a graphic representation of the points, lines, and planes used in frontal cephalometric analysis.

Dental midline: The horizontal distance between the maxillary and mandibular incisor midlines

Clinical norm: 0 mm

Clinical deviation: 1.5 mm

Interpretation: Determines dental midline asymmetry.

Maxillomandibular width: The horizontal distance between the jugal process of the maxilla and the frontal facial plane

Clinical norm: 10 mm for patient of average size at 8½ years of age. Needs to be corrected for size.

Interpretation: Determines if a crossbite is skeletal in nature. Large values are associated with skeletal lingual crossbites, whereas lesser values indicate skeletal buccal crossbites.

Maxillomandibular midline: The angle formed by the ANS-Me plane through ANS and perpendicular to the zygomatic frontal suture plane

Clinical norm: 0 mm

Clinical deviation: 2 mm

Interpretation: Determines whether facial asymmetry is attributable to total size discrepancy or a functional shift of the mandible.

Denture to jaw midlines: The horizontal distance between the midlines of the mandibular incisors and maxilla and mandible

Clinical norm: 0 mm

Clinical deviation: 1.5 mm

Interpretation: Aids differential diagnosis between denture shift and mandibular shift.

Occlusal plane tilt: Measures the degree of parallelism between the occlusal plane and a line through the zygomatic frontal sutures

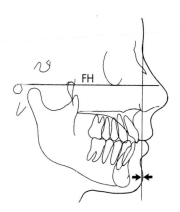

ZERO MERIDIAN

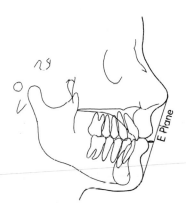

LIP PROTRUSION

Clinical norm: 0 mm

Clinical deviation: 2 mm

Interpretation: A skeletal asymmetry in addition to a tilt in occlusal plane is usually a signal of possible temporomandibular joint dysfunction.

Maxillary width: The horizontal distance between the jugal processes of the maxilla

Clinical norm: 61.9 mm at 9 years of age. Increases 0.6 mm per year.

Clinical deviation: 3 mm

Interpretation: Indicates the width of the maxilla. The change in value is useful in cases involving sutural expansion of the palate.

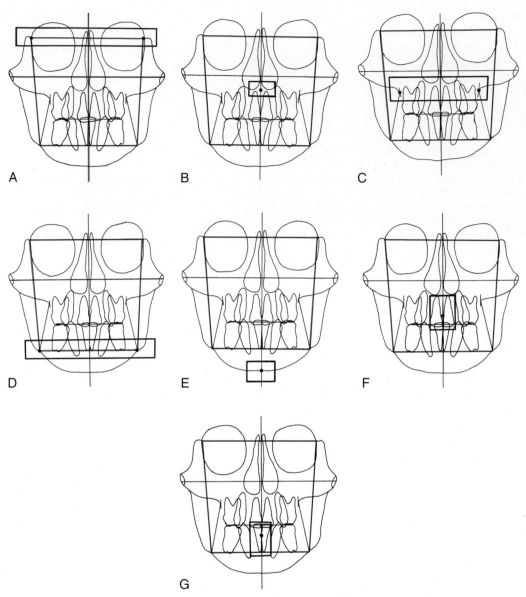

Figure 26-10 Frontal reference points (see also Fig. 26-7). **A,** LZF/RZF, bilateral points on the medial aspect of the zygomaticofrontal sutures at the intersections of the orbits. **B,** ANS, tip of anterior nasal spine. **C,** LJ/RJ, bilateral points on the jugal processes and the intersection of the maxillary tuberosities and the zygomatic buttresses. **D,** LAG/RAG, points at the lateral inferior margin of the antegonial protuberances of the mandible. **E,** Me, menton, point of the inferior border of the mandibular symphysis directly inferior to the mental protuberance. **F,** I point, a point selected at the interdental papilla of the upper incisors at the junction of the crowns and gingiva. **G,** I point, a point selected at the interdental papilla of the lower incisors at the junction of the crowns and gingiva.

DIRECTIONS OF GROWTH

The constructed gonial angle is formed by the intersection of the ascending ramus and the body of the mandible. This angle can be used as an initial assessment of future mandibular growth. The direction of growth is very important in the selection of a functional appliance if that method of treatment is indicated. In cases such as mandibular prognathism, the information would lead one to the conclusion that treatment might best be delayed due to the possibility of latent mandibular growth.

The gonial angle is divided into two parts to determine the angular relationship between the ascending ramus and the body of the mandible. A line is constructed between nasion and the constructed gonial angle (facial depth line), dividing the gonial angle into upper and lower compartments. As a general rule, the upper angle with a normal range of 52 to 55 degrees indicates horizontal or counterclockwise growth. The lower angle with a range of 70 to 75 degrees is an indicator of vertical or clockwise growth. The astute clinician needs to keep in mind that growth is rarely in a straight line, but rather exhibits more of a curve (Fig. 26-11).

When the upper angle is large, the growth will be more forward, whereas a large lower number would indicate

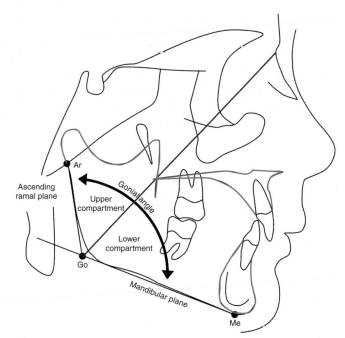

Figure 26-11 Facial growth vector assessment and the gonial angle.

downward growth. A small upper number would be indicative of clockwise growth. Counterclockwise growth is likely when the lower number is small.

Another method of assessing the direction of growth is to divide the upper angle by the lower angle, resulting in a percentage. The numerical value can then be compared with the numbers in the following list to give an idea of the growth vector. A more in-depth analysis may be indicated in more difficult musculoskeletal discrepancies.

Ideal growth: 70% to 78%
Clockwise tendency: 69.9% to 68.1%
Clockwise growth: ≤68%
Excessive clockwise growth: <60%
Counterclockwise tendency: 78.1% to 79.9%
Counterclockwise growth: ≥80%
Excessive counterclockwise growth: >88%

COMPUTERIZED CEPHALOMETRIC DIAGNOSIS AND TREATMENT PLANNING

The availability of inexpensive and powerful computers in the dental office has made comprehensive cephalometric software a reliable tool for the practitioner. These computer programs, in addition to providing accurate models of the skeletal and soft tissue anatomy, allow an accurate prediction of esthetic results by evaluation of the soft tissue changes secondary to orthodontic and orthopedic alterations in the hard tissues. One can also evaluate multiple treatment plans and examine the changes that would result relative to the soft tissue before actually initiating a specific treatment plan.

DIGITAL IMAGING

Imaging has been an important aspect of dental care since the early 1900s. The x-ray was discovered by Wilhelm Conrad Roentgen in late 1895. This discovery

resulted in how dental anatomy would be evaluated. Dr. Otto Walkoff took the first dental radiographs in 1896 with an exposure time of 25 minutes. Later that same year, advances were made in the field such that the exposure time was reduced to 9 minutes. The first dental radiographs were obtained in the United States that same year by the Eastman Kodak Company. Finally in 1919, Kodak produced the first dental x-ray films designed for direct exposure. F-speed film introduced in 2000 required 1/60th of the radiation of the 1919 films.

Over the years, dentistry has been on the cutting edge of radiology. Dentistry entered a new era of diagnostic imaging when French dentist Francis Mouyen introduced digital imaging in 1987. This method creates images with the use of a computer. In recent years, cone beam computed tomography (CT) has come into play. This digital imaging system can produce both two-and three-dimensional images.

Digital imaging provides high resolution and reduced radiation to the patient when compared with conventional radiography. Additionally, these digitally generated images provide an accurate and reproducible method of analysis. Digital radiographs used in conjunction with the appropriate software can generate three-dimensional images and allow an accurate evaluation of anatomic structures. Improved image sharpness in, for example, the central incisor region can be accomplished by digitally eliminating the shadows cast by the cervical vertebrae. A more relevant image results in a more accurate diagnosis.

In 2001, the TOM OR-DVT-9000, the first dentomaxillofacial dedicated cone beam CT machine, was dedicated in the United States. Virtually every practitioner can benefit from this new technology. In the past few years, image centers have been established that allow clinicians in larger cities to have access to these facilities. Stand-alone software packages placed at office workstations enable dentists to view a full range of sophisticated views. Software programs such as Dolphin (www.dolphinimaging.com), In-Vivo Dental (www.anatomage.com), and V-Works (www.cybermed.co.kr) allow dentists to view the data from the CT machines.

ANTEROPOSTERIOR INTERARCH DISCREPANCIES

CLASS I

A class I occlusion is one in which the mesiobuccal cusp tip of the maxillary first molar aligns with the buccal groove of the mandibular first molar (Fig. 26-12). Because of this sagittal relationship, most class I occlusions demonstrate reasonably normal skeletal and soft tissue profiles.

CLASS II DIVISION I

In class II division I malocclusion, the mesiobuccal cusp tip of the maxillary first molar is positioned anterior to the buccal groove of the mandibular first molar (Fig. 26-13). The sagittal molar relationship of these patients is referred to as a *disto-occlusion* as opposed to a *neutro-occlusion* in patients with class I occlusion. The exact reason for this relationship may be skeletal, dental, or a combination of the two. The nature of the problem can be more accurately determined by the use of cephalometric analysis. This type of malocclusion is often characterized by excessive overjet in the anterior region. Unlike the patient with class I occlusion, these patients often exhibit more downward growth, abnormal muscle pressure, and a convex soft and hard tissue profile.

In vertical growth patterns in which the upper molars are erupting along the facial axis and the upper incisors are erupting in a protruded direction, space between the upper molars and incisors is increased, which results in the typical dental characteristics of the class II division I malocclusion.

CLASS II DIVISION II

The molar position observed in patients with class II division II malocclusion is similar to that of those with class II division I malocclusion, although the excessive overjet associated with the latter is not seen (Fig. 26-14). The anterior relationship of a class II division II malocclusion is characterized by lingual tipping of the central incisors and labial flaring of the lateral incisors. Whereas patients with class II division I malocclusion show a weak chin, patients with division II malocclusion tend to have a square jaw, skeletal deep bite, and a short lower facial height. Class II division II malocclusions demonstrate strong growth patterns in which the upper molar grows down the facial axis while the upper incisor moves down with a retroclination. In this case, there is a diminution of space between the molar and incisor. This results in a pinching or closing of the arch, which gives the characteristic flaring of the

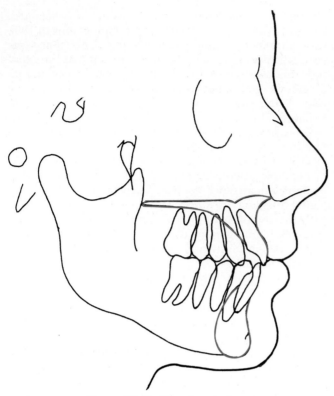
Figure 26-12 Class I occlusion.

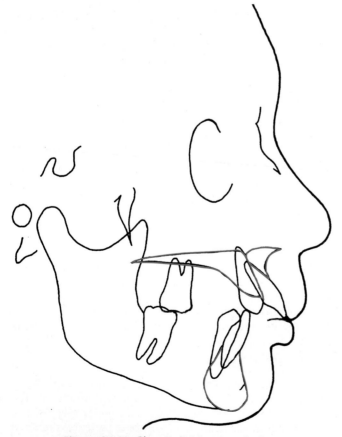
Figure 26-13 Class II division I occlusion.

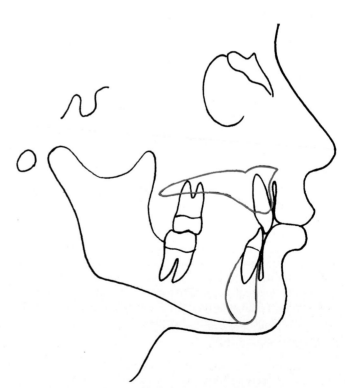
Figure 26-14 Class II division II occlusion.

upper lateral incisors and linguoversion of the centrals. In severe cases, an hourglass-shaped upper arch form may result.

CLASS III

In class III malocclusion, the mesiobuccal cusp tip of the maxillary first permanent molar is posterior to the buccal groove of the mandibular first permanent molar (Fig. 26-15). The most common cause of class III malocclusions is excessive growth of the mandible. The molar position of these patients is referred to as *mesio-occlusion,* whereas the anterior relationship shows a negative overjet. Many cases demonstrate dental compensations in which the maxillary incisors are excessively flared and the mandibular incisors are severely tipped to the lingual. These patients typically show concave facial profiles and steep mandibular plane angles attributable, in part, to an obtuse gonial angle.

FACIAL TYPES

Classification of the face by one of the three general facial types is imperative even though no definitive correlation between malocclusion and facial types has been demonstrated. It should be obvious that the prognosis for a pleasing facial result in treatment of a class II malocclusion associated with a retrognathic mandible would be more uncertain than that in treatment of a class II malocclusion occurring with an orthognathic mandible.

The three basic facial types or patterns are dolichofacial (vertical), mesofacial (ideal), and brachyfacial (horizontal). The determination of the patient's facial pattern is important in growth prediction as well as in treatment planning. Therefore one of the first assessments necessary for an accurate craniofacial diagnosis is classification of the patient's facial type.

Although all facial types may be observed in association with different malocclusions, a statistically significant higher incidence of specific types does occur with certain types of malocclusion, such as the association of class II malocclusions with retrognathic mandibles and of class III malocclusions with prognathic mandibles. On the other hand, an orthognathic facial type is not always associated with an ideal class I occlusal relationship. As the clinician becomes more familiar with the different types of malocclusion, it will become obvious that certain facial patterns are commonly associated with each classification of malocclusion.

MESOFACIAL PATTERN

The mesofacial pattern is most often associated with class I occlusions because these patients are characterized by a relatively normal maxillary and mandibular relationship that results in good facial balance (Fig. 26-16).

DOLICHOFACIAL PATTERN

The faces of patients with the dolichofacial pattern are usually long and of weak musculature because of the tendency for vertical growth. The molar occlusion is often of the class II division I variety. The protruded dentition of

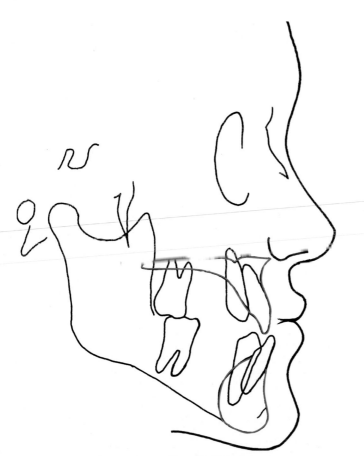

Figure 26-15 Class III occlusion.

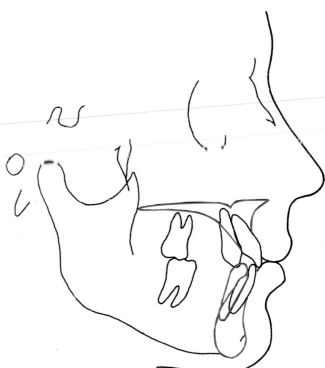

Figure 26-16 Mesofacial pattern.

these patients often results in facial grimacing and disharmony. Reduction of the interincisal angle will result in a more pleasing facial profile (Fig. 26-17).

BRACHYFACIAL PATTERN

The short faces and wide, square mandibles of patients with a brachyfacial pattern are most often associated with class II division II malocclusions. The mandibular growth of these patients is usually forward rather than downward. Consequently, these patients typically exhibit excessive anterior overbites and strong chins (Fig. 26-18). Esthetically the brachyfacial patient can generally accommodate a fuller dentition with a more acute interincisal angle. The fuller dentition helps balance the strong chin and the shorter lower facial height by giving more forward projection to the midfacial region.

VERTICAL ARCH DISCREPANCIES

OPEN BITE

Open-bite relationships are characterized by failure of the teeth in both arches to meet properly (Fig. 26-19). Open bites may be observed in the anterior or posterior region and may be attributable to supraeruption of the adjacent teeth or infraeruption of the teeth in the area of question. Open bites may be caused by abnormal habits, deviant growth patterns, or an abnormal tongue position.

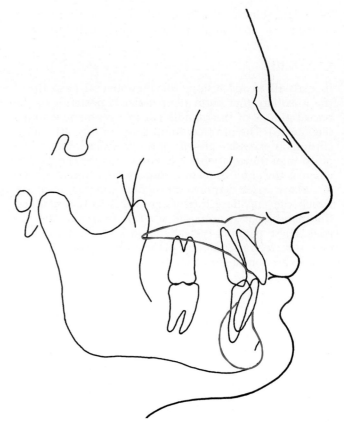

Figure 26-18 Brachyfacial pattern.

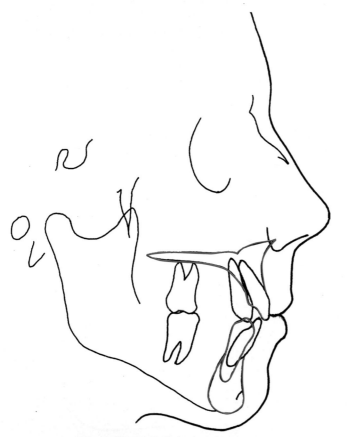

Figure 26-17 Dolichofacial pattern.

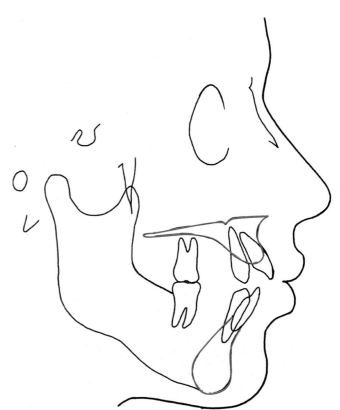

Figure 26-19 Open-bite pattern.

DEEP BITE

Deep bites are most often observed in class II division I malocclusion in which, because of the excessive overjet, the mandibular incisors supraerupt until they come into contact with the hard palate (Fig. 26-20). The class II division II malocclusion is also associated with a deep bite, although in these patients the cause may be infraeruption of the posterior teeth or supraeruption of the maxillary anterior teeth. In many deep-bite cases, the condition results in overclosure of the mandible leading to labial movement of the upper incisors and, in some cases, generalized spacing of the maxillary anterior teeth. The correction leading to opening of the bite is determined by the type of malocclusion, the esthetic goals, and the philosophical approach of the clinician. A comprehensive case analysis is therefore necessary to define the etiologic factors.

ANGLE CLASSIFICATION OF OCCLUSION

Orthodontists are concerned with facial form, function, oral health, and beauty. The primary criteria for classifying the occlusion were developed in 1899 by Edward Angle, the father of modern orthodontics, to evaluate the sagittal relationship of the canines and molars. Angle was a non-extractionist who considered the bust of Apollo Belvedere to be the epitome of facial balance, and consequently it served as a guide to his treatment objectives. Angle contended that dental arch expansion was necessary for proper orthodontic treatment. With this method of treatment, Dr. Angle rarely removed teeth. Insightful orthodontists such as Charles Tweed, Hays Nance, and P. R. Begg refuted Angle's approach to treatment, which often resulted in poor facial esthetics, instability, and periodontal problems. These latter orthodontists often recommended

the removal of teeth to improve facial esthetics and avoid double protrusion. Over the years the pendulum has swung back and forth between extraction and nonextraction. The fear of creating a "dished-in" profile has been reported. The statement has been made that the removal of premolars in orthodontic therapy will result in flat facial profiles and temporomandibular joint dysfunction. A study carried out at Washington University evaluated 160 extraction cases. The findings of the study indicate that, if proper diagnostic criteria are used in the treatment evaluation, the removal of teeth is not detrimental to good facial balance. The Angle system of classification (described earlier) is a simple analysis that allows one to classify a patient's occlusion into one of three different categories (class I, II, or III). Although this system allows ease of understanding and communication, it should be augmented with further data to develop an appreciation of facial form. It has been our experience that better and more gratifying results are achieved when the original diagnosis and treatment plan correlate the sagittal, dental, and skeletal relationships with facial form.

The Angle description of the sagittal relationship of the maxillary and mandibular dental units does not take into account their spatial orientation with respect to the patient's facial type. For example, Figs. 26-21 and 26-22 show examples of two patients who both demonstrate Angle class III malocclusion. From the photographs it is apparent that the overall relationship of the bony bases and the teeth to the face are quite dissimilar, even though both examples are given the same Angle classification. Fig. 26-21 depicts an example of maxillary deficiency (retrognathism), whereas Fig. 26-22 is representative of a case demonstrating mandibular prognathism. Even though the Angle relationship is the same, the comprehensive diagnosis and treatment plan should be quite different if the most favorable result for each patient is to be achieved. Therefore, further supplementation of the Angle system of classification is in order.

DESCRIPTIVE SKELETAL AND DENTAL EVALUATION

Before the basic steps involved in comprehensive analysis are outlined, five descriptive terms must be defined and clearly understood. They are as follows:

Orthognathism. A skeletal term indicating the ideal balance between the cranial base, the maxilla, and the mandible from a sagittal view.

Prognathism. The anterior positioning of either one or both bony jaws relative to the facial skeleton and soft tissues. Hence the following entities may exist: maxillary prognathism, mandibular prognathism, or bimaxillary (maxillary and mandibular) prognathism.

Retrognathism. The posterior placement of either one or both jaws relative to the face. Similar entities can be demonstrated as were mentioned in the previous category.

Protrusion. A forward positioning of the dental units (teeth) relative to their bony base. Again, protrusion may occur with maxillary or mandibular teeth or both.

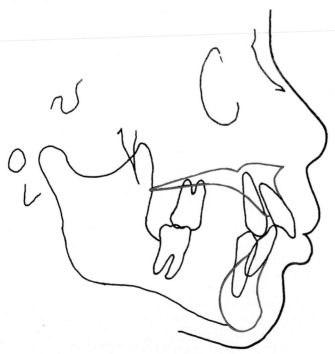

Figure 26-20 Deep-bite pattern.

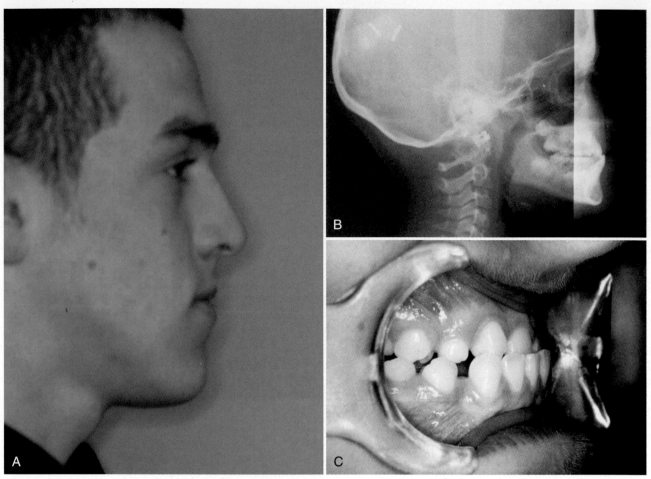

Figure 26-21 A, Maxillary retrognathism (clinical appearance). **B**, Maxillary retrognathism (cephalometric radiograph). **C**, Class III occlusion.

Retrusion. A posterior placement of either one or both dentoalveolar units relative to their respective bony bases.

Although the terms *prognathism* and *retrognathism* describe improper skeletal relationships of the jaws and the face, protrusion and retrusion simply indicate the relation of the dentoalveolar unit with respect to its supporting jaw.

Thus four components exist that can occur in any one of three possible sagittal positions (anterior, posterior, and ideal). These constitute 81 possible combinations.

By supplementing the Angle classification with additional analyses to determine the relative maxillary and mandibular skeletal, dental, and facial relationships, the clinician can obtain a more detailed diagnosis. The specific components of the craniofacial complex responsible for the discrepancy are also more clearly identified. Cephalometric analysis also must be correlated and compared with other diagnostic records and clinical findings, because the former cannot be expected to provide all the necessary information for an accurate treatment analysis.

The accuracy of the diagnosis is dependent on a thorough and systematic evaluation of several of the morphologic components in combination; individual measurements are of little value by themselves. Isolated measurements may demonstrate clinical deviation from the norm, but when these dimensions are combined with others, they may show collective compensation yielding a normal occlusal relationship. In contrast, a malocclusion may also be the result of individual dimensions that are considered within normal limits yet in combination result in an abnormal arrangement.

Any cephalometric measurement may be misleading at one time or another. There are no specific groups of factors that provide 100% accuracy. It is important to realize that the fewer factors used in the analysis, the greater the risk of misdiagnosis.

It is the borderline cases that often require a more detailed analysis. Obvious cases involving severe skeletal dysplasia often can be diagnosed using relatively few factors.

To properly analyze a cephalometric tracing, one must evaluate the interarch as well as the patient's facial characteristics.

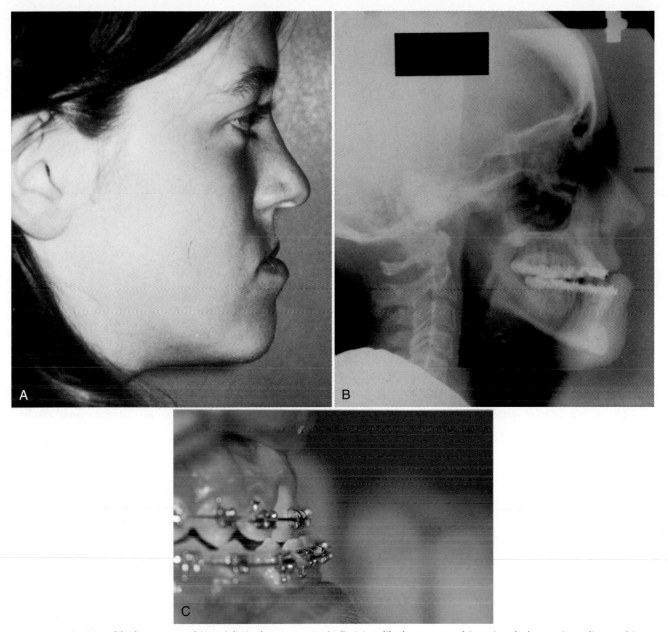

Figure 26-22 A, Mandibular prognathism (clinical appearance). **B**, Mandibular prognathism (cephalometric radiograph). **C**, Class III occlusion.

EVALUATION OF FACIAL ESTHETICS

A thorough and systematic evaluation of a patient's facial structures forms the basis for an accurate diagnosis and subsequent treatment. Too often the lateral cephalometric radiograph and diagnostic casts are used as substitutes for a complete clinical examination of the patient's facial characteristics. Lines, angles, and numbers should not be used as the only diagnostic tools, but rather should be viewed as an adjunct to what the clinician visually assesses about the patient's facial form. To develop the clinical ability to observe variations from the normal facial structure, the practitioner must have a firm grasp of what constitutes an ideal face (complete with ideal variations). This section deals with the facial examination of the ideal face. The guidelines are directed at the adolescent and teenaged patient and do not have complete application to patients 5 to 10 years of age, because facial proportions generally change with the approach of puberty.

To properly evaluate the patient, the clinician should have the patient stand in a relaxed position. The patient's head should be positioned with the Frankfort horizontal plane parallel to the floor (Fig. 26-23). Patients should not be asked to simply "look straight ahead," because patients tend to place their head in the position that is habitually

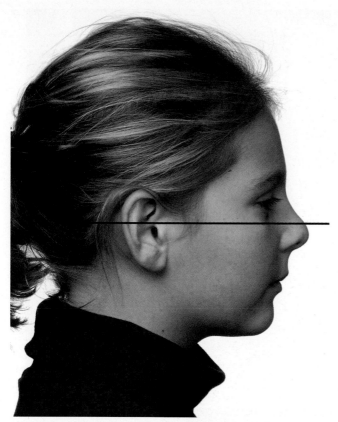

Figure 26-23 Patient's head positioned with the Frankfort horizontal parallel to the floor.

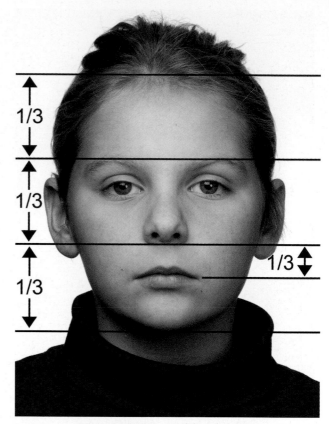

Figure 26-24 Frontal facial thirds.

preferred. It is also important to position the patient's occlusion in centric relation rather than centric occlusion. The patient's lips should be in repose during the examination. Patients frequently mask lip incompetence by forcing their lips together.

FRONTAL VIEW

The evaluation begins with the frontal view. This is the view people most often see of themselves. The balance between the upper, middle, and lower thirds of the face is analyzed (Fig. 26-24). The upper third is bounded by the hairline (when combed back) and glabellar area. This area is least informative and is not the area to which corrections would normally be directed. More emphasis is placed on the proportions and symmetry of the middle third (from the glabellar region to subnasale) and the lower third (subnasale to menton).

In the middle third of the face, when the patient is looking straight ahead, the sclera of the eye is not seen superior or inferior to the pupil. Normal intercanthal distance is 30 to 32 mm (CD, ±2 mm). Normal interpupillary distance is 60 to 65 mm. The inner and outer canthal tendons should fall close to a straight horizontal axis through the palpebral fissures (the fissures created when the eyelids are closed). The distance between the semilunar folds in the intercanthal area should approximate the alar base width (Fig. 26-25). Deviations from these

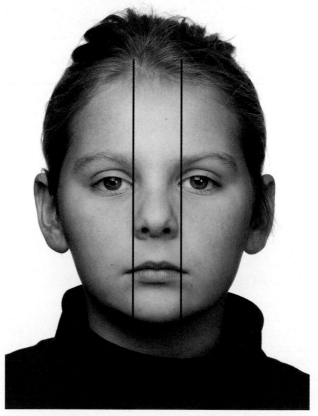

Figure 26-25 Comparison of the intercanthal distance and alar base width.

general guidelines could indicate some deformity of the middle facial third.

Evaluation of the lower facial third is then carried out. The ratio of the middle and lower facial thirds in vertical height should be approximately 5:6. The upper lip and its relationship to the teeth are noted with the lips in repose and also during smiling. The distance between the medial limbus of the eyes should equal the width of the mouth when it is relaxed (Fig. 26-26). Interlabial distance is measured with the lips at rest; up to 3.5 mm of interlabial distance is considered acceptable. The upper lip length from subnasale to stomion (lip commissure) should represent one third of the lower third facial height (see Fig. 26-24). Normal upper lip length should be 22 mm (CD, ±2 mm) in males and 20 mm (CD, ±2 mm) in females. Ideally, with the lips in repose, 2 to 4 mm of the upper incisor should be visible. More than this amount could indicate a vertical maxillary excess. One important characteristic that is often missed is that the incisal edges should approximate the lower lip line. Next, the patient's smile is assessed. Another important aspect of a well-balanced smile is the height, uniformity, and contour of the gingival margins. Grafts and gingival recontouring may be an important treatment modality in selected cases. In addition, the facial surfaces of the anterior teeth should converge toward the facial midline; the long axis (direction of the anterior teeth) in an esthetic smile also follows a progression as the teeth move away from the midline. The separations between the maxillary anterior teeth help to define an attractive smile. The spaces between the edges of the teeth are known as embrasure spaces. These spaces follow a pattern that begins between the central incisors and progresses as one moves away from the dental midline. Smile patterns vary with individuals, but esthetically, when a person smiles, the upper lip vermilion should rest on or near the cervicogingival margin of the incisors (Fig. 26-27). The position of the lower lip is also noted. Excessive eversion of the lower lip is seen in patients with mandibular retrognathism (Fig. 26-28). The mentalis muscle can be hyperactive during forced closure of the lower lip (Fig. 26-29); such muscle hyperactivity is frequently seen in patients with mandibular retrognathia, vertical maxillary excess, apertognathia (open-bite deformity), and lip incompetence.

The last evaluation of the full face is that of facial symmetry. The face is divided in half by a line that bisects the glabella, nasal tip, upper lip, and chin (Fig. 26-30). The face is also divided vertically into equal fifths (Fig. 26-31).

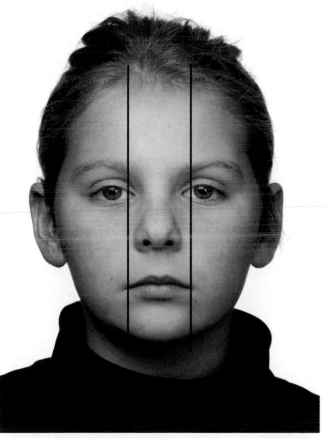

Figure 26-26 Comparison of the medial limbus width and the width of the mouth.

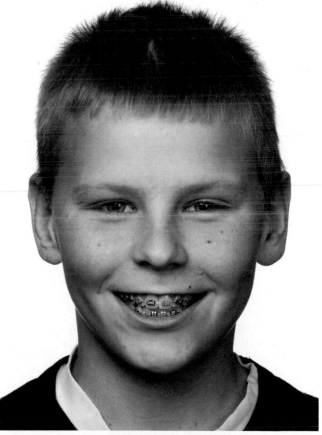

Figure 26-27 Ideal smile pattern.

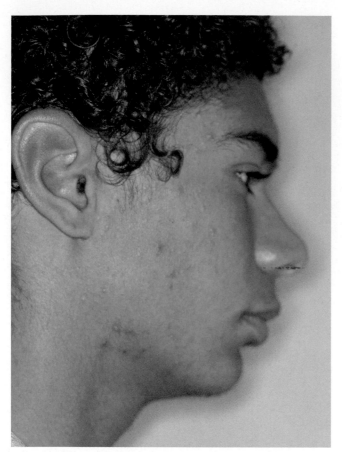

Figure 26-28 Excessive eversion of the lower lip.

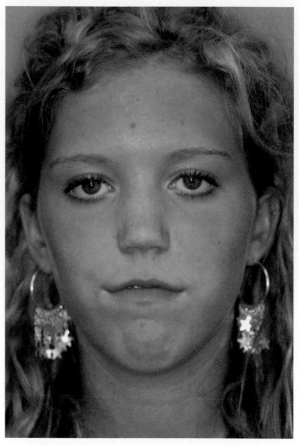

Figure 26-29 Hyperactive mentalis muscle during forced lip closure. Patient has lip incompetence.

PROFILE VIEW

The patient is next evaluated from the profile view. The examination considers many of the same features noted in the frontal examination. The face is divided into thirds (Fig. 26-32). A comparison of the vertical facial heights and the AP relationship of the facial thirds constitutes the initial assessment. The vertical relationships are the same in the profile view as they are in frontal views.

The upper facial third profile establishes the relationship between the forehead and superior orbital rim. The further the forehead protrudes beyond the superior orbital rim, the less esthetically acceptable it is. The globe of the eye and its relationship to the superior orbital rim is assessed. The superior orbital rim is normally 8 to 16 mm anterior of the globe.

The evaluation of the middle facial third involves an assessment of the relationship between the globes, inferior orbital rims, cheekbones, nose, and upper lip. The nasal bridge should project anterior to the globe by 5 to 15 mm. A reference line dropped from the most anterior projection of the globe and perpendicular to the Frankfort horizontal plane should fall on, or slightly behind, the soft tissue of the cheek.

In evaluation of the lower facial third, the vertical dimensions as described in the frontal view need to be

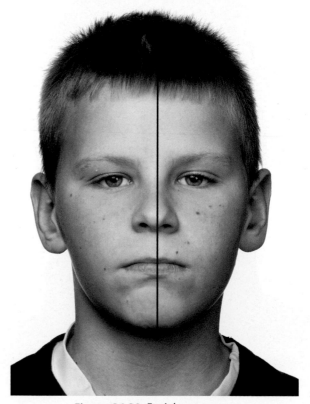

Figure 26-30 Facial symmetry.

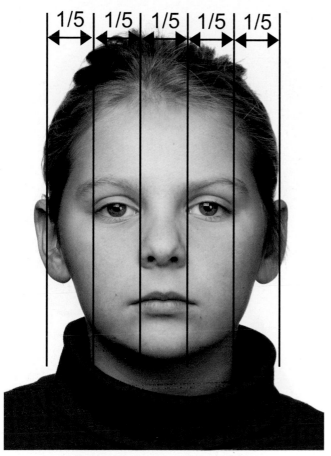

Figure 26-31 Vertical facial fifths.

considered. In addition, AP assessments are done. Projection of the upper lip is clinically evaluated by measuring from the nasolabial fold to the subnasale and comparing that numeric value to the distance from the subnasale to the tip of the nose. Ideally this ratio should be 1:1 (Fig. 26-33). The relationship of the nose and upper lip is determined by measuring the nasolabial angle (Fig. 26-34). This value can range from 90 to 110 degrees.

The lower facial third is compared with the middle and upper thirds. The zero meridian is a straight line constructed by placing a line through the soft tissue nasion, perpendicular to the Frankfort horizontal plane. The lips and chin should fall near this line. (Fig. 26-35). During the profile evaluation of the lower facial third, any AP discrepancies between the maxilla and mandible (i.e., prognathism and retrognathism) are noted. The upper and lower lip positions are also assessed. The shape and size of the chin button are appraised. In some cases, apparent mandibular retrognathism is in reality a flat or deficient chin button (microgenia). Conversely, too prominent a chin may be visualized as a pseudoprognathism and may be esthetically unacceptable.

The evaluation of the patient's face constitutes an important portion of the initial diagnosis and treatment plan phase of orthodontics. A systematic approach to examining the face is essential (Fig. 26-36). Basic guidelines of facial form have been reviewed. The values discussed are normal values for whites, but these must be used as relative guidelines only. The clinician must look at the patient's face and assess the overall harmony that

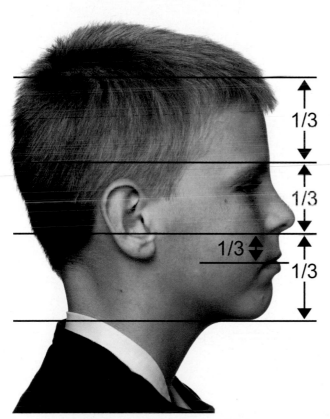

Figure 26-32 Profile facial thirds.

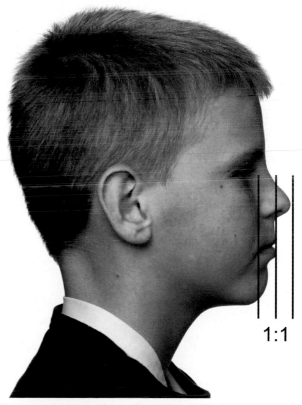

Figure 26-33 Ratio shows 1:1 relationship between nasolabial fold to subnasale, and subnasale to tip of the nose.

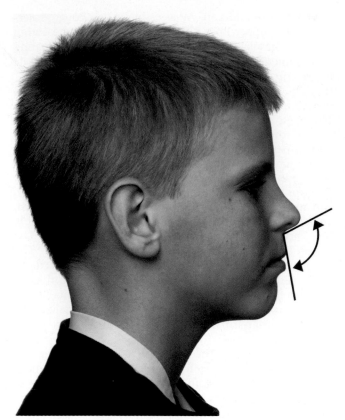

Figure 26-34 Nasolabial angle.

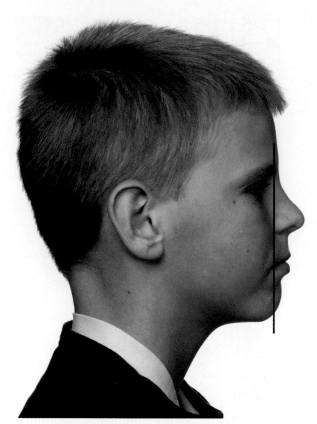

Figure 26-35 Zero meridian.

Lateral View

1. Frankfort Horizontal Plane: (FH)
   This plane is constructed from superior porion:
   (Po) to inferior orbitale (O) and represents the basic
   horizontal plane of the head.

2. Zero Meridian:
   The horizontal distance from the chin to a line
   perpendicular to (FH) and tangent to soft tissue nasion.

3. Maxillary Depth:
   The angle formed by the intersection of (FH) and N-A
   point planes.

4. Nasolabial Angle:
   The angle formed by the intersection of the lines tangent
   to the columella of the nose and the upper lip.

Lateral View Lip Measurements

1. Interlabial Gap:
   0-3.5 mm with lips in repose.

2. Upper Lip Length:
   Measured from (SN) to the inferior border of the upper lip.

3. Upper Incisor relative to the Upper Lip:
   The amount of upper incisor relative to the inferior border
   of the upper lip in repose.

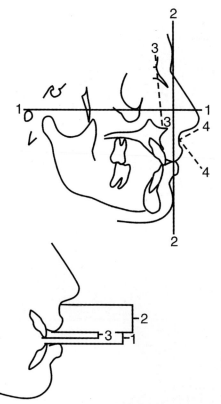

Figure 26-36 Summary of lateral dentofacial measurements.

exists. When deviations from normal facial form are detected, variations in treatment modalities must be considered to achieve better facial harmony. The main treatment objective is always to provide the patient with the best functional and esthetic result possible.

SUGGESTED READINGS

Angle EH. Classification of malocclusion, *Dent Cosmos* 41:248-264, 350-357, 1899.

Arnett GW. Facial keys to diagnosis and treatment planning—part I, *Am J Orthod Dentofacial Orthop* 103:299-312, 1993.

Arnett GW. Facial keys to diagnosis and treatment planning—part II, *Am J Orthod Dentofacial Orthop* 103:395-411, 1993.

Bell WH, Proffit WR, White RP. *Surgical correction of dentofacial deformities*, vol 1, Philadelphia, 1980, WB Saunders.

Boley JC. Serial extraction revisited: 30 years in retrospect, *Am J Orthod Dentofacial Orthop* 112:575-577, 2002.

Broadbent BH. A new x-ray technique and its application to orthodontia, *Angle Orthod* 1:45-66, 1931.

Broadbent BH. The face of the normal child, *Angle Orthod* 7:183-208, 1937.

Brodie AG et al. Cephalometric appraisal of orthodontic results: a preliminary report, *Angle Orthod* 8:261-351, 1938.

Burstone CJ. Lip posture and its significance in treatment planning, *Am J Orthod* 53:262-284, 1967.

Downs WB. Variations in facial relationships: their significance in treatment and prognosis, *Am J Orthod* 34:812-840, 1948.

Dugoni SA et al. Early mixed dentition treatment: posttreatment evaluation of stability and relapse, *Angle Orthod* 65:311-332, 1995.

James RD. A comparative study of facial profiles in extraction and nonextraction treatment, *Am J Orthod Dentofacial Orthop* 114:265-276, 1998.

Katz MI. Angle classification revisited. Is current use reliable? *Am J Orthod Dentofacial Orthop* 102:173-179, 1992.

Klocke A, Nanda RS, Kahl-Nieke B. Skeletal class II patterns in the primary dentition, *Am J Orthod Dentofacial Orthop* 112:596-601, 2002.

Lines PA, Lines RR, Lines CA. Profilemetrics and facial esthetics, *Am J Orthod* 73:648-657, 1978.

Long RE, McNamara JA. Facial growth following pharyngeal flap surgery: skeletal assessment on serial lateral cephalometric radiographs, *Am J Orthod* 87:187-196, 1985.

McNamara JA. Influence of respiratory pattern on craniofacial growth, *Angle Orthod* 51:269-300, 1981.

Morley J. The role of cosmetic dentistry in restoring a youthful appearance, *J Am Dent Assoc* 30:1166-1172, 1999.

Owen AH 3rd. Diagnostic block cephalometrics, part 1, *J Clin Orthod* 18:400-422, 1984.

Owen AH 3rd. Clinical interpretation of diagnostic block cephalometric analysis, *J Clin Orthod* 20:710-715, 1986.

Reidel RA. The relation of maxillary structures to cranium in malocclusion and in normal occlusion, *Angle Orthod* 22:142-145, 1952.

Ricketts RM. Cephalometric analysis and synthesis, *Angle Orthod* 31:141-156, 1961.

Ricketts RM, Schulhof RJ, Bagha L. Orientation—sella-nasion or Frankfort horizontal, *Am J Orthod* 69:648-654, 1976.

Rody WJ Jr, Araujo EA. Extraction decision-making Wigglegram, *J Clin Orthod* 36:510-519, 2002.

Sarver DM. Video cephalometric diagnosis (VCD): a new concept in treatment planning? *Am J Orthod Dentofacial Orthop* 110:128-136, 1996.

Schulhof RJ. When S-N is abnormal, *J Clin Orthod* 11:343, 1977.

Simon PW. *Fundamental principles of a systematic diagnosis of dental anomalies*. Boston, 1926, The Stratford.

Steiner C. Cephalometrics for you and me, *Am J Orthod* 39:729-755, 1953.

Tweed CH. The Frankfort-mandibular incisor angle (FMIA) in orthodontic diagnosis, treatment planning and prognosis, *Angle Orthod* 24:121-169, 1954.

CHAPTER 27

Managing the Developing Occlusion

▲ **Ronald A. Bell, Jeffrey A. Dean, Ralph E. McDonald,** and **David R. Avery**

CHAPTER OUTLINE

*I*t should be the goal of every practitioner providing oral health care for children and adolescents to assess and guide the developing occlusion toward optimal outcomes. The Clinical Guidelines of the American Academy of Pediatric Dentistry[1] on "Management of the Developing Dentition and Occlusion in Pediatric Dentistry" illustrates this responsibility with the following statement:

> Guidance of eruption and development of the primary, mixed and permanent dentitions is an integral component of comprehensive oral healthcare for all pediatric dental patients. Such guidance should contribute to the development of a permanent dentition that is in a stable, functional, and esthetically acceptable occlusion. Early diagnosis and successful treatment of developing malocclusions can have both short-term and long-term benefits while achieving the goal of occlusal harmony, function, and dental facial esthetics.

Ngan and colleagues[2] illustrate this responsibility regarding contemporary practice in stating "Pediatric dentistry has increasingly shifted from a conservative-restorative approach toward a concept of total pediatric patient care. Thus all aspects of oral health care including diagnosis, prevention, oral medicine, restoration, and correction of malocclusion are increasingly the responsibility of the pediatric dentist." In the context of these statements, clinical decisions are presented daily that challenge pediatric practitioners in affecting outcomes in management of the developing occlusion. As defined by Moyers,[3] space supervision is "when the judgment of the dentist determines that the individual patient's occlusion will

have a better chance of obtaining optimum development through supervised intervention of the transitional dentition than without clinician directed intervention." Space supervision encompasses procedures such as preventive orthodontics, guidance of eruption, interceptive orthodontics, and phased "early" orthodontic treatment that should be understood in terms of its diagnostic parameters, treatment basis, and clinical applications.

DEVELOPMENT OF OCCLUSION AND TIMING OF INTERVENTIONS

A review of studies by Baume,[4] Moorrees,[5,6] Bishara and colleagues[7] and Moyers and Wainwright[8] provides an understanding of the biogenetic course of the primary, transitional, and permanent dentitions that is critical to management of the developing dentition. Evaluating study models of the primary dentitions of 30 children obtained sequentially at various developmental stages, Baume[4] reported two consistent morphologic arch forms of the primary dentition: either generalized spaces between the teeth were present (type I) or the teeth were in proximal contact without spacing (type II). The archform in both types appears congenital rather than developmental as the original pattern exhibited upon eruption was maintained from ages 3 to 6 years. Spaced arches frequently exhibit two distinct diastemas, referred to as *primate spaces* — one between the mandibular canine and first primary molar and the other between the maxillary lateral incisor and primary canine. Baume[4] observed that until eruption of the permanent first molars, the sagittal dimension of the primary dental arches remained essentially unchanged with the possible exception of a slight decrease as the result of the development of dental caries on the proximal surfaces of the molar teeth. Only minor changes in the transverse dimension of the primary dental arches occurred during the 3- to 6-year age period unless negatively influenced by deleterious functional patterns. Given these findings, orthodontic intervention during the primary dentition up to 6 years of age is mostly directed toward maintaining inherent arch dimensions and arch integrity with preventive and restorative services. Space maintainers when primary teeth are lost prematurely are the next major consideration in maintaining arch dimensions. Control of functional problems such as elimination of deleterious thumb-sucking habits and correction of functional crossbites may also receive attention during the primary dentition years. While desirable, treatments for these factors are often deferred depending upon cooperation of the child in appliance protocols.

The early mixed dentition (6 to 9 years of age) is a period much more prone to localized factors that may result in severe malocclusion problems if undetected. In addition to a continuation of basic preventive and space maintenance issues, problems encountered in this period include dentoalveolar anterior crossbites, ectopic eruption of permanent incisors and/or first permanent molars, posterior crossbites, open-bite and flared maxillary incisors associated with deleterious oral habits, and developmental anomalies (e.g., ankylosis, supernumerary teeth, missing teeth). Baume,[4] comparing models of 60 children before and after eruption of the permanent molars, found three distinct kinds of molar adjustment (Fig 27-1) "Early" mesial shift during first permanent molar eruption occurs at the expense of any posterior spacing that might have been present to include breakdown spaces resulting from interproximal caries. Moyers,[8] agreeing that the pattern of transition involving the straight terminal plane is normal, suggested that the occlusion forming a mesial step (distal surface of the lower second primary molar is mesial to the same surface of the maxillary molar) is most ideal for class I development. A distal step (distal surface of lower second primary molar is distal to the same surface of the maxillary molar) is indicative of a developing class II malocclusion. Proper permanent molar occlusion was achieved from a straight terminal plane by a second mesial shift of the molars as second primary molars are exfoliated. This "late" shift of the mandibular first molar, often under the additional influence of the emerging second permanent molar, occurs at the expense of the leeway space with an attendant arch length decrease of 2 to 3 mm on average.

Further evaluation by Baume indicated a transverse widening of the intercanine width of the upper and lower dental arches occurred during eruption of the permanent incisors. The increase represented a physiologic widening by lateral and frontal alveolar growth to provide space for the erupting permanent incisors and their greater mesiodistal widths. The mean increase in intercanine width was greater in the maxillary arch (3 to 4 mm) than in the mandibular arch (2 to 3 mm). In the mandibular arch, the greatest tendency to increased width was during the eruption of the lower lateral incisors, whereas in the maxillary arch it occurred primarily during eruption of the

maxillary central incisors. Whereas the increase was slightly greater in nonspaced primary arches than in spaced arches, the arches with spaces generally resulted in favorable alignment of the permanent incisors. About 40% of the arches without primary dental spacing resulted in crowded anterior segments. Moorrees reported similar dimensional changes concurrent with incisor transitional periods.[5]

Bishara and colleagues[7] also reported arch dimensional changes in their studies of patients from age 6 weeks

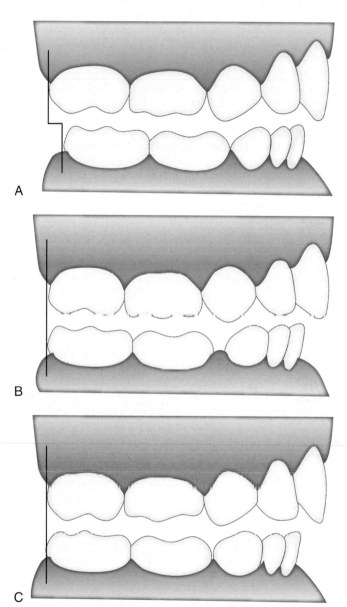

Figure 27-1 A, Diagram showing mesial step terminal plane that allows the first permanent molar to erupt directly into proper class I occlusion. **B,** Straight terminal plane with primary spacing. "Early mesial shift" of mandibular molars closing primary spaces will help establish proper first permanent molar occlusion. **C,** Straight terminal plane without primary spacing. Permanent molars erupt into end-on position in the mixed dentition. Proper first permanent molar occlusion may be attained when the second primary molars exfoliate and a "late mesial shift" of the mandibular first permanent molar occurs.

to 45 years of age, noting that (1) significant maxillary and mandibular arch width increases occurred between 6 weeks and 2 years of age, (2) the mandibular intercanine width was established by 8 years of age (i.e., after eruption of the four incisors), (3) although arch width increased between 3 and 13 years of age, there was a slight decrease in width, more in the intercanine than intermolar area, after complete eruption of the permanent teeth. In sum, incisor alignment patterns and intercanine arch dimensions are essentially established by age 8 years of age. Interceptive procedures receive significantly more emphasis in this period to allow a harmonious transition directed toward achieving alignment of the permanent incisors and 6-year molars with symmetrical arch development and coincident midlines. Additionally, early recognition and elimination of deleterious oral habits or deviant functional patterns should enhance normal patterns of development while diminishing the long-term effects of atypical growth.

In addition to malocclusion factors identifiable during first molar and incisor transition, corrective measures to align and position the erupting buccal segments come into play during the late mixed dentition (9 to 12 years of age) when primary canines and molars are exfoliating in conjunction with eruption of the permanent canines and premolars. Epidemiologic studies demonstrate that crowding and malalignment become significantly more prevalent and exhibit greater severity between the mixed dentition period (6 to 12 years of age) and the adolescent young permanent dentition (12 to 18 years of age). This suggests that normal transitional changes do not compensate for anterior malalignment and crowding in that late mesial shift of the buccal segments upon exfoliation of second primary molars results in decreased arch length and arch circumference. Nance[9] observed that in the average patient's mandibular arch, a leeway size difference of +1.7 mm per side exists with the combined mesiodistal widths of the primary canine, first primary molar, and second primary molar being larger than the mesiodistal widths of the corresponding permanent canine and premolars. The difference between the total width of the corresponding three primary teeth in the maxillary arch compared with the three permanent teeth that succeed them is +0.9 mm per side of leeway space. The control of this leeway space in terms of arch dimensional change through space supervision may offer opportunities to significantly improve tooth size–arch size adjustments for the relief of typical levels of crowding. Gianelly[10,11] and others have shown that the control of leeway space will accommodate typical levels of lower incisor crowding in approximately 75% of mixed dentition patients presenting for orthodontic treatment. As applied to the late mixed dentition, a positive excess leeway space to an overall deficiency of less than 2 mm per quadrant may be considered potential situations for space supervision programs. Lower arch length deficiencies of more than 2 to 3 mm per quadrant should be considered a discrepancy beyond simple guidance procedures.

In keeping with supervision of leeway space as a fundamental concept, the vast majority of patients should be evaluated around the time of the clinical emergence of the lower canine, lower first premolars, and upper first premolars. These teeth erupt about 1 to 1½ years ahead of the final buccal segment transition. This leaves time to assess overall dimensional needs and plan treatment interventions for the relief of crowding, manage space to minimize future permanent tooth extractions, coordinate the transverse widths of the dental arches, and guide teeth into favorable positions that provide more stable long-term results. A second advantage for this timing in diagnosis and treatment planning is that it precedes the pubertal growth spurt in females, which in turn is approximately 2 years ahead of the pubertal growth spurt in males. If a skeletal malocclusion is noted, the opportunity for growth modification with dentofacial orthopedics to take advantage of peak growth velocities is available for influencing in a positive manner skeletal discrepancies, arch development, and facial balance. Consultation with an orthodontist is critical for children in whom skeletal considerations, severe growth problems, extensive crowding with pronounced tooth mass–arch length discrepancies, and dental anomalies are present that significantly compromise the child's orofacial development. Coordination will lead to more accurate identification of problems, aid in appropriate treatment decisions, and offer the potential for optimal results without having to resort to compromised treatment options in the full permanent dentition. Psychological aspects of treatment in terms of patient motivation, improved and dramatic dentofacial change, a social desire for treatment, and generally cooperative age group results in improved well-being for the child and parents as well as a good practice-builder with timely coordinated management.

One should recognize that certain disadvantages involved in "early" treatment must be factored into the equation on whether to intervene in an individual patient. These include the reality that overall treatment time is likely prolonged, multiple problems often arise in individual patients, untoward responses may occur given the variability of growth dynamics, there is potential for iatrogenic damage to the developing teeth, some children cannot cope with treatment demands, and patient and parent burnout often occur given that overall management is rarely a one-shot operation. Parents must have realistic perspectives of treatment goals and be willing to assume financial and appointment obligations involved in treatment. While things happen slowly during the development of the occlusion, timing is critical for certain procedures, in that there are many problems that can occur and jeopardize successful outcome. In the decision-making process for an individual patient, the clinician involved in early orthodontic procedures should ask two key questions, each with their own subset of questions to be asked:
1. *What is the specific problem?* How did it happen? Is the etiology resolved? What will happen without treatment? Will it stay the same, get worse, or go away on its own? Simply put, not every child can or should be treated using interceptive procedures. Roughly half of patients fall into an area of real or absolute need in requiring corrective treatment for functional and esthetic problems that will potentially lead to deterioration of the occlusion if untreated. Even though some children

may benefit from interceptive treatments, there should be understanding that later comprehensive treatments will be necessary to achieve acceptable results.

2. *What will the likely result of interceptive treatment be?* The remaining estimate of up to 50% of children is the population group that might benefit from early orthodontic interventions in the developing occlusion years. This group involves malocclusion factors in which treatment intervention will potentially eliminate or minimize the need for future orthodontic treatment. At the least, interceptive treatments should enhance long-term treatment options and outcomes without compromising future needs. So a subset of questions should be asked. Is treatment justified in terms of improvement in esthetics and function while eliminating or minimizing the need for future treatment? Will the intervention correct a problem at the optimal time to enhance later options and outcomes? Can treatment methods be used to advantage such that the skill and experience of the clinician intersects with patient needs? Does treatment meet socioeconomic issues? Does the treatment present an outcome that can be easily realized in conjunction with later comprehensive care that will be required anyway?

In answering these questions, a thorough clinical examination supported by appropriate diagnostic records should be obtained before initiating treatment interventions. The clinical examination should assess the patient's overall health status, extraoral facial patterns (profile, facial symmetry, area of discrepancy), occlusion from an esthetic and functional standpoint, temporomandibular joint function, neuromuscular patterns, growth patterns, and nasopharyngeal airway patterns. A form similar to the one depicted in Fig. 27-2 is helpful in composing clinical findings and formulating the patient's diagnosis, problem list, and treatment plan summary. In terms of diagnostic records beyond clinical findings, necessary records may range from simple photos or study models when treating a functional posterior crossbite to a complete set of orthodontic records for a patient with a skeletal malocclusion or severe crowding. More comprehensive records may include an eight-film series of extra and intraoral photographs, appropriately trimmed orthodontic study models, a full-mouth series or panoramic radiograph, lateral and anteroposterior cephalograms, and when indicated temporomandibular diagnostic views such as corrected axis tomograms or magnetic resonance imaging. Supplemental diagnostic procedures can also include a detailed tooth-size arch-size space analysis (Chapter 25) and a cephalometric analysis (Chapter 26). And finally, cone beam computed tomography should be considered in special cases, such as impacted teeth or craniofacial patients.

EARLY LOSS OF TEETH AND SPACE MAINTENANCE

If arch integrity is disrupted by early loss of primary teeth, problems may arise that affect the alignment of the permanent dentition. Opposing teeth can supraerupt, more distal teeth can drift and tip mesially, and more forward teeth can drift and tip distally (Figs. 27-3 and 27-4). Altered tooth positions may include a "symptomatic" space deficiency with loss of arch length and circumference, blocked or deflected eruption of permanent teeth, unattractive appearance, food impaction areas, increased caries and periodontal disease, and other negative aspects of malocclusion. The altered occlusal relationships may evidence traumatic interferences and untoward jaw relationships. When early primary tooth loss occurs, corrective measures such as passive space maintenance, active tooth guidance with space regaining, or a combination of both may be needed to optimize the normal process of occlusion development.

Miyamoto and colleagues[12] observed the effects of the early loss of primary teeth by measuring crowding and malalignment in the permanent dentition of 255 schoolchildren aged 11 years or older. Children who had premature loss of one or more primary canines or molars were more likely to receive orthodontic treatment in the permanent dentition with the need more than three times greater in children who had lost one or more primary teeth through 9 years of age than the control group. Premature loss of primary molars was especially associated with major malalignment of permanent teeth. No differences were observed in effects between loss of first and second primary molars. Crowding of anterior teeth was directly affected by the premature loss of primary canines. A review of the clinical literature by Owen[13] revealed the following general factors should be considered in assessing the implications of premature loss of primary teeth to arch development, the development of a malocclusion, and the need for a space maintainer.

1. *Incidence of space loss.* Almost all cases of early primary molar loss show some decrease in arch length (i.e., mesial movement of permanent molars, distal movement of anterior teeth). The amount of closure is affected by numerous variables (e.g., tooth involved, time of loss).

2. *Time elapsed since loss.* Most of the space loss usually takes place during the first 6 months after the primary tooth is lost with a tendency for space closure to occur more rapidly in the maxillary arch than in the mandible. This indicates that when a primary tooth is removed and factors indicate need for space maintenance, it is best to insert an appliance as soon as possible after the extraction.

3. *Stage of development/dental age of the patient.* In general, more space loss is likely to occur if teeth are actively erupting adjacent to the area left by the premature loss of the primary tooth. Significant space loss is most influenced by the stage of eruption of the first permanent molars with the potential particularly high if a primary molar is lost just before or during eruption of the first permanent molars. The amount of space closure is usually less if the permanent molars are fully erupted into occlusal interdigitation at the time of primary tooth loss. A similar situation exists if the first primary molar has been lost prematurely and the permanent lateral incisor is in an active state of eruption. The eruption of the permanent lateral incisor may result in distal movement of the primary canine and

ORTHODONTIC DIAGNOSIS, TREATMENT, AND MECHANICS PLAN

Name _____   Race ___ Sex ___   Birthdate _____   Age _____   Chart No. _____

Resident's Name: _____   Records Date: _____

1. Patient History

A. Significant Medical History: _____
_____

B. Patient's and/or Parents' Chief Complaint: _____
_____

C. Attitude Toward Treatment: _____
_____

2. Clinical Examination

A. Soft Tissue

Profile _____ Lip Competence _____ Lip/Incisor at Rest _____ Smiling _____
Oral Hygiene _____ Periodontal Status _____ Other _____

B. Occlusion Class: I   II   III   Division: I   II

Overjet _____ mm   Overbite _____ mm   Midline _____ mm
Crossbite _____
Molar Relation: Left _____   Right _____
Cuspid Relation: Left _____   Right _____

C. Dental Development Stage and Eruption Sequence:

D. Habits and/or Other Significant Clinical Findings:

E. TMJ and Function:

Opening Path: Normal Deviated: _____
Closing Path: Normal Deviated: _____
Range of Motion: Vertical _____ mm   Protrusion: _____ mm
          Left Deviation: _____ mm   Right Deviation: _____ mm
Joint Sounds   None   Left   Right
          Opening   _____   _____
          Closing   _____   _____
          Crepitus   _____   _____
Muscle Tenderness: None   _____
Tongue Function: Normal   _____

3. Model Analysis   Static Tanaka and Johnston Analysis (JADA 1974)

Total M-D Width of Upper Incisors _____ mm "A"   Total M-D Width of Lower Incisors _____ mm "B"

Maxillary Arch Length Discrepancy (From $\underline{6|}$ to $|\underline{6}$)   Mandibular Arch Length Discrepancy (From $\overline{6|}$ to $\overline{|6}$)
Total Predicted Tooth Mass: Total Predicted Tooth Mass:
  [("B" ÷ 2) + 11 mm] × 2 + "A" = _____ mm   [("B" ÷ 2) + 10.5 mm] × 2 + "B" = _____ mm
Total Measured Arch Length   =   _____ mm   Total Measured Arch Length   =   _____ mm
          Difference   _____ mm   Difference   _____ mm

A

Figure 27-2 "Orthodontic Diagnosis and Treatment Plan" form. **A,** Front side.

4. Attach computerized cephalometric tracing and appropriate analysis.

5. Diagnostic and Arch Length Analysis Summary and Problem List

6. Treatment Plan or Objective Sequence

7. Mechanics Plan–Appliance Selection—Retention

8. Projected Treatment Time (With Good Compliance), Treatment Fees

9. Faculty Authorization to Start Treatment:

_____   _____
Signature   Date

B

Figure 27-2 cont'd **B**, Back side. IUSD Pediatric Dentistry.

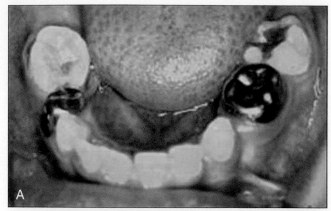

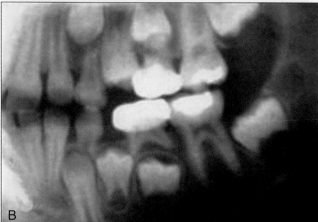

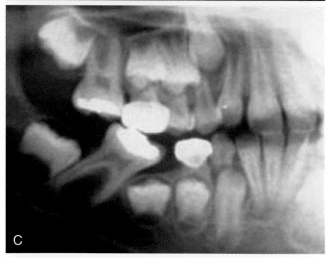

Figure 27-3 A, Space loss and occlusion changes associated with early loss of lower primary molars. **B,** Radiograph of left segment with loss of first primary molar. Note some distal movement of primary canine. **C,** Radiograph of right segment with loss of mandibular second primary molar and associated space loss approximating 4 to 6 mm. Note pronounced mesial tipping of permanent first molar crown without notable bodily movement.

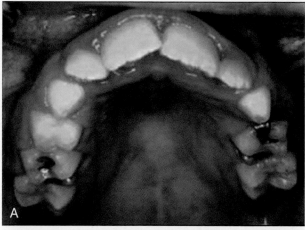

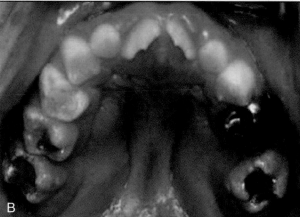

Figure 27-4 Loss of upper primary molars in association with eruption of first permanent molars and space loss. **A,** Loss of upper left first primary molar with space loss approximating 4 to 6 mm. **B,** Loss of upper left second primary molar with space loss approximating 6 to 8 mm. Note rotation of first molar in conjunction with more bodily movement.

Another factor is in terms of available abutments for securing a space maintainer at the time of the primary tooth loss. A second primary molar lost at 5 years of age requires different abutment considerations than one lost during the mixed dentition when first permanent molars have erupted. Also, teeth actively erupting adjacent to the edentulous area have a greater effect on the amount of space lost than do fully erupted teeth. For example, if the first primary molar is lost during the time of active eruption of the first permanent molar, a strong forward force will be exerted on the second primary molar that causes it to tip into the space required for eruption of the first premolar. Changes may extend anteriorly with shift of the dental midline and retrusion of the anterior segment after early loss of a first primary molar.

4. *Amount of space closure.* Loss of maxillary second primary molars results in the greatest amount of closure, up to 8 mm of space loss in a quadrant (see Fig. 27-4B). Loss of mandibular second primary molars show the next greatest amount with space loss measured up to 4 mm in a quadrant (see Fig. 27-3A, C). Loss of upper or lower first primary molars show almost equal amounts

encroachment on space available. This condition is frequently accompanied by a shift in the midline toward the area of the loss. In the mandibular arch, a lingual "collapse" of the anterior segment may occur with a resulting increased overbite.

of space closure when compared with one another—the amount is most impacted by timing of the first primary molar loss (see Fig. 27-4A). Space loss potential is particularly high if the primary molar loss occurs in approximation to first permanent molar eruption regardless of which primary molar is lost and in which arch the loss occurs. After first permanent molars have erupted into occlusion, loss of second primary molars may still result in significant space closure. Loss of a first primary molar with retention of the second primary molar shows minimal amounts of space closure as the second primary molar serves to buttress first permanent molar positions after occlusion is established.

5. *Direction of closure.* Maxillary posterior spaces close predominantly by mesial bodily movement and mesiolingual rotation around the palatal root of the first permanent molars. Only minimal mesial crown tipping of the first molar is usually noted. In contrast, mandibular spaces close primarily by mesial tipping of the first permanent molars along with distal movement and retroinclination of teeth anterior to the space (see Fig. 27-3C). Bodily movement of first molars is not typically notable in the lower arch as seen in the upper arch. Lower molars also tend to roll lingually in conjunction with their mesial crown tipping during space loss movements.

6. *Eruption timing of permanent successors.* Grøn,[14] in evaluating the emergence of permanent teeth, found that teeth normally erupt when three fourths of the root is developed, regardless of the child's chronologic age. However, the eruption timing of a permanent successor may be delayed or accelerated after premature loss of a primary tooth depending on the developmental status, bone density of the area, and nature of the primary

tooth loss. Very early loss before significant root formation of the permanent successor usually results in delayed eruption timing that may alter normal transitional adjustments in arch length, arch width, and arch circumference. Several studies have indicated that loss of a primary molar before 7 years of age leads to delayed emergence of the succedaneous tooth, whereas loss after 7 years of age leads to early emergence. The magnitude of any timing change in eruption is affected by age at time of tooth loss; if a primary molar is lost at 4 years of age, the emergence of the premolar could be delayed by as much as 1 year, with emergence occurring at root completion. If the loss occurs at 6 years of age, a delay of about 6 months is more likely, with emergence seen when root development approaches completion. Primary tooth loss within 6 to 12 months of normal exfoliation time may result in acceleration in eruption timing of the underlying permanent tooth.

Individual permanent teeth are often observed to be delayed in their development and consequently in their eruption timing. Impacted permanent teeth or deviations in eruption paths may be reflected with abnormally delayed eruption times. In cases of this type it is generally necessary to extract the primary tooth, construct a space maintainer, and allow the permanent tooth to erupt and assume its normal position (Fig. 27-5). The exact timing of permanent tooth eruption is less important in the overall occlusion development compared with greater significance related to sequencing, site of eruption, and adequate space for subsequent eruption.

7. *Amount of bone covering the nonerupted tooth.* Prediction of eruption based on timing of primary tooth loss and stage of root development is not reliable if the bone

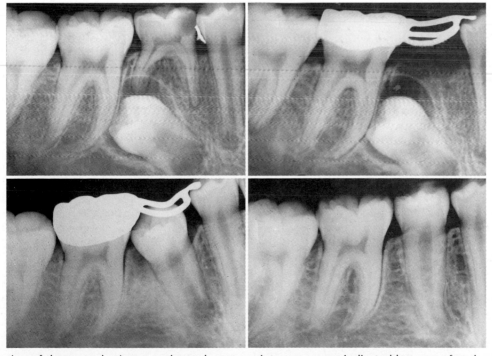

Figure 27-5 Extraction of the second primary molar and space maintenance were indicated because of prolonged retention of the primary tooth and impaction of the second premolar. The second premolar eventually erupted into its normal position.

covering the permanent tooth has been destroyed by infection. Emergence is then usually accelerated. If there is bone covering the tooth, it can be predicted that eruption will not readily occur. A guide is that premolars usually require about 4 to 6 months to move through 1 mm of bone as measured on bite-wing radiographs.

8. *Abnormal oral musculature.* Strong mentalis muscle patterns may have a pronounced negative effect after loss of mandibular primary molars or canines with collapse of the arch and distal drifting of the anterior segment that is often exhibited. Thumb or finger habits may similarly produce abnormal forces in initiating collapse of the dental arches after untimely loss of primary teeth.

9. *Congenital absence of the permanent tooth.* Before space maintenance, the presence of a normal successor must be ensured before space maintenance through radiographic evaluation. Should the succedaneous tooth be congenitally absent or significantly malformed, the decision is a challenging one, whether to hold the space for many years until a permanent prosthesis can be provided or to allow space closure with the likelihood of orthodontic treatment to achieve proper alignment.

When utilized, a space maintainer must fulfill the fundamental role of preventing untoward mesial migration of buccal segments and lingual collapse of anterior segments in maintaining the mesiodistal dimension of the prematurely lost primary tooth. The appliance should not interfere with masticatory function, nor should it inhibit or deflect normal growth changes. It should be simple to construct and maintain; durable, strong, and stable; passive in not imposing pressures on remaining teeth that might affect orthodontic movements; and easily cleanable without enhancing dental caries or soft tissue pathology. Beyond these fundamental roles, space maintainers may be designed to prevent supraeruption of teeth opposing the space, improve esthetics, and assist in speech (i.e., anterior space maintainers in control of oral habits).

When a primary tooth is lost prematurely, it does not follow that a space maintainer is automatically necessary or desirable. The decision to place a space maintainer and which design to use is affected by the specific tooth that was lost, from which arch, at what time, whether the permanent successor is present and developing normally, the patient's overall oral health status and motivation, and the status of existing arch length to accommodate the permanent teeth. If analysis indicates a positive arch length or deficiency of less than 1 to 2 mm per quadrant, the use of a space maintainer to hold tooth positions may be considered potentially beneficial. If the space is not held, the total arch length may be further decreased and lead to possible premolar extractions requirements. Holding the space may allow the permanent premolars and canines to erupt and utilize leeway space to alleviate anterior crowding. However, if the arch length deficiency is 2 to 3 mm per quadrant or more, a significant discrepancy exists where space regaining, serial extraction, and/or comprehensive orthodontic treatment may be indicated. If there is no question that permanent teeth will have to be removed to obtain a favorable occlusion, space maintenance may not be desirable as the space would need to be closed during orthodontic treatment anyway. In less obvious extraction cases, holding the space to allow teeth to erupt and prevent impactions can be a valuable service. As related to the premature loss of specific primary teeth, the arch involved, and developmental timing, the following recommendations are made with regard to placement and design of space maintainers.

Loss of Primary Incisors

Early loss of lower primary incisors is generally due to ectopic eruption of the permanent incisors in reflecting excessive incisor liability. Given the potential for increased intracanine width during permanent incisor eruption, the clinician should monitor development in the lower incisor area and generally not intervene. Individual circumstances may indicate extraction of the antimere primary incisor to enhance incisor positioning and midline symmetry. The loss of lower incisors in other circumstances such as trauma, advanced caries, or extraction of a neonatal tooth may result in anterior space loss if it occurs before primary canine stabilization is realized.

Premature loss of maxillary primary incisors does not generally result in decreased upper intracanine dimensions if the incisor loss occurs after the primary canines have erupted into occlusion at approximately 2 years of age. The support of the mandibular occlusion "holds" the maxillary anterior intracanine width dimensions. Baume type I spaced primary dentitions have significant latitude to resist arch dimensional changes. If the anterior primary teeth were in contact before the loss or there is evidence of an arch-length inadequacy in the anterior region, space adjustments in alignment after the loss of one of the primary incisors is a potential factor in space maintenance (Fig. 27-6). The major consequence of early loss of maxillary primary incisors is most likely delayed eruption timing of the permanent successors as reparative bone and dense connective tissue covers the site. In addition, unattractive appearance and potential development of deleterious habits (e.g., tongue-thrust swallow, forward resting posture of the tongue, improper pronunciation of fricative sounds—"s," "f") may be of concern following premature loss of primary maxillary incisors. An anterior appliance incorporating artificial primary teeth may be considered to satisfy esthetic and functional needs. Acrylic partial dentures have been successful in the replacement of single (Fig. 27-7) and multiple (Fig. 27-8) maxillary primary incisors. Given the demands of cooperation in wear and frequent appliance loss or damage, such removable appliances can be problematic in preschool-age children.

A fixed option using primary incisor denture teeth secured from a rigid steel wire (0.036 or 0.040) extended to bands or stainless steel crowns on the primary molars, a so-called "Hollywood" bridge, may be a more predictable option (Fig. 27-9). One can obtain additional stabilization in keeping the wire from flexing by placing an occlusal rest on the first primary molar, using a Nance button, or by covering the ridge with acrylic resin. Use of such an appliance incorporating artificial primary anterior teeth is elective to primarily address esthetic demands rather than specific space management concerns.

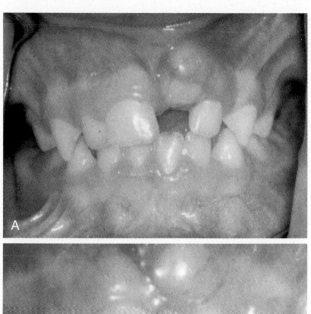
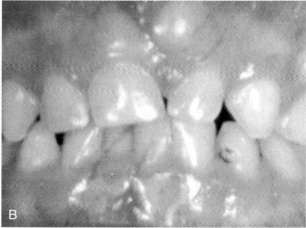

Figure 27-6 A, Child with some loss of space in the primary incisor area that was observed at the time of the first examination. **B,** Space closure continued and was accompanied by drifting of teeth throughout the anterior area, including the canines.

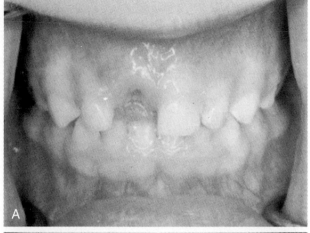
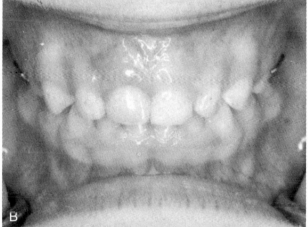

Figure 27-7 A, This 3½-year-old child has lost a primary incisor as the result of trauma. **B,** A removable palatal retainer with a primary central incisor pontic has been constructed to prevent space closure and to restore normal appearance.

Loss of Primary Canines

Most often due to ectopic eruption of permanent lateral incisors, early loss of a mandibular primary canine is a significant indicator of a tooth size-arch size discrepancy. Unilateral loss of a lower primary canine is frequently followed by a shift in the dental midline toward the side of loss, lingual collapse of the incisor segment, and possibly deepening of the bite (Fig. 27-10A, B). The asymmetric disruption in arch integrity complicates normal eruption of the permanent canines and premolars toward the affected side. If ectopic eruption involves bilateral loss of both lower primary canines, pronounced lingual inclination and distal drifting of the permanent incisors, deepening of the overbite, increased overjet, and significant loss of arch perimeter is likely to be the alignment result (see Fig. 27-10C, D).

If one primary canine is lost during incisor eruption, it may be desirable to extract the contralateral primary canine to help maintain arch symmetry. Whereas extraction of the contralateral primary canine may improve the appearance of incisor alignment and midline integrity, crowding problems requiring such intervention are a strong indicator of a significant arch length deficiency

that will likely become grossly evident upon permanent canine and premolar eruption. Some clinicians recommend a lingual holding arch with spur attachments to control incisor positioning and prevent encroachment on permanent canine eruption positions when primary canines are lost prematurely. Even though this may be feasible in some cases, the asymmetric positioning and displacement of the incisors typically contradicts simple placement of a lingual holding arch at this stage without first aligning the incisors with active appliance therapy. The inherent questionable prognosis relative to arch length-tooth size considerations brings into question simple appliance therapy at this point in development. Regardless of the individual decision, the prognosis related to ectopic loss of primary canines is generally not good concerning the long-range occlusion status.

The ectopic loss of maxillary primary canines occurs less frequently than mandibular loss given more favorable space adjustments for incisor liability. When it occurs, ectopic loss of a maxillary primary canine typically reflects a very distal eruptive displacement of the permanent lateral incisor and not necessarily a significant tooth mass problem. Atypical upper anterior alignment may

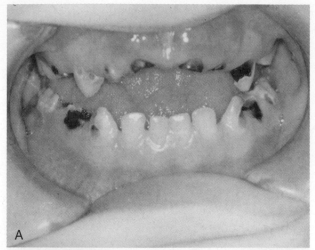

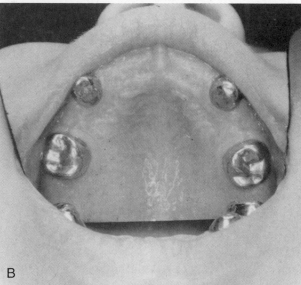

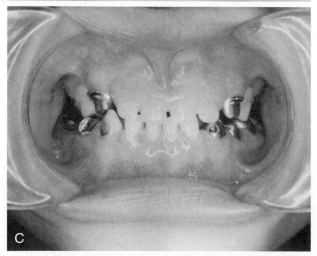

Figure 27-8 A, This 4-year-old child required removal of nonrestorable maxillary primary incisors and first primary molars. **B,** Stainless steel crowns were placed on the primary canines and second molars. **C,** A maxillary removable partial retainer with incisor pontics maintains space, improves appearance, and reduces the possibility of a tongue-thrust.

occur with resultant crowding and blockage of the permanent canine because it erupts so late in normal transition. Early loss of maxillary primary canines is an indicator for early orthodontic treatment with an understanding the child is a definite candidate for comprehensive orthodontic intervention.

Loss of First Primary Molars

The effect of premature loss of first primary molars in both arches is mostly dependent on the state of eruption of the first permanent molars. If the primary first molar is lost during the primary dentition from ages 3 to 5 years, there should be little or no space loss associated with mesial movement of the second primary molar. However, as first permanent molars erupt at age 5 to 7 years, a strong force is exerted that pushes the second primary molar forward into the first primary molar space (see Fig. 27-3B). This results in a loss of posterior arch length within the quadrant that can lead to crowding as the canines and premolars erupt in later stages. In addition to posterior effects, mandibular arch length may be further compromised by distal and lingual shifting of anterior teeth toward the side of first primary molar tooth loss. Therefore loss of a first primary molar in either arch approximating eruption of first permanent molars indicates use of a space maintainer is generally desirable to stabilize second primary molar and canine positioning.

If the first primary molar is lost after first permanent molars have erupted into occlusion and the second primary molar is still in position, minimal space loss should be evidenced in either arch. This is particularly applicable when first permanent molars are positioned in a full class I or class II cuspal interdigitation. If first permanent molars are in an end-to-end relationship, the location by arch of the missing first primary molar may be a factor in potential molar adjustments. If loss of the first primary molar occurs in the upper arch, untoward shifting from the end-to-end occlusion may result in class II molar positioning. To ensure this will not happen, a space maintainer for the upper arch may be considered. If the first primary molar loss occurs in the lower arch, any molar shift would be in the direction of a class I relationship. Space maintenance would be less likely unless absolute preservation of leeway space was indicated until permanent canines and premolars erupt.

A unilateral fixed space maintainer called a *band* or *crown and loop* is usually the appliance of choice for early loss of first primary molars. The appliance incorporates a band or crown on the second primary molar with a soldered wire-loop extension extending forward to contact the distal-cervical surface of the primary canine in the quadrant (Fig. 27-11). The loop uses 0.036 or 0.040 stainless steel wire strong enough to withstand biting forces while ensuring a rigid abutment contact in stopping forward movement of the second primary molar and distal movement of the primary canine. Wire design approximates the gingival contour of the extraction space to avoid occlusal interferences and is wide enough to allow the permanent tooth to erupt. A modification of the design is use of a single-wire extension "arm" rather than a full loop from the posterior abutment to contact

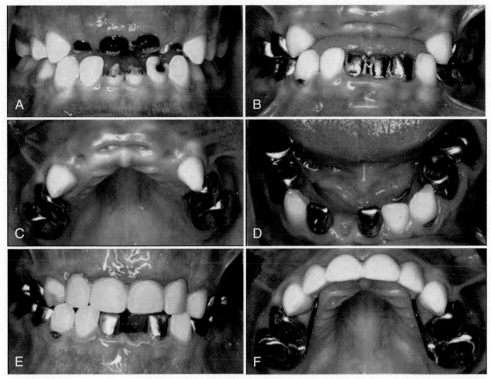

Figure 27-9 Early loss of maxillary primary incisors in 4½-year-old child. **A,** Pretreatment caries with non-restorable maxillary primary incisors. **B, C,** and **D,** Postrestorative appearance with multiple stainless steel crowns. While interdigitation should hold anterior intercanine space, the parents and patient requested cosmetic incisor replacement. **E** and **F,** A fixed space maintainer with a "Hollywood" bridge fulfills esthetic demands as an elective treatment. Appliance used one-size-larger crowns fitted over restorative crowns on second primary molars as abutments.

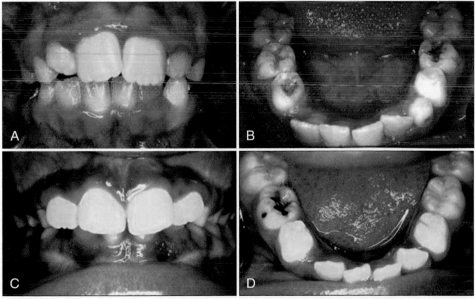

Figure 27-10 Ectopic loss of lower primary canines in association with permanent lateral incisor eruption. **A** and **B,** Unilateral canine loss results in asymmetric arch dimensions as the incisors shift toward the side of loss and lingualize their positioning. **C** and **D,** Bilateral ectopic loss of canines allows maintenance of arch symmetry, but results in significant lingual retroclination and supraeruption of lower incisors, increased overjet, deepened overbite, and reduction in lower arch dimensions.

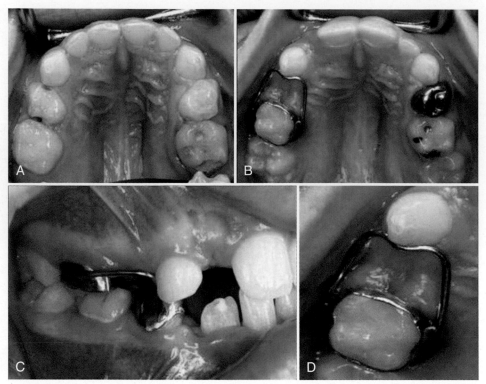

Figure 27-11 A and **B,** Pre-treatment at 4½ years of age and follow-up at 7 years showing value of properly fitted and designed band and loop appliance to hold space for an extracted first primary molar. **C,** Buccal occlusion showing proper relationship of erupted first permanent molars. **D,** Close-up of design shows loop is sufficiently large to allow the eventual eruption of the permanent tooth.

the anterior abutment (Fig. 27-12). The single arm of 0.036 or 0.040 wire is rigid enough to hold the space while reducing by half possible interferences to eruption of the underlying tooth. Neither the loop nor the arm design restores chewing function or prevents eruption of opposing teeth, a possible consideration in some cases. In addition, the wire may inhibit primary canine distolateral movement as permanent incisors erupt, particularly in association with lower lateral incisor eruption. For this reason, the status of permanent incisor eruption sequencing, symmetry, and positioning should

be monitored and guidance steps taken to optimize normal incisor eruption. The clinician must recognize these limitations and prepare for modifications in the overall space supervision planning.

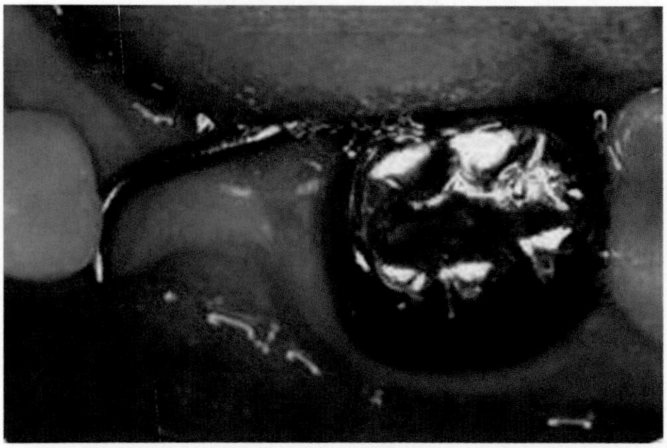

The use of a band as the abutment attachment makes it easy and economical to construct, takes little chair time, and adjusts readily to accommodate the changing dentition. The use of a stainless steel crown as the abutment base (Fig. 27-13) offers the advantage of increased stability and retention. A crown is used if the second primary molar has extensive caries or if the tooth has had vital pulp therapy. The steel crown should be prepared as described in Chapter 18. An impression is made, the crown removed from the tooth and seated in the impression, and a working model prepared on which to fabricate the loop. Because it is difficult to remove the crown (converted to a band) to make adjustments, adapting a band or one size larger crown over a cemented crown restoration and constructing a conventional band and loop appliance is another alternative to address unilateral space maintenance (Fig. 27-14).

If first primary molars are lost bilaterally within a lower arch and the second primary molars are retained, two separate unilateral loop appliances are generally indicated until first permanent molar and incisor eruption are complete. Bilateral lingual holding arch designs should not be placed before eruption of the permanent incisors as the lingual wire may interfere with incisor positioning during eruption. Additionally, primary incisors as anterior stops do not offer sufficient anchorage to prevent loss of arch length in most cases. Either of the loop or arm designs is relatively

Figure 27-12 Close-up of unilateral crown and arm space maintainer.

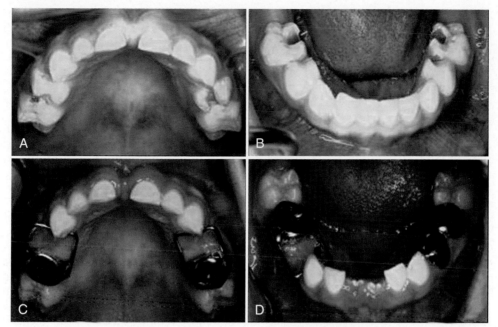

Figure 27-13 A and **B,** Pretreatment of upper and lower arches with caries and pulp involvement of primary molars. **C** and **D,** Same upper and lower arches with crown and loops placed for early loss of three first primary molars. Note erupted first permanent molars with proper positioning.

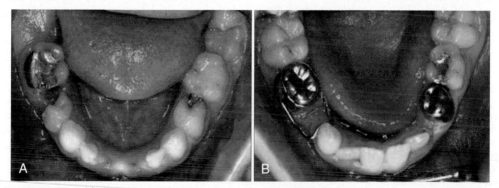

Figure 27-14 A, Pretreatment of lower arch with caries and pulp involvement of primary molars. **B,** Same lower arch with band and loop placed over a restored crown on the second primary molar for early loss of right first primary molars. The band was fabricated from the next larger sized crown by removing the occlusal surface and shortening the cervical portion of the crown. Note erupted first permanent molars with proper positioning.

effective as long as the clinician realizes the appliances are dependent on abutment teeth that may exfoliate before the need for space maintenance is complete. After the permanent incisors have fully erupted and as the primary canines and molars exfoliate, a second appliance that stabilizes final permanent molar position and arch length may be necessary to prevent subsequent space loss.

Loss of Second Primary Molars

If a second primary molar is lost in a child 2 to 5 years of age, no space loss should occur while the first permanent molar is in basal bone. The options in managing such early loss are very limited due to lack of retention elements for fixed appliances and patient cooperation in the use of appliances at this age. As first permanent molars erupt, however, considerable loss in arch length can occur if no second primary molar is present as an eruptive guide

(Fig. 27-15). Space loss of as much as 8 mm in a maxillary quadrant has been documented as the first permanent molar displaces forward through bodily crown-root movement and mesiolingual rotation around the palatal root. Early loss of lower second primary molars in conjunction with first permanent molar eruption timing results in up to 4 to 6 mm of space loss during transition. The lower first molars move forward by pronounced mesial tipping of the crown with more modest bodily tooth movement expressed in molar adjustments. Distal movement and retroclination of teeth anterior to the space is also a likely consequence to early loss in the lower arch. If the loss of the second primary molar occurs after the first permanent molars have fully erupted and normal cuspal interdigitation has been established, the degree of space loss should be less dramatic than earlier during molar transition regardless of arch involved. However, mesial

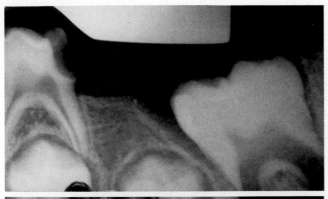
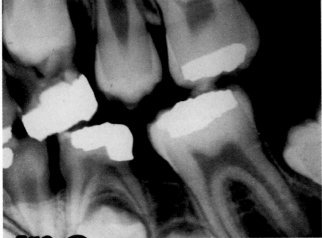
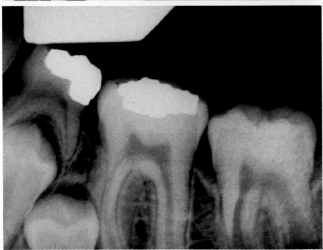

Figure 27-15 A sequence of three radiographs showing early loss of a lower second primary molar and mesial movement of the first permanent molar before eruption. Eventually there was complete closure of the space needed for the second premolar.

movement of the permanent molar through lack of buttressing support from the missing second primary molar usually results in space loss that may be significant in amount. Quadrant space loss on the order of 2 to 3 mm without the buttressing support of the second primary molar may be realized—easily enough to compromise positioning of the permanent canines and premolars.

Given the findings regarding space loss with second primary molars, a space maintainer is generally indicated in most patients to control permanent molar positions. If the loss occurs just before eruption of the first permanent molar, that is, when the first molar crown is still covered with oral mucosa and a thin partial covering of bone, a space maintainer to guide the positioning of the first permanent molar into normal occlusion is desirable. The appliance of choice is a distal shoe for both the maxillary (Fig. 27-16) and mandibular arches. The appliance incorporates a posterior wire-loop extension from the first primary molar that supports a vertical tissue blade positioned to contact and guide the erupting permanent molar into normal position. The depth of the intragingival extension should be about 1.0 to 1.5 mm beyond the mesial marginal ridge of the molar to "capture" the surface as the tooth erupts vertically. Gauged in length to represent the missing second molar, accurate placement is critical to insure that the distal shoe does not extend too far distally over the first molar and block its eruption, nor be too short and not maintain the space occupied by the lost second primary molar. It has been observed that the soft tissue tolerates the blade extension well, although a small metallic "tattoo" in the gingiva may result.

The first primary molar is first prepared with a stainless steel crown or well-adapted band that provides a retentive base for the distal shoe. An impression is made to prepare a working model. If the primary second molar has not yet been extracted, it is cut off the model and a hole made with a bur that simulates the position of the distal root of the tooth. If the second primary molar has been removed previously, the positioning of the tissue extension may be determined with measurements on bite-wing or periapical radiographs or by measuring the mesiodistal width of the contralateral second molar. The extension blade is contoured, extended distally into the prepared opening on the model and the loop soldered to the band or crown. An alternative in design is the use of an adjustable Gerber extension employing a trombone-type attachment with the sleeve portion tach-welded or soldered to the band or crown (see Fig. 27-16). The sliding extension can be positioned into the tube sleeve and the posterior length adjusted to the proper spacing with the blade extension positioned directly into the extraction space or a surgical incision made just at the mesial contact area of the erupting first permanent molar. Crimping of the sleeve tube holds the length of the established extension loop. The tach-welded area should ideally be supported with additional solder to reinforce the appliance from occlusion forces. Before final placement, a radiograph of the distal shoe in position should be made to determine whether the extension is in proper relationship with the unerupted first permanent molar. Final adjustments in length and contour may be made to make sure mesial contact of the first permanent molar is provided. Brill,[15] in describing chair-side fabrication procedures, presents the distal shoe as an efficient and cost-effective appliance for guiding the unerupted permanent first molar into position with success rates relatively equal to studies looking at the longevity of other space maintainers.

Several conditions contraindicate the use of distal shoe appliances. Given the extent of caries involvement, there

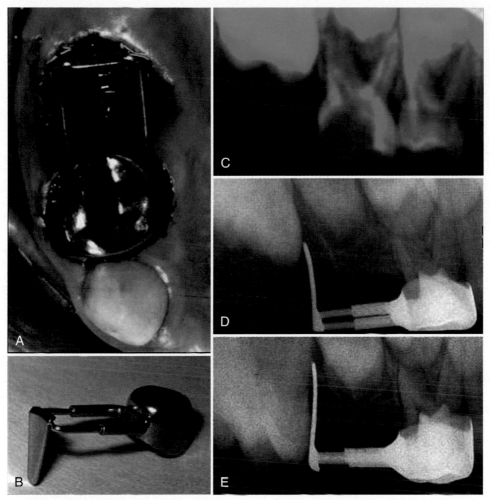

Figure 27-16 A, The second primary molar is non-restorable and must be extracted. A crown with a distal shoe extension to help guide the first permanent molar has been placed. **B,** Picture of a prefabricated crown with Gerber-type distal shoe extension as used in case. **C, D,** and **E,** Progress can be seen on radiographs in guiding the eruption of the permanent molar over 12 months.

may be lack of abutments to support a cemented appliance. Poor oral hygiene or lack of patient and parental cooperation greatly reduces the possibility of a successful clinical result. Histologic studies show that the distal shoe does not become lined with epithelium and is associated with a chronic inflammatory response. Therefore certain medical conditions such as blood dyscrasias, immunosuppression, congenital heart defects, history of rheumatic fever, and diabetes contraindicate the use of the appliance. If the distal shoe is contraindicated, two possibilities for treatment exist: (1) allow the tooth to erupt and regain space later, or (2) use a removable or fixed appliance that does not penetrate the tissue but places pressure on the ridge mesial to the unerupted permanent molar (Fig. 27-17). Carroll and Jones[16] reported on a pressure-type appliance successfully used to guide the permanent molar as it erupted. Given the fact that the first permanent molars are guided in their eruption by the distal-cervical aspect of the second primary molar, the acrylic or pressure extension usually serve as an ineffective guide for eruptive positioning. The removable extension is more likely to work in the lower arch if the eruption bulge area of the first permanent molar can be

engaged with the acrylic. If several teeth are missing, the removable appliance can serve to restore function and prevent super-eruption of opposing teeth.

After the first permanent molar has been guided into position, a distal shoe is usually indicated for replacement with a different appliance. Continued vertical development will usually result in tipping of the permanent first molar over the top of the blade extension with resulting space loss and tissue complications. One option is to remove the intragingival extension and replace it with a reverse band and loop employing an occlusal directed extension to prevent the molar from tipping over the wire. Exfoliation of the first primary molar as an abutment may also occur before eruption of the second premolars. So a more preferred option to replace a distal shoe once the first permanent molars have erupted adequately to be banded is the use of a bilateral space maintainer such as a mandibular lingual holding arch, maxillary transpalatal bar, or maxillary Nance appliance. These same bilateral space maintainers are the method of choice to provide stability to first permanent molar positions whenever the second primary molars are lost and first

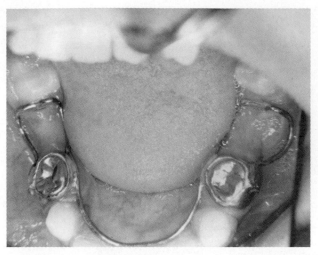

Figure 27-17 A modified distal shoe "pressure" appliance to provide bilateral space maintenance and eruption guidance for the first permanent molars. The permanent molars are erupting properly, and the intragingival extensions may be removed.

permanent molars have erupted into occlusion. Even after first permanent molar occlusion is established, the loss of second primary molars will potentially result in significant amounts of closure without the buttressing effect of the primary second molar.

The classic bilateral mixed dentition space maintainer in the mandibular arch is the soldered lingual holding arch (Figs. 27-18). With bands fitted to the first permanent molars, a 0.036- or 0.040-inch steel wire is contoured to the arch and extended forward to make contact with the cingulum area of the incisors (Fig. 27-19). The design stabilizes lower molar positions from moving mesially and incisor relationships from retroclining lingually in sustaining the canine-premolar segment space (i.e., leeway space). The lingual wire must simply be contoured to not interfere with normal eruption paths and provide an anterior arch form so that the incisors have an opportunity for alignment. In the mixed dentition, the soldered lingual holding arch should present minimal problems with breakage, minimal oral hygiene concerns, minimal interference in eruptive movements of permanent canines and premolars, and no concerns about whether the child is wearing the appliance. Importantly, the bilateral design and use of permanent teeth as abutments allows application during the full transitional dentition period of the buccal segments. As stated earlier, lower lingual arches should not be placed before the eruption of the permanent incisors because of their frequent lingual eruption path. The lingual wire may interfere with normal incisor positioning if the appliance is in position before lateral incisor eruption. Additionally, abutting against primary incisors as anterior stops does not offer sufficient anchorage to prevent significant loss of arch length.

Used in the maxillary arch to stabilize molar positions bilaterally, the soldered transpalatal bar incorporates a transverse palatal wire of 0.036 or 0.040 stainless steel wire

soldered to molar abutments (Fig. 27-20A). The rigid transverse wire prevents the two main space loss patterns of upper first permanent molars: mesiobuccal rotation and anterior bodily displacement. While the appliance may allow some minor mesial tipping of the upper molars, this is generally considered insignificant as to overall space loss in the maxillary arch. The simple transpalatal contour of the connector wire offers the main argument for this appliance: It is easy to fabricate and offers minimal irritation to the palatal tissue or tongue. The Nance appliance uses a contoured rigid wire with an acrylic "button" contacting the palatal shelf as an anterior stop for bilateral molar stabilization in the maxillary arch (see Fig. 27-20B). Providing the same molar rotation and bodily movement control as transpalatal bars, the added bracing of the acrylic button against the anterior palatal vault offers some additional resistance against forward tipping movements of the molars. Whereas the bilateral stability of the transpalatal appliance appears adequate in most situations, the resistance of the Nance with its acrylic palatal stop is preferred by some clinicians. Tissue irritation beneath the button does not appear to be a clinical problem in most cases if proper hygiene is followed.

The fixed space maintainers as described have the distinct advantage that they are stable, not easily broken, and wear is not dependent on the child. Ensuring the appliance is passive and does not cause unwanted tooth movement is generally the greatest concern. Proper design should minimize eruption interferences and the effects of unfavorable abutment loss or impingement of soft tissues. Poor band fit or defective cement may serve as a locus for debris accumulation and subsequent decalcification. Steps to prevent this include adapting a band that contours tightly to the tooth surface and extends beneath the gingival margins, providing a thorough prophylaxis before cementation, keeping the tooth thoroughly dry during cementation, using glass ionomer cements, and teaching the child and parent proper oral hygiene practices to include the use of fluoride rinses. Closely checking the appliance at 6-month intervals to monitor potential problems is standard protocol.

Areas of Multiple Primary Molar Loss
Loss of multiple primary molars may lead to mutilation of the developing dentition unless an appliance is constructed to maintain relationships of remaining teeth and to guide eruption of the developing teeth. In addition to arch dimension concerns, reduced masticatory function is undesirable from a nutritional standpoint. Removable acrylic partial dentures have been used successfully in either arch after the loss of multiple teeth. If artificial teeth are included, an essentially normal degree of function and acceptable esthetics can be restored. The disadvantages lie in their unpredictability outside the clinicians control because the appliances require patient cooperation and can be easily lost or broken during wear. During the transitional stages of exfoliation and eruption, stability of removable appliances is often difficult to sustain with the loss of abutments. The wire clasps and resin contact areas may present "food-traps" for plaque

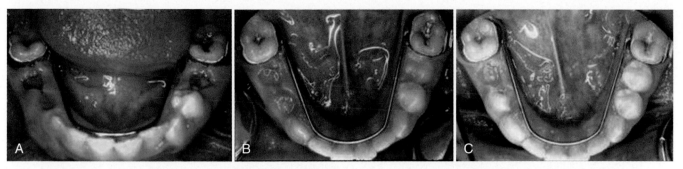

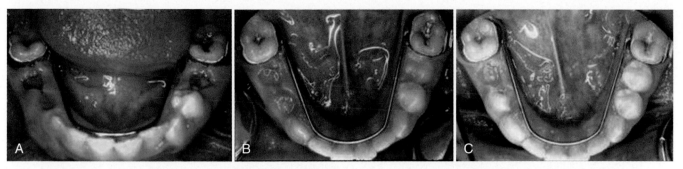

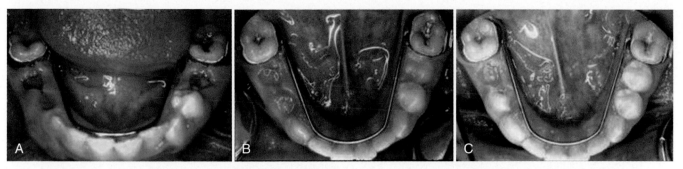

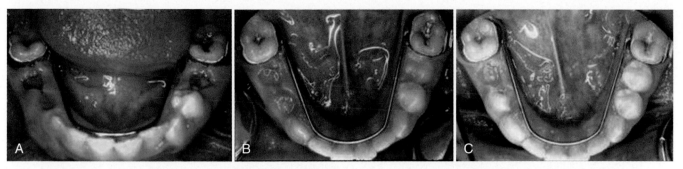

Figure 27-18 Lingual holding arch for bilateral space maintenance and guidance of buccal segment eruption patterns. **A,** Initial appliance placement in conjunction with primary molar extractions. **B,** Eruption transition at 6 months after extractions. **C,** Eruption status at 1 year. Note improvement in anterior and buccal segment alignment.

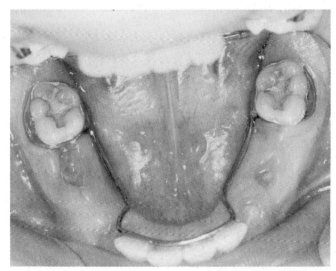

Figure 27-19 Proper design of a passive mandibular soldered lingual holding arch positioned with wire contact at the cingulum area of the permanent incisors. Note the wire offsets and contours to position the wire away from the eruption path of buccal segment teeth and to avoid tongue irritation. (Courtesy Dr. Theodore R. Lynch.)

accumulation, with increased potential for soft tissue irritation and dental caries.

If the loss of one or both of the second primary molars occurs a short time before the eruption of the first permanent molars, the acrylic removable appliance may be considered in preference to one of the distal shoe maintainers described previously. An acrylic partial denture with a distal extension to guide first permanent molars into position may be used (Fig. 27-21). The teeth to be extracted are cut away from the stone cast and a depression is cut into the stone model to allow the fabrication of the acrylic extension. The acrylic will extend into the alveolus after removal of the primary teeth. The extension may be removed after eruption of the permanent tooth. It is occasionally necessary to recommend extraction of all the primary teeth in a preschool child. Although this was more common in the prefluoridation era, some children even today must have all of their teeth removed because of widespread oral infection and because the teeth are nonrestorable. Preschool children can wear complete dentures successfully before the eruption of permanent teeth (Fig. 27-22).

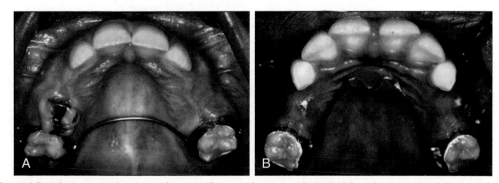

Figure 27-20 Bilateral fixed space maintainers for maxillary molar control. **A,** Soldered transpalatal bar using 0.036 wire contoured to traverse the palatal contour. The appliance prevents forward bodily movement and rotation of molars around palatal roots. **B,** Nance appliance incorporates an 0.036 wire that traverses the arch with a midline acrylic button positioned against the anterior palatal contour. The design prevents molars from forward bodily movement, rotation around the palatal roots, and mesial tipping.

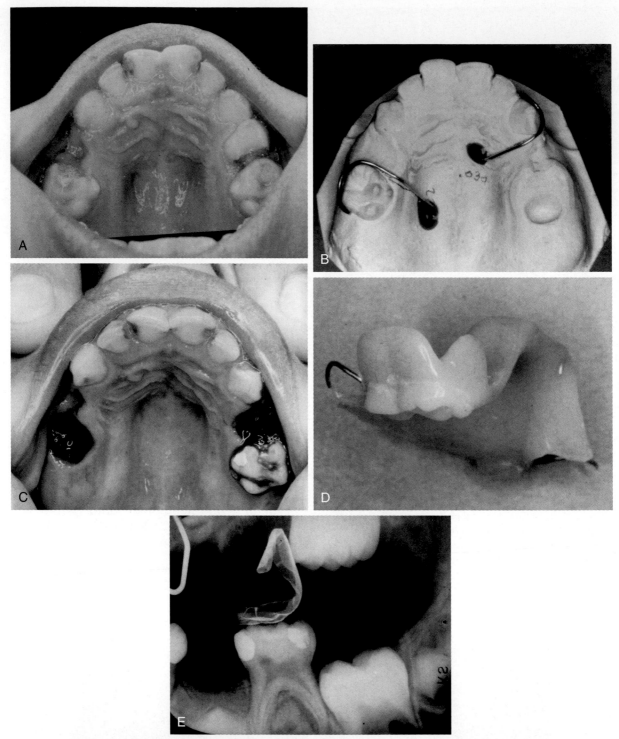

Figure 27-21 A, Clinical and radiographic examination revealed need to extract both maxillary first primary molars and the left second primary molar at age 6 years. **B,** The teeth indicated for extraction are cut away from the stone model and a depression is made in the second molar area for an acrylic distal shoe-type extension. **C,** The primary teeth have been extracted in preparation for the placement of the partial denture. **D,** The acrylic distal shoe extension. **E,** Lead foil has been placed over the tissue extension to determine, with the aid of a radiograph, whether the acrylic is positioned properly to guide the eruption of the first permanent molar. (Courtesy Dr. Paul E. Starkey.)

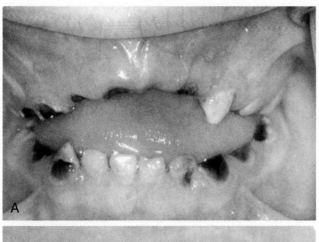

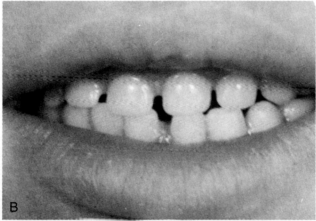

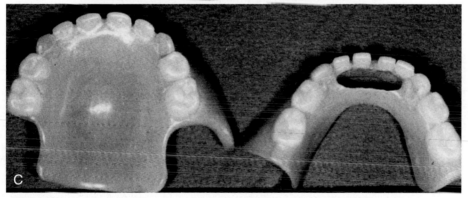

Figure 27-22 A, Primary teeth with rampant gross caries and pulpal involvement. **B,** Complete dentures in place after the extraction of all primary teeth. **C,** Modification of the dentures after eruption of upper first permanent molars and lower permanent incisors.

Loss of First Permanent Molars

The first permanent molar is unquestionably the most important unit of mastication and is essential in the development of functionally desirable occlusion. A carious lesion may develop rapidly in the first permanent molar and occasionally progress from an incipient lesion to a pulp exposure in a 6-month period. The loss of a first permanent molar in a child can lead to changes in the dental arches that can be traced throughout the life of that person. Unless appropriate corrective measures are instituted, these changes include diminished local function, drifting of teeth, and continued eruption of opposing teeth.

The second molars, even if unerupted, start to drift mesially after the loss of the first permanent molar. A greater degree of forward bodily movement will occur with loss of the first permanent molar in children in the 8- to 12-year age group. In older children, if the loss occurs after eruption of the second permanent molar, more exaggerated mesial tipping of the second molar can be the expected outcome. Although the premolars undergo the greatest amount of distal drifting, all the teeth anterior to the space, including the central and lateral incisors on the side where the loss occurred, may show evidence of movement. Contacts open and the premolars, in particular, rotate as they fall distally. There is a tendency for the maxillary premolars to move distally in unison, whereas those in the lower arch may move separately. When the maxillary first permanent molar loses its opponent, it erupts at a faster rate than the adjacent teeth. The alveolar process is also carried along with the molars and causes problems when prosthetic replacements are needed. The treatment of patients with the loss of first permanent molars must be approached on an individual basis. A superimposed existing malocclusion, abnormal musculature, or the presence of deleterious oral habits can affect the result, as in the case of the premature loss of primary molars.

Loss of a first permanent molar before the eruption of the second permanent molar presents problems in both anteroposterior space control and vertical eruption control of opposing molars. Although it is possible to prevent overeruption of a maxillary first permanent molar by placing a lower partial denture, there is no completely effective way to influence the path of eruption of the developing second permanent molar other than the use of an acrylic distal shoe extension on a partial denture as described previously. The second molar drifts mesially before eruption when the first permanent molar has been extracted. Repositioning this tooth orthodontically is possible after its eruption. However, the child must then be considered for prolonged space maintenance until the time when a more permanent tooth replacement can be inserted. The removal of the opposing first permanent molar, even when the tooth appears to be sound and caries free, is sometimes recommended in preference to allowing it to extrude or to subjecting the child to prolonged space maintenance and eventual fixed replacement.

If the first permanent molars are removed several years before eruption of the second permanent molars, there is an excellent chance that the second molars will erupt in an acceptable position (Fig. 27-23). However, the axial inclination of the second molars, particularly in the lower arch, may be greater than normal.

The decision whether to allow the second molar to drift mesially or to guide it forward in an upright position may be influenced by the presence of a third molar of normal size. If there is a question regarding the favorable development of a third molar on the affected side, repositioning the drifted second molar and holding space for a replacement prosthesis is usually the treatment of choice.

When the first permanent molar is lost after the eruption of the second permanent molar, orthodontic evaluation is indicated, and the following points should be considered: Is the child in need of corrective treatment other than in the first permanent molar area? Should the space be maintained for a replacement prosthesis? Should the second molar be moved forward into the area formerly occupied by the first molar? The latter choice is often the more satisfactory, even though there will be a difference in the number of molars in the opposing arch. A third molar can often be removed to compensate for the difference. Without treatment the second molar will tip forward within a matter of weeks (Fig. 27-24).

Another option to consider is autotransplantation of a third molar into the first molar position (Fig. 27-25). According to Bauss and colleagues, autotransplantation has become a well-established treatment modality in cases of early tooth loss or aplasia.[17] For third molars with partly developed roots, transplantation success rates have been reported in the range of 74% to 100%.

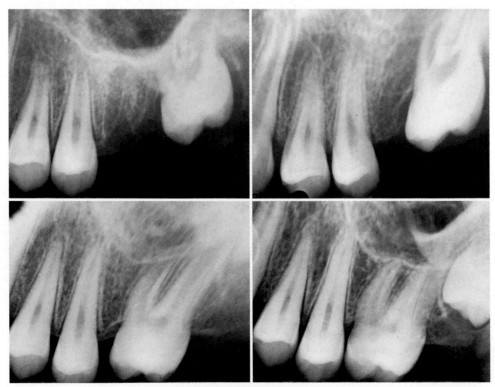

Figure 27-23 Radiographs taken at 6-month intervals after a maxillary first permanent molar was lost before the eruption of the second permanent molar.

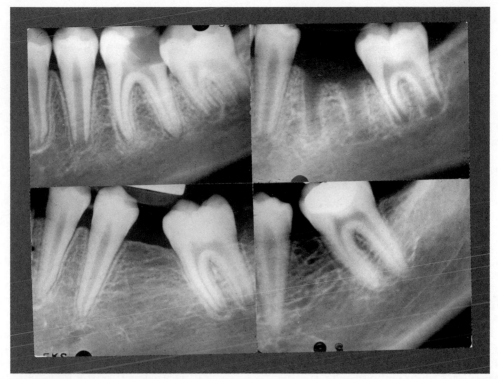

Figure 27-24 Radiographs taken at 6-month intervals after the loss of a mandibular first permanent molar. Notice the degree of tipping of the second molar and distal drifting of the premolars.

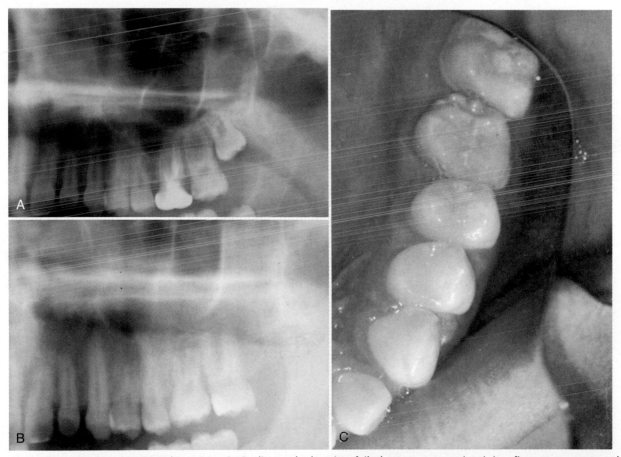

Figure 27-25 Third molar autotransplantation. **A,** Radiograph showing failed attempt at maintaining first permanent molar and minimal root development of third permanent molar. Radiographic **(B)** and clinical view **(C)** of third molar 15 months after autotransplantation. Note continued root development.

ORAL HABITS IN CHILDREN

Bruxism

Defined as nonfunctional grinding or gnashing of teeth, bruxism has been reported in up to 15% of children and young adults. Usually occurring at night, bruxism can result in significant abrasion of primary and permanent teeth if continued over a prolonged period (Fig. 27-26). A vinyl bite-guard that covers occlusal surfaces of all teeth can be worn at night to prevent continued abrasion. The occlusal surface of the bite-guard should be flat to avoid occlusal interferences. A mouth guard of the type described in Chapter 22 may also help in overcoming the habit. Ramfjord[18] believes occlusal interferences may trigger bruxism if combined with nervous tension. Therefore occlusal equilibration can be used to help the problem if obvious interferences are present. Sheppard[19] recommends construction of an anterior bite plate that allows for continued eruption of the posterior teeth if they have been abraded by the habit. When bruxism continues into adulthood, periodontal disease and/or temporomandibular joint disturbances can be a resulting factor.

Digit Sucking Habits

Many children suck their thumbs or fingers for short periods during infancy or early childhood with the habit considered normal during the first 2 years of life. If present at such an early age, parents should be advised to periodically observe the nature and intensity of the habit. If the child demonstrates gradually diminishing activity, it is probable the habit will cease without intervention. Traisman and Traisman[20] reported the average age at which digit-sucking stopped was 3.8 years, although other studies indicate a persistent incidence of up to 20% at age 4 years. These studies indicate changes in the anterior occlusion caused by digit-sucking are temporary with little likelihood of long-term effects if the habit is discontinued by age of 3 to 4 years.

If the intensity of the habit persists or increases and adverse dental and skeletal changes are noted beyond age 4 years, corrective measures may be needed to avoid undesirable occlusion problems (Fig. 27-27). By the age of 6 to 7 years, estimates indicate approximately 10% to 15% of children have a persistent digit-sucking habit that run the gamut from incidental sucking at bedtime to pronounced habits that seems to be almost constant. Almost all authorities recognize persistent digit-sucking habits extending into the incisor transition period can cause a malocclusion or aggravate an already existing one. Pressure generated from the habit can produce changes in the anterior segments of the dental arches with labial flaring and protrusive spacing of maxillary anterior teeth and increased overjet. Remodeling of the maxillary alveolar process and vertical displacement of the maxillary anterior teeth can result in an open-bite relationship. In addition, the digit positioning can interfere with eruption of the lower incisors to exaggerate the open-bite appearance in the incisor segment. Intense patterns may contribute to pronounced lingual inclination of the mandibular incisors that further increases the overjet situation. The increased open-bite and overjet may lead to abnormal muscle activities where the tongue protrudes during swallowing as an adaptation to the anterior space. Subtelny,[21,22] in evaluating 34 digit-sucking children using cineradiography, reported that 82% exhibited tongue-thrust activity during swallowing. Dental findings included protruded maxillary incisors, anterior open-bite, and increased maxillary arch length as a result of atypical muscular forces from the thumb, the perioral musculature, and forward positioning of the tongue. The child with a persistent digit-habit that results in an open-bite typically exhibits a convex profile with hypotonic upper lip, lower lip hypertonicity with marked mentalis muscle activity, and tongue-thrusting. These patterns maintain and possibly intensify the developing anterior open-bite and overjet discrepancy.

The effect of prolonged digit-sucking on posterior relationships is less clear. Strong muscle contractions of the circumoral musculature with the highest force levels approximating the maxillary canine area have been documented with extraoral habits. These may result in a relative constriction in maxillary arch width that has been associated with an increased development of functional posterior crossbites in children whose habits persist past the age of 4 to 5 years. While not as profound, associations between distal-step primary molars and class II permanent molars have been suggested in children whose habits extend into the transitional dentition period. Popovich and Thompson[23] observed 1258 children at the Burlington Growth Centre, the group represented approximately 90% of the pediatric population of Burlington, Ontario.

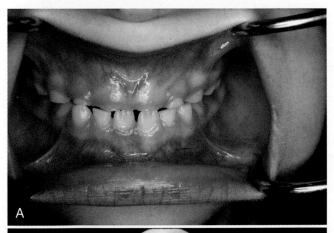

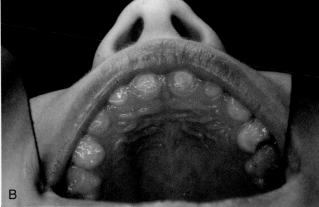

Figure 27-26 Bruxism resulting in severe abrasion of the maxillary primary anterior teeth.

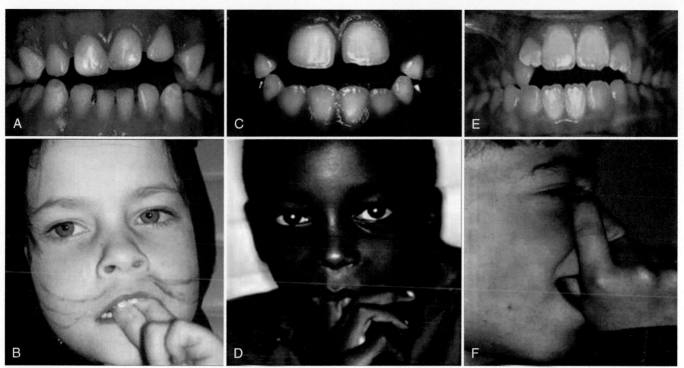

Figure 27-27 Occlusion of three children with different patterns of digit-sucking habits. **A** and **B,** An open-bite in the primary dentition caused by the child placing two fingers between the anterior teeth. **C** and **D,** An open-bite with flared maxillary incisors in the mixed dentition caused by an index finger-sucking habit. **E** and **F,** An open-bite with maxillary constriction produced by sucking the thumb as presented. The maxillary constriction resulted in a posterior crossbite with a functional shift of the mandible on closure.

Many of the children were seen annually from 3 to 12 years of age with their oral habits and occlusion status recorded at 3, 6, 9, and 12 years of age. There was a significant association between the prevalence of class II malocclusion and persisting digit-sucking in the different age groups. Class II malocclusion increased from 21.5% at 3 and 4 years of age to 41.9% at 12 years of age with the probability of a class II malocclusion increased as the duration of the habit increased. If the habit was stopped before 6 years of age, the effects on occlusion were often transitory. In contrast, no child who stopped a habit after 6 years of age had a normal occlusion at age 12. An interesting observation was that children who had used a pacifier had a significantly lower rate of digit-sucking. However, Zardetto and others[24] point out that similar occlusal and myofunctional alterations are detected among children who have prolonged pacifier habits (either conventional or physiologic pacifiers), when compared with those with no sucking habits. Children who were pacifier users were significantly more likely to show open-bite, posterior cross-bite, increased overjet, and alteration in cheek mobility than habit-free children.

Interceptive treatments to stop a digit-sucking habit depend upon the patient's age, emotional and psychological state, cooperative motivation of the parents and child, nature of occlusion changes, and associated functional adaptations. An age-based approach provides a foundation for treatment, although individual patient findings may result in a more aggressive approach to intervention or, more likely, cause greater caution and actually delay or defer treatment. These age-based concepts are:

Before Age 4 If one accepts the premise that a digit-habit will usually stop by age 4 years and the effects on the occlusion are probably not permanent, then direct intervention before this age has questionable merit. Additionally, the understanding of the child complicates cooperation with any of the intervention options.

4- to 6-Year Age Group Psychological ploys and reward systems may help some children to cease digit-sucking in this age group. In conversation with the child, the dentist discusses the problem and its effect on the teeth. The child is asked to keep a daily record of each episode of digit-sucking and to report on their progress in stopping the habit. A decrease in the number of times the habit is practiced is evidence of progress and indicates the child will likely discontinue the habit. A positive approach involves cooperation of the parents who are often overanxious about the habit. This anxiety may result in nagging or punishment that often creates greater tension and may even intensify the habit. The parents should consent to disregard the habit and not mention it to the child for a more successful outcome. A timed reward system may help. For each day the child refrains from the habit, a "star" is placed on a calendar. In month 1, the child receives some reward or prize predetermined by the parent if the monthly calendar has 28 stars (i.e., two bad days allowed). In month 2, the goal is 29 stars to receive a reward. Month 3 should present a calendar completely filled with stars. The prizes are progressively enhanced as to value for the child. If the child ceases the habit for 3 months, the long-term chances of stopping the habit and enhancing occlusal development are good (Fig. 27-28).

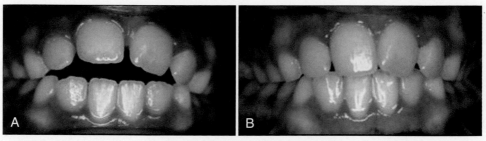

Figure 27-28 A, Open-bite with some maxillary constriction evident in the mixed dentition of an 8-year-old child with a persistent thumb-sucking habit. **B,** The child was encouraged to discontinue the habit through a positive rewards system. There was self-correction of the open-bite and transverse relationships by 9 years of age when the dysfunctional habit was discontinued.

Negative reinforcers such as mittens, bandages, and bitter tasting medicaments applied directly to the offending digit can occasionally affect a stoppage of the habit. Many practitioners have been successful using "thumb-guard" gadgets that the child wears on their thumb as a reminder not to use the thumb. These approaches meet greater success in children who express a desire to quit and just need a little help—the "reinforcers" are viewed as reminders rather than punishment.

The School-Age Years Although reward techniques may work in some children aged 6 years or older, the persistent habit may be so ingrained as to present unlikely successful stoppage with such ploys. This is the kid who has "tried to stop, but just cannot get it done." The transition of the permanent incisors and the ingrained nature of the habit often require direct appliance therapy to not only stop the habit but also enhance proper tooth eruption and alignment by influencing any acquired muscular patterns. A palatal crib appliance that prevents the offending digit from being placed in the sucking position and acts to restrain the tongue from forward positioning is a valuable adjunct in habit therapy during the mixed dentition years (Fig. 27-29). Palatal crib designs generally use the first permanent molars as anchorage abutments with a major connecting wire of standard 0.040 stainless steel orthodontic wire ensuring a strong and stable appliance that is resistant to both digit and tongue pressures. The crib approximates the cross-arch level

of the upper canines with the "fence" extending vertically to about the level of and just lingual to the lower incisors. Positioning should ensure no occlusal interferences in all functional excursions and allow clearance for upper incisors to lingualize into normal inclinations. The posterior transpalatal wire provides further rigidity and prevents constriction of maxillary intermolar width through pressures placed on the "fence" by the tongue or digit.

Palatal crib appliances are particularly effective in promoting a favorable environment for self-correction of incisor open-bite if applied when incisors are in active eruption phases. Labial flaring of the incisors should be reduced by the action of the upper lip when the digit and the tongue are no longer acting as opposing forces. Most children accommodate to the palatal crib in a short time and rarely are any problems lasting ones. Haryett and associates[25,26] reported that upon insertion of palatal crib appliances, nearly 80% of patients stopped sucking their thumbs within 7 days after insertion of the appliance. They also reported if the appliance was removed 3 months after insertion, the chance of the habit recurring was likely. The best chance of lasting success occurred when the appliance was left in place for 6 to 10 months. Therefore it is recommended that the fixed palatal crib be treatment planned to be worn for a period of 6 to 8 months.

The child's cooperation should be obtained when placing a palatal crib appliance. The function of the appliance

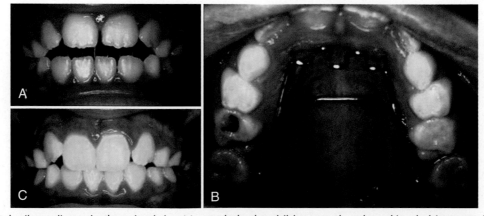

Figure 27-29 Palatal crib appliance in the mixed dentition to help the child stop a thumb-sucking habit, control forward tongue positioning, and allow eruptive "self-correction" of the anterior open-bite. **A,** Pretreatment incisor open-bite at time of appliance placement. Note crib appliance's vertical extension to level of lower incisors. **B,** Palatal crib appliance of 0.040 stainless steel. **C,** Posttreatment closure of open-bite after 6 months of crib therapy. The habit stopped within 1 week of appliance placement.

is to "help" and to "remind" the patient—the appliance cannot break the habit by itself without the child's cooperation. Failure to gain at least tacit cooperation will usually result in failure because the child resorts to new habit postures, complains, and causes such a commotion that the parent demands removal, or the child even physically removes or distorts the appliance purposefully. Because cooperation and motivation are critical to success, the child should be told that the appliance is being used to help him/her to stop sucking the thumb that has affected the position of the teeth. Some temporary difficulty with speech and eating should also be anticipated upon placement with most children accommodating in a short time. Some patients present with palatal irritation of the crib at about a month into appliance wear. This is usually attributable to pressures from the tongue pushing the appliance upward and is more common if second primary molars are used as anchorage abutments. A simple intraoral three-pronged pliers adjustment can be used to bend the anterior crib away from the tissue. This adjustment is usually only necessary at the initial first month check because the tongue soon adapts and "reprograms" from forward positioning.

Positive changes in open-bite and overjet should be notable by 3 months into treatment and self-correction should be achieved by the sixth month of the appliance protocol. If protrusion of the maxillary incisors and anterior open-bite have not "self-corrected" after the habit and tongue thrust are controlled, the discrepancy should be reevaluated to ensure that other problems (e.g., lip sucking) are not factors. In these situations, additional orthodontic treatment may be indicated to align the protruded and flared incisors into normal overbite and overjet positions. Older children in the late mixed or young permanent dentition with more established occlusal relationships, prolonged atypical functional patterns, and less eruptive potential are less likely to demonstrate self-correction. They usually require corrective orthodontic treatment using Edgewise techniques.

Variations of the palatal crib ranging from simple wires contoured to the palate without vertical extensions, to appliances incorporating reminder aspects (e.g., rollers on the Bluegrass appliance, a removable Hawley-type appliance), to the use of "rakes," "spurs," or "spikes" extending from the crib-wire or bands, have been advocated by various clinicians. A removable partial retainer with a series of smooth loops placed lingual to the incisors has proved successful in helping overcome a habit (Fig. 27-30). However, because a child may have a strong physical and emotional urge to continue the habit and not a strong resolve to quit, the use of a removable crib appliance is much less likely to succeed when compared with a fixed crib approach. The Bluegrass appliance (Fig. 27-31) incorporates a modified, six-sided roller constructed to spin around a 0.045-inch stainless steel wire when rolled by the tongue. Haskell and Mink[27] reported successful stoppage of thumb-sucking in children using the appliance with a program of positive reinforcement. The use of rakes and spurs in habit therapy have also been reported with success, although Haryett and associates[25,26] found 27% of children wearing a "rake" had transitory sleep disturbances compared with only 8% of children wearing a palatal crib. They also found that 14

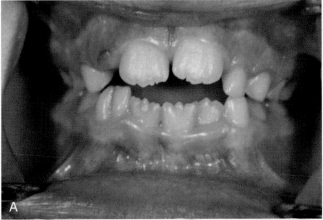
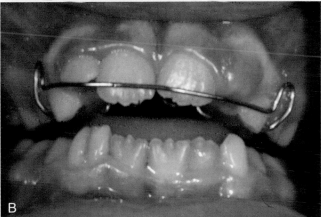
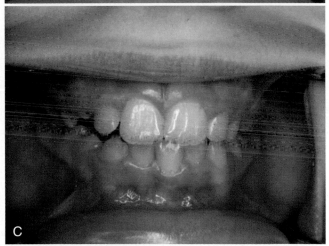

Figure 27-30 A, Anterior open-bite caused by a thumb-sucking habit. **B,** A Hawley-type reminder appliance was constructed after other problems in the patient's life were recognized and treated. **C,** The occlusion 18 months after the child had overcome the habit.

children (21.2%) of 66 children being treated developed mannerisms that persisted even after appliance therapy was discontinued. These included nail biting, chewing of hair or cloth, scratching of the body, and cracking of knuckles, but no enuresis. Davidson and associates[28] reported 36% of thumb-sucking children who received no treatment and were still actively thumb-sucking also developed other mannerisms. Thus there was no greater substitution of

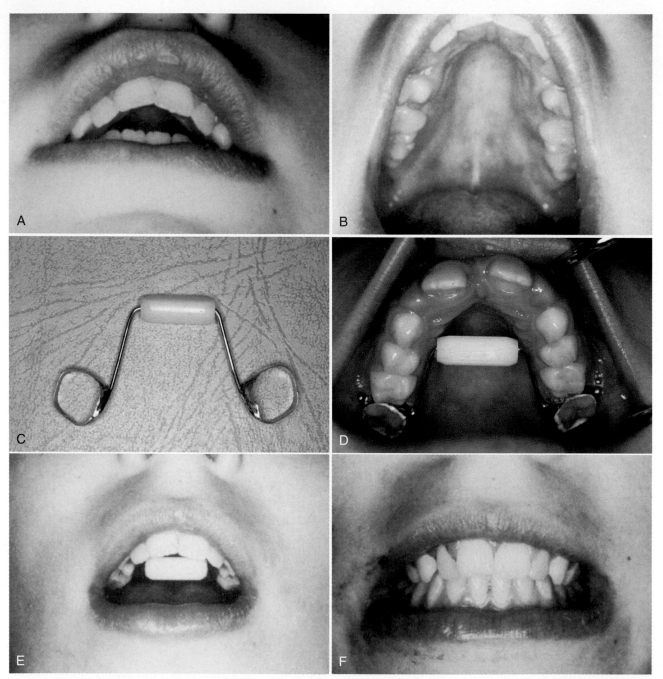

Figure 27-31 A and **B,** Anterior open-bite and palatal configuration in the mixed dentition associated with a thumb-sucking habit. **C,** Bluegrass appliance with occlusal view of the appliance in place. **D,** Anterior view of the appliance in place. **E,** Correction of the anterior open-bite. (Courtesy Dr. John R. Mink.)

mannerisms when a habit is treated with an appliance than when a habit is not treated. With no significant advantages in treatment effectiveness seen by other designs in the context of early intervention, the basic palatal crib appliance remains the recommended appliance design of choice for treating digit-habits in the transitional dentition.

Tongue-Thrust Swallowing Habits

Three major problems are usually associated with abnormal forward tongue positioning—anterior open-bite, protrusion of the incisors, and lisping. Proffit[29] suggests two

major reasons for a relatively high prevalence of anterior tongue positioning in children and relates to physiology (maturation) and to anatomy (growth). Infants normally position the tongue forward and down in the mouth at rest and during swallowing to help establish an airway for respiration. An infant's swallow is characterized by strong lip activity, placement of the tongue tip against the lower lip, and relaxation of the elevator muscles of the mandible. Physiologic transitions in swallowing patterns begin during the first year of life as teeth erupt and continue over the next several years as oral function matures. There is a gradual activation of the elevator muscles of the mandible in swallowing so that a mature swallowing pattern is characterized by relaxation of the lips, placement of the tongue behind the maxillary incisors, and elevation of the mandible until posterior teeth contact in occlusion. This is usually observed before a child is 4 or 5 years of age.

A prolonged abnormal swallowing pattern into the mixed and permanent dentitions is characterized by protrusion of the tongue between the anterior dentition, lack of molar contact, and excessive circumoral muscle activity. Studies have shown the prevalence of tongue-thrust is much greater than the prevalence of anterior open-bite. Subtelny[21,22] demonstrated using cineradiography that tongue-thrust activity between the incisors with incomplete contact of the molars during swallowing occurs in as many as 40% of adults with clinically acceptable occlusion. Fletcher[30] reported that in 1615 children ages 6 to 18 years, 52.3% of the 6- and 7-year-old children thrust their tongue. The incidence rates were reduced to 34% at age 10 years, while almost 25% of the 16- to 18-year-olds showed tongue-thrust patterns. Hanson and Cohen[31] found a similar incidence and age distribution of the tongue protruding between the teeth during swallowing. Despite these high numbers for tongue-thrust patterns, random samples of 8000 school-age children show an overall open-bite incidence of 5.7 % in US school children. Blacks have a much higher prevalence than whites of an open-bite greater than 2 mm (9.6% to 1.4%, respectively). From the data, it becomes obvious that tongue thrust does not necessarily coincide with open-bite malocclusion and deviations from "normal" swallowing are not necessarily detrimental to the occlusion.

Given the high percentages of tongue-thrust in children, the decreasing prevalence in older age groups, and the lack of direct cause and effect relationships with open-bite malocclusions, it seems reasonable to conclude that most tongue thrust patterns are normal transitional occurrences. The adaptation to the more typical adult swallowing pattern appears to be related to an increase in the functional space for tongue activity during adolescent growth changes. The mandible follows skeletal growth patterns that allow space for a downward and backward accommodation of the tongue. Concurrently, tonsillar and adenoid lymphoid tissue mass is reduced to allow greater oropharyngeal air space. Vertical growth of the dentoalveolar structures of the mandible and maxilla contribute to an increase in oropharyngeal space that allows the tongue to assume a more posterior position as the child proceeds through puberty.

Transition towards adult swallowing patterns appears to be affected by a prolonged digit-habit or by a skeletal malocclusion in which anterior open-bite or incisor protrusion exists between the dental arches (e.g., class II division 1). In these individuals, continued functional tongue protrusion during deglutition is viewed as an adaptation that maintains the anterior open-bite and is not a primary etiological factor in causing the open-bite. Studies by Profitt[32] and others have shown there is no "equal balance" of forces on the dentition produced by the tongue versus the lip musculature during functional activity. The expansive forces of the tongue are significantly greater

than and not balanced by the containing forces of the lips. The shape of the dental arches and position of the teeth do not appear to be overwhelmingly influenced by the horizontally directed pressures of the lips and tongue during normal functional activities such as swallowing and speaking. Profitt[32] reported tongue pressures decrease as the size of the arch increases, patients with protruding incisors have less lingual tongue pressures than do normal occlusions, and when incisors are retracted the tongue pressures increase to normal values. These findings are the reverse of what would be expected if tongue pressure had pushed the teeth into protruded positions. However, stronger relationships with the patient's arch form and the resting pressures of the tongue and lips have been found. An anterior positioned tongue "at rest" can impede vertical eruption of the teeth and result in an open-bite. This may be reflected in the findings that most habit related open-bites are self-correcting when digit-sucking is eliminated and tongue positioning controlled.

The controversy concerning tongue thrust swallowing extends into treatment approaches that include palatal crib-type appliances, full orthodontic therapy, myofunctional therapy, or combinations of the above. The occurrence of an open-bite is often initially related to a thumb- or finger-sucking habit and then retained by the tongue being thrust forward or the tongue merely occupying the space. In appliance therapy for digit-habits, a vertical crib "fence" helps modify forward tongue positioning associated with the anterior open-bite. With stoppage of the habit, the tongue assumes more normal swallowing patterns as muscular functions reflect adaptation to the corrected anterior open-bite. But what about the child who presents with an anterior open-bite and does not have a history of a digit-habit? Will this child benefit from a palatal crib appliance to restrain the tongue? Or should other approaches be taken in managing the open-bite? The answer lies in understanding our previous discussion on normal swallowing patterns and the implications of tongue-thrust to occlusion. Without a documented digit-habit, palatal crib therapy directed specifically toward tongue-thrust swallowing as a "causative" factor seems questionable in the school-age child. This is based on the reasoning that without a documented extraoral habit, the most likely causative factors would be either a significant airway obstruction with habitual mouth-breathing or a skeletal open-bite pattern. Both of these situations require a much more comprehensive approach than simple interceptive appliance therapy. In fact, placement of a tongue-restricting palatal crib appliance could exacerbate airway problems by forcing the child to posture the mandible open to accommodate the appliance. The palatal crib design could actually make things worse. The same applies to a skeletal open-bite with the usual implications of a vertical growth pattern. In addition, the variability of normal swallowing patterns in relation to malocclusion and the spontaneous improvement in tongue-thrusting patterns and anterior open-bite that is evidenced in 80% of children by age 12 years argues against tongue-thrust directed therapy as a standalone treatment for open-bite.

Myofunctional therapy is the conscious retraining of the tongue and strengthening of the lip muscles through a specially designed exercise program. Promoted with the expectation that training muscles to function properly will reduce abnormal pressures, successive steps in the training program include acquainting the patient with the abnormal swallowing pattern, teaching the correct pattern of swallowing using various exercises, and reinforcing the correct patterns. Training exercises involve proper tongue-tip placement against the roof of the mouth and not between the teeth, masseter muscle isometrics to ensure swallowing with the molar teeth in contact, and lip exercises to correct mentalis and facial muscle activities. One technique has the patient practice swallowing correctly 20 times before each meal. Holding a glass of water in one hand and facing a mirror, the child takes a sip of water, closes the teeth into occlusion, places the tip of the tongue against the incisive papilla, and swallows. This is repeated and followed each time by the relaxation of the muscles until the swallowing progresses smoothly. The use of a sugarless mint may also help in muscle training. The child is instructed to use the tip of the tongue to hold a mint against the roof of the mouth until it melts. As the mint is held, saliva flows and makes it necessary for the child to swallow. Treatments are usually programmed to take from 7 to 10 weeks of exercises until the oral environment is stabilized. Most therapists prefer to wait until the child is about 9 years of age before beginning treatment as normal developmental changes occurring around this same time allow more favorable positioning of the tongue. After the patient has trained the tongue and muscles to function properly during swallowing, an acrylic palatal retainer with a "fence" may be constructed as a reminder to position the tongue properly during swallowing (Fig. 27-32).

In patients with tongue-thrust swallowing and a speech problem, referral to a speech therapist is the most appropriate course of action. If a malocclusion is also present, the coordinated use of myofunctional therapy by the speech therapist and orthodontic treatment may be undertaken to take advantage of each service. Generally, any therapy aimed at altering the tongue positions during swallowing and speech should be done in conjunction with or after the orthodontic treatment rather than preceding it. If mouth-breathing postures are identified with clinical symptoms of airway blockage, the dentist should refer the child to an otolaryngologist for appropriate medical consideration. Patients who are obligate mouth-breathers secondary to hypertrophic adenoid tissue or allergic conditions can have corresponding poor postural relationships that can influence the developing skeletal face. With proper diagnosis and management, the airway interferences may be reduced or eliminated to influence the occlusal development and orofacial musculature in a positive direction. In patients with tongue-thrust alone and no malocclusion, speech, or airway problems, there is no reason to recommend any interceptive orthodontic treatment.

ANTERIOR CROSSBITE IN THE PRIMARY AND MIXED DENTITIONS

Dentoalveolar anterior crossbite represents a linguoversion of one or more maxillary anterior teeth with resultant "locking" behind the opposing mandibular teeth in

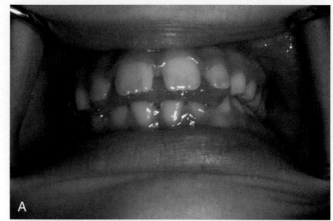

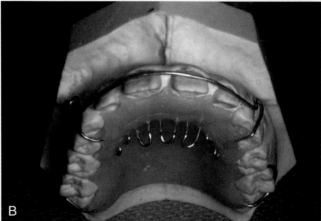

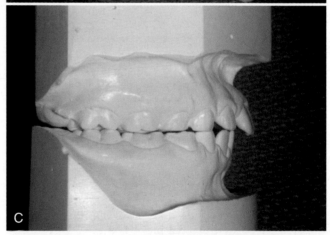

Figure 27-32 A, Anterior open-bite resulting from a tongue-thrust swallowing pattern. **B,** A removable retainer with a crib-like component helped "retrain" the tongue from being thrust forward during the swallowing process. **C,** The tongue-thrust pattern has been overcome and the occlusion is greatly improved.

full closure (Fig. 27-33). The anterior crossbite is usually an acquired malocclusion resulting from local etiological factors (e.g., over-retained primary incisors) that interfere with the normal eruptive positioning of the maxillary anterior teeth. In some cases during closure movements, premature contacts due to the lingual malpositioning may result in a forward mandibular deviation to effect full closure that "locks" the anterior segment in a crossbite

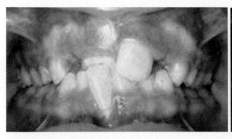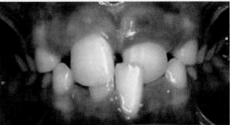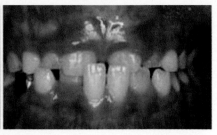

Figure 27-33 Examples of dentoalveolar anterior crossbites with lingually locked maxillary central incisors. The malpositioning with traumatic occlusion results in forward displacement of the lower incisor and stripping of the gingival tissues.

posture involving multiple teeth. Such an acquired muscular pattern is referred to as a pseudo-class III malocclusion as the mandible shifts from class I to class III relationships during closure (Fig. 27-34). In most cases, localized dentoalveolar anterior crossbites with or without mandibular displacement should be treated as soon as it is discovered. Delayed treatment can lead to serious complications such as loss of arch dimensions and asymmetric midlines, traumatic occlusion with stripping of gingival tissue on the labial aspect of the lower tooth, wear facets on involved incisors, and untoward growth patterns if a functional shift is involved. Importantly, at later developmental stages, differential diagnosis not only becomes more difficult, but the mechanics for correction become more complex with less predictable results. Diagnosed with consideration of the following clinical findings, simple appliance designs are usually adequate to achieve correction of dentoalveolar anterior crossbites.

1. *Number of teeth involved.* Involvement of one or two incisors usually represents a dental crossbite, although the chance of functional displacement is increased as more teeth are involved. Suspicion of a skeletal malocclusion grows in proportion to the number of teeth in crossbite.
2. *Inclinations of maxillary and mandibular incisors.* Dentoalveolar and functional crossbites usually exhibit lingual inclination of the maxillary incisors and normal to slight labioversion of the lower incisors in response to incisal interferences. Lower incisors are retroclined while maxillary incisors usually exhibit normal to proclined inclinations in a true skeletal class III malocclusion.
3. *Mandibular closure pattern and facial profile.* In a dentoalveolar crossbite, the facial profile and buccal occlusion

should present a neutroclusion at rest, first contact, and full closure with the soft tissues masking the dental malpositioning. Any displacement of the mandible should be observable as a shift from neutroclusion to class III buccal patterns "worsens" a normative profile at rest to an apparent prognathism in full closure. If the child can readily bite to an edge-to-edge incisor position without directed jaw manipulation, evidence of a forward shift of the mandible is confirmed. A class III skeletal malocclusion should close in a smooth pattern without anteroposterior disruption. A mesiocclusion of molar positioning and prognathism of the profile should persist at all times.
4. *Familial appearance.* If similar dentofacial conditions exist, the probability increases that the case involves a skeletal problem that is genetic in origin rather than a localized malocclusion.
5. *Cephalometric analysis.* Assessment of lateral cephalograms can usually confirm impressions of the clinical examination (See Chapter 26). Realizing that anterior displacement may demonstrate cephalometric measurements indicating mandibular prognathism when the cephalogram is obtained in full occlusion, analysis of centric relation cephalograms or overlay analysis of rest position and full occlusion tracings should be used to demonstrate true skeletal relationships. The inclination pattern of the upper and lower incisors is a key factor in this assessment.

Diagnosed in the transitional dentition, dentoalveolar anterior crossbites with or without mandibular displacement are usually approached from the viewpoint that the primary discrepancy involves one or more maxillary anterior teeth in linguoversion. Any labial inclination of

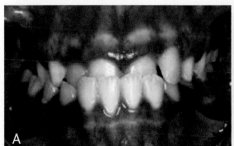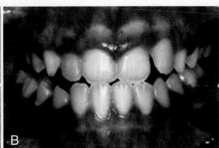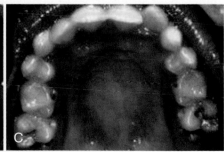

Figure 27-34 Lingually displaced central incisors may produce occlusal interferences on closure that result in a functional anterior shift of the mandible (pseudo-class III malocclusion). **A,** Maximum intercuspation after anterior shift of mandible. **B,** First contact with edge-to-edge incisor interferences. **C,** Maxillary incisors malpositioned lingual to arch form.

lower incisors is in response to the upper malpositioning. This simplifies treatment in that correction is directed toward labial movement of displaced maxillary incisors to "jump" the bite. After normal maxillary incisor positions are achieved, the proclination of lower incisors is usually self-correcting with the establishment of normal overbite and overjet. Studies have shown that gingival recession in the lower anterior segment improves spontaneously after crossbite correction. Removal of the traumatic occlusion allows normal attachment levels to be sustained without specific periodontal treatment procedures needed in the majority of cases. Assuming local etiologic factors such as over-retained primary incisors have been eliminated, one of several treatment methods may be selected. This is done after an evaluation of biomechanical decision factors such as the following:

1. *Incisor positioning and space available.* If space is available, options can be directed toward simple labial directed tipping movements of involved maxillary incisors. This particularly applies if the root of the lingual tooth is in the same relative position as it would occupy in normal occlusion. If space is not available or with greater bodily tooth displacement, Edgewise appliances may be required to create space and provide controlled orthodontic movements.

2. *Stage of eruption.* If the displaced maxillary incisor is in active eruption, the treatment may use simple leveraging techniques to redirect the tooth forward into acceptable position. If fully erupted, the forces of occlusion will usually not allow simple leveraging of eruption paths. Directed forces to effect labial repositioning of the involved maxillary anterior teeth will be required.

3. *Degree of overbite.* During treatment, occlusal bite planes are often proposed to remove overbite interferences during labial movement. Whereas this is desirable in the use of removable appliances and those incorporating labial bracketing of involved teeth, the 3- to 4-mm freeway space at rest position and use of directed lingual applied forces from fixed appliances negates the need for bite-opening in achieving successful labial movement in most clinical situations. Exceptions involve cases exhibiting more than 5 mm of overbite extending beyond freeway space. The overbite has greater impact on retention, in that positive overbite will maintain positioning of the incisors once corrected.

In addition to these factors, cooperation of the patient and parent as well as personal preference of the clinician are considerations in treatment mechanics. Treatment approaches are of two general types: (1) passive incisal guides that during mandibular closure redirect or "leverage" maxillary anterior inclinations in a labial orientation, and (2) active appliances that use directed orthodontic forces to achieve labial repositioning of the maxillary anterior teeth.

TONGUE BLADE/POPSICLE STICK THERAPY

Cooperative children can often correct a localized anterior crossbite using the wedging effect of a tongue blade or popsicle stick (Fig. 27-35). Teeth in initial eruption with a minimal degree of locking can often be repositioned

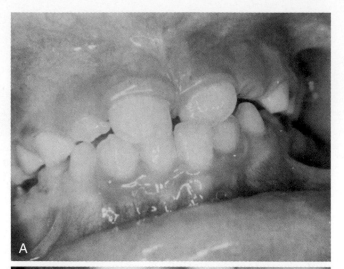

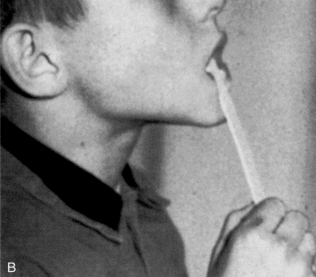

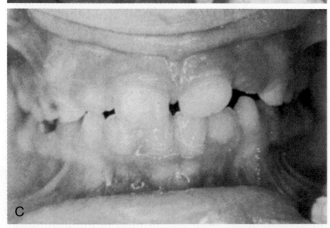

Figure 27-35 A, Partially erupted central incisor with a minimal degree of overbite and lingual locking. **B,** A tongue blade was used to exert labial directed pressure on the lingually locked incisor. **C,** Correction of the crossbite accomplished with the tongue blade.

within 24 to 72 hours. The child is instructed to place the stick behind the locked tooth and, using the chin as a fulcrum, exerts pressure on the tooth toward the labial. The procedure is done in 15- to 30-minute increments at a time for at least several hours of engagement. The obvious advantage of the technique is "self-correction" in avoiding the expense and time involved with appliance therapy. The technique is highly dependent upon the frequency, duration, and accuracy with which the child uses the leverage stick against an erupting incisor. While it is still possible to correct an established crossbite with intense tongue blade therapy, the treatment is very unlikely if the tooth is erupted into full crossbite.

LOWER INCLINED PLANE

An acrylic extension from the lower anterior teeth designed to engage the incisal edge of lingual displaced maxillary teeth during closure applies pressure upon patient closure that will direct the engaged tooth labial into normal bite position (Fig. 27-36). Prerequisites for an inclined plane are adequate space in the maxillary arch, a normal or excessive overbite, and sufficient mandibular teeth for retention of the acrylic. The inclined plane is constructed using self-curing resin on a working model to enclose the lower canine to canine anterior segment. This maximizes stability while preventing excessive lingual movement of the lower incisors. The acrylic should engage only the upper tooth or teeth in crossbite and incorporate approximately a 45-degree incline to the long axis of the lower incisors. The incline portion should extend about ¼ inch posteriorly such that the patient cannot readily bite behind the inclined plane.

At placement, the inclined plane is tried in the child's mouth before cementation to ensure only the locked upper incisor is in contact with the acrylic and the plane does not touch palatal tissue. The posterior "bite opening" should be slightly beyond rest position (not more than 2 to 3 mm) to avoid excessive muscle fatigue. This bite opening limits the time the appliance can be worn as eruption of posterior teeth may occur within 2 weeks and a tendency to an anterior open-bite may result. The physical activities of children with bite planes should be restricted to minimize the possibility of avulsion or luxation of the teeth that occlude on the plane from a blow to the chin. Follow-up should be made at 1 week with adequate bite jumping usually achieved within this time. If not "jumped" after 1-week, the inclined plane may be continued no more than an additional week. The appliance design and upper spacing should be evaluated for any interference to correction before continuing. The

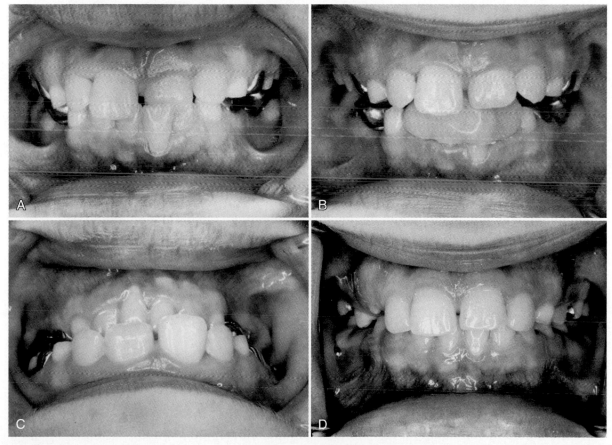

Figure 27-36 A, Essentially normal occlusion except for the central incisor crossbite. **B,** A lower cemented acrylic bite plane was used to reposition the lingually locked incisor. **C,** The tooth has moved into correct position with sufficient overbite to maintain the new relationship. **D,** Four years after the correction of the crossbite. Notice improvement in the appearance of the tissue on the labial surface of the lower left central incisor.

inclined plane should not be applied beyond this 2-week period due to the danger of overeruption of the posterior teeth and opening of the bite. If not corrected in this time, the original diagnosis may be in error or more controlled mechanics are indicated. Once achieved, the appliance should be carefully removed to allow final positional adjustments with the natural vertical overlap providing retention of the corrected positions.

The advantages of the inclined plane lie in ease of fabrication, simplicity of action, rapid correction time, and possible use when there is insufficient eruption to engage active appliances. Disadvantages include discomfort associated with forced bite opening, poor esthetics, limitations on diet, potential for gingival irritation, possibility of creating an open-bite, and, of particular concern, the risk of traumatic injury if the child hits their chin while the inclined plane is positioned in the mouth. In addition, the inclined plane may be dislodged by occlusal stress and require recementation. Given these disadvantages and the availability of other options that more predictable and safer, the use of acrylic inclined planes is generally to be avoided except when other options are simply not feasible.

PALATAL-SPRING APPLIANCES (REMOVABLE HAWLEY OR FIXED PALATAL WIRE)

A fixed or removable appliance incorporating palatal springs provides the best option for dental anterior crossbites that are not amenable to tongue-blade guidance. Properly oriented springs exert targeted labial directed pressures against the teeth from the palatal side and are not impacted by the reverse overjet. The major disadvantages are technical in nature - the finesse needed in engaging the spring to the involved tooth or teeth, adjustments if breakage occurs, modification for retention if overbite is not adequate, and untoward movements. These disadvantages may be readily overcome with proper fabrication and management of the appliance.

A removable Hawley-type retainer modified with auxiliary springs can reduce lingual displacement of maxillary incisors with correction usually achieved in 6 to 12 weeks (Fig. 27-37). A conventional Hawley retainer incorporating a labial bow and Adams clasps on the molars provides the base for the spring component. Although usually not necessary, the use of full posterior occlusal coverage enhances

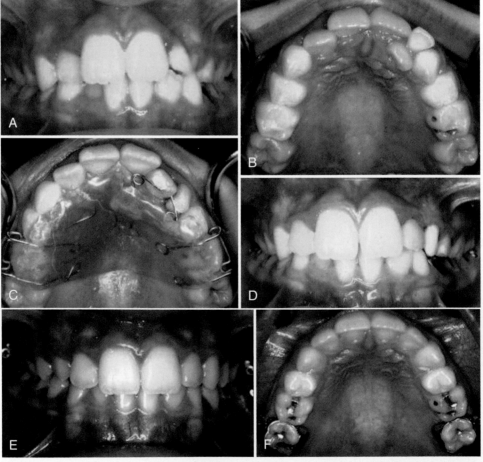

Figure 27-37 Removable Hawley-type finger-spring appliance **A** and **B,** Lingual locked permanent lateral incisor with retained primary lateral incisor and insufficient space for the lateral to move forward. **C,** A removable Hawley-type appliance with finger-spring designed to correct the condition. Note that the retained primary incisor was extracted and the mesial surface of the primary canine was disked to allow space for tooth movement. Activation of the spring with engagement under the lingual composite "button" resulted in labial movement of the tooth. **D,** The corrected occlusion at the time the appliance was discontinued. **E** and **F,** Same patient 3 years later without any intervening retention or other treatments. Bands have just placed in preparation for phase 2 braces.

effectiveness of a removable approach by minimizing any overbite interference to labial movement. Appliance action is enhanced by seating the appliance when in occlusion to more fully engage the finger-spring in counterbalancing displacement effects of spring engagement.

Incorporating a helical-loop finger-spring of 0.020 or 0.022 stainless steel wire, activation should represent 2 to 3 mm of helical loop closing from passive spring positioning that approximates the incisal edge of the contacted tooth. The spring tends to slide along the sloping lingual surface of the incisor to exaggerate tipping effects when activated. This problem can be overcome by bonding a small "button" of flowable composite on the lingual surface to create a retentive undercut for maintaining a cervical orientation of the spring. This optimizes labial movement with less tipping by orienting the force vector closer to the center of rotation of the engaged tooth. The composite should not interfere with vertical closure after the malposed tooth is moved out of crossbite (i.e., not placed too far incisally) while ensuring spring engagement by extending the mesiodistal width of the tooth.

FIXED TRANSPALATAL WIRES WITH SPRINGS

A transpalatal connector wire of 0.036 or 0.040 stainless steel soldered to banded molars that incorporates a helical-loop spring of 0.020 stainless steel wire provides a very effective method to labialize maxillary incisors involved in anterior crossbite (Fig. 27-38). The orientation of the spring essentially mirrors the procedures outlined for the removable Hawley appliance. Using the lingual composite button to engage the spring, the increased stability and rigidity of the fixed anchorage system

dramatically enhances directed forces toward the center of rotation of the engaged incisors. The fixed approach results in significantly less tooth tipping in offering a more bodily applied tooth movement and provides continuous force application that is not dependent on the child's cooperation. These factors combine to effect correction of dental anterior crossbites using a fixed spring approach with average treatment times of 1 to 3 weeks.

Abutment support may be from either second primary molars or first permanent molars depending on developmental and eruptive status, condition of the crown, and clinician choice. After fitting bands to selected abutments and preparing a working model, the anchor wire is bent to approximate the palatal arch form about 5 mm lingual to the anterior teeth in crossbite. This positioning provides accurate space for bending a compact double-helical loop spring as the active component. The maxillary incisors to be engaged should be cut off horizontally on the working model at the cingulum level to create a "table" to position the spring horizontally with proper length. Passively the helical loop extends from the anchor wire to rest on the cut-off incisal table with the free end of the spring at the labial surface. The original positioning of the palatal anchor wire about 5 mm behind the crossbite teeth provides this distance using a double-helical design. Careful soldering of the spring to the palatal wire completes the appliance in preparation for polishing.

Labial Edgewise Archwires

Edgewise brackets and labial archwire mechanics are used when multiple incisors are in crossbite, palatal displacement and rotations are severe, and adjacent tooth movements

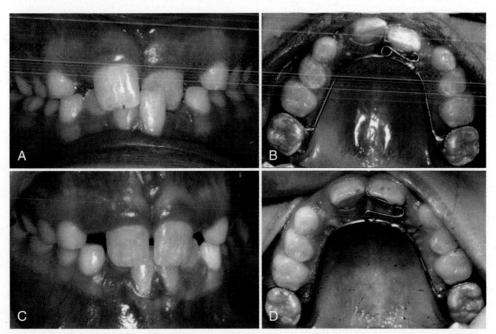

Figure 27-38 Fixed palatal finger-spring appliance. **A,** Lingual locked permanent central incisor with significant overbite. **B,** Fixed palatal appliance at delivery with double helical loop finger-spring designed to labialize the single incisor. Initial activation of the spring from a passive position at the labial surface to engage the lingual composite "button" resulted in directed movement of the tooth. **C,** The corrected occlusion at 17 days treatment time. **D,** The appearance of the spring at completion with the incisor out of crossbite. The lingual composite had been removed at 10 days treatment time to eliminate vertical interference with positioning.

are needed to adjust anterior spacing. While the clinician who wisely applies Edgewise techniques can achieve greater control in tooth positioning, their use presents major disadvantages in the early mixed dentition when most anterior crossbites are corrected. Disadvantages include increased chair-time in placement, adjustment, and removal, need for special equipment and supplies, increased soft tissue irritation, decalcification of teeth, risk of injury to developing teeth with excessive biomechanical movements, and the expectations and expenses associated with "braces." Discussion of Edgewise archwire techniques fall beyond the concepts of interceptive management and are illustrated in the section on Comprehensive Orthodontics.

POSTERIOR CROSSBITE IN THE PRIMARY AND MIXED DENTITIONS

Differential diagnosis and treatment of posterior crossbites in children must determine whether the discrepancy is a localized problem in tooth eruption (dental crossbite), a gross basal disharmony between the maxilla and mandible (skeletal crossbite), or a transverse discrepancy in upper to lower arch width that produces a lateral shift of the mandible on closure (functional crossbite). Dental posterior crossbites involve atypical eruption and alignment with localized displacement of individual teeth into crossbite configurations. Most often involving isolated permanent maxillary first molars or premolars, dental crossbites are usually corrected in conjunction with comprehensive Edgewise orthodontics. Within an interceptive context, isolated first permanent molar crossbites can be corrected by use of cross-arch elastics (Fig. 27-39). A hook or button (either bonded to enamel or welded onto bands) on the lingual surface of the upper molar and the buccal surface of the lower molar are employed to secure elastics. The elastics should be changed by the child or parent each day until the crossbite has been corrected. Typically, a crossbite involving isolated first molars can be corrected with cross-arch elastics in 4 to 8 weeks. If either of the opposing molars are in correct alignment before treatment, an anchorage appliance (lower lingual arch or upper Nance/Trans Palatal Bar) may help prevent movement of that tooth. The corrected cuspal interdigitation usually holds the teeth in their new relationship, so there is no need for a retentive appliance.

Skeletal posterior crossbites present as gross discrepancies in basal relationships of the maxilla and mandible, usually presenting a full bilateral crossbite with severe constriction of the maxilla (Fig. 27-40). Midlines are generally coincident to the facial midline in occlusion with no functional deviations observed on closure. The skeletal dysplasia is often complicated by other factors such as crowding of the maxillary teeth, anterior open-bite, and environmental factors that impede normal growth patterns (e.g., severe airway problems, cleft palate). Kurol and Berglund[33] found 4 of 86 crossbites in children, a relatively low frequency, presented as full bilateral crossbite. Modeer and associates[34] reported a similar 2% incidence of bilateral crossbites in children.

Functional posterior crossbites involve a lateral shift of the mandible during closure in response to transverse

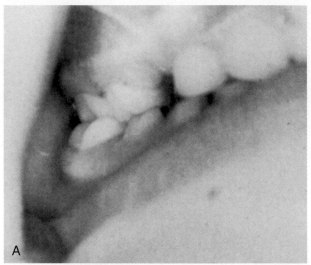

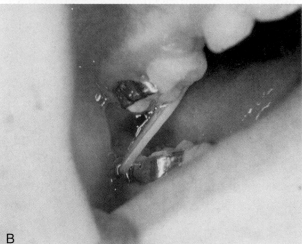

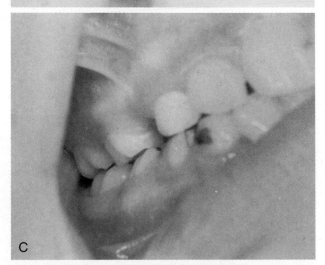

Figure 27-39 A, Buccal crossbite limited to the first permanent molars on the right side. **B,** Molar bands with hooks and cross-arch elastics from lingual of upper to buccal of lower are used to correct the crossbite. **C,** The crossbite has been corrected in a 4-week period.

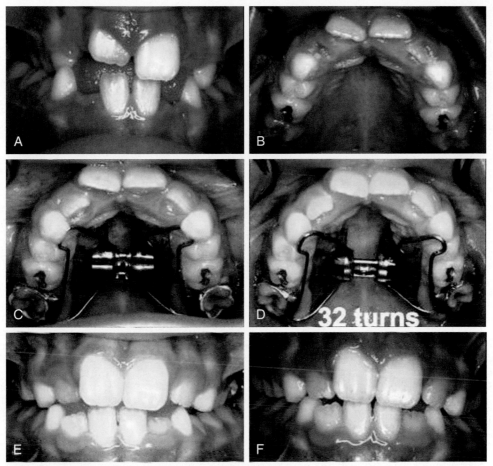

Figure 27-40 An acrylic jackscrew rapid palatal expander (Haas RPE) in the mixed dentition with bands on the permanent first molars and bonded composite on the primary canines. **A** and **B**, The pretreatment bilateral posterior crossbite with constricted and tapering maxillary archform. **C** and **D**, The rapid palatal expansion appliance appearance at cementation and after expansion involving 32 turns on a once-a-day schedule. **E**, The occlusion at 3 months with the appliance maintained for retention. **F**, The occlusion 1 year after appliance removal.

occlusal interferences between the maxillary and mandibular arch-widths. The deviation of the mandible presents as a unilateral crossbite in centric occlusion involving multiple posterior teeth on one side, normal buccolingual occlusion of the contralateral side, and a deviation of the lower midline and chin toward the crossbite side (Figs. 27-41 and 27-42). While presenting a unilateral appearance in occlusion, functional posterior crossbites show cusp-to-cusp transverse contacts bilaterally with a constricted maxillary arch of insufficient width to enclose the lower dentition at initial contact. Factors contributing to constriction in maxillary width include upright primary canine interferences, thumb and finger habits, and mouth-breathing/airway problems. Studies demonstrate a direct linear progression between prolonged digit and pacifier habits beyond the age of 4 years and a higher incidence of posterior crossbites.

Functional posterior crossbites are one of the more common occlusion problems observed in the primary and mixed dentitions with an incidence rate of 5% to 8% of children. Lindner and Modeer,[35] documenting patterns in 76 primary dentition children, reported three or more teeth (canines back) were involved in 85% of the crossbites

with two-thirds extended to include the primary lateral incisors. A lateral shift of the mandible was seen in 97% of the children, resulting in a lower midline discrepancy of about 2 mm on average. Other studies support the impression that more than 90% of posterior crossbites in children exhibit functional shifting of the mandible on closure as a component of the crossbite pattern. As a result of the functional shift, dental, skeletal, and neuromuscular adjustments likely result in further constriction of the maxillary arch, maldistribution of erupting teeth and alveolar bone, and asymmetric growth of the contralateral sides. Kutin and Hawes,[36] in a study of 35 children with posterior crossbite in the primary dentition followed into the mixed dentition, reported 32 of the children showed persistent crossbite of the first permanent molars after their eruption. Other studies also suggest posterior crossbites are generally not self-correcting as consistent incidence rates are shown in children 3, 6, 8, 10, and 12 years of age. It appears that less than 10% of posterior crossbites present in the primary dentition self-correct into the mixed dentition.

In conjunction with functional posterior crossbites, asymmetric condylar positioning has been demonstrated on tomograms and transcranial radiographs. Hesse and

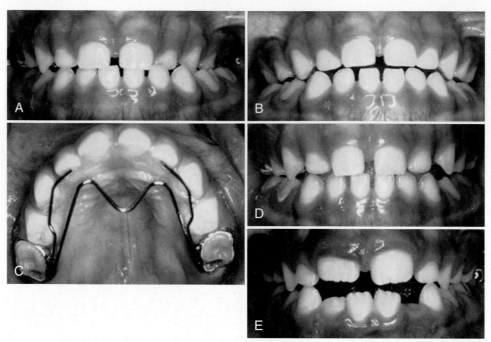

Figure 27-41 W-arch appliance. **A,** Functional posterior crossbite in the primary dentition in maximum intercuspation occlusion. Crossbite extends through buccal segment from the lateral incisor with a 2.5-mm mandibular midline shift to the affected side. **B,** In rest to first contact position, the dental midlines are normal with the posterior segments edge-to-edge bilaterally in transverse width. **C,** Soldered W-lingual arch appliance at cementation. **D,** The crossbite was corrected in 6 weeks with 2- to 3-mm overexpansion; the appliance was left in place for 3 months. Notice that the dental midlines are properly aligned with the functional shift eliminated. **E,** Two years posttreatment, the transverse posterior widths are in proper relationship with no mandibular shift evident during closure.

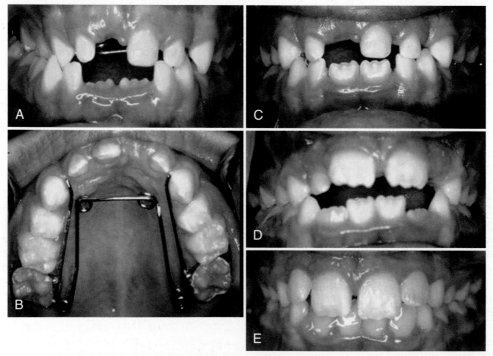

Figure 27-42 Quad-helix appliance. **A,** Functional posterior crossbite in the early transitional dentition in maximum intercuspation occlusion. Crossbite extends through buccal segment with a 1.5-mm mandibular midline shift to the affected side. **B,** Soldered quad-helix appliance at cementation. Note symmetrical and horizontal loop design for optimum expansion with minimal buccal tipping of molars. **C,** Occlusion 2 weeks after appliance removal. The crossbite was corrected in 4 weeks, the appliance left in place for 2 months. Dental midlines are properly aligned with the functional shift eliminated. **D,** Six months posttreatment, the transverse posterior widths remain in proper relationship with no mandibular shift evident during closure. **E,** Two years after treatment into mid mixed dentition with proper transverse relationships and no functional shift of mandible noted.

colleagues[37] documented condylar positioning using temporomandibular joint tomograms in 22 functional posterior crossbite patients corrected with maxillary expansion at a mean age of 8.5 years. The condyle on the noncrossbite side was positioned more anterior before treatment and moved posteriorly and superiorly after treatment. The condylar position was similar at pretreatment and posttreatment stages on the crossbite side. Importantly, correction of the crossbite with maxillary expansion established symmetry of condylar relationships in all planes of space. Myers and associates[38] similarly reported that joint spaces were asymmetric in pretreatment functional cross-bite children while correction led to symmetry of condylar joint spaces. Pirtiniemi and colleagues,[39] comparing condylar path and mandibular length in nine unilateral posterior crossbite children treated using maxillary expansion between the ages of 5 to 8 years with a group of 13 subjects with untreated crossbites into young adulthood, reported the condylar path evidenced asymmetry in both treated and untreated subjects with greater steepness and condylar rotation on the crossbite side. The eminence was flatter in both groups on the noncrossbite side while mandibular length was shorter on the crossbite side. In comparing the groups, the degree of mandibular asymmetric length was twice as great in untreated subjects versus children with treated posterior crossbites. Other studies confirm displacement of the mandible in growing children produces asymmetric mandibular length with the crossbite side shorter than the noncrossbite side. The mandibular rotation also results in a sagittal asymmetry of contralateral sides with the crossbite side expressing a more distal step–class II relationship and the noncrossbite side a more class I to class III pattern. Even though correction with maxillary expansion improved molar positioning toward class I positions on the crossbite side and reduced the midline discrepancy, full establishment of symmetrical relationships after correction is not a consistent finding. The continuation of some degree of asymmetry after correction suggests unbalanced growth occurred to the time of correction, after correction more balanced symmetry of the growth patterns was expressed, and any acquired pretreatment morphological asymmetry remains after correction.

Early correction of posterior crossbites has been shown to enhance developmental patterns by redirecting teeth into more normal positions, correcting asymmetries of condylar position, allowing normal vertical closure without functional deviations, making beneficial dentoskeletal changes during periods of dynamic growth, and eliminating factors detrimental to dentofacial development. Early treatment also allows simplified approaches that are less complex, less time consuming, and more physiologically tolerable to structural tissues than treatment demands in older patients. Delaying correction until the permanent dentition requires more complex mechanics to achieve basal arch corrections and may necessitate surgical approaches to achieving maxillary expansion.

Selective Equilibration

Selective equilibration of deflective interferences, usually the primary canines, may enhance differences between intercanine widths and offer some potential for functional crossbite correction without appliances. The equilibration involves selective reduction (i.e., slanting) of the lingual aspects of the upper primary canines and labial reduction of the lower primary canines. Selective grinding, according to Lindner,[40] is successful when the maxillary intercanine width difference is larger than the mandibular intercanine width by a positive 2 to 3 mm before the selective grinding. When the upper-to-lower intercanine width approximates the same width or the lower is greater, selective grinding is not effective and upper canine expansion is required. In most full primary or mixed dentition cases, equilibration procedures alone are insufficient to eliminate a functional discrepancy associated with a constricted maxillary dentoalveolar width.

MAXILLARY EXPANSION

Appliances employed for maxillary expansion in the correction of posterior crossbites include fixed palatal wire designs (e.g., W-arch, quad-helix), fixed jackscrew expanders (e.g., Hyrax, RPE of Haas) and removable split-acrylic plate appliances (e.g., Schwarz Plate). Successful treatments during the primary and mixed dentitions have been documented for the fixed approaches at greater than a 90% success rate and for removable appliances at 70% success. Dimensional changes have documented that early expansion techniques to correct posterior crossbites in children require an average final overall increase of about 3 to 4 mm in intramolar width and 2 to 3 mm of intracanine width change for successful correction. The clinical reports further indicate that expansion protocols, regardless of appliance used, should incorporate an overexpansion of about 2 to 3 mm beyond these final desired increments during the active phase to accommodate settling adjustments after treatment.

Transverse expansion of the maxillary arch is directed at a combination of dentoalveolar expansion and orthopedic separation of the midpalatal suture. It is considered desirable to optimize opening of the midpalatal suture to provide more stable basal arch expansion than orthodontic oriented lateral expansion. The nature of orthodontic and orthopedic movements is closely related to the rate of expansion, the magnitude of force application, and the patient's developmental stage in considering the appliance options. Fixed palatal jackscrew appliances, such as the RPE of Haas (see Fig. 27-40) and the Hyrax (Fig. 27-43), are applied bilaterally to maxillary posterior teeth with the midline screw generally expanded at a rate of one to two turns per day (one turn equals 0.25 mm of screw widening) during an active treatment time of 1 to 4 weeks. Single activations of fixed jackscrews produce high magnitude forces in the 3- to 10-pound range that maximize orthopedic separation by overwhelming suture tissues before substantial orthodontic movement can occur. The relative skeletal and dental components produced by rapid palatal expansion have been evaluated using standardized non-anatomic reference points (e.g., implants) and frontal cephalograms. Krebs[41] reported average arch-width increases of 6 mm (range, 0.5 to 10.3 mm) for 23 subjects aged 8 to 19 years with the total dental arch increase twice that of the skeletal segments. Analyzing the Krebs data, Hicks[42] estimated skeletal separation accounted for

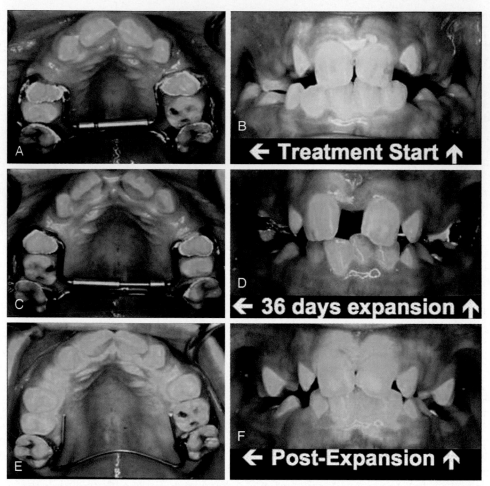

Figure 27-43 Hyrax appliance in late transitional dentition with bands on the permanent first molars and first premolars. **A,** The Hyrax appliance at cementation **B,** The pretreatment bilateral posterior crossbite with symmetrical but constricted maxillary archform. **C** and **D,** Appliance and occlusion appearance after expansion involving 36 turns on a once-a-day schedule. The large midline diastema reflects orthopedic separation of the mid-palatal suture. **E** and **F,** The occlusion at 6 months postexpansion. The Hyrax was maintained for 5 months, then replaced with fixed the transpalatal appliance for retention.

approximately one half of increased arch width in 8- to 12-year-olds and about one third of the increase in 13- to 19-year-old subjects. Retention periods using fixed appliances of 3 to 6 months (e.g., expanded appliance, transpalatal bar) are recommended to allow reorganization and stabilization of rapidly expanded maxillary sutures.

Fixed palatal wire appliances (e.g., W-arch, quad-helix) accomplish maxillary expansion following "low-force" and "slow-expansion" procedures compared with the jackscrew appliances. Thomas and colleagues[43] determined W-arch (see Fig. 27-41) and quad-helix (see Fig. 27-42) designs with 6 to 8 mm of expansion produced lateral forces in the range of 400 to 600 g (approximating 1 pound) at the molar positions and from 200 to 300 g at the canine level. Some degree of sutural separation has been documented during the primary and mixed dentition stages using forces in these ranges. Hicks, using less than 2-pound forces in achieving maxillary arch width increases from 3.8 to 8.7 mm during treatment, estimated skeletal changes represented 24% to 30% of the total arch width increase in 10- to 11-year-old subjects and 16% in 14- to 15-year-old patients. Although they did not

document the relative ratios of orthopedic versus orthodontic change, Harberson and Myers[44] reported radiographic evidence of suture opening during the deciduous and early mixed dentition in 8 of 10 successfully corrected posterior crossbites using a W-arch appliance. Bell and Lecompte[45] reported suture separation on each of 10 subjects (x age = 6 y. 9 m.) using quad-helix appliances with mean increases of maxillary intermolar width of +5.3 mm and maxillary intercanine width of +4.1 mm in successfully correcting functional posterior crossbites The conceptual model of fixed palatal wire appliances in the primary and mixed dentitions is that favorable orthopedic and orthodontic ratios of expansion are realized with less disruption than rapidly expanded sutures. Because of the "physiologic" nature of the expansion, the integrity of tissue elements is sustained to allow enhanced stabilization of the changes with retention periods of 3 months or less appearing adequate.

The palatal wire W-arch and quad-helix designs offer the advantages of increased molar rotational ability, relative comfort, minimal effect on speech and deglutition, reduced soft tissue irritation, and removal of adjustment responsibility from the patient-parent. Posterior crossbites in the full primary dentition are usually treated at ages 4 to 5 years with banding of the deciduous second molars. In the mixed dentition period (i.e., age 6 to 11 years), the first permanent molars are generally banded for posterior crossbite correction. During the active eruption stage of the first permanent molars, from about 6 months before emergence until opposing occlusion is established, maxillary expansion procedures should usually be delayed. The first permanent molars may not be affected by expansion of the deciduous dentition during this transitional stage and may erupt into crossbite, thus requiring additional treatment. Delaying expansion until the first permanent molars are in occlusion results in no significant technical problems related to treatment. The Hyrax jackscrew appliance becomes the priority choice for maxillary expansion when gross discrepancies in basal relationships present as full bilateral crossbites, when there is pronounced maxillary constriction with severe crowding of the maxillary teeth, and when other factors suggest the use of a rapid palatal expansion to exaggerate orthopedic over orthodontic movements. True bilateral posterior crossbites require twice as much incremental expansion as needed in functional crossbites, bringing into play the greater increments achievable with fixed jackscrew appliances. Older patients in the late mixed and young permanent dentition (i.e., the 10- to 16-year-old) require higher force systems of rapid palatal expanders given an increasing resistance to sutural separation. Additionally, the transitional status of exfoliating primary and erupting permanent teeth in the late mixed dentition may complicate anchorage options in using palatal wire appliances. The Hyrax is used until growth is complete (girls 16 to 17 years; boys 18 to 21 years) with sutural separation anticipated during the earlier stages of this developmental period. After retention, regardless of whether jackscrew or palatal wire-type appliances were used in treatment, the laterally tipped dental elements will upright. This dental relapse must be factored into the active expansion and retention phases.

The soldered W-arch uses a 0.036 or 0.040-inch steel wire contoured to the arch from bands on the most distal teeth involved in the crossbite. The wire is expanded to the bilateral width of the central fossae of the banded molars before cementation such that the appliance must be compressed 2 to 3 mm bilaterally to place it on the banded teeth. It is reactivated by being removed for additional adjustment every 3 or 4 weeks if necessary until the crossbite has been corrected (see Fig. 27-41). The appliance may be used as a retainer for 3 to 6 months after active treatment. The soldered W-arch is very stable with its primary use in situations that require 4 to 5 mm of maxillary buccal expansion such as typically required in functional posterior crossbites. Some palatal expansion may occur with the W-arch.

The quad-helix appliance, by incorporating four helical loops into the W-arch design, provides refined adjustment capability in providing a longer range of force application (see Fig. 27-42). For that reason, quad-helix treatment is emphasized, although the basic W-arch design follows similar protocols. The quad-helix is fabricated from 0.036 stainless steel wire with the loops equal in size to optimize symmetrical expansion and the "cosmetic" look of the appliance. The anterior loops should be at the level of the canines and approximate the palatal width to minimize the space between the crossbar and the palatal contour. All loops should be as horizontal as possible with the anterior loops circling toward the palate at the level of the primary canines and the posterior loops away from the palate. This places the helical loop section and the lateral expansion forces in a more palatal position for enhanced expansion effects. The posterior loops should extend approximately 2 to 3 mm distal to the molar bands for enhanced molar rotation and expansion.

The progress of expansion is followed as described for the W-arch appliance using a 2- to 3-week appointments interval. Adjustments are made only when progress between successive appointments is static and the amount of increased arch width is inadequate. Expansion is considered adequate when the occlusal aspect of the maxillary lingual cusps contact the occlusal slope of the mandibular buccal cusps in representing approximately 2 to 3 mm of overexpansion to compensate for later uprighting of laterally tipped teeth once appliances are removed. Successful expansion with slight overcorrection is usually achieved in 4 to 6 weeks. If an adjustment is necessary, the appliance should be removed for activations to ensure appropriate expansion increments both in amount and location. Activations consist of again opening with finger "accordion" type action or incorporating strategic bends along the wire lengths to increase lateral expansion. Bends can be done intraorally, but tend to create compensating adjustments such that multiple intraoral activations frequently produce untoward movements. The appliance is left in the expanded position to serve as a retainer with a recommended minimum retention period of at least 3 months. Longer periods are suggested if the patient has a history of oral habits (e.g., thumb sucking, mouth-breathing, tongue thrusting) or exhibits continued functional inconsistencies in mandibular closure. While using the appliance as its own retainer is convenient, the possibility of continued expansion into buccal crossbite must be realized. Thus supervision during "retention" with a monthly monitoring schedule is desirable. Heat annealing of the appliance may also be considered or the clinician may use a follow-up Hawley-type retainer.

Fixed Hyrax jackscrews are preferred for bilateral posterior crossbites with pronounced maxillary constriction that require 6 to 8 mm of expansion to correct the transverse discrepancy and in older patients where sutural integrity requires greater force magnitudes to achieve basal arch changes (see Fig. 27-43). Expansion effects with the Hyrax appliance are closely related to the rigidity of the appliance, positioning of the jackscrew relative to the palatal archform, and resistance of the maxillary complex. Banded designs reinforced with buccal and lingual connector wires between multiple abutments demonstrate the most rigidity in design. If employed in the mixed dentition, the first permanent molars and second primary molars provide excellent anchorage for the appliance. In the adolescent dentition, anchorage usually involves first permanent molars and either first or second premolars. These appliances have been shown to generate the greatest orthopedic response when positioned high in the palatal contour and as far posterior toward molar positions as possible. Given the force levels generated, an activation rate of one turn per day is advised to achieve expansion on the order of 6 to 8 mm (24 to 32 turns) during an active treatment time approximating 1 month. After sufficient expansion is obtained, the appliance is left in place for 6 months to allow reorganization of the expanded suture and enhanced stability of achieved arch width.

ERUPTION PROBLEMS AND ERUPTION "GUIDANCE"

Abnormal eruption patterns with resultant ectopic displacement, asymmetry of alignment, disruption in arch integrity and crowding are all benchmarks of a tooth size–arch size discrepancy. In addition, local factors such as supernumerary teeth, congenital absence or malformation of permanent successors, necrosis or dystrophic calcification of a primary tooth secondary to trauma or caries, and ankylosis of primary molars may present barriers to normal eruption and alignment. The watchword for evaluation should be in monitoring the sequence and symmetry of eruption patterns with a basic rule that the transition should be about the same for contralateral segments.

ECTOPIC ERUPTION OF FIRST PERMANENT MOLARS

First permanent molars may be positioned too far mesially in their eruption path with resultant ectopic resorption of the distal root of the second primary molar. Bjerklin and Kurol[46] distinguished two types of ectopic eruption—reversible and irreversible. In the reversible type, the molar frees itself from the ectopic position and erupts into normal alignment with the second primary molar remaining in position (Fig. 27-44). Most permanent molars in children with reversible patterns had freed themselves by 7 years of age. In the irreversible type, the maxillary first molar remains unerupted and in contact with the cervical root area of the second primary molar (Fig. 27-45). By the age of 7 and 8 years, any ectopic eruption of a permanent first molar should be considered irreversibly locked. Young[47] observed that ectopic eruption of first permanent molars occurred 52 times in 1619 children (3%), with the problem seen more frequently in boys (33 times) than in girls (19 times). The ectopic molar often occurred in more than one quadrant, and was most often observed in the maxilla (only two ectopic lower first molars were noted). Young[47] further observed that two thirds of ectopic molars erupted into their essentially normal position without corrective treatment (reversible). Bjerklin and Kurol[46] also reported that children with irreversible ectopic eruption patterns had significantly larger permanent first molars, a more pronounced mesial angle path of eruption, and a tendency toward a shorter maxilla in relation to the cranial base. No significant differences in these variables were found between sides with reversible ectopic eruption and sides with normal eruption. Ectopic molars also show a significant familial tendency with a prevalence of 19.8% in

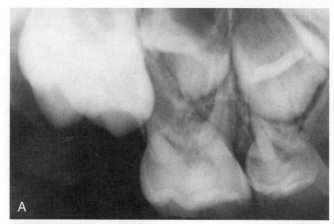

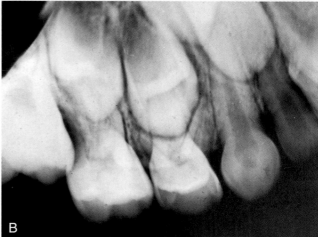

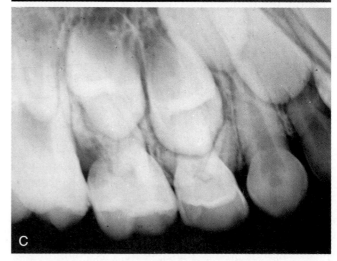

Figure 27-44 A, Ectopic eruption of a maxillary first permanent molar with evidence of resorption of the distal buccal tooth of the second primary molar. **B** and **C,** Subsequent radiographs show continued resorption of the primary molar, but "self-corrective" eruptive positioning of the first permanent molar. Approximately two thirds of ectopic molars are reported to exhibit such a "reversible" pattern.

affected siblings versus the overall 2% to 3% general occurrence. A frequent occurrence rate of ectopic first permanent molars at 25% in cleft lip and cleft palate children again implicates maxilla positioning and basal arch size as etiologic factors.

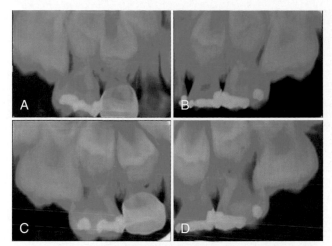

Figure 27-45 A and **B,** Periapical radiographs demonstrating bilateral ectopic eruption of maxillary first permanent molars with resorption of the distal aspect of the second primary molars. **C** and **D,** Subsequent radiographs obtained at 6-month recall showing "irreversible" pattern of ectopic eruption with continued resorption of the primary molars and greater mesial displacement of the first permanent molars.

Irreversible ectopic molars that remain locked, if untreated, can lead to premature loss of the primary second molar with a resultant decrease in quadrant arch length, asymmetric shifting of the upper first molar toward class II positioning, and supraeruption of the opposing molar with distortion of the lower curve of Spee and potential occlusal interferences. Early assessment with intraoral or panoramic films approximating first permanent molars eruption timing is thus critical to identify the problem and provide the opportunity to intercept potential sequelae. If detected at 5 to 6 years of age, an observation approach of "watchful waiting" with appropriate monitoring may be indicated given the two thirds potential for self-correction. With self-correction being unlikely approaching 7 years of age, continued "locking" of the first molar with advanced resorption of the primary second molar usually warrants intervention. Another timing clue is that when the opposing molar reaches the level of the lower occlusal plane, intervention is indicated to establish proper vertical control and prevent supraeruption. Because the anomaly often occurs bilaterally in conjunction with a tooth mass discrepancy, the finding should result in careful examination of other areas for similar conditions.

Interceptive correction involves guidance of the ectopic molar into normal position, retention of a favorable eruption sequence, and maintenance of arch length. Importantly, the resorptive process of the primary molar generally stops once the ectopic positioning is corrected and the tooth remains to stabilize arch integrity. One option is to restore the second primary molar with pulpotomy and a stainless steel crown supplemented with band material extending subgingivally to rest mesial to the ectopic molar. Designed to serve as a guide for eruption positioning, the extension must be carefully placed so as not to exaggerate

molar entrapment. The technique seems simple, but is actually very difficult to do and should generally be avoided. A number of other corrective procedures have been reported with treatments varied by the extent of blockage, degree of primary tooth resorption, direction of displacement, timing, arch length status, and patient cooperation. Approaches include separators and distalizing appliances.

Orthodontic elastic separators are the first choice if access is sufficient to allow insertion for engagement in the contact areas of entrapment. The first placement is the most difficult and often requires a modified separator and floss engagement. This is done by looping floss through the separator, passing the floss through the contact area, pulling the doubled separator into the cervical area of contact, and then pulling one side of the separator through the contact with the floss. Progressive use of larger separators placed conventionally—from smaller, stretchier elastic types to more rigid plastic types—at subsequent visits facilitates this approach. Replacement at 1- to 2-week intervals usually accomplishes correction within 2 months. Separating springs can also be used provided sufficient eruption for insertion between the contact areas. However, separating springs tend to impinge upon tissues and are easily displaced with concerns as to swallowing or aspiration. If used, insertion is most easily achieved by grasping the active arm of the spring with How or Weingardt pliers. Floss looped through the helix serves as a safety device if the spring slips out of the pliers. The head of the spring is placed on the marginal ridge while the active arm is directed below the contact point of the teeth. The spring may be inserted from the buccal or lingual side (whichever provides the greatest access); the buccal approach is usually easier. The spring is left in place until the tooth has freed contact with the adjacent tooth and is erupting. The patient should be seen every 2 to 3 weeks for evaluation of eruption progress and reactivation of the spring.

Brass ligature wire threaded between the contact areas of the affected teeth may facilitate distal movement of the permanent molar through periodic tightening of the looped wire as a separating force. The wire should be twisted or a new one placed at approximately 3- to 5-day intervals until the desired separation is achieved. Brass wire usage is uncomfortable and local anesthetic is often required; the brass wire usually has to be replaced one or more times before correction is achieved, relapses easily, and in essence is vastly overrated. Treatment with any of the separator techniques requires that only a minimal lock be evidenced and that minimal resorption of the primary second molar has occurred. Of the three, elastic separators are much easier to employ and are much less problematic for minimal locks than either separating springs or brass wire.

Irreversible ectopic eruptions may require the use of distally directed forces from the second primary molars to disengage and allow eruption of the first permanent molar. The Humphrey appliance employs a distally directed S-shaped loop that is actively engaged onto the occlusal surface of the ectopically erupting permanent molar (Fig. 27-46). In original usage, it was often necessary to

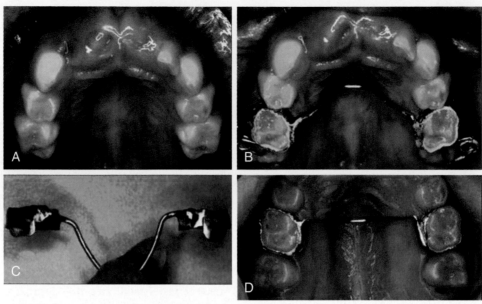

Figure 27-46 Distalizing spring (Humphrey) appliance. **A,** Bilateral ectopic eruption of the maxillary first permanent molars. **B,** A Humphrey-type banded appliance with distalizing springs has been fabricated to reposition the ectopic first permanent molar. The ectopic molars were uncovered at the time of band fitting. At placement, composite ridges were bonded to the occlusal surfaces for spring engagement. **C** and **D,** After distal repositioning of the first permanent molar was achieved, the appliance was removed, springs were cut off, and band material tach-welded to provide extensions to maintain first permanent molar eruption into favorable positions.

remove the appliance for activations of the loop and a restoration was required in the first molar after correction. The advantages were stability and ability to correct severe locks of the 6-year molar. Subsequent modifications to the original Humphrey design include the use of helical springs (0.018 to 0.022 wire) to provide more continual force and easier reactivations, added stability by anchoring banded molars bilaterally with a palatal wire, using springs from buccal and lingual aspects to minimize rotations of the permanent molar, and using bonded composite resins to engage the distalizing springs. Problems in activation and adjustment of the spring, possible occlusal interferences distorting the wire, need for access to the occlusal surface of the first permanent molar, and possible reciprocal movement of primary molars are all disadvantages. Once distalized, the spring needs to be removed to allow vertical eruption of the molar to ensure correction. To prevent relapse of the molar back into the undermined area, band extensions are tack-welded to the distal aspect of the band and the appliance is recemented.

The Halterman appliance uses elastomeric chains rather than springs as the distalizing force (Fig. 27-47). Using a rigid 0.036 stainless steel wire "hook" extended distally from the lingual aspect of bands on the second primary molars, stretching of elastomeric chains from bonded buttons on the ectopic molar essentially "slingshots" the molar distally. Extending the wire from the lingual of the primary molar avoids wire impingement with the anterior border of the ramus during opening. The wire should approximate the palatal contour with the hook positioned horizontally to approximate the buccolingual midpoint of the desired molar location and about 5 mm beyond the distal marginal ridge of the involved permanent molar. This position provides adequate stretch of the elastic forces in a vertical and parallel orientation to normal arch alignment. An occlusal button, cleat, or bracket is bonded to the central fossae area of the ectopic first molar as far mesially as accessible. Clinician-preferred (i.e., self or light-cured) resin bonding is used with success dependent on avoidance of moisture contamination. Hybrid glass ionomer cements that allow moisture exposure and do not require acid etching are an alternative if isolation is compromised. In placement, the elastomeric chain should already be secured to the button during the bonding process to ensure composite material does not extend into undercut areas and block elastic engagement. After bonding the button, the appliance is cemented and the elastomeric chain stretched to the distal hook. Closed-loop chain is recommended for enhanced force application. Being relatively simple to apply as well as predictable and effective, the Halterman distalizing technique is currently the preferred method when elastic separators are not applicable.

ERUPTION GUIDANCE IN THE LOWER INCISOR SEGMENT

Developmental patterns often find permanent lower incisors erupting into a lingual position behind the primary incisors as a "double-row" of teeth. While the majority of these cases self-correct via eventual exfoliation, if not self-corrected by age 8 years, extraction of the primary incisor may be necessary (see Chapter 9). The tongue usually positions the permanent incisor forward into normal alignment. In conjunction with eruption of lower lateral incisors, there is a normative increase in lower intercanine width of 2 to 3 mm with a range from 0 to 5 mm. This

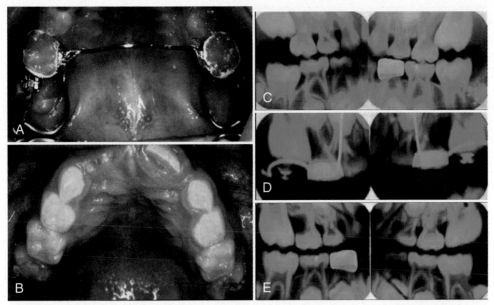

Figure 27-47 Fixed Maxillary Halterman appliance. **A,** Bands on second primary molars with distal engagement arms for engaging elastomeric chains to bonded attachments on bilateral ectopic first permanent molars. **B,** The first permanent molar has erupted into a favorable position after six weeks treatment time. Radiographs showing distal repositioning of the first permanent molar from pretreatment **(C)**, at 2 weeks of treatment **(D)**, to 1 year posttreatment **(E)**.

"growth" in lower anterior space helps compensate for the inherent tooth mass liability. After the lower permanent incisor transition is complete by 7 to 8 years of age, the "normative" finding presents almost 2 mm of incisor crowding. Studies document no future increase in lower intercanine width for relief of crowding will occur after this stage of incisor eruption is complete. However, extra space is available within the overall arch as represented by the size difference between the primary canines and primary molars versus the permanent canines and premolars. This "leeway space" represents a plus 1.7 mm on average in each lower quadrant and provides potential for the relief of lower incisor crowding. Gianelly,[11] reporting on 100 consecutive mixed dentition children presenting for orthodontic needs, found that 85 of the children presented lower incisor crowding, with an average crowding discrepancy of −4.4 mm, a discrepancy significantly greater than population averages of approximately 2 mm. When leeway space was calculated into a space analysis, adequate room to accommodate an aligned dentition was indicated in 72% of the subjects with crowding. Given this potential, if an overall space analysis indicates a child's arch perimeter is adequate to accommodate or be within 2 to 3 mm of relieving any incisor mal-alignment, the clinician should consider options to facilitate adjustments through guidance of eruption and timely use of the available leeway space.

A first option when incisor crowding is less than 3 to 4 mm involves disking the primary canines on their mesiolingual surfaces. Timely disking provides a "sluiceway" for lingual displaced incisors to slide forward toward the anterior arch form under the muscular pressure of the tongue (Fig. 27-48). Bilateral disking can provide up to 2 to 3 mm of space for "unraveling" of lingual displaced incisors. With proper slicing of the mesiolingual corner at the gingival contact area, there is actually no measurable encroachment on overall leeway space in the individual quadrant. Movement of the incisors under tongue pressure potentially increases midline arch length and overall arch circumference as the arch is rounded out in a forward direction. In the case of labial malpositioned incisors, while disking may provide additional room for alignment, the lips are a more significant factor in the balance between muscular forces. The result is lingual flattening of the anterior segment and a decrease in overall arch space. Disking must involve slicing the canine subgingivally to completely free the contact area. Disking just the crown is not enough. The use of a tapered bur of a size to allow access without injury to adjacent permanent teeth is required (#699 or #169). Local anesthesia or nitrous oxide support is frequently required as dentin exposure and periodontal insult are necessary to adequately disk primary canines. Placement of a wedge is sometimes necessary to protect the lateral incisor. Timing is critical to allow optimal tooth positioning and ease of access. Given normative intercanine width increases of 2 to 3 mm during lateral incisor eruption, disking should be delayed until eruptive "wedging" effects of the incisors are realized. If indicated, disking of lower primary canines is therefore recommended around 7 to 8 years of age in proximity to completion of the lateral incisor eruption.

While excessive incisor liability may result in ectopic loss of lower primary canines (reviewed earlier in this chapter), more often the primary canines remain and the permanent incisors erupt significantly malpositioned. If disking of the canines is not an option due to the level of crowding or positioning of the incisors, elective extraction of the primary canines to maintain arch symmetry, coincident midlines, and incisor integrity may be considered (Fig. 27-49). Such intervention becomes more viable when the incisor liability and crowding is greater than

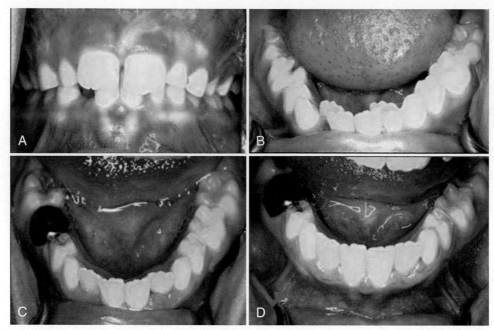

Figure 27-48 Incisor guidance with disking of lower primary canines. **A** and **B,** Presentation of approximately 4.5 mm of lower incisor crowding with lingual malpositioning of lateral incisors, retained lower left primary lateral, and 80% overbite. Given significant overbite and positioning of incisors, decision made to disk the lower primary canines bilaterally in conjunction with restorative appointments. **C,** Same patient at 6-month recall appointment after disking. Slight additional disking of canines was done at recall. **D,** Same patient at 1 year from start of first disking. Archform is established as the tongue pressures positioned the lingual displaced incisors forward into the spaces created by disking.

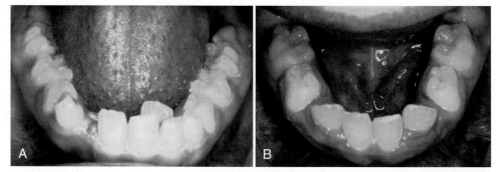

Figure 27-49 Elective extraction of lower primary canines. **A,** Significant lower incisor crowding and malpositioning evidenced by advanced lower right primary canine resorption with ectopic positioning of adjacent lateral incisor, lower dental shifting toward right, and retained lower left primary lateral. Due to imminent loss of the lower right canine and malpositioning, a decision was made to extract the primary canines bilaterally. **B,** Same patient 1 year later with symmetry and integrity of lower incisor alignment. Patient is on course for either serial extraction protocol or setup for arch development dependent upon other variables.

4 mm in the anterior segment. However, the clinician must remember early loss of lower primary canines will likely result in significant lower arch collapse. Therefore the extraction of primary canines should not be undertaken without parental understanding of the consequences and, ideally, orthodontic consultation. Given the long-term implications, such intervention goes beyond a first step in guidance of eruption and actually represents the start of either a phased early treatment program or a serial extraction program.

ERUPTION GUIDANCE IN THE MANDIBULAR CANINE AND PREMOLAR SEGMENT

Between 10 and 12 years of age, radiographic evaluation of the buccal segments provides particular considerations in eruption guidance as to primary resorption patterns, eruption sequencing, molar adjustments to achieve class I relationships, and usage of leeway space. Because the lower canine and first premolar often erupt in approximate timing to one another and are larger than their primary predecessors, they often take a mesial eruption path with the canine over-lapping the lateral incisors. To minimize such malpositioning, their timely transition along with concurrent disking of the mesial surface of the second primary molar may provide up to 2 to 3 mm of space for their distal positioning (Fig. 27-50). The second premolars usually erupt about a year later, frequently taking a path of eruption along the distal root of the second primary molar. Extraction of the second primary molar is sometimes indicated to allow normal eruption of the second premolar if such an atypical pattern is noted. In addition to assessing eruption of the second premolars, consideration should be given to placement of a lingual holding arch concurrent with removal or exfoliation of the second primary molars (see Fig. 27-18). If the available buccal segment space is tight, the optimal use of leeway space for crowding is desirable, and/or the second permanent molars are erupting before the second premolars, the lingual arch may be a critical element in controlling overall arch dimensions.

Treatment-based articles have documented positive alignment effects in the use of passive lingual holding arches for control of leeway space when employed in the late mixed dentition. DeBaets and Chiarini[48] reported on arch changes in 39 mixed dentition cases with lower anterior crowding treated with passive lingual arch therapy and selected removal of primary molars over a 4 year period as compared with a matched group of 60 untreated children with similar crowding. In untreated subjects, lower canine and premolar mesial displacement occurred with overlap of already crowded lower incisors. In contrast, lingual arch subjects showed decreased lower anterior crowding of 3 to 4 mm on average through the time of second permanent molar eruption. The permanent canines and premolars erupted with an average of 1.5 mm more distal positioning per side in lingual arch subjects than in controls. Dugoni and associates[49] published similar findings in 25 mixed dentition patients with reductions in lower incisor crowding greater than 3 millimeters after placement of passive lingual arches and selected primary molar extractions. After an average post-retention period of 10 years, 19 of the 25 patients continued to show clinically satisfactory lower anterior alignment. When compared with 10-year follow-up studies of orthodontic aligned patients, these results suggest stability of the alignment with lingual arch therapy was greater than or at least equal to active orthodontic treatments. Reballato et al[50], using cephalograms, study models, and tomograms of the mandibular body, reported dimensional changes in 14 mixed dentition patients with incisor crowding of 3 millimeters or more that were treated with passive lingual arches in comparison to 16 untreated control subjects. In lingual arch patients, arch length did not measurably change through eruption of the succedaneous teeth. This compared with an average arch length decrease of 2.5 mm per side in the untreated controls. Arch length changes were related to first molars moving forward + 1.7 mm in the control group compared with only + 0.3 mm in the lingual arch group. Concurrently, incisors tipped forward slightly in the lingual arch group (+ 0.4 mm) while up-righting of incisors in the controls reduced arch length 0.65 mm. In sum, the lingual arch reduced mesial molar migration and incisor lingual movement in controlling arch length with concurrent

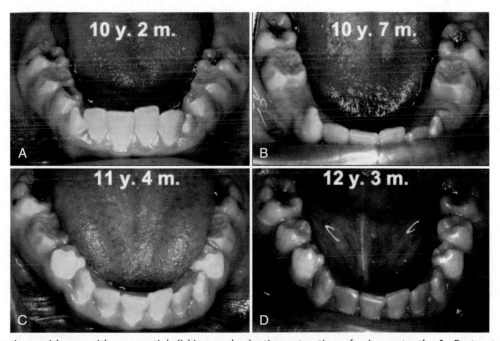

Figure 27-50 Eruption guidance with sequential disking and selective extraction of primary teeth. **A,** Pretreatment alignment with mesial eruption path of permanent canines to overlap incisors. **B,** Alignment at 5 months after elective extraction of primary first molars and disking of the mesial surface of the second primary molars. **C,** Permanent canines and first premolars have erupted in distal orientation with reduction in anterior crowding. **D,** After eruption of second premolars, nice arch form is established with overall adequate space and easily correctible minor rotations.

relief of 3 to 4 mm of lower incisor crowding in the treatment subjects. Brennan and Gianelly[51] quantified dimensional changes in 107 consecutive mixed dentition patients treated with passive lingual arches through eruption of all succedaneous teeth with occasional extraction of second primary molars being the only other intervention. Arch length decreased an average of 0.4 mm while width increased slightly in lingual arch patients. The resultant average +4.4 mm of total available leeway space produced an average decrease in lower incisor crowding from a pretreatment of −4.8 mm to +0.2 mm of space after treatment. The space adjustments were enough to resolve incisor crowding completely in 65 subjects (roughly 60%). An additional 16 subjects (one in six) had a final discrepancy of less than 1 mm, and 13 subjects (1 in 10) had a final discrepancy less than 2 mm. Only 14 patients (13%) had crowding greater than 2 mm after full buccal segment eruption was complete. Of note, the majority of patients with higher levels of postlingual arch crowding presented with initial ectopic loss of the lower primary canines. In sum, a passive lingual arch with selected removal of primary teeth provided adequate space and eruption guidance to relieve significant lower incisor crowding in 105 of the 107 subjects.

These studies consistently confirm arch length remains relatively constant or decreases minimally in patients treated with a passive lingual arch by reducing forward movement of molars and lingual movement of lower incisors. Timely treatment not only maintains arch length, but allows distal eruptive positioning of canines and premolars as a positive influence on relief of mixed dentition crowding in the 2- to 4-mm range, enough to relieve lower crowding in about two thirds to three fourths of patients.

ERUPTION GUIDANCE IN THE MAXILLARY CANINE AND PREMOLAR SEGMENT

In the 7- to 8-year-old child, maxillary permanent canine positioning approximates the distal aspect of the root of the lateral incisor. This is associated with a normative distal tipping of the lateral incisor crowns under the fulcrum pressure of the canine at the lateral root area. The maxillary canine then normally deflects toward a more vertical positioning toward the primary canine root area as eruption continues with a concurrent more labial orientation of the canine. This labial orientation can be noted clinically by bulging in the vestibular aspect of the alveolar process. As resorption of the primary canine proceeds in normal patterns, the adjacent maxillary lateral incisor crown should tip mesially as vertical eruption of the permanent canine continues down the primary canine root length. With exfoliation of the primary canine, the maxillary permanent canines typically emerge with a slight labial orientation that tends to lingualize into the archform as eruption proceeds under the balancing forces of the perioral tissues.

Given this tortuous and long journey, permanent maxillary canine eruption disturbances resulting in severe displacement and/or impaction are reported in 2% of the population with females affected three times more frequently than males. As the final succedaneous tooth to erupt in the maxilla, mesiolabial displacement of the permanent canine is usually due to an arch length deficiency as the canine assumes whatever space is left over in the quadrant. In contrast to labial displacement, arch length deficiency appears to be less of a factor in palatal impactions as 85% demonstrate adequate arch length in the involved quadrant. An etiologic factor in true palatal impactions may actually be excessive space in the canine area rather than a lack of arch length. When maxillary lateral incisors are absent, peg-shaped, or smaller than the lower incisors, palatally displaced maxillary canines are noted in approximately 40% to 45% of patients. When the ectopic permanent canine is in close proximity to the root of the lateral incisor, notable displacement of the incisor and idiopathic root resorption of the incisor may occur. The resorption is often difficult to diagnose because most of the lesions are located palatally toward the middle and apical third of the incisor with the overlapping canine crown concealing radiographic visualization of the resorptive process. It has been reported that up to 12.5% of ectopic palatal positioned canines cause resorption of the adjacent incisors. In about half of cases analyzed, the resorption extends into the pulp of the involved teeth with the degree of resorption ranging from loss of one fourth of the root to almost complete loss of root structure. The actual percentage of resorption occurrence may be much higher than reported due to inherent limitations of two-dimensional radiographs used by most clinicians.

Screening for potential displacement and impaction of maxillary canines should start at 10 to 11 years of age with clinical and radiographic examination to include evaluation of eruption trajectory, symmetry of positioning, status of root development, and orientation to the adjacent lateral incisor and primary canine. In cases of mesially displaced maxillary canines with overlap of adjacent permanent lateral incisor roots beyond age 10 years, timely removal of the adjacent primary canines greatly enhances the possibility for more distal and vertical eruptive directions. This timing coincides with when eruptive forces are optimal as the permanent canine attains approximately two-thirds root development. Once the apices of the canine are three-fourths or more formed, the eruptive force is reduced and the tooth will more likely have to be actively moved into the mouth. The clinical examination should involve palpation of the buccal aspect of the alveolar bone in the canine region slightly above the primary canine. A canine bulge should be evident, indicating the presence of the canine in a normal path of eruption at this stage of development. Although presence of the buccal bulge does not necessarily preclude the possibility of impaction, the absence of such a clinical indicator by 10 to 11 years of age should warrant exploration. A major clinical clue to significant canine malpositioning involves excessive distal and labiolingual tipping of the lateral incisor crown. This suggests the erupting canine is placing a fulcrum-type pressure on the lateral root "pushing" the root mesially to tip the crown in a distal direction. If the lateral crown is tipping labially, the permanent canine is probably displaced in front of the lateral root. If the lateral crown is tipping in a lingual direction, the canine crown is more likely to be displaced behind the lateral root. Other clinical signs include delayed eruption of the canine beyond 13 to14 years of age with prolonged retention of primary canines and soft tissue bulging either too high in the vestibule or palatally.

Radiographic evaluation of the maxillary canine area should be particularly emphasized when lateral incisor inclinations are pronounced as noted before, small maxillary (pegged) lateral incisors are present, primary canines are not appropriately mobile, and the eruptive bulging of the canines is atypical. Although excessive mesial inclination resulting in overlap of the canine crown with the lateral incisor roots on radiographs may suggest potential impaction, this prognostic sign can only be applied reliably if the overlapping is present after root development of the lateral incisors is almost complete and the canine has attained approximately two-thirds root development (i.e., around 10 to 11 years of age). At that point, the degree of overlap of the canine crown with the lateral incisor root and the resorption pattern of the primary canine and first primary molars are key indicators for potential canine impaction and for the prognosis of successful interceptive guidance. Localization of the labial or lingual positioning of the tooth by special radiographic technique is essential—the procedure described in Chapter 5 helps in this localization. Studies indicate that if the displaced permanent canine overlap of the adjacent permanent lateral incisor is not beyond the midline long axis of the lateral (still toward the "distal" half of the root), the chances for the canine repositioning and erupting into normal position after primary canine extraction shows roughly 85% to 90% success. If the canine overlap is beyond the lateral incisor's long axis (toward the mesial half of the root or beyond), successful repositioning drops to approximately 60% of cases with extraction of the primary canine.

Follow-up at 1 year after the primary canine extraction should evidence significant improvement in canine positioning. If not improved, the canine is probably positioned to the palate and will require complicated treatment options to include surgical exposure with removal of obstructing structures to allow "hoped-for" passive eruption, surgical exposure with active orthodontic traction to move the tooth into position, autotransplantation of the impacted canine into the proper position, or extraction of the impacted canine and substitution by the first premolars. Surgical exposure that allows natural eruption is dependent on the displaced tooth having a reasonable axial inclination and incomplete root development to achieve eruptive potential. When conditions for "passive" eruption are not met, an active approach involving surgical exposure followed by active orthodontic traction applied to the tooth may be necessary. Beyond our level of discussion, orthodontic traction involves complex biomechanical force parameters of direction, duration, amount, and method of activation in positioning the tooth.

Maxillary Anterior Diastemas
Parents are often concerned about anterior spacing that presents during eruption of the maxillary dentition. Unless there is a valid reason to intervene early, active

treatment should be postponed until the complete eruption of the permanent canines because anterior spaces often close spontaneously as the lateral incisors and particularly the permanent canines erupt. After the canines erupt, the condition can be reevaluated and appropriate treatment taken as needed. Fig. 27-51 shows a patient whose parent wanted the diastema closed and was concerned about the high position of the canines. No treatment was begun. The follow-up image shows closure of the diastema 24 months later. Notice that the canines are in reasonably good alignment.

Valid reasons for early closure of excess maxillary spaces may be in consideration of atypical or asymmetric eruption patterns. Lateral incisors may be erupting lingually without sufficient space to be aligned labially into the arch. The maxillary incisors may be excessively flared and "splayed" with lip interpositioning that puts the teeth at risk for traumatic injury. Adjusting the symmetry of alignment, consolidating spaces, and retracting excessively proclined incisors may be indicated to facilitate

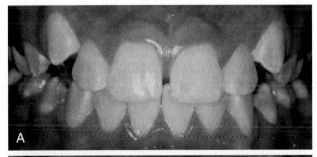
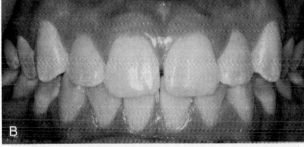
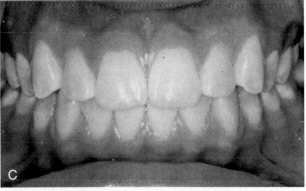

Figure 27-51 A, Patient with midline diastema and highly positioned canines. No treatment was instituted. **B,** Twenty-four months later, the diastema has closed significantly and the canines are erupting into a more favorable position. **C,** Thirty-six months later, the diastema has closed completely, and the canines have assumed a near-ideal position.

long-term development. An extremely heavy labial frenum may prevent natural closure of a diastema. If orthodontic closure is advocated, it should occur before the frenectomy to reduce the chance of scar tissue impeding tooth movement. If there is sufficient arch space for the eruption of incisors and canines, it is best to delay frenum surgery until these teeth have fully erupted.

Supernumerary Teeth

Supernumerary teeth can be associated with delayed eruption of permanent teeth, overretention of primary teeth, deflection of roots with unusual inclinations, and displacement of teeth, diastemas, abnormal root resorption, and formation of follicular or dentigerous cysts (Fig. 27-52). Occurring approximately eight times more frequently in the maxilla than in the mandible, supernumerary permanent teeth have been reported in up to 3.6% of children. The occurrence of supernumerary teeth in several members of the same family has been observed, indicating a familial pattern. The most frequent site is the maxillary anterior segment where atypically shaped accessory teeth of a conical tuberculated form, known as *mesiodens*, occur between the maxillary central incisors (Fig. 27-53). Reported in boys twice as often as in girls, 80% of mesiodens have a single occurrence while 20% have two or more supernumerary teeth. The mesiodens usually presents a peg- or cone-shaped crown with a single root. More than 90% are palatally positioned. Approximately three of four mesiodens remain unerupted and commonly need surgical removal at some point during treatment because they often prevent eruption of adjacent permanent teeth or cause their ectopic eruption. Supernumerary primary teeth (Fig. 27-54) are apparently less common than supernumerary permanent teeth.

If a supernumerary tooth is identified through radiographic techniques (see Chapter 5), the decision whether to intervene surgically or keep the tooth under observation must be made. If not interfering with symmetric development of adjacent teeth and there is no evidence of cyst formation, the correct decision may be to observe the tooth until the child is old enough to better tolerate the surgical procedure. Watchful waiting until the development of the permanent incisors reaches approximately two-thirds to three-quarters root formation allows for less risk to the incisor development in the surgical procedures. Possible eruption of the supernumerary tooth and avoidance of surgical exposure are also potential benefits in delaying intervention. However, in the case of severe exfoliation and eruption irregularities, earlier removal of a supernumerary tooth and the overretained primary teeth may be desirable to lessen potential sequelae. The clinician must still consider the status of the adjacent permanent teeth and may prefer to wait until root development is preferably two-thirds established before surgically removing the supernumerary tooth.

When surgical removal is accomplished, exposure of the unerupted permanent tooth or teeth with provision of an eruption channel is recommended (Fig. 27-55). Reports suggest up to 80% of permanent maxillary teeth will spontaneously erupt after the supernumerary is removed. During surgery, the bone and soft tissue should be

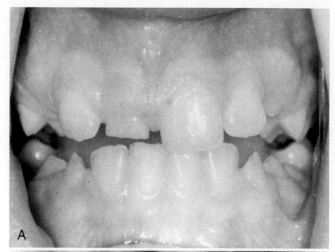

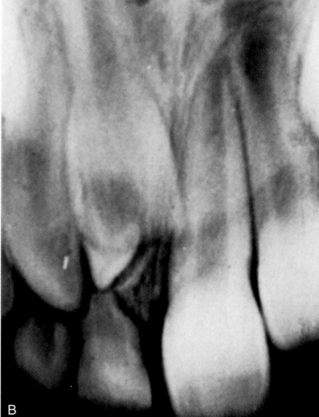

Figure 27-52 A, Patient with an unerupted maxillary permanent central incisor and retained primary central incisor. Permanent laterals are erupting. **B,** Radiograph shows a supernumerary tooth (mesiodens), which has delayed the eruption of the permanent incisor.

removed from the incisal third of the tooth or teeth that are delayed in their eruption. If the permanent teeth are positioned extremely high, a prolonged period of watchful waiting may be necessary until they have migrated within the bone to a position that would allow surgical intervention. An open pathway should be maintained, if possible, to hasten the eruption of the delayed tooth. A thin covering of dense scar tissue can delay eruption indefinitely. Ultimately, orthodontic treatment is often necessary to

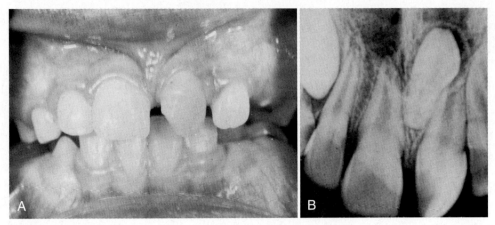

Figure 27-53 A, Rotation and labioversion of a maxillary central incisor with midline diastema. **B,** Radiographic assessment revealed a well-developed midline supernumerary tooth (mesiodens) with an inverted eruption path. Surgical removal of the tooth is indicated.

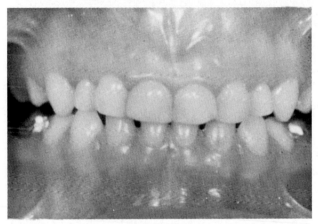

Figure 27-54 Supernumerary maxillary primary incisors positioned distal to the lateral incisors. There may be corresponding supernumerary permanent teeth. The teeth should be counted at the time of the clinical examination so that erupted supernumerary teeth will not be overlooked.

make adequate room for the unerupted tooth and to position it properly in the arch. Because of these considerations and the frequency with which supernumerary teeth are observed, radiographic surveys that include maxillary anterior views are essential for children 5 to 7 years of age to allow for early detection and planning.

Congenitally Missing Teeth

Studies have reported an incidence rate of congenitally missing permanent teeth (excluding third molars) in 2.3% to 9.6% of the population with no significant gender differences. Oligodontia affects two or more teeth in about one half of cases, frequently in a symmetrical pattern involving antimeres. The most frequently missing permanent teeth are third molars (one to four wisdom teeth are absent in up to one third of the population), mandibular second premolars, maxillary lateral incisors, and maxillary second premolars. Morphologic changes such as cone-shaped teeth are characteristically seen in association with missing

permanent teeth—agenesis and peg-shaped maxillary lateral incisors approximates a 1:1 ratio. The congenital absence of primary teeth demonstrates a much lower prevalence than absence in the permanent dentition. The prevalence of missing primary teeth ranges between 0.1% and 0.7% with absence usually located in the maxillary or mandibular incisor areas. When a number of primary teeth fail to develop, other ectodermal deficiencies are usually evident (e.g., ectodermal dysplasia). If the absence is localized to only one or two primary teeth, no specific treatment is generally needed. However, the long-term implications are significant because the analogue of the permanent tooth is derived from the primary tooth bud. Therefore a missing primary tooth almost always means the associated permanent tooth will be missing with attendant occlusion factors.

The management of congenitally missing permanent teeth requires a thorough evaluation of arch length, occlusion, and facial growth patterns given the long-term consequences to esthetic and functional arch alignment in terms of which specific tooth is missing, adjacent teeth drifting into the space, the distribution of the space, and supraeruption of opposing teeth. Early consultation with the orthodontist and prosthodontist is important in determining appropriate care. If one or both of the permanent maxillary lateral incisors are missing, the dentist must decide whether to hold space for prosthetic replacements or to encourage the permanent canine to erupt mesially into the lateral incisor position. In the latter instance, the mesial eruption path of the adjacent permanent canines may erupt fully forward into the lateral space and naturally compensate for the missing lateral incisors. This pattern of "canine replacement" is particularly beneficial when the patient presents with excessive maxillary overjet and dental protrusion or a significant tooth size discrepancy that would benefit from an extraction protocol. Consolidation of the maxillary archform with canine "replacement" leads to reduction of the protrusive overjet and compensation for a tooth mass discrepancy. Orthodontic treatment is generally needed to place the canine in the correct axial inclination before the

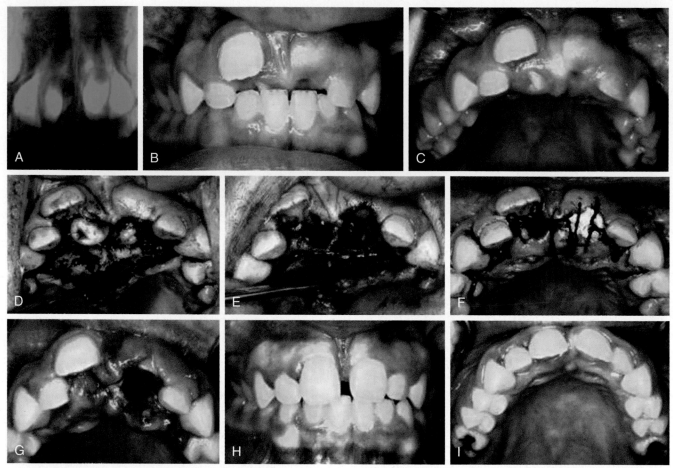

Figure 27-55 Surgical removal of supernumerary incisors with uncovering of blocked permanent incisors allows normative eruption positioning of the involved incisors. **A,** Radiograph showing two mesiodens associated with retained primary central incisors and delayed eruption of permanent central incisors at age 9 years and 6 months. The primary incisors were extracted at this time. **B** and **C,** Same patient at age 11 years and 10 months. **D, E,** and **F,** Surgical removal of two mesiodens with uncovering of unerupted incisor. **G,** One week after surgery. **H** and **I,** Same patient at age 13 years and 1 month. One year after surgical uncovering, no orthodontic appliances.

crown is reshaped to resemble the lateral. In some instances the shape of the canine may not be favorable to use as a lateral, even with extensive recontouring. In contrast, a patient with class I or class III relationships and more normal alignment spacing usually benefits from having the canines in their normal A-P positions and restoration of the missing lateral incisors with prosthodontic treatment (Fig. 27-56). If the canines are erupting too far forward from their normal positions in this case, timely removal of the primary canines may enhance a more distal eruption path toward normal canine positions. However, with the advent of implants for replacement of lateral incisors, that recommendation has changed. According to Kokich[52], the ideal situation is to encourage the canine to erupt adjacent to the permanent central incisor. After it has erupted, it can be moved distally into its normal position. By moving the tooth distally, bone is maintained in forming an alveolar ridge with adequate buccal lingual width to facilitate proper implant placement.

When one or more permanent premolars, usually the seconds, are congenitally missing, should the space be maintained for fixed prostheses later, or should the space

be closed? Many factors influence the decision, including the degree of arch length deficiency, facial and skeletal patterns, molar relationships, vertical aspects of the malocclusion, anteroposterior incisor positioning, and stage of transitional dentition are all factors in deciding whether to retain or extract the overlying second primary molar. For example, if just one premolar is absent and the rest of the occlusion is esthetically and functionally sound, long-term retention of the primary molar is usually encouraged until growth is complete and prosthodontics can be used to replace the missing premolar. However, the larger mesiodistal width of the primary molar may cause incorrect occlusal relationships with the permanent teeth. Slicing the mesial and/or distal surfaces of the primary molar may allow improved interdigitation, but often the bulbous, divergent roots of the primary molar prevent mesial movement of the permanent molar. Also, the roots of the primary molar may be resorbed, and the tooth may be lost eventually. To summarize, if the primary molar is maintaining vertical occlusion and arch length stability, then it should be retained for alveolar bone integrity and to set up for implant prosthetics. An exception would be in a

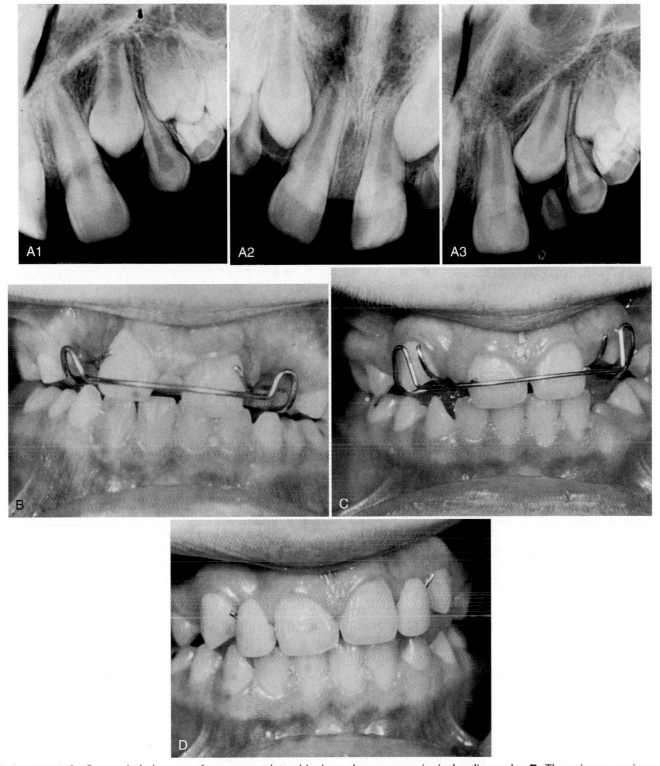

Figure 27-56 A, Congenital absence of permanent lateral incisors shown on periapical radiographs. **B,** The primary canines were extracted to encourage a more distal eruption path of the permanent canines. A Hawley-type appliance with springs was constructed to close the diastema between the central incisors. **C,** Auxiliary wires were added to the appliance to guide the permanent canines into a more favorable position. **D,** Space has been regained for eventual fixed prostheses to replace the lateral incisors. Meanwhile the removable retainer with lateral pontics is worn.

child with a significant tooth size-arch size discrepancy where a serial extraction protocol would provide successful esthetic and functional outcomes. Early extraction would provide positive alignment factors without compromising long-term results because later orthodontic tooth movements will bring alveolar bone support.

The general concept of the primary molar being maintained when the underlying premolar is missing applies except when the retained primary molar exhibits significant ankylosis. Restorative coverage (i.e., composite build-ups, stainless steel crowns) of the ankylosed primary molar may help maintain occlusal harmony if the vertical discrepancy is not extreme. In most cases, however, early extraction of the affected primary molar may enhance occlusal outcomes by avoiding excess vertical collapse and loss of alveolar bone height that occurs secondary to early ankylosis. Even in cases of ankylosed second primary molars over missing premolars where future prosthetic replacement is planned, early extraction of the primary molar may be advisable. The consequence of leaving severely displaced ankylosed primary molars when the premolars are absent will likely result in vertically compromised alveolar heights of adjacent teeth because there is no erupting premolar to maintain alveolar ridge integrity. For these reasons, the early extraction of ankylosed second primary molars when the second premolars are congenitally absent should be an early treatment planning decision and is usually desirable. If extracted early, the majority of alveolar ridge reduction secondary to the extraction will occur in the first year after removal, will represent about an overall one-third loss in width, and is not progressive. Adjacent tooth movements usually maintain adequate alveolar width for subsequent implant placement and establish better arch length adjustments for proper occlusion. Planning must also consider whether to hold the space for future prosthetic replacement or allow "driftodontics" to start closing the space of the missing premolar. Early extraction is particularly indicated if the case can be handled long-term with a premolar extraction protocol and where multiple premolars are absent symmetrically. Given long-term considerations, the treatment options available, and the multiple disciplines potentially involved, the clinician must take the lead role in coordinating treatment and using the expertise of specialists.

COMPREHENSIVE ORTHODONTICS FOR THE DEVELOPING OCCLUSION

Comprehensive orthodontics can be defined as an in-depth evaluation of a patient's entire orofacial complex and the corrective treatments necessary to achieve optimal dental esthetics, facial esthetics, skeletal balance, and functional harmony. Comprehensive orthodontic treatment recognizes broader based malocclusion factors than those cited in interceptive orthodontics and guidance of eruption. Diplomates of the American Board of Orthodontics (ABO) listed the correction of skeletal class II and class III malocclusions, excess vertical development, and severe tooth size-arch size discrepancies presenting displaced permanent teeth as complex problems indicated for comprehensive levels of early treatment intervention.[53] The achievement of functional and esthetic

harmony requires the coordination of a multitude of factors, from the fine details of tooth positioning to the relationships of the maxilla and mandible. With an awareness of normality as a variable range, the fundamental goals of comprehensive orthodontic management of the occlusion may be delineated as the possession of:

1. *Dental esthetics.* The tooth alignment and arch form are generally consistent with orthognathic class I molar positioning, normal anterior overbite and overjet, integrity of dentitional alignment, and symmetric arches positioned over basal bone. The details of these dental esthetic descriptors are best defined in the context of the Six Keys of Occlusion as delineated by Andrews[54] to include proper molar relationship, proper crown angulation and inclination, no rotations, tight contacts, and a flat occlusal plane.

2. *Facial esthetics.* Balanced facial profile and frontal symmetry with harmonious relationships between the jaws, teeth, and soft tissues are realized within the context of normal facial developmental patterns relative to patient age, ethnic/racial differences and growth patterns.

3. *Optimally functional occlusion.* The interplay of gnathologic factors allows comfortable and efficient actions of the orofacial components in a harmonious neuromuscular environment without deleterious stress on the teeth, periodontal structures, and temporomandibular joints.

4. *Stability of occlusion.* When applied to postorthodontic treatment, the interrelationships of the teeth, jaws, and soft tissues should not only meet the esthetic and functional goals of treatment, but are also sustained with long-lasting stability and retention of achieved goals.

Comprehensive orthodontic treatment usually requires complete fixed Edgewise appliances to achieve final positioning of all or nearly all of the permanent teeth into optimal esthetic and functional harmony within alveolar basal bone. If a practitioner decides to initiate comprehensive levels of orthodontic care, it is important that he or she accept responsibility to provide the treatment to full completion standards. It is not appropriate to provide only one phase of treatment with the intention of referring the patient for the final and definitive phases of care unless the separate treatments were predetermined between consulting providers. If the practitioner recognizes the need for, but is unwilling or unable to provide comprehensive care, it is appropriate to refer the patient to a practitioner able to address all of the orthodontic needs.

The interventions necessary to achieve comprehensive goals may be accomplished in one single phase or in specifically planned phases of treatment. To determine the approach in most patients, the preferred time for evaluating comprehensive orthodontic needs and implementing treatment is from the transitional mixed dentition into the young permanent (adolescent) dentition. The ABO Diplomates stated that there are numerous advantages for both the patient and the practitioner in terms of early orthodontic treatment and, importantly, that the final results of early treatment tend to be better. The basis for these statements lies in the fact that the clinician has the ability with mixed dentition timing to control arch length adjustments in terms of leeway space and late mesial molar shifts for the relief of most levels of crowding, to employ space gaining and arch expansion procedures in reducing extraction needs, to control incisor and buccal segment eruption patterns for adjustments in overbite, open-bite, and leveling of the curve of Spee, to control deleterious habits and functional deviations in occlusion, and to use growth modification with dentofacial orthopedics for skeletal discrepancies. Most of the January1998 and June 2002 issues of the *American Journal of Orthodontics and Dentofacial Orthopedics* are dedicated to a broad range of topics related to the rationale for common procedures employed in early orthodontic treatment. These issues serve as excellent reference sources for review.

A convenient way to look at comprehensive orthodontics in the context of "early" treatment is to relate it in terms of the developmental stage of the dentition. The dental stages in which comprehensive treatments are considered for growing patients involve the full primary to the mid mixed dentition through transitional eruption of the first molars and incisors (4 to 10 years of age), the mid to late mixed dentition overlapping the transition of the buccal segments (10 to 12 years of age), and the early permanent dentition (12 to 16 years of age). The general scope of interceptive orthodontic interventions in these stages is outlined earlier in this chapter. They serve as a focus for the presentation of case examples that illustrate more comprehensive treatments necessary to address more complex needs in growing patients.

THE PRIMARY TO MID MIXED DENTITIONS (AGE 4 TO 10 YEARS)

Abnormal dental, skeletal, and functional relationships that are notable in the primary dentition may have profound effects on orofacial growth patterns if not corrected early. Additionally, they can become increasingly difficult to correct as the child transitions toward the permanent dentition. Some of the more significant problems that can be treated effectively in the primary dentition involve functional and bilateral posterior crossbites along with deleterious oral habits. As illustrated in earlier sections, significant orthodontic and orthopedic changes can be affected with various "interceptive" appliances in this period. A further example of primary dentition intervention that potentially extends into more comprehensive concepts is shown in Fig. 27-57 with correction of a pseudo-class III malocclusion. Without such early treatment, the functional aspects of the malocclusion could carry over into much more complex skeletal problems as growth continues to compensate for the deviations. It is not necessarily the intent of an early phased treatment to prevent the need for full Edgewise appliances in the permanent dentition. The goal is to establish normal vertical, transverse, and sagittal relationships of the dentition with functional perioral balance. However, as illustrated in this interceptive case, it is possible to establish such a harmonious relationship of the dental units that further treatment is unnecessary. Such an outcome is also illustrated in Fig. 27-58 where more involved early treatment mechanics were employed. Each of these cases support the idea that the real goal of such treatment in developmental stages should be to minimize or

eliminate the amount of orthodontic treatment needed in the permanent dentition with more ideal outcomes. The remaining cases presented involve just such comprehensive treatments where Edgewise appliances are used to finish the treated occlusion toward optimal functional and esthetic outcomes.

Correction of class II skeletal relationships in the primary and early mixed dentition stages using functional appliances and extraoral headgear has been reported in the literature. In contemporary practice, however, class II malocclusions are generally managed from the mid to the late mixed dentition extending on into the young permanent dentitions with positive outcomes. This later timing coincides with the pubertal growth period for enhanced dentofacial orthopedics and the transition of the buccal dentition to optimally affect sagittal dentoalveolar corrective changes. In addition, later timing simplifies retention considerations of any achieved correction by reducing the time between the early treatment phase, the full Edgewise phase, and the completion of growth. In contrast, skeletal class III relationships should ideally be addressed in the primary and incisor transition period to establish normative overbite and overjet relationships into the mixed and permanent dentitions. Class III corrections in this time frame have been consistently shown to present efficient and effective treatment outcomes compared with later treatment timing. This particularly applies if the class III pattern involves a retruded maxillary complex as the causative factor or if the anteroposterior discrepancy is the result of a functional anterior displacement of the mandible (pseudo-class III). If the major component of the class III pattern is a severe skeletal overgrowth of the mandible, attempts at correction are more variable and often require retreatment as the lower jaw outgrows the correction. This is especially true if there is a strong genetic/familial component to the mandibular prognathia.

Vertical growth abnormalities can also be successfully managed in this early transitional period. Patients with deep overbites and a horizontal growth pattern (low mandibular plane angle) may benefit from a removable anterior bite plane to allow supracruption of the posterior dentition.

Because the permanent incisors and first molars have erupted by age 8 to 9 years in both arches, fixed Edgewise appliances can be placed in a segmental fashion to accomplish specific dental orthodontic movements. Molar to incisor bracketing treatments (2 × 4 setup) generally last from 6 to 12 months and are designed to correct severe and detrimental displacements in establishing normative overbite and overjet of the incisor segments. After the 2 × 4 mechanics, the patient is typically placed in a resting retention phase until full eruption of the permanent dentition is established around age 12 to 13 years. A first-phase approach using a 2 × 4 setup with a transpalatal bar for anchorage to help correct a class II division 2 deep-bite malocclusion at age 9 years and 4 months is presented in Fig. 27-59. Lower arch development was enhanced with a mandibular lip bumper during the upper retention phase.

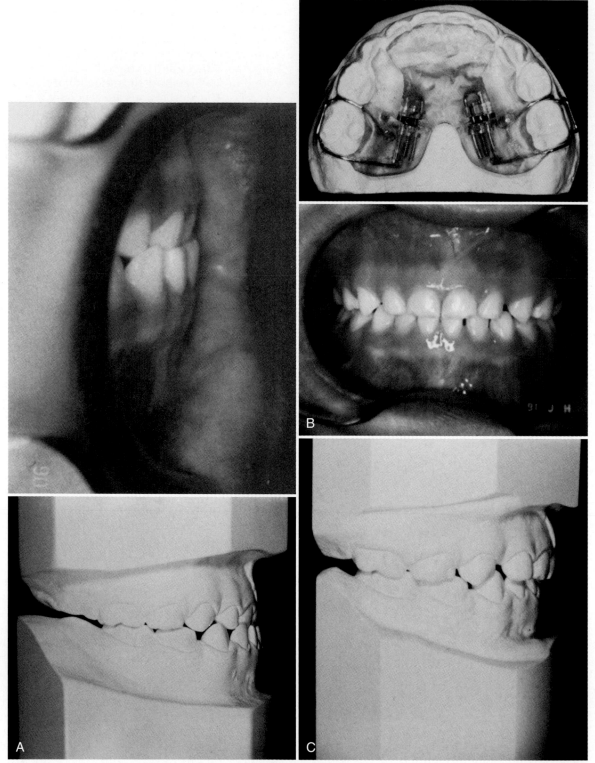

Figure 27-57 Primary dentition anterior crossbite with functional shift of mandible. **A,** Pretreatment clinical and model view of occlusion. **B,** Anterior sagittal appliance designed to labialize the primary incisors. **C,** Posttreatment clinical and model view of occlusion.

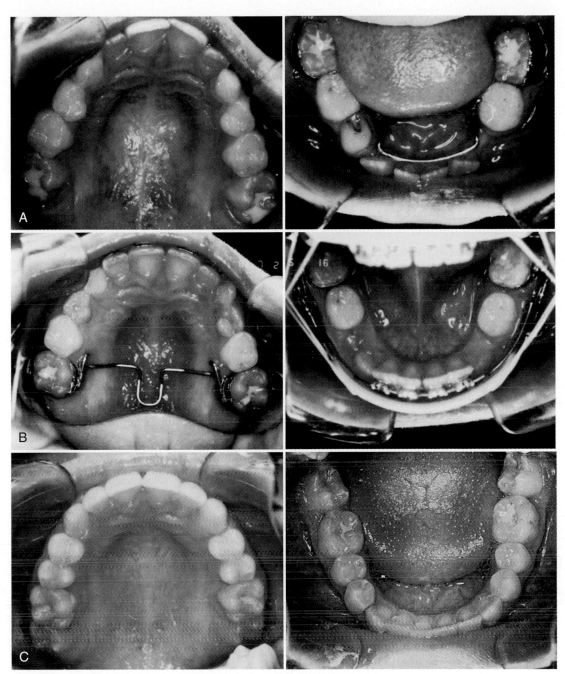

Figure 27-58 Patient treated with phase I orthodontics only. **A,** Pretreatment occlusal views; note tapered maxillary arch and arch length insufficiency in the mandibular arch. **B,** Phase I treatment with fixed 2 × 4 Edgewise appliances, maxillary transpalatal bar, and mandibular lip bumper. Note arch length development, particularly in the lower arch. **C,** Posttreatment occlusal views in permanent dentition without additional full edgewise bracketing.

Full Edgewise appliances followed in the permanent dentition to finalize alignments (age 12 years and 10 months).

THE MID TO LATE MIXED DENTITION (AGE 10 TO 12 YEARS)

Given that the majority of patients present with class I skeletal relationships and any malocclusion requiring treatment most likely involves crowding, the incorporation of space supervision concepts with the control of leeway space is a major component of treatment in the late mixed dentition. Addressed in a sequential consideration of guidance in an earlier section of this chapter, Fig. 27-60 illustrates the value of a mandibular lingual holding arch in the relief of lower anterior crowding at 11 years and 8 months of age in controlling leeway space. Class I molar relationships were maintained with the lingual arch and selective primary extractions over 18 months of space supervision. Seventeen months of full Edgewise appliances completed the alignment (15 years and 5 months).

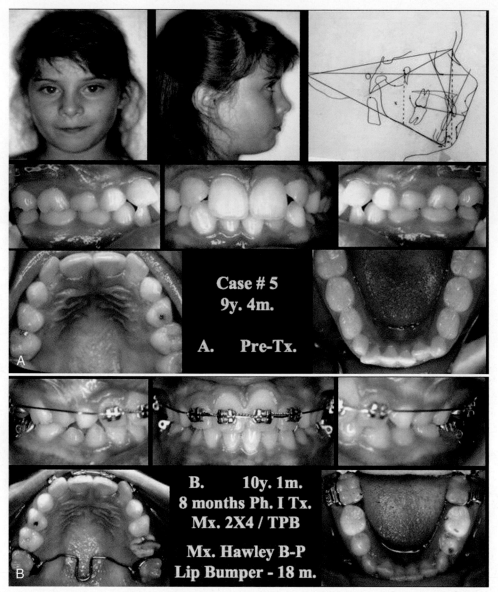

Figure 27-59 A, Class II division 2 deep-bite malocclusion at age 9 years and 4 months with mesofacial growth pattern, retrognathic mandible, ANB = +6 degrees, moderate incisor crowding. **B,** A maxillary 2 × 4 with a transpalatal bar was used along with a mandibular lip bumper for 8 months of phase I treatment. The upper was retained with a Hawley bite plane; the lip bumper was continued for an additional 18 months.

Patients who present with skeletal class II malocclusions often benefit from dentofacial orthopedics employing directed extraoral headgear mechanics and/or mandibular advancement (functional) appliances during the late mixed dentition period. The growth modification appliances timed with pubertal growth enhances maxillary to mandibular skeletal and dental relationships in preparation for full Edgewise appliances to finish and detail final alignment.

Mid to late dentition treatments in managing the occlusion with full Edgewise appliances to follow in the permanent dentition typically involve:

Space supervision. To hold lower leeway space (lingual holding arch), hold upper leeway space, and derotate permanent first molars (transpalatal bar).

Expansion appliances. Transpalatal arch bars, Hyrax, lip bumpers.

Fixed Edgewise appliances and archwires. Banded molars and bracketed incisors for 2 × 4 mechanics. Allows for molar derotation and uprighting, incisor leveling, incisor alignment, and incisor protraction or retraction

Extraoral headgear. Directed cervical-pull, high-pull, or protraction reverse-pull headgear applications with selection dependent on the vertical and sagittal facial growth pattern as well as stage of development. Often used with anterior bite planes.

Functional appliances. Removable (e.g., Bionator) and fixed (e.g., Herbst) mandibular advancement appliances serve as examples of many options. The type

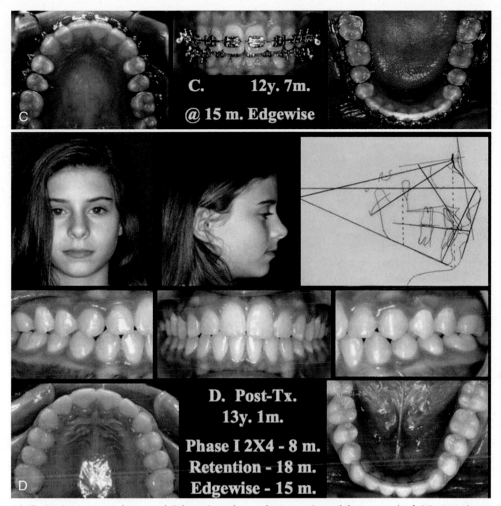

Figure 27-59 cont'd C, Patient started second Edgewise phase that continued for a total of 15 months until age 12 years and 7 months. **D,** Final records obtained 3 months after removal of Edgewise appliances at age 12 years and 10 months.

of functional appliance and its design vary significantly depending on the facial growth pattern.

Selected extractions. Timely removal of both primary teeth and selected permanent teeth in guidance and serial extraction protocols optimizes the use of available space. The patient's diagnosis influences which of the "early" treatment modalities would be appropriate to employ. One pervasive philosophy in early orthodontic treatment is that the simplest biomechanics necessary to achieve the desired treatment outcome is the best.

EARLY PERMANENT DENTITION (AGE 12 TO 16 YEARS)

Comprehensive orthodontic care in the adolescent permanent dentition again includes both orthopedic and orthodontic components. Orthopedic components might involve continued applications of palatal expanders, headgears, and functional appliances. Fig. 27-61 illustrates the correction of a class II malocclusion employing a functional appliance into the permanent dentition.

An Activator for mandibular advancement worn in combination with a high-pull headgear for restraint of maxillary growth addressed the skeletal class II problem. The orthodontic component included full fixed Edgewise appliances to establish as near "ideal" occlusal relationships as possible. Extraction of a single maxillary first premolar was used in the full Edgewise phase to camouflage the midline asymmetry in finishing with a good buccal occlusion.

Localized tooth displacements such as maxillary canine impactions and significant genetic tooth size-arch size discrepancies not manageable with space supervision procedures are also commonly addressed in this period. The removal of selected permanent teeth in cases of significant tooth size-arch size discrepancies with severe tooth displacements or to camouflage class II or class III dental malocclusions often offers good options as part of a comprehensive treatment plan.

If a patient has undergone an earlier phase of treatment successfully, the Edgewise phase of treatment might take as little as 12 to 18 months and hopefully

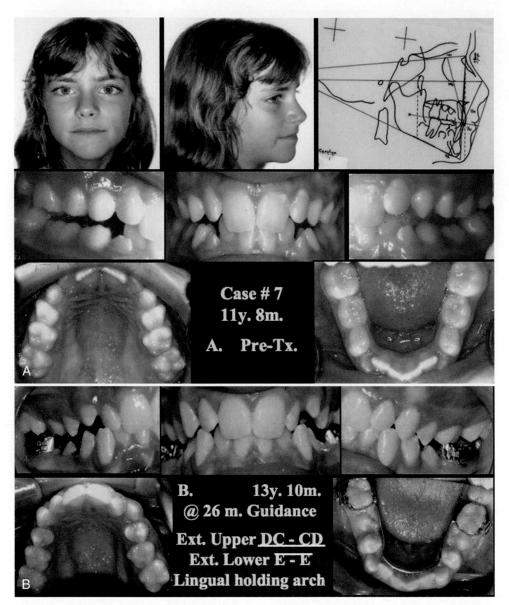

Figure 27-60 A, Class I mixed dentition at 11 years and 8 months with notable anterior crowding, delayed dental developmental timing, mesofacial growth pattern, and bilateral ankylosed lower primary molars. **B,** Patient at age 13 years and 10 months after 26 months' guidance with selective extraction of upper primary canines and first molars, lower first and second primary molars, and passive lingual holding arch.

will involve little, if any, orthopedic needs. However, if this is the start of comprehensive care, more treatment time will likely be needed. Treatment with full Edgewise appliances includes leveling and alignment of the dentition, space consolidation, transverse coordination of upper to lower archforms, sagittal arch coordination (class II or III elastic wear), establishment of root parallelism over basal bone, finishing and detailing of intraarch and interarch positioning (i.e., first-, second-, and third-order archwire bends), and buccal or anterior segmental finishing procedures to establish maximum interdigitation between arches. In selected patients, the Edgewise treatment may be more

limited in nature, unnecessary as determined by the dental practitioner, or unwanted as determined by the patient and/or parent. Limited treatment can involve segmented arch therapy in which only the teeth or arch needing attention is addressed. Occasionally the practitioner may be so satisfied with the result after an earlier phase that no further treatment is recommended. However, this is fairly uncommon. A more likely occurrence is that the patient and/or parents decide that they are satisfied with the result, even though some finishing details are needed. It is critical to stress to parents before initiating early treatments that most children will benefit from a final period of

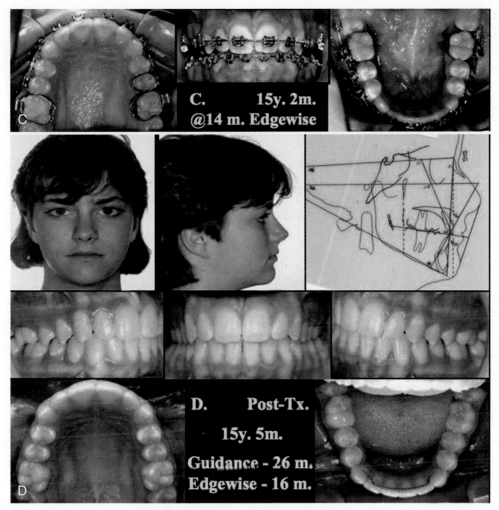

Figure 27-60 cont'd C, Full upper and lower Edgewise appliances were used for a total of 15 months. **D,** Final records obtained after removal of Edgewise appliances at age 15 years and 5 months.

full orthodontic appliances (phase II) to optimize esthetic and functional outcomes. It is particularly important to allow for final tooth positioning of the permanent second molars.

Retention following the definitive stage of comprehensive Edgewise treatment should involve the philosophy of "retention for a lifetime." There are many different types of retention schemes. Although no perfect retention scheme has been developed and periodic observation is warranted for all, the following retention schedule seems to provide for stable results:

1. Maxillary and mandibular Hawley retainers worn 24 hours a day for 4 to 6 months, followed by 6 to 8 months of at-night-only wear.
2. After 1 year, reassess if wear can be reduced to 1 or 2 nights per week with the patient increasing wear as needed if the retainers become tight from tooth movement.
3. Continue wear as above for "retention for a lifetime," or at an absolute minimum, until age 21 years, at which time the craniofacial growth rate has been reduced to that of an adult.

The use of a backup set of thin acrylic overlay retainers is a very useful way of inexpensively giving the patient an emergency set of retainers if the Hawley retainers are lost or damaged. As an added benefit, they can be used for home bleaching of the teeth for those patients who are interested. Fixed retention may be necessary in special circumstances. A lower canine-to-canine fixed, bonded wire can be helpful for severe rotations and an upper lateral-to-lateral fixed, bonded wire is useful to prevent space opening for patients with initial diastemas.

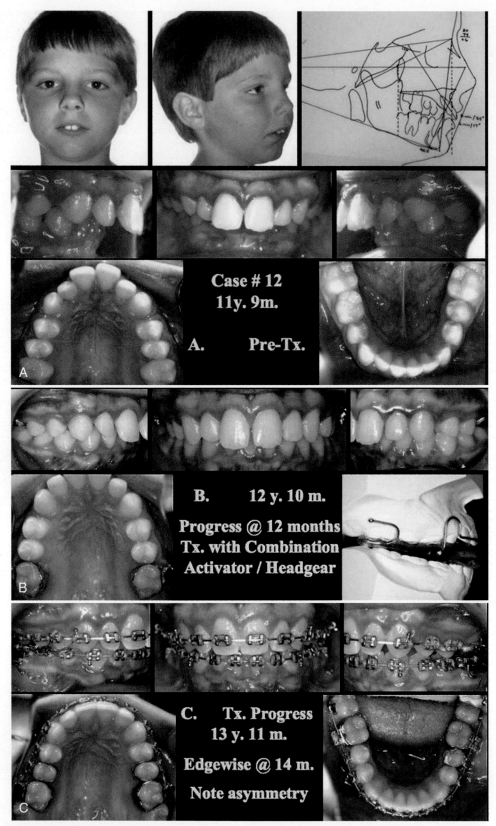

Figure 27-61 A, Class II division 1 mixed dentition with convex profile, lip interpositioning, mesofacial growth patterns, ANB = +10 degrees, mandibular retrognathia, and maxillary dental protrusion at age 11 years and 9 months. **B,** Patient after 12 months of wearing a mandibular functional advancement appliance (i.e., Activator) and cervical-pull headgear in combination following a regimen of 12 to 14 hours of wear per day. **C,** Patient started full Edgewise phase at age 12 years and 10 months. The treatment progress at 14 months of Edgewise illustrates midline asymmetry with class I right and class II left buccal occlusion.

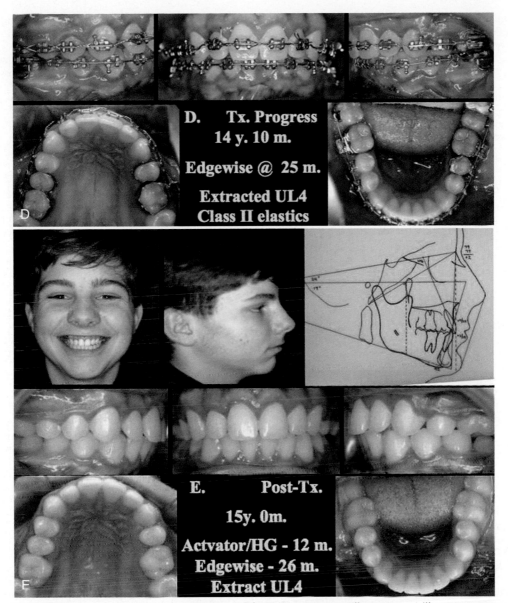

Figure 27-61 cont'd D, Treatment progress at 25 months of Edgewise treatment illustrates midline symmetry attained in conjunction with selective extraction of the upper left first premolar. **E,** Final records obtained at age 15 years and 0 months after 12 months of growth modification and 26 months of Edgewise appliances.

REFERENCES

1. American Academy of Pediatric Dentistry. Reference manual: Guideline management of the developing dentition and occlusion in pediatric dentistry, *Pediatr Dent* 31(6): 196-208, 2009/2010.
2. Ngan PW, et al. Orthodontic treatment in the primary dentition, *J Am Dent Assoc* 116:336-340, 1988.
3. Moyers RE. *Handbook of Orthodontics*, 4th ed. Chicago, 1988, CV Mosby.
4. Baume LJ. Physiological tooth migration and its significance for the development of occlusion, *J Dent Res* 29: 123-132, 331-348, 440-447, 1950.
5. Moorrees CFA. Growth changes of the dental arches: A longitudinal study, *J Can Dent Assoc* 24:449-457, 1958.
6. Moorrees CFA. *Dentition of the Growing Child*. Cambridge, 1959, Harvard University Press.
7. Bishara SE, et al. Arch width changes from 6 weeks to 45 years of age, *Am J Orthod Dentofacial Orthop* 111: 401-409, 1997.
8. Moyers RE, Wainwright RL. Skeletal contributions to occlusal development. In McNamara JA, *The Biology of Occlusal Development, Craniofacial Growth Series*, 1977, Monograph, p 89-111.
9. Nance HN. The limitations of orthodontic treatment. I. Mixed dentition diagnosis and treatment, *Am J Orthod* 33:177-223, 1947.
10. Gianelly AA. Crowding—timing of treatment, *Angle Orthod* 64:414-418, 1994.
11. Gianelly AA. Leeway space and the resolution of crowding in the mixed dentition, *Semin Orthod* 1:188-194, 1995.
12. Miyamoto W, et al. Effect of premature loss of deciduous canines and molars on malocclusion of the permanent dentition, *J Dent Res* 55:584-590, 1976.

13. Owen DG. The incidence and nature of space closure following the premature extraction of deciduous teeth—a literature survey, *Am J Orthod* 59:37-49, 1971.

14. Grøn AM. Prediction of tooth emergence, *J Dent Res* 41:573-585, 1962.

15. Brill WA. The distal shoe space maintainer: Chairside fabrication and clinical performance, *Pediatr Dent* 24:561-565, 2002.

16. Carroll CE, Jones JE. Pressure-appliance therapy following premature loss of primary molars, *J Dent Child* 49:347-351, 1982.

17. Bauss O, et al. Autotransplantation of immature third molars: Influence of different splinting methods and fixation periods, *Dent Traumatol* 18(6):322-328, 2002.

18. Ramfjord SP. Bruxism: A clinical and electromyographic study, *J Am Dent Assoc* 62:21-44, 1961.

19. Sheppard IM. The treatment of bruxism, *Dent Clin North Am* 207-213, 1960.

20. Traisman AS, Traisman HS. Thumb- and finger-sucking: A study of 2,650 infants and children, *J Pediatr* 52:566-572, 1959.

21. Subtelny JD. Oral habits—studies in form, function, and therapy, *Angle Orthod* 43:349-383, 1973.

22. Subtelny JD. Oral respiration: Facial maldevelopment and corrective dentofacial orthopedics, *Angle Orthod* 50:147-164, 1980.

23. Popovich F, Thompson GW. Thumb and finger sucking—its relation to malocclusion, *Am J Orthod* 63:148-155, 1973.

24. Zardetto CG, et al. Effects of different pacifiers on the primary dentition and oral myofunctional structures of preschool children, *Pediatr Dent* 24:522-560, 2002.

25. Haryett RD, et al. Chronic thumb-sucking: Psychologic effectiveness of various methods of treatment, *Am J Orthod* 53:569-585, 1967.

26. Haryett RD, et al. Chronic thumb-sucking—a second report on treatment and its psychologic effects, *Am J Orthod* 57:164-178, 1970.

27. Haskell BS, Mink JR. An aid to stop thumb sucking— the "Bluegrass" appliance, *Pediatr Dent* 13:83-85, 1991.

28. Davidson PO, et al. Thumb-sucking: Habit or symptom? *J Dent Child* 34:252- 259, 1967.

29. Proffit WR. *Contemporary Orthodontics*, 4th ed. St Louis, 2007, Mosby.

30. Fletcher BT. Etiology of finger-sucking: Review of literature, *J Dent Child* 42:293-298, 1975.

31. Hanson ML, Cohen MS. Effects of form and function on swallowing and the developing dentition, *Am J Orthod* 64:63-74, 1973.

32. Proffit WR. Equilibrium theory revisited—factors influencing position of the teeth, *Angle Orthod* 48:175-185, 1978.

33. Kurol J, Bergland L. Longitudinal study and cost-benefit analysis of the effect of early treatment of posterior crossbites in the primary dentition, *Eur J Orthod* 14:173-179, 1992.

34. Modeer T, et al. Sucking habits and their relation to posterior crossbite in 4 year old children, *Scand J Dent Res* 90:323-328, 1982.

35. Lindner A, Modeer T. Relation between sucking habits and dental characteristics in preschool children with unilateral crossbite, *Scand J Dent Res* 97:278-283, 1989.

36. Kutin G, Hawes RR. Posterior cross-bites in the deciduous and mixed dentitions, *Am J Orthod* 56:491-504, 1969.

37. Hesse K, et al. Changes in condylar position and occlusion associated with maxillary expansion for correction of functional unilateral posterior crossbite, *Am J Orthod Dentofac Orthop* 111:410-418, 1997.

38. Myers DR, et al. Condylar position in children with functional posterior crossbites before and after correction, *Pediatr Dent* 2:190-194, 1980.

39. Pirtiniemi P, et al. Relationship between craniofacial and condyle path asymmetry in unilateral crossbite patients, *Eur J Orthod* 12:408-413, 1990.

40. Lindner A. Longitudinal study on the effect of early interceptive treatment in 4-year-old children with unilateral cross-bite, *Scand J Dent Res* 197:432-441, 1989.

41. Krebs AA. Rapid expansion of mid-palatal suture by fixed appliance. An implant study over a 7- year period, *Trans Eur Orthod* 131-132, 1964.

42. Hicks EP. Slow maxillary expansion—a clinical study of skeletal versus dental response to low magnitude force, *Am J Orthop* 73:121-141, 1979.

43. Thomas GG, et al. Experimentally determined forces of maxillary lingual arch expansion appliances, *J Pedod* 7(1):3-7, 1982.

44. Harberson VA, Myers DR. Mid-palatal suture opening during functional posterior crossbite correction, *Am J Orthod* 74(3):310-313, 1978.

45. Bell RA, Lecompte EJ. The effects of maxillary expansion using a quad-helix appliance during the deciduous and mixed dentitions, *Am J Orthod* 79:152-157, 1981.

46. Bjerklin K, Kurol J. Ectopic eruption of the maxillary first permanent molar: Etiologic factors, *Am J Orthod* 84:147-155, 1983.

47. Young DH. Ectopic eruption of the first permanent molar, *J Dent Child* 24:153-162, 1957.

48. DeBaets J, Chiarini M. The pseudo class I: A newly defined type of malocclusion, *J Clin Orthod* 29:73-88, 1995.

49. Dugoni SA, et al. Early mixed dentition treatment— post-retention evaluation of stability and relapse, *Angle Orthod* 65:311-320, 1995.

50. Rebellato J, et al. Lower arch perimeter preservation using the lingual arch, *Am J Orthod Dentofac Orthop* 112:449-456, 1997.

51. Brennan MM, Gianelly AA. The use of the lingual arch in the mixed dentition to resolve incisor crowding, *Am J Orthod Dentofac Orthop* 117:81-85, 2000.

52. Kokich VG. Congenitally missing teeth—orthodontic management in the adolescent patient, *Am J Orthod Dentofac Orthop* 121:594-595, 2002.

53. Bishara SE, et al. Proceedings of the workshop discussions on early orthodontic treatment. College of Diplomates of the American Board of Orthodontics, *Am J Orthod Dentofac Orthop* 113:5-6, 1998.

54. Andrews LF. The six keys to normal occlusion, *Am J Orthod* 62:296-309, 1972.

SUGGESTED READINGS

Bacetti T, Franchi L, McNamara JA. Treatment and post-treatment craniofacial changes after rapid maxillary expansion and facemask therapy, *Am J Orthod Dentofac Orthop* 118:404-413, 2000.

Bishara SE. Impacted maxillary canines, *Am J Orthod Dentofac Orthop* 101:159-171, 1992.

Dincer M, et al. Space maintainer effects on intercanine arch width and length, *J Clin Pediatr Dent* 21:47-50, 1996.

Ericson S, Kurol J. Resorption of incisors after ectopic eruption of maxillary canines—a CT study, *Angle Orthod* 70:415-423, 2000.

Foley TF, Wright GZ, Weinberger SJ. Management of lower incisor crowding in the early mixed dentition, *J Dent Child* 63:169-174, 1996.

Halterman CW. A simple technique for the treatment of ectopically erupting permanent first molars, *J Am Dent Assoc* 105:1031-1033, 1982.

Humphrey WP. A simple technique for correcting an ectopically erupting first permanent molar, *J Dent Child* 29: 176-178, 1962.

Kennedy DB, Turley PK. Clinical management of ectopically erupting first permanent molars, *Am J Orthod Dentofac Orthop* 96:336-345, 1987.

Kluemper GT, Beeman CS, Hicks EP. Early orthodontic treatment—what are the imperatives? *J Am Dent Assoc* 131: 613-620, 2000.

Koroluk LD, Tulloch JF, Phillips C. Incisor trauma and early treatment for Class II Division I malocclusion, *Am J Orthod Dentofacial Orthop* 123:117-126, 2003.

Moorrees CFA, Chadha JM. Available space for the incisors during dental development: A growth study based on physiologic age, *Angle Orthod* 35:12-24, 1965.

Moorees CFA, et al. Growth studies of the dentition—a review, *Am J Orthod* 55:600-613, 1969.

Ngan P, Alkire RG, Fields H. Management of space problems in the primary and mixed dentitions, *J Am Dent Assoc* 130:1330-1339, 1999.

Rajab LD. Clinical performance and survival of space maintainers—evaluation over a period of five years, *J Dent Child* 69:156-160, 2002.

Tulloch JF, et al. Outcomes in a 2-phase randomized clinical trial of early Class II treatment, *Am J Orthod Dentofac Orthop* 125:657-667, 2004.

Vargo J, et al. Treatment effects and short-term relapse of maxillomandibular expansion during the early to mid-mixed dentition, *Am J Orthod Dentofac Orthop* 131:456-463, 2007.

Vizzotto MB, et al. The Quad-helix appliance in the primary dentition—orthodontic and orthopedic measurements, *J Clin Pediatr Dent* 32(2):165-170, 2007.

CHAPTER 28

Multidisciplinary Team Approach to Cleft Lip and Palate Management

▲ James E. Jones, Alan Michael Sadove, Jeffrey A. Dean, and Donald V. Huebener

CHAPTER OUTLINE

Cleft lip and palate, the most common of the craniofacial anomalies, are severe congenital anomalies that have an incidence of 0.28 to 3.74 per 1000 live births globally. In the United States, cleft lip and palate occur in approximately 1 in 1000 newborns. The incidence varies widely among races. Cleft lip and palate occur in about 1 in 800 white newborns, 1 in 2000 black newborns, and 1 in 500 Japanese or Navaho Indian newborns. Isolated cleft palate occurs in about 1 in 2000 newborns and demonstrates less racial variation. Cleft lip and palate together account for approximately 50% of all cases, whereas isolated cleft lip and isolated cleft palate each occur in about 25% of cases. Many of these congenital anomalies appear to be genetically determined, although the majority are of unknown cause or are attributable to teratogenic influences (see Chapter 6).

CLASSIFICATION OF CLEFT LIP AND PALATE

There is a tendency to conceptualize cleft lip and palate as a homogenous anomaly. If that was true, a treatment plan applicable to all cases could be formulated. However, the reality is that clefts vary widely in their clinical presentations (Fig. 28-1).

To standardize reporting of cleft lip and palate, the Nomenclature Committee of the American Association of Cleft Palate Rehabilitation devised a classification system that later was adopted by the Cleft Palate Association. The complexity of this system, however, has made its acceptance less than overwhelming. Veau proposed the most frequently used system.[1] He classified clefts of the lip as follows:

- Class I—a unilateral notching of the vermilion not extending into the lip
- Class II—a unilateral notching of the vermilion border, with the cleft extending into the lip but not including the floor of the nose
- Class III—a unilateral clefting of the vermilion border of the lip extending into the floor of the nose
- Class IV—any bilateral clefting of the lip, whether it be incomplete notching or complete clefting

Veau divided palatal clefts into four classes as follows (Fig. 28-2):
- Class I—involves only the soft palate
- Class II—involves the soft and hard palates but not the alveolar process
- Class III—involves both soft and hard palates and the alveolar process on one side of the premaxillary area
- Class IV—involves both soft and hard palates and continues through the alveolus on both sides of the premaxilla, leaving it free and often mobile

Veau did not include submucous clefts of the palate in his classification system. Submucous clefts may frequently be diagnosed by the following physical findings: bifid uvula, palpable notching at the posterior portion of the hard palate, and a zona pellucida (thin, translucent membrane). Submucous clefts of the palate may be associated with an incomplete velopharyngeal mechanism or eustachian tube dysfunction.

MULTIDISCIPLINARY CLEFT LIP AND PALATE TEAM

Children born with cleft lips and palates have many problems that need to be solved for successful habilitation. The complexity of these problems requires that

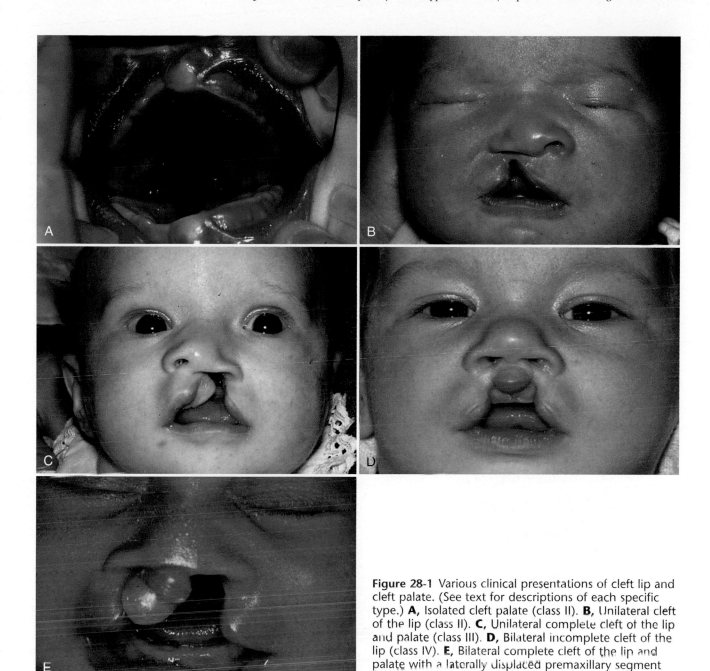

Figure 28-1 Various clinical presentations of cleft lip and cleft palate. (See text for descriptions of each specific type.) **A,** Isolated cleft palate (class II). **B,** Unilateral cleft of the lip (class II). **C,** Unilateral complete cleft of the lip and palate (class III). **D,** Bilateral incomplete cleft of the lip (class IV). **E,** Bilateral complete cleft of the lip and palate with a laterally displaced premaxillary segment (class IV).

numerous health care practitioners cooperate in providing the specialized knowledge and skills necessary to ensure comprehensive care. The cleft palate team concept has evolved from that need.

To address the many treatment regimens and different care protocols, the American Cleft Palate– Craniofacial Association (http://www.cleftpalate- craniofacial.org) convened a consensus conference on recommended practices for the care of patients with craniofacial anomalies. This conference produced the document "Parameters for Evaluation and Treatment of Patients with Cleft Lip/Palate or other Craniofacial Anomalies."[2] This serves as a guide for implementing the multidisciplinary approach to cleft and craniofacial care and is used by teams in the United States and Canada.

Because optimal care is best achieved by multiple types of clinical expertise, the teams may be composed of individuals in (1) the dental specialties (orthodontics, oral surgery, pediatric dentistry, and prosthodontics), (2) the medical specialties (genetics, otolaryngology, pediatrics, plastic surgery, and psychiatry), and (3) allied health care fields (audiology, nursing, psychology, social work, and speech pathology).

These care providers assess the patient's medical status and general development, dental development, facial esthetics, psychological well-being, hearing, and

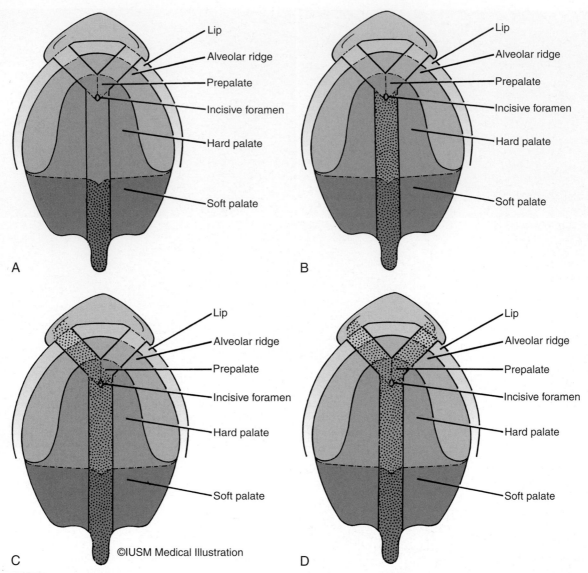

Figure 28-2 Veau's classification of cleft lip and palate. Shaded area, Extent of the cleft. **A,** Class I cleft of the soft palate only. **B,** Class II cleft of the soft and hard palate but not involving the alveolar process. **C,** Class III unilateral complete cleft of the lip and palate. **D,** Class IV bilateral complete cleft of the lip and palate.

speech development (Fig. 28-3). Team members must communicate effectively among themselves, with the child and parents, and with the primary care physician and dentist. Individuals on the team must respect one another's opinions and be flexible in planning and carrying out therapy. Periodic evaluation is necessary to assess the effect of previous therapy and to determine whether an alternative approach may be necessary. A team conference immediately after patient examination is a desirable way to discuss current problems and plan timely therapy.

Whitehouse describes the clinical team as a "close, cooperative, democratic, multiprofessional union devoted to a common purpose—the best treatment of the fundamental needs of the patient."[3]

GENERAL RESPONSIBILITIES OF TEAM MEMBERS

DENTAL SPECIALTIES

The pediatric dentist is responsible for the overall dental care of the patient. Numerous dental anomalies and malocclusions occur with a cleft lip or palate. These may be attributed to the congenital clefting itself or may be secondary to the surgical correction of the primary defects. A high correlation is found between the number and severity of dental problems and the type and severity of the cleft.

The pediatric dentist should discuss with the patient and parents the traditional dental problems associated with clefting. Any one, or several, of the following

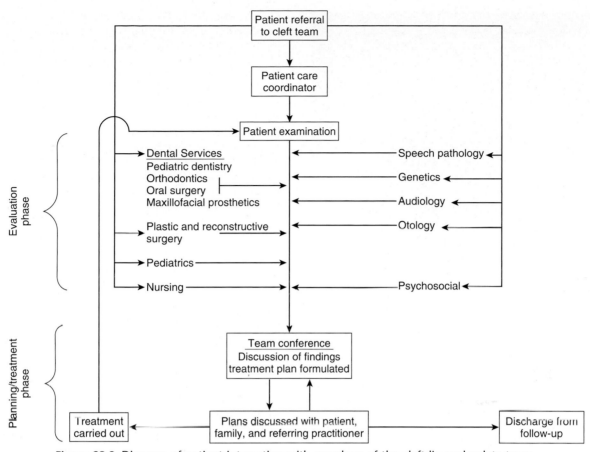

Figure 28-3 Diagram of patient interaction with members of the cleft lip and palate team.

conditions may occur with a significantly greater frequency than in the general population:

1. Natal, or neonatal, teeth are usually maxillary central incisors observed in patients with a complete unilateral or bilateral cleft palate (Fig. 28-4).

2. There is a high incidence of congenitally absent teeth, especially the primary or permanent lateral incisor area adjacent to the alveolar cleft. There is also an increased incidence of congenitally missing premolars.

3. There is a significant increase in the frequency of supernumerary teeth (Fig. 28-5), which are often seen in those with complete unilateral or bilateral clefts. Again, the primary lateral incisors are most frequently absent. Occasionally, there can be supernumerary teeth and congenitally missing teeth in patients with cleft lip only with or without notching of the alveolus.

4. It is common to find ectopic primary lateral incisors located palatally, adjacent to, or within the cleft site. In the permanent dentition, canines on the side of the complete alveolar cleft may erupt palatally into the cleft.

5. Various anomalies of tooth morphology are frequently seen in association with complete unilateral and bilateral clefts of the palate. These include enamel hypoplasia, microdontia or macrodontia, fused teeth, and aberrations in crown shape. The teeth most often affected are the primary and permanent maxillary incisors.

6. Permanent teeth that erupt adjacent to a cleft of the alveolar ridge usually have a deficiency of supporting

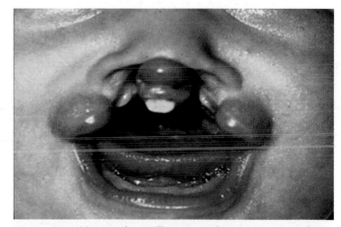

Figure 28-4 Neonatal maxillary central incisor in a newborn infant with a bilateral complete cleft of the lip and palate.

alveolar bone about the root surfaces. These teeth are susceptible to premature loss. A decrease in alveolar bone support may be accentuated when periodontal disease is present or when orthodontic appliance therapy is used indiscriminately.

7. With great frequency, permanent central incisors adjacent to an alveolar cleft erupt in a rotated position and with deviations of axial root inclination.

8. With a complete cleft of the palate and alveolus there is no longer a contiguous maxillary arch. External forces applied to the maxilla (e.g., by muscles of

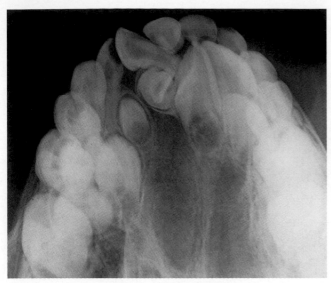

Figure 28-5 Maxillary occlusal radiograph demonstrating supernumerary maxillary central incisors.

mastication or by the contraction of scar tissue after surgical repair of the cleft palate) can result in medial collapse of the posterior segments. A posterior crossbite may be observed unilaterally or bilaterally.

9. In an infant with a complete bilateral cleft of the lip and palate, the premaxilla is often protuberant and mobile. There may be a greater than 100% overbite with subsequent stripping of the labial-attached gingiva overlying the mandibular incisors (Fig. 28-6). Traumatic anterior end-to-end occlusion, or an anterior crossbite, is also common.

10. In a patient with a complete unilateral or bilateral cleft of the palate, the lateral facial profile may appear noticeably convex (Fig. 28-7). This may become more perceptible as the child grows older. The appearance may be attributed to a true mandibular or pseudomandibular prognathism. In pseudomandibular prognathism, the maxilla is in spatial disharmony with

the mandible. This may be caused by a retrognathic maxilla or an attenuation of the anteroposterior and vertical growth of the maxilla.

Parents are often so overwhelmed by other aspects of the cleft that they give dental care a low priority or even neglect it altogether. Preventive dental care is extremely important in these cases. The intact dental occlusion is the foundation around which future orthodontic therapy takes place. For this reason, optimum dental health is essential for total habilitation of the patient. Any compromise will lead to a less than optimal result. Routine prophylaxis and fluoride treatments are mandatory. Referral for preventive dental care should be made during the first year of life. Fluoride supplements, dentifrices, and rinses are indicated if the patient lives in a nonfluoridated community. The parents and patient should be instructed in proper dental hygiene techniques, especially around the defect. Close communication between the primary care dentist and the cleft team is important to ensure the continuity of care necessary during the extended treatment of such patients. Routine periodic reports from the cleft team should be forwarded to the child's primary care dentist, especially during orthodontic or surgical treatment. Pediatric dentists often are involved in the presurgical and postsurgical treatment phase of maxillary orthopedics. Both active and passive appliances are used to bring the cleft segments into a more ideal alignment and thereby promote a more favorable initial surgical outcome.

The orthodontist plays a key role in the diagnosis and treatment of a cleft condition by obtaining records

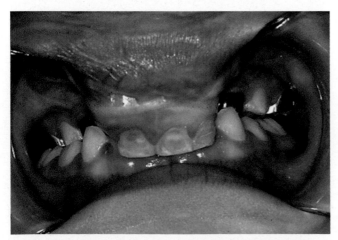

Figure 28-6 Bilateral complete cleft of the lip and palate demonstrating a greater than 100% overbite. Stripping of the labial attached gingiva of the mandibular central and lateral incisors is common in this presentation.

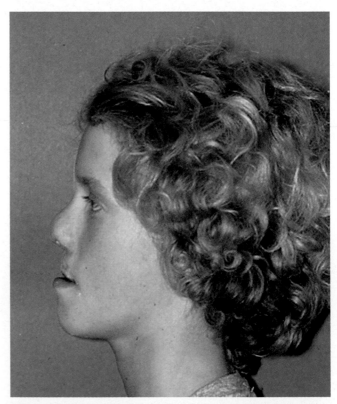

Figure 28-7 Lateral facial profile of an adolescent boy with a repaired bilateral complete cleft of the lip and palate. Maxillary hypoplasia, secondary to the cleft defect, often produces a greatly concave lateral facial profile.

necessary for diagnosis and treatment planning. These include cephalometric and panoramic radiographs, study models, and diagnostic photographs. Analysis of these records enables the orthodontist to describe and quantitate the facial skeleton and soft tissue deformities. Using expertise in the growth and development of the facial skeleton, this specialist can identify problem areas and, with some limitations, predict growth and development. Many team members depend on the orthodontist's analysis and quantitations of the cleft anomaly for treatment planning.

The orthodontist also provides comprehensive orthodontic care for patients. Most orthodontic care can be considered conventional, but for difficult dental configurations, innovation and imagination are required for treatment. If surgical treatment is indicated, the orthodontist works closely with the surgeon to plan the most appropriate procedure. Immediate postoperative function, esthetic result, and long-term stability are factors considered before surgery.

The ability to surgically alter skeletal relationships of the maxillomandibular complex is the basis for participation by the oral and maxillofacial surgeon on the cleft team. This specialist evaluates all patients for facial form and function and jaw position. Many patients have significant skeletal malocclusions that cannot be treated by conventional orthodontics and require surgical correction.

The surgical placement of primary and secondary alveolar cleft bone grafts is another important role of the oral and maxillofacial surgeon. These grafts aid in dental habilitation. The grafted bone supports the teeth adjacent to the cleft site and provides bone through which teeth may erupt. A detailed discussion of these grafts follows later in this chapter.

The maxillofacial prosthodontist replaces, restores, or rehabilitates orofacial structures that may be congenitally missing or malformed. Nonliving materials are used to restore and enhance form and anatomy. There is a special commitment to the oral cavity because this specialist fabricates prosthetic appliances to rehabilitate mastication, deglutition, speech, and oral esthetics.

Many patients with clefts have congenitally missing teeth or malformed teeth that may need to be removed. In these cases, masticatory function, speech, and orofacial esthetics are compromised, and successful habilitation dictates that these missing teeth be replaced to achieve as near normal a condition as possible (Fig. 28-8). The maxillofacial prosthodontist may do this with fixed or removable appliances or with a combination of the two.

Occasionally, patients demonstrate aberrant speech patterns caused by failure of the soft palate to elevate properly. In such cases, a palatal lift appliance is fabricated to aid the speech mechanism. In other cases the maxillofacial prosthodontist may fabricate a speech bulb prosthesis to aid or augment the velopharyngeal mechanism. In patients with considerable escape of air through persistent palatal fistulas, the fistulas can be obturated (Fig. 28-9).

MEDICAL AND ALLIED HEALTH SPECIALTIES

The patient care coordinator arranges appointments, maintains patient records, and monitors the interaction of the patient and family with the various team members.

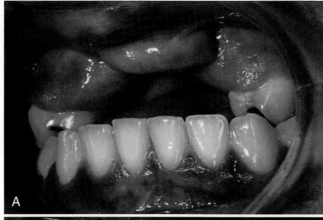

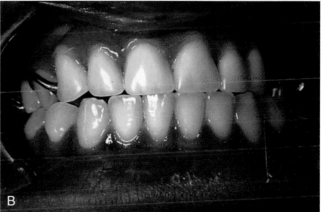

Figure 28-8 A, Bilateral complete cleft of the lip and palate in which the maxillary six permanent anterior teeth have been removed. **B,** Removable prosthodontic appliance providing acceptable occlusal and esthetic results.

The coordinator corresponds with health and school personnel near the patient's home to help provide continuity of care for the cleft patients within the community. The coordinator is the most convenient point of contact with team members for the patients, their families, and health care practitioners outside the medical center complex.

The pediatrician, often the patient's own pediatrician or family physician, is responsible for maintenance of the patient's overall health. This specialist performs complete physical evaluations and helps assess the patient's physiologic status. Close attention is also directed to growth status and other developmental milestones.

The medical geneticist examines the patient to find characteristics of syndromes associated with cleft lip and palate. Consideration is given to the genetic basis for the anomaly, and this information is related to the parents. Genetic counseling is a very important function of the geneticist. Parents are vitally interested in risk assessment relative to future offspring, and other family members who may be at risk are often counseled (see Chapter 6).

The role of the plastic and reconstructive surgeon usually begins with a determination of the timing and method of lip closure. With complete clefts, the plastic surgeon may next be responsible for obtaining bone grafts to be used in closing defects of the maxillary dental alveolus. This specialist is also involved in cleft palate repair.

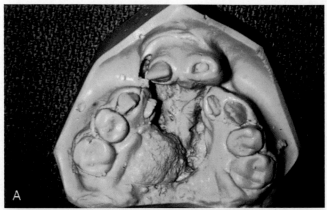

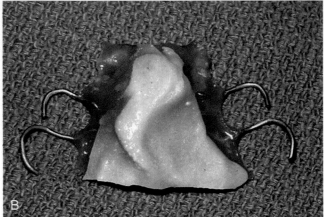

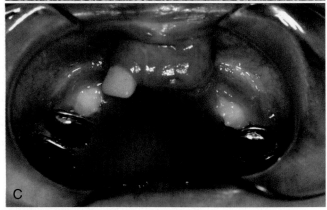

Figure 28-9 A, Diagnostic maxillary model of a bilateral complete cleft of the lip and palate. Notice the large patent oronasal fistula that resulted after several attempts to close the defect surgically. **B,** Maxillary prosthesis constructed for the patient to obturate the palatal defect. **C,** Palatal prosthesis in place. This closure provides a reduction in the amount of fluids and foods that enter the nasal cavity during eating. The closure also facilitates more normal speech production.

An additional responsibility may be to conduct a naso-pharyngoscopic examination of the speech mechanism. If a defect is identified, the plastic surgeon may perform a pharyngoplasty to improve velopharyngeal function. The final role is to correct internal or external cleft nasal deformities.

The social worker acts as the patient's advocate in many cases and aids in psychosocial assessment. This team member assists the family by making referrals to persons or agencies at the local, county, and state levels for guidance regarding financial resources for medical care. During hospitalization, the social worker provides supportive counseling and facilitates communication between the family and medical or hospital personnel. The focus is on helping the family cope with stress during and after surgery and on dealing with emotional factors involved in forming realistic expectations of surgical outcomes and in adapting to problems of body image.

The psychiatrist and psychologist evaluate the patient for strengths and weaknesses in cognitive, interpersonal, emotional, behavioral, and social development. Emphasis is placed on the patient's ability to cope with the emotional and physical stress created by the cleft defect. Consultation with the parents and school regarding educational or behavioral management occurs when indicated.

The speech pathologist functions essentially as a monitor of speech output. All speech sounds are analyzed to determine deviations from normal, and the cause of any deviation is evaluated. To the extent that anatomic variations are corrected, the speech pathologist offers therapeutic options to enhance maturation of speech or to achieve satisfactory compensation in motor production for optimal speech.

The audiologist performs tests to identify any hearing difficulties. When neither the child nor the parents recognize hearing problems, the result can be a delay in speech and language development and poor performance in school. When hearing tests or impedance measures are abnormal, a referral is made to an otolaryngologist for an ear examination. The otolaryngologist coordinates audiologic tests and any special studies that may be needed to evaluate middle ear structures. Any middle ear surgery that is to be done is performed by this member of the team. He or she also may perform a nasopharyngoscopic examination in coordination with the speech pathologist.

Nurses provide varying functions that are valuable to the cleft lip and palate team. They actively communicate with other disciplines in passing on information regarding the special needs of each child and family. Nurses emphasize total family involvement, not just treatment of the patient. They prepare patients and families for either outpatient or inpatient surgery and assist in the overall management process. Above all, they are extremely important in assessing the initial feeding issues and advising parents with ongoing nutritional concerns.

The presence of more complex craniofacial anomalies, such as Crouzon syndrome, Treacher-Collins syndrome, or hemifacial microsomia, require additional specialists on the team because there is more deformity. Some of these care providers include anesthesiologists, diagnostic medical imaging radiologists, neurologists, neurosurgeons, and ophthalmologists in addition to those cleft team providers already mentioned.

MULTIDISCIPLINARY SEQUENCING OF TREATMENT IN CLEFTS

The following discussion focuses on major treatment procedures performed by members of the cleft team. For convenience, treatment is divided into four stages, which generally correspond to stages in the child's dental development.

STAGE I (MAXILLARY ORTHOPEDIC STAGE: BIRTH TO 18 MONTHS)

Management of the patient with a cleft begins with immediate attention to the needs of the newborn. Feeding problems are often associated with cleft anomalies, which make it difficult for the infant to maintain adequate nutrition. These problems include insufficient suction to pull milk from the nipple, excessive air intake during feeding (requiring several burpings), choking, nasal discharge, and excessive time required to take nourishment.

McNeil in the 1950s[4,5] and other authors since then have advocated various prosthetic appliances, both active and passive, for the treatment of infants born with unilateral and bilateral clefts of the lip and palate. One such prosthesis, an intraoral maxillary obturator, has proved beneficial by providing an artificial palate. The advantages of this prosthetic therapy include the following:

1. Provides a false palate against which the infant can suck, reduces the incidence of feeding difficulties in newborns, and helps maintain adequate nutrition
2. Provides maxillary cross-arch stability and prevents arch collapse after definitive cheiloplasty (surgical closure of the lip)
3. Provides maxillary orthopedic molding of the cleft segments into approximation before primary alveolar cleft bone grafting

In a study by Jones, maxillary obturators were constructed to facilitate feeding for 51 infants with unilateral or bilateral cleft lip and palate.[6] From birth, each infant had continuously experienced feeding difficulties before obturator therapy. After the infants had worn the obturator for at least 8 months, parents reported that they were more comfortable while feeding their infants and that nasal discharge was reduced. The time required for feeding and the difficulty experienced by the parents were also reduced. Of particular importance was the reported reduction of parental apprehension during feeding. All parents recommended the obturator for others who have infants with cleft lips and palates. It was also reported that the weights of the infants at 1, 3, and 6 months of age consistently remained at, or above, the 50th percentile compared to normative growth data. No fluctuation in weight was noted even after primary lip closure at about 3 months of age.

Not all clinicians who work with infants with cleft lips and palates advocate use of prosthetic feeding appliances. Some believe that such appliances are not effective in facilitating feeding. Pashayan and McNab recommend using a standard nipple that has been crosscut.[7] This enlarged cut provides improved ejection of the milk into the infant's mouth with a minimum of effort. Although this recommendation is appropriate for infants born with isolated clefts of the palate, obturator construction is generally indicated for those born with complete clefts of the lip and palate. This is especially important in consideration of the maxillary orthopedic molding of the alveolar segments after surgical closure of the lip. In a recent survey, it was reported that approximately 32% of cleft teams in the United States and Canada use this prosthetic feeding appliance.

Impression Technique and Obturator Construction

An alginate impression of the infant's maxillary arch is made with a modified stock tray. Ideally, this is accomplished as soon after birth as possible. The infant is held upright during the impression process to prevent aspiration of excess material (Fig. 28-10). Appropriate emergency equipment, including forced oxygen, suction, and standard airway management equipment, should be available. The impression should exhibit good anatomic detail with coverage of the entire maxillary arch (Fig. 28-11). A stone model is then produced. The steps in obturator construction are as follows:

1. Block out excessive undercuts with modeling dough or wax. Modeling dough is preferred because it is easy to remove from the finished prosthesis.
2. Apply a tinfoil substitute over the entire surface of the maxillary model and let it dry.
3. If necessary, place a dam of modeling dough on the back of the model to hold the resin in the palatal defect while curing.
4. Pour a mixture of soft, autopolymerizing acrylic resin into the cleft to the level of the palate. This provides retention for the prosthesis by gently contouring into the available undercuts (Fig. 28-12).

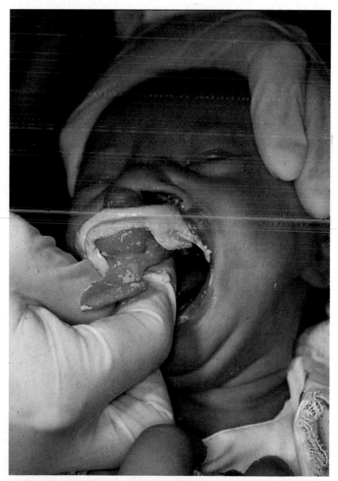

Figure 28-10 Maxillary impression for obturator construction on a newborn with a cleft lip and palate. The infant is held in an upright position to prevent aspiration of excess material.

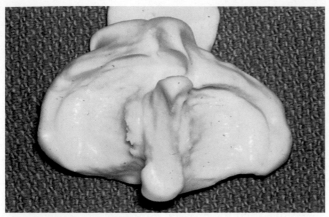

Figure 28-11 Final impression of the infant's maxillary arch. Notice the extension of the material into the cleft defect, as well as the roll produced in the buccal fold. Attention to such detail ensures an excellent reproduction of the intraoral architecture for obturator construction.

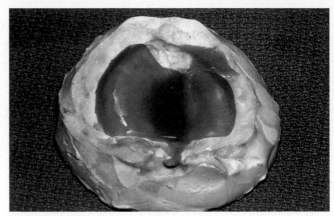

Figure 28-13 Maxillary model at the completion of the application of autopolymerizing acrylic resin. The obturator is allowed to cure for 20 minutes and then is trimmed and polished. Notice the extension of the resin into the mucobuccal fold. This extension further increases the retention of the prosthesis.

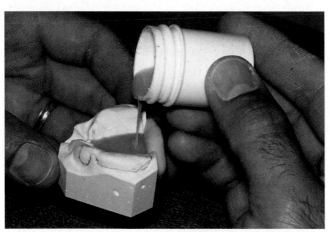

Figure 28-12 Application of soft, autopolymerizing resin into the cleft to the level of the palate. This material provides increased retention of the obturator by contouring into the cleft. Notice the dam of modeling dough, which aids in the placement of the resin.

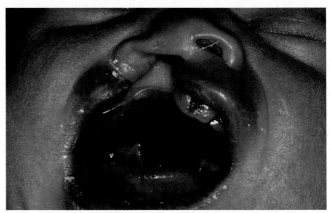

Figure 28-14 Obturator in place on the infant's maxillary arch. Notice the extension of the soft resin into the cleft defect, which provides increased retention. (From Jones JE, Kerkhof RL. Obturator construction for maxillary orthopedics in cleft lip and palate infants, *Quintessence Dent Technol* 8:583-586, 1984.)

5. Place the model in a warm, moist environment to cure for 20 minutes.
6. Add autopolymerizing acrylic resin to the palate using a "salt and pepper" method, making sure the acrylic resin extends well into the mucobuccal fold area (Fig. 28-13).
7. Remove the appliance from the model, and rinse the wax and modeling dough off with hot water. Then trim and polish the appliance.

Clinical Management of Initial Obturator Therapy (Birth to 3 Months)

The appliance is positioned in the infant's mouth (Fig. 28-14). Areas of excessive pressure on any intraoral tissues by the acrylic resin are identified by observation and then reduced. Care is taken to keep the acrylic resin from impinging on muscle attachments or extending to the depth of the buccal vestibule. Parents are instructed in placement and removal of the appliance and its daily cleaning. Infants are usually seen for adjustments 2 days after appliance delivery. Monthly observations are then scheduled. In most cases, this appliance will serve until the time of initial lip closure at approximately 3 months of age. The major advantage of obturator use during this stage is to enhance the child's ability to obtain nourishment.

Premaxillary Orthopedics (Birth to 4 or 5 Months)

In some cases of bilateral cleft lip and palate, the infant has a premaxillary segment positioned severely anterior to the maxillary arch segments or deviated laterally to one side of the cleft defect (Fig. 28-15). This presents a difficult clinical challenge for the surgeon before surgical closure of the lip. If lip surgery is undertaken with the premaxilla in such an abnormal position, the chances of lip dehiscence (lip separation caused by increased pressure at the suture lines) are increased.

As early as 1686, Hofman described the use of a head cap and premaxillary strap to reposition the premaxilla.[8] This type of apparatus is useful for anteroposterior and

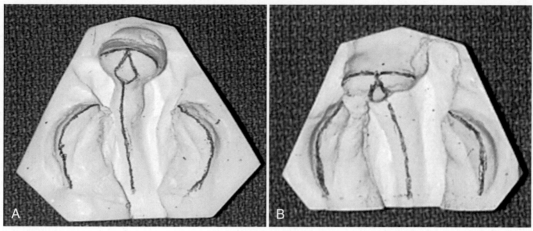

Figure 28-15 Representative diagnostic models of two clinical presentations in bilateral complete cleft of the lip and palate. **A,** Severe anteroposterior protrusion of the premaxillary segment. **B,** Severe anteroposterior protrusion of the premaxillary segment with a lateral deviation.

vertical repositioning. The following describes the construction and orthopedic management of the typical clinical presentations: an anteriorly positioned maxilla and a laterally displaced premaxilla.

As soon as possible (usually within 2 weeks of birth), an impression is made of the infant's maxillary arch for construction of an intraoral obturator in the manner previously described. After delivery of the obturator, the infant is allowed to become accustomed to the appliance for 1 week. At the second appointment, the infant is fitted with a premaxillary retraction appliance.

Appliance Construction for Premaxillary Retraction
A baby bonnet is made to provide "headgear" anchorage for a premaxillary retraction strap. An elastic strap is placed over the protruding premaxilla and anchored to the infant's head using the bonnet. By the application of sequentially increasing equal forces to the premaxilla, the premaxilla is retropositioned into a more normal position relative to the maxillary segments. This bonnet-and-strap appliance is worn 24 hours a day and is removed only for feeding. The desired movement can usually be accomplished within 6 to 8 weeks (Fig. 28-16).

In many cases the use of soft, elastic tape (Microfoam Tape; 3M, St. Paul, Minn.) can be used to retract the premaxillary segment in a simpler manner than with the bonnet retraction system (Fig. 28-17). The advantages are its ease in fabrication; however, it does not afford the same control of the force direction and therefore cannot be used in all instances.

In the case of a laterally deviated premaxilla in an infant with a bilateral cleft lip and palate (Fig. 28-18A), a straight extraoral force would not place the premaxilla in the facial midline. Therefore the premaxilla must be positioned in the midline before premaxillary retraction. In this clinical presentation, an impression is made of the infant's premaxilla for construction of an external acrylic "bulb" prosthesis. This appliance is fitted over the protruding and laterally displaced premaxilla and anchored to the infant's head

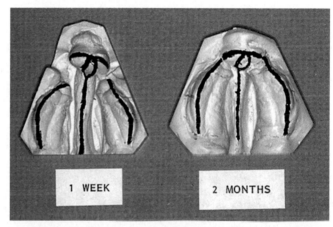

Figure 28-16 Diagnostic models for an infant with a complete bilateral cleft of the lip and palate at 1 week of age (before premaxillary retraction therapy is begun) and at 2 months of age (at the completion of premaxillary retraction therapy). Notice the essentially normal position of the premaxillary segment within the lateral palatal segments.

with a bonnet appliance (see Fig. 28-18B). By the application of sequentially increasing differential forces to the premaxilla with elastic straps attached to the bulb prosthesis, the premaxilla is brought into the facial midline (see Fig. 28-18C). Depending on parental compliance with therapy (the appliance should be in place 24 hours a day), the laterally displaced premaxilla can be repositioned to the facial midline in 3 to 4 weeks. After the premaxilla is in the midline, the bulb appliance is replaced by a single elastic strap (see Fig. 28-18D). Over the next 1 to 2 months, equal pressure is applied on the still protruding premaxilla to reposition it into a more normal position between the lateral segments (see Figs. 28-18E and F).

The rationale for use of a bulb prosthesis before elastic strap retraction includes the following considerations:
1. The bulb prosthesis affords greater control over the differential forces applied to the premaxilla.

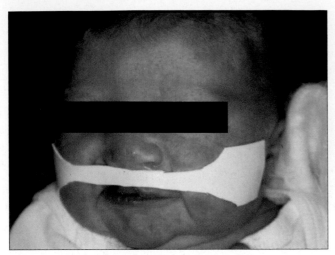

Figure 28-17 Premaxillary retraction using soft elastic tape (Microfoam Tape, 3M).

2. Movement of the premaxilla into the facial midline before retropositioning (rather than into a laterally deviated position) decreases the risk of distorting a vomer stalk.
3. The need for a surgical premaxillary setback (a procedure known to be associated with possible growth attenuation and other complications) is eliminated.
4. Optimum premaxillary positioning may eliminate the need for a staged lip closure (adhesions before definitive lip repair) and thereby decrease total hospitalization time and cost.
5. The appearance of the nose and lip is improved because the lip can be surgically closed under less tension and the alveolar segments have an underlying symmetric alignment.

Airway Obstruction
Infants with airway obstruction secondary to Pierre Robin sequence (micrognathia, glossoptosis, and cleft palate) may require intervention to aid breathing (Fig. 28-19A). An obturator with a posterior palatal extension should be used to reposition the tongue downward and forward out of the cleft site (see Fig. 28-19B). If a nonsurgical approach is unsuccessful, lip-to-tongue adhesion (thus positioning the tongue anteriorly and opening the oral airway) or tracheostomy may be necessary.

Cheiloplasty
The appearance of an unrepaired wide cleft lip can be distressing. Some parents feel anxiety, depression, guilt, or rejection. Lip surgery will significantly improve the infant's appearance and may thereby relieve parental apprehensions and enhance acceptance.

Surgical closure of the cleft lip may be accomplished shortly after birth. However, most surgeons defer closure to allow the infant to be followed by the primary care physician, who assesses early growth and development

and rules out the presence of any other congenital anomaly. Surgical closure is usually accomplished at 10 weeks of age. At the time of lip closure, when the infant is under general anesthesia, an impression is made of the maxillary arch for construction of a new obturator. This is necessary to accommodate craniofacial growth during the first few months of life.

Maxillary Orthopedics (3 to 9 Months)
After definitive lip closure at about 3 months of age, maxillary arch collapse in unilateral or bilateral complete cleft is common. It is attributed to the increased tension placed on the segments by the repaired lip. To prevent this collapse, the obturator is used to provide cross-arch stability and support. As pressure is exerted on the anterior segments of the maxilla by the repaired lip, orthopedic molding of the segments can be achieved. In unilateral cases, the force applied to the greater segment by the intact lip molds that segment around to approximate the lesser segment (Fig. 28-20). This molding is facilitated by the obturator, which provides a fulcrum around which the anterior portion of the greater segment rotates. At the same time the appliance resists any tendency for the greater and lesser segments to collapse toward the midline. In bilateral cleft cases, the repaired lip provides further retraction at the premaxilla, positioning it between the two lateral maxillary segments. When the maxillary segments are in good alignment and abutted across the cleft sites, the patient is ready for the primary cleft bone graft. This generally occurs by 6 to 9 months of age.

Bone Grafting of Alveolar Cleft Defects
Bone grafting of alveolar cleft defects has been a confusing issue to many patients and practitioners. This stems in part from the lack of unanimity concerning terminology and technique. The following definitions, which have been reasonably accepted by practitioners, will be used in this discussion.

Primary bone grafting refers to bone-grafting procedures involving alveolar cleft defects in children younger than 2 years of age; this term implies nothing about technique. Early secondary bone grafting refers to bone-grafting procedures performed between 2 and 4 years of age. *Secondary bone grafting* is done between 4 and 15 years of age, and *late secondary bone grafting* refers to reconstruction of residual alveolar cleft defects in the adult.

Primary Alveolar Cleft Bone Grafting
Primary alveolar cleft bone grafting is controversial. The concept fell into disfavor in the early 1970s amid numerous reports of significant attenuation in midfacial growth. Robertson and Jolleys used an orthodontic appliance for the first 3 months of life when the lip, anterior palate, and soft palate were closed.[9]

A retention device was then fitted until closure of the hard palate at 11 months. Primary bone grafting was carried out at 12 to 15 months when bone was inserted with little dissection through a horizontal incision in the buccal sulcus. After a 5-year follow-up, the authors noted

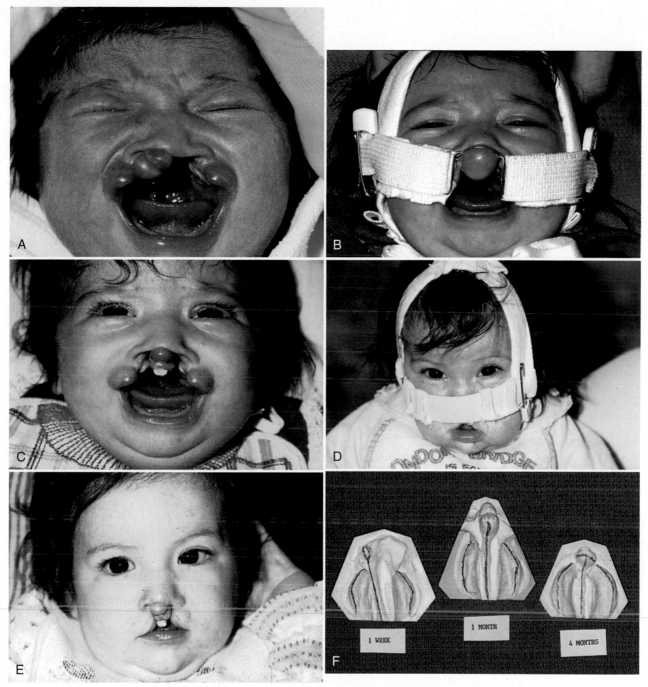

Figure 28-18 A, A bilateral complete cleft of the lip and palate in a newborn infant. Notice the severely anteriorly protruded and laterally deviated premaxillary segment. **B,** Placement of "bulb" prosthesis over the premaxillary segment; bulb is anchored to the bonnet. **C,** Patient at the end of bulb therapy to position the laterally deviated premaxillary segment to the facial midline. **D,** Strap therapy to improve the anteroposterior relationship of the protruding premaxillary segment before definitive lip closure. **E,** Premaxillary segment at the completion of strap therapy. Notice the improvement in position (compare with A) at this time. **F,** Sequential models at 1 week (initial presentation), 1 month (completion of bulb therapy), and 4 months (completion of strap therapy). Notice the improving position of the premaxillary segment at these various times. (**D** and **F** from Jones JE, et al. Three dimensional premaxillary orthopedic technique for improved position and symmetry prior to cheiloplasty in bilateral cleft lip and palate patients, *Quintessence Int* 16:229–231, 1985.)

that patients in the grafted group showed a clear deterioration of the dental-base relationship and development of pseudoprognathism, whereas among those in the nongrafted group the dental-base relationship remained stable. Limitation of growth occurred in the maxillae of the grafted patients and was manifested by reduced anteroposterior development, an increased incidence of crossbite, and a reduced area of the upper jaw. These authors, as well as others, recommended that bone grafting in young patients be abandoned.

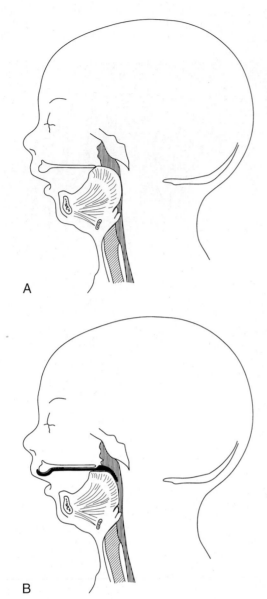

Figure 28-19 A, Infant with airway obstruction secondary to Pierre Robin sequence. Notice the closure of the oral airway related to the retroposition of the tongue. **B,** Infant with obturator in position. Notice the anterior placement of the tongue, which allows the oral airway to remain open.

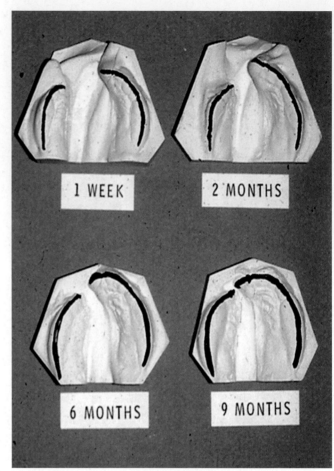

Figure 28-20 Sequential maxillary arch dental models demonstrating maxillary orthopedic molding in an infant with a unilateral complete cleft of the lip and palate. Notice that, as the cleft defect closes with time, lateral arch dimension is maintained, which produces optimal maxillary arch symmetry. (From Jones JE, et al. Maxillary arch expansion in cleft lip and palate infants prior to primary autogenous alveolar bone graft surgery, *Quintessence Int* 17:245-248, 1986.)

These negative reports led to nearly universal cessation of primary alveolar cleft bone grafting on the basis that the procedure, performed at such an early age, significantly attenuates maxillary and midface growth. However, certain interesting facts emerge when these reports are carefully analyzed. None of the reporting groups used the same surgical technique. Although the techniques may appear similar at first glance, there are differences that make each approach unique. Therein lies a problem with the categorical statement that primary cleft bone grafting should be abandoned because it impedes maxillary and midfacial growth. What is primary cleft bone grafting? How broad is its definition? As discussed earlier, the term primary cleft bone grafting implies nothing about technique, only timing. The term is applied to any cleft bone grafting technique used between birth and

2 years of age. Because the techniques vary, sweeping statements that condemn or condone primary cleft bone grafting should be viewed with suspicion. Each technique should be judged on its merits, without any bias traceable to the popular view that primary cleft bone grafting retards maxillary and midfacial growth.

Many of the negative reports have used techniques involving extensive dissection in areas adjacent to and including the vomeropremaxillary suture. Friede reported that surgery in the area of the vomeropremaxillary suture may lead to impaired maxillary and midfacial growth in individuals with unilateral and bilateral clefts.[10] He stated that techniques that disturb the vomeropremaxillary suture would never have been introduced if surgeons had realized the significant role that this suture apparently plays in the postnatal growth of the face in the cleft patient.

For more than 40 years, although primary cleft bone grafting has been generally held in disfavor, one group in particular, Rosenstein and colleagues, has championed the cause of primary cleft bone grafting. As might be expected, their technique differs significantly from the others used. In their approach, a newborn with a cleft was fitted with a maxillary orthopedic appliance. The lip was repaired at approximately 6 weeks of age. Through the orthopedic appliance and pressure of the repaired lip on the alveolus, the maxillary segments were molded into alignment so that the segments abutted across the cleft site. Premaxillary orthopedics was used as necessary with a bilateral cleft to position the premaxilla before lip closure. With the segments well aligned, a minimal dissection technique was used at 6 to 9 months of age to develop a pocket at the level of the alveolus across the cleft site (Fig. 28-21). A 2-cm segment of rib was harvested and split longitudinally. Half was inserted into the pocket in an on-laid fashion over the alveolus, bridging the cleft. Palatoplasty (surgical closure of the palate) was typically completed at 1 year of age.

Preliminary results were encouraging, and in 1982 Rosenstein and colleagues reported on a series of 32 patients who were followed up for up to 15 years.[11] They found no significant attenuation of maxillary or midfacial growth in patients who had received primary cleft bone grafts compared with cleft patients who had received no grafts. In 1991, they reported on another 37 patients (20 with unilateral and 17 with bilateral clefts) and reached the same conclusions.[12] In 2003, they described an additional 82 cases and reported on secondary surgical need and the status of teeth adjacent to the cleft.[13] The authors stated that the growth in their sample was as good as that in other similar samples that did not receive the primary bone grafting. In addition, the authors reported the incidence of orthognathic surgery to be 18.29%; of pharyngoplasty, 3.65%; and of surgical closure of oronasal fistulas, 29.27%.

In cases of unilateral complete clefts, 53.13% of the lateral incisors present adjacent to the cleft area were usable, and in bilateral cases, 57.77% were usable.

The apparent success of their technique can be attributed to the following departures from previous methods:
1. Lip repair was separated from bone grafting.
2. The bone graft was inserted only when the two halves of the maxilla abutted in the alveolar region where there was no great gap to bridge.
3. The limited dissection was carried out only on the anterior surface of the maxilla and alveolus, with no dissection performed in the area of the vomeropremaxillary suture.

Experience demonstrated that in nongrafted clefts, maxillary arch collapse was common after palatoplasty in unilateral and bilateral cases. When the palate was repaired, pulling the tissue together in the midline created transpalatal forces that moved the lesser segment or, in the case of bilateral clefts, the lateral maxillary segments toward the midline. This often resulted in a maxillary arch form that led to crossbite situations and compromised masticatory function. These problems were not always easily correctable. Reestablishing a reasonable arch form through orthodontic and surgical means presented a challenge because scar tissue that had formed across the palate often prevented desired segmental movement. If segmental movements could be accomplished, it was often at the expense of soft tissue form and function. Palatal fistulas frequently persisted or reopened. Periodontal compromises because of stretching of tissue were common. Primary grafting

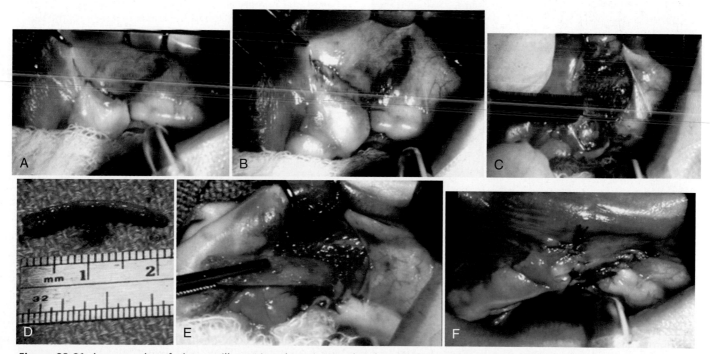

Figure 28-21 A composite of pictures illustrating the primary alveolar cleft bone graft technique. **A,** Abutted maxillary segments with initial incisions outlined. **B,** Development of a small mucosal flap from the lip that will be used to cover the labial surface of the graft. **C,** The development of the subperiosteal pockets on the labial aspect of the alveolus. **D,** Section of rib that has been split longitudinally and contoured slightly to conform to the curvature of the maxillary anterior alveolus. **E,** Insertion of the rib segment into the labial pockets. **F,** Tissue closure over the graft.

establishes maxillary arch continuity early in life by producing a one-piece maxilla rather than two or three segments (Figs. 28-22 and 28-23) and thus facilitates future treatment. Often these patients can be treated like any conventional orthodontic patient. In many instances, primary lateral incisors erupt into and through the graft.

Use of a primary alveolar cleft bone graft does not necessarily preclude the later accomplishment of a secondary alveolar cleft bone graft if it is indicated. The objectives of a secondary cleft bone graft can be somewhat different, as will be seen. Although a recent survey of cleft and craniofacial teams of the American Cleft Palate–Craniofacial Association reported that only 3% of teams perform primary alveolar cleft bone grafting, in our experience it provides excellent results. Continued critical evaluation of our results is being accomplished to document the benefits of the procedure.

A different approach to normalizing the cleft alveolar segment relationships has been advocated by Huebener and Marsh.[14] In their treatment protocol, which uses the forces created by either lip adhesion or primary lip closure, a passive alveolar molding appliance similar to that used by

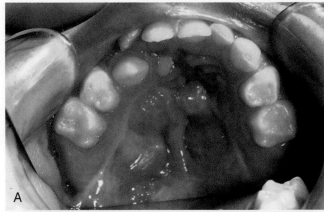

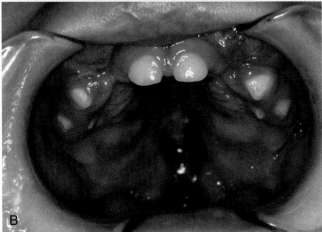

Figure 28-23 **A,** Intraoral view of a unilateral complete cleft of the lip and palate after primary alveolar cleft bone graft. **B,** Intraoral view of a bilateral complete cleft of the lip and palate after primary alveolar cleft bone graft. Because the premaxillary segment is fixed to the lateral maxillary segments, the arch form is expected to remain in good relationship.

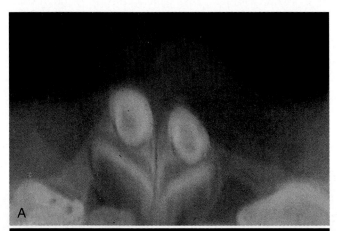

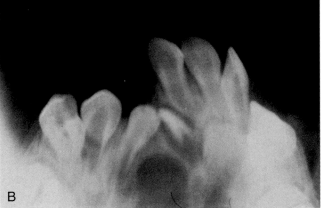

Figure 28-22 **A,** Radiograph of bilateral complete cleft of the lip and palate after primary alveolar cleft bone graft. Notice the grafted bone bridging the cleft sites, which provides stabilization of the premaxillary segment. **B,** Radiograph of unilateral complete cleft of the lip and palate after primary alveolar cleft bone graft. Notice the grafted bone bridging the cleft site and the migration of the primary lateral incisor through the graft.

Rosenstein is employed.[15] The passive appliance does not have an acrylic extension over the alveolar ridges and it is placed on the day of the lip surgery. The tension created by lip closure acts over time on the anterior alveolar cleft segments (in both unilateral and bilateral cleft) and shapes these cleft segments around the anterior portion of the molding appliance. The appliance is worn by the infant until palatoplasty. Usually at that time the cleft segments are abutting and the torqued maxillary frenum has returned to the midsagittal plane. In this protocol, no primary alveolar bone grafting is performed.

Some researchers have recommended the use of active appliances for the normalization of the infant cleft alveolar segments before initial lip surgery. Latham and colleagues use a dentomaxillary advancement appliance to bring unilateral cleft segments into approximation.[16] In bilateral clefts, they expand collapsed lateral cleft segments and actively retract the premaxilla into a more ideal arch form. They postulate that such presurgical maxillary orthopedic procedures make lip surgery easier and result in less soft tissue tension following closure.

More recently, Grayson and Cutting have promoted the use of a nasoalveolar molding (NAM) appliance with a nasal labial extension to shape the nasal cleft cartilage.[17] The objective of this presurgical effort is to reduce the severity of the cleft deformity, approximate the alveolar and lip segments, decrease the nasal base width, and attempt to achieve symmetry of the nasal cartilages. (Fig. 28-24). They indicate that if these treatment objectives are achieved, the esthetic and functional outcome of the primary lip and nose surgery should be more favorable. In addition, an additional presurgical treatment objective in bilateral cleft patients is columella lengthening. With the use of bilateral nasal stints and taping techniques, the almost absent columella in bilateral clefts can be nonsurgically elongated before initial lip and nose surgery.

Palatoplasty

Closure of the palate is accomplished between 12 months and 2 years of age. The primary purpose of completing palate closure by 2 years of age is to facilitate the acquisition of normal speech, because this correlates with the age at which most children begin to talk. The procedure may also improve hearing and swallowing by aligning the cleft palatal musculature.

After primary closure of the cleft palate, approximately 25% of patients demonstrate some velopharyngeal insufficiency. A persistent inability to close the nasopharynx may result in unsatisfactory speech (nasality and articulation problems), regurgitation of fluids from the nose, and facial grimacing. Of the various surgical approaches to correct velopharyngeal insufficiency, the pharyngeal flap is most commonly used at Indiana University. The procedure is generally performed when velopharyngeal insufficiency is documented in an attempt to normalize the speech of the child before he or she begins school.

One of the most important aspects of stage I is the beginning of infant oral health care. It is during this time that the American Academy of Pediatric Dentistry advocates the "age one" dental visit.[18] During this visit,

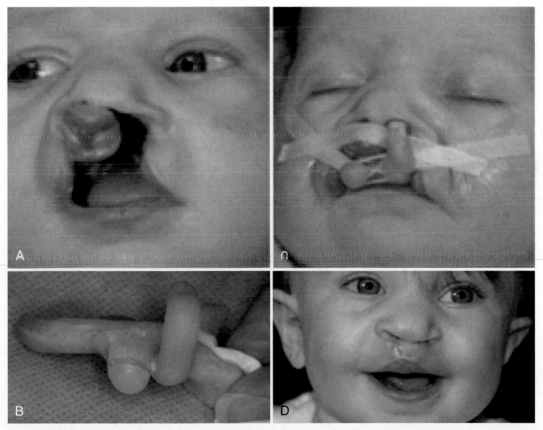

Figure 28-24 A, A 6-week-old infant with a bilateral cleft lip and palate. There is complete bilateral clefting of the palate, an incomplete cleft lip on the right side, and complete cleft lip on the left side. The premaxilla is displaced anteriorly and to the right side. **B,** A nasoalveolar molding (NAM) that has a left nasal extension designed to give better shaping to the left nares. The acrylic portion that fits over the palate and premaxilla is designed to bring the premaxilla to center, and back into alignment with the right and left alveolar segments. This is accomplished with selective addition and removal of acrylic. **C,** The infant with the NAM appliance in place and active at almost 3 months of age. **D,** The infant at post lip repair. The premaxilla has been brought into good arch alignment with the alveolar segments. (Photos courtesy of Jennifer Kugar, DDS, MSD, James Whitcomb Riley Hospital for Children, Craniofacial Anomaly Team.)

the pediatric dentist examines the oral cavity, notes any abnormalities in the soft and hard tissues, and provides anticipatory guidance to the parents regarding oral health care. Also during this visit emphasis is placed on the prevention of oral disease. In particular, this first visit offers parents an opportunity to discuss the many developmental issues unique to the cleft deformity. The pediatric dentist explains the role of each specialist on the cleft team and outlines the treatment benchmarks to be accomplished for their child during specific intervals.

STAGE II (PRIMARY DENTITION STAGE: 18 MONTHS TO 5 YEARS OF AGE)

Treatment during the primary dentition stage of dental development is initially focused on establishing and maintaining oral health. Meticulous daily oral hygiene for the child, with emphasis on direct assistance from the parents, is established to reduce the possibility of devel-

opment of dental caries. Ectopic eruption of the primary maxillary anterior dentition is common around the cleft defect.

Special care should be taken to keep these teeth free from caries because food often is lodged in and around the cleft defect. An increase in the frequency of periodic recall examinations, possibly to 3- to 4-month intervals, enables the dentist to intercept areas of decalcification. This preventive regimen is continued throughout all subsequent stages in the management of the cleft.

In some extensive cases of unilateral and bilateral complete clefts of the lip and palate, surgical closure is postponed beyond the usual 18 to 24 months of age. In these cases, because of the development of speech at this age, maxillary prosthetic appliances are constructed to provide normal maxillary arch integrity (Fig. 28-25). As the child grows, more tissue will become available to close the palate when doing so is surgically appropriate.

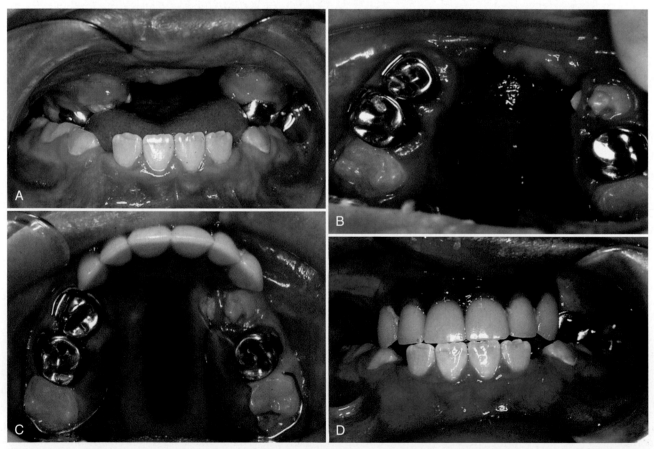

Figure 28-25   A, Intraoral view of a unilateral complete cleft of the lip and palate. Because of the extensive cleft of the hard and soft palate, the treatment of choice was prosthodontic obturation of the defect until growth was sufficient to allow definitive surgical closure. **B,** Maxillary arch demonstrating extensive cleft of the palate requiring an interim prosthesis. **C,** Interim maxillary prosthesis in place. This effectively closes the oral from the nasal cavities and facilitates mastication and speech. The appliance is removed daily for cleaning. **D,** Interim prosthesis in occlusion. The prosthetic anterior teeth provide support of the upper lip and improves esthetics.

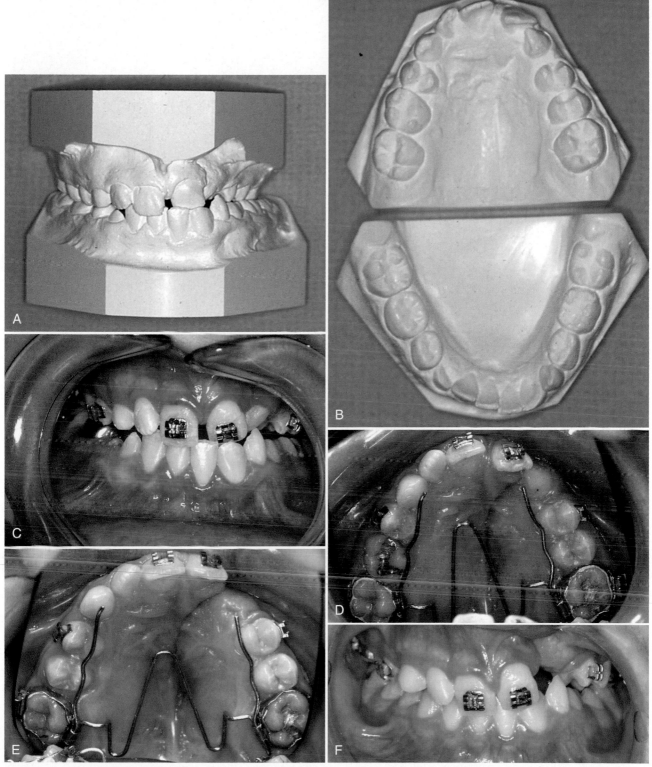

Figure 28-26 Interceptive correction, in the mixed dentition, of a full maxillary left crossbite in a complete unilateral cleft of the lip and palate. **A,** Diagnostic models for a unilateral complete cleft of the lip and palate. Notice the presence of a crossbite extending from the maxillary left central incisor to the maxillary first permanent molar. **B,** Occlusal views of maxillary and mandibular models. Notice the pronounced asymmetry of the maxillary arch. **C,** Occlusion with fixed appliances in place on the maxillary arch. **D,** Occlusal view demonstrating removable W arch to correct the posterior segmental crossbite. **E,** Occlusal view demonstrating correction of posterior crossbite and improved alignment of the maxillary anterior segment. Notice the improved maxillary arch symmetry. **F,** Occlusion at the end of interceptive therapy. Notice the correction of the anterior and posterior crossbites. At this time, the patient team ready for secondary alveolar bone grafting (see text for description of secondary bone-grafting procedure).

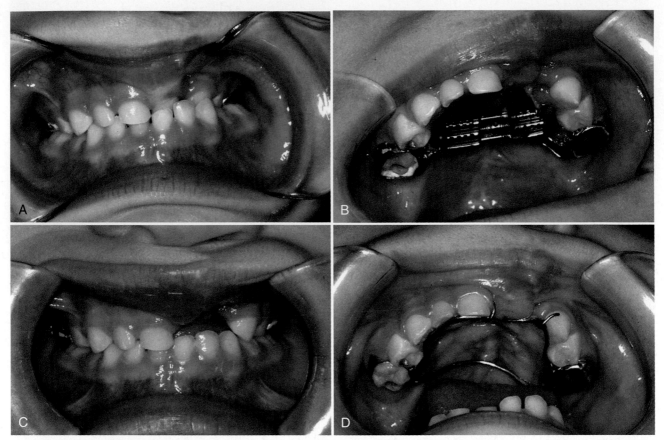

Figure 28-27 Interceptive correction, in the primary dentition, of a full maxillary left crossbite in a complete unilateral cleft of the lip and palate. **A,** Occlusion demonstrating a crossbite from the maxillary left primary incisor extending to the second primary molar. **B,** Fixed palatal expander in place on the maxillary arch at the completion of expansion. The left primary central incisor, loosened by traumatic occlusion before initiation of therapy, exfoliated during treatment. **C,** Occlusion at the completion of interceptive therapy. Notice the correction of the posterior crossbite. **D,** Placement of a passive maxillary arch-holding appliance to maintain optimal arch symmetry until the time of secondary alveolar bone grafting.

STAGE III (LATE PRIMARY OR MIXED DENTITION STAGE: 6 TO 10 OR 11 YEARS OF AGE)

Many problems encountered during the late primary and mixed dentition stage of dental development arise from ectopically erupting permanent central and lateral incisors or crossbites of the posterior dental segments. Treatment therefore concentrates on correction of a developing traumatic occlusion and posterior segmental alignment. Interceptive correction of a traumatic occlusion is essential to prevent destruction of enamel in the involved dentition (Fig. 28-26). Maxillary expansion to correct posterior segmental collapse is accomplished by routine palatal expansion (Fig. 28-27). This is especially important in patients who have not undergone primary alveolar cleft bone grafting. Once the condition is corrected, retention can be maintained by passive holding appliances.

Secondary Alveolar Cleft Bone Graft

A successful alveolar cleft bone graft satisfies several objectives. In addition to giving bony support for the teeth adjacent to the cleft and providing bone through which

teeth can erupt, it offers maxillary arch continuity and aids in closure of the oronasal fistula. It also supports the alar base of the nose.

Conceptually the technique is not difficult, but technically it can be tedious. There are several approaches to developing the required soft tissue flaps, but all seem to be variations of the technique described by Boyne and Sands.[19] The soft tissue in and adjacent to the cleft side is incised and elevated so that labial and palatal mucosal leaflets are everted to obtain labial and palatal closure. The tissues lining the cleft are elevated and inverted into the nose for nasal floor closure. Particulate marrow and cancellous bone harvested from the iliac crest is placed into the cleft defect, filling it from the piriform rim to the alveolar crest before closure of the labial tissues (Fig. 28-28).

Providing bony support to teeth adjacent to the cleft site is of paramount importance (Fig. 28-29). In most cases, bone should be grafted into the cleft before orthodontic tooth alignment is begun. When the cleft is filled with normal, viable bone, the orthodontist can proceed with tooth alignment without fear of exposing a root surface into the cleft site. In fact, after a 2-month healing

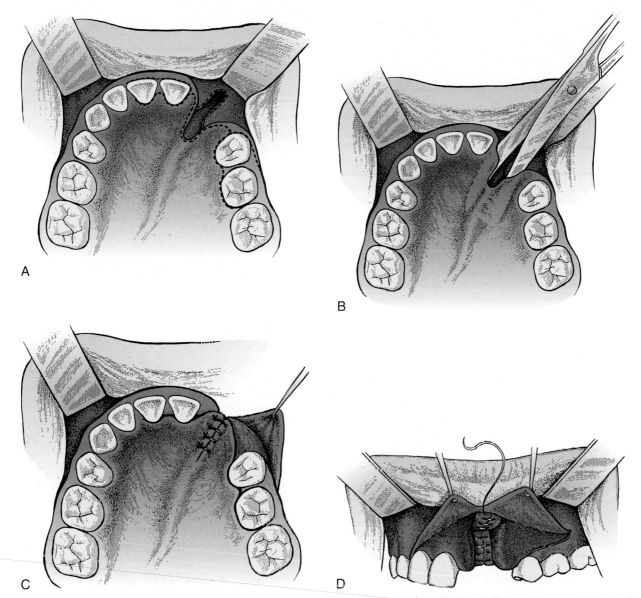

Figure 28-28 Technique for secondary alveolar cleft bone graft. **A,** Mucosal incisions outlined. **B,** Development of palatal mucoperiosteal flap. **C,** Closure of palatal mucosa. **D,** Closure of nasal mucosa within cleft site.

period, a tooth can be moved into the newly grafted bone with the expectation that the bone will respond to the tooth movement as any normal bone would. Any tooth movement undertaken before the graft is placed could jeopardize the bony support of the teeth adjacent to the cleft.

As a related consideration, grafted bone that obliterates the alveolar cleft also provides bone through which teeth can erupt. When canines and, in some cases, central incisors are allowed to erupt before bone grafting, they often lack adequate periodontal bone support. When the bone graft precedes permanent tooth eruption, compromised periodontal situations can often be prevented. El Deeb and colleagues studied the eruption patterns of canines through grafted bone in alveolar cleft defects.[20] They found that canine teeth erupt spontaneously through the grafted bone but that this eruption may be later than normal and

that it takes longer. In their study, 27% of the canines erupted spontaneously. The remainder required surgical uncovering and orthodontic forces to accomplish eruption and alignment in the arch. Turvey and associates found the rate of spontaneous eruption to be 95%, which represents a significant difference.[21] However, the point is that canines can and do erupt through the grafts. If eruption seems greatly delayed, surgical and orthodontic intervention is appropriate.

El Deeb and colleagues have recommended that the graft be placed between 9 and 12 years of age when the canine root is one quarter to half formed.[20] They reported that the canine subsequently has normal root development and that morphologic conditions will be unaffected by the surgical procedure.

Restoring maxillary arch continuity and stabilizing the maxillary segments represent other major objectives.

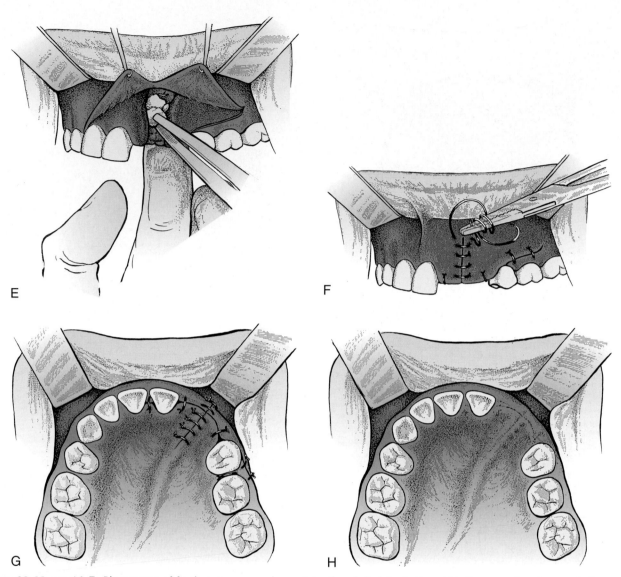

Figure 28-28 cont'd **E,** Placement of fresh autogenous bone into the cleft defect. **F** and **G,** Reapproximation and closure of mucoperiosteal flaps. **H,** The reconstructed maxillary alveolus.

In the bilateral cleft case, the premaxilla is stabilized as the bone grafts are incorporated between the premaxilla and the lateral maxillary segments. In the process, the alveolar ridge contour is restored so that the ability to provide a stable, esthetic prosthesis is enhanced. There is often some degree of collapse of the maxillary arch form. It is possible to expand the arch after grafting, as pointed out by Boyne and Sands[22]; however, it is preferable to expand these collapsed segments to as optimal an arch form as possible before grafting. Pregraft expansion also widens the cleft site, which allows better access for nasal floor closure. After the arch expansion has occurred, the bone graft can be placed. After the graft has been incorporated, it can be expected to maintain a good arch form.

Closure of the oronasal fistula is often the most significant result of bone graft surgery, according to patients. They often have fluid regurgitation into the nose and mucus drainage from the nose into the oral cavity through the fistula. Depending on its size, the fistula can produce significant speech problems because air escapes when the patient phonates. Although closure of this fistula can be effected with only soft tissue closure, Enemark and associates have indicated that closure is more successful when combined with a bone graft.[23]

With a cleft maxilla the cleft extends through the piriform rim beneath the alar base of the nose. As a result, the alar base on the cleft side is often depressed because of lack of underlying bony support. Filling the cleft with bone provides underlying bony support that often elevates the alar base of the nose. Although this may not entirely correct any existing nasal deformity, it does provide good support over which nasal reconstructive and revision surgery can be accomplished.

Secondary alveolar cleft bone grafting has been widely accepted. According to several researchers,[19,24-28]

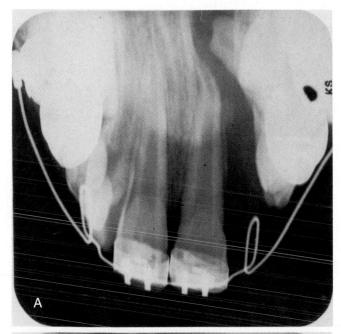

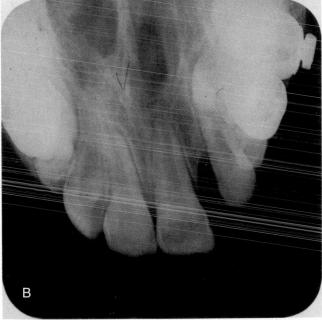

Figure 28-29 A, Pregraft maxillary occlusal radiograph demonstrating cleft defect with thin layer of bone over the distal root surface of the maxillary left central incisor. The canine has not started to erupt at this time. **B,** Postgraft maxillary occlusal radiograph demonstrating consolidation of bone across the cleft defect. Preliminary orthodontic alignment has been completed. The canine can be expected to erupt through the grafted area. (From Nelson CL, et al. Indiana's craniofacial anomalies team: Dentists play an important role, *J Indiana Dent Assoc* 65[6]:9-13, 1986.))

success rates are generally in the 90% range. Morbidity has included pain in the donor site, dehiscence of mucosal flaps, and partial or complete loss of grafted bone. Infection in the donor or recipient sites has been rare. An unpublished survey by Huebener indicated that secondary alveolar bone grafting (grafting performed in the mixed dentition) is routinely performed by all teams.

Secondary alveolar cleft bone grafting is an important procedure that greatly facilitates total habilitation. Not only is speech improved but dental, esthetic, and psychosocial benefits are to be gained. It is necessary again to emphasize the different objectives of primary and secondary grafting and to reiterate that they are not mutually exclusive procedures. The primary graft, over time, may satisfy some or all the objectives of secondary grafting. However, to the extent that it does not, augmenting the primary graft with particulate marrow and cancellous bone from the iliac crest may be recommended as a secondary procedure.

Effect of Facial Esthetics on Self-Concept

Appearance helps determine how an individual interacts with society and, in turn, how society perceives and accepts that individual. Facial esthetics is especially important to the development of self-concept. A child born with a serious congenital facial anomaly may find adaptation difficult. For example, Striker and associates have stated that the psychological sequelae of cleft lip and palate may have as great an impact on the individual as the physical aspects.[29] MacGregor stressed that, because of society's emphasis on physical attractiveness and conformity, the role of the face in interactions with others is such that many problems associated with cleft lip and palate involve considerations of mental health.[30]

Of special importance in the comprehensive dental management of cleft lip and palate is the dentist's ability to provide the young patient with interim prostheses to improve facial appearance (Fig. 28-30). These can be periodically adjusted to allow eruption of the developing dentition. Such treatment, when possible, should begin before the child starts formal education.

STAGE IV (PERMANENT DENTITION STAGE: 12 TO 18 YEARS OF AGE)

The majority of persons with cleft lips and palates require some degree of orthodontic management and can be treated in a conventional manner. Some cleft patients, however, will require a combined orthodontic-surgical approach in the permanent dentition to achieve optimal outcome. Before initiating the indicated therapy, the orthodontist completes a full diagnostic examination to determine the status of the patient's craniofacial development.

Most orthognathic surgical procedures involving the maxilla and mandible are deferred until the teenage years, when maximum growth of the jaws has been attained and all permanent teeth except the third molars have erupted. In boys, surgeons usually delay osteotomies until approximately 17 to 18 years of age; in girls, because of earlier maturation, surgery sometime after 15 years of age is possible. The manner in which the maxilla and mandible relate to each other spatially after growth is frequently difficult to predict based on the patient's appearance as a child. An example is the patient with a complete bilateral cleft lip and palate who has a protuberant premaxilla at birth. In childhood, the lateral

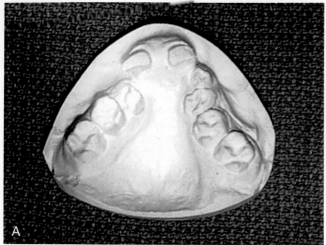

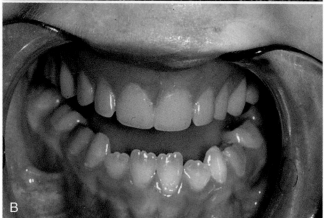

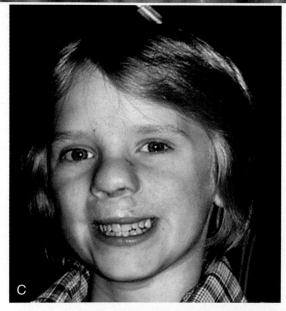

Figure 28-30 A, Plaster model of patient's maxillary arch ready for construction of the interim denture. **B,** Transitional maxillary complete overdenture. Such appliances may be used several years without replacement. **C,** Transitional maxillary overdenture in place. The patient's self-esteem is greatly enhanced by his essentially normal facial esthetics.

profile may appear severely convex, and the initial impression is that the patient will require a premaxillary segment surgical setback. This could be an erroneous assumption, and corrective surgery could be potentially deleterious if it is performed at an early age. With time, many of these persons acquire an essentially normal lateral facial profile. By the time maximum growth has been attained, a surprising number of these persons acquire a more normal convex profile.

In some instances, children with a cleft with a severely retrusive maxilla cannot undergo orthodontic correction with conventional therapy. In these cases the surgical procedure often used is the LeFort I maxillary advancement. This procedure is not technically feasible until the patient has a full complement of permanent dentition. The horizontal cuts to free the maxilla must necessarily be made above the apexes of the permanent dentition. Unerupted cuspids or bicuspids would make this procedure impractical. Therefore surgery must be deferred until the permanent dentition has erupted.

Cosmetic Surgery

Major nasal bone surgery may be deferred until the patient is in the early teens. However, cartilaginous nasal tip asymmetries may be corrected at any time. Additional tip-cartilage revisions may be performed as needed.

Common secondary deformities of the repaired unilateral or bilateral cleft lip include an upper lip that is too long or short, a tight upper lip, a deficiency of the vermilion tissue, and residual clefts (or notching) of the lip. Accurate predictions of how such deformities will manifest themselves are impossible until growth of the tissues is complete. Consequently, final surgical revision is frequently deferred until the mid to late teens. It is also prudent to defer final lip revisions until any surgical or orthodontic treatment that will change the osseous or dental support of the upper lip is complete.

REFERENCES

1. Veau V. Treatment of the unilateral hairlip. International Dental Congress Eighth Transaction, 1931, Paris, pp 126-1311.
2. Parameters for the evaluation and treatment of patients with cleft lip/palate or other craniofacial anomalies. American Cleft Palate-Craniofacial Association, *Cleft Palate–Craniofacial J* 30(Suppl 1); 2000, revised 2007.
3. Whitehouse FA. Treatment as a dynamic system, *Cleft Palate J* 2:16-27, 1965.
4. McNeil CK. *Oral and facial deformity.* London, 1954, Pittman.
5. McNeil CK. Congenital oral deformities, *Br Dent J* 101:191-198, 1956.
6. Jones JE. The use and clinical effectiveness of the maxillary obturator appliance in cleft lip and palate infants: birth through six months of age. Doctoral dissertation. San Jose, Costa Rica, Empresarial University, 2003.
7. Pashayan HM, McNab M. Simplified method of feeding infants with cleft palate with or without cleft lip, *Am J Dis Child* 133:145-147, 1979.
8. Hofman JP. De labiis leoporinis/von Hasen-Scharten. Heidelberg, 1686, Bergmann.

9. Robertson NRE, Jolleys A. Effects of early bone grafting in complete clefts of the lip and palate, *Plast Reconstr Surg* 42:414-421, 1968.

10. Friede H. The vomero-premaxillary suture: a neglected growth site in midfacial development of unilateral cleft lip and palate patients, *Cleft Palate J* 15:398-404, 1978.

11. Rosenstein SW, et al. The case for early bone grafting in cleft lip and cleft palate, *Plast Reconstr Surg* 70:297-302 1982.

12. Rosenstein SW, et al. The case for early bone grafting in cleft lip and palate: a second report, *Plast Reconstr Surg* 87:644-654, 1991.

13. Rosenstein SW, et al. A long-term retrospective outcome assessment of facial growth, secondary surgical need, and maxillary lateral incisor status in surgical-orthodontic protocol for complete clefts, *Plast Reconstr Surg* 111(1):1-13, 2003.

14. Huebener DV, Marsh JL. A survey of early management of cleft lip and palate—the first 18 months. Unpublished data presented at the American Cleft Palate–Craniofacial Annual Meeting, 2002.

15. Rosenstein SW. Orthodontic and bone grafting procedures in a cleft lip and palate series: an interim cephalometric evaluation, *Angle Orthod* 45:227-237, 1975.

16. Latham RA, et al. An extraorally activated expansion appliance for cleft palate infants, *Cleft Palate J* 13:253-261, 1976.

17. Grayson BH, Cutting CB. Presurgical nasoalveolar orthopedic molding in primary correction of the nose, lip, and alveolus of infants born with unilateral and bilateral clefts, *Cleft Palate Craniofac J* 38:193-198, 2001.

18. American Academy of Pediatric Dentistry, Guideline on Infant Oral Health Care. In *American Academy of Pediatric Dentistry Reference Manual 2008-9*. Chicago, 2009, American Academy of Pediatric Dentistry, pp 90-92.

19. Boyne PJ, Sands NR. Secondary bone grafting of residual alveolar and palatal clefts, *J Oral Surg* 30:87-92, 1972.

20. El Deeb M, et al. Canine eruption into grafted bone in maxillary alveolar cleft defects, *Cleft Palate J* 19:9-16, 1982.

21. Turvey TA, et al. Delayed bone grafting in the cleft maxilla and palate: a retrospective multidisciplinary analysis, *Am J Orthod* 86:244-256, 1984.

22. Boyne PJ, Sands NR. Combined orthodontic surgical management of residual palato-alveolar cleft defects, *Am J Orthod* 70:20-37, 1976.

23. Enemark H, et al. Secondary bone grafting in unilateral cleft lip and palate patients: indications and treatment procedure, *Int J Oral Surg* 14:2-10, 1985.

24. Bertz JE. Bone grafting of alveolar clefts, *J Oral Surg* 39:874-877, 1981.

25. Hall HD, Posnick JC. Early results of secondary bone grafts in 106 alveolar clefts, *J Oral Maxillofac Surg* 41:289-294, 1983.

26. Kortebein MJ, et al. Retrospective analysis of 135 secondary alveolar cleft bone grafts, *J Oral Maxillofac Surg* 49:493-498, 1991.

27. Kwon HJ, et al. The management of alveolar cleft defects, *J Am Dent Assoc* 102:848-853, 1981.

28. Troxell JB, et al. A retrospective study of alveolar cleft grafting, *J Oral Maxillofac Surg* 40:721-725, 1982.

29. Striker G, et al. Psychosocial aspects of craniofacial disfigurement: a "state of the art" assessment conducted by the Craniofacial Anomalies Program Branch, the National Institute of Dental Research, *Am J Orthod* 76:410-422, 1979.

30. MacGregor FC. Social and psychological implications of dentofacial disfigurement, *Angle Orthod* 40:231-233, 1970.

CHAPTER 29

Practice Management

▲ Ann Page Griffin and Jasper L. Lewis, Jr.

CHAPTER OUTLINE

The practice of modern dentistry requires delivery of quality care combined with adherence to excellent business principles. Dentists traditionally trained in the art and science of dentistry must also become skilled in techniques of sound business management. Today's practitioner must be clinically astute and knowledgeable about all aspects of managing a small business, consumer needs and demands, government regulations, and third-party participation—aspects of dentistry not often addressed thoroughly in the clinical setting of dental school.

The transition from a role of dental student or resident to business owner and manager is an enormous challenge. That transition often begins when the young dentist enters practice and suddenly realizes that dentistry encompasses more than clinical and technical competence. A successful dentist must be concerned with many management concepts, including leadership, delegation, interpersonal relationships, personal style, community image, and time management, as well as the day-to-day operation and fiscal management of a business.

The primary responsibility of a dentist is to provide quality patient care. However, private practice—and, in today's environment, many school, hospital, and government dental facilities—like any other business, must make a profit to survive. The practitioner must maintain a balance between patient care and business requirements while keeping moral, ethical, legal, familial, and professional responsibilities in proper perspective.

While maintaining this balance, a pediatric dentist must provide a place where children can feel safe, loved, and well cared for; where parents can be educated about how to help their children have a lifetime of good oral health; where the staff know that they are an integral part of the practice, that they are important and appreciated, and that their opinions count. Furthermore, the successful pediatric dental practice is one where other practitioners and health care providers choose to refer patients or call for information concerning young people's oral health issues; where the community as a whole knows, respects, and appreciates the practice; and where needed changes can be made in any area with better, innovative ideas and methods endorsed and implemented.

Every new dentist begins practice expecting to be successful. Those satisfied with their level of achievement after several years realize that a successful dental practice is composed of three systems: personnel, patient, and operational.

PERSONNEL SYSTEMS

PERSONNEL NEEDS

A personable, professional staff is vitally important for practice success. The dentist must invest time, effort, and money to hire, train, and retain quality individuals who can be developed into a team. A team of committed professionals, working together, focused on the patients and the practice, can make the difference between an excellent and a mediocre practice. Therefore, staff development is a sound investment in any practice.

Before becoming an employer, the dentist must be aware of state and federal regulations concerning hiring; employment policies, including Occupational Safety and Health Administration (OSHA) requirements; employee records maintenance and retention; employee discipline and dismissal; and so on. All employment applications, other forms and tests used in the hiring process, and employment policies described in the office manual should be reviewed by an attorney for the practice who is familiar with state and federal laws.

The number of employees in a dental office varies according to the type of practice and patient volume. Pediatric and orthodontic practices usually require more team members than other types of practices.

Initially, the new practitioner may need to hire only one or two staff members. If only one individual is hired at first, a second employee should be added when patient flow increases to the point that this person can no longer assist at the chair and handle the business desk (e.g., collect fees, make appointments, answer the telephone by the third ring, prepare and mail statements on time, and pursue broken appointments). The first employee, who is already knowledgeable about scheduling and practice flow, may move to the business desk. The second employee may serve as a full-time clinical assistant.

The third office employee may be a second clinical assistant or a dental hygienist. When the dentist treats hygiene patients more than 8 hours per week and the state practice act limits the performance of some hygiene duties by a certified dental assistant, a hygienist may be hired. This will allow the dentist to concentrate on other treatments and procedures. Depending on patient volume, the hygienist may be full time or part time. Other employees may then be added as needed.

Additional help may be gained through the use of part-time employees. These employees may *job share,* a term used to describe the splitting of a full-time position between two people, or a position may need to be filled only part time (i.e., a few hours per day or week).

PRACTICE ADMINISTRATOR

The business of managing and administering a dental practice has become complex and time consuming for the dentist, even with a well-trained staff. Some larger dental practices now hire well-educated, trained practice administrators. "The key responsibilities of a Practice Administrator could be compared to those of a Chief Executive Officer (CEO) of any corporation[1]:

1. Strategic planning and positioning—chief strategist
2. Team building—culture, positioning, performance contracts, empowerment
3. Monitoring all departments, making adjustments/changes as needed
4. Chief deal maker"[1]

Once a practice administrator is on staff, the doctor's position becomes similar to that of the chairman of the board of directors of a corporation or company, a major policy voice as well as owner of the right of refusal or veto authority. In some cases, several practices may share the services of a practice administrator.

COORDINATORS

Two of the key positions in a practice with several staff members may be a Clinical Coordinator and a Business Coordinator. A Coordinator is an experienced senior staff member who shows leadership skills and enjoys using her or his initiative. The following outlines may be edited to fit the need of any office.

Clinical Coordinator Responsibilities

- Overall coordination of clinical area.
- Meet regularly with the doctor.
- Suggest clinical staffing needs.
- Help evaluate clinical staff performance.
- Maintain clinical staff employee records.
- Coordinate office-wide OSHA training.
- Direct and maintain clinical staff work schedules.
- Assign collateral duties to clinical staff.
- Direct the "morning huddle," a brief meeting to plan/review the day.
- Help schedulers with scheduling questions.
- Direct flow of patients through the clinical area.
- Make certain all systems are consistent, e.g., data entry, paperwork, laboratory delivery, etc.
- Help plan and maintain clinical area budget.
- Supervise clinical supply inventory and ordering.

Business Coordinator Responsibilities

- Overall coordination of the business desk.
- Meet regularly with the doctor.
- Suggest business area staffing needs.
- Help evaluate business staff performance.
- Maintain business staff employee records.
- Administer and interpret employee benefits.
- Maintain updated personnel/office manual.
- Answer parents' or patients' questions concerning office procedures, financial matters, etc.
- Help the doctor monitor practice statistics.
- Manage accounts payable.
- Monitor daily deposits and reconcile monthly bank statements.
- Manage ordering of business supplies.
- Maintain office calendar.

Note: If a Practice Administrator is employed, a number of these duties may be delegated to her or him, thereby releasing the Business Coordinator to focus on duties at the business desk.

- Work to free the dentist from administrative details.
- Handle correspondence for the dentist when requested.

COLLATERAL DUTIES

Every office has a myriad of duties which must be completed on schedule but may not fall into one specific category. The schedule for every office may be different, but among these collateral duties are the following.

Daily
- Check to see that laboratory work is on schedule.
- Stock units.
- Clean sinks, countertops, and treatment chairs.
- Empty sterilizers.
- Take out trash.
- Clean and sterilize impression trays.
- Check x-ray processor.
- Clean consult room.
- Clean staff lounge/kitchen area.
- Check/tidy patient bathroom.
- Duplicate x-rays.
- Straighten reception area.

Weekly
- Order office supplies; check packing slip against items received; put away.
- Order clinical supplies; check packing slip against items received; put away.
- Clean various equipment such as ultrasonic, x-ray processor, air, and suction
- Collect time sheets.

Monthly
- Check emergency kit contents, drug expiration dates, etc.
- Shred confidential papers and forms.

Odd Times
- Change sterilization fluids.
- Clean plaster trap.
- Inactivate charts.

In the well-managed office, these and other miscellaneous tasks are assigned to staff members, perhaps on a rotating basis, to be done regularly as time allows.

INTERVIEWING AND HIRING

Mastery of the interviewing process is difficult but necessary. Hiring begins with attracting well-qualified applicants. Potential employees may come from personal recommendations made by current staff; area technical schools, colleges, and universities; or classified advertisements.

Interviewing becomes easier and more enlightening with repetition. The more opportunities an interviewer has to conduct interviews, the smoother and more productive the sessions. Use of a set of interview questions standardizes the process. These questions should explore the following traits: initiative, organization, conscientiousness, effective communication, ability to work well with others, technical or business training and experience, and the ability to apply previous training and experience to the job. If questions are skillfully posed, an applicant's answers will indicate strengths or weaknesses in these areas.

The following steps should make the interview more effective:

1. Read the resume or job application to learn about the person before the interview. Chat a few moments to put the interviewee at ease as the interview begins.
2. Have a written set of questions that will elicit strengths or weaknesses in the areas mentioned above.
3. Tell the interviewee that some specific questions will be asked and notes will be taken.
4. Listen well. Note body language and eye contact because they often speak louder than words.
5. The interviewer should talk less than 25% of the time. The purpose of the interview is to understand the applicant and his or her potential for the job. Excessive talking by the interviewer limits the time and opportunity that the applicant has to tell about personal abilities and experiences.
6. Do not help the interviewee answer questions. Let pauses happen. The applicant may be thinking during the silences, and the interviewer can see how well and quickly the person responds.
7. Do not ask questions that can be answered with "yes" or "no." If the interviewee begins answering "yes" or "no," ask him or her to explain or expound on the answer.
8. Never argue with an applicant. Maintain poise and remember that you, the interviewer, are in control.

Two of the most desirable traits in a dental team member are (1) a warm, empathetic personality and (2) cognitive ability, defined as aptitude for learning and capacity to draw from past experience in new situations. Several excellent instruments are on the market to measure cognitive ability and various aspects of personality and behavioral style (e.g., Cognitive Ability Testing Instrument — Wonderlic Personnel Test, Wonderlic, Inc., Libertyville, IL, www.wonderlic.com; Personality and Behavioral Style Instrument — DiSC Classic [Personal Profile System], Inscape Publishing, Minneapolis, MN, www.inscape.com.)

To maximize efficiency, a well-trained staff member may conduct the first interview. If the candidate is promising, employment tests, a tour of the office, an introduction to other staff members, and a brief conversation with the dentist should be a part of the first interview. References should be checked between the first and second interviews.

The second interview should include a longer conversation with the dentist and office observation or work time. The dentist should pay the applicant for time spent observing and/or working in the office. Inviting the prospective employee to work in the office for a few hours allows staff members to form an opinion about the person's potential. Likewise, the applicant will better understand office ambiance and patient flow before accepting the job.

Although the final hiring decision rests with the dentist, it is a good idea for certain key staff members to concur. Current employees significantly affect the success or failure of a newly hired staff member because they help train and interact closely with him or her.

An offer may be made after the working interview. If the applicant will not be hired following the first or second interview, he or she may be told at that time or notified by mail within 1 week of either interview. If an applicant is rejected, maintain all applications, test forms, and other paperwork for at least 1 year in case a complaint concerning unfair hiring practices is filed by the rejected applicant.

If testing is part of the application and interviewing process, testing must be standardized, that is, all applicants must be given identical tests. If an applicant is hired, all interview and employment records must be kept for the duration of employment plus 30 years. Employment records and employee medical records should be maintained separately in identical folders or binders and kept in a locked file or kept off site by the dentist.

If the applicant is to be hired, the dentist should offer the job using the term *full-time* or *part-time* employment and should avoid using the word permanent, either orally or in writing. Use of the term *permanent* connotes continuous work with a contractual understanding, regardless of problems that might develop later. If dismissal should become necessary, the employee might claim wrongful dismissal if promised permanent employment.

ORIENTATION AND TRAINING

In *The One Minute Manager,* a book long-favored by business managers, Blanchard and Johnson wrote, "Most companies spend 50% to 70% of their money on people's salaries. And yet spend less than 1% of their budget to train their people. Most companies, in fact, spend more time and money on maintaining their buildings and equipment than they do on maintaining and developing people."[2]

The comments of Blanchard and Johnson are equally appropriate concerning training of dental auxiliaries. Adequate training, a requisite for productive staff, is often slighted in busy dental offices.

A new employee must be made to feel welcome and a part of the team. Orientation on the first day of employment and a written training schedule to be followed the first 6 to 8 weeks should be part of this process.

The most effective way to orient new employees is to follow a checklist, which ensures that each new staff member will receive similar information. Fig. 29-1 is an example of an orientation checklist for new employees.

Orientation should include a review of the office manual. An up-to-date office manual (policy and procedural manual) can prevent misunderstandings with current and new staff members and reduce training time for new auxiliaries. An office manual outlines the duties, obligations, and mutual expectations of the employee and employer, and clarifies office policies, employment procedures, benefits, training methods, and office paperwork. Preferably, the dentist writes the manual with input from experienced senior staff members. Prototypes of office manuals are available in print or in software versions to assist in the process. The attorney for the practice should review the manual before implementation.

A training/benefit waiting period may be the first 60 to 90 days of employment, during which time the dentist

Orientation Checklist
An employee record should be set up, containing the following:

- Resume _____
- Application form _____
- Interviewing notes and test forms _____
- Tax and employment forms, including the often-overlooked Employment Eligibility Verification (I-9) form from The Bureau of Citizenship and Immigration Services _____
- Copies of licenses _____
- Personal data about emergency contact, family names, etc. _____
- Salary and benefits _____
- OSHA-required training records _____

Office tour provided, including review of work hours, dress code, personal item storage, parking, brief hisory of practice. _____
Introduced to other staff (written list of names and brief job descriptions) _____
Job description reviewed _____
Training procedures and expectations reviewed _____
Beginning and end of day procedures explained _____
Office security, lock-up, housekeeping, etc. explained _____
Safe work procedures reviewed _____
Emergency procedures reviewed _____
Confidentiality emphasized concerning
- Salary _____
- Patient data _____
- Production, collection, and any other practice financial data _____

Insurance forms completed and submitted (at end of training period) _____
Office manual reviewed _____

Note: Medical information/records should be maintained in separate files. These include records such as hepatitis vaccine (administered within 10 days of beginning employment) or declination thereof, accidents at work; sick leave reasons, etc.

Figure 29-1 Example of orientation checklist for new team members.

determines whether there is a match between office needs and a new employee's skills and personal style. Use of the term *training/benefit* waiting period rather than *probationary* or *trial* period connotes the importance of performance to the new employee, emphasizing that this is considered a time to work diligently, to strive to learn as much as possible.

Much of the responsibility for training new employees can be delegated to current staff. A well-trained veteran staff member may become a Training Coordinator, available to instruct the new employee, answer questions, and check progress. Although one person may efficiently coordinate training, all other team members and the dentist should be involved in the process also. Additionally, the Training Coordinator can maintain training and continuing education (CE) records for the entire staff, thereby assuring CE requirements for licensing recertification are fulfilled.

In the most successful practices, the dentist and team members realize that training is an ongoing process; dental professionals continue to learn about new methods and materials in order to better care for patients and maintain professional licenses. Attendance at CE courses, review of current literature and journals, and group study using audiotapes, DVDs, CDs, and so on are appropriate for continuous training. A portion of each staff meeting can be used for additional training and discussions of new treatment methods and materials. Also, the establishment of an office library makes books, journals, and audiovisual aids easily available to all team members. Learning together strengthens a dental team and encourages pride in personal and professional growth.

WAGE AND BENEFIT ADMINISTRATION

Wage and benefit administration is an aspect of practice management lacking clear-cut rules and guidelines. Therefore, many dentists find it a particularly difficult task. There must be a balance between managing payroll costs, sharing practice income and profits equitably with staff members, and maintaining careful control of expenses.

The most successful dentists and managers set high standards for their practice, including top-notch performance and productivity from all team members. In return, these dentists compensate team members well, sharing increased profits with staff members who helped produce the growth. As a result, auxiliaries realize that the better the practice does financially, the better they will do. They also understand that if the practice has an unproductive period in which production, collections, and profits decline, raises and some other benefits may be delayed. Benefiting from growth and increased profits or, conversely, experiencing the pinch of fiscal decline allows auxiliaries to feel responsibility toward the practice that they might not otherwise sense.

Employees receive more than wages; net pay is only one part of a complete compensation package. Although higher take-home pay with fewer benefits may attract some employees, fair wages with expanded benefits generally help retain team members. Each employee should be given an annual total compensation statement listing gross wages, employer-paid taxes, and the dollar value of benefits such as vacation, personal leave, insurance, uniform allowance, and free or reduced-cost dental care. Fig. 29-2 is an example of an individual total compensation statement. Receiving an actual statement of wages and benefits lets employees perceive their full value. The dentist should communicate to staff members how valuable they are to the practice rather than how much they cost the practice. Although it is a subtle difference, such phrasing can boost staff members' professional pride, dedication, and loyalty to the practice. Auxiliary personnel who are made to feel valued and appreciated are generally more productive than those told what they "cost" the practice.

Wage and benefit administration requires careful planning. A comprehensive salary plan helps retain employees by offering salaries commensurate with community wage scales. It also allows the dentist to evaluate relative pay among employees and to review wages and benefits in a timely and organized manner. If planning is neglected, a dentist may give raises that are too large or too frequent or, conversely, forget about salary reviews for an

---

Total Compensation Statement for the Calendar Year _____

Employee Name _____

Gross wages	$ _____
Social Security contribution	$ _____
Medicare contribution	$ _____
Unemployment insurance	$ _____
Worker' compensation insurance	$ _____
Health insurance	$ _____
Retirement plan contribution	$ _____
Vacation: _____ days	$ _____
Personal leave: _____ days	$ _____
Continuing education/travel/expenses	$ _____
Uniform allowance	$ _____
Dental care	$ _____
Other (Such as bonus, medical reimbursement, cafeteria plan, health savings account, etc.)	$ _____
Total wages and benefits	$ _____
Hours worked	$ _____
Total compensation per hour	$ _____

Thank you. We realize how valuable you are as a member of our dental team, and it is a pleasure to see the full scope of wages, taxes, and benefits you receive. Together we can make next year, _____, the best year yet for our practice and our patients.

Figure 29-2 Individual total compensation statement.

---

extended period. The former condition results in excessive wage costs; the latter may cause good employees to quit. A common problem expressed by many dentists in practice for 15 to 20 years is that a long-term staff member's total compensation package is excessive. The young practitioner can avoid this problem by establishing a salary plan.

To begin a salary plan, the dentist first lists the staff positions in the office, including business positions (e.g., receptionist, scheduling coordinator, patient accounts coordinator), and clinical positions (e.g., clinical assistant, hygienist, sterilization/laboratory assistant). The relative worth of each position to the practice is determined using the following questions:

1. How long would it take to find a replacement?
2. Are there specific certification, education, or training requirements?
3. What is the value of longevity in this position?
4. How skilled is a certain individual?

The more competent, valuable, and difficult to replace the employee is, the higher the wage should be.

The dentist should survey similar jobs in other practices in the area to determine minimum and maximum pay ranges. The survey might also include similar businesses such as other health care offices, law offices, banks, and real estate firms. In summary, wages should be commensurate with the community standard and an employee's value to the office.

Salaries should be evaluated at least yearly; raises are based on merit (positive behavior and work deserving praise), increases in cost of living (inflation), and the overall economic status of the practice.

Pediatric dental practices often employ more personnel than general or some other specialty practices because a number of patients may be scheduled simultaneously, and many children cannot be left alone while in the treatment chair. Generally, labor costs in pediatric dental practices, including payroll taxes, require about 22% to 26% of gross collections. Benefits may add another 2% to 5%, closer to 5% if a retirement plan is funded.

Fair salaries and good benefits are necessary to avoid job dissatisfaction; however, salary and benefits do not necessarily motivate an employee to perform better. Motivated staff members are most often those to whom responsibility is delegated. Their personal and professional growth is encouraged and recognized by the dentist. They are appreciated and told how valuable they are to the office, the dentist, and the patients. In short, motivated staff members are recognized for the contributions they make to the practice, and money is only one way appreciation is shown.

PERFORMANCE APPRAISALS

Potentially effective staff members are often dismissed because of poor job performance, which may be the result of the dentist's failure to define expectations. Employees can be expected to perform optimally only if requirements are clear. Team members must know what they are expected to do, how to do it, and what the criteria are for an acceptable or, better yet, outstanding job performance.

The purpose of performance reviews is to recognize past growth and accomplishments while setting new goals and standards of achievement. Periodic performance appraisals allow the dentist and team members to evaluate personal attributes, job strengths, and areas to be improved so that goals for personal and professional growth can be set. Appraisals should be honest but positive, resulting in better job performance and improved efficiency.

Each staff member should be evaluated according to similar criteria, including competence in performing tasks, work habits, contributions to the team, and behavior toward patients, coworkers, the dentist, and the office. Nebulous topics, such as attitude, poor mannerisms, or personality conflicts should be addressed by listing specific examples of positive or negative instances involving the person. Evaluation forms that can be completed by the staff member and dentist are helpful but not absolutely necessary. Simple notes about strengths, growth opportunities, and the employee's needs as they match or conflict with the needs of the practice are sufficient for the evaluation conversation. Discussing the staff member's opinion of his or her own performance often makes the appraisal more meaningful. Performance appraisals should be given regularly to improve job performance and encourage personal growth. An appraisal should be given after completion of the training/benefit waiting period and at least annually thereafter. All appraisal forms and notes should be dated at the time of the appraisal and signed by the dentist and the auxiliary. If the auxiliary refuses to sign, the dentist should so note on the form.

Job skills and work performance should be reviewed separately from salary. A conversation that combines performance review with news of a raise interferes with the staff member's concentration. An employee may be so interested in hearing about a salary increase that setting goals for performance improvement is relegated to a secondary level of importance.

During the review, strengths should be enumerated first. People listen better when they feel that the appraiser recognizes their strengths rather than only their deficiencies. Use of the term *development areas* or *opportunities for growth* rather than *weaknesses* when discussing areas to be improved connotes positive potential.

Most people respond best when asked to concentrate on no more than three or four areas for development. Hearing about more than three or four points to be improved is overwhelming and may delay the employee's responsiveness and improvement.

The dentist may offer to help the employee improve in certain areas through additional training, CE courses, and such, thereby giving the staff member a sense of support. The dentist and staff member should agree on realistic goals to be met by a certain date, with regular discussions during the interim to evaluate progress and establish other objectives.

PERSONNEL RECORDS

Personnel records are important documents. They are a history of the employee-employer relationship, just as a patient's chart is a documentation of the patient-dentist relationship. If a problem arises with an employee (e.g., a charge of wrongful dismissal in case of termination), the record will serve as proof that the dentist correctly discharged employer responsibilities.

Records, including job application, interviewing notes, testing forms, performance appraisals, wage and benefit information, training records, unsafe incident logs, and so on, should be maintained for the duration of employment plus at least 30 years following an auxiliary's departure. Records for OSHA-mandated training must be maintained from the date the training occurred and must include dates of training, contents of the session, and the name and qualifications of the trainer. Check with your state OSHA office for information concerning the number of years that these records must be maintained. Medical records must be maintained in individual locked files separate from other personnel records for the duration of employment plus 30 years and include all appropriate forms with pertinent data.

Personnel records for all employees should be identical in appearance, consistently maintained, and kept confidential, preferably in locked files. A comprehensive employee record could include the following:
• Employee's name
• Address and telephone number
• Social Security number
• Completed job application and resume if submitted during the application process

- Employment tests given as part of the hiring process
- Date of employment
- Licenses or certifications
- Completed tax forms, including federal and state income tax and Employment Eligibility Verification (I-9 form available from the Bureau of Citizenship and Immigration Services)
- Spouse's name, employer, and telephone number
- Person to contact in case of emergency
- Salary record and summary of benefits
- Training records, including OSHA training and cardiopulmonary resuscitation training
- Performance appraisal forms and notes from one-on-one discussions signed and dated by the employee and the dentist
- Absentee records
- CE course records
- Record of termination, including last date of employment, and the employee's letter of resignation or notes from the dismissal conversation if the employee was fired

Medical records, including injury or exposure to harmful substances, and record of hepatitis inoculation, or signed and dated refusal of the vaccine, must be maintained in separate locked files.

DISMISSAL

Dismissal of an employee is one of the most difficult tasks a dentist may face. Whereas interviewing becomes easier with experience, firing someone does not. There are, however, processes that can make a dismissal less stressful.

Dismissal usually happens because of incompetence in job performance or unacceptable behavior such as patient abuse, sabotage, theft, harassment or substance abuse on the premises. Problems arise often when an employee loses interest and, therefore, effectiveness and/or efficiency in her or his responsibilities. Behavior and performance problems must be addressed; simply ignoring the situation will not make it go away. The dentist and staff member should discuss the problems and ways they can be rectified. After an initial discussion with the employee, it should be absolutely clear to the employee that improved attitude and/or job skill is a requirement for continued employment. The employee and dentist should sign and date notes from the initial and subsequent meetings. A specific date by which behavior and/or skills must improve should be set with the dentist and the staff member meeting frequently in the interim to assess improvements.

When coaching an employee who is trying but is incompetent, a combination of the following procedures may be used. The dentist should write a description of acceptable performance criteria, including skills needed for the job. It is more effective to name specific characteristics and skills needed for the particular position than to enumerate only negatives; i.e., what the person is not doing. The goal is to have the staff member understand the requirements of the job, the ways that she or he fails to meet them, and ways that expectations can be fulfilled.

The dentist then establishes a time frame for improvements; between 1 and 3 months is usually appropriate.

The auxiliary and the dentist should discuss, sign, and date the agreement about performance improvements. The dentist should review progress with the employee each week, making notes of these discussions in the employee's record. If the employee reaches the goal of acceptable job performance within the time allowed, new goals should be set. In this way, a staff member can be coached into continuously improved performance.

If an employee will not or cannot improve behavior or achieve required skill levels, dismissal will probably be necessary. In the dismissal conversation, failure to meet performance improvement may be discussed. The dentist must try to dismiss the person without causing anger and resentment. Although the employee's skills do not match office needs, often the person can leave without negative feelings if the dismissal conversation is conducted properly.

If an employee is behaving in an unacceptable way (e.g., consistently arriving late, abusing sick leave, or breaching confidentiality requirements), a serious warning may rectify the problem. If an employee is given serious disciplinary warnings before dismissal, the dentist should put the warnings in writing and include a statement to this effect: "Continuation of these actions by this employee may lead to disciplinary measures, up to and including dismissal." After this statement is explained, the employee and the dentist should sign and date the statement, and it should be retained in that individual's personnel file.

If an employee refuses to sign and date notes from any discussion, the dentist should so note on the statement and sign and date the document himself/herself. Such a note is an acceptable record that the discussion occurred.

In most states no notice is necessary for dismissal related to unlawful behavior such as stealing, patient mistreatment, or deliberate property damage. The staff member committing such actions can be dismissed immediately if such actions can be proved indisputably. It should be clearly stated in the office manual that such conduct will not be tolerated and will result in immediate dismissal.

Preferably, a dismissed employee leaves immediately after the termination conversation. The dentist may pay severance wages, but payment is not mandatory in all states. (The dentist should check with an attorney about state law and write the policy in the office manual.) It is unwise for an employee who was fired to remain on the job. The dismissed person may sabotage the practice, even unconsciously, and bother other staff members with the details of termination. Thus a dentist may pay a penalty for being kind-hearted enough to let a fired employee keep working until he or she finds another job. If a dismissed employee remains employed while searching for another job, a departure date should be set; otherwise, the job search may be prolonged.

If the dentist is unclear about the proper way to discipline or dismiss an employee, he or she should seek advice from a lawyer versed in labor relations. It is much less costly to pay an attorney than to be involved in a wrongful dismissal lawsuit with a disgruntled employee.

COMMUNICATION

Concern with intraoffice communication is not a novel phenomenon since all human relationships depend on it. Relationships with team members, patients, other health care professionals, family, and friends depend on the ways in which one communicates. Even if the clinical dentistry is superlative, patients can perceive problems and stresses among the staff and/or with the dentist. If the dentist and team members are not functioning as a unit, patients may feel that the entire practice, including the care delivered, is below average. The following steps can be taken to strengthen intraoffice communications:

1. Write a practice mission statement with input from the team. Have the finished statement framed and hung in the reception room.
2. Survey team members about the state of communications among staff. Address problem areas and set standards for improvement.
3. Use personality inventories to learn more about your own and coworkers' styles, their impact on others, and how individuals react when stressed. Hire a psychologist or other trained professional to administer and interpret personality surveys. Greater understanding and cooperation among staff is well worth the cost.
4. Schedule regular staff meetings, at least monthly, on office time. The dentist may choose to rotate leadership of meetings among the group so that staff members, as well as the dentist, feel responsible for productive meetings.
5. A morning huddle is an excellent way to begin each day. Scheduled about 15 minutes before the first patient appointment, a huddle assures all staff members arrive on time, provides time to share personal important happenings among staff, allows review of the day's schedule, any changes or particular patient needs, and generally starts the day on a positive note, calm and organized. Figure 29-3 is a suggested agenda for an effective morning huddle.
6. Schedule a planning retreat at least annually. A retreat is an away-from-the-office session involving the dentist and all team members, usually one day, during which every aspect of the practice is assessed and improvements are planned. Goals in production, collections, new patients per month, recare system effectiveness, and such can be set for the next 6 to 12 months until another retreat is scheduled and the process is repeated.
7. Attend CE courses together. Use ideas and materials from the courses to enrich staff meetings and improve office processes.
8. Encourage one-on-one discussions, dentist to team member and team member to team member. Write intraoffice memos as needed. Memos are particularly helpful in a practice employing part-time people who may miss staff meetings. Post a central calendar to note staff meetings, vacation schedules, and CE course dates.
9. Post a bulletin board out of sight of patients for staff use. Pertinent professional information, personal news, and amusing items may be displayed.
10. Plan fun events involving the entire team. Groups that learn to enjoy one another are more productive, work more synergistically, and are more capable of handling stressful situations in the practice.

Agenda for Morning Huddle

Operative
1. Number of sedations, on whom? previous experience? special needs?
2. Any medical alerts today? If so, prescriptions? special needs?
3. Any medical alerts tomorrow? If so, prescriptions? special needs?
4. Special needs or setups for today? tomorrow?
5. Time for emergencies?

Hygiene
1. Number of hygiene appointments scheduled?
2. Number of new patients? special needs?
3. Any medical alerts today? If so, prescriptions? special needs?
4. Any medical alerts tomorrow? If so, prescriptions? special needs?
5. Special needs or setups for today? tomorrow?

Orthodontic
1. Bandings? debandings? on whom? time? assistants involved?
2. Appliances? retainers? problems?
3. Impressions? on whom? for what?
4. Records? on whom?
5. Consults within next three days? with whom? times? workups done?
6. Appliances due tomorrow? for whom? type? Are they ready? problems?
7. Any unusual needs today?
8. Follow-ups from yesterday?

Activities Report
1. Yesterday's production and percent of goal
2. MTD production vs MTD goal
3. MTD new patient count
4. Today's projected production
5. Tomorrow's projected production
6. Collection problems with individual patients today? tomorrow?
7. Number of broken appointments yesterday? number reappointed?
8. Concerns with schedule, today, tomorrow, and through five days hence.

Business Desk
1. Any missing charts for today? solution?
2. Any missing charts for tomorrow? solution?
3. Information about today's new patients

Figure 29-3 Huddle agenda.

PATIENT SYSTEMS

FIRST APPOINTMENT

A good first appointment experience provides the foundation for an enjoyable, long-term relationship with patients and parents. The impression given on that visit is lasting.

Although walk-in emergencies occur occasionally, most initial contacts with a practice are by telephone.

Because a caller frequently judges the entire practice by a voice on the telephone, the business staff should be trained in correct telephone etiquette and procedures. A wealth of information and resources about telephone skills training can be found by searching the Internet for "Phone Etiquette Training."

During the initial telephone conversation, certain information should be gathered from the parenting adult. Use of a form can help standardize the procedure.

Completed by the receptionist and used during the first visit, such a form is an invaluable aid in patient registration and can be kept permanently in the patient chart. Fig. 29-4 is an example of such a form.

A packet mailed before the first examination is an excellent introduction to the practice. The packet might contain the following items:

1. A brochure that provides information about the practice, the practice web address, a list of services offered,

John L. Doe, D.D.S.
222 Ash Street
Greenville, NC 27834
(919) 752-5183

NEW PATIENT TELEPHONE INTERVIEW

Date of call _____   Appointment _____
Taken by _____   Call for earlier appointment _____
                                     New patient packet mailed _____

Patient's name _____ Age (if minor) _____
Parent's name (if minor) _____
Phone (home) _____ (work) _____
Address _____ City _____ Zip _____
Other family members who are patients: _____
Referral _____
First dental visit: Yes   No
If no, are there current radiographs to be requested from another office?   Yes   No
If yes, name of dentist _____
Address _____ City _____ Zip _____
Phone _____ Date called _____ Date received _____
Special dental concerns _____
Special medical concerns _____

Emergency (circle)

Lost filling   Fractured tooth   Toothache, how long?
Bumped tooth   Knocked-out tooth   _____

Other symptoms: Sensitive to hot/cold/sweet
                   Bleeding
                   Constant pain
                   Swelling
                   Apprehension
                   Awake at night
                   Other _____

Dental insurance   Yes   No   or other coverage: (circle)   Medicaid
                                                                       Special health services

_____ Patient informed that fee for first examination is due at time of the examination.

_____ Patient informed we will be happy to file insurance for subsequent visits.

Comments _____

Figure 29-4 New patient telephone interview form.

general advice about how parents can best help children prepare for the first dental appointment, a map to the office, and a reminder of appointment date and time.

2. A health history form stamped in red ink in an upper corner, "Please complete and bring with you."
3. A note of welcome addressing the young patient.

The physical layout of the reception area and business desk must allow staff members a full view of the reception room. On arrival, the patient and parents should be greeted by a team member whether or not a sign-in sheet is used.

A well-trained team member should escort new patient arrivals to a conference room or the operatory. At this time, the staff person should review the child's health history with parents, recording pertinent notes for the dentist. The patient and parents may be given a brief tour of the office, and the tour guide can reinforce information given in the practice brochure.

The dentist should then be introduced by the staff member who interviewed the new patient and parents. After a short conversation addressed mainly to the patient, the dentist should again review the health history with the parents, reading notes made by the staff member during the interview. This routine provides two opportunities to ensure that the health history has been correctly completed and that the review with parents is documented. If the initial conversation occurred in a conference room, the dentist should leave while the team member prepares to take the child to the operatory. In this way, if the child is upset, the dentist who must gain full cooperation during the dental examination is not involved.

In many offices, parents accompany their child to the operatory. Although this often adds stress and causes the child's behavior to be worse, the presence of parents in the operatory is a reality in many pediatric dental offices in today's litigious society. The dentist can, however, wisely limit the number of adults accompanying each patient to the operatory. Fig. 29-5 is an example of information given

to parents about this limit. Note that the statement also forbids the use of cell phones in the operatory, which can be a most annoying problem.

After the examination, the dentist should present the case to the parents who usually want answers to the following questions: What is wrong? Can it be fixed? How much will it cost? The practitioner should keep these questions in mind and plan case presentations accordingly. Many new-to-practice dentists overtalk during case presentations, confusing parents and patients with excessive clinical terminology. The dentist may wish to rehearse case presentations with staff members, seeking their critique and suggestions.

At some point during the first appointment, an assistant or hygienist should give home care instructions. The patient and parents are then escorted to a checkout area. The next appointment is usually scheduled before the fee is collected. After checkout, a staff member should express thanks to the parents for choosing the office and remind them that the practice appreciates referrals. The child and parents should leave the office feeling that the dentist and staff are extraordinarily caring, thorough, skilled, and efficient. The first appointment should make parents eager to recommend the practice to other family members and friends.

PATIENT FLOW

For appointments subsequent to the initial examination visit, visualizing the overall pattern by which patients move through an office can make each appointment more productive and valuable for the patient and practice. All appointments have the following phases: Stage 1 is telephone contact, usually initiated by the parent or guardian. Stage 2 includes arrival, check-in and greeting, and escorting of the patient and parents to the conference room or operatory. During stage 3, the patient is seated in the operatory, with instruments and supplies placed for efficient treatment delivery. Stage 4 includes the clinical treatment procedures. During stage 5, dismissal, the parents make the next appointment. The patient's treatment plan, whether the next appointment is restorative or hygiene, must be entered into the computer before the chart is refiled. If treatment plans are entered consistently following each examination, new patient or recare, treatment plans, even for those patients not scheduled that day, are never lost.

Stage 6 includes collection of the fee. Staff members must receive training in collection procedures so that collection efforts are handled properly and professionally.

During stage 7, the staff member thanks the parents and patient with a smiling, cheerful farewell that will leave a lasting impression. Stage 8 involves recontact, including the recare system, special correspondence with the patient and parents, and other forms of ongoing communication.

The dentist and team should discuss all eight phases, set standards and procedures for each, plan ways to welcome patients and parents, provide service that will be perceived as extraordinary, ensure reappointment, and encourage referrals. In a practice committed to total quality of patient care, such concepts are worked and improved continuously.

Explanation to Parents about Patient Safety and Privacy

For your comfort both parents, or **one** adult, are welcome but not required to accompany your child to the operatory. However, for the safety and privacy of other patients **all others,** including children who are not scheduled at this appointment, are asked to remain in the reception room. Young children in the reception room will need a supervisory adult.

In addition, the use of cell phones is prohibited in the operatory. The conversations carried on by others present in the clinical area can be most distracting to children, preventing us from close, careful communication with each young patient.

Thank you for your understanding. Your cooperation in these matters helps us to serve your child better.

Figure 29-5 Explanation to parents about patient safety and privacy.

PATIENT DISMISSAL

Properly managed dismissal of problem patients or families from your practice can be as important as properly dismissing an employee. Each state and/or Dental Board has certain laws that govern the dismissal of a patient. It behooves the dentist to become acquainted with these laws and closely follow them. Furthermore, the dentist should know what the state laws are as far as transferring patients, including charging for radiographs and records. The dentist must weigh the advantages and disadvantages of his or her actions and responses in each individual case and seek legal advice if necessary. Everything should be documented, knowing that any notes written into a patient's chart could, in case of a lawsuit, be read aloud in court. And, neither the dentist nor a staff member should argue with or belittle a patient or parent, because such actions may well cause the patient to leave the practice or could trigger a lawsuit.

PREVENTIVE PROGRAM

Offering preventive information and oral health counseling is an important part of dental service, appealing to increasingly sophisticated health care consumers. Intraoffice educational efforts can include topics such as home care, thumb sucking, diet, oral health during pregnancy, the dangers of smokeless tobacco, and infant oral health. Information should be shared with individuals at their levels of need and comprehension. A well planned and executed preventive education program can be a dynamic marketing tool.

An excellent way to offer educational and preventive services is through a dental health educator–marketing coordinator. The educator may be developed from among current staff members, or a new person may be employed. An invaluable resource, the educator must be given proper training and sufficient time to perform intraoffice teaching responsibilities, patient-relations tasks, and community-wide educational activities.

MARKETING AND PRACTICE GROWTH

Professional marketing goes beyond just efforts to bring more patients into the practice. Through marketing, parents, patients, and others in the community (i.e., prospective patients) can be educated about the value of dental health and ways that it can be achieved.

There are two aspects to marketing a dental practice. Internal marketing includes activities within an office that affect current patients. New-patient packets mailed before the first appointment, special correspondence to patients, giveaways, and improved office ambiance with, for example, a comfortable area for parents, play areas with electronic games and special toys for young patients and, perhaps, a separate area for teenage patients, are all forms of internal marketing.

External marketing activities are targeted at current and prospective patients. A website, a telephone on-hold message system, schoolchildren tours of the office, lectures to educational, civic, and social organizations about disease prevention, the latest dental techniques and

infant oral health, and career counseling with youngsters interested in learning more about the dental profession are forms of external marketing.

Internal and external marketing efforts must be well planned, coordinated among staff, included in the budget, reviewed periodically, and evaluated for effectiveness. Successful programs should result in improved oral health habits among patients and in the attraction of many new patients.

Although opinions vary among management consultants concerning appropriate numbers of new patients monthly for a well-established general practice, 20 to 40 seems to be an accepted range. However, most experts agree that, after 5 to 7 years in practice, a pediatric dentist might realistically set a goal of 50 to 60 new patients monthly. Typically, this number is needed to compensate for attrition as children grow older and transfer to a general dentist, move away, or leave the pediatric practice for some other reason.

COMMUNICATIONS WITH PARENTS AND PATIENTS

A sense of trust must be developed between parents, patients and the dental team. This rapport comes from skillful communications. Like communication among office team members, communication with parents and patients includes listening, speaking, writing, reading, and using nonverbal language.

Listening with empathy and patience to the questions and concerns of parents and patients is a must. Although the dentist must spend sufficient time with parents to fulfill professional responsibilities, ensure that informed consent is given, and establish trust; a well-trained auxiliary can deepen the parent-patient-practice relationship. A staff member can listen to problems, interpret concerns, reiterate answers to parents' and patients' questions, give home care instructions, and help parents and patients understand office procedures.

Dentists and auxiliary personnel should speak in layperson's terms so that parents and patients can understand the diagnosis and recommended treatment. Informed consent may require that forms and instructions be read aloud to parents who cannot read English or comprehend adequately. Many offices now employ a bilingual staff member to facilitate communication with non-English speaking parents and patients.

Written health history forms, health status updates, patient instructions, preventive literature, and other paperwork must look impeccable and be easily read and understood. All paperwork should be reviewed annually to make certain it remains pertinent and legally worded. Completed forms (including parents' comments) must be read and understood by the dentist and team members. Diagnoses previously recorded on the patient's chart and treatment notes from the last appointment should be read by the dentist and auxiliary personnel before beginning treatment at each appointment.

Unspoken (body language) messages from parents such as facial gestures and other body language must be interpreted with sensitivity. Surprisingly, parents typically judge a practice, accept treatment, and refer others based more on good feelings than on the quality of dentistry received. Skillful communications by the dentist and staff members and clean, attractive, well-organized office ambiance help generate these good feelings.

OPERATIONAL SYSTEMS

SCHEDULING

Proper scheduling controls the activity and flow of the dental office, increases productivity and efficiency, and allows the dentist to work at a comfortable pace. Efficient appointment scheduling makes the office pleasant, whereas poor scheduling creates a hectic, stressful environment for patients and staff members.

The telephone links patients to the practice, and it must be answered in a cheerful and genial manner. The attitude of the appointment secretary can give a positive impression, making scheduling a pleasant experience, or create a negative one, resulting in no appointment being made. The appointment secretary should listen carefully to each parent or patient and try to be accommodating while offering two choices of appointment times. If neither time is convenient for the parents, the secretary offers two more until one is accepted. It is inefficient to ask when the patient would like to come because treatment often dictates the length of an appointment and the time of day it can be scheduled.

Because appointment scheduling is complex, it is essential for a dentist to develop an ideal schedule, a plan toward which the appointment secretary can work. In most situations, a pediatric dental office functions more efficiently when *block scheduling* is used. With block scheduling, patients with similar treatments are given appointments in a particular period. For example, new patient examinations may be scheduled at a time when no restorative cases are scheduled. In this way, several new-patient appointments can be staggered throughout an hour or two when the dentist and most clinical staff can give their undivided attention to the new patient and parents. Sealant applications might be scheduled at the same time as new patients in this scheduling scenario if an assistant or hygienist can do the sealants with little or no help or, perhaps, recares (periodic oral examinations) could be scheduled in one chair.

Furthermore, more difficult and lengthy procedures, such as pulpotomies, crowns, composite restorations, orthodontic bandings, and procedures for preschool children 5 years of age and younger, are scheduled early, when the dentist, auxiliary personnel, and patients are fresh. Less difficult procedures such as simple operative procedures, orthodontic adjustments, and hygiene appointments for older children may be scheduled in the afternoons. Appointments just before lunch and in late afternoon should be reserved for the simplest procedures such as suture removals, simple extractions, eruption checks, and posttrauma examinations.

Sedated and difficult patients and those needing hospitalization require the dentist's undivided attention, so their treatment should be scheduled during specific periods weekly. Once a month or as the need arises, a period should be set aside for oral health appointments for infants. Infants can be checked for evidence of nursing caries or developmental problems while parents receive instructions about preventive care and diet. Teenagers' appointments may be scheduled together, perhaps one, two, or more afternoons weekly, depending on the number who need to be seen.

As part of the checkout process, the next appointment should be made. Although it may seem efficient to schedule a series of visits for the patient who needs several restorative appointments, it is preferable to schedule only one appointment at a time. Scheduling several appointments may cause some parents or patients to disregard keeping one or more in the series. Also, scheduling serial appointments can fill the appointment book for weeks and months, and thus allow little time for booking new patients or patients with emergencies.

Despite the best efforts of the appointment secretary, a few individuals will refuse to keep appointments for treatment or hygiene. These patients should be contacted periodically and invited to reschedule. As mentioned previously, entering a treatment plan for every patient at every visit or, if no treatment is needed, entering the next hygiene appointment, assures that patients are not lost.

SURGICAL REFERRALS

Some pediatric dentists have instituted a section of their practice entitled Surgical Referrals, indicating care for patients who need dental treatment and meet American Academy of Pediatric Dentistry Guidelines for General Anesthesia. This particular program is one in which a patient is treated under general anesthesia and then sent back to the referring doctor, mimicking the approach frequently used by some other specialties such as oral surgery.

These patients may be seen for an initial examination by the pediatric dentist, treated in the proper setting while under general anesthesia, seen for at least one postoperative visit, and if appropriate, returned to the referring doctor.

RECARE SYSTEM

The foundation of any successful dental practice is the recare system. The recare system provides a constant source of patients in a structured maintenance program that safeguards their oral health and emphasizes the fact that the dentist and staff care a great deal about them. The term *recare* is preferable to the frequently used word *recall*. *Recare* connotes ongoing, continual attention, whereas *recall* suggests an occasional check for problems (e.g., the recall of an automobile for repair or replacement of faulty parts).

The most effective and efficient recare systems that retain the most patients are those in which the next hygiene appointment is scheduled 6 months in advance at the conclusion of the present appointment. A reminder postcard or e-mail reminder may then be sent 3 to 4 weeks before the appointment. Conversely, recare systems in which a message is sent to the parents requesting them to call the office to schedule an appointment are often ineffective. People forget to respond, and the messages are frequently lost. Systems that rely on the appointment secretary to call all recare patients to schedule an appointment can be productive but are inefficient because it can take many hours to reach all patients.

There are two types of preappointed recare systems: *preselected* and *preassigned*. When implementing either system, the appointment secretary should emphasize to parents and patients that the preappointed recare system is for their convenience and is more likely to allow them to choose an appointment 6 months hence at the time that they prefer.

In preselected systems, at checkout, the parent chooses the next recare appointment. In 5 to 5½ months, a notification with the day, date, and time is generated and mailed or an e-mail message is sent.

In preassigned systems, the patient may be told at checkout that a notice will be mailed 3 to 4 weeks before the next appointment with the day, date, and time included. The appointment may be at approximately the same time as the present visit or it may alternate to be during or after school. The parents are encouraged to call if they have questions when they receive the recare appointment notice, but the staff member should avoid offering to change the appointment because that terminology invites parents to make changes. After the patient leaves, the next appointment is assigned, with the time needed for prophylaxis, behavioral management, medical complications, and time of the current appointment taken into consideration. This method is especially helpful in a busy practice because it speeds the checkout process and allows more scheduling flexibility.

For either a preselected or preassigned system, the appointment date is entered in the computer so that notifications can be generated when needed. Approximately 3 to 4 weeks before an appointment, recare reminders are sent. If the recare appointment must be changed for any reason, such as a change in the dentist's schedule, the change can be made before the notification is mailed or e-mailed. Hence, if the appointment was preassigned, no call is necessary; the time is simply corrected by staff before sending the reminder. If the parent preselected the recare appointment time, rescheduling should be done by telephone.

On receipt of the recare card, parents who find the time inconvenient usually call to reschedule. A confirmation telephone call should be made 1 or 2 days before the appointment. The staff person calling to confirm should be prepared to reschedule appointments if changes are requested.

The wording of the recare message must emphasize the importance of regular hygiene appointments. Box 29-1 is an example of an appropriate message for a recare card in a pediatric dental office.

Flexibility to accommodate appointment changes initiated by the office can be built into the preappointed system by leaving 1 or 2 days unscheduled toward the end of each month. If the time is not needed for changed appointments, it may be booked 1 or 2 weeks ahead with regular restorative appointments, new

---

Box 29-1

Example of a Recare Postcard Message

Patient Name: _____
Hygiene appointment: _____   (time)   (date)
   At this time, we will thoroughly examine all hard and soft tissue for dental disease, check for proper growth and development, clean teeth and apply special fluoride. Remember, if sealants are in place, regular 6-month examinations are necessary for proper maintenance.
   Changed appointments affect many people. If you cannot keep this appointment, please call at least 24 hours in advance so that this time may be given to another patient. We look forward to seeing you and your child on the above date.

---

examinations, and rescheduled appointments initiated by patients.

CHECKING RECARE SYSTEM EFFECTIVENESS

The recare program is the life-support system for any practice. The recognized minimum goal is for at least 8 of 10 active patients to return regularly at the prescribed frequency for hygiene appointments (i.e., 80% effectiveness). The effectiveness of the recare system should be checked at least quarterly.

Accuracy of the check depends on a close count of charts of patients who have been seen in the previous 18 months (active patients), except those whose treatments could be classified as single-visit emergencies (Clinical Dental Terminology [CDT] code No. DO140) who are not enrolled as regular patients.

The following example illustrates a quick, easy way to check the effectiveness of a recare system:

4000 active patients ÷ 6 months (recare frequency) = 667 recare appointments per month for 100% effective system

Actual average for 3 months = 300 recare appointments per month

300 actual ÷ 667 potential = 45% effective system

Goal = 80% or more of active patients returning for regular recare appointments

4000 active patients × 0.80 = 3200 patients

3200 patients ÷ 6 months (recare frequency) = 533 recare appointments per month as 80% goal

533 recares per month as 80% goal

−300 recares per month actual average
233 additional recares per month

233 × $$ average recare fee × 12 months = thousands of dollars additional income generated from current patients—plus better care and service to patients

After the current effectiveness rate is determined, the dentist and staff can work toward the goal of 80% of active patients returning regularly for recare. Problems with the system should be listed and analyzed, and ways to improve the system must be planned and implemented. Many practitioners find that 60% or more of restorative and orthodontic treatment needs are diagnosed during hygiene examinations, which reinforces the importance of an effective recare system in any office.

BROKEN APPOINTMENTS AND PURGING PATIENT CHARTS

A phrase frequently used in dental offices is "patients who drop between the cracks." This phrase describes patients whose treatment is diagnosed and presented but who leave the office without scheduling and fail to call back for an appointment. It can also apply to patients whose treatment is not rescheduled after a broken or canceled appointment. Patient care suffers, and a great deal of money may be lost in a practice that lacks a viable system for contacting these patients.

If a patient fails to keep an appointment, a staff member should telephone the parents within 10 to 15 minutes. If unsuccessful, call again within 24 hours. If the parents cannot be reached by telephone, a message, perhaps by email or, failing that, by regular mail, should be sent asking them to contact the office. If the appointment cannot be rescheduled, the patient must be listed or flagged in the computer. At the end of each month, a broken appointment list can be printed so that patients with failed appointments can be recontacted.

A patient who has not completed treatment or who has an appliance or prosthesis should receive a letter explaining the dental consequences of not completing treatment or not having periodic adjustment and examination of a device. Such letters should be mailed to the patient's last known address after obtaining a Certificate of Mailing (PS Form 3817) from the U.S. Post Office. A copy of the letter should be kept in the patient's chart with the Certificate of Mailing attached, which provides proof that the letter was mailed and that the dentist's professional responsibility was fulfilled. A Certificate of Mailing adds nominal cost to first class postage.

It is important to purge patients' charts regularly, at least once a year, preferably in September or October. This is a relatively simple matter if the charts whether hard copies or electronic are marked with a yearly date indicating that the patient had a recare appointment within that year. The appointment secretary can pull the charts of patients who have not been seen during that year and telephone or e-mail the parents to stress the importance of regular hygiene appointments. Parents of children with incomplete treatment should be informed of the treatment yet to be rendered and the importance of completing it. Parents with dental insurance should be reminded that benefits for that year will be lost unless they schedule an appointment for their child before year's end. Many people will schedule an appointment to avoid losing insurance benefits. Individuals who refuse

to reschedule should be contacted once more, so noted in the patient chart, before their charts are placed in the inactive file.

Active files, maintained in the accessible office chart shelves or on computer, are charts of patients who have received care within the previous 18 months. Inactive files consist of charts of patients seen before the previous 18 months who have been contacted but refuse to reschedule. Some state laws specify a minimum period after the last treatment date that dental records must be maintained. Regardless of the statutory requirement, it is best to maintain records for as long as possible but certainly no less than 10 years from the last treatment date for adults and up to age 28 for patients treated when they were children. Charts should be kept as evidence against malpractice claims and to answer medical or dental questions that may arise in later years. If storage becomes a problem, records can be scanned into digital files. Such records are admissible in most state courts. Of course, a proper backup system for storage of inactive charts must be maintained if the office has only computerized charts.

Some dental offices prefer to create and maintain charts on computer, a "paperless office." In this case, the dentist must be certain that he or she, at least two staff members, and, if necessary, an off-site computer resource expert are completely knowledgeable about the hardware, software and backup system. One or more of these individuals must be available for immediate assistance in case of computer problems, electrical failure or some other crisis that causes computer malfunction. "Our computers are down" is not an acceptable excuse for having no charts, treatment plans, or health history when patients telephone to make an appointment or present for treatment.

PRODUCTION AND COLLECTIONS

A dental practice is a small business, and like any business, it must be profitable. For the practice to operate profitably, high-quality dental treatment must be provided in an efficient manner, and the office must be administered according to recognized sound business principles and procedures.

Every successful business establishes goals. A production goal is one of the most important in a dental practice. It determines the amount of money that must be charged at the current collection rate to reach the break-even point and enjoy a profit above and beyond that point.

The best way to calculate a production goal is to determine the break-even point, the amount of money needed each year to pay all office expenses, the dentist's compensation (salary or draw plus benefits and retirement funding), and a profit (return on investment) for the owner-dentist. The dentist in an incorporated practice takes a "salary" as an employee of the corporation; in a sole proprietorship (unincorporated practice), the dentist takes a "draw." An example of the calculation of the break-even point follows:

Break-even point = Total fixed costs ÷ (1.0 minus % variable costs are of gross collections)

Fixed costs include office overhead (staff salaries and benefits, occupancy costs, administrative costs, taxes, insurance, etc.), the dentist's salary or draw and benefits, and repayment of money borrowed to finance the practice startup or purchase. Variable costs usually include laboratory fees and dental supplies (costs that vary according to patient load) and are typically 8% to 13% of gross collections in pediatric dental practice and 15% to 20% in general practice.

If total fixed costs are $750,000 and variable costs are 10%, calculate the break-even point as follows:

$$\text{Break-even point} = \$750,000 \div (1 - 0.10) = \$750,000 \div$$
$$0.90 = \$833,333 \text{ per year}$$

In this example, to pay fixed costs of $750,000 plus variable costs of 10%, the office must collect $833,333 for the year. That, however, is not the end of the calculation. Assuming the average collection rate is 97% of production (97¢ of every $1 charged as fees is collected), the practice would have to produce $859,106 to collect $833,333. If the dentist wishes a profit/bonus of $100,000 above and beyond salary or draw, the practice would need to produce an additional $103,093 (97% of which would be collected) to cover costs plus profit/ bonus, a total production of $962,199. At 97% collection rate, $933,333 would be collected ($833,333 to pay fixed and variable costs plus $100,000 profit/ bonus).

To establish an accurate production goal, the dentist must know the break-even point plus desired profit, the number of days worked per year, the collection percentage rate (the percentage of production collected), and the show rate (the percentage of patients who keep appointments as scheduled).

For example, if the break-even point plus profit is $933,333 per year, the dentist works 190 days per year, the collection rate is 97%, and the show rate is 85%:

$$\$933,333 \div 190 \text{ days} = \$4912 \text{ per day collection goal}$$

$$\$4912 \div 0.97 \text{ collection rate} = \$5064 \text{ per day}$$
$$\text{production goal}$$

$$\$5064 \div 0.85 \text{ show rate} = \$5958 \text{ scheduled to produce}$$
$$\$5064 \text{ to collect } \$4912 \text{ per day}$$

Note in this example: $5958 worth of treatment must be scheduled daily because on average, 15% of scheduled patients will not keep their appointment. Typically, 97% of fees produced that day on patients who do keep appointments will be collected. The dentist has 190 patient days during the year in this example to produce/collect to meet that year's goal of $933,333.

This concept of treatment scheduled vs. production vs. collections is key to managing the financial health of a practice. The method for setting scheduling, production and collection goals *must* be understood and used.

Many dentists are more concerned with production than with collections; however, collections control cash flow. One can spend only collected dollars. A very productive practice can have serious financial difficulties if collections do not provide sufficient cash flow to cover the expenses and generate a profit. Collections, therefore, must be monitored constantly. Most offices find that a 97% collection rate is the minimum acceptable level for private-pay and insurance patients. Of these collections, the over-the-counter portion, collected on the day treatment is rendered, should be a minimum of 30% and preferably as much as 50% to maintain an adequate cash flow.

PAYMENT POLICY

A clearly stated payment policy presented to parents in a professional manner facilitates collections. Although all team members should be familiar with payment procedures, one staff person should be designated as the patient account coordinator. The patient account coordinator should clarify payment methods with parents, process insurance forms and other third-party payments, and handle billing and delinquent accounts.

The most effective way to familiarize parents with payment procedures is to review methods of payment with them, preferably at checkout after the initial examination. Having a written policy ensures that there are no misunderstandings. Box 29-2 is an example of a payment policy.

DENTAL INSURANCE

The new-to-practice dentist should realize that dental insurance coverage does not necessarily mean that parents will seek regular dental care for their children or accept all recommended treatment. Parents and patients tend to accept services they have been taught to value from practitioners they trust. Dentists and team members must work with all parents and patients to build rapport and to educate them about the value of good oral health beginning in infancy. Only in this way will comprehensive care be accepted so that a practice can grow to full potential. Even though filing insurance claims can be time consuming and, at times, annoying, remember that dental insurance is beneficial for a practice because it allows many patients to accept treatment they could not otherwise afford.

The dentist and staff members should refer to dental insurance as "assistance" and should never allude to "full benefit coverage." In this way, parents are taught to think of dental insurance as a partial payment, help with the cost of their child's dental care, never meant to pay fees in full. A written explanation is an excellent way to help parents understand their coverage. For those who have dental insurance, the information can be enclosed with the new-patient packet mailed prior to the first examination. Box 29-3 is an example of a brief explanation of how dental insurance works.

The dentist should not discount or disregard the portion of fees not paid by an insurance company; i.e., the patient's copayment. Doing so may constitute insurance

Box 29-2

Payment Procedures

We appreciate your allowing us to provide dental care for your child. Because we value our relationship with you and believe that the best relationships are based on understanding, we offer these explanations of payment for services.

- We ask that you pay the cost of the initial examination on the day of that appointment. Since most insurance policies have an annual deductible amount, it is likely that the fee for the examination will not be covered. We will promptly refund your payment if your insurance carrier pays.
- Payment in full by cash, check, or charge at each appointment as service is rendered is requested. We accept _____, _____, and _____ credit cards.
- For patients with dental insurance, after receipt of a predetermination of benefits from your insurance carrier, we will accept payment for treatment in excess of $_____ directly from the company. However, if we do not receive payment from the company within 5 weeks after the submission of a claim, you will be expected to pay for all dental services. In the event of duplicate payment, you will be reimbursed. We ask that fees totaling less than $____ be paid as treatment is rendered. Your insurance carrier may then reimburse you directly. (If the office files all insurance claims for patients, this sentence might be, "We will then file a claim for you and your insurance carrier may reimburse you directly.")
- Even if you have insurance coverage, you are responsible for payment of your account. We will be happy to help you receive the maximum benefits available under your policy; however, please realize that the relationship is between you, the insured, and your insurance company.

- Payment plans may be set up for our patients without dental insurance. If more than $_____ of treatment is required, payment may be made in four parts:
- One fourth at the initial appointment
- One fourth 30 days after the initial payment
- One fourth 60 days after the initial payment
- One fourth 90 days after the initial payment
- If a payment plan is agreed on, you will be asked to sign a financial agreement, and receive a book of coupons, one of which is to be mailed with each monthly payment. Payments are due by the 10th of each month.
- Statements are mailed monthly, usually by the 25th of the month. If there is a balance on your account, you will receive a statement regardless of the date on which treatment was rendered unless a signed payment plan allows extended payments.
- If insurance is pending, you will receive an interim statement to let you know that the account has not been paid.
- If you require credit for longer than described above, personal arrangements should be made with your bank or credit union.
- Half the cost of an appliance or prosthesis must be paid when impressions are taken. This is necessary because our office must pay a portion of laboratory costs when appliances are ordered. The remainder of the cost of the appliance is due when the appliance is placed.
- Please be aware that the parent bringing the child to our office is legally responsible for payment of all charges.

We look forward to years of close association with you as we work together to maintain your child's oral health. Thank you!

---

fraud because the dentist has misrepresented actual charges. For example, if a fee for a procedure is $100 and an insurance company pays only $80, do not submit a claim for the full $100 fee if $80 is accepted as payment in full. Submit the $100 claim only if the parent is expected to pay the $20 that is not covered.

INSURANCE ASSIGNMENT

A basic decision to be made concerning collections is whether the office will wait for payment of fees from insurance carriers or ask that fees be paid as treatment progresses. An office that waits on payment from insurance carriers is said to "accept insurance assignment." An office that requires fees be paid as treatment is delivered is a "cash practice."

Many new dentists decide between accepting insurance or requesting full payment by determining the prevailing method in their communities. However, several other factors should also be considered when making the decision. For example, a mature pediatric dental practice with a patient load of 40 to 50 or more patients daily may have to process 175 or more insurance claims weekly. This amount of paperwork may necessitate hiring an additional staff person. Furthermore, accepting insurance assignment may delay cash receipts for 6 to 8 weeks or longer when paper claims are filed and 2 to 3 weeks when electronic claims are submitted. The beginning practitioner who decides to accept assignment of benefits must, therefore, plan for another source of operating cash while waiting for initial insurance claims to be paid.

On the other hand, many dentists and management experts agree that the acceptance of assignment can be a good marketing tool because parents are more likely to accept recommended treatment for their child if they have to pay only the difference between the actual fee and the amount their dental insurance covers. In addition, parents who are pleased that their insurance benefits

Box 29-3

For Our Patients with Dental Insurance

The best dental service is based on friendly, mutual understanding. Therefore we invite you to discuss any aspects of your child's dental care or the level of assistance your dental insurance provides you.

Your insurance is a contact between your employer and the insurance company. We cannot influence how much of our fees your insurance will cover. Your benefits are determined by the policy your employer purchased.

You will need to bring the insurance claim form, with your portion of the form completed and signed, to the first visit. We will file the insurance for you. If you have any questions about completing your portions of the claim form, please call our office.

We will appreciate your bringing your insurance benefits booklet also. By reading the booklet together, we can understand your dental benefits (i.e., what your insurance will cover).

We ask that the cost of the initial examination be paid on the day of that visit. Since most insurance companies have an annual deductible amount per family or insured person, the cost of the examination probably will not be covered.

Because there are certain fees or procedures most dental insurance policies do not allow, please expect to pay the portion of the fee not covered at each visit. We will refund any duplicate payment your insurance company makes.

Please sign the space provided on your insurance form for payment to be made directly to our office. Otherwise, we will not receive payment, and you will be billed for treatment.

One copy of the insurance form is a receipt for your records and tax purposes. Please keep copies of all office correspondence for reference with insurance claims.

Please be aware that the parent bringing the child for dental care is legally responsible for payment of all charges. Your obligations are:

- To certify to the insurance company that your treatment was received
- To understand that *you*, not your insurance company, are responsible to our office for the services rendered.

We appreciate your selecting our practice for your child's dental care.

Thank you!

---

substitute for cash are more likely to tell others about this service and the office.

Some offices work with a hybrid system in which parents pay full fees for treatments up to, for example, $500, and insurance assignment is accepted for fees in excess of $500. In this case, a predetermination of how much the insurance will pay should be obtained from the insurance carrier so the office knows how much copayment to collect from the parents as treatment progresses.

For the office that accepts insurance assignment, the most important information to obtain about each patients' insurance is the insurance company's name, telephone number, and plan number; the employer's name, telephone number, and contact person; deductible requirements and amount; maximum annual and lifetime benefits; preestimate requirements; percent or scheduled amount paid on various procedures, including preventive and orthodontic treatment; and any exclusions.

INSURANCE REFERENCE GUIDE

An insurance reference guide, a synopsis showing deductible amounts and fees not covered, is an invaluable aid to offices that accept insurance assignment. Using such a guide allows the patient account coordinator to quickly determine at each visit the portion of the fee to be paid by the parents. Fees not covered and deductibles can then be collected as treatment is rendered. Collecting fees on the day of service increases cash flow and saves preparing and mailing statements for unpaid account balances after insurance payment has been received.

Many dental computer systems have software features that can record insurance payment schedules for

numerous carriers. Whether a guide is maintained manually or as part of the computer software, business staff must obtain and annually update information about the schedule of benefits for insurance carriers most frequently dealt with by the office.

PREDETERMINATION

Many insurance carriers request the submission of a treatment plan (predetermination) for procedures that will cost $300 to $350 or more. Usually the choice of whether to file a predetermination and the task of doing it rests with the dental office. The insurance company determines the amount to be paid according to the contract with the parent's employer and responds to the dental office. The parents can then be informed about the amount of assistance available from their insurance carrier.

A copy of the submitted predetermination form should be kept in either an electronic or a hard copy "tickler" file so that the patient's treatment can be scheduled immediately when clarification of benefits is received from the insurance company. The file must be checked monthly by a staff member. Any predeterminations submitted but not returned by an insurance company should be pursued, because the patient will be waiting to begin treatment.

FILING CLAIMS

Third-party claims may be filed manually or electronically. Electronic claims usually result in a significantly shorter turnaround time. The faster a claim is paid, the better the cash flow for the dental office. Details of electronic filing should be available from any computer vendor whose system allows such filing.

The staff member who handles insurance and other third-party claims must be trained in filing and follow-up of claims because requirements and procedures vary among third-party payers. This person should attend seminars about dental benefits, read management journal articles on the topic, and keep up with the latest CDT (Current Dental Terminology) codes. CDT codes are typically revised every 2 years. The ADA's current handbook on CDT codes is available from www.ada.org. Another useful manual to complement the *ADA Handbook* is *Coding with Confidence: The "Go To" Guide for CDT 2009/2010* by Dr. Charles Blair, which says, "In many cases thousands of dollars are recovered by proper coding usage, documentation, and truthful narratives. Both the practice and the patient 'win' through proper documentation and correct and accurate reporting for maximum legal reimbursement. Many offices will find that they are leaving 'money on the table' by not properly understanding and applying properly the official CDT – 2009/2010 code set."[3]

Filing claims as treatment progresses rather than waiting to file the total claim after a series of appointments improves cash flow. In this way, the dentist receives payment as work is performed. Claims should be filed only for treatment delivered.

A master copy of the insurance form should be signed by the parents and kept in the patient's chart, so that insurance claims can be filed using "signature on file."

PENDING INSURANCE CLAIMS

Toward the end of each month, an outstanding insurance claims report should be generated so that each overdue claim can be pursued. If time permits, the patient account coordinator may call the insurance company to inquire about payment. Alternatively, the parent may be called to pursue the overdue claim. Parents should have been informed as treatment began that they would be expected to pay all noncovered fees as well as claims not paid by 5 to 6 weeks after treatment.

WELFARE DENTAL SERVICES

Practitioners must decide how much dental service their practice can provide for welfare patients. The positive for doing so is the personal and professional satisfaction of knowing you, the dentist, have cared for some of the neediest patients in your community and have met some of your moral and ethical obligations as a professional. The negative for doing so is that many states' program reimbursement levels fall short of covering the actual cost of dentistry delivered to welfare patients. In this case, the dentist loses money on the services rendered to every welfare patient he or she treats. Some pediatric dentists solve this quandary by treating a limited number of welfare patients who meet criteria set for their practice.

Medicaid (known by other titles in some states) is a state-administered program in which each state sets its own guidelines regarding eligibility and services, including reimbursement rates. The wise practitioner investigates his or her state program thoroughly before deciding to become a welfare provider. One might begin seeking information at a variety of websites available through the U.S. Department of Health and Human Services.

HEALTH INSURANCE PORTABILITY AND ACCOUNTABILITY ACT OF 1996

Historically, the protection of patient privacy has been expected and accepted as an ethical standard in the health care professions. Effective April 2003, it became a legal requirement. The United States Department of Health and Human Services has issued comprehensive privacy regulations that apply to all health care providers who transmit (or authorize a third party to transmit on their behalf) protected health information electronically (such as electronic claim forms). The health care provider may use and disclose a patient's protected health information only as the patient permits or as allowed under the privacy rules. In addition, the privacy rules give patients certain rights, such as the right to amend their protected health information. Further details on this act are available on the U.S. Department of Health and Human Services website.[5]

DIRECT REIMBURSEMENT

Direct reimbursement, a benefit gaining support among employers and employees nationwide, is an excellent alternative to dental insurance. Under direct reimbursement, the dentist receives payment from the parents as services are rendered. The parent then submits a paid statement directly to his or her employer and is reimbursed for a portion of the fee. Implementation of a direct reimbursement plan and the amount of reimbursement is decided by the parents' employer. Information about active direct reimbursement plans in any state should be available from the state dental society.

MANAGED CARE

Dental benefit organizations fit under the umbrella term *managed care,* which is an insurance industry term for a system that curbs expenditures in benefit plans by cutting reimbursement levels and transferring financial risk to those providing care (in this case, the dentist).

In managed care, it is the payment methods rather than the actual dental treatment modalities that are different. Each managed care system has a specific mechanism of payment for treatment, usually accompanied by some form of utilization review. Dentists who participate in managed care organizations surrender control of their fees for that part of their patient population enrolled in the managed care organization.

The two most widely used types of dental managed care are the preferred provider organization (PPO) and capitation contract dentistry (CCD). A PPO is a network of private practitioners who contract with a plan to provide specific services to a particular patient population at reduced fees. Patients enrolled in a certain PPO must choose a dentist from the organization's list of providers. In CCD plans, the dentist contracts with a plan to provide specific services to enrollees in return for a monthly capitation amount whether or not the enrollees-patients actually make and keep appointments. In other words, the dental office receives a monthly lump capitation payment based on the enrolled number of patients eligible for treatment in that office.

Dentists must weigh many issues, options, and fiscal matters regarding managed care. The ADA has a comprehensive array of resources to help dentists understand and analyze the positive and negative aspects of managed care. Among the services offered is contract analysis, which is available from the ADA through individual state dental societies. Any dentist who is considering signing a contract with a dental benefit organization is well advised to consult with the ADA and his or her own attorney, financial advisor, and management consultant.

FISCAL MANAGEMENT

Fiscal management concerns the way in which the finances of a business are controlled. Fiscal aspects of a dental practice include accounts receivable (money owed to the practice), fee structure, accounts payable (money owed by the practice), budgeting, and monitoring methods. In a well-managed practice, the dentist carefully administers each of these aspects.

BILLING AND ACCOUNTS RECEIVABLE

The dentist and business staff members should establish a regular routine for handling billing; receipt of mail payments from individuals, insurance companies, and other third-party organizations; and pursuit of delinquent accounts. Consistency in following these procedures is extremely important to ensure effective collection of fees.

At checkout, polite but direct effort should be made by business staff to collect payment for treatment rendered that day. If the office files insurance claims for patients, the noncovered portion of the fee or at least 30% of that day's charges should be collected. If insurance pays more than 70% of that claim, a refund can be made to the parents.

When parents do not pay on the day of treatment, a statement with an envelope addressed to the office should be presented at checkout. Regular monthly statements should be mailed by the 25th of the month to be received before the first, when many people pay bills. Statements should be sent to every account, including those waiting on insurance payments, regardless of when the service was rendered. Receipt of a statement reminds parents that they have an outstanding balance. Some dentists prefer to have a fourth of the statements mailed each week of the month to better manage cash flow. With this method, patients whose last names begin with A through F receive statements the first week of the month, those whose last names begin with G through L receive them the second week, and so on.

Accounts receivable are fees billed but not collected, that is, all money owed to a practice by patients. In offices that accept assignment of insurance or allow patients to pay dental fees on a payment plan, 1 to 1½ months' gross production is the recommended guideline for total accounts receivable. When the accounts receivable total is more than 1½ months' production, cash flow suffers and many accounts become uncollectible.

Many practices have excessive accounts receivable because there is no system and no one staff member (patient account coordinator) responsible for processing overdue (delinquent) accounts. These accounts must be separated into categories of over 30, 60, 90, or 120 days late in payment to organize the collection of fees and to determine which accounts need priority collection action. Laws concerning collection techniques and do's and don'ts for collecting overdue accounts vary from state to state. Therefore, the dentist must make certain his or her patient accounts coordinator is well trained in the legalities of pursuing delinquent accounts in that state.

Each dentist must determine when accounts are considered overdue or delinquent. An account on which no payment has been made for 30 to 60 days may be considered overdue. The staff member acting as patient account coordinator should pursue payment using telephone calls and letters. If there is no response or payment by 90 to 120 days, the account may be forwarded for outside collection action (i.e., sent to a collection agency or an attorney) after the dentist reviews the account and gives approval.

If the patient's treatment is incomplete or the patient has an appliance or prosthetic device, the dentist should seek legal counsel before designating the patient's chart inactive and sending the account for outside collection action. An attorney can best advise on patient abandonment issues, so that potential legal problems are avoided.

Another excellent source of information concerning patient chart inactivation is the American Dental Association. The ADA has a variety of publications pertinent to this subject as well as other practice management issues. Of particular interest is *Frequently Asked Legal Questions* available through ADA Member Services are helpful in locating specific publications that address particular practice management issues.[6]

FEES

The following factors must be considered when setting proper fees:
1. The dentist's and assistant's time required to do a procedure or the hygienist's time for hygiene procedures
2. Cost of operations per hour (overhead), including salaries, benefits, rent, supplies, laboratory costs, insurance, taxes, and infection control, among others
3. Prevailing professional fees in the area, although collusion with other dental practices is illegal
4. Profit after debt service

Fees must be reviewed at least annually and, if necessary, raised more than the inflation rate to continue to generate an adequate margin of profit. Most patients expect, accept, and may not even notice small adjustments in fees. Problems may arise, however, when a dentist who is reluctant to increase fees does not do so for several years and then must implement a significant increase. A hiatus in raising fees while costs of operations continue to increase means lower profits. If this pattern is allowed to continue, a practice can have significant financial difficulties that force a fee increase of 20% to 30% or more in one year. Because many patients notice and complain about such a large increase, it is better to raise fees gradually year to year to adjust for inflation and to cover increases in expenditures.

Fee increases should not be announced to patients; an increase simply is made effective on a certain date. The dentist and staff who have pride in the quality of their care and service will seldom feel defensive about fee increases, and that feeling will be imparted to patients and parents. Most people are willing to pay for care that they value and service that exceeds the norm.

Staff members need some information about why regular fee increases are necessary. With no concept of overhead costs, the staff may assume that all fee increases go directly into the dentist's pocket, which is far from true. Sharing information about expenses such as laboratory fees, clinical and office supplies, utilities, and taxes allows team members to understand the necessity of regular fee increases.

Fee increases or fee cuts have significant impact on practice income and profit as demonstrated in Tables 29-1 and 29-2.

ACCOUNTS PAYABLE

Accounts payable is the total amount of money the practice owes for goods and services received. Bills should be paid no more frequently than twice a month after statements are checked against invoices.

Whereas an invoice is an itemized list of goods received with each supply shipment, a statement is a summary of all invoices for that month. Paying accounts regularly from statements rather than from invoices can help avoid mistakes, such as paying the same bill twice, and ensure that the practice maintains an excellent credit rating.

INVENTORY CONTROL

A well-organized inventory system can prevent running out of necessary supplies and materials or being oversupplied and thus tying up excess cash. Whether the practice is computerized or not, the basics are the same. *Central Supply* maintains predetermined maximum and minimum levels for each item. *Working Inventory* is withdrawn from the designated Central Supply

Table 29-1

Impact of Fee Increase on Profitability

Current Overhead %	% Fee Increase	Increase in Net Income %
65	5	14.3
65	10	28.6
65	20	57.2
60	5	12.5
60	10	25
60	20	50
55	5	11.1
55	10	22.2
55	20	44.4

Courtesy Dr. Charles W. Blair.

Table 29-2

Impact of Fee Cut on Production Required to Maintain Same Net Income

Current Overhead %	Fee Cut %	% of Production Increase Required to Maintain Same Net
65	5	16
65	10	40
65	20	233
60	5	14
60	10	33
60	20	200
55	5	13
55	10	29
55	20	80

Courtesy Dr. Charles W. Blair.

area and distributed to the appropriate places in the practice.

Purchase orders for Central Supply may be generated on a designated day each week to help prevent frequent disruptions during work hours, or they may be generated whenever needed. One or two staff members may be responsible for submitting purchase orders to suppliers. Upon receipt of supplies, all invoices and packing slips should be checked against items received for accuracy. The new supplies should be entered into the inventory software or onto the manual list, and then placed in the Central Supply area. Upon moving items from Central Supply to Working Inventory, enter the withdrawal to ensure maintenance of maximum and minimum level counts. An annual or semiannual manual inventory count is recommended to maintain accuracy.

WRITING A BUDGET

Sound fiscal management includes making certain that the business is profitable. As Dunlap and Wagner wrote in *Knowing the Numbers*, "Business and profits are not dirty words. They are legitimate terms to describe activities directed towards the attainment of a livelihood. Quality cannot exist in the absence of profit. The attaining of profits is an essential part of a dentist's professional responsibility."[7]

Stated another way, James F. Parker, former CEO of Southwest Airlines, says, "In the free enterprise system, the most basic measure of success by a private business is profitability—not just one quarter or one year of profits, but a sustainable basis for consistent and growing profits."[8]

There are two ways to increase profitability in any practice: earn more or spend less. Control of expenses (savings) is one of the most underused yet valuable tools to increase profitability. Unspent dollars can go directly to the bottom line in the form of profit.

The most effective way to save is to control spending through budgeting. A budget is the translation of the future plans of a business into dollars; also defined as the financial portion of the business plan. Basically, it is a plan for the income and expenses of the practice.

Budgeting begins when the annual gross production goal is established. The break-even point should be calculated, and the desired profit added to determine the total annual production-collection goal. (See section on Production and Collections for information on calculating the break-even point.)

Remember that the collection percentage rate must be considered when forecasting annual production and collection goals. If, for example, the practice collection rate is 95%, $736,842 must be produced to collect $700,000. As previously mentioned, the minimum collection goal should be 97% (i.e., for every $1 of dentistry produced, 97¢ is collected).

Next, each expense should be scrutinized. Increases must be predicted based on inflation, increases in practice productivity, additional staffing needs and equipment additions or upgrades. Savings should also be planned and worked.

After income goals and expenses are calculated, annual totals should be divided by 12 months to determine the monthly production-collection goal and the allowance for each expense category, including personnel, occupancy, administrative, equipment and furnishings, clinical supplies, laboratory costs and marketing.

In summary, a budget should project income, propose maximums for each category of expense and forecast the year's profit. Figures should be monitored monthly, quarterly, and annually.

A monthly journal of income (collections) and expenses should show each category of expense as a percentage of collections. Box 29-4 gives average expenses commonly seen in pediatric dental practices. Obviously, expenses vary from practice to practice; therefore this list is only a guideline.

PRACTICE MONITORS

Well-managed businesses use numbers as management tools so that business decisions are based on facts and figures, not guesswork or emotions. Well-managed dental practices should use the same criteria. Vital statistics needed for good management include the following:

- Production: per day, week, month, and year to date compared with the same period last year
  - Goal and actual practice production per hour, day, month, and year
  - Dentist's actual production
  - Hygienist's actual production
- Collections: per day, week, month, and year to date compared with the same period last year
  - Goal of 97% or more of production
  - Collection percentage rate (collections for a period divided by production for the same period)
- Number of hours and days worked per month and per year
- Number of active patients (Patients seen within past 18 months, not including those seen for single-visit emergencies. Count individual patients, *not* patient

---

Box 29-4

Categories of Expenses in a Pediatric Dental Practice

Personnel
Salaries—22% to 26% including payroll taxes
Benefits—approximately 2% to 5%

Occupancy—5% to 10%

Lease or note payment	Repairs and
Insurance on building	maintenance to
and contents	facility
Janitor/grounds/security	Utilities (except
	telephone)

Administrative—6% to 10%

Accounting, legal—under 2%	Laundry
Advertising—for staff	Licenses/permits
Answering service	Meals for business
Collection costs/bank charges	Office supplies,
	printing
Computer expenses	Postage
Continuing education - staff	Taxes
Dues and subscriptions	Telephone
Insurance	Miscellaneous
Malpractice	
Business	
Disability for doctors	

Equipment, furnishings, contingency—4% to 6%
Note for purchase or lease payments; 3 months operating money as contingency

Clinical supplies—4% to 8%

Off-site laboratory—under 2% for pediatric dentistry only; up to 4% if significant orthodontics is done

Marketing—2% to 5%

Advertising, yellow pages	Practice brochures
Giveaways	and other literature
Web site	

Note: depreciation and amortization do not directly affect cash flow and are, therefore, not listed. If the dentist prefers, depreciation on the office building can be monitored in the "occupancy" category; depreciation on equipment and amortization for software can be monitored as part of the "equipment, furnishings, contingency" category.

---

visits because one patient may have had three or more appointments in an 18-month period.)
- Number of hygiene patients seen per month and year
  - Goal: 80% or more of active patients enrolled in the recare system
- Number of patient appointments scheduled in a day, week, and month
- Number of patient appointments kept in the same day, week, and month
- Show rate (percentage of kept appointments, calculated by dividing the number of patients who kept appointments as made by the number scheduled for that same period)

- Show rate goal: 85% or higher in pediatric dental offices
- Accounts receivable each month
  - Total accounts receivable (A/R) and increase or decrease since previous month
  - A/R at 30 days
  - A/R at 60 days
  - A/R at 90 days
  - A/R at 120 days and over
  - Bad-debt write off
  - Welfare and other third-party adjustments/write-offs
  - Professional courtesy adjustments/write-offs
- Overhead: per month, per year (average: 50% to 60% in pediatric dental practices, not including compensation for doctors) Additionally, the percentage of collections spent for each of the following categories of expense should be monitored:
  - Personnel costs
  - Occupancy costs
  - Administrative costs
  - Equipment, furnishings, and contingency fund
  - Clinical supplies

- Laboratory fees
- Marketing
- Total compensation for dentists in actual dollars and as a percentage of collections

DAILY STATISTICS

A short form completed daily by the business staff keeps the dentist informed of daily activities. Fig. 29-6 illustrates the information to be monitored daily.

MONTHLY STATISTICS

Monthly practice statistics can be collected in a single-sheet format. Assembly of these numbers on a single sheet allows quick evaluation and comparison with previous similar time periods. Fig. 29-7 is an example of a monthly monitoring form.

FISCAL FACTS, AVERAGES, MEDIANS, AND GOALS IN A PEDIATRIC DENTAL PRACTICE

The following facts and statistics are gleaned from scores of private pediatric dental practices. The practices range in age from a few years to 30 years or more. Regional

---

Daily Activities

Date: _____

	Restorative	Orthodontic
No. patients scheduled	_____	_____
No. patients seen	_____	_____
% patients seen (show rate)	_____	_____

Combined total no. scheduled for restorative and for orthodontic _____
Combined total no. seen for restorative and for orthodontic _____
Combined % seen, not including emergencies (show rate) _____

| No. broken appointments | _____ | _____ |
| No. rescheduled | _____ | _____ |

Hygiene Activity

No. patients scheduled	_____
No. patients seen	_____
% patients seen (show rate)	_____

| No. broken appointments | _____ |
| No. rescheduled | _____ |

Production $_____
Daily goal adjustment $_____
Collection/deposit $_____

Figure 29-6 Daily activities form.

Monthly Practice Monitor for _____

Monthly statistics collected in single-sheet format allow quick evaluation and comparison to previous similar time periods.

Pediatric Dentistry Statistics

	This Mo.	Last Mo.	Year to Date	Same Mo. Last Year	Last Year to Date
Days worked					
Hours worked					
Dentist production plus hygiene production					
Private and insurance production					
Welfare and other reduced fee production					
Welfare production to total production ratio (%)					
Production per day					
Production per hour					
Total collections					
Private and insurance collections					
Welfare and other reduced fee collections					
Collection to production ratio (%)– private and insurance					
Collection to production ratio (%)– welfare and reduced fee					
No. and date statements mailed					
Accounts receivable (A/R) total					
A/R aging $ — Current					
30 days					
60 days					
90 days					
120 days					
In collections					
Total adjustments (write-offs)					
New patient appointments					
Recare patient appointments					
Total patient appointments					
Show rate (% of kept appointments)					
Total patients leaving practice					
If full-banded orthodontics is part of the practice, complete this section also.					
Orthodontic production					
Orthodontic collections					
Contracts receivable C/R total					
C/R aging $ Current					
30 days					
60 days					
90 days					
120 days					
In collections					
No. new patient exams					
No. recall for revaluation					
No. records taken					
No. bands and bonds					
No. periodic adjustments					
No. debandings					
No. leaving incomplete					

Figure 29-7 Monthly practice monitor form.

differences are not specified. The following figures, as the title of this section suggests, represent averages and goals typical of the specialty in most, but not all, regions of the country.

Production
• Goal: Dentist plus hygiene department per-hour charges—$650 to $750 or more per hour without full banded orthodontics; $850 to $900 or more per hour with orthodontics
• Average production per day—$5000 to $7500

• Average production per year—$950,000 to $1,250,000
• Gross production = every dollar charged at full fees
• Net production = gross production minus amount adjusted off for welfare, managed care, professional courtesy, and so on

Collections
• Minimum goal: 97% of net production (collections for a period divided by net production for that same period)
• Over-the-counter goal: 30% to 50% of daily charges

- At $950,000 annual production, every 1% that collections is increased = $9500
- Gross collections = every dollar collected
- Net collections = gross collections minus amount adjusted off for returned checks due to nonsufficient funds (NSF), patient refunds, and so on

Accounts Receivable
- Goal: not more than 1 to 1½ months' gross production
- Current—50% to 60% of total
- 30 days—15% to 20% of total
- 60 days—10% to 15% of total
- 90 days—under 10% of total
- 120+ days—to outside collection

Appointments in a Mature Practice (Restorative, Hygiene, and Orthodontic)
- Average patients per day = 50 to 65
- Average patients per month = 900 to 1150
- Average new patients per month = 55 to 70. Count DO150 (Comprehensive Oral Examination) and DO145 (Oral Evaluation, for a patient younger than 3 years of age and counseling with primary care giver). Do not count DO140 (Emergency Examination) unless the patient returns for a comprehensive examination.
- Average recare patients per month = 425 to 500

Average Work Times per Week, Month, and Year
- Office hours—phone covered by staff 36 to 38 hours per week
- Dentist's hours with patients—32 to 36 hours per week
- Days per month—17 days
- Hours per month—130 to 138 hours
- Days per year—190 to 195 days

Treatment and Hygiene Minimum Goals
- Show rate: 85% or higher (number of patients who come as scheduled during a certain period divided by number of patients scheduled for that period, not counting last-minute fill-ins or emergencies)
- Goal: case acceptance/case presentations = 80% to 90% (treatment delivered divided by treatment proposed)
- Goal: treatment completion/treatment scheduled = 88% to 93% (treatment completed divided by treatment scheduled)
- Goal: 70% to 80% of active patients enrolled in recare system

Example of Checking Recare System Effectiveness
- 4000 active patients ÷ 6 months = 667 recares per month for 100% effective system
- Actually averaging 350 recares per month
- 350 ÷ 667 = 52% effective system
- Goal: 80% effective system
- 4000 × 0.80 = 3200 active patients
- 3200 ÷ 6 months = 553 recares per month for 80% effective system

Effects of 80% Effective Recare System on Practice Income

553 recares per month = 80% goal

$$\underline{-350 \text{ actual recares per month}}$$
183 more recares per month if goal is met

183 × $135 average recare fee (child and adult; with and without BWX) = $24,705 per month increased production

$24,705 per month production × 12 months = $296,460 per year increased production

ADVISORS

The new and long-term dentist should have a group of experienced advisors with whom he or she is comfortable. These may include an accountant, attorney, banker, insurance advisor, practice management consultant, computer expert, and investment counselor/retirement planner. If the young dentist joins a practice as an associate, many experts advise him or her to retain an attorney other than the one used by the current owner/dentist(s). Doing so should assure that each lawyer maintains loyalty, confidentiality and best advice for his or her client only. Other advisors to the young dentist may be those already used by the practice.

RETIREMENT PLANS

The time for a dentist to begin planning retirement is the day he or she begins practice. For those who choose to be employees or associates in state and federal institutions, dental schools, hospitals, and some private practices, retirement plans and other benefits may be part of the employment package. However, even then it is wise to evaluate whether the retirement package will allow the new dentist to maintain present or desired lifestyle when retirement comes. A financial advisor/retirement planner can help determine if the dentist might need to supplement offered retirement by, for example, regular savings, investments, or an IRA. If retirement funding is inadequate, one may not be financially able to retire when the time comes.

For those who enter private practice, it is imperative to begin a retirement plan as soon as possible because the only financial benefits you can expect in retirement will be those you have amassed plus Social Security.

A financial advisor can help the dentist choose between many plans with varying tax benefits, such as an IRA, a 401K, pension plan, pension and/or profit sharing plan, and so on. The earlier one begins, the greater the accumulation of wealth at retirement due in large measure to compound interest. Compound interest is the concept of adding accumulated interest to the principal.[8]

The rule of 72, a simple way of illustrating the growth potential of compound interest, is a useful tool for calculating an approximation of the time needed to retain an investment before it doubles in value. You can find an example of the rule online.[9]

REFERENCES

1. Lewis JL. What a practice administrator can do for you. Pediatr Dent 2002;24(1):50-52.
2. Blanchard K, Johnson S: The One Minute Manager. New York, 2003, Harper Collins, 2003.
3. Blair C. Coding with Confidence: The "Go To" Guide for CDT 2009/2010. Mt. Holly, NC, Dr. Charles Blair & Associates, Inc, 2006.
4. Centers for Medicare and Medicaid Services. General Information. Available at: http://www.cms.hhs.gov/home/medicaid.asp. Click on Medicaid Program – General Information.
5. U.S. Department of Health and Human Services. HIPAA Privacy Regulations. Available at: http://www.os.dhhs.gov/ocr/hipaa.
6. American Dental Association. Member Services. Available at: http://www.ada.org; by telephone 1-800-947-4746; or reference librarians at the ADA Library, 312-440-2653.
7. Dunlap JE, Wagner JB. Knowing the Numbers: Gain and Retain Control of Your Practice. Tulsa, Okla, PennWell. 1989.
8. Parker JF. Do the Right Thing. Upper Saddle River, NJ, Pearson Education Inc, 2008.
9. Rule of 72. The Rule of 72: Double Your Money, Reduce Your Debt. Available at: http://ruleof72.org/.

CHAPTER 30

The Child in Contexts of Family, Community, and Society

▲ Karen M. Yoder and Burton L. Edelstein

CHAPTER OUTLINE

The preceding chapters delineate the range of options and opportunities available to practitioners to promote and ensure individual children's oral health through clinical interventions. This chapter turns to the larger question of how all children's oral health can be promoted and ensured through family, community, and society-wide population-level interventions, including governmental interventions (Fig. 30-1).

This shift from thinking of individual children as "patients" to thinking about the oral health of all children is inherent to a shift from "clinical-think" to "population-think" or "public health-think." Just as clinical dentistry uses standard approaches to assessing the individual child's oral health status through complete examination, providing needed services through clinical care, and assuring oral health promotion through ongoing preventive care, so too does population-oriented public health dentistry conduct surveillance to assess population health, attend to the adequacy and availability of dental care delivery systems to provide care, and conduct oral health promotion activities that maximize the totality of a society's oral health.

Pediatric dentistry and public health dentistry share common origins, because society, most often through its governmental structures, has long attended to the needs and interests of vulnerable populations, whether those populations are made vulnerable by social or physical liabilities or dependencies that result from age or special needs. Pioneers in community dentistry who were motivated by concern for children's oral health include photography giant George Eastman who developed school-based dental programs at the turn of the twentieth century, Alfred Fones who founded the dental hygiene profession's first school in 1913, and American Academy of Pediatric Dentistry (AAPD) founders who created an organization with a mission that today affirms its commitment to "advocate policies, guidelines and programs that promote optimal oral health and oral health care for children."

Just as the range of potential interventions for clinicians is wide, so too is the range of potential interventions for dentists who commit their work to improving all children's oral health. At the family level, oral and general health behaviors and environmental conditions, including availability and use of fluoridated water, are key oral health determinants. At the community level, the availability of oral and general health educational programs, school-based and school-linked dental sealant programs, school nutrition and "junk-food" policies, and even school-based dental care programs exemplify oral health and dental care determinants that address groups of children rather than individual children. At the societal level, state and federal policies on licensure regulate the availability of dental workforce, policies on financing of public insurance programs like Medicaid and the State Children' Health Insurance Program (SCHIP) influence the availability of care, and fluoridation policies impact disease burden. Questions of who can provide what components of care with what financing under what conditions and to which children are the "mega" systems questions of public health and public policy that directly impact the practice of dentistry for children.

Conceptually, pediatric dentistry and public health dentistry share a unique niche within the spectrum of dental disciplines. They are the only two recognized specialties of dentistry that are essentially holistic in nature. Unlike other recognized areas of dental specialization that attend to a particular tissue, such as periodontics and endodontics, or a set of clinical techniques, such as orthodontics, prosthodontics, and oral and maxillofacial surgery, or to a diagnostic domain, such as oral pathology and oral radiology, both pediatric dentistry and public health are defined by those they serve—children in the case of pediatric dentistry and entire populations in the case of public health dentistry. For this reason, the required knowledge and skill sets needed to well manage the target population's oral health are broad.

Care of children requires a working knowledge of all core dental disciplines with a particular application to patients who are simultaneously growing and developing. Care of populations similarly requires a working knowledge of all core public health disciplines. Epidemiology is the study of disease prevalence, distribution, and correlates across groups of people and is analogous to diagnostic modalities in clinical dentistry. Biostatistics is the discipline of measurement whose theories and techniques are used for describing, analyzing, and interpreting health data. It is analogous to skills used to interpret clinical data. Environmental health is the branch of public health that deals with all aspects of the natural, built, and social environment as it impacts human health. It is analogous to the clinician's assessment of individual children's home conditions that impact oral health behaviors, care seeking, compliance, and health outcomes. Nutrition is the study of foods and nutrients and their effect on health and plays the same role in population health as it does in individual health. The public health discipline of health policy and management deals broadly with the conditions under which care is provided across populations by dealing with issues as wide ranging as care financing, health care workforce, safety-net health facilities, systems of care, resource allocations, and governmental and professional regulation. It is analogous to the wide range of issues that clinical dentists deal with in managing their practices. Just as in dentistry, children and families have their own unique holistic niche within public health in the discipline of maternal and child health (MCH)—the field that deals with children, including those with special health care needs, in the context of their parents, families, communities, and societies. As dentistry for children uses all of the clinical disciplines, so too does MCH use all of the disciplines of public health to focus attention on children's health. The essential need for both pediatric dentistry and MCH was well stated by child health leader Grace Abbott in the 1930s when she asserted that "children are not pocket editions of adults" but need to be attended to with special consideration of their vulnerabilities and served through an approach that is "not merely an adaptation of the program for adults."

With this perspective, it is clear that public health dentistry is of direct relevance to the daily practice of dental care for children. This chapter describes many of the opportunities, options, resources, and possibilities available to the dental professions to assess, improve, promote, and manage the oral health of children.

A quote attributed to the classical Roman poet Virgil, "as the twig is bent, the tree inclines" provides a paradigm for public health's concern for children and their oral health. After following a cohort of 980 people from birth to age 26, researchers noted that "adult oral health is predicted by not only childhood socioeconomic advantage or disadvantage, but also by oral health in childhood."[1] Research techniques in MCH, including "social determinants of health," "lifecourse studies," and "common determinants of health modeling," all suggest that conditions impacting children play out consequentially throughout life. This is particularly true of oral health in that having childhood caries, particularly early childhood caries, is the strongest indicator of lifelong caries risk. This is because the presence of early childhood caries signifies the presence of a well-established caries process that remains stable as the primary teeth exfoliate and are replaced by permanent teeth and as periodontal diseases cause recession that exposes root surfaces to caries as children age into adulthood and senescence. Similarly, genetic, environmental, behavioral, and even psychological factors strongly impact periodontal health, dental development, occlusion, the occurrence and effects of trauma, susceptibility to soft tissue lesions, and every other aspect of a child's oral health.

CHILDREN'S ORAL HEALTH AND DENTAL CARE

While dental care is an essential component of oral health attainment and maintenance, its contribution is relatively modest compared with other oral health determinants. One effort to model the relative importance of various determinants of general health suggests that only about 10% of health status can be explained by access to health care. The remaining 90% can be attributed primarily to health behaviors and secondarily to environmental and hereditary factors.[2] Such conceptual modeling has been applied to children's oral health status to clarify the relative importance of various oral health determinants. The model shown in Fig. 30-1 lists the "use of dental care" as only one of six "child-level" factors influencing oral health along with eight "family-level influences", eight "community-level influences," and the ongoing impacts of time and environment on each level of influence.[3] An analogous approach to explaining oral health disparities in children considers four levels of influence: (1) "macro" factors as wide ranging as the natural environment and dental care systems that are available to children; (2) "community" factors that include the social/cultural environment and availability of dental services; (3) "interpersonal" factors involving social stressors, integration, and support; (4) "individual" factors of biology, health behaviors, care-seeking behaviors, and psychological considerations.[4]

Such models help clinicians understand the range of factors that they can, and cannot, manage or influence in seeking to help each child and each child's family obtain and maintain excellent oral health. The technical content of clinical care is entirely within the scope of clinical dental practitioner. However, key approaches to children's dental care, including anticipatory guidance, primary prevention through modification of health behaviors, disease suppression through individually tailored disease management plans, and encouraging compliance with professional recommendations, all move the clinician away from the biologic sciences and their technical

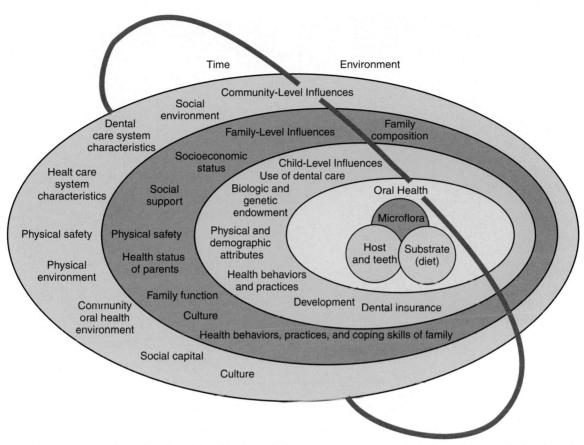

Figure 30-1 The promotion of children's oral health through family, community, and society wide population-level interventions, including governmental interventions. (Reproduced with permission from *Pediatrics,* vol. 120, pages 510-520, 2007 by the AAP.)

correlates and into the realms of social and behavioral sciences and their roles in health education and health promotion. These "soft" disciplines have equal relevance for the oral health of individuals and populations. The dentist who seeks to improve children's oral health must therefore rely equally on clinical and public health interventions that are based on both "hard" and "soft" science.

DISEASE BURDEN

The term *disease burden* implies the volume and distribution of disease within a population as well as its consequences in terms of morbidity and mortality. Dental caries remain highly prevalent worldwide (Fig. 30-2). In the United States and other countries, it is the most prevalent childhood chronic illness. It is disproportionately a disease of poverty, minority, and social disadvantage (Fig. 30-3). In the United States, for example, information prepared for the U.S. Surgeon General's Workshop on Children and Oral Health in 2002 reported profound disparities in both oral health status and access to dental care by age, income, race, and parental education[5] (Table 30-1). That report predicted that epidemiologic and demographic trends would drive childhood caries experience higher and would lead to additional stress on the dental delivery system that attends to poor and low-income children. Since that time, disease burden and

inequities in its distribution have increased among young children. More U.S. children were born in 2007 than at the peak of the "baby boom" and further growth is anticipated to be disproportionate among minority, poor, and single-parent families whose children also experience higher caries rates and lower treatment rates. While caries experience among older children has declined, caries experience among 2- to 5-year-olds is at a record level of 28%, suggesting additional future stress on dental care capacity. Possible explanations for increasing disease burden among young children include nonclinical factors, among which are demographic changes, lesser availability of fluoride exposure because of increased use of nonfluoridated bottled water, changes in parenting styles and practices, and temporal changes in dietary practices. Dental service rates continue to be highest for children from higher income families while the publicly funded dental programs for poor and low-income children (Medicaid and the State Child Health Insurance Program), despite improvements, continue to reach only about a third of enrolled low- and modest-income children with dental services.

Not only is childhood caries the most common chronic disease of U.S. children,[6] but it is consequential at many levels—from mild dysfunction to death. A morbidity–mortality pyramid constructed for early childhood caries (ECC) and its consequences would include a wide base

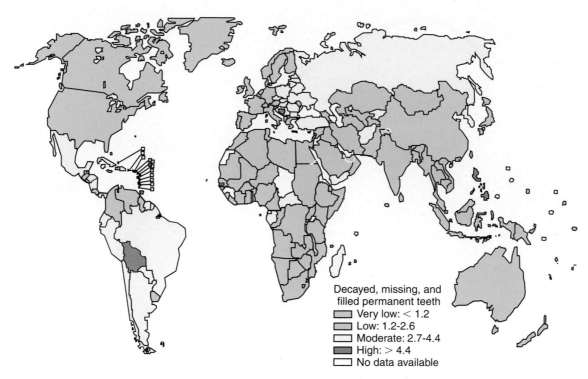

Decayed, missing, and
filled permanent teeth

Very low: < 1.2
Low: 1.2-2.6
Moderate: 2.7-4.4
High: > 4.4
No data available

The designations employed and the presentation of material on this map do not imply
the expression of any opinion whatsoever on the part of the World Health Organization
concerning the legal status of any country, territory, city or area or of its authorities, or
concerning the delimitation of its frontiers or boundaries. Dashed lines represent
approximate border lines for which there may not yet be full agreement.

Figure 30-2 World Health Organization map of childhood dental caries. (Petersen PE. The World Oral Health Report 2003, Geneva, Switzerland: World Health Organization; 2003. Available at http://www.who.int/oral_health/media/en/orh_report03_en.pdf. Accessed Feb 10, 2009.)

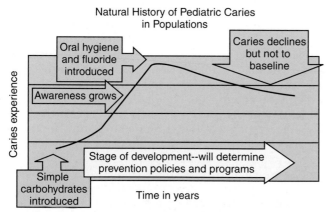

Natural History of Pediatric Caries
in Populations

Oral hygiene
and fluoride
introduced

Caries declines
but not to
baseline

Awareness grows

Caries experience

Stage of development--will determine
prevention policies and programs

Simple
carbohydrates
introduced

Time in years

Figure 30-3 Natural history of pediatric caries in populations. (Edelstein BL. Pediatric caries worldwide: Implications for oral hygiene products, *Compendium* 26[5]:Suppl 1, 2005.)

representing high prevalence of dysfunctions related to intermittent pain and infection. These include difficulties that children encounter in daily functions of eating, sleeping, and attending to learning. With greater distraction from more intense dental pain, additional disruptions, including lost school time and increases in family stress, occur along with family-level disruptions in lost work as parents seek care for their affected child. In the

aggregate, these family-level disruptions result in lost productivity and performance and take a societal toll that is of concern to public policy makers. More severe impairment from ECC further disrupts normal childhood functions while natural sequelae of cavities, including localized and generalized infections, constitute acute illness requiring intensive pharmacologic and surgical management. Such infections occasionally extend to adjacent and distant vital structures, leading to critical impairment, hospitalization, and occasional death. The death of a 12-year-old residing near Washington, DC, from a brain abscess secondary to an infected first permanent molar led to extensive Congressional investigations of the oral health and dental care of socially disadvantaged children and resulted in greater policy-maker attention to public health strategies for improving children's oral health. These included attention to insurance coverage for dental services, workforce competency and capacity, safety-net adequacy, and promotion of dental prevention through community water fluoridation, school-based sealant programs, and public information efforts. These federal efforts are mirrored in a host of state oral health planning initiatives that are evidenced in oral health plans developed by most states. These plans, like all governmental efforts, focus most tightly on children and other vulnerable populations. Common public health interventions called for by these plans include all of the

TABLE 30-1

Prevalence of Dental Caries in Primary Teeth Among Youths 2 to 11 Years of Age by Selected Characteristics*

Characteristic	1988-1994		1999-2004		Difference
	Percent	Standard error	Percent	Standard error	
Age					
2 to 5 years	24.23	1.32	27.90	1.29	3.67[†]
6 to 11 years	49.90	1.79	51.17	1.96	1.27
Sex					
Male	39.50	1.73	44.43	1.90	4.92
Female	40.24	1.44	39.80	1.79	-0.44
Race and ethnicity					
White, non-Hispanic	35.84	1.46	38.56	1.90	2.72
Black, non-Hispanic	40.99	1.65	43.34	1.83	2.35
Mexican American	53.61	2.15	55.40	1.75	1.78
Poverty status					
Less than 100% FPL	51.18	2.02	54.33	2.47	3.15
100% to 199% FPL	44.50	1.94	48.75	2.43	4.24
Greater than 200% FPL	31.10	1.74	32.30	1.62	1.20
Total	39.97	1.16	42.17	1.44	2.20

*Unites States, National Health and Nutrition Examination Survey, 1988-1994, 1999-2004.
[†] $P < .05$
FPT, federal poverty threshold or level.
From Dye BA ,et al. Trends in oral health status: United States, 1988-1994 and 1999-2004. National Center for Health Statistics, *Vital Health Stat* 11(248), 2007.

aforementioned Congressional interests as well as calls for greater surveillance, engagement of non–dental health professionals in promoting children's oral health, promoting early care, building partnerships and coalitions with others concerned with child health and welfare, developing case management and disease management systems in communities, and reducing tobacco initiation and prevalence. Many of these proposed public-level interventions mirror AAPD policies that call for engagement of medical practitioners in oral health promotion, early establishment of dental care in a "dental home," and maximal use of anticipatory guidance based on risk assessment. Similarly, the federal Maternal and Child Health Bureau, the Centers for Disease Control and Prevention, the National Institutes of Health, Head Start, the Food and Nutrition Service, the Department of Defense, and other federal agencies have long promoted population-level interventions that hold promise to improve children's oral health.

DENTAL CARE DELIVERY IN DEVELOPING COUNTRIES

Population-level interventions in many developing countries lack adequate resources; consequently, throughout the world, oral health problems continue to adversely affect health and quality of life. In many developing countries, access to oral health services is extremely limited and carious teeth are typically left untreated or extracted because of pain. In many locations, the ratio is often one dentist to tens of thousands of residents. For these circumstances, the World Health Organization (WHO) commissioned a report on the establishment of priorities in oral health care for developing countries, calling for treatment that is affordable for governments and focuses on community-oriented promotion of oral health.[7] There is no single model that is suitable for universal application; however, the basic components of the Basic Package for Oral Care (BPOC) include (1) Oral Urgent Treatment (OUT), (2) Affordable Fluoride Toothpaste (AFT), and (3) Atraumatic Restorative Treatment (ART). OUT can be provided by appropriately trained personnel in primary care facilities, such as rural medical aides and primary care nurses. Their responsibilities include providing relief of oral pain, first aid for oral infections and dentoalveolar trauma, and referral of complicated cases. The second component, making affordable fluoride toothpaste available, attempts to overcome the infrastructure, technology, and resources needed to provide optimal fluoridation of water, especially in highly rural populations that lack central water supplies. In many developing countries, there have been substantial reductions in dental caries over the past few decades, which have been attributed to the widespread use of fluoride dentifrice. In some countries, toothpaste is classified as a cosmetic product and subject to higher taxation; therefore, this recommendation is encouraging governmental support of this preventive measure through local manufacturing and elimination of taxes. The third component, ART, is an innovative approach for the management of dental caries that involves no dental drill, running water, or electricity, and usually no anesthetic. Dentinal lesions are cleaned using hand instruments and are filled with an adhesive fluoride-releasing restorative material. Appropriately trained dental auxiliaries can provide ART, making restorative treatment more affordable and accessible in medical clinic, community, and school settings. The average annual failure rate is about 4% to 5% for the first 3 years and is comparable to amalgam restorations using conventional methods.

THE STRUCTURE OF DENTAL PUBLIC HEALTH IN THE UNITED STATES AND ITS ROLE IN CHILDREN'S ORAL HEALTH

The public health infrastructure consists of the agencies, institutions, and people who are charged with assessment of the status of conditions related to oral health, policy development to assure science-based prioritization of resources, and the assurance of adequate systems for the provision of essential public health services. A wide range of entities, both governmental and nongovernmental, are included in the U.S. public health system: more than 3000 local health departments and 59 state and territorial health departments, as well as tribal health departments, laboratories, federal departments and agencies, hospitals, other health care providers, and volunteer organizations. There are approximately 450,000 employed public health workers distributed, almost evenly, at the local, state, and national levels. Funding for public health comes from local, state, and federal government, grants from foundations, reimbursement from insurance companies, and a variety of patient and regulatory fees.[8]

Goals of the federal Health Resources and Services Administration (HRSA), parent agency of the Maternal and Child Health Bureau , typify public health interventions.

HRSA's oral health goals are (1) to improve the health infrastructure and systems of care for all, especially the underserved, vulnerable, and special needs populations, to ensure access to comprehensive, quality oral health services, (2) to improve oral health status and outcomes (and their measurement) in seeking to eliminate health disparities, (3) to improve the quality of oral health services (preventive and curative) for all, especially underserved, vulnerable, and special needs populations, and (4) to promote oral health through building public-private partnerships, including strengthening the dental public health infrastructure.[9] HRSA accomplishes these tasks by establishing oral health programs at health centers, providing grants for access programs that sometimes include dental education and community-based partnerships,

and providing incentives to increase workforce in underserved areas.

The foundation for current public health roles was delineated by the Institute of Medicine in 1988 in *The Future of Public Health*.[10] This landmark publication identified public health's core functions as assessment, policy development, and assurance. Examples of "proven and promising" practices in oral health for each of the three public health core functions can be accessed at the website of the Association of State and Territorial Dental Directors (ASTDD).[11] Assessment examples include state-based oral health assessment systems. Policy development includes models of state oral health coalitions and collaborative partnerships. Assurance programs include workforce development and school-based and school-linked service delivery models. A second report of the Institute of Medicine, *The Future of Public Health in the 21st Century*, identified the six main responsibilities of the federal government in public health as policy-making, financing, public health protection, collecting and disseminating information about U.S. health and health care delivery systems, capacity building for population health, and direct management of services.[12] Each of these roles can be applied to programs and services that help maintain and improve the oral health of children. Dental public health is defined by the specialty's certification body, American Board of Dental Public Health, as "The science and art of preventing and controlling dental diseases and promoting dental health through organized community efforts. It is that form of dental practice that serves the community as the patient rather than the individual. It is concerned with the dental education of the public, with applied dental research, and with the administration of group dental care programs as well as with the prevention and control of dental disease on a community basis." Dental public health is one of nine specialties recognized by the American Dental Association. Board certification requires specific competencies that encompass the skills that enable dental public health professionals to develop and administer programs to ensure the oral health of children and adults[13] (Box 30-1).

Community dentistry and dental public health personnel and programs are guided by science-based health objectives that were first developed in 1979, the Healthy People National Health Objectives. At 10-year intervals, the U.S. Department of Health and Human Services builds on new scientific information, current data, and innovations to update and revise the objectives.[14] The two overarching goals of Healthy People objectives are to (1) increase quality and years of healthy life, and (2) eliminate health disparities. One of the Healthy People objectives focus areas is oral health. Several objectives point to goals to be achieved for children (Box 30-2).

COMMUNITY ORAL HEALTH PROGRAMS WITH IMPACT ON CHILDREN'S ORAL HEALTH

The Healthy People Oral Health Objectives have helped shape innovative programs aimed at improving access to care and overall oral health status of children. Following

Box 30-1

Board Certification Competencies

Dental public health professionals must be competent in these skills:

- Plan oral health programs for populations
- Select interventions and strategies for the prevention and control of oral diseases and promotion of oral health
- Implement, manage, and develop resources for oral health programs for populations
- Incorporate ethical standards in oral health programs and activities
- Evaluate and monitor dental care delivery systems
- Design and understand the use of surveillance systems to monitor oral health
- Advocate for, implement, and evaluate public health policy legislation and regulations to protect and promote the public's oral health
- Critique and synthesize scientific literature
- Design and conduct population-based studies to answer oral and public health questions

Source: American Dental Association, Commission on Dental Accreditation and Licensure. Accreditation Standards for Advanced Specialty Education Programs in Dental Public Health. http://www.ada.org/prof/ed/accred/standards/dph.pdf. Accessed October 15, 2008.

Box 30-2

Healthy People 2010 Oral Health Goals Specifically Affecting Children

21-1 Reduce the proportion of children and adolescents who have dental caries experience in their primary or permanent teeth (Target: 11%)

21-2 Reduce the proportion of children, adolescents, and adults with untreated dental decay (Target: varies by age groups)

21-8 Increase the proportion of children who have received dental sealants on their molar teeth (Target for children 8 years and adolescents 14 years: 50%)

21-9 Increase the proportion of the U.S. population served by community water systems with optimally fluoridated water (Target: 75%)

21-10 Increase the proportion of children and adults who use the oral health care system each year (Target: 56%)

21-12 Increase the proportion of low-income children and adolescents who received any preventive dental service during the past year (Target: 57%)

21-13 (Developmental) Increase the proportion of school-based health centers with an oral health component

21-15 Increase the number of states and the District of Columbia that have a system for recording and referring infant and children with cleft lips, cleft palates, and other craniofacial anomalies to craniofacial anomaly rehabilitative teams

Source: Healthy People 2010, vol. 2, second edition, Part B, pages 11-34. Available at: http://www.healthypeople.gov/document/HTML/Volume 2/21Oral.htm. Accessed October 15, 2008

are some of the most effective population-level interventions and programs that affect children's oral health.

COMMUNITY WATER FLUORIDATION

Although many water supplies contain some naturally occurring fluoride, adjusting the fluoride concentration to the optimal level for caries prevention is a highly effective method of preventing and controlling the effects of the dental caries process. The first adjustment of water fluoride levels in the United States occurred in Grand Rapids, Michigan, in 1945. Twenty-five states and the District of Columbia have met or exceeded the national objective of 75% of the U.S. population served by community water systems with optimally fluoridated water.[15] In 2000, 65% (MMWR July 11, 2008), and in 2008 nearly 70% of U.S. residents using water from a communal water system had access to fluoridated water.[16] Achieving higher levels of fluoridation are expected to require (1) recognition by policy makers and the public that dental caries remains an important public health problem and that fluoridation is an equitable and cost-effective method of addressing the problem, even in smaller populations where the per-capita cost of fluoridation is higher; (2) continuing science-based education of the public about the established safety of fluoridation; (3) the political will to adopt new fluoridation systems in communities that are not currently served. To overcome the challenges facing fluoridation, public health professionals at the national, state, and local levels will need to enhance their promotion of fluoridation and commit the necessary resources for equipment, personnel, and training.[16]

SCHOOL-BASED AND SCHOOL-LINKED DENTAL SEALANT PROGRAMS

Population interventions that deliver pit and fissure sealants for school children are especially important because dental caries in school children occurs predominantly in the pits and fissures of molars.[17] School-based services are delivered onsite at schools using portable equipment or a self-contained mobile dental clinic. School-linked sealant programs can be coordinated with school personnel and delivered at a dental clinic site in proximity of the school. Fig. 30-4 reflects the use of a mobile dental clinic serving children in a rural area of Indiana. In this setting the mobile clinic also enabled use of dental equipment powered by a generator in an Amish community that does not

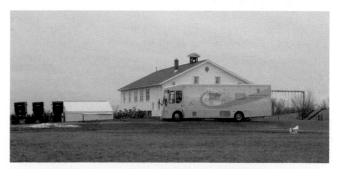

Figure 30-4 A mobile dental clinic provides dental services for children in a rural school without electricity.

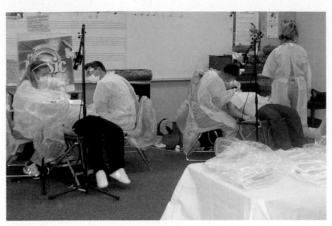

Figure 30-5 Portable dental equipment is used for a sealant program in an elementary school.

supply electricity. Fig. 30-5 shows a typical setup using portable dental equipment for a sealant program inside a school or community health center site. These programs, particularly when they target schools with high concentrations of children from poor and low-income families, are particularly effective in extending this key preventive modality to children who are least able to access routine dental care.[18] Sealants are considered such an essential component of care at the interface between public health and clinical dentistry that their prevalence is a key national MCH indicator that is annually tracked in every state.

INFANT ORAL HEALTH EARLY CHILDHOOD CARIES PREVENTION PROGRAMS

ECC is defined by the AAPD as the presence of one or more decayed, missing, or filled tooth surfaces in any primary tooth in a child 71 months or age or younger. Young children typically see a pediatrician or family physician many times before they have their first dental appointment. Although dental professional associations recommend that children should have their first dental appointment by age 1 year, that goal is far from being met. Neither parents nor dentists have universally adopted this recommendation; therefore interventions by medical personnel can enable a level of professional oral health oversight. Medicaid programs in an increasing number of states reimburse primary pediatric medical care providers, including pediatricians, family physicians, and nurse practitioners, for oral health counseling, screening, and fluoride varnish application. Experience has confirmed that oral health anticipatory guidance and fluoride varnish can be successfully adopted into medical practices with appropriate training, staff commitment, and resources for professional dental care referrals.[19]

HEAD START PROGRAMS

Although the focus of Head Start encompasses all aspects of enrollees' health, federal "Performance Standards" include requirements that directly affect the oral health of millions of children. Head Start is a federally funded, comprehensive child development program that serves preschool-aged children and families with low income. Head Start began in 1965 as an 8-week summer program for children from impoverished families as a part of President Lyndon B. Johnson's War on Poverty. It grew to a year-round program with more than 1 million children enrolled in Head Start and Early Head Start during the 2006-07 school year. The 18,145 grantee sites and 49,038 classrooms are found in most communities and cities in the United States. Head Start directors, teachers, and health coordinators are responsible for ensuring daily supervised classroom-based tooth brushing with fluoride dentifrice and comprehensive dental services for the children who are enrolled. Figure 30-6 demonstrates active teaching and learning taking place in a Head Start classroom where dental students are attempting to inspire very young children to form good oral health habits. Federal Performance Standards require, within 90 day of enrollment, that each child receive a dental examination that fulfills that State's Medicaid Early and Periodic Screening, Diagnosis and Treatment (EPSDT) standards. Comprehensive follow-up services to address unmet oral health needs must be completed by the parents or by the Head Start grantee organization within the academic year.[20] The health policy council, which is a required entity for each Head Start grantee, provides an excellent opportunity for dental health professionals to become members of Head Start leadership groups and to be effective advocates for promoting oral health for enrolled children and their families. The impact of assuring oral health services for a significant number of children from low-income families nationwide qualifies Head Start as an important stakeholder in the goal of optimal oral health for children.

PUBLIC FINANCING OF ACCESS TO DENTAL CARE

Public health also concerns itself with children's access to dental care through two primary approaches that are both longstanding. The first is the provision of

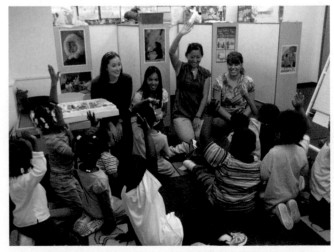

Figure 30-6 Dental students engage children in an oral health lesson at a Head Start Program.

insurance coverage through Medicaid and SCHIP for children who do not have access to commercial coverage. This strategy is intended to increase the odds that a child will gain access to private dental care. The second approach is the direct provision of dental services in a variety of "safety net" settings that include governmentally subsidized care in community health centers, dental training programs, hospital dental clinics, and school-based dental facilities.

CONCLUSIONS

Public health and pediatric dentistry share common concerns, goals, and interventions. Both recognize that children's oral health must be promoted and assured through policies and programs that impact children within the contexts of their families, communities, and society. Effective collaborations between clinicians who care for individual children and public health authorities who care for populations of children are essential if oral disease burden among children is to be reduced and children's health and welfare are to be assured. A Workshop on Children and Oral Health sponsored by the U.S. Surgeon General developed a set of recommendations for improving children's oral health. Distilled from expert perspectives offered by many different disciplines, they are:

1. Start early in children's lives and involve all who come in contact with young children and their families.
2. Assure the needed competencies of all who work to improve children's oral health.
3. Be accountable to children's oral health outcomes and to resources committed to oral health programs in order to ensure that efforts are most effective and worthwhile.
4. Take public action through health education, public policy formulation, removal of barriers to oral health and dental care, and enhancement of the social environment to promote oral health.
5. Maximize the utility of science—both biologic and behavioral science—in order to ensure efficiency and effectiveness.
6. Fix public programs when they fail to meet their objectives by ensuring sufficient resources, management, and accountability.
7. Grow an adequate workforce of health professionals, child care workers, nutritionists, behaviorists, and others who can promote children's oral health and wellbeing.
8. Empower families and enhance their capabilities and opportunities to ensure their children's oral health.

These eight approaches are synergistic and cross clinical and public health domains. Effective dentistry for children requires that all concerned with children's oral health subscribe to the full array of these recommendations. The resulting improvement in children's oral health will secure a future in which oral health disparities are eradicated, oral health is assured, and oral function is guaranteed. No longer, will it be observed that too many children suffer too much from preventable dental and oral conditions.

REFERENCES

1. Thomson WM, et al. Socioeconomic inequalities in oral health in childhood and adulthood in a birth cohort, *Commun Dent Oral Epidemiol* 32:345-53, 2004.
2. McGinnis JM, et al. The case for more active policy attention to health promotion, *Health Aff* 21(2):78, 2002.
3. Fisher-Owens SA, et al. Influences on children's oral health: a conceptual model, *Pediatrics* 120;e510-e520, 2007.
4. Patrick DL, et al. Reducing oral health disparities: a focus on social and cultural determinants, *BMC Oral Health* 6(Suppl 1):4-21, 2006.
5. Edelstein BL. Disparities in oral health and access to care: findings of national surveys, *Ambulat Pediatr* 2(Suppl): 141-147, 2002.
6. Oral Health in America. Report of the U.S. Surgeon General, 2002. Available at: http://www.nider.nih.gov.
7. Frencken JI, et al. Basic Package of Oral Care. WHO Collaborating Centre for Oral Health Care Planning and Future Scenarios, College of Dental Science University of Nijmegen, The Netherlands. Available at: http://www.globaloralhealth-nijmegen.nl.
8. Harvey H. An Overview of the U.S. Public Health System in the Context of Bioterrorism. Report for Congress. Congressional Research Service, The Library of Congress. January 17, 2003. Washington, DC.
9. Duke EM. Remarks to the Oral Health Network of Missouri and the Missouri Primary Care Association, April 2, 2004 Lake Ozark, Missouri. Available at: http://newsroom.hrsa.gov. Accessed on February 10, 2009.
10. Institute of Medicine. The Future of Public Health. Washington DC, 1988, National Academy Press.
11. Association of State and Territorial Dental Directors. Proven and promising practices. Available at: http://www.astdd.org/index.php?template=bpfulllisting.php.
12. Institute of Medicine (IOM). The Future of Public Health in the 21st Century. The National Academy of Science, 2002.
13. American Dental Association, Commission on Dental Accreditation and Licensure. Definitions of Recognized Dental Specialties. Available at: http://www.ada.org/prof/ed/accred/standards/dph.pdf.
14. Healthy People National Health Objectives. Available at: http://www.healthypeoplegov/hp2020.
15. Centers for Disease Control and Prevention. Available at: http://www.cdc.gov/fluoridation/statistics/cwf_status.htm.
16. Populations receiving optimally fluoridated public drinking water—United States, 1992-2006. July 11, 2008. *MMWR Morb Mortal Wkly Rep* 57(27);737-741, 2008.
17. Kaste LM, et al. Coronal caries in the primary permanent dentition of children and adolescents 1-17 years of age: Unites States, 1988-1991, *J Dent Res* 75(Spec No):631-641, 1996.
18. Siegal MD, et al. Impact of targeted, school-based dental sealant programs in reducing racial and economic disparities in sealant prevalence among schoolchildren—Ohio, 1998-99. August 31, 2001, *MMWR Morb Mortal Wkly Rep* 50(34);736-738, 2001.
19. Lewis C, et al. Fluoride varnish use in primary care: What do providers think? Pediatrics 2005;115(1): e69-e76. Available at: http://pediatrics.aappublications.org/cgi/content/full/115/1/e69.
20. National Head Start Association. Available at: http://www.nhsa.org.

CHAPTER 31

Oral Surgery for the Pediatric Patient

▲ Elie M. Ferneini, Charles E. Hutton, and Jeffrey D. Bennett

CHAPTER OUTLINE

O ffice-based pediatric oral surgical procedures include dentoalveolar surgery (primarily consisting of exodontia), intraoral soft tissue procedures (e.g., frenectomy), medical and surgical management of odontogenic infections, and intraoral surgical procedures involving the alveolar ridge (e.g., enucleation of an odontoma). The basic principles employed in the management of these surgical conditions are essentially identical to those used by the pediatric dentist in management of the various other dental diagnoses encountered.

The initial step in patient management is to develop a diagnosis. The diagnosis is developed through a process involving taking a history, physical examination, and imaging. Once the decision to do surgery is made, the practitioner should visualize the various steps and their sequence as well as the potential complications and their management before administering local anesthetic.

For the pediatric patient there must be consideration to the patient's ability to cooperate. Depending on the patient's age, systemic health, and planned surgery, the practitioner may consider using nitrous oxide inhalational sedation, oral sedation, intramuscular sedation, intravenous sedation, or a combination of these modalities. Regardless of the route of agent administration or the selection of pharmacologic agent, the primary consideration in sedating a pediatric patient is the depth of sedation achieved. Oral sedation and nitrous oxide are the agents most commonly used in the pediatric dental office. Nitrous oxide is advantageous in that it can be titrated achieving both rapid onset and recovery from the effect of the nitrous oxide. The practitioner must be aware that nitrous oxide when combined with an oral agent (e.g., benzodiazepine or chloral hydrate) can potentiate the effect of the oral agent, producing a more profound depth of sedation and at times producing a depth of sedation equal to general anesthesia.[1, 2]

General principles that apply to both the adult and pediatric patient include profound anesthesia, aseptic technique, visibility, and surgical site stability. Achieving profound anesthesia is dependent on knowledge of the anatomy of the second and third division of the trigeminal nerve. This is discussed in Chapter 13.

Most office-based oral surgical procedures do not dictate adherence to sterile technique, but require a clean technique. The clean technique requires that the dentist scrubs his or her hands with an antiseptic soap. The hands may be dried off using a nonsterile disposable towel. The hands are then gloved. The dentist does not need to wear a sterile gown but should wear a gown covering his or her arms. A mask and eye protection are also used by the dentist. The gown, mask and eye protection are as much for the protection of the dentist as they are for the protection of the patient. The perioral region and oral cavity do not need to be decontaminated for a clean technique. However, only sterile water or sterile saline should be used for irrigating a surgical wound. Surgical drills that are self-irrigating can accommodate the use of sterile irrigating solutions. Last, the dentist may opt to drape the patient and place protective eyewear on the patient. Draping and eyewear maintain sterility in the sterile surgical field, as well as protect the patient from soiling of clothes or from having debris or a suture injure the eye. The clean technique strives to achieve the basic premise of a sterile technique, which is to prevent any organism from the surgical staff, other patient, instrumentation, or equipment from contaminating the patient.

Adequate visibility is required for all dental procedures. For oral surgical procedures this entails adequate access, adequate light, and a good suction to create a debris-free surgical field. Adequate access requires appropriate mouth opening. Opening the patient's mouth and maintaining its opening can be facilitated with a bite block (Fig. 31-1) or a Molt mouth prop. A small bite block may be used and the degree of mouth opening varied by its placement in the mouth. For maximal mouth opening

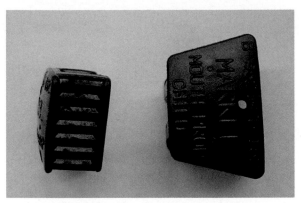

Figure 31-1 Two views of a bite block.

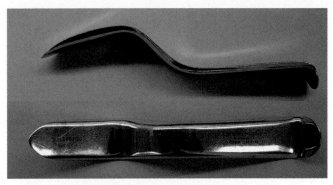

Figure 31-3 Minnesota retractor.

the bite block is placed more posteriorly. A piece of floss may be attached to the bite block. The knot securing the floss to the bite block must be secure so that it does not loosen. If the bite block is displaced into the pharynx, the floss attached to the bite block extends out of the mouth, assisting in retrieval of the bite block. The Molt mouth prop has a ratchet-type action and can be used to assist in opening the patient's mouth. This can be beneficial when managing the uncooperative patient. Excessive force could be applied with the Molt mouth prop causing iatrogenic injury, such as displacement of teeth or injury to the temporomandibular joint. In addition to keeping the mouth open for the surgical procedure, the bite block stabilizes the mandible. When extracting a mandibular tooth, using the bite block minimizes mandibular movement and the resultant transmission of excessive forces to the temporomandibular joint.

Adequate access also requires appropriate retraction. Commonly used retractors in oral surgery include the Austin retractor (Fig. 31-2), the Minnesota retractor (Fig. 31-3), and the Weider retractor (Fig. 31-4). The Austin and Minnesota retractors are usually used to retract the cheek and surgical flaps. Tongue retraction is usually performed using a Weider retractor. The Weider retractor is a

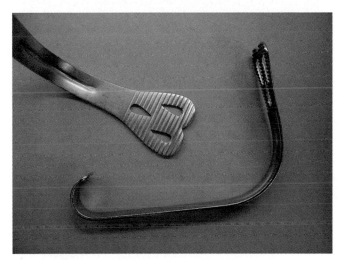

Figure 31-4 Weider "sweetheart" retractor.

heart-shaped retractor with a serrated edge. Retraction of the tongue with the Weider retractor is best achieved by placing the lateral aspect of the retractor firmly against the alveolus. A gauze or sponge packing may be placed just medial to the retractor. This packing provides a barrier between the surgical site and the pharynx preventing the tooth, surgical debris, or irrigating solution from potentially being swallowed, aspirated or irritating the pharynx. If the tongue is retracted medially, the pharyngeal barrier is displaced medially, opening up a passage between the mouth and the pharynx and there is the potential to stimulate the gag reflex. Care must also be taken not to position the retractor too far posteriorly into the pharynx, which also stimulates the gag reflex. Retraction may be performed either by the dentist using his or her nondominant hand or by the assistant.

Adequate visibility depends on establishing a debris-free surgical field. This requires a good surgical assistant using high-speed surgical suction. The surgical tray should have a Fraser suction tip (Fig. 31-5), which are available in various sizes. The Fraser tip has an opening in the handle that allows regulation of the suction power. The operator of the suction places his or her thumb over the hole in the handle when the suction is placed on bone and maximal suction power is desired. When less suction power is desired (e.g., when

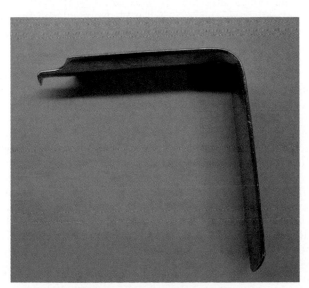

Figure 31-2 Austin retractor.

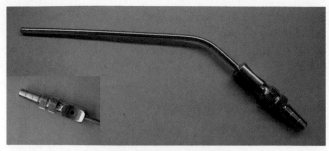

Figure 31-5 Fraser suction tip.

suctioning soft tissue), the operator leaves the opening in the handle open, which decreases the suction power. The practitioner should also have a Yankauer or tonsillar suction available (Fig. 31-6). This suction removes significant quantities of debris and with its blunt tip can be passed blindly down the throat.

SIMPLE EXODONTIA

Indications for extractions for children are much the same as for the adult patients: nonrestorable caries, apical disease, fractures of crowns or roots, prolonged retention of primary teeth because of improper root resorption or ankylosis, impacted teeth, and supernumerary teeth. The dentist must have an understanding of the growth and development of the pediatric patient in order to assess and diagnose the situations that will be encountered in the pediatric patient. For example, the dentist should have knowledge of the eruption pattern of the primary and permanent teeth. Delayed eruption, especially when asymmetric, is frequently an indication of an abnormality.

Radiographic surveys of teeth to be extracted are of prime importance. The dentist should observe the size and contour of the primary roots, the amount and type of resorption, the relation of the roots to the succedaneous teeth, and the extent of disease (Fig. 31-7).

Simple exodontia in the pediatric patient requires minimal modification from that used in the adult. Concepts that may dictate slight modification include the following: (1) the dentist must be cognizant of the proximity of the deciduous tooth to the succedaneous tooth; (2) the roots on primary teeth with nonresorbed roots will be long, slender and potentially divergent.

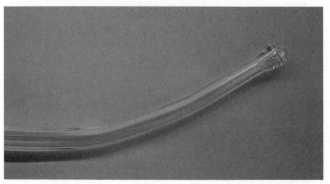

Figure 31-6 Yankauer or tonsillar suction.

The patient must be positioned appropriately for the surgical procedure. For the extraction of a maxillary tooth, the patient is positioned in the dental chair such that the maxillary occlusal plane is at an angle between 60 and 90 degrees to the floor. For the extraction of a mandibular tooth, the patient is positioned in the dental chair such that the mandibular occlusal plane is parallel to the floor. The height of the chair should be such that the patient's mouth is at or slightly below the level of the dentist's elbow level. The surgeon's elbow of their dominant arm should be against their body. When performing surgery in the dental office in a dental chair (compared with the operating room on an operating room bed), the patient is usually semisupine rather than completely supine. Patients are generally more reclined for extractions of maxillary teeth. There is an advantage for the sedated patient to be positioned more upright and not fully supine. The pediatric patient's ribs are angled more horizontally relative to the vertebral column and the accessory muscles are less developed, resulting in less effective thoracic expansion and a greater dependence on diaphragmatic breathing. Diaphragmatic breathing is compromised when the patient is supine; thus maintaining a more upright position is respiratorily favorable, especially in the sedated patient.

The basic details are eloquently illustrated in more detail in the fifth edition of *Contemporary Oral and Maxillofacial Surgery*.[3] The first step in extracting a tooth is to separate the soft tissue attachment from the cervical aspect of the tooth. A #9 Molt elevator (Fig. 31-8) is most commonly used. The Molt elevator is a dual-ended instrument; one end is sharply pointed and is used to initiate the separation of the soft tissue attachment from the tooth. The sharp pointed end of this instrument is placed interproximally on the mesial aspect of the papillae. The concave aspect of the instrument faces the tooth. Using a twisting motion, the dentist elevates the papillae. The tip of the elevator is then slid through the sulcus along the crest of the alveolar bone completely separating the buccal soft tissue attachment from the tooth. The same can be done on the lingual or palatal aspect of the tooth. If a flap is reflected, the broad, rounded end of the instrument may be used in a pushing (concave aspect of instrument against bone) or a pulling motion (instrument more perpendicular to bone with the concave aspect of the instrument facing the direction of movement) to reflect a full-thickness mucoperiosteal flap.

Extracting a tooth is an exercise in administering a controlled force in a slow and deliberate fashion to expand the alveolus and disrupt the periodontal ligaments, such that the tooth can be atraumatically removed from the jaw. The second step in extracting a tooth is to use a dental elevator to luxate the tooth. A straight elevator (Fig. 31-9) is most commonly used. The straight elevator has a concave blade that is placed toward the tooth being luxated. The blades are available in various sizes. The edge of the blades may be serrated to better grasp the tooth. The separation and reflection of the dental papillae facilitates placement of the elevator such that it rests on the alveolus. The elevator is initially inserted perpendicular to the tooth in the axial plane, and either parallel

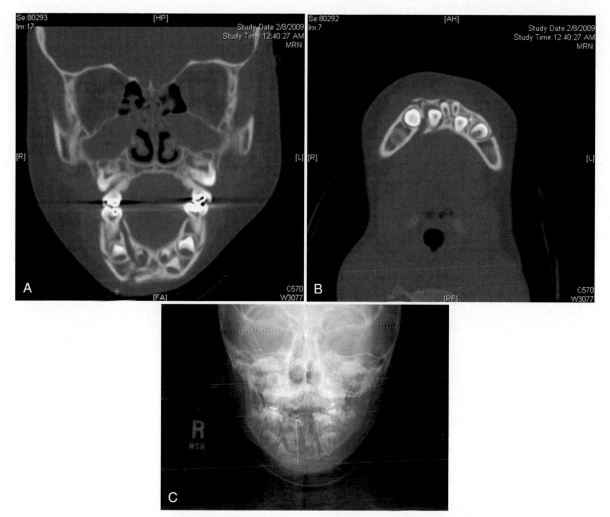

Figure 31-7 Proximity of succedaneous teeth to roots of deciduous teeth.

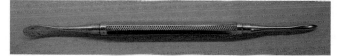

Figure 31-8 #9 Molt elevator.

or with the blade of the elevator angled toward the alveolar crest up to 45 degrees from the alveolar crest in the coronal plane. The elevator is then turned such that the portion of the blade resting on the alveolus acts as a fulcrum and the coronal portion of the blade rotates toward the tooth being extracted. This action expands the alveolus, disrupts the periodontal ligament, and establishes initial mobility of the root. The degree of mobility need not be great to achieve benefit from an elevator. Indeed, only limited movement can be achieved when there are adjacent teeth. Excessive force can fracture the tooth being extracted, converting a simple, closed extraction into an open extraction, or damage adjacent teeth or restorations. The straight elevator may in selected situations be used as a wedge. In this situation, once a space has been created between the bone surrounding the tooth socket and the tooth, the elevator is "wedged" between the alveolar bone and the tooth. Wedging the elevator inferiorly expands the alveolus, which facilitates extracting the tooth with forceps. Alternatively, as the elevator is "wedged" apically into the space between the bone and the tooth, the tooth is displaced coronally.

The last step in extracting a tooth is to remove the tooth with forceps, which must be appropriately selected. Several forceps are available in smaller sizes for the pediatric patient. (Fig. 31-10). The basic principles in selecting forceps are as follow:

1. The beaks of the forceps should adapt to the root surface of the tooth.
2. The beaks of the forceps when positioned and engaging the tooth should be parallel to the long axis of the tooth.
3. The size of the beaks of the forceps should be small enough not to engage the adjacent teeth during luxation and removal of the tooth. The beaks of the forceps should be placed under the separated and reflected soft tissue and the tooth firmly engaged.

The first force applied by the dentist when using forceps is apically directed. The apically directed force positions the

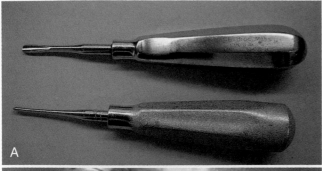

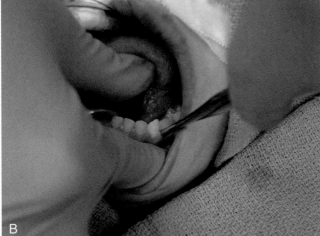

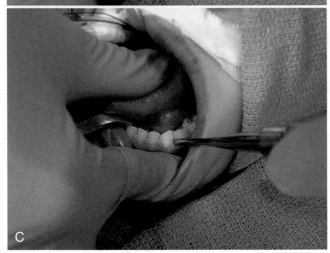

Figure 31-9 A, Straight elevator. The straight elevator can be placed at 45 degrees to the occlusal plane **(B)** or parallel to the occlusal plane **(C).**

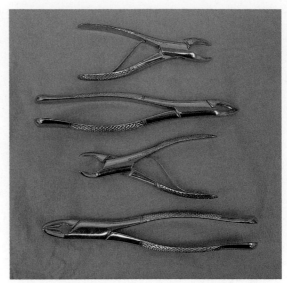

Figure 31-10 The armamentarium for exodontic procedures in pediatric patients is much the same as for adults, even though all anatomic structures are smaller. Several forceps for primary teeth offer some convenience; however, they are not necessary to perform any of the extractions. Large adult forceps, such as the "cowhorn" are contraindicated in the pediatric patient.

center of rotation as close to the root apex of the tooth as possible. The more apical the center of rotation and the closer it is to the apex of the tooth, the less the apical third of the root is subjected to translational movement, and the less likely an apical third root fracture will occur. The apically directed force also disrupts the periodontal ligaments. With apically directed force maintained, the tooth is luxated toward the buccal and lingual/palatal aspect. Luxation is slow. Movement is in one direction, and then stopped while the alveolus is allowed to expand before movement begins in the opposite direction. With each deliberate movement, the force is increased expanding the alveolus. Rapid, jerky movements are ineffective and not recommended. Rotational forces may be applied for selected roots that are conical (anterior teeth, mandibular premolars, maxillary second premolar). The opposite hand may be placed such that the index finger or thumb is positioned on either the buccal and/or lingual/palatal aspect of the alveolus and can feel the expansion of the alveolus. Finally, once the alveolus is sufficiently expanded and the periodontal ligament disrupted, slight coronal tractional forces are applied and the tooth is removed.

In general, anterior teeth should be luxated to the labial aspect during the extraction procedure because of the lingual position of the permanent teeth, and posterior teeth should be luxated with buccal and lingual pressures. However, the dentist may know the direction of least resistance and may deliver the tooth based on the individual situation. Although rare, the dentist may know when the roots of the deciduous molars are configured such that they could engage the succedaneous tooth and possibly cause the succedaneous tooth to be extracted with the deciduous tooth. If this is recognized radiographically or becomes noted during the extraction, then sectioning the deciduous tooth with a surgical handpiece may be indicated.

A traditional dental drill should not be used for surgical procedures. The surgical drill must vent its air away from the surgical field. If a drill vents its air toward the surgical site, there is significant risk for development of air emphysema or an air embolism. Air emphysema is the result of air being forced into the tissue planes under the periosteal flap. This can cause a significant dissection of the tissue planes, resulting in crepitus and swelling that could infringe fascial spaces and cause airway problems.

When drilling on bone, air could be forced into the vascular channels within the bony canals. Air that is forced into these vascular channels can travel through the bloodstream and cause an embolus in more distant and vital organs.

A root tip from a primary tooth may fracture during the procedure. The dentist should attempt to remove the root tip. Proper use of an elevator will ideally have loosened the root of the tooth, which facilitates root tip removal. However, if the dentist thinks that the attempt to remove the root tip poses a significant risk to the adjacent tooth or the succedaneous tooth, then the residual root tip should be left in the bone. Usually these root tips do not cause adverse sequelae. They may eventually resorb or migrate toward the gingiva and become exposed with the eruption of the permanent tooth. A post-treatment radiograph should be obtained and the child's parent should be informed. Informing the parent before the extraction and obtaining a written consent listing the various potential complications avoids having to present the complication as an unlikely and unexpected sequelae of surgery with the perception of "poor quality" treatment.

A primary tooth may be submerged or ankylosed. Ankylosed teeth may be slightly out of occlusion (Fig. 31-11) or they may be completely within the alveolar process yet show evidence of having once been in the mouth. A submerged tooth may have nonresorbed divergent roots, or may have all or nearly all the root resorbed. Despite having the root significantly resorbed, the tooth may show no signs of mobility when pressure or leverage is applied and exhibit a solid sound on percussion. These teeth may be virtually welded to the surrounding bone. The radiographic and clinical examination may not entirely predict the considerable difference in the degree of ankylosis and what difficulties may be encountered in the removal of the tooth. The basic principles pertaining to extraction are followed. A tooth with nonresorbed divergent roots in which the potential for a root fracture is high and the path of draw is inadequate may be best extracted by sectioning the tooth. If luxation is not accomplished with reasonable forceps pressure when extracting the ankylosed tooth, a surgical approach is required.

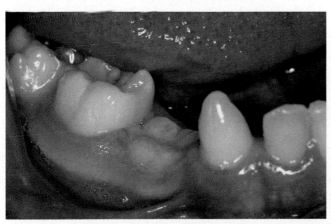

Figure 31-11 Ankylosed tooth.

One such technique to surgically remove an ankylosed tooth entails making a horizontal cut just below the cervical margin of the crown with a fine fissured cross cut bur. A straight elevator is inserted to fracture and remove the crown. The remaining portion of the tooth is then removed. Depending on the clinical and radiographic examination, this can be accomplished by either (1) using a bur to judiciously and conservatively remove bone around the tooth until it can be removed or (2) using a bur to carefully "drill away" the tooth. Frequently the difference between tooth structure and bone cannot be determined clinically. Care must be taken to minimize excessive bone removal and avoid injury to another tooth. An intraoperative or postoperative radiograph may be indicated to assess the situation. The dentist may decide to leave a portion of the residual root. This rarely is associated with any adverse sequelae.

IMPACTED TEETH

An impacted tooth is one that fails to erupt. This may be secondary to insufficient space in the dental arch (e.g., dental crowding or aberrant tooth development), mechanical obstruction secondary to a pathologic lesion (e.g., odontoma), a supernumerary tooth, or malposed tooth germs. Failure of a tooth to erupt may also be associated with genetic abnormalities.

IMPACTED THIRD MOLARS

The extraction of third molars is the most common surgical procedure in dentistry. It is therefore, critical for the pediatric dentist to understand the standard of care for the treatment of the impacted third molar. Refer to *Contemporary Oral and Maxillofacial Surgery* for a review on surgical principles and technique for extracting third molars. There are multiple reasons for extracting a third molar; however, the primary reason for the pediatric dentist to refer the patient to a surgeon for the extraction of an impacted third molar is to limit the progression of periodontal disease. Even though Ash and colleagues raised this issue almost 50 years ago, the concept of prophylactically extracting third molars to prevent disease versus extracting them when pathology develops remains a controversial subject.[4]

The extraction of third molars in the young patient, however, is not necessarily deemed as *preventive*. Several publications from the Oral and Maxillofacial Surgery Foundation and American Association of Oral and Maxillofacial Surgeons jointly sponsored Third Molar Clinical Trials have demonstrated that "absence of symptoms does not indicate absence of disease or pathology." Data from these studies has "demonstrated that periodontal pathology initiates in the mandibular third molar region" and spreads throughout the mouth.[5,6] Additionally, caries in erupted third molars increases in prevalence with increasing age. Recent literature has also demonstrated an association of periodontal disease with systemic manifestations, further supporting the indications for extracting third molars. One controversial issue regarding mandibular third molars is the issue of their influence on anterior crowding of mandibular teeth, especially after orthodontic therapy. Multiple studies have been reported that support both sides of this controversy. Even though it is likely that third molars play an etiology in crowding, their role may not be clinically significant.[7]

If it is advantageous to extract third molars, the timing of this procedure should be such that optimize health and minimize potential risks and complications. Optimal bone healing with improvement of intrabony defects on second molars adjacent to third molars has been shown to occur when surgery is performed in individuals younger than 25 years of age.[8] Risks associated with surgery, such as, alveolar osteitis, injury to the inferior alveolar nerve, and oroantral communication, have also been demonstrated to be higher in individuals 25 years of age and older.[9] Health Related Quality of Life indicators are also better for younger individuals.[10]

IMPACTED TEETH OTHER THAN THIRD MOLARS

The most commonly impacted tooth is the third molar. Whereas any tooth could be impacted, other commonly impacted teeth (in this frequency) seen by the dentist include the maxillary canine, second premolar, mandibular second molar, and maxillary incisors. Rare is the impaction or failure to erupt of a deciduous tooth. The latter is commonly associated with pathology, such as an odontoma or supernumerary tooth. Commonly impacted supernumerary teeth managed by the pediatric dentist include the mesiodens and supernumerary mandibular premolars.

The prevalence of impaction of the permanent maxillary canine is up to 2% (Fig. 31-12). Eight percent of the time the impaction occurs bilaterally. The occurrence of an impacted canine is greater in female patients and has a predilection of occurrence in individuals with a familial history.[11] The impacted maxillary canine is labially positioned 15% of the time and palatally positioned 85% of the time. Arch length deficiency probably contributes to the impaction of the labially positioned canine while it may not be a contributing factor with the palatally positioned canine.[12]

Most commonly, the second premolar is reported as the next most frequently impacted tooth. The mandibular premolar is more commonly impacted than the maxillary premolar. The impacted mandibular premolar is usually located lingually or midalveolus and the maxillary premolar is located palatally. Kaban and Troulis, however, report the maxillary incisors as the tooth impacted most frequently after the maxillary canine.[13] They believe that the frequency of impaction of the maxillary incisors is most likely secondary to injury, infection, or loss of the deciduous incisors. If the deciduous incisors are lost prematurely, a dense, hyperplastic, fibrous tissue may form over the alveolus, which impedes eruption and contributes to the impaction of the permanent maxillary incisors.

The incidence of impaction of the mandibular second molar is estimated to be 3 in every 1000 patients.[14] It tends to be unilateral with a slight predilection for female patients. Several different etiologies have been described. The etiology may be secondary to arch length discrepancy with the developing third molar tooth providing a mechanical obstruction. Alternatively, impaction of a mandibular second molar can occur when there is sufficient arch length. In this situation, it has been proposed that there is a lack of guidance of eruption of the second molar by the distal root of the first molar. A more mesial inclination of the second molar during its development and eruption results in its being trapped below the distal height of contour of the first molar crown.[15] The latter concept is similar to what has been described as a contributing factor in the impaction of a maxillary canine and a lack of guidance by the lateral incisor root.

Ideally early recognition of an altered eruption pattern and if possible interceptive serial extractions of deciduous teeth and/or orthodontics can facilitate eruption. However, regardless of early recognition, a tooth may become impacted. Once an altered eruption pattern is recognized, the dentist must perform a clinical and radiographic

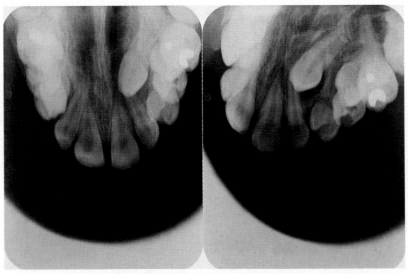

Figure 31-12 Impacted cuspid.

examination. Palpation of the buccal, lingual, or palatal aspects may reveal a bulge, suggesting the location of the impacted tooth. When the tooth is not palpable, radiographic imaging is indicated to determine the location of the impacted tooth. Several radiographic techniques can be used to assist in locating an impacted tooth. These are discussed in Chapter 5.

Management of an impacted tooth may include (1) observation, (2) extraction of the impacted tooth, (3) surgical exposure and assisted eruption, (4) surgical uprighting, or (5) autotransplantation. Several factors need to be taken into consideration in deciding the management of the impacted tooth. These include age and health of the patient, the potential pathology associated with the impacted tooth, location and angulation of the impacted tooth, the benefit of surgery, the frequency and severity of the risks of surgery, the risks and consequences of no surgical intervention, as well as the economic consequences of surgical versus nonsurgical intervention and the quality of life associated with each of these decisions.

This chapter does not discuss the treatment planning decisions pertaining to whether to perform an extraction versus a surgical exposure or surgical uprighting. If the decision is made to surgically expose the tooth and facilitate eruption, care must be coordinated between the appropriate dental colleagues. The first step is to create and ensure that there is adequate space to accommodate the eruption of the impacted tooth. Surgical exposure should not be performed until adequate space is obtained. For example, if a premolar is to be extracted to establish space for the exposure and eruption of a canine, the orthodontic appliances should be in place before the extraction of the premolar tooth. Although it is likely that orthodontic tooth movement may not be initiated until after the premolar tooth is extracted, the application of orthodontic appliances establishes a commitment by the patient to the planned treatment before the irreversible extraction of the premolar tooth.

Surgical Exposure

The ideal time to surgically intervene to expose an impacted tooth is when the root of the impacted tooth is almost completely formed and the apex is not yet closed. Exposure of a palatally impacted tooth is frequently accomplished by making a sulcular incision between the palatal tissue and the teeth and reflecting a full-thickness mucoperiosteal flap. The anterior and posterior extent of the mucoperiosteal flap is dependent on the access required. Frequently a prominence or bulge is evident where the impacted tooth's crown lay. The bone overlying this bulge may be thin and easily removed with a curette or periosteal elevator. For thicker bone, a surgical handpiece with bur and copious irrigation or a chisel is used to remove bone in a controlled manner, with care taken not to damage the tooth. Bone is removed to expose enough of the palatal surface of the tooth's crown to which an orthodontic bracket can be attached to aid in eruption. Depending on the impaction and path of eruption, additional bone may be removed to facilitate eruption. The exposed dental follicle is removed with a curette. Care must be exercised to maintain the integrity of bone around the crestal margins of the adjacent teeth. Additionally, an impacted tooth may be in close proximity to the roots of the adjacent teeth and care must be exercised not to damage or devitalize these adjacent roots. The mucoperiosteal flap is repositioned into its original position and the soft tissue overlying the impacted tooth's crown is excised, exposing the crown and orthodontic bracket. The gold chain attached to the orthodontic bracket is passed through this window of soft tissue and frequently secured to the orthodontic arch wire with silk suture. The palatal mucoperiosteal flap is anatomically aligned and secured with a resorbable suture. The soft tissue window overlying the crown of the impacted tooth can be left open or packed with a periodontal dressing for approximately 4 days. If the tooth is deeply impacted within the palate, no overlying tissue may be excised and the gold chain is brought through the soft tissue at the crestal margin, frequently corresponding with the incision.

When exposing a labially impacted canine, a critical component of the surgery outcome is the maintenance of a cervical margin of attached mucosa on the erupted impacted tooth. Two surgical techniques exist: (1) apical positioned flap and (2) closed technique. The apical positioned flap technique consists of a horizontal crestal incision that is made in the edentulous region with two vertical releasing incisions on the mesial and distal aspects of this edentulous region. The flap is reflected and the tooth is exposed removing bone as necessary to the cervical margin. The bracket is attached and the flap is repositioned apical to the bracket ideally at the level of the cervical margin of the tooth. The premise of the apical positioned flap is to maintain a collar of attached gingiva that will advance coronally as the tooth erupts (Fig. 31-13). The closed technique consists of a crestal-sulcular incision with or without a vertical release that allows the development of a full thickness mucoperiosteal flap. The tooth is exposed, removing necessary bone, and a bracket is attached. The gold chain attached to the bracket is attached to the orthodontic arch bar generally with silk suture and the flap is closed with resorbable suture. The gold chain generally exits the wound through the crestal incision. The closed technique can be used for all labially impacted canines; however, it is indicated for high impactions or midalveolar impactions when the apical positioned flap is contraindicated. There may also be a disadvantage with the apical positioned flap technique in

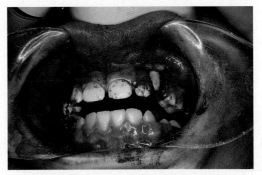

Figure 31-13 Apically positioned flap.

that it can contribute to increased crown length and intrusive relapse.[16] These basic principles are used for surgical exposure of most impacted teeth.

Autotransplantation is an alternative to positioning the impacted tooth into occlusion when surgical exposure and orthodontic assisted eruption of a canine tooth is not a viable option. This technique should only be used in the pediatric patient as an alternative to an extraction and not as a routine alternative to surgical exposure and orthodontic assisted eruption. The autotransplantation technique has also been used when a nonrestorable first molar is extracted and a third molar is transplanted into the first molar site. The technique entails first creating a recipient site that can accommodate the transplantation and then atraumatically extracting the impacted tooth. Damage to the periodontal ligament of the extracted impacted tooth must be avoided. Optimal results mandate that the transplanted tooth be inserted into the recipient site within minutes. The tooth once positioned into the recipient site is stabilized with a segmental orthodontic arch wire. Endodontic treatment with calcium hydroxide is initiated between 6 and 8 weeks and definitive root canal therapy is performed at 1 year.[17] The success rate for a transplanted tooth is reported to be between 70% to 95%.[18]

Surgical uprighting is a technique that has most commonly been used for bringing an impacted mandibular second molar into occlusion (Fig. 31-14). The optimal time for performing the procedure is when the root is two-thirds formed and the apex is open. The tooth should have a mesial inclination not to exceed 90 degrees and should be neither labially or lingually inclined for optimal results.[19] Excessive mesial inclination has an increased risk for devascularizing the tooth. In this situation the surgical procedure would be more consistent with an autotransplantation than a surgical uprighting. Excessive labial or lingual inclination is associated with diminished crestal bone on the respective surface, compromising initial stability and ultimate bone height on that respective surface of the tooth.

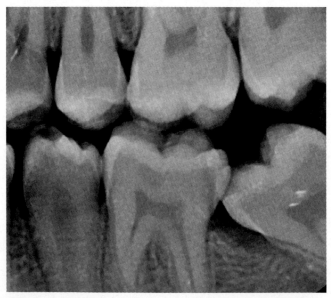

Figure 31-14 Mesially impacted mandibular second molar.

The surgical technique entails making a sulcular incision that extends from the mesial of the first molar to the distal buccal of the second molar. The incision is then extended distally along the alveolar crest angling into the buccal sulcus along the external oblique ridge. A full-thickness mucoperiosteal flap is reflected. Adequate space must be created distal to the impacted second molar tooth. Prophylactic removal of the third molar is commonly performed. Using a surgical drill with a bur, it may be necessary to remove bone on the distal aspect of the second molar to the level of its greatest concavity. This ensures that there is adequate space for the impacted second molar to be moved into. An elevator is then used to elevate and reposition the tooth. The repositioned tooth should be slightly out of occlusion. Most frequently the surgically uprighted tooth is stable in its new position and requires no additional stabilization. If the tooth is mobile it should be splinted with an orthodontic arch wire for approximately 2 weeks. The mucoperiosteal flap is approximated into position, taking into consideration the newly uprighted tooth, and sutured. Antibiotics are generally prescribed for the first week. Prophylactic endodontic therapy generally is not required.

Extraction of Impacted Teeth Other Than Third Molars

The extraction of a non-third molar impacted tooth entails many of the techniques described pertaining to the exposure of the impacted tooth. However, a few critical points may differ. The supernumerary impacted tooth or the unerupted succedaneous tooth that is scheduled to be extracted may be deeply impacted. Complications associated with extraction may include injury to adjacent tooth roots or vital structures, such as the inferior alveolar nerve. Localization of the deeply impacted tooth may be achieved with cone beam computed tomography (CT). The cone beam CT may provide a better image, demonstrating the exact location of the tooth and its proximity to adjacent roots and vital structure. Cone beam CT imaging may also be beneficial for localizing teeth that will be exposed. The technique cannot be considered standard of care at this time and probably should not become standard of care for many impacted teeth that are readily palpable.

A full-thickness mucoperiosteal envelope flap is created with or without a vertical release. If a vertical release is used to facilitate access, the vertical releasing incision should be made away from the planned extraction. Usually the crown of the tooth is exposed. When extracting the impacted tooth, the objective is to minimize the amount of bone removal. To facilitate extraction of the tooth with minimal bone removal, the tooth may be sectioned such that the crown and root are removed separately.

ASSOCIATED HARD TISSUE LESIONS

ODONTOMA

Odontomas are the most frequently occurring odontogenic tumors seen in pediatric patients (Fig. 31-15). They are frequently discovered when the patient presents for

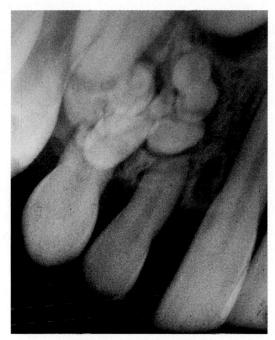

Figure 31-15 Odontoma.

evaluation of an unerupted tooth or incidentally during routine radiographic examination. There are two types of odontomas: compound and complex. A compound odontoma represents multiple toothlike structures. A complex odontoma has irregularly shaped masses of enamel with no anatomic resemblance to a tooth. Treatment for an odontoma involves simple enucleation and curettage.

Enucleation is usually carried out intraorally. A mucoperiosteal flap of sufficient size is elevated to expose the tumor. If required, the overlying bone is removed using a round or tapered fissure bur. The odontoma is well encapsulated and can be curetted from the surrounding bone. The specimen is sent for biopsy. The surgical site is irrigated with normal saline and the wound is reapproximated using resorbable sutures.

ODONTOGENIC CYSTS

The dentigerous cyst is the most common odontogenic cyst in the pediatric population. It is usually associated with an unerupted permanent tooth or with a supernumerary tooth. Traumatic cysts are also common, especially in active young patients. They are usually unilateral and solitary. Appropriate imaging should be obtained when the dentist suspects a cyst or lesion in the pediatric patient. A biopsy is preferable before definitive surgery. However, if a general anesthetic is required to manage the pediatric patient for a lesion in which the dentist is most confident about the diagnosis, it is usually preferable to perform the definitive procedure and obtain histological evaluation on this specimen with the intent that only one general anesthetic will be necessary. Aspiration is always advised before biopsy to rule out a vascular lesion.

The initial step in managing a cystic lesion is to aspirate the wound. Aspiration of the cystic cavity assists the dentist with differential diagnosis and allows the dentist

to rule out a vascular lesion. The treatment of a dentigerous cyst involves complete enucleation of the cyst and its epithelial lining. If an impacted third molar is involved with the cyst, removal of the tooth is indicated. Otherwise, an effort should be made to save the involved permanent tooth to help preserve the integrity of the dental arch. Although a dentigerous cyst is a benign cyst lined by squamous epithelium, this epithelium has a potential to undergo neoplastic change (e.g., ameloblastoma). Postoperative observation should continue until the permanent tooth has erupted and complete healing has occurred.

An eruption cyst is a cystlike lesion caused by eruption trauma of either primary or permanent teeth. Usually seen in erupting molar areas, it usually resolves spontaneously when the involved tooth penetrates the gingival tissue.

SOFT TISSUE PROCEDURES

The pediatric dentist frequently is involved in the management of several minor intraoral soft tissue lesions. This section discusses commonly seen soft tissue pathologic conditions: mucocele, ranula, fibroma, and pyogenic granuloma. Lingual and labial frenectomies are discussed in Chapters 20 and 7, respectively.

MUCOCELES AND RANULAS

A mucocele or mucous retention cyst is a benign pathologic lesion. The lesion is a result of the extravasation of saliva from an injured minor salivary gland. The collection of extravasated fluid develops a fibrous wall around itself forming a pseudocyst. The lesion can fluctuate in size depending on its fluid-filled state. A decrease in lesion size is frequently associated with a history of drainage of a thick viscous fluid. The lesion is nonpainful, soft, doughy, and fluctuant to palpation. Clinically the overlying mucosa may have the same coloration as the lower lip or have a bluish hue. Lesions of longer duration may appear firmer and fibrotic and be difficult to distinguish from a fibroma. A mucocele most likely results secondary to a traumatic event that in most situations goes unrecognized. The lower lip is the most common location.

The basic premise in excising a mucocele is to remove the fibrous capsule and any associated minor salivary glands. For a lesion within the lip, the lip is frequently everted and stretched. This stabilizes the lesion. A Kazanjian retractor can be used to isolate and stabilize the lesion. An elliptical incision (staying within the confines of the lesion) is made in the lip perpendicular to the fibers of the orbicularis oris muscle. Using a combination of sharp and blunt dissection, the fibrous capsule of the lesion is separated from the surrounding tissue. If done properly, the mucocele can be removed intact. All minor salivary glands surrounding the lesion and within the surgical field should be removed. Removal of the surrounding minor salivary glands minimizes the potential for recurrence. Hemostasis is controlled and closure is accomplished with a 4-0 resorbable suture. The lip is a prominent area and it may be challenging for the smaller child to not disturb the wound during healing. The suture knots should be buried, and an extra suture to ensure integrity of the closure may prevent the wound from dehiscing (Fig. 31-16).

A ranula is a mucous retention cyst that occurs in the floor of the mouth and is associated with the sublingual gland. A ranula in a young pediatric patient needs to be differentiated from a lymphatic malformation. A ranula may be managed by marsupialization or excision of the sublingual gland. Many surgeons initially manage a ranula with marsupialization and perform an excision of a sublingual gland secondarily if the ranula recurs, although some surgeons think that there is a high incidence of recurrence with marsupialization and choose excision of the sublingual gland as their primary surgical intervention. The first step before performing either of the two procedures is to identify and cannulate the ipsilateral submandibular duct. The mucosa overlying the lesion is then excised. When performing a marsupialization, the lining of the pseudocyst cavity is then sutured to the overlying mucosa of the floor of mouth. A Penrose drain may be sutured in place to maintain the definitive communication between the pseudocyst and the oral cavity. If the intent is to excise the sublingual gland, once the overlying mucosa is excised, blunt dissection is used to identify and isolate the sublingual gland. Extraoral pressure elevating the floor of mouth can facilitate this process. Anterior traction of the gland may also facilitate dissection. The lingual nerve and submandibular duct, which are in close proximity to the deep surface of the sublingual gland, should be identified before definitive excision to minimize iatrogenic injury. The wound is loosely closed.

FIBROMA AND PYOGENIC GRANULOMA

The pediatric patient may present with other soft tissue lesions. Common lesions found in the pediatric patient include both the fibroma and the pyogenic granuloma. Oral pathology is discussed elsewhere in this text. If the lesion is small, it may be excised completely and the specimen submitted for histological evaluation. This can usually be accomplished by making an elliptical incision within normal tissue around the lesion. The depth of the dissection is determined by the appearance and feel of the lesion. Minor modifications to this basic technique are dependent on the differential diagnosis. For example, removal of interproximal tissue and scaling of teeth may be indicated when excising a pyogenic granuloma to ensure complete removal and minimize recurrence.

INFECTION OF THE HEAD AND NECK REGION

This section focuses on infections of odontogenic etiology. However, whereas the etiology of head and neck infections may be odontogenic, the etiology may also be secondary to sinus, salivary gland, skin, or middle ear conditions. Defining the etiology is critical to the management of the infection because the infection may persist and potentially worsen if the cause is not removed and the appropriate antibiotic is not selected based on the etiology. Infections can progress rapidly in both the pediatric patient and the adult patient; however, the pediatric patient is especially susceptible to rapidly becoming dehydrated and systemically ill from what may appear to be a relatively minor infection.

This discussion provides a protocol for management of the pediatric patient with a head and neck infection. Similar to CPR/BLS, which provides an algorithm and a sequence for managing the airway, breathing, and circulation, this section provides a logical sequence for assessing and treating the patient. An experienced individual can assess the situation and perform CPR simultaneously; likewise, the experienced dentist may perform several of these assessments and interventions simultaneously.

The first step in managing the pediatric patient with a head and neck infection is to obtain a history. The history includes details about both the patient's present illness and the patient's past medical and surgical history. The history of the present illness must include (1) onset, (2) rate of progression, (3) history of preceding odontogenic pain, upper respiratory infection, sinus pain, otitis media, (4) airway compromise (dysphagia, dyspnea, change in voice), (5) trismus,

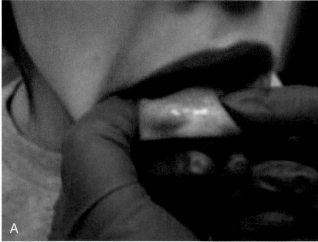

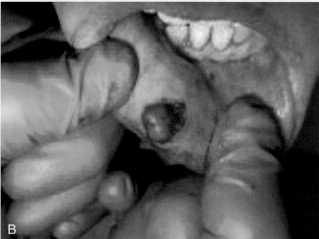

Figure 31-16 Mucocele and stages of surgical excision. **A,** An elliptical incision made with a combination of blunt and sharp dissection. **B,** The mucocele sac is separated from the surrounding mucosa.

and (6) ophthalmic complaints (e.g., photophobia, changes in visual acuity). It may be difficult to elicit a complete history from a younger patient when neither the patient nor the parent is able to provide a history of preceding odontogenic pain. The dentist must obtain a complete past medical history. In managing a patient with an infection it is important to identify diseases that compromise the immune system (e.g., diabetes) as well as diseases that compromise the patient's ability to withstand stress (e.g., congenital heart disease). The latter is important because a severe infection can impose a severe physiologic stress on the patient and the patient's ability to respond to the infection may be dependent on his or her systemic reserve.

The second step in managing the pediatric patient with a head and neck infection is to examine the patient. The clinical examination includes visual inspection identifying the (1) patient's respiratory compromise, distress, or lack of distress, (2) involved swelling and the severity of the swelling, (3) palpation of the tissues discerning their tenderness, and consistency (cellulitic or fluctuant), (4) assessment of maximal mouth opening, and (5) examination of the dentition. The radiographic examination may consist of a periapical or panoramic radiograph, which can be obtained in the office. The panoramic radiograph is a good screening radiograph. A periapical radiograph may provide more discerning information; however, this may be difficult to obtain if the child's head and neck is swollen. Severe fascial space infections require a CT scan with contrast to delineate the full involvement of the infection. A differential diagnosis is developed from the history and examination.

The dentist must be knowledgeable with the anatomic spaces of the head and neck and the routes in which infection can spread. The routes of dissemination of an infection are dependent on the position of the roots of the teeth relative to anatomic considerations such as muscles, maxillary sinus, and root angulation relative to their respective jaws. For example, a vestibular space infection is the result of an infection dissecting through the lateral maxillary or mandibular bone and perforating the buccal bone inferior (maxilla) or superior (mandible) to the buccinator muscle attachment. The maxillary teeth can result in a canine space infection, which can extend and ultimately involve the periorbital tissues. The proximity of the maxillary teeth to the maxillary sinus can produce a maxillary sinusitis. Posterior spread of a maxillary infection can involve the infratemporal space and have direct spread into the orbital tissues through the inferior orbital fissure. Mandibular molar infections can spread above or below the mylohyoid muscle resulting in a sublingual space or submandibular space infection, respectively. An infection of the sublingual space displaces the tongue superiorly and posteriorly. Posteriorly a mandibular infection may spread either lateral to the ramus or medial to the ramus resulting in either a submasseteric space or a pterygomandibular and/or lateral pharyngeal space infection, respectively. The submasseteric space, the pterygomandibular space, and the infratemporal space make up the masticator space. Infections of the masticator

space result in trismus. Infections of the sublingual, submandibular, submental, and masticator space can compromise airway integrity. Although rare, infections of the head and neck may have hematogenous spread via the valveless veins of the face and cause central neurologic infections.

The third step in managing the pediatric patient with a head and neck infection is to develop a plan of intervention. The first step in this interventional plan entails an assessment of the airway. Because airway assessment is so critical, it is a step unto itself. Urgent airway intervention may be indicated based on the involved fascial spaces, their severity, the patient's signs and symptoms, and the progression of the infection. Managing a patient with a compromised airway requires a team approach between the surgeon (capable of performing a tracheostomy, if necessary) and the anesthesiologist. This is a challenging situation in the adult wherein inducing a sedative state or general anesthetic may worsen an already compromised airway. In situations where the airway is compromised, the adult patient may be fiberoptically intubated with minimal sedation. The fearful pediatric patient lacks the ability to cooperate, necessitating a more profound depth of sedation, which potentially makes airway management a more challenging and dangerous situation.

Once the airway is assessed and controlled, the practitioner must continue with the interventional plan development. The components of intervention include (1) determining whether the infection should be treated in an outpatient or inpatient setting, (2) establishing the appropriate antibiotics to use, and (3) undertaking surgery (incision and drainage and removal of the etiology). Indications for admitting a pediatric patient to the hospital include fever (temperature $\geq$ 101.5°F), lymphadenopathy, elevated white blood cell count (WBC), poor oral intake, dehydration, involved fascial spaces, associated findings (e.g., dysphagia), and the appearance of being ill (i.e., looking sick). The latter item should not be disregarded; this is one situation in which the general appearance of the patient provides significant guidance.

Odontogenic infections are polymicrobial. There is a significant increase in resistance to antibiotics that has developed over the past couple of decades, especially to beta lactamase–producing organisms. The antibiotic for a less severe odontogenic infection that is to be managed in an outpatient setting is penicillin VK (25 to 50 mg/kg per day in divided doses every 6 to 8 hours) or clindamycin (10 to 20 mg/kg per day in divided doses every 6 hours).[20] Because of the increase in beta lactamase–producing organisms, the first-line antibiotics for infections requiring hospitalization are intravenous ampicillin-sulbactam (Unisyn) or intravenous clindamycin. Hospitalization facilitates supportive care, such as providing hydration, nutritional support, and fever management.

Surgery includes incision and drainage and removal of the source of infection (which may involve pulpectomy or extraction). In our opinion, if hospitalization is required, the offending tooth should be extracted. The following are basic principles for performing an incision and drainage. If the patient is not going to have a general anesthetic, the site must be anesthetized with local anesthesia. Regional block anesthesia without infiltrating the infective site is recommended. A Gram stain and culture and sensitivity (C&S) test is indicated for all fascial space infections (this does not include a vestibular space infection), immunocompromised patients, or infections that have failed multiple courses of antibiotic treatment. Ideally, an aspirate for a Gram stain and C&S is obtained before making the incision and drainage. Before incising the infection, a needle on a syringe is inserted into the wound and its contents aspirated. The aspirate is submitted for Gram stain and C&S. When draining a vestibular space infection, an incision is made frequently centered within the swelling. The incision is carried through the mucosa down and through the periosteum. There must be knowledge of the anatomy to avoid vital structures, such as the mental nerve and facial artery. A small hemostat (mosquito) is inserted with the beaks closed. Blunt dissection is performed with the beaks closed. The beaks are opened and withdrawn. The hemostat beaks are never blindly closed when the instrument is in the wound to prevent injury to vital structures. A Penrose drain may be placed into the incision and drainage site and secured with a nonresorbable suture for a few days. The drain keeps the wound open and patent, facilitating irrigation (if necessary) and spontaneous drainage of the wound and preventing a recurrent collection from developing. Refer to a surgical text for more detailed information pertaining to draining fascial spaces.[20]

FRACTURE OF THE MANDIBLE

The pediatric dentist may encounter pediatric patients who have suffered a traumatic event and injured the soft and/or hard tissue of the face. These injuries can include soft tissue lacerations, dentoalveolar injuries, and facial fractures of the maxilla, mandible, nose, and cheek. Probably the most common injury that the pediatric dentist sees is the dentoalveolar injury, which includes intrusion and avulsion of teeth, crown and tooth fractures, and alveolar fractures. Diagnosis and assessment of these injuries is discussed elsewhere.[21] The mandibular fracture is the most common skeletal injury that occurs in the pediatric age group that is seen within the hospital. However, the patient with a mandibular fracture may initially present to the pediatric dentist and the pediatric dentist must be able to recognize the injury and make the appropriate referral.

When assessing a patient who presents with a facial injury, the treating doctor must recognize that the patient can have associated injuries. A history of the events contributing to the event and a comprehensive physical evaluation is important and must be completed. The treating doctor must also be cognizant that the force required to cause a facial fracture is directed to the head and neck, and could result in neurologic or cervical injury. Understanding the mechanism of injury may present some insight. The doctor should inquire as to loss of consciousness or symptoms suggestive of neurologic injury (e.g., dizziness, lightheadedness, amnesia of the event, nausea and vomiting). In the awake adult individual, cervical trauma is assessed frequently by clinical examination and the patient's ability to relate whether or not neck pain is present. In the younger patient who cannot reliably relate whether or not neck pain is present, radiographic assessment may be indicated. The pediatric dentist must be cognizant that the pediatric patient may sustain cervical injuries as well as other injuries secondary to the mechanism of injury and manage the patient to minimize those potential adverse consequences. For example, if there is any question that the patient has sustained a cervical injury, the patient should be supinely positioned and EMS contacted for transportation to the emergency department.

The first step in assessing the patient who presents with a facial injury is to obtain a comprehensive history. The younger patient may be less able to provide reliable answers. These questions include:
1. "Where does it hurt?" "What makes it hurt?"
2. "Can you open your mouth?" (Does the patient have any limitation of jaw movement? Is the bite different?)
3. "Do you have any loose teeth?"
4. "Do your lips feel different?" "Are your lips numb?"

The answer to these questions may reveal the patient's diagnosis. A patient may complain of pain in the temporomandibular joint. This is suggestive of a hemarthrosis or a fracture of the condyle. On clinical examination the patient may have a chin abrasion or laceration. The force of a blunt trauma to the region of the chin that results in an abrasion or laceration may be transmitted to the condylar region. Thus a chin abrasion or laceration in a patient complaining of pain in the temporomandibular joint may support the suspicion of an injury to the joint. Alternatively, a patient who presents with a chin abrasion or laceration secondary to blunt force should be assessed for pain in the joint that may be suggestive of a condylar fracture.

Bony or muscular injury can result in limited mobility of the jaw because of pain, bony mechanical obstruction, joint or soft tissue swelling, or muscular inflammation or irritability. A unilateral condylar injury may result in deviation to the ipsilateral side with opening in the occlusion secondary to the action of the contralateral lateral pterygoid muscle.

Fractures of the mandible can result in a malocclusion. Unilateral condylar fractures usually result in an ipsilateral premature bite. Bilateral condylar fractures may result in bilateral shortened rami with a resultant anterior open bite and mandibular retrognathia. A hemarthrosis of the condyle may result in an ipsilateral posterior open bite secondary to the joint swelling and inferior displacement of the rami. Because of the elasticity of the pediatric mandible, a fracture may not always result in displacement and a resultant malocclusion. The practitioner must be diligent and assess for tenderness of the region which may be an indication of an injury. Hemorrhage into the tissue associated with the fracture may result in localized ecchymosis in the buccal or lingual vestibule. A fracture may result in gingival tearing. The findings may be more subtle with slight evidence of sulcular blood along the teeth adjacent to the fracture. Teeth adjacent to the fracture may be loose. This must be distinguished from an avulsive type injury, an alveolar fracture, or the normal resorptive pattern present in a mixed dentition. Palpation of the mandible may identify a step along the inferior border. Bimanual palpation may demonstrate segmental mobility or elicit discomfort.

The bony canal of the inferior alveolar nerve traverses the rami and the body of the mandible. A fracture of the mandible may result in hemorrhage into the canal with a resultant compressive type injury, or the nerve may sustain a contusion, a stretching type lesion, or a partial or complete transection. Paresthesia occurs as a result of the nerve injury. In most situations in which the fracture segments are not grossly displaced, the paresthesia is transient and recovery occurs over the next several weeks to months. Pediatric patients are less able to report various symptoms and may not be able to express that they are paresthetic.

Radiographic examination of the mandible in the office usually includes a panoramic radiograph. This image is useful and reliable in visualizing the entire mandible, including the condyles, rami, angle, body, and symphysis. Radiographic assessment ideally should occur in two planes. A condylar/subcondylar fracture may not always be recognized on a panoramic radiograph. Additionally, the panoramic radiograph does not demonstrate the lateral/medial displacement of the fracture segments in the coronal plane as demonstrated on a Towne's view. A fracture that is not clearly visualized on the panoramic radiograph may be identified on the Towne's view. The symphysis may be outside the ideal trough of the panoramic radiograph and a nondisplaced or greenstick fracture may not be clearly seen on a panoramic image. A mandibular occlusal radiograph at 90 degrees to the mandible should be obtained when a mandibular symphyseal fracture is suspected and is not seen on a Panorex. For the patient who presents to the emergency department, CT imaging is becoming more regularly used and is replacing more traditional flat plane imaging. The CT scan provides images in the axial, coronal, and sagittal views. Three-dimensional reconstruction is also available and should be requested. It is important to have all of these images available because a fracture may be easily visible and recognized on only one of the views.

The discussion of managing the pediatric patient focuses on the patient with a mixed dentition. Treatment of a mandible fracture includes reduction of the fractured segments, reestablishment of a stable occlusion, and stabilization of the fractured segments. Fractures in pediatric patients can heal rapidly and treatment should ideally be initiated within the first days. If for various medical conditions or associated injuries fracture reduction is not initiated within the first few days, the bony segments may begin to heal and reduction may become difficult, if not impossible. One advantage in managing pediatric patients with mixed dentition is that minor malocclusions usually self-correct with growth.

Condylar fractures can be classified as either intracapsular or extracapsular. A pediatric patient who has sustained an intracapsular fracture or injury is at increased risk of ankylosis or growth disturbance. Treatment is frequently dictated by the degree of malocclusion and jaw opening/function. If the occlusion is grossly normal, the fracture may be managed with a blenderized diet, analgesics if necessary, and observation. Physiotherapy to ensure symmetric opening may be indicated. If the pediatric patient has a malocclusion or significant pain, a short period of 7 to 10 days of maxillomandibular fixation may be warranted. The risk of rami shortening and an anterior open bite is a concern in a patient who has sustained a bilateral condylar fracture and the practitioner may more readily consider a period of maxillomandibular fixation. Guiding elastics for a period of 1 to 2 weeks after the release of maxillomandibular fixation may be beneficial to facilitate symmetric opening. Open reduction and fixation, even for a displaced condylar fracture in the pediatric patient, is rarely indicated. Slight malocclusions usually self-correct with growth.

Management of a nondisplaced body or symphysis fracture may also be managed with a blenderized diet and observation. When maxillomandibular fixation is required (for either a nondisplaced or displaced fracture), the patient is frequently placed into fixation for a period of approximately 3 weeks. An alternative to maxillomandibular fixation for a body or symphysis fracture is to place a lingual splint which is secured to the teeth with either circumdental or circumandibular wires. The advantage of the splint is that it does not require the patient's jaws to be wired closed. This facilitates respiratory care as well as nutritional support in the seriously injured patient. A disadvantage of a lingual splint is that it may require a separate anesthetic to take the impression in order to make the splint. If the patient is having multiple injuries managed during the same operation the dental surgical team may take the maxillary and mandibular impression at the beginning of the operation, fabricate the splint, and have it ready to be placed before termination of the anesthetic. Angle fractures or fractures posterior to the teeth require maxillomandibular fixation for a period of 3 weeks. Open reduction and internal fixation (ORIF) is an option in managing the pediatric patient. Care must be taken to avoid succedaneous developing teeth. The authors have rarely found it necessary to perform an ORIF of a pediatric mandible fracture. Slight malocclusions usually self-correct with growth.

Maxillomandibular fixation is traditionally achieved by ligating an arch bar to the teeth in each arch with circumdental wires placed around the cervical collars of the teeth. The shape and shortness of the deciduous teeth may make this difficult at times. The arch bar provides hooks (with the opening apically positioned) that can be used to secure wires or elastics to achieve either tight maxillomandibular fixation with absolute lack of movement or place elastics that allow limited function and guide the patient's opening and occlusion. If the patient's dentition does not facilitate circumdental wiring, the practitioner may opt to use skeletal wiring either alone or in combination with circumdental wiring. Skeletal fixation consists of circumandibular wires, piriform wires, and zygomatic buttress wires. A circumandibular wire is placed around the mandible. The wire is inserted extra-orally using a Keith needle or an awl. The inferior border of the mandible is palpated and the first end of the wire is passed along the lingual aspect of the mandible and enters the mouth in the lingual vestibule adjacent to the mandible. Care must be taken to pass the wire along the lingual surface of the mandible; if the wire is passed too far medially it may injure various structures, such as Warthin's duct. The other end of the wire is passed through the same extraoral puncture site in the skin inferior to the border of the mandible. This end of the wire is passed buccally and enters the mouth in the depth of the vestibule just adjacent to the buccal surface of the mandible. Each wire end is grabbed individually and the wire is sawed back and forth until the inferior aspect of the looped wire passes through the soft tissue and lies firmly against the inferior aspect of the mandible. The pediatric mandibular cortex is thin and aggressive sawing action can result in pulling the wire through the mandible, resulting in a new fracture. Piriform and buttress wires are achieved by making an incision over the respective site and creating a hole to pass a wire through with a bur. The practitioner must be cognizant where the developing tooth buds are.

This discussion focuses on management of the mandible fracture in the pediatric patient with mixed dentition. Patients with permanent dentition have less capacity for the bone to adapt and remodel.

SUMMARY

This chapter outlines basic principles used in the management of basic oral and maxillofacial surgical procedures. Many of the principles discussed can be used in various aspects of dental practice.

REFERENCES

1. Litman RS, et al. Breathing patterns and levels of consciousness in children during administration of nitrous oxide after oral midazolam premedication, *J Oral Maxillofac Surg* 55:1372-1377, 1995.
2. Litman RS. Airway obstruction after oral midazolam, *Anesthesiology* 85:1217-1218, 1996.
3. Hupp JR. Principles of uncomplicated exodontia. In Hupp JR, Ellis E III, Tucker MR, eds. *Contemporary oral and maxillofacial surgery*, 5th ed. Philadelphia, 2008, Mosby/Elsevier, pp 95-126.
4. Ash MM, et al. A study of periodontal hazards of third molars, *J Periodont* 33:208, 1962.
5. Blakey GH, et al. Changes in third molar and non-third molar periodontal pathology over time, *J Oral Maxillofac Surg* 65:1577-1583, 2007.
6. Blaket GH, et al. Progression of periodontal disease in the second/third molar region in subjects with asymptomatic third molars, *J Oral Maxillofac Surg* 64:189-193, 2006.
7. Harradine NW, et al. The effect of the extraction of third molars on later lower incisor crowding: a randomized controlled trial, *Br J Orthod* 25:117, 1998.
8. Kugelberg CF, et al. Periodontal healing after impacted lower third molar surgery in adolescents and adults. A prospective study, *Int J Oral Maxillofac Surg* 20:18, 1991.
9. Chipasco M, et al. Germectomy or delayed removal of mandibular third molars: the relationship between age and incidence of complications, *J Oral Maxillofac Surg* 53:418-422, 1995.
10. Phillips C, et al. Risk factors associated with prolonged recovery and delayed healing after third molar surgery, *J Oral Maxillofac Surg* 61:1436, 2003.
11. Bishara SE. Impacted maxillary canines: a review. *Am J Orthod Dentofacial Orthop* 101:159-171, 1992.
12. Jacoby H. The etiology of maxillary canine impaction, *Am J Orthod* 84:125-132, 1983.
13. Kaban LB, Troulis MJ. Dentoalveolar surgery. In Kaban LB, Troulis MJ, eds. *Pediatric oral and maxillofacial surgery.* Philadelphia, 2004 WB Saunders, pp 131.
14. Yehoshua S, et al. Second molar impactions, *Angle Orthod* 68:173-178, 1999.
15. Alling C, et al. *Impacted teeth.* Philadelphia, 1993, WB Saunders, pp 210-227.
16. Kokich VG. Surgical and orthodontic management of impacted maxillary canines. *Am J Orthod Dentofac Orthop* 126:3, 2004.
17. Sagne S, Thilander B. Transalveolar transplantation of maxillary canines. A follow up study, *Eur J Orthod* 12:140-147, 1990.
18. Pogrel MA. Evaluation of over 400 autogenous tooth transplants, *J Oral Maxillofac Surg* 45:205-211, 1987.
19. Pogrel MA. The surgical uprighting of mandibular second molars, *Am J Orthod Dentofac Orthop* 108:180-183, 1995.
20. Topazian RG, et al. *Oral and maxillofacial infections*, 4th ed. Philadelphia, 2002, WB Saunders.
21. Fonseca RJ, et al. *Oral and maxillofacial trauma*, 2nd ed. Philadelphia, 1997, WB Saunders.

INDEX

Note: Page numbers followed by *f* indicate figures; *b* indicates box; *t* indicates table.